OCCUPATIONAL THERAPY

Practice Skills for
Physical Dysfunction

OCCUPATIONAL THERAPY

Practice Skills for Physical Dysfunction

FOURTH EDITION

Edited by

Lorraine Williams Pedretti, MS, OTR
Professor Emeritus
Department of Occupational Therapy
San José State University
San José, California

with 50 contributors and 679 illustrations

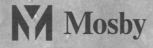 Mosby

St. Louis Baltimore Boston Carlsbad Chicago Naples New York Philadelphia Portland
London Madrid Mexico City Singapore Sydney Tokyo Toronto Wiesbaden

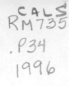

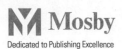

Dedicated to Publishing Excellence

Editor: Martha Sasser
Associate Developmental Editor: Amy Dubin
Project Manager: Carol Sullivan Weis
Designer: Sheilah Barrett
Manufacturing Supervisor: David Graybill
Cover Illustrator: Video Impact Productions Corp.

Printed in the United States of America
Composition by Progressive Information Technologies
Printing/binding by Von Hoffman, Inc.

Mosby-Year Book, Inc.
11830 Westline Industrial Drive
St. Louis, Missouri 63146

Library of Congress Cataloging in Publication Data

Occupational therapy: practice skills for physical dysfunction / edited by
 Lorraine Williams Pedretti; with 50 contributors. — 4th ed.
      p.   cm.
  Rev. ed. of: Occupational therapy / Lorraine Williams Pedretti, Barbara
Zoltan. 3rd ed. 1990.
  Includes bibliographical references and index.
  ISBN 0-8151-6812-8
  1. Occupational therapy.   2. Physical handicapped — Rehabilitation.
I. Pedretti, Lorraine Williams, 1936 –   .
  [DNLM: 1. Occupational Therapy.   2. Disabled.   WB 555 0149 1996]
RM735.P34   1996
615.8'515 — dc20
DNLM/DLC
for Library of Congress   95-41859
                                                              CIP

00 01 02 03 / 10 9 8 7 6 5

Contributors

Carole Adler, BS, OTR
Clinical Supervisor
Department of Occupational Therapy
Santa Clara Valley Medical Center
San José, California

Rebekah Reishus Allely, OTR/L
Occupational Therapist
Department of Burn Rehabilitation
Washington Hospital Center
Washington, DC

Pat Atchison, OTR
Senior Occupational Therapist II
Department of Occupational Therapy
Fairmont Hospital
San Leandro, California

Diane J. Atkins, OTR, FISPO
Assistant Professor/Coordinator
Amputee Program
The Institute for Rehabilitation and Research (TIRR)
Department of Physical Medicine and Rehabilitation
Baylor College of Medicine
Houston, Texas

Julie Belkin, OTR, CO, MBA
Director of Product Development
North Coast Medical, Inc.
San José, California

Elizabeth Maria Bianchi, BS, MS, OTR
Formerly: Senior Occupational Therapist
Stanford University Hospital
Stanford, California

Helen Bobrove, OTR
Formerly: Clinical Specialist, Orthopedics
Stanford University Hospital
Stanford, California

Karin Berglund Bonfils, OTR
Certified Affolter Instructor, Consultant/Lecturer;
Therapist and Consultant
Placer Therapy Center
Auburn, California
Formerly: Staff Therapist and Clinical Educator
The Rehabilitation Institute
Santa Barbara, California

Cynthia M. Burt, MS, OTR
Assistant Director
Department of Rehabilitation Services
University of California – Los Angeles
Los Angeles, California

Gordon Umphred Burton, PhD, OTR
Associate Professor
Occupational Therapy Department
San José State University
San José, California

Albert M. Cook, PhD, PE
Professor and Dean
Faculty of Rehabilitation Medicine
University of Alberta
Edmonton, Alberta
Partner
Assistive Technologies 2000
Sacramento, California

Jan Zaret Davis, BS, OTR
NDT Occupational Therapy Instructor in Adult
Hemiplegia
President, International Clinical Educators, Inc.
Port Townsend, Washington

Jeanette Engle-Ramirez, MRA, OTR
Director of Rehabilitation
Mount Diablo Medical Center
Concord, California
Lecturer
Department of Occupational Therapy
San José State University
San José, California

Carroll B. English, MA, OTR
Senior Occupational Therapist
Orthopedic and Neurological Rehabilitation Inc., (ONR)
Los Gatos, California
Formerly: Application Specialist
North Coast Medical, Inc.
San José, California

Fred Feuchter, PhD
Associate Professor of Anatomy and Physiology
Department of Occupational Therapy
Samuel Merritt College
Oakland, California

Denise Foderaro, OTR, CHT
Menlo Park, California
Formerly: Senior Occupational Therapist
Cardiac Rehabilitation
Santa Clara Valley Medical Center
San José, California

Diane Foti, MS, OTR
Occupational Therapist/Lecturer
Department of Occupational Therapy
San José State University
San José, California
Senior Occupational Therapist
Kaiser Permanente Medical Center
Redwood City, California

Jean Hietpas, OTR, LCSW
Clinical Specialist for the Multiple Sclerosis Center
Department of Rehabilitation Services
University of California, San Francisco
San Francisco, California

Jocelyn M. Hittle, OTR, CHT
Director
The Hand Center
Gilroy and Los Gatos, California

Merry Lee Hooks, OTR/L
Director of Occupational Therapy
Parkview Acres Convalescent Center
Department of Rehabilitation
The Hill Haven Corporation
Dillon, Montana

Susan M. Hussey, MS, OTR
Lecturer
Department of Biomedical Engineering
California State University – Sacramento
Partner
Assistive Technologies 2000
Sacramento, California

Janet L. Jabri, MBA, OTR, FAOTA
National Director of Rehabilitation
GCI Rehabilitation Division
Pan Care, Inc.
San José, California

Cheryl Leman Jordan, OTR/L, MA, FAOTA
Burn Rehabilitation Research Coordinator
Department of Burn Rehabilitation
Washington Hospital Center
Washington, DC

Mary C. Kasch, OTR, CHT, FAOTA
Director
Hand Rehabilitation Center of Sacramento
Sacramento, California

Sheri L. Lieberman, OTR
Carmel, California
Formerly: Clinical Coordinator of Occupational Therapy
Department of Rehabilitation Services
Stanford University Hospital
Stanford, California

Susan M. Lillie, OTR
Senior Occupational Therapist
Adaptive Driver Evaluation Program
Santa Clara Valley Medical Center
Guest Lecturer, Department of Occupational Therapy
San José State University
San José, California
Member, State of California Department of Motor
Vehicles Medical Advisory Board

Maureen Michele Matthews, BS, OTR
Clinical Supervisor Occupational Therapy
Department of Occupational Therapy
Santa Clara Valley Medical Center
San José, California

Guy L. McCormack, OTR, PhC
Chairperson/Associate Professor
Department of Occupational Therapy
Samual Merritt College
Oakland, California

Deborah Morawski, BS, OTR
Supervisor
Occupational Therapy Department
Community Hospital and Rehabilitation Center of
Los Gatos-Saratoga
Los Gatos, California

Karen L. Nelson, MS, OTR
Clinical Supervisor, Rehabilitation
Home Health Plus
Santa Clara, California
Lecturer
Department of Occupational Therapy
San José State University
San José, California

Jan Polon Novic, OTR
Santa Cruz, California
Formerly: Clinical Coordinator of Neurological and
Intensive Care Units
Stanford University Hospital
Stanford, California

Stephanie O'Leary, MS, OTR
Program Manager
Veterans Affairs Palo Alto Health Care System
Palo Alto, California
Formerly: Occupational Therapist
Cardiac Rehabilitation
Santa Clara Valley Medical Center
San José, California

Sharon Pasquinelli, MS, OTR
Manager
Division of Occupational Therapy
Department of Rehabilitative Services
The Medical Centers at the University of California, San Francisco
San Francisco, California

Lorraine Williams Pedretti, MS, OTR
Professor Emeritus
Department of Occupational Therapy
San José State University
San José, California

Heidi McHugh Pendleton, MA, OTR, PhD (cand.)
Assistant Professor
Department of Occupational Therapy
San José State University
San José, California

Karen Pitbladdo, MS, OTR
Clinical Specialist, Occupational Therapy Department
Brigham and Women's Hospital
Boston, Massachusetts
Formerly: Clinical Coordinator of Occupational Therapy in Orthopedics
Stanford University Hospital
Stanford, California

Sara A. Pope-Davis, MOT, OTR/L
Staff Occupational Therapist
Laurel Regional Hospital
Laurel, Maryland

Lynda M. Rock, MOT, OTR
Unit Coordinator
OT/PT Outpatient Services
The Institute For Rehabilitation and Research
Houston, Texas

Katie Schlageter, OTR
Assistant Manager, Out Patient Rehabilitation Program
Alta Bates Medical Center
Berkeley, California

Kathleen Barker Schwartz, EdD, OTR, FAOTA
Professor
Department of Occupational Therapy
San José State University
San José, California

Jerilyn A. Smith, OTR
Director of Occupational Therapy
Pacific Hills Manor
Morgan Hill, California;

Lecturer
Department of Occupational Therapy
San José State University
Formerly: Senior Occupational Therapist
San José Medical Center
San José, California

Patricia Smith, MS, OTR, CVE
Founder and Director
Occupational Assessment and Modification
San José, California

Joan Smithline, BS, PT
Clinical Specialist
Stanford Health Services, Department of Rehabilitation Services
Stanford, California
Founder, Back On-Line
Work Place Design
Menlo Park, California

Michelle Tipton-Burton, BS, OTR
Senior Occupational Therapist, Head Injury and Pediatric Services
Department of Occupational Therapy
Santa Clara Valley Medical Center
San José, California

Darcy Ann Umphred, PhD, PT
Professor and Vice Chairperson
Department of Physical Therapy
University of the Pacific
Stockton, California

Maureen Forte Undzis, BS, OTR
Highlands Ranch, Colorado
Formerly: Assistant Director
Clinical Services
Department of Occupational Therapy
Rancho Los Amigos Medical Center
Downey, California

Ingrid E. Wade, BSOT, OTR, CHT
Clinical Director
R.L. Petzoldt Memorial Center for Hand Rehabilitation
San José, California

Mary Warren, MS, OTR
Director
Occupational Therapy Department
Visual Independence Program
The Eye Foundation of Kansas City
Department of Ophthalmology-School of Medicine
University of Missouri-Kansas City
Kansas City, Missouri

Carol J. Wheatley, MS, OTR/L
Assistant Supervisor of Occupational Therapy
Maryland Rehabilitation Center
Division of Rehabilitation Services
Maryland State Department of Education
Baltimore, Maryland
Instructor
Department of Occupational Therapy
Towson State University
Towson, Maryland

Elizabeth J. Yerxa, EdD, LHD (Hon.), OTR, FAOTA
Distinguished Professor Emerita
Department of Occupational Therapy
University of Southern California
Los Angeles, California

Barbara Zoltan, MA, OTR
Consultant in Private Practice
Saratoga, California

Preface

This is an exciting era in which to enter health care. Occupational therapists have professional skills, equipment, technology and resources undreamed of just a few years ago. Knowledge of human function and dysfunction continues to increase rapidly. Significant advances in medical science, rehabilitation, and technology have made independence more feasible for those with severe physical impairments. Occupational therapists make critical contributions to the achievement of successful rehabilitation outcomes for persons with physical dysfunction.

The fourth edition of this text book reflects this progress in health care and rehabilitation. The reader is introduced to important changes in clinical technology, and increases in the scope of occupational therapy practice that have occurred in recent years. A cadre of expert contributors has added several new chapters and changed or expanded others to reflect current practice. Some of the new information in this edition especially worthy of note is trends in health care reform, documentation of occupational therapy services, motor learning, evaluation of motor control, evaluation and treatment of visual deficits and cognitive deficits, the social and psychological experience of disability, sexuality and disability, an introduction to the use of physical agent modalities, a problem solving approach to hand splinting, neurodevelopmental treatment, the Affolter approach, driver evaluation and training, assistive technology in practice, work evaluation and work hardening, the Americans with disabilities act and its implications for occupational therapy, upper extremity amputations and prosthetics, and low back pain.

This book is intended for use by occupational therapy students in baccalaureate and entry-level master's degree programs and as a reference for occupational therapy practitioners. Its purposes are: 1) to introduce the reader to occupational therapy practice in physical dysfunction; 2) to support the preparation of the student for occupational therapy practice with adults who have acquired physical disabilities; 3) to teach skills necessary for beginning practice in occupational therapy for physical dysfunction; and 4) to provide a foundation for the development of clinical reasoning skills. It is assumed that the reader using this text has had academic preparation in general psychology, anatomy and physiology, neuroanatomy and neurophysiology, kinesiology, human growth and development, medical terminology, conditions of orthopedic and neurological dysfunction, and theories of occupational therapy.

The content of the book is arranged according to the occupational therapy process within the context of the occupational performance model. Part I is concerned with the foundations for treatment: a model for practice, history, trends in health care, evaluation, treatment planning, documentation, and teaching activities. Part II covers methods of evaluation and treatment for the performance components: range of motion, muscle strength, motor control, dysphagia, visual deficits, sensory dysfunction, perceptual motor deficits, cognitive dysfunction, social and psychological factors, and issues of sexuality. Treatment approaches and their specific evaluation procedures for the performance components and performance areas are covered in Part III. These include therapeutic modalities, orthotics, the sensorimotor approaches to treatment, activities of daily living, wheelchairs, assistive technology, the Americans with Disabilities Act (ADA), and work evaluation and hardening. The final segment of the book, Part IV is concerned with treatment applications for selected physical dysfunctions. These include upper and lower extremity amputations, burn injuries, rheumatoid arthritis, hand injuries, cardiac dysfunction, low back pain, hip fractures, motor unit dysfunction, spinal cord injury, cerebral vascular accident, traumatic brain injury, and degenerative diseases of the central nervous system. Since it is not possible to cover all of the physical disabilities that may be acquired in adult life, these were chosen because they are often encountered in practice and the principles of treatment are applicable to similar dysfunctions.

Each chapter concludes with review questions and in some chapters learning activities are suggested as well. The purposes of the questions and activities are to assist the student to master the content, begin to develop clinical reasoning skills, achieve learning objectives, and prepare for evaluation of learning. Instructors may wish to use the questions for assignments or construction of examinations, and the learning activities for structuring laboratory experiences.

Sample case studies and treatment plans are presented at the end of each chapter in Part IV. These are *not* comprehensive treatment plans nor are they intended to present the only approach to treatment for the particular patient or physical dysfunction. Rather they are intended to serve as models for the novice. The student is encouraged to add objectives and methods to these treatment plans and to generate new treatment plans for real or hypothetical patients encountered in the academic program.

Both the terms *patient* and *client* have been used in this book to designate the consumer of occupational therapy services. Whether one or the other was used depends on the preference of the particular contributing author.

Lorraine Williams Pedretti

Acknowledgments

With this edition several new chapter contributors are introduced. Many are nationally and internationally known experts in their disciplines. Administrators, educators, researchers, and master clinicians are represented. They are from all regions of the United States and one lives in Canada. Of forty-two contributors to the fourth edition, nine contributed to the third edition and thirty-three are first time contributors. Nine of the forty-two were faculty colleagues during my tenure as an educator at San José State University, Department of Occupational Therapy. Three of those were also my former students. Of the remaining thirty-three contributors, thirteen were once my students. It gives me great pleasure to witness their professional achievements and clinical expertise and to be able to call upon them to contribute their knowledge to this work. Material that remained from the third edition was credited to former contributors as well as the individual who revised the chapter for this edition. All of the chapter authors are gratefully acknowledged for their expertise and contributions to this fourth edition.

Sincere appreciation is extended to Martha Sasser, Executive Editor, and Amy Dubin, Associate Developmental Editor, for their guidance and support through the manuscript preparation process. Carol Sullivan Weis, Project Manager, Mosby-Year Book, Inc., and Donna King, Project Manager, Progressive Information Technologies, are also gratefully acknowledged.

Barbara Zoltan, MA, OTR, co-editor for the third edition, and Janet Jabri, MBA, OTR, FAOTA, are acknowledged with gratitude for their assistance in initiating this project and especially for securing so many outstanding contributors.

Gratitude is extended to consultants and readers Lela A. Llorens, PhD, OTR, FAOTA, Amy Killingsworth, MA, OTR, Heidi McHugh Pendleton, MS, OTR, Ginny Polito Hasboun, OTR, Laurie Effersen, OD, MS, OTR, and Darcy A. Umphred, PhD, RPT and to Mr. Stephen Schmidt, PT, who executed art work for Chapters 1, 17, and 26.

For their assistance with computer technology, Gordon Burton, PhD, OTR, and Mr. Gary Del Monte, Technical Support Assistant, are gratefully acknowledged.

The American Occupational Therapy Association, Membership Department, is acknowledged for its assistance in locating contributing authors.

To the publishers, vendors, health care facilities, and individuals who permitted us to use material from their publications, we extend our sincere gratitude. The patients and models who posed for photographs are also gratefully acknowledged.

Finally, special appreciation is extended to my professional colleagues in education and in clinical practice, to my students, and to my family who offered their approval, support, encouragement, patience, and love.

Lorraine Williams Pedretti

Contents

OCCUPATIONAL THERAPY
Practice Skills for
Physical Dysfunction

PART I

Foundations for Treatment of Physical Dysfunction

Occupational Performance: A Model for Practice in Physical Dysfunction

Lorraine Williams Pedretti

The practice of occupational therapy in physical dysfunction should be guided by a unifying conceptual system. Theories, models, and frames of reference can be used as conceptual systems. These three terms are sometimes used interchangeably and there is no universal agreement on their meanings.[15] Christiansen[15] defined a model as a way of "structuring or organizing knowledge for the purpose of guiding thinking." The purpose of a model is to help the practitioner analyze situations, determine methodologies, and conceive alternatives. The use of a model in practice can be the basis for theory development.[15]

Frames of reference are based on models and have a methodological focus. They are mechanisms to link theory to practice and must meet certain criteria to be considered frames of reference. A theory encompasses principles and relationships that predict or explain phenomena under specified conditions.[15] Theories, models, and frames of reference have been articulated for occupational therapy by Fidler,[25] Mosey,[25,26] Reilly,[25] Kielhofner,[19,20,25] Ayres,[25] Llorens,[25] Gilfoyle and Grady,[17] King,[21] Allen,[1] and Schkade and Schultz.[30] It is suggested that the reader consult the referenced material.

According to the definitions just stated, occupational performance is a model for practice that can serve as a unifying conceptual system, and treatment of physical dysfunction can be carried out in its context. This chapter describes the model, defines its terminology, and traces its evolution. The scope of practice is described on a continuum within the context of the occupational performance model. The compatibility of the model with the philosophy of occupational therapy is discussed, and its relationship to three main treatment approaches is presented.

THE OCCUPATIONAL PERFORMANCE MODEL

The occupational performance model describes the domains of concern of occupational therapy and the content of the occupational therapy process.[4,12] It consists of three performance areas, three performance components, and two performance contexts. The performance areas are the following: (1) activities of daily living, (2) work and productive activities, and (3) play or leisure activities. Fundamental to these performance areas are the performance components, as follows: (1) the sensorimotor component, (2) the cognitive/cognitive integration components, and (3) the psychosocial/ psychological components. Function in the performance areas takes place in the contexts in which tasks are performed. Thus the model reflects temporal and environmental performance contexts[12] (Fig. 1-1).

OCCUPATIONAL PERFORMANCE

Occupational performance refers to the ability to perform those tasks that make it possible to carry out occupational roles in a satisfying manner that is appropriate to the individual's developmental stage, culture, and environment.[3-5,24] *Occupational roles* are the life roles that the individual holds in the society. These may include roles such as preschooler, student, parent, homemaker, employee, volunteer, or retired worker.[4,24]

Occupational performance requires learning and practice experiences with the role and developmental state-specific tasks, and the utilization of all performance components. Deficits in task learning experiences, performance components, and/or life space may result in limitations in occupational performance.[4]

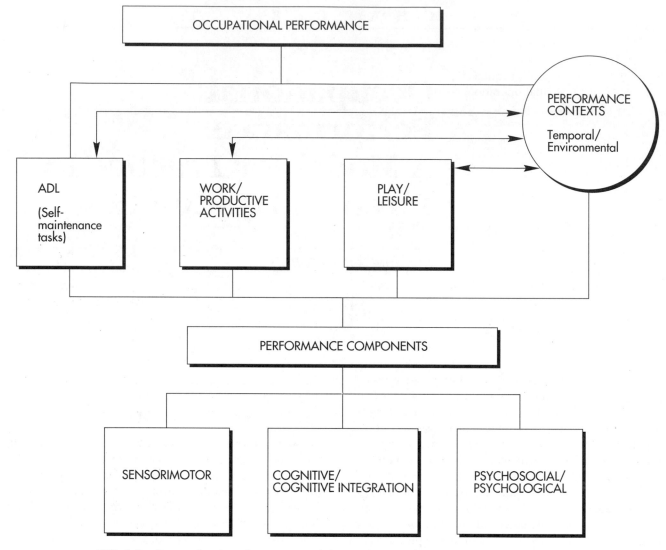

FIG. 1-1 Occupational performance model. Based on Uniform Terminology for Occupational Therapy, ed 3, *Am J Occup Ther,* 48:1047-1054, 1994. (Diagram adapted from the American Occupational Therapy Association, Inc.: A curriculum guide for occupational therapy educators, 1974.)

PERFORMANCE AREAS

Activities of daily living (ADL), work and productive activities, and play and leisure activities are referred to as performance areas. Activities of daily living are the self-maintenance tasks of grooming, hygiene, dressing, feeding and eating, mobility, socialization, communication, and sexual expression. Work and productive activities include home management, care of others, educational activities, and vocational activities. Play and leisure include play exploration and play or leisure performance in age appropriate activities.[3,12,22]

PERFORMANCE COMPONENTS

Performance components are "the learned developmental patterns of behavior which are the substructure and foundation of the individual's occupational performance."[3-5] Performance components include the (1) sensorimotor component, (2) cognitive/cognitive integration components, and (3) psychosocial/psychological components.[3,4] Adequate neurophysiological development and integrated functioning of the performance components are basic to an individual's ability to perform occupational tasks or activities in the performance areas.[24]

The *sensorimotor component* includes three function types: sensory, neuromusculoskeletal, and motor. Sensory functions include sensory awareness and processing and perceptual processing. Neuromusculoskeletal functions include reflex responses, range of motion, muscle tone, strength, endurance, postural control, postural alignment, and soft-tissue integrity. Motor functions include gross coordination, crossing the midline, laterality, bilateral integration, motor control, praxis, fine coordination/dexterity, oral motor control.[12]

The *cognitive/cognitive integration component* refers to the ability to use higher brain functions. Included are the following: level of arousal, orientation, recognition, attention span, initiation of activity, termination of activity, memory, sequencing, categorization, concept formation, spatial operations, problem solving, learning, and generalization.[12]

The *psychosocial/psychological component* encompasses the abilities for social interaction and emotional processing. In this category are values, interests, self-concept, role performance, social conduct, interpersonal skills, self-expression, coping skills, time management, and self-control.[12]

PERFORMANCE CONTEXTS

Successful occupational performance occurs in the context of the individual's cultural requirements and is consistent with age and developmental stage.[22] When assessing function in performance areas, it is important for the occupational therapist to consider the performance contexts in which the patient must operate. The selection of appropriate interventions is determined, in part, by the performance context.[12]

Performance contexts may be temporal or environmental. *Temporal contexts* include the individual's age, developmental stage or phase of maturation, and the individual's stage in important life processes such as parenting, education, or career. Disability status (acute, chronic, terminal,[12] improving, or declining) requires consideration.

Environmental contexts are of three kinds: physical, social, and cultural. The physical environment includes home, buildings, outdoors, furniture, tools, and other objects. The social environment includes significant others and social groups. The cultural environment includes customs, beliefs, behavior standards, political factors, and opportunities for education, employment, and economic support.[12]

EVOLUTION OF THE OCCUPATIONAL PERFORMANCE MODEL

In 1973 the American Occupational Therapy Association (AOTA) published *The Roles and Functions of Occupational Therapy Personnel.*[4] This publication referred to occupational performance as a frame of reference that included three performance skills, later named areas, and five performance components, later combined to become three. The purpose was to describe the areas of expertise of the occupational therapist and the domains of concern within the profession.

The AOTA Task Force on Target Populations, in its publication in April 1974, stated that . . . "the generic foundation, or frame of reference [of occupational therapy] is to be found in the concept of occupational performance." It further stated that "the goal . . . of

occupational therapy . . . is the improvement of occupational performance regardless of the target population."[6]

In 1974 the concept of the occupational performance frame of reference appeared in *A Curriculum Guide for Occupational Therapy Educators,* published by the AOTA.[4] Figure 1-2, from this publication, shows Dimension Two of a two-dimensional frame of reference,* and its purpose was to diagram the content of occupational therapy practice and to identify the areas of concern of occupational therapy, which could guide curriculum content. The occupational performance frame of reference was presented, with some modification, by Mosey[26] in 1981. She called it the "domain of concern for occupational therapy" and described it as "consisting of performance components within the context of age, occupational performance and an individual's environment." She defined "domain of concern" as "those areas of human experience in which practitioners of the profession offer assistance to others."[26]

In 1979 the AOTA published *Occupational Therapy Product Output Reporting System and Uniform Terminology for Reporting Occupational Therapy Services.*[9] This document presented a national system for reporting on hospital-based occupational therapy services. It defined the terminology in the occupational performance frame of reference. It also defined all of the elements of ADL including dressing, grooming, hygiene, mobility, communication, object manipulation, emotional and coping skills, work, and play/leisure. In addition, it defined the elements of sensorimotor, cognitive, and psychosocial components as well as other treatment-related terminology.[9]

In 1989 the second edition of *Uniform Terminology for Occupational Therapy* was published.[10] Its purpose was to define occupational peformance areas and components addressed in occupational therapy direct service. It defined and described the tasks and activities included in performance areas (ADL, work activities, and play or leisure activities) and sensorimotor, cognitive/cognitive integration, and psychosocial/psychological performance components.

In 1994 the third edition of *Uniform Terminology* was published.[12] It defined and described occupational performance areas and performance components and added temporal and environmental performance contexts.

Thus the concept of the occupational performance model was developed from a series of task forces and committees of the AOTA. It was generated from professional conceptualizations of practice and originally described as a frame of reference for practice and for curriculum design in education.[23] Subsequently the terminology was used and standardized in official docu-

---

* Dimension One (not shown) diagrammed the processes in occupational therapy practice.

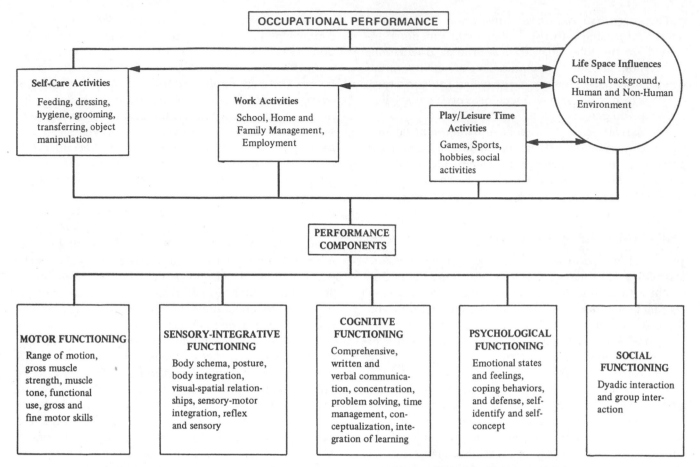

FIG. 1-2   Occupational performance frame of reference. (From the American Occupational Therapy Association, Inc.: *A curriculum guide for occupational therapy educators,* 1974.)

ments of the AOTA[9,10,12] and intended to describe the domains of concern in occupational therapy practice across specialty areas.

THE OCCUPATIONAL PERFORMANCE MODEL AND OCCUPATIONAL THERAPY PHILOSOPHY

The philosophy of occupational therapy is reflected in its definition and in its philosophical base statement. The definition of occupational therapy and the philosophical base statement support the occupational performance model.

Definition of Occupational Therapy

. . . the art and science of directing man's participation in selected tasks to restore, reinforce and enhance performance, facilitate learning of those skills and functions essential for adaptation and productivity, diminish or correct pathology, and to promote and maintain health. Its fundamental concern is the development and maintenance of the capacity throughout the life span, to perform with satisfaction to self and others, those tasks and roles essential to productive living and to the mastery of self and environment.*

* American Occupational Therapy Association: Occupational therapy: its definition and functions, *Am J Occup Ther* 26:204-205, 1972.

In the definition just quoted *occupation* refers to the goal-directed use of time, energy, and interest and active participation in ADL, work and productive activity, and play and leisure.[2,11] The concept of occupation, then, includes all of the performance areas outlined in the occupational performance model. Another key phrase in the definition of occupational therapy is "participation in selected tasks." This phrase implies that the patient's active involvement in his or her treatment is essential to effective occupational therapy. Selected tasks include not only those tasks that will best help meet the therapeutic objectives but also those that will help the patient in environmental contexts, which are also important in the occupational performance model. The performance of tasks and roles essential to productive living throughout the lifetime is also central to the definition of occupational therapy. Role performance is the unifying theme of the occupational performance model.

The Philosophical Base of Occupational Therapy

In 1979 the Representative Assembly of the AOTA adopted a philosophical base for occupational therapy.[7] This philosophical base states:

Man is an active being whose development is influenced by the use of purposeful activity. Using their capacity for intrinsic motivation, human beings are able to influence their physical and mental health and their social and physical environment through purposeful activity. Human life includes a process of continuous adaptation. Adaptation is a change in function that promotes survival and self-actualization. Biological, psychological and environmental factors may interrupt the adaptation process at any time through the life cycle. Dysfunction may occur when adaptation is impaired. Purposeful activity facilitates the adaptive process.

Occupational therapy is based on the belief that purposeful activity (occupation), including its interpersonal and environmental components, may be used to prevent and mediate dysfunction, and to elicit maximum adaptation. Activity as used by the occupational therapist includes both intrinsic and therapeutic purpose.*

In addition to the adoption of this philosophical base, the Representative Assembly affirmed that

. . . there be universal acceptance and implementation of the common core of occupational therapy as the active participation of the patient/client in occupation for the purposes of improving performance [and that] the use of facilitating procedures is only acceptable as occupational therapy when used to prepare the patient/client for better performance and prevention of disability through self-participation in occupation.*

The philosophical base states that people can improve or influence their health through participation in purposeful activity (occupation). The term *purposeful activity* is a central theme of this philosophical base and was apparently used to mean occupation as defined previously. It also implies that purposeful activity characterizes the tools of occupational therapy and points to the influence of environment on performance.

The affirmations accompanying the philosophical base emphasized that the active participation of the patient in purposeful activity is the core of occupational therapy and placed adjunctive and enabling procedures in perspective as preparatory for purposeful activity. It is clearly stated that such procedures are acceptable as occupational therapy only if they are used as the means to occupational performance in life roles.

THE CONCERNS OF OCCUPATIONAL THERAPY

In this model the concerns of occupational therapy are the performance areas and components.[4,12,22,26] Therefore, the occupational therapy program may include treatment methods designed for the remediation of deficits or for the compensation for deficits in performance areas and performance components.[4] For work on a per-

*American Occupational Therapy Association: Resolution 532-79(1979), Occupation as the common core of occupational therapy, Representative Assembly minutes, April, 1979, Detroit, Mich, *Am J Occup Ther* 33:785, 1979.

formance component (for example, motor skill development), the methods *must* be directed to the patient's ability in the performance areas; functional independence is a core concept of occupational therapy theory and the goal of the occupational therapy process.[29]

ASSUMPTIONS ABOUT THE OCCUPATIONAL PERFORMANCE MODEL

In an effort to interpret occupational performance, the following assumptions have been made:

1. Occupational performance subserves satisfactory occupational role fulfillment.
2. Occupational performance of human beings can be categorized into the areas of ADL, work and productive activities, and play or leisure activities.
3. Development, performance, and maintenance of occupational performance are influenced by intrapersonal and extrapersonal elements. Intrapersonal elements include the temporal aspects of performance contexts as well as genetic, neurophysiological, and pathological factors. Extrapersonal elements include the physical environment, objects/tools, and social, cultural, and familial elements.
4. An appropriate balance in occupational performance is essential for the maintenance of health.
5. Appropriate balance changes with chronological/developmental age, life cycle, and life events and circumstances.
6. Failure in development of occupational performance or loss, disruption, or change of occupational roles can be caused by intrapersonal and/or extrapersonal factors.
7. Adequate occupational performance is dependent on intact neurophysiological development[24] and the integrated functioning of the sensorimotor, cognitive/cognitive integration and, psychosocial/psychological subsystems of the individual.
8. Defect, disease, or injury affecting any performance component causes a failure of integration of the performance components subsystem and results in a failure or disruption in the performance areas and, thus, a failure or disruption in satisfying fulfillment of occupational roles.
9. The role of the occupational therapist is to facilitate both an appropriate balance and optimum occupational performance toward the resumption of occupational roles.
10. The occupational therapist is concerned with remediation of and compensation for defects in the performance components and performance areas.
11. The primary tool of the occupational therapist for the remediation of performance areas and performance components is purposeful activity.
12. The occupational therapist is also concerned with preparing the patient for performance of purposeful activity and may use adjunctive and enabling methods as steps in the treatment continuum. These in-

clude but are not limited to exercise, facilitation and inhibition techniques, physical agent modalities, splints, sensory stimulation, and assistive devices.[32]

13. Exclusive use of adjunctive and enabling methods out of context of the patient's occupational performance is not considered occupational therapy.

THE TREATMENT CONTINUUM BASED ON THE OCCUPATIONAL PERFORMANCE MODEL

As occupational therapy has become less dependent on medical direction, its role has expanded considerably. Occupational therapists have developed and demonstrated competence in many specialized practice areas associated with physical dysfunction. The occupational therapist's concern, from the onset of the illness or injury, is for the patient to become as independent as possible in the performance areas and to resume previous occupational roles or to assume new and satisfying occupational roles. In many dysfunctions occupational therapy intervention may begin at the time of surgery or in the early stages of acute care; thus occupational therapy can make an important contribution at every stage in the treatment continuum.[27]

Figure 1-3 is a model for the treatment continuum in physical disabilities practice. A particular occupational

therapist may be responsible for only one or two stages on the continuum, but treatment is always within the context of occupational performance.

The stages in this treatment continuum overlap or can occur simultaneously. The treatment continuum is not a strict step-by-step progression. It addresses the performance components and performance areas in the occupational performance model and takes the patient through a logical progression from dependence to occupational performance to resumption of life roles. The treatment continuum identifies the concerns of occupational therapy practice within the context of occupational performance. The paragraphs that follow describe the four stages in the treatment continuum.

Stage One: Adjunctive Methods

Procedures that prepare the patient for occupational performance but are preliminary to the use of purposeful activity are concerns of occupational therapy.[13] Stage one procedures may include exercise, facilitation and inhibition techniques, positioning, sensory stimulation, selected physical agent modalities, and devices such as braces and splints.[32] Stage one methods and devices are often used in (but are not limited to) the acute stages of illness or injury. During this stage the occupational therapist is likely to be most concerned with assessing and

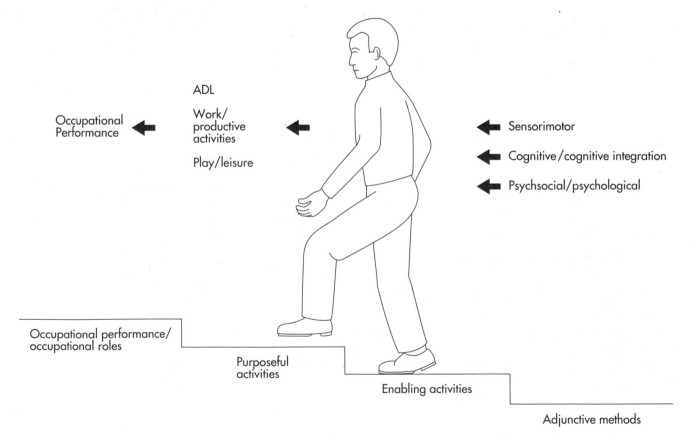

FIG. 1-3 Treatment continuum within occupational performance model. (From a poster by Karin Boyce, OTS.)

remediating performance components. It is important for occupational therapists to plan the progression of treatment so that adjunctive modalities are used as preparation for purposeful activity and are directed toward maximum independence in the performance areas.

Stage Two: Enabling Activities

Purposeful activity has been defined as one that has an autonomous or inherent goal beyond the motor function required to perform the task.[13] Engagement in purposeful activity also requires the active participation of the patient and requires and elicits coordination of sensorimotor, psychosocial, and cognitive systems.[8,11] By these criteria, many methods used in occupational therapy may not be directly purposeful but may be a step toward purposeful activities. Such methods are referred to as *enabling methods.*

Occupational therapists have created many enabling devices and methods that simulate purposeful activities. Examples are sanding boards, skate boards, stacking cones or blocks, practice boards for mastery of clothing fasteners and hardware, driving simulators, work simulators, and table-top activities such as pegboards for training perceptual-motor skills. Such devices and activities are not likely to be as meaningful to the patient or to stimulate as much interest and motivation as purposeful activities. They may be needed, however, as a preparatory or ancillary part of the treatment program to train specific sensorimotor, perceptual, or cognitive functions necessary for activities in the performance areas.

Special equipment, such as wheelchairs, ambulatory aids, special clothing, communication devices, environmental control systems, and other assistive devices may also be used. These devices can be important in enabling independence in the performance areas and assumption of occupational roles.

In stage two the therapist is still concerned with assessment and remediation of performance components. Now, however, the therapist also begins to assess and teach activities in the performance areas.

Stage Three: Purposeful Activity

Purposeful activity has been the core of occupational therapy since its inception. Purposeful activity includes activities that have an inherent or autonomous goal and are relevant and meaningful to the patient.[13] It is part of the daily life routine and occurs in the context of occupational performance.[11] Examples are feeding, hygiene, dressing, mobility, communication, arts, crafts, games, sports, work, and educational activities.

The purposefulness of an activity is determined by the individual performing it and by the context in which it is performed. Occupational therapy practitioners use purposeful activities to evaluate, facilitate, restore, or maintain a person's ability to function in life roles.[11] Purposeful activity is used to enhance functioning in the performance areas. It is carried out by the occupational

therapy practitioner in a health care facility or in the patient's home. At this stage the occupational therapist is primarily concerned with assessing and remediating deficits in the performance areas.

Stage Four: Occupational Performance and Occupational Roles

In the final stage of the treatment continuum, the patient resumes or assumes occupational roles in his or her living environment and in the community. Appropriate tasks of ADL, work and productive activities, and play and leisure are performed to the patient's maximum level of independence, which is defined for each individual according to capacities and limitations. Formal occupational therapy intervention is decreased and ultimately discontinued. As a consequence of earlier therapy, the individual is performing in occupational roles at this stage.

THE RELATIONSHIP OF THE OCCUPATIONAL PERFORMANCE MODEL TO TREATMENT APPROACHES
BIOMECHANICAL APPROACH

The biomechanical approach to the treatment of physical dysfunction applies the mechanical principles of kinetics and kinematics to the movement of the human body.[28] These mechanical principles deal with how forces acting on the body affect movement and equilibrium.[14] Methods of treatment in this approach use principles of physics related to forces, levers, and torque.

Examples of biomechanical techniques include joint measurement, muscle strength testing, kinetic activity, therapeutic exercise, and orthotics. The purposes of the biomechanical approach are to (1) assess specific physical limitations in range, strength, and endurance; (2) restore function of range, strength, and endurance; and (3) reduce deformity.

The biomechanical approach is most appropriate for patients who have motor unit or orthopedic disorders but whose central nervous system (CNS) is intact. These patients can control isolated movement and specific movement patterns, but have weakness, low endurance, or joint limitation. Examples of such disabilities are orthopedic dysfunctions, including rheumatoid arthritis, osteoarthritis, fractures, amputations, hand trauma, burns, and motor unit disorders, such as peripheral nerve injuries, Guillain-Barré syndrome, spinal cord injuries, and muscular dystrophy.

Biomechanical methods of evaluation and treatment are primarily directed at restoration of elements of the sensorimotor component in the occupational performance model. Many of the adjunctive or enabling techniques and modalities are also biomechanical, and biomechanical principles can also be applied to purposeful activity in the performance areas. Biomechanical principles are used in sawing wood, rolling out dough, and vacuuming carpets, for example.

SENSORIMOTOR APPROACHES

Before the sensorimotor approaches to treatment evolved, therapists tried to apply biomechanical principles to patients with damaged central nervous systems and met with many problems as a result. Because biomechanical treatment demanded controlled voluntary movement, it was inappropriate for patients who lacked such control.

Sensorimotor approaches are used with patients who have CNS dysfunction. They are based on theories of motor recovery.[16] The normal CNS produces controlled, well-modulated movement. In the damaged CNS, coordination and well-modulated, controlled movement are not possible. All sensorimotor approaches to treatment use neurophysiologic mechanisms to normalize muscle tone and elicit more normal motor responses.[16,33] Some approaches use reflex mechanisms, and the sequence of treatment may be based on the recapitulation of ontogenetic development.[31] Chapters 21 through 25 describe the sensorimotor approaches of Rood, Brunnstrom (movement therapy), Knott and Voss (proprioceptive neuromuscular facilitation), Bobath (neurodevelopmental treatment), and Affolter.

All of the sensorimotor approaches are directed to motor recovery and improvement of motor performance. They do not consider motivation, arousal, attention, role dysfunction, or temporal adaptation and the influence of these factors on motor behavior.[16]

If the sensorimotor approaches are to be considered part of the armamentarium of the occupational therapy practitioner, they must be applied to purposeful activity, as described in Chapters 21 through 25. The application of an approach, not associated with purposeful activity, may be used "to prepare the client or patient for better performance and prevention of disability through self-participation in occupation."[7] When used to precede and enable purposeful activity, and as part of purposeful activity, the sensorimotor approaches can be valuable methods in the occupational performance model, addressing the sensorimotor and cognitive/cognitive integration components and the performance areas.

REHABILITATION APPROACH

The term *rehabilitation* means a return to ability, that is, the return to the fullest physical, mental, social, vocational, and economic usefulness that is possible for the individual. It means the ability to live and work with remaining capabilities.[18] Therefore the focus in the treatment program is on abilities rather than on disabilities.[28] Rehabilitation is concerned with the intrinsic worth and dignity of the individual and with the restoration of a satisfying and purposeful life. The rehabilitation approach uses measures that enable the patient to live as independently as possible with some residual disability. Its goal is to help the patient learn to work around or compensate for physical limitations.[28]

The rehabilitation approach is a dynamic process and requires that the patient be a member of the rehabilitation team. It requires ongoing assessment and follow-up to maintain maximum function and, therefore, must keep pace with advances in methods and equipment (rehabilitation technology), social change, and community resources to provide the best services and opportunities for each patient.[18]

In this approach occupational therapy focuses on performance areas more than on performance components. The aim of the occupational therapy program is to minimize disability barriers to role performance. The occupational therapist must assess the patient's capabilities and determine how to overcome the effects of the disability. The treatment methods of the rehabilitation approach include modalities such as the following:

1. Self-care evaluation and training
2. Acquisition and training in assistive devices
3. Adaptive clothing
4. Homemaking and child care
5. Work simplification and energy conservation
6. Work-related activities
7. Leisure activities
8. Prosthetic training
9. Wheelchair management
10. Home evaluation and adaptation
11. Community transportation
12. Architectural adaptations
13. Acquisition and training in the use of communication aids and environmental control systems.

Frequently the methods of the rehabilitation approach are used in combination with biomechanical or sensorimotor approaches. First, biomechanical or sensorimotor principles can be applied during rehabilitation activities to enhance and reinforce the restoration of the sensorimotor and cognitive components. Second, the treatment program often focuses on performance areas and performance components simultaneously. Thus the restoration of sensorimotor, cognitive, and psychosocial functions are combined to improve functioning in the performance areas.

In an examination of the treatment approaches just described, the cognitive/cognitive integration, and psychosocial/psychological performance components in the occupational performance model are not explicitly considered. The occupational performance model demands the consideration of temporal and environmental aspects of performance contexts. Di Joseph urges occupational therapists to consider not only motor control but motor behavior, that is, "a person acting purposefully within and upon his or her environment." She stated further that ignoring the emotive and cognitive aspects of motor behavior is a reductionistic approach that fails to consider all factors in the production of purposeful action.[16] Treatment goals for patients must be based on a combination of mind, body, and environment; these goals should be reached through the use of activities that are compatible with the needs and values of the person and not necessarily with those of the therapist.[16] Interaction between the person and the environment is essential to the development of functional independence.[29] The person is mind and body, not just a motor system to be evaluated and treated.[16]

The occupational performance model is holistic in its application to treatment of the patient. It demands consideration of the performance areas, performance components, and performance contexts for its application.

SUMMARY

The occupational performance model serves as a conceptual system for occupational therapy practice in physical dysfunction. The treatment continuum, conceptualized on the basis of this model, accommodates the wide range of modalities in use in occupational therapy practice and integrates them into the occupational performance framework. Using the occupational performance model, the occupational therapy practitioner identifies the individual's occupational roles and role dysfunction and assesses performance areas, performance components, and performance contexts by identifying assets, skills, and deficits. Treatment goals and intervention strategies are selected based on the assessment. The general goal of the treatment program is to restore the patient to his or her maximum level of performance in valued occupational roles through remedial or compensatory treatment approaches.

REVIEW QUESTIONS

1. Define model, theory, and frame of reference.
2. What is the purpose of a model?
3. Briefly outline the elements in the occupational performance model.
4. What is the difference between a performance area and a performance component? How are they related?
5. Define "occupational role." Give some examples.
6. Select one of your occupational roles and list all of the tasks in each of the performance areas that are necessary to fulfill that role.
7. List the stages in the treatment continuum and give examples of treatment modalities that might be used in each.
8. Define "enabling activities" as used in this chapter.
9. What is a key concept in the definition of occupational therapy? How is it related to the occupational performance model?
10. Define "purposeful activity.'"
11. Which treatment modalities can be thought of as primarily biomechanical in nature?
12. With which diagnoses is a biomechanical approach most likely to be used? Why?
13. How does the biomechanical approach fit into the occupational performance model?
14. For which diagnoses are the sensorimotor approaches most likely to be effective?
15. How can the sensorimotor approaches be integrated in an occupational performance framework?
16. Describe what is meant by "rehabilitation approach."
17. List six treatment modalities that are part of the rehabilitation approach.
18. How is the rehabilitation approach integrated with the other approaches to treatment discussed in this chapter?

REFERENCES

1. Allen C: Activity, occupational therapy's treatment method, *Am J Occup Ther* 41:563-565, 1987.
2. American Occupational Therapy Association: Occupational therapy: its definition and functions, *Am J Occup Ther* 26:204-205, 1972.
3. American Occupational Therapy Association: *The roles and functions of occupational therapy personnel*, Rockville, Md, 1973, The Association.
4. American Occupational Therapy Association: *A curriculum guide for occupational therapy educators*, Rockville, Md, 1974, The Association.
5. American Occupational Therapy Association: Project to delineate the roles and functions of occupational therapy personnel, Rockville, Md, 1972. Cited in *A curriculum guide for occupational therapy educators*, Rockville, Md, 1974, The Association.
6. American Occupational Therapy Association: Task force on target populations, Association report II, *Am J Occup Ther* 28:231, 1974.
7. American Occupational Therapy Association: Resolution 532-79 (1979), Occupation as the common core of occupational therapy, Representative Assembly minutes, April 1979, Detroit, Mich, *Am J Occup Ther* 33:785, 1979.
8. American Occupational Therapy Association: Purposeful activities, a position paper, *Am J Occup Ther* 37:805, 1983.
9. American Occupational Therapy Association: Occupational therapy product output reporting system and uniform terminology for reporting occupational therapy services. In *Reference Manual of the official documents of the American Occupational Therapy Association*, Rockville, Md, 1989, The Association.
10. American Occupational Therapy Association: Uniform terminology for occupational therapy, ed 2, *Am J Occup Ther* 43:808-815, 1989.
11. American Occupational Therapy Association: Position paper: purposeful activity, *Am J Occup Ther* 47:1081-1082, 1993.

12. American Occupational Therapy Association: Uniform terminology for occupational therapy, ed 3, *Am J Occup Ther* 48: 1047-1054, 1994.
13. Ayres AJ: Basic concepts of clinical practice in physical disabilities, *Am J Occup Ther* 12:300, 1958.
14. Brunnstrom S: *Clinical kinesiology,* ed 3, Philadelphia, 1972, FA Davis.
15. Christiansen, C: Occupational therapy, intervention for life performance. In Christiansen C, Baum C: *Occupational therapy, overcoming human performance deficits,* Thorofare, NJ, 1991, Slack.
16. Di Joseph LM: Independence through activity: mind, body, and environment interaction in therapy, *Am J Occup Ther* 36:740, 1982.
17. Gilfoyle E, Grady A: *Children adapt,* ed 2, Thorofare, NJ, 1989, Slack.
18. Hopkins HL, Smith HD, Tiffany EG: Rehabilitation. In Hopkins HL, Smith HD, editors: *Willard and Spackman's occupational therapy,* ed 6, Philadelphia, 1983, JB Lippincott.
19. Kielhofner G, editor: *A model of human occupation,* Baltimore, 1985, Williams & Wilkins.
20. Kielhofner G, Burke JP: A model of human occupation. I. Conceptual framework and content, *Am J Occup Ther* 34:572, 1980.
21. King LJ: Toward a science of adaptive responses, *Am J Occup Ther* 32:429, 1978.
22. Llorens LA: *Application of a developmental theory for health and rehabilitation,* Rockville, Md, 1976, American Occupational Therapy Association, Inc.
23. Llorens LA: Personal communication, July 6, 1988.
24. Llorens, LA: Performance tasks and roles through the life span. In Christian C, Baum C: *Occupational therapy, overcoming human performance deficits,* Thorofare, NJ, 1991, Slack.
25. Miller BR and associates: *Six perspectives on theory for the practice of occupational therapy,* Rockville, Md, 1988, Aspen Publishers.
26. Mosey AC: *Occupational therapy: configuration of a profession,* New York, 1981, Raven Press.
27. Pedretti LW: The compatibility of treatment methods in physical disabilities with the philosophical base of occupational therapy. Paper presented to the American Occupational Therapy Association National Conference, Philadelphia, May 13, 1982.
28. Reed KL: *Models of practice in occupational therapy,* Baltimore, 1984, Williams & Wilkins.
29. Rogers JC: The spirit of independence: the evolution of a philosophy, *Am J Occup Ther* 36:709, 1982.
30. Schkade JK, Schultz S: Occupational adaptation: toward a holistic approach for contemporary practice. I. *Am J Occup Ther* 46:829-837. II. *Am J Occup Ther* 46:917-925, 1992.
31. Stockmeyer SA: An interpretation of the approach of Rood to the treatment of neuromuscular dysfunction, *Am J Phys Med* 46:900, 1967.
32. Trombly CA: Include exercise in purposeful activity, *Am J Occup Ther* 36:467, 1982 (letter).
33. Willard HL, Spackman CS, editors: *Occupational therapy,* ed 4, Philadelphia, 1971, JB Lippincott.

History and Trends in Treatment Methods

Sharon Pasquinelli

The clinical practice of occupational therapy is a dynamic process shaped by many factors. Development of theories, refinement of frames of reference, generation of models, and research activities are some of the factors that characterize internal professional growth and development. Additionally, as members of society at large, occupational therapists and patients are influenced by external environmental factors such as cultural and social attitudes, economic realities, political opinions, and technological advances. These internal and external factors may act separately or synergistically to influence clinical practice.

In the area of adult physical dysfunction, there is evidence that treatment techniques are included in, or excluded from, practice based on the factors just mentioned.[48] This chapter presents an historical overview of the development of occupational therapy for physical dysfunction. It also discusses the impacts of cultural, social, economic, political, and technical influences on the development of the profession.

HUMANITARIANISM

MORAL TREATMENT

Occupational therapy's philosophical roots extend to the period of moral treatment in early nineteenth-century Europe. Dr. Philippe Pinel, a French physician, and Samuel Tuke, an English Quaker, were two of the leaders in promoting the practice of moral treatment.[49] Moral treatment was based on a humane philosophy that evolved from the cultural, political, and religious beliefs of the time. Society valued humanitarian principles and practices, and these values influenced the treatment of the mentally ill. Main features of this philosophy included respect for human individuality, acceptance of the unity of mind and body, and belief in the ability of mentally ill patients to function and adapt to their environments as a result of participating in activities.[9,11,19]

American advocates of moral treatment included Dr. Benjamin Rush, Dr. Amariah Brigham, and Dr. Thomas Story Kirkbride. These physicians were among the first Americans to use moral treatment concepts in psychiatry. Patients engaged in structured daily routines and activities or occupations, which included work and recreation. Occupations, according to Rush, should "engage the mind, and exercise the body: as swinging, riding, walking, sewing, embroidery, bowling, gardening, mechanic arts; to which may be added reading, writing, conversation, etc. the whole to be performed with order and regularity."[49]

As superintendent of the Pennsylvania Hospital for the Insane in the mid 1800s, Kirkbride stressed the use of moral treatment and occupations in treatment of the mentally ill. He described moral treatment as daily efforts to provide "system, active movements and diversity of occupation". Structured daily routines were organized to engage patients in what were thought at the time to be gender-specific occupations. "Men engaged in agricultural pursuits, carpentry, painting and general maintenance. Women performed domestic chores and manual crafts."[45]

Adolf Meyer[38] summarized the philosophy of moral treatment by stating that the unique feature of people is their ability to organize time through activity. Meyer believed that even under difficulty, people maintain a balance through actual doing or practice.[38]

Moral treatment represented a shift in 19th century thinking from a pessimistic viewpoint that labeled the mentally ill as "insane and incurable" to an optimistic one. This humanistic philosophy promised positive outcomes for the mentally ill, who became viewed as capable of reason and "curable".[45] Moral treatment was thus the response of the medical community to the prevailing social attitudes regarding mental illness.

Moral treatment was practiced successfully for many years. Concepts of moral treatment, including the therapeutic value of occupation, however, gradually declined after the American Civil War. The demise of moral treatment was due in part to the overcrowding of mental hospitals, economic difficulties, and a shift in medical opinion regarding mental illness. At the time, mental illness was widely thought to have an emotional and psychological basis, but this theory gradually yielded to a competing scientific school of thought that sought to explain mental illness in terms of brain pathology.[11]

ARTS AND CRAFTS MOVEMENT

The rise of the arts and crafts movement, circa 1890, was society's reaction to dealing with the perceived social ills created by the Industrial Revolution. The economy was changing from an agrarian society to a manufacturing one, and people who moved from the farms to the city struggled to adapt to city life. Factories mass-produced machine-made products that were previously handmade. American life was often characterized by dissatisfaction that stemmed from monotonous and repetitive work conditions prevalent in the work place. The number of people with disabilities requiring treatment increased because of industrial accidents, and further increased when a severe polio epidemic occurred in the eastern United States in 1916.[54]

Medical advances in the treatment of tuberculosis, injuries resulting from widening use of the automobile, and the increase in industrial accidents contributed to a need for new methods to treat disabilities.[60] As a reaction to these conditions, a social lay health movement known as the arts and crafts movement gained popularity. The use of arts and crafts as therapeutic media in occupational therapy stems from this movement that blossomed in the early 20th century.

John Ruskin, an English philosopher, and William Morris, an English artist and architect, promoted and popularized the concepts of the arts and crafts movement. Morris, a student of Ruskin, emphasized the values of good design and quality craftsmanship.[33,49] Craft work was believed to improve physical and mental health through exercise and the satisfaction gained from creating a useful or decorative article with one's own hands.

Over time people adapted and adjusted to the changes brought about by the Industrial Revolution. City life, industrial work, factory systems, and machine-made goods became socially and culturally acceptable. The arts and crafts movement began to lose its purpose and soon was overshadowed by the onset of World War I. Additionally, the philosophy of humanitarianism was being challenged by the medical community as unscientific and unmeasurable.[48]

FORMAL BEGINNINGS OF THE PROFESSION

In 1914 George Edward Barton opened Consolation House in Clifton Springs, New York, to treat the sick and disabled. Barton, an architect diagnosed with tuberculosis, assisted his recovery from hysterical paralysis through the use of manual work. His experiences convinced him to devote his life to rehabilitating the disabled

and to study medicine and occupations. In his studies he became acquainted with Dr. William Rush Dunton, Jr, a Maryland psychiatrist. Barton wrote Dunton to organize a group of people interested in discussing "occupation". Dunton was interested in forming a national society. Through their correspondence, Dunton recommended to Barton the appointment of several people who would form the founding committee of such an organization.[34]

Occupational therapy formally began in March, 1917, in Clifton Springs with the first meeting of the National Society for the Promotion of Occupational Therapy. In addition to Barton and Dunton, the committee members were the following: Eleanor Clarke Slagle, a social service worker; Thomas Bissell Kidner, an architect; Susan Cox Johnson, an arts and crafts instructor; and Isabel G. Newton, Barton's secretary.[34] Although these individuals were of varied backgrounds, they shared common beliefs and interests in the therapeutic use of occupation and in the therapeutic relationship of the patient, the therapist, and occupations.[46,47]

WORLD WAR I

In November, 1917, the United States entered World War I. A conference of physicians who specialized in the reeducation of soldiers disabled in the war recommended that reconstruction hospitals be established in which the rehabilitation of soldiers could begin as early as possible.[23] In 1918 civilian women were appointed to provide therapy for the wounded. To meet the demand caused by the vast number of wounded soldiers, short War Emergency Courses were set up in Boston, Philadelphia, St. Louis, Baltimore, and New York City. The women receiving this training, who later became known as reconstruction aides, played an important role in the development of occupational therapy for physical disabilities. After completing their training, many reconstruction aides were sent overseas to treat the wounded.[36,47]

In military hospitals at home and abroad, occupational therapy reconstruction aides developed programs for rehabilitation of injured soldiers. The aides used therapeutic activities to treat orthopedic and neurological conditions and stress disorders.[36,52]

World War I resulted in rapid growth of occupational therapy for physical dysfunction. The value of occupational therapy reconstruction aides in the rehabilitation of disabled soldiers was recognized by the public and the medical profession, leading to the establishment of occupational therapy schools.

Toward the end of the war, veterans with complex rehabilitation needs were returning home, and Army and Navy hospitals expanded to meet their needs. A Department of Occupational Therapy was established at Walter Reed General Hospital in Washington, D.C., and came under the direction of Bird T. Baldwin, a psychologist, in April, 1918. Baldwin and the occupational therapy reconstruction aides developed a scientific and holistic rehabilitation program for soldiers with physical disabilities.[8,59] The aides were assigned to the orthopedic ward where methods of systematically recording range of motion and muscle strength were established. Activities were selected based on an analysis of the motions involved, including joint position, muscle action, and muscle strengthening. Methods of adapting tools were suggested, and splints were fabricated to provide support during the recovery process. According to Baldwin, the purpose of occupational therapy is "functional restoration" to "help each patient find himself and function again as a complete man physically, socially, educationally, and economically."[7]

After the war there was little carry-over of occupational therapy concepts into civilian hospitals because of a lack of personnel. Reconstruction aides were not granted military status and most left the service after the war ended. Treatment techniques developed during the war to treat physical dysfunction were not sufficiently documented in occupational therapy literature and were lost. Occupational therapy practice in physical dysfunction diminished while practice in mental health and psychiatry continued.

In 1923 the National Society for the Promotion of Occupational Therapy changed its name to the American Occupational Therapy Association (AOTA).[50] The association became increasingly involved with establishing educational standards, recognizing qualified trainees, and publishing articles of interest to occupational therapy.

DEPRESSION YEARS

The Great Depression of the 1930s had a substantial economic impact on the medical professions, including the practice of occupational therapy. Budgets were cut, staff layoffs occurred, and supplies and equipment were limited. Many occupational therapy clinics and schools closed.[50]

Treatment of physical disabilities focused on restoring function and developing strength for patients to return to work. Typical caseloads included fractures, residual hand disabilities, tuberculosis, and poliomyelitis. Few cases of hemiplegia, quadriplegia, and paraplegia were treated, because most of these patients died of infections.[54]

In the mid 1930s most occupational therapists did not believe that occupational therapy could stand alone as an independent profession. Occupational therapists sought alliance with the American Medical Association (AMA) to implement minimum standards of training to "establish standards for training institutions, and to accredit each new school." ". . . the powerful AMA came to the rescue." The profession became a medical ancillary.[50]

Occupational therapy also came under increasing pressure from the medical profession and society to change from a holistic philosophy to a reductionistic one. Reductionism refers to a scientific process of understanding function by analyzing small, discrete parts.[30]

WORLD WAR II

As in World War I the second World War brought an increased recognition of the value of and need for occupational therapy services. The profession was not prepared to meet the rapid increase in demand for trained personnel. The Army once again developed war emergency courses to meet the need.[14]

In Army and Navy hospitals, departments of rehabilitation medicine emerged and clinical programs flourished. Occupational therapists were considered part of the interdisciplinary team and specialized in the treatment of peripheral nerve injuries and amputations. Clinical practice included activities of daily living (ADL), work simplification, functional performance, therapeutic exercise, and training in the use of prosthetics.[54]

Occupational therapists negotiated with the Army to raise their status from subprofessional to professional. The Army agreed and demanded that graduates of the war emergency courses be eligible for full registration with AOTA. After some debate AOTA decided to support the short training courses.[49]

The war served to crystallize concepts of treatment and to expand the body of practical and theoretical knowledge used by occupational therapists. In 1947 the first text on occupational therapy was written, Willard and Spackman's *Principles of Occupational Therapy*. According to Clare S. Spackman, the goals of occupational therapy in physical dysfunction were, "(1) to improve the motion of joints and the strength of muscles; (2) to develop co-ordination, motor skills and work tolerance; and (3) to prevent the building up of unwholesome psychologic reactions or to correct them if they are already established." Therapeutic activities and exercises were prescribed, analyzed, graded, and adapted to obtain specific motions. Attention was paid to the patient's posture, bed and wheelchair position, muscle substitution patterns, range of motion, and muscle strength.[53]

REHABILITATION MOVEMENT

By the 1940s the profession had practiced under at least two philosophies: holism and reductionism. Whereas holism had provided a broad humanistic approach to therapy, reductionism had led to a precise and extensive technology for the treatment of a wide range of physical disabilities. Emphasis was placed on acquiring clinical skills such as progressive resistive exercises, neuromuscular facilitation, ADL, prosthetic training, and fabrication of orthoses. The advantage of this trend was that therapists became proficient in the use of a variety of treatment techniques. As a result, therapists' values and ideas were altered, and these new attitudes were reflected in the therapeutic activities prescribed for the disabled.[39]

This technical orientation resulted in a gradual erosion of the earlier humanistic philosophical base as a foundation for the profession. Instead occupational therapy became increasingly focused on technique acquisition. These techniques were practiced without integrating them into a philosophical base, theory, or frame of reference.

Shannon[52] later called the profession's movement away from the traditional humanistic philosophy "the derailment of occupational therapy." He stated that a new philosophy had developed, which viewed man "as a mechanistic creature susceptible to manipulation and control via the application of techniques." This "technique philosophy" contradicted the philosophy on which the profession was founded. According to Shannon the profession faced two alternatives. The first alternative was to ignore the crisis between the original humanistic philosophy and the contemporary "technique philosophy." The second alternative was to reinstate the traditional "values and beliefs on which the profession was founded and thereby arrest the process of derailment."[52]

RETURN OF HUMANISM

The decade of the 1960s was an era of change, when society once again began to embrace humanistic ideals. Social movements, such as civil rights activities and the war on poverty, reflected the values and beliefs of the time.[17] The profession of occupational therapy also explored the need for change. By the 1960s the profession recognized that therapists had not only accepted reductionist thinking but also that this mode of thinking had replaced the original emphasis on purposeful activity or occupation. There was growing concern over the inadequacies of the philosophical base supporting occupational therapy. As a result the founding principles of humanism received increased attention.[30]

According to Kielhofner[28], there are two viewpoints regarding purposeful activity or occupation as the philosophical foundation of the profession. The first viewpoint sees the development of occupational therapy as a process of continuous adaptation. In adapting to meet changing times and health care needs, the profession adopted the "technique philosophy" and disavowed "activity . . . as a generic philosophy."[28] Proponents of this first perspective consider purposeful activity or occupation to be an impractical philosophical premise.

Proponents of the second viewpoint argue that purposeful activity or occupation offers an accurate perspective that has characterized occupational therapy throughout its history. Since its conception, occupational therapy has been based on the idea that activity (1) restores health in individuals suffering from either mental or physical dysfunction and (2) maintains the well-being of the healthy individual.[16] Activity is viewed not only as the core of occupational therapy but also as

the unique feature of the profession. Reductionistic occupational therapy practice is viewed as seriously deviating from the early philosophical premises of the field.[31,52] This second viewpoint holds that technique-based practice must be reunited with the earlier activity-oriented philosophy of occupational therapy.

A study by Bissell and Mailloux[10] in 1981 explored the use of crafts in occupational therapy for the physically disabled. This study surveyed 250 occupational therapists in the United States who chose physical disabilities as their specialty. The results of this study showed that, although most of the respondents used crafts as a treatment modality, the majority only used crafts a small percentage of the treatment time. The greatest amount of treatment time was devoted to self-care activities and therapeutic exercise. The authors concluded that "if therapeutic crafts are no longer considered a central concept of occupational therapy, there may be a need to revise the curricula pertaining to craft use."[10]

Fidler[22] stated that many occupational therapists have disclaimed activities and identified with the modalities of other professions to achieve credibility. These modalities "eliminate the self as the doer-agent and place the causative agent outside the self."[22] According to Fidler, "when occupational therapists are comfortable labeling a significant part of their practice as unproductive activity, the fundamental principles of occupational therapy are denied."[22]

Since the 1960s newer sensorimotor and neurophysiological treatment approaches have developed. Clinical emphasis on these approaches has increased, whereas emphasis on activities has decreased. According to Cynkin,[16] occupational therapists have incorporated these newer techniques into practice without looking at how they relate to an activity-oriented philosophical base for treatment. In the process of acquiring these techniques, occupational therapists have disavowed the use of activities as the core of occupational therapy.

TREND REVERSAL

In an effort to establish a single philosophical base of occupational therapy, the Representative Assembly of the AOTA adopted Resolution No. 531-79 in April, 1979. This philosophical base states:

Man is an active being whose development is influenced by the use of purposeful activity. Human beings are able to influence their physical and mental health and their social and physical environment through purposeful activity. Human life is a process of continuous adaptation. Adaptation is a change in function that promotes survival and self-actualization. Biological, psychological and environmental factors may interrupt the adaptation process at any time throughout the life cycle, causing dysfunction. Purposeful activity facilitates the adaptive process. Purposeful activity (occupation), including its interpersonal and environmental components, may be used to prevent and mediate dysfunction and to elicit maximum adaptation. Activity as used by the occupational therapist includes both an intrinsic and a therapeutic purpose.[4]

As written, purposeful activity (occupation) is the key concept in the philosophical base. The term "occupation" or "occupational" was suggested to reestablish a continuity between current trends and the historical beliefs of the profession.[5,24,28,29] Despite the historical use of the term, purposeful activity was not officially defined by the profession until several years later.

In 1981 an AOTA task force was charged to look at occupational therapy and physical therapy. Among the recommendations included in the task force report were to "define purposeful activity" and to "develop a policy on the use of modalities."[27]

In April, 1983, the AOTA adopted a position paper to clarify the use of the term "purposeful activities." This document was revised in 1993.[26] The original position paper defined purposeful activities as tasks or experiences in which people actively participate as part of their daily life routines.[25] In the 1993 revision, purposeful activities were further described as "goal directed behaviors or tasks that comprise occupations."[26] Both editions of the position paper stated that, when engaged in purposeful activity, an individual's attention is focused on the goal of the activity rather than the process needed to achieve the goal.[25,26] Although open to interpretation, this definition of purposeful activity appears to be in concert with both the traditional philosophy of occupational therapy and the concept of human occupation. Other key concepts in the position papers are that purposeful activity (1) is a legitimate tool of occupational therapy, (2) requires and elicits coordination of the sensorimotor, cognitive, and psychosocial systems, and (3) has unique meaning to each person. Furthermore, occupational therapists analyze, adapt, and grade activities to promote restoration of function and to assist individuals in achieving competence in the occupational performance areas of ADL, work, and play/leisure.[25,26]

Following the publication of the original official position paper on purposeful activity in 1983, several experts further defined the terms "purposeful activity" or "occupation." Gilfoyle[24] defined *occupational* as "a process of action in which the person is the action agent or 'doer.'" To clarify the term further, Evans[21] defined *occupation* as "the active or 'doing' process of a person engaged in goal-directed, intrinsically gratifying and culturally appropriate activity." Inherent in these definitions are the underlying concepts of biopsychosocial unity, developmental sequence, and adaptive capacities. Evans suggested that occupation is the core concept of occupational therapy, and as such, it determines the boundaries of the profession's domain.

Brienes[12] stated that all activities requiring both mental and physical involvement can be assumed to be purposeful activities. Llorens[35] suggested that the profession be based upon and committed to a holistic philosophy that uses purposeful activity or occupation to remedy occupational dysfunction. Rogers[51] called for a study of human occupation. She stated that occupation is the medium of therapy and that occupational therapists need to understand the health-enhancing nature of occupation. West[58] recommended that the term "occupation" be used as the common core of occupational therapy, that the profession speak in terms of "serving the occupational need of human beings" rather than "treating the whole person", and that the profession define and organize itself around occupational performance dysfunction.

Mosey[40] stated that the profession is too diverse to adhere to a monistic professional identity and suggested that a pluralistic approach be considered. In a monistic perspective occupational therapy is defined by one basic principle that governs all other principles. Some bases for monistic approaches to occupational therapy are purposeful activity, occupation, human growth and development, occupational behavior, adaptive responses, and the systems model. In contrast, a pluralistic approach defines a profession by many principles. Gilfoyle[24] suggested that professional unity may not mean adhering to a single theory but, rather, to a set of theories.

THERAPISTS RESPOND

In response to AOTA's attempt to promote the use of purposeful activity as the core of occupational therapy practice, many therapists expressed concern about the restrictions that purposeful activity or occupation would place on practice in the treatment of physical disabilities.* These restrictions include, but are not limited to, (1) jeopardizing reimbursement, (2) negating the skills and knowledge achieved by experienced clinicians, (3) jeopardizing referrals, and (4) excluding methods, such as exercise, splinting, and inhibition-facilitation techniques.

The concerns stem from an unclear or unacceptable definition of purposeful activity that excludes exercise. These therapists believe that tying treatment methods to purposeful activity is not always appropriate or effective. Many patients receiving occupational therapy services are not yet at an appropriate level of motor activity to participate in purposeful activity. In such circumstances, it is argued, clinicians must use adjunctive treatment techniques to assist in the development of motor skills needed to participate in purposeful activity. Adjunctive techniques, as described by Trombly,[56] include exercise, electrical stimulation, biofeedback, massage, whirlpool, and thermal application. Therapists holding this viewpoint do not believe that the profession's historical use of *purposeful activity* should be denied. They believe, however, that the definition of purposeful activity needs

---

* References 10, 13, 15, 20, 32, 43, 56, 57

to be expanded to incorporate contemporary treatment techniques. It is believed that, instead of attempting to redirect the focus of the profession, the profession needs to include current clinical practices that have proved effective on an empirical and practical basis.[6,56]

Other therapists expressed concern that although purposeful activity may have been one of the unifying concepts of occupational therapy in the past, this philosophical base no longer promotes cohesiveness among the profession. Pedretti[42] stated that purposeful activity "may have served to identify, define and articulate a disunity that has existed . . . for years." Lyons[37] reaffirmed this viewpoint by stating that although purposeful activity "has been one of the unifying concepts of occupational therapy in the past . . . today the use of this term seems more divisive than unifying." The phrase purposeful activity "has become an umbrella for a heterogeneous bag of human endeavors." For some therapists, *purposeful activity* means crafts, games, or activities of daily living. Other therapists include exercise and physical modalities in their own personal definitions of purposeful activity. Lyons[37] warned that by allowing the term to "mean all things to all people," purposeful activity is losing "its power to direct and influence" the profession. Lyons also encouraged therapists to examine the concepts of Soviet activity theory, which contends that activity is better described neither as purposeful nor as purposeless, but rather as human occupation.

In 1984 Pasquinelli conducted a study to describe the relationship and relevance of occupational therapy's philosophical base to the treatment methods used in physical disabilities practice. The results of this study supported the view that occupational therapists who specialize in physical dysfunction use a wide variety of treatment techniques. Some of these techniques agreed with the philosophical base but others did not. Facilitation techniques and nonactivity-oriented techniques appeared to be least consistent with the concept of purposeful activity. This incongruity had not prevented occupational therapists from using these techniques. In fact, some passive techniques were used just as frequently, and in some cases more frequently, than traditional activity-oriented techniques. All these treatment techniques were viewed as legitimate professional tools regardless of whether or not a technique agreed with the philosophical base.[41]

New techniques and modalities have been integrated into the occupational therapy philosophical base by means of the continuum of health care services provided by occupational therapists. Llorens[35] reviewed clinical practice in nine sites serving a variety of patient populations. The clinicians at these sites valued purposeful activity or occupation as part of the treatment process. Occupation did not account for the entire therapy program, however. A continuum of occupational therapy services was described, from occupational dysfunction to occupational function.

In an attempt to resolve the conflict of activity versus exercise, Dutton[18] suggested viewing activity and exercise not as mutually exclusive and philosophically opposed treatment techniques, but as complements that provide a continuum of therapy. She examined the biomechanical and sensorimotor frames of reference and developed guidelines and criteria for when to use biomechanical and sensorimotor activities and when to incorporate purposeful activities into the treatment plan. Exercise and sensorimotor activities were viewed as techniques to prepare patients for purposeful activity or occupation. Dutton advocated both activity and exercise within a treatment plan. Patients need to engage in occupation to make the transition from simple to complex movements and to function in the environment.[18]

Pedretti conceptualized a four-stage treatment continuum that is consistent with the occupational performance frame of reference. (See Chapter 1.) The model depicts a continuum of treatment activities from the use of modalities to occupation or purposeful activity. The model consists of four stages: adjunctive methods, enabling activities, purposeful activity, and occupational performance and community reintegration. Occupational therapy intervention contributes to the patient's progress from the early, acute stages of occupational dysfunction to the desired outcome of occupational performance.[43] The debate over the use of physical agent modalities is viewed as a debate over the incorporation of these modalities into adjunctive methods, the first stage of this model.[44]

In 1991 AOTA's Physical Agent Modality Task Force report defined physical agent modalities as those modalities that "use the properties of light, water, temperature, sound, and electricity to produce a response in soft tissue. Physical agent modalities include, but are not limited to: paraffin baths, hot and cold packs, Fluidotherapy, contrast baths, ultrasound, whirlpool, and electrical stimulation units."[2] Later that year AOTA approved an official statement on physical agent modalities. The statement read:

Physical agent modalities may be used by occupational therapy practitioners when used as an adjunct to or in preparation for purposeful activity to enhance occupational performance and when applied by a practitioner who has documented evidence of possessing the theoretical background and technical skills for safe and competent integration of the modality into an occupational therapy intervention plan.[1]

Taylor and Humphry[55] surveyed occupational therapists in physical disabilities regarding their use of, training in, and opinions regarding use of physical agent modalities. Of the occupational therapists surveyed, those in hand rehabilitation were the most frequent users of these modalities and held the most positive opinions regarding their use. Hot and cold packs were the most commonly used modalities, whereas ultrasound was the least frequently used. These results confirmed the findings of the member data survey conducted by the Physical Agent Modality Task Force.[55]

In 1992 AOTA's Representative Assembly approved a physical agent modalities position paper to clarify the parameters for the appropriate use of physical agent modalities in occupational therapy. As a result, AOTA's Policy 1.25 was amended to state that the use of physical agent modalities in occupational therapy is appropriate "only in preparation for, or as an adjunct to, purposeful activity to enhance occupational performance."[3]

SUMMARY

In the formative years of the profession, occupational therapy adhered to holistic and humanistic philosophies regarding patient care. The philosophies and the treatment techniques used were consistent with the professional beliefs and the external political, sociocultural, and medical environments of the time. As external environments changed, occupational therapists responded and adapted by using and refining a wide variety of treatment techniques. Later these techniques became viewed as reductionistic and deviating from the original holistic foundation. Therapists thus worked toward a resolution whereby the holistic foundation and a variety of techniques could be integrated and acknowledged as occupational therapy.

Although treatment techniques have evolved over the years, the holistic values and beliefs established in the formative years of the profession continue to be upheld. These beliefs include that occupation as prescribed by occupational therapy practitioners promotes health, prevents and remedies dysfunction, and elicits adaptation to the environment. Even as new treatment techniques and technologies are developed in the future, occupational therapy intervention that promotes occupational function will remain consistent with the philosophical base of the profession.

REVIEW QUESTIONS

1. What factors influence professional development?
2. Describe moral treatment. How did moral treatment concepts affect occupational therapy?
3. What factors led to the advent and demise of the arts and crafts movement?
4. When did occupational therapy formally begin? Which individuals were involved? What were some of their beliefs?
5. How did World War I influence the profession?
6. Describe the role of the occupational therapy reconstruction aides in hospitals.
7. What impact did the depression have on the profession?
8. Define *reductionism*.
9. Define *occupations* according to Rush.
10. State one outcome of World War II.
11. State one advantage of reductionism.
12. What factors led to the return of humanism?
13. Describe the controversy that resulted from practicing under two opposing philosophies.
14. What key concepts are included in the philosophical base? Why?
15. What events happened following the establishment of AOTA Resolution No. 531-79 in 1979? Why?
16. Describe three ways that treatment techniques and modalities have been integrated into our holistic philosophical base.
17. Define *physical agent modalities*.
18. According to AOTA, when may physical agent modalities be used by occupational therapy practitioners?

REFERENCES

1. American Occupational Therapy Association: *Official: AOTA statement on physical agent modalities,* Rockville, Md, 1991, The Association.
2. American Occupational Therapy Association: *Physical agent modality task force report,* Rockville, Md, 1991, The Association.
3. American Occupational Therapy Association: *Association policy 1.25: registered occupational therapists and certified occupational therapy assistants and modalities,* Rockville, Md, 1992, The Association.
4. American Occupational Therapy Association: Association policy 1.11: the philosophical base of occupational therapy, *Am J Occup Ther* 47:1119, 1993.
5. American Occupational Therapy Association: Association policy 1.12: occupation as the common core of occupational therapy, *Am J Occup Ther* 47:1119, 1993.
6. Ayres AJ: Basic concepts of clinical practice in physical disabilities, *Am J Occup Ther* 12:300, 1958.
7. Baldwin BT: Occupational therapy, *Am J of Care for Cripples* 8:447, 1919.
8. Baldwin BT: *Occupational therapy applied to restoration of function of disabled joints,* Washington, DC, 1919, Walter Reed General Hospital.
9. Bing R: Occupational therapy revisited: a paraphrastic journey: 1981 Eleanor Clark Slagle lecture, *Am J Occup Ther* 35:499, 1981.
10. Bissell JC, Mailloux Z: The use of crafts in occupational therapy for the physically disabled, *Am J Occup Ther* 35:369, 1981.
11. Bockoven JS: Legacy of moral treatment: 1800s to 1910, *Am J Occup Ther* 25:223, 1971.
12. Breines E: The issue is: an attempt to define purposeful activity, *Am J Occup Ther* 38:543, 1984.
13. Clopton JS: Craft use with physically disabled questioned, *Am J Occup Ther* 35:669, 1981 (letter).
14. Colman W: Evolving educational practices in occupational therapy: the war emergency courses, 1936-1954, *Am J Occup Ther* 44:1028, 1990.

15. Courtsunis DG and associates: Purposeful activity restricts practice, *Am J Occup Ther* 36:468, 1982 (letter).
16. Cynkin S: *Occupational therapy: toward health through activities,* Boston, 1979, Little, Brown.
17. Diasio K: The modern era: 1960 to 1970, *Am J Occup Ther* 25:237, 1971.
18. Dutton R: Guidelines for using both activity and exercise, *Am J Occup Ther* 43:573, 1989.
19. Engelhardt HT: Defining occupational therapy: the meaning of therapy and the virtues of occupation, *Am J Occup Ther* 31:666, 1977.
20. English C and associates: On the role of the occupational therapist in physical disabilities (the issue), *Am J Occup Ther* 36:199, 1982.
21. Evans KA: Nationally speaking: definition of occupation as the core concept of occupational therapy, *Am J Occup Ther* 41:627, 1987.
22. Fidler GS: From crafts to competence, *Am J Occup Ther* 35:567, 1981.
23. The future of disabled soldiers: recommendations of the conference called by the General Medical Board of the Advisory Commission of the Council of National Defense, *Modern Hospital* 9:124, 1917.
24. Gilfoyle EM: Transformation of a profession: 1984 Eleanor Clark Slagle lecture, *Am J Occup Ther* 38:575, 1984.
25. Hinojosa J and associates: Purposeful activities, *Am J Occup Ther* 37:805, 1983.
26. Hinojosa J and associates: Position paper: purposeful activity, *Am J Occup Ther* 47:1081, 1993.
27. Huss AJ: Nationally speaking: whither thou goest? Report of the AOTA task force on OT/PT issues, *Am J Occup Ther* 38:81, 1984.
28. Kielhofner G: A heritage of activity: development of theory, *Am J Occup Ther* 36:723, 1982.
29. Kielhofner G: *Health through occupation: theory and practice in occupational therapy,* Philadelphia, 1983, FA Davis.
30. Kielhofner G, Burke JP: A model of human occupation. I. Conceptual framework and content, *Am J Occup Ther* 34:572, 1980.
31. Kielhofner G, Burke JP: Occupational therapy after 60 years: an account of changing identity and knowledge, *Am J Occup Ther* 31:675, 1977.
32. Leffler JS: Derailment of occupational therapy, *Am J Occup Ther* 32:53, 1978 (letter).
33. Levine RE: Looking back—the influence of the arts-and-crafts movement on the professional status of occupational therapy, *Am J Occup Ther* 41:248, 1987.
34. Licht S: The founding and founders of the American Occupational Therapy Association, *Am J Occup Ther* 21:269, 1967.
35. Llorens LA: Changing balance: environment and individual, *Am J Occup Ther* 38:29, 1984.
36. Low JF: The reconstruction aides, *Am J Occup Ther* 46:38, 1992.
37. Lyons BG: The issue is: purposeful versus human activity, *Am J Occup Ther* 37:493, 1983.
38. Meyer A: The philosophy of occupational therapy, *Am J Occup Ther* 31:639, 1977.
39. Mosey AC: Involvement in the rehabilitation movement: 1942-1960, *Am J Occup Ther* 25:234, 1971.
40. Mosey AC: A monistic or a pluralistic approach to professional identity? 1985 Eleanor Clark Slagle lecture, *Am J Occup Ther* 39:504, 1985.
41. Pasquinelli S: The relationship of physical disabilities treatment methodologies to the philosophical base of occupational therapy, unpublished thesis, San Jose State University, 1984.
42. Pedretti LW: The compatibility of treatment methods in physical disabilities with the philosophical base of occupational therapy. Paper presented to the American Occupational Therapy Association National Conference, Philadelphia, May 13, 1982.
43. Pedretti LW: Occupational performance: a model for practice in physical dysfunction. In Pedretti LW: *Occupational therapy practice skills for physical dysfunction,* ed 4, St Louis, 1995, Mosby-Year Book.
44. Pedretti LW, Smith RO, Hammel J and associates: Use of adjunctive modalities in occupational therapy, *Am J Occup Ther* 46:1075, 1992.
45. Peloquin SM: Looking back—moral treatment: contexts considered, *Am J Occup Ther* 43:537, 1989.
46. Peloquin SM: Looking back—occupational therapy service: individual and collective understandings of the founders. I. *Am J Occup Ther* 45:352, 1991.
47. Peloquin SM: Looking back—occupational therapy service: individual and collective understandings of the founders. II. *Am J Occup Ther* 45:733, 1991.
48. Reed KL: Tools of practice: heritage or baggage?—1986 Eleanor Clark Slagle lecture, *Am J Occup Ther* 40:597, 1986.
49. Reed KL: The beginnings of occupational therapy. In Hopkins HL, Smith HD, editors: *Willard and Spackman's occupational therapy,* ed 8, Philadelphia, 1993, JB Lippincott.
50. Rerek MD: The depression years: 1929 to 1941, *Am J Occup Ther* 25:231, 1971.
51. Rogers JC: The spirit of independence: the evolution of a philosophy, *Am J Occup Ther* 36:709, 1982.
52. Shannon PD: The derailment of occupational therapy, *Am J Occup Ther* 31:229, 1977.
53. Spackman CS: Occupational therapy for patients with physical injuries. In Willard HS, Spackman CS, editors: *Occupational therapy,* ed 1, Philadelphia, 1947, JB Lippincott.
54. Spackman CS: A history of the practice of occupational therapy for restoration of physical function: 1917-1967, *Am J Occup Ther* 22:67, 1968.
55. Taylor E, Humphry R: Survey of physical agent modality use, *Am J Occup Ther* 45:924, 1991.
56. Trombly CA: Include exercise in purposeful activity, *Am J Occup Ther* 36:467, 1982 (letter).
57. Walker JK and associates: Against crafts emphasis, *Am J*

Occup Ther 36:469, 1982 (letter).

58. West W: A reaffirmed philosophy and practice of occupational therapy for the 1980s, *Am J Occup Ther* 38:15, 1984.

59. Wish-Baratz S: Looking back—Bird T. Baldwin: a holistic scientist in occupational therapy's history, *Am J Occup Ther* 43:257, 1989.

60. Woodside HH: The development of occupational therapy: 1910-1929, *Am J Occup Ther* 25:226, 1971.

Occupational Therapy and Health Care Reform

Kathleen Barker Schwartz, Jeanette Engle-Ramirez

HISTORY OF HEALTH CARE REFORM IN THE UNITED STATES

To comprehend today's health care system and occupational therapy's role within it, it is necessary to understand the events and ideas that have contributed to shaping American health care. This chapter begins with a description of three periods in the history of United States health care. It examines key ideas that have led to the current health care system and discusses current and future trends in health care.

SCIENTIFIC MEDICINE (1900-1920)
Scientific Reforms

By 1920 the image of medical care had been transformed to one of efficiency and science.[46] The noisy, dirty asylum of the 19th century was replaced by that of the clean, efficient hospital of the twentieth century. This transformation was in part due to discoveries of antiseptic procedures for surgical and nursing care. Medical care was also influenced by the reforms of the progressive era,[31] which combined the social obligation of relieving poverty and illness with the emphasis on national efficiency and science. Edward T. Devine, a reformer of that period, wrote that it was in society's interest to promote medicine, including medical education and laboratory research "to improve general levels of efficiency and skill in the population."[19]

The ideology of efficiency and science had its roots in the ideas of scientific management first proposed by Frederick Taylor,[49] an engineer. He proposed that the engineering values of rationality, efficiency, and systematic observation could be applied to management and other areas of life to address society's ills.[49] The idea that knowledge could be developed through research and observation and applied to patient care became an underlying tenet of the science of medicine. By 1920 medicine was a scientific discipline concerned with the identification and cure of diseases.[51] Doctors were viewed as people of science and hospitals were where cures were effected.

Scientific medicine and the education of its practitioners required reliable standards. When Abraham Flexner, executive director of the Carnegie Foundation for the Advancement of Teaching, toured medical schools in 1910 with the American Medical Association (AMA) Council on Medical Education he found great disparities among the schools. His report provided the basis for substantial reform in medical education.[23] By 1920 medical schools had consolidated, raised educational standards, and revised curricula.

While Flexner[23] emphasized the notion of accountability in medical education, Dr. E.A. Codman,[14] a scientific management enthusiast, campaigned for accountability in medical treatment. He proposed that physicians and hospitals should be responsible for quality and developed a system using detailed medical record entries to examine effective therapeutic interventions. His work pioneered today's quality improvement efforts.

The movement for compulsory health insurance between 1915 and 1920 was built on the ideal of the social efficiency to be achieved by guaranteeing a healthy population: healthy workers would be productive contributors to society. In 1919 it was estimated that $600 million was lost in pay because of sickness, and families spent more than $1 billion a year on medical care.[43] The AMA's initial response to the idea of compulsory coverage was positive.[36] As time passed, however, doctors formed negative opinions based on their experience with the newly passed workmen's compensation legislation. The first movement for compulsory health insurance was defeated by (1) the weakness of the bills and (2) division within the medical profession, business, and labor over determining what health services would be provided, who would pay, and how services would be provided. It appears that similar concerns defeated President Clinton's 1993-94 health reform effort.

The emphasis on efficiency promoted deference to medical authority and provided a rationale whereby physicians could argue for control of the health care system.[45] From this viewpoint patients were part of the production system and nurses were helpers to doctors, who possessed the scientific knowledge and thus the authority. Bayard Holmes, a prominent Chicago physician, wrote in the AMA Journal: "The hospital is essentially part of the armamentarium of medicine . . . If we wish to avoid the fate of the tool-less wage worker, we must control the hospital."[32] By 1920 the medical profession had gained considerable strength and prestige through successes in surgery, claims to expertise based on science, and through the strength of its professional organizations.[46]

Emergence of Occupational Therapy

The founders of occupational therapy first met in Clifton Springs, New York, on March 15, 1917, against the backdrop of World War I. Indeed 21 days later the United States would enter the war. Thus much of the profession's early years were spent on the war effort as follows: negotiating a role for its practitioners, preparing the "reconstruction aides" for service at the front, and educating the occupationalists to treat the returning war-wounded in the United States.[39] Surgeon General William Gorgas, in planning for the physical restoration of disabled servicemen, recommended "work, mental and manual . . . during the convalescent period"[25] and saw occupational therapy as a profession that could assist in that process.

A second important area of practice was with individuals who suffered industrial accidents. Elizabeth Upham[50] estimated that industrial accident patients exceeded the war casualties. Social concern for the victims of the Industrial Revolution was great during the progressive era, and occupational therapy's potential to return these individuals to productive societal roles was promising.[1] A third major area of practice was with patients with mental illness. Indeed the profession traced its roots to the humane treatment movement in the United States in the 1800s.[11]

During its early years the profession emphasized its work with individuals having both physical and mental disabilities, war-wounded as well as civilians. The profession portrayed itself as working with patients throughout the three stages of recovery.[29] During convalescence they would do bedside, diversional treatment. Once patients were strong enough, they would be engaged in occupations that would strengthen both mind and body. Finally, once patients were ready to return to the community, they were engaged in occupations that would prepare them for vocational success. By 1920 the profession had adopted *occupational therapy* as its name and promoted the notion of the "science" of occupation by calling for "the advancement of occupation as a therapeutic measure, the study of the effects of occupation upon the human being, and the dissemination of scientific knowledge of this subject."[16] At the same time it maintained a broad definition of practice: "The duties of the occupational therapist are broad and far-reaching, including as they do something of arts and crafts, social

services, trades and industries, and humanity."[2] These actions were consistent with the progressive reformers' social concerns and enthusiasm for science. Such a broad definition, however, while humanistic in spirit, did not fit well within the scientific medicine model that advocated narrow specialties. As competing health professions developed, the breadth of this definition would make overlap and conflict inevitable.

While the profession defined itself in broad social terms, it also seemed to accept the notion of its place as helper to the physician. This stance in part reflected the views of its founders, particularly Dr. William Rush Dunton, a psychiatrist. Dunton wrote that in the same way the physician relies upon the nurse to give medication, "so must he rely upon the therapist to administer the practical part of occupational therapy. . . . The occupational therapist, therefore, has the same relation to the physician as has the nurse, that is, she is a technical assistant."[20] This view placed the doctor at the top of the hierarchy within the medical system.[28]

ADVANCEMENT OF REHABILITATION (1945-1955)
Development of Rehabilitation Model

World War II revived the need for the United States to provide medical care for its wounded soldiers. Recent scientific discoveries had resulted in much higher survival rates than for World War I. Such laboratory discoveries as sulfa drugs and penicillin confirmed the importance of medicine as a science that could make a great contribution to society. The demand for medical services also increased in the civilian population as workers migrated to the industrial areas. The promise of further medical breakthroughs plus increased demand for military and civilian medical care generated pressure to build hospitals and public health centers. The 1946 Hill-Burton Act provided for federal aid to states for construction of additional facilities. This legislation provided funding for the construction of rehabilitation centers.

With the increase in centers for medical care came growing awareness of the need for health insurance. President Truman came to power in 1948 with the campaign promise of instituting national health insurance. This effort was defeated, in large part by opposition from the AMA, which mounted a heavily financed campaign that linked national health insurance to socialism and communism. One pamphlet asked, "Would socialized medicine lead to socialization of other phases of American life?" and it answered, "Lenin thought so. He declared: Socialized medicine is the keystone to the arch of the Socialist state."[45] The defeat of national health insurance left a predominantly private system as the obvious alternative. The next ten years would establish Blue Cross and Blue Shield as the winners among rivals for national recognition.[4] An interesting alternative was proposed by Henry J. Kaiser, who believed he could provide prepaid and comprehensive services at affordable prices.

Ten years after the war Kaiser-Permanente had a growing network of hospitals with a half million people enrolled. Kaiser's prescience is acknowledged today as health maintenance organizations (HMOs) have become predominant health care providers.

Following World War II a major effort was launched to reorganize and revitalize the Veterans Administration (VA) hospital system. Departments of physical medicine and rehabilitation were created within the VA to bring together all the services needed to care for the large number of war injured. This interdisciplinary approach to care led to the development of comprehensive rehabilitation centers in the private sector as well: "The theory that handicapped persons can be aided by persons who understand their special needs originated during World War II. The armed services established such hospitals for disabled veterans as the one for paraplegics in Birminham Calif. They helped the morale and physical condition of the patients so much that others were built for civilians."[41]

A prominent voice in the development of rehabilitation medicine was Howard Rusk, head of rehabilitation and physical medicine at New York University. In an article written in *The New York Times* Rusk cited the shortage of trained personnel to work with the "5,300,000 persons in the nation who suffer from chronic disability".[35] The article discussed a study by the Commission on Chronic Illness. Their findings were: (1) Medicine and its related fields do not have specific answers for the control of many of the diseases that cause long-term illness. The social, economic, medical, and emotional effects of long-term disability, however, can be eliminated or substantially reduced through comprehensive, integrated rehabilitation services. (2) The greatest single factor in preventing more rapid expansion of urgently needed rehabilitation services is the shortage of trained personnel.[35] Rusk stated that meeting the needs of the aged, chronically ill, and disabled citizens depended on national commitment to these needs. He cited occupational therapy as one of the necessary services.

The Specialization of Occupational Therapy

Like World War I, World War II provided a great impetus for occupational therapy services. The war highlighted the value of occupational therapy: "Although occupational therapy started during the last World War, it developed slowly and now the doctors are finding this aid to the sick and wounded invaluable as a needed part of the medical profession. A local orthopedist, Dr. Browne, said when he spoke to the group of occupational therapy students, 'This war will bring occupational therapy into its own. . . .' "[40]

The war also played a role in defining occupational therapy. Emphasis was put on physical disabilities and therapy that would "aid in restoring function to injured limbs and muscles and wounds received in the different theatres of war. . . ."[40] The focus on physical disabilities was accompanied by a shift from activities common in World War I, such as needlepoint, to those perceived as more manly occupations: "The Army is death on the old-time invalid occupations of basket weaving, chair caning, pottery and weaving. These are 'not believed to be interesting occupation for the present condition of men in military service,' says an officer from the Surgeon General's office. The stress now is on carpentry, repair work at the hospital, war-related jobs like knitting camouflage nets, and printing."[26]

The growth of the rehabilitation industry, itself a product of the war, led to development of occupational therapy services. A proviso of the Hill-Burton Act was that rehabilitation centers must "offer integrated services in four areas: medical, including occupational and physical therapy, psychological, social and vocational."[54] Although occupational therapy was defined as part of the rehabilitation team, conflicts arose with other professions that were also vying to establish themselves. A conflict between occupational therapists and physical therapists over amputation cases resulted in the Surgeon General mandating that after fitting, those with upper extremity amputations would be handled by occupational therapists and those with lower amputations by physical therapists. Another conflict developed within the VA system with physiatrists who advocated moving occupational therapy under their aegis as part of physical medicine, rather than neuropsychiatry or orthopedics.[28] In addition, a small group of OT educators successfully resisted physical medicine's attempts to control OT registry and entry-level education programs.[15] Less serious conflicts also developed with art therapy and related groups. These conflicts were predictable, given the broad nature of occupational therapy's definition. They came at a time when each discipline tried to establish its predominance within the health field.[45]

As the rehabilitation movement helped to establish the importance of occupational therapy, it further positioned the profession within the medical model. Occupational therapy was urged to specialize and separate into two distinct fields, physical disabilities and psychiatry. The head orthopedist at Rancho Los Amigos Hospital in Downey, California, argued that the separation would result in "strengthened treatment techniques" and thus more credibility among medical doctors. He asserted that "the medical profession in general does not recognize your field as an established necessary specialty."[30] The American Occupational Therapy Association sought closer ties with the American Medical Association in order to gain more credibility. The following quote indicates the difficulties the profession faced in defining and promoting itself:

Both occupational and physical therapy have taken some selling—to the medical profession as well as to the public. Many hospitals have still to discover occupational therapy. Some die-hard MDs, reluctant to see its medical implication, still think a lot of it is boondoggling, and there's been a lot of confusion about its function. Occupational therapy is not giving someone something to do just to keep him happy. It is not vocational training. It is not making pretty things to sell. All of these have therapeutic value as morale builders but they're not occupational therapy. As defined by the American Medical Association, occupational therapy is treatment for illness or disability through remedial work activity prescribed by a doctor and directed by trained technicians.[26]

The closer relationship with medicine probably helped the profession gain credibility, at least within the medical model. The negative aspects of the alignment included greater loss of autonomy and a lessening focus on the broader aspects of care entailed by its original definition.

GROWTH OF HEALTH CARE INDUSTRY (1965-1985)
Business of Health Care

The legislation to create Medicare was passed in 1965. For President Johnson it was the highest priority among the Great Society programs. The legislation combined two areas: Part A, compulsory hospital insurance, and Part B, insurance for physician fees. In addition, Medicaid was created to give expanded assistance to the states for medical care for the poor.

Medicare and Medicaid were very successful, indeed too successful. By 1970 the country was seeing sharp increases in medical care expenses caused by high demand and generous funding formulas.[17] The mood in Congress changed from concern about medical policy for the elderly and poor to concern with controlling spiraling health care costs. The government intervened with several attempts to control costs, the most effective being 1983 legislation to reform the funding formula for Medicare, using prospective payment as the basis for reimbursement. The intent was that the government would reimburse using a set fee varying by diagnostic related group (DRG), that is, type of diagnosis. The approach supported the scientific management view that the patient is a standardized product and the hospital a factory.

The creation of new models of health care delivery was encouraged. Congress passed legislation in 1973 requiring employers to offer at least one HMO plan. This legislation also financially supported the development of more HMOs. The idea originally proposed by Kaiser was now viewed as one of the most promising ways to deliver care and control costs. Investor-owned hospital chains such as Hospital Corporation of America appeared on the scene. These for-profit enterprises marketed their idea that they could deliver superior health care focused on financial management, efficiency, and productivity. The role played by third party insurance payers became a critical one. By 1980 more than 92% of hospital expenditures were represented by third parties: the Government, Blue Cross, and major insurance corporations.[46]

The decade since the introduction of Medicare saw a sharp rise in costs followed by efforts to control and regulate health care. Health care became an important industry, and third party insurers became a critical force. Interest in private enterprise and HMOs represented a shift away from the country's former confidence in the government's role in health care. As scientific management, with its focus on efficiency and productivity, became a critical tenet of the medical care system, critics asked how well the standardization of medical practice fit with the realities of clinical judgment.[45]

Expansion of Occupational Therapy

The boom of the 1970s in the health care industry helped occupational therapy develop both within the hospital and beyond. Occupational therapy services were now available to private homes, public schools, nursing homes, community mental health centers, and the work place. Medicare legislation provided reimbursement for occupational therapy services; these services had to be provided in conjunction with physical therapy, speech therapy, or nursing, however, all considered to be primary services.[28] Concerns about reimbursement were expressed by the president of AOTA, in her address to the Delegate Assembly in 1976. She read a letter from an unidentified AOTA member which stated in part: "Unless we can . . . solv[e] the gigantic problems of reimbursement for our services, we shall cease to exist."[33]

Substantial effort was made in the 1970s to redress this issue. The AOTA moved to Washington in 1972, hired public relations staff and lobbyists, and formed a government affairs department to follow legislative events. The association launched an extensive marketing campaign targeted toward physicians and third party payers as well as consumers. The Association revised its negative view of licensing and assisted state organizations in securing licensing for occupational therapy practice. In succeeding years the profession gained coverage for occupational therapy services so that currently, occupational therapy is reimbursed in in-patient and out-patient settings, rehabilitation, and skilled nursing facilities. For Medicare reimbursement for home health, however, occupational therapy can be referred only in conjunction with nursing, physical, or speech therapy, although once services are initiated they can continue even if the other services are terminated.[48]

Medicare defined occupational therapy as "medically-prescribed treatment" concerned with improving or restoring functions impaired by illness or injury. To qualify for reimbursement by Medicare, occupational therapy must be prescribed by a physician, performed by a qualified occupational therapist or certified occupational therapy assistant (COTA) under supervision, and be "reasonable and necessary."[7] Because Medicare was national, it provided a model by which other third parties could define occupational therapy services, one tied explicitly to the medical model. At the same time leaders within the profession called for occupational therapy to lessen its ties with the medical illness model and to adopt a theoretical base drawn from the behavioral sciences as well as the medical sciences.[42] Therapists were urged to reclaim the early definition of occupational therapy rooted in humane treatment.[12] The passage of PL 94-142 Education for All Handicapped Children in 1975 increased pediatric practice within an educational rather than a medical setting. Thus tension developed between practice in physical disabilities, which required adherence to the medical model for reimbursement, and practice in other areas that were not as closely bound to the medical model.

In summary, the two decades after Medicare saw substantial efforts to advocate for the profession. The AOTA responded to reimbursement concerns by marketing occupational therapy as a cost-effective, necessary service. The American Occupational Therapy Foundation (AOTF) was created to conduct research to establish the profession's legitimacy and efficacy. A strong public relations staff was established within the national office to enable the profession to participate in legislation and to promote the fast-growing field. The growth of the health care industry meant a substantial increase in the need for occupational therapists in a variety of settings. Those working in physical disabilities found their practice circumscribed by the new Medicare regulations that tied reimbursement to the medical model.

This history lays the groundwork for consideration of current and future trends in health care. These trends are discussed in the remainder of this chapter.

CURRENT TRENDS IN HEALTH CARE REIMBURSEMENT
THEMES IN CHANGING PATTERNS OF HEALTH CARE REIMBURSEMENT

Since the mid1980s the national economy and its increased debt have spurred an examination of the cost and quality of the U.S. health care system[18] (Box 3-1).

Although most agree that the United States has excellent health care, it is expensive and is not equally available to all citizens.[5]

Occupational therapy in physical disabilities is affected by shifting reimbursement patterns of health care. The outcome of health care reform and health care reimbursement is still unclear but some themes prevail in current patterns of changing reimbursement. These themes include the following: (1) a primary care/managed care model, (2) an effort to achieve low cost with high quality, (3) the rationing of health care, (4) an emphasis on outcome over process, (5) patient and caretakers assume more responsibility, (6) an emphasis on wellness, (7) a desire to provide basic coverage for as many Americans as possible, (8) reimbursement by grouping charges/cross training, and (9) networks of providers.[5]

Primary Care/Managed Care Model

Many Americans choose their physician based on the health problem they are experiencing. For example, for an injured knee the patient may see an orthopedic surgeon; for blurred vision the patient might go to an ophthalmologist. In a primary health care model, one physician oversees the provision of all health care needs. When a specialist is needed the patient first sees the primary care physician (PCP), who then refers him or her to the appropriate specialist. This PCP becomes the "gatekeeper" of health care.

The managed care plan usually assists the PCP by providing case managers. The PCP or service provider calls the case manager to determine what is a usual and customary service, or who in the network provides the care needed. Authorization must be obtained before treatments or procedures except for emergencies. This model is meant to decrease costs by limiting specialty visits. A

BOX 3-1

ISSUES PUSHING HEALTH CARE REFORM IN THE 1990S

A review of the issues associated with health care reform in the 1990s demonstrates that these are not new issues. The United States continues to struggle with the cost and provision of health care to all Americans.

- 37 million Americans (10 million of whom are children) are uninsured or underinsured (i.e., one illness away from bankruptcy).
- So-called safety-net institution type care cost taxpayers $1 trillion in 1993.
- ". . . health care costs have quadrupled since 1980. Costs are projected to double by the year 2000 . . . ."

- ". . . bureaucracy and administrative overhead cost nearly 23 percent of every health care dollar as compared to 8 percent to 9 percent in Canada and 6 percent to 7 percent in Hawaii."
- "More than 2 million Americans lose their health insurance every month."
- "Many insured Americans don't really have a choice because they belong to a plan chosen by their employer."
- "Differences in patient outcomes and quality of care are not being adequately addressed."

From Anderson R: The challenge of healthcare reform, *Advance/Rehab* 3:13-14, 1994.

physician group may monitor quality by reviewing referral patterns and use of various services including occupational therapy.[44] Occupational therapy may see more referrals from PCPs, specifically those in family practice, internal medicine, or pediatrics. They may also be included in case management for certain types of patients.

Low Cost with High Quality

Providing more services with fewer resources (lower costs) is central to making health care reform work. The goal of achieving the same outcomes with different, low-cost treatment requires defining quality care and determining how to provide it while keeping costs down. Standardization of care is proposed as one way to achieve this goal.[44] One method of standardizing care is through clinical pathways-of-treatment protocols that enable patients with similar diagnoses to receive similar care. Variations in patient treatment would be promptly noted, and a new treatment initiated to maintain consistency in quality and cost. A system to compare quality across different pathways or various components of services will be necessary to ensure that low cost does not reduce quality.[8] Occupational therapy should be involved in the development of clinical pathways and quality monitors.

Rationing Health Care

It is believed that one of the reasons for the high cost of health care in the United States is the technological imperative that every patient is entitled to any advanced medical procedure, regardless of the cost or the benefit from the procedure.[9] A health care system that includes rationing of care by providing criteria for when a service is appropriate is one approach to combat these costs. The goal of achieving lower costs has led to the idea of adapting a formal system of rationing health care services.[52] States that use rationing have had to determine under which conditions a patient will be able to receive a service. It is yet to be determined how criteria will be developed if national health care is rationed.[47] Should such an approach become popular, occupational therapy will also be rationed. The profession should position itself so that it can have input into key decisions about who gets what type of care.

Emphasis on Outcome over Process

Much of the current health care system is designed to monitor quality by reviewing processes. That is, it examines who has the clinical skills and training to do a procedure, determines where it is safest to have this procedure done, and monitors safety of the equipment. These monitoring systems have been developed in response to mandates from the states and accreditation agencies such as the Joint Commission on Accreditation of Hospital Organizations.[34]

To encourage lower costs and high quality, a shift from process monitoring to outcome monitoring is advo-

cated to determine whether the delivery of care has resulted in beneficial treatment for the patient.[27] Using this approach, if occupational therapy is found to be too costly and the benefit to the patient is determined to be low, then occupational therapy will not be a treatment of choice. Licensing, which has been used to preserve specialty areas of practice, may no longer play that role. Licensing for occupational therapists may not be needed in all states. Emphasis may shift to monitoring outcomes while decreasing the number of visits and to supervising COTAs or aides in the provision of care.[38]

Patient and Caretakers Assume More Responsibility

As costs decline along with the number of outpatient visits and length of inpatient stays, reliance on the physician, therapist, or other health care provider will decrease because the patient will not see the provider as frequently.[24] Discussions about the use of the telephone to monitor progress and perform case management have started. Pilot programs now monitor patients via the phone lines while exercising.[8] Individuals and their caretakers may be assuming more responsibility for continuing their own care and progress than in the current system, in which the therapist is seen as the "coach" who assists the patient to move forward. This coaching may be done more from a distance.[24] If this trend continues, occupational therapy will need to develop more and different coaching techniques and continue to emphasize home programs.

Emphasis on Wellness

In addition to individuals taking more responsibility for their care after illness, an emphasis on prevention of illness has been discussed as a method of controlling cost. Providing vaccinations, emphasizing patient education, and encouraging people to practice healthy lifestyles are some ways to implement wellness. With the focus on prevention, there is debate on whether health care should be provided to people who knowingly follow a lifestyle that causes an illness requiring costly treatment (for example, cigarette smoking that causes lung cancer). Questions are being raised whether treatment should be covered by health care dollars or should the individual who chooses this unhealthy lifestyle be responsible for payment of that treatment.[47] Thus part of health care reform involves determining how wellness and prevention will be integrated and to what extent individuals will be held responsible for their lifestyles. A focus on prevention helps occupational therapy promote education and wellness as part of treatment and to enhance its role. Training by occupational therapists in body mechanics to prevent injury is one example.[10]

Basic Coverage for Everyone

With 37 million Americans uninsured or underinsured, basic coverage for everyone is a real challenge. At the center of the health care debate is the definition of "basic." One only need look at the difference in service coverage for occupational therapy under individual state Medicaid Acts to determine that this is not a new debate. This debate may result in a new definition of basic coverage as treatment for a specific illness rather than as type of service provided, as it is defined by most insurers now. It is difficult to predict how and if basic coverage for everyone will be achieved and to determine how this could affect occupational therapy.[44]

Reimbursement by Grouping Charges/ Cross Training

The current reimbursement system recognizes and encourages different disciplines by reimbursing individually for each service. A new proposal advocates grouping charges, that is, paying one fee regardless of who delivers the care and how much care is provided. This system would share reimbursement across physician specialties, across entities such as hospitals and physician groups, and across allied health professionals such as occupational and physical therapists. This sharing would encourage the specialist to become a generalist because the provider has an incentive to provide more care under one entity than to send the patient to other service providers and have to share the grouped charges. Occupational therapy may see changes in the rate of increase of salaries as groupings of charges is shared across disciplines. Occupational therapists may see other providers such as COTAs or certified athletic trainers (ATCs) involved in areas that traditionally belonged to occupational therapy.[24] Occupational therapists may become more generalists than specialists, and training may expand to include some areas of other specialties (cross-training) or even a merging of two professions.

In cross-training, an individual prepared in one profession is trained to perform skills typically associated with another profession. The aim of cross-training is to deliver optimal service while containing costs. It is consistent with trends to increase quality and efficiency while decreasing costs in health care reimbursement. In January, 1995, AOTA adopted a White Paper called *Occupational Therapy and Cross-Training Initiatives.*[3] Its purpose is to "provide AOTA members with a basis for evaluating and responding to cross-training initiatives at the institutional, local, state, or national level."[3] According to AOTA the consumer's well-being and interests are central to any decisions about the delivery of OT services, and the OT practitioner is accountable for the quality of services delivered. There is a legal and ethical responsibility for OT practitioners to receive training, or to train others, only in those skills appropriate to the individual's level of expertise and that can be safely performed and supervised. State and federal laws that regulate health care delivery and the policies of third party payers must be considered when any cross-training initiative is considered. Inappropriate cross-training as a result of admin-

istrative pressures for cost containment or shortage of personnel must be avoided.[3]

Networks of Providers

Managed care and HMOs (Box 3-2) are in the forefront of provider networks.[21] Even Medicare is offering to older Americans, on a voluntary basis, the ability to join a managed care network through "HMO-style" plans.[13] Because a flat rate is given regardless of how much care is provided, there is a financial risk that the provider takes when entering these networks. Many different disciplines may be grouped together to share reimbursement and the responsibility to treat a patient group.[8] OT may be part of these networks and therefore share the risk with other providers.

Also emerging are groups called Health Insurance Purchasing Cooperatives (HIPCs) and Independent Practice Associations (IPAs) (Box 3-2). These HIPCs contract with provider networks formed by HMOs or IPAs. Exactly how networks will be formed and how many HMOs, HIPCs, or IPAs a region will have is unknown. It appears, however, that they may have a role in health care reform in some states.[6]

Health care reform also addresses the issue of choice of providers. It has been argued that the patient should be able to choose among many providers. The decisions are yet to be made as to how choice may be accomplished and may vary by region or by state.[44]

TYPES OF REIMBURSEMENT

Reimbursement from an HMO, HIPC, or IPA may be by reduced rate, case rate, or capitation.

Reduced Rate

This method has been a traditional way of cutting costs by asking providers to give a percentage off their prices. In some instances a fee schedule has been established, and providers agree to take a certain reimbursement for a particular service or procedure. This method reimburses services based on the number of sessions or procedures done.[24]

Case Rate

A case rate is a specific amount of money contracted with a provider or set of providers to take a patient from point A to point B. For example, a Worker's Compensation HMO may contract with a physician and therapy service together to treat any repetitive motion injury for the first 60 days of care. The case rate may be $540, which would include physician visits, x-ray films, medications, splints, therapy, and any other service or supply provided to that patient. It is up to the network or provider to manage costs of the case so that a profit is made. Case rates shift the incentives from wanting to do more to wanting to do less.

The benefits of such a system to the provider are that collection problems are decreased and cash flow is im-

BOX 3 - 2

HEALTH CARE REFORM DEFINITIONS

MANAGED CARE

A general term for organizing networks of doctors and hospitals in order to give people access to quality, cost-effective health care. HMOs were the earliest form of managed care.

HMOs (HEALTH MAINTENANCE ORGANIZATIONS)

Prepaid health plans that provide a range of services in return for fixed monthly premiums. Virtually any organization can sponsor an HMO, including the government, medical schools, hospitals, employers, labor unions and insurance companies.

HIPCs (HEALTH INSURANCE PURCHASING COOPERATIVES)

Regional consumer groups, who would shop for the highest-quality plan at the lowest price on behalf of a large number of people, including employees of small businesses.

IPAs (INDEPENDENT PRACTICE ASSOCIATIONS)

A type of HMO that contracts with individual doctors to provide services to its members. IPA physicians see HMO patients in their own offices. Most physicians are free to contract with more than one HMO at a time, unless they work directly for a specific HMO, as well as see fee-for-service patients.

CAPITATION

Under this system, a managed-care plan pays a doctor, hospital or other service provider, a fixed amount to care for a patient over a given period. Health-care providers don't get extra reimbursement even if the costs of care exceed that amount.

Adapted from Words to live by: a reader's guide, *Newsweek*, 121:33, 1993. Newsweek, Inc. All rights reserved. Reprinted by permission.

proved. Payment is received at the beginning of the treatment. It allows independence for practitioners to provide care in the manner they see fit rather than relying on the managed care network, but input and oversight may come from the network to help ensure monitoring of quality. One way to monitor quality may be for case rate contracts to require the contractor to provide data on quality, amount, and type of services provided, which would be reviewed by the network.[8]

Capitation

Under capitation (Box 3-2), a fixed amount is usually prepaid at a set rate, per member, per month regardless of how many of the members use the service.[37] For example, a certain HMO health plan has 20,000 members in a provider's service area. They have offered to contract with this provider (an outpatient therapy center) at the rate of $.45 per member per month (including both physical and occupational therapy services). Should the provider take this contract? To decide the provider needs the following information: (1) use of therapy for this particular member group and (2) the frequency of visits (the average number of treatment visits per therapy referral for this group).[37]

In this example, 1 in every 40 members is referred for therapy a year. Each referral has on average 6.5 visits. Total annual income: $.45 × 20,000 members per month × 12 months = $108,000.

Total visits per year: 20,000 divided by 40 = 500 × 6.5 = 3250. The provider knows that the cost of each treatment is $33.00 so the total cost is 3250 × 33 = $107,250/year. Profit or loss: 108,000 − 107,250 =

$750 profit. In this example the provider will make a profit, but it may be difficult in the future to make a profit if costs increase for salaries, supplies, or overhead. It will also be important to monitor how many treatments are being given and to be sure use does not change.[37]

OPPORTUNITIES FOR OCCUPATIONAL THERAPY

Occupational therapy has undergone many transitions as patients' needs and reimbursement for the service has changed. To position for the future, occupational therapy can (1) emphasize function, (2) continue to be resourceful and creative, (3) network with primary care physicians, (4) decrease the barriers across disciplines, (5) assist with case management, (6) carve out unique areas and types of services, and (7) conduct research to demonstrate cost effectiveness.[22]

Occupational therapy must stay focused on function and the specific priorities of the individual patient. A key to occupational therapy has been motivation of the patient while treating the physical dysfunction. Linking motivation and increased responsibility of the patient could assist in lowering cost, while achieving high quality.

Occupational therapy has always been resourceful with equipment needs and uses. Assisting the patient in purchasing only equipment that will be functional and will move the patient toward independence is one example. This resourcefulness and creativity to decrease number of visits to lower costs in service delivery could be a very important and useful tool, making the occupational therapist a valuable member of the health care provider network.[24]

Although occupational therapy has received referrals from primary care physicians, a majority of the occupational therapist's referrals come from specialist physicians such as orthopedic surgeons, physiatrists, and neurologists. With primary care physicians becoming the "gate-keepers" of the patient's care under primary care and managed care models, it will be important to continue marketing occupational therapy to primary care physicians and IPAs working closely with them on pathways of care to ensure that occupational therapy remains a part of the system.

Occupational therapy has always striven to differentiate itself from other disciplines such as physical therapy or speech pathology. If insurers do not recognize physical and occupational therapy as different entities (as noted under capitation), it will be important for occupational therapy to work to remove barriers of differences between disciplines or to work to define the needs of both disciplines to continue to offer an array of services to the patient.[22]

Some occupational therapists are case managers within managed care networks. Occupational therapists are skilled at looking holistically at the patient and therefore can be excellent case managers. Because it is necessary to manage services more cost effectively, occupational therapists should consider phone monitoring of patient progress or oversight of a case while being treated by a COTA or aide.

Research is needed in rehabilitation to document the most effective and efficient ways to provide rehabilitation services and to outline these pathways. Data are needed to determine when services should be discontinued and which services save money in the course of treatment. It is imperative that occupational therapists be involved in and conduct this research in order to provide a sound future for the profession.[24]

SUMMARY

The history of health care reform in the U.S. from 1900–1985 is a story of the vast growth of the health care industry and the science of medicine and how that growth has created a reliance on a public-private third party payer insurance system. It is a story of the government's success and failure in trying to create and manage health care policy, and the uneasy partnerships that must be maintained within the private-public health care system of the United States. From 1917-1985 occupational therapy developed from a small gathering of founders to a profession of respectable size. The history illustrates occupational therapy's struggle to advance the profession by positioning itself as a cost-effective, necessary service within the medical system while trying to maintain a broad definition and area of practice.

Occupational therapy has seen many changes in reimbursement over the years and has adapted service provision to these changes. As the current reimbursement of occupational therapy service changes from fee-for-service to case rates and capitation under a new managed care type model, occupational therapy will again need to adapt to the changing systems of reimbursement.

REVIEW QUESTIONS

1. How did the progressive era influence changes in health care in the early 1900s?
2. What influence did Abraham Flexner have on medical education in the early 1900s?
3. What physician introduced the concept of quality improvement efforts in patient care in the early part of the century?
4. When was the idea of compulsory health insurance first introduced?
5. When did occupational therapy emerge and how did the profession view itself in relation to the physician in its early days?
6. When was the rehabilitation model developed? What important historical event led to its development and expansion?
7. Which president in the post

World War II era promised to institute national health insurance? Why were his efforts defeated?

8. Who founded a network of hospitals that served as a model for the development of health maintenance organizations (HMOs)?

9. How did the two world wars influence the growth and development of occupational therapy?

10. When and how did the specialization of occupational therapy come about?

11. What were the pros and cons for occupational therapy aligning itself with the medical model?

12. Outline the history of health care as an industry beginning with the advent of Medicare in 1965.

13. What is the role of the primary care physician in a managed care plan?

14. List at least 4 factors that are pushing health care reform in the 1990s.

15. If health care rationing occurs, how will it be determined who gets health care?

16. What is meant by outcome monitoring to reduce the costs of health care?

17. How would grouping charges affect delivery of occupational therapy services?

18. What is meant by cross-training?

19. What are the general AOTA guidelines for cross-training initiatives?

20. What are networks of providers? How does the network share costs of health care?

21. Define the following: PCP, HMO, IPA, HIPC, managed care, capitation, case rate.

22. Discuss ways that occupational therapy can become a competitive service in the new health care systems.

REFERENCES

1. Ambrosi E, Schwartz K: The profession's image, 1917-1925. I. Occupational therapy as represented by the media, *Am J Occup Ther* (in press).

2. American Occupational Therapy Association, *Bulletin No 1,* Towson Md, 1923, Sheppard Pratt Hospital Press.

3. American Occupational Therapy Association: White paper: occupational therapy and cross-training initiatives, *OT Week* 9(10): 32-33, March 9, 1995.

4. Anderson O: *Blue cross since 1929,* Cambridge, 1975, Ballinger.

5. Anderson R: The challenge of healthcare reform, *Advance/Rehab* 3:13, 1994.

6. Anderson, R: New models of health care delivery, *Advance/Rehab* 3:47, 1994.

7. Article 3101.9 Medicare guidelines for occupational therapy services, Health Care Financing Administration. In Scott S, editor: *Payment for occupational therapy services,* Rockville, Md, 1988, American Occupational Therapy Association.

8. Barnett A, Gilbert Mayer G: *Ambulatory care management and practice,* Gaithersburg, 1992, Aspen Publications.

9. Belkin L: The high cost of living, *The New York Times Magazine* 1:31, 1993.

10. Bernstein D: Cost-containment push will usher in prevention, return-to-work programs, *Rehab Today* 2:227, 1994.

11. Bing R: Occupational therapy revisited: a paraphrastic journey, *Am J Occup Ther* 35:499, 1981.

12. Bockoven JS: Legacy of moral treatment: 1800s to 1910, *Am J Occup Ther,* 25:224, 1971.

13. Buterbaugh L: Medicare meets managed care, *Medical Work News* 34:40, 1993.

14. Codman EA: *A study in hospital efficiency as demonstrated by the case reports of the first two years of a private hospital,* Boston, 1914, published privately.

15. Colman W: Maintaining autonomy: the struggle between occupational therapy and physical medicine, *Am J Occup Ther* 46:63, 1992.

16. *Constitution of the National Society for the Promotion of Occupational Therapy,* Baltimore, 1917, Sheppard Pratt Hospital Press.

17. Davis K: Economic theories of behavior in non-profit private hospitals, *Econ and Bus Bull* 24:1, 1972.

18. Davy JD: Nationally speaking: status report on reimbursement for occupational therapy services, *Am J Occup Ther* 38(5):295, 1984.

19. Devine E: *The principles of relief,* New York, 1904, Macmillan.

20. Dunton WR: *Prescribing occupational therapy,* Springfield Ill, 1928, Charles C Thomas.

21. Evans M: HMO is the way to go, *Industry Week* 243:64, 1994.

22. Evert M: Value in a changing environment, *Am J Occup Ther* 47:1063, 1993.

23. Flexner A: *Medical education in the United States and Canada,* New York, 1910, Carnegie Foundation for the Advancement of Teaching.

24. Foto M: Managing changes in reimbursement patterns. II. *Am J Occup Ther* 42:629, 1988.

25. Fourteen hospitals chosen for war's disabled, *The New York Times,* p 7, April 1, 1918.

26. The gift of healing, *Mademoiselle,* pp 114-15, 177-178, 1943.

27. Greenspun B: Putting outcome data to use, *Advance/Rehab* 3:47, 1994.

28. Gritzer G, Arluke A: *The making of rehabilitation,* Berkeley, 1985 University of California Press.

29. Hanson C, Walker K: The history of work in physical dysfunction, *Am J Occup Ther* 46:56, 1992.

30. *Higher status near, doctor tells therapists: department scrapbooks, 1955-63,* Archives of the Department of Occupational Therapy, San José State University, San José, Calif.

31. Hofstadter R: *The age of reform,* New York, 1969, Knopf.

32. Holmes B: The hospital problem, *JAMA* 47:320, 1906.

33. Johnson J: Delegate assembly address, April 9, 1976, *Am J Occup Ther* 30(7):444-449, 1976.

34. *The joint commission 1994 accreditation manual for hospitals,* Vol 1, Library of Congress catalog #93-78938, pp. xi-xiii, 1993.

35. Lack of trained personnel felt in rehabilitation field, *The New York Times,* Jan 25, 1954.

36. Lambert A: Report of the committee on social insurance, *JAMA* 66:1951-85, 1916.

37. Lanute D: Capitation, *Advance/ Rehab* 3:29, 1994.

38. Larkins P: Playing hardball in a managed competitive environment, *Advance/Rehab* 3:17, 1994.

39. Low J: The reconstruction aides, *Am J Occup Ther* 46:38, 1992.

40. *Occupational therapy classes have outstanding guest speakers from various army and civilian hospitals: department scrapbook, 1943-54,* Archives of the Department of Occupational Therapy, San José State University, San José, Calif.

41. OT instructor says San José needs rehabilitation center, *Spartan Daily,* San José, Calif, Feb 9, 1953, San José State College.

42. Reilly M: Occupational therapy can be one of the great ideas of 20th century medicine, *Am J Occup Ther* 16:1, 1962.

43. Schweiniz K: Sickness as a factor in poverty, 1919, Proceedings of the National Conference on Social Work, p 156.

44. Smith L: The coming health care shakeout, *Fortune* 127:20, 1993.

45. Starr P: *The social transformation of American medicine,* New York, 1982, Basic Books.

46. Stevens R: *In sickness and in wealth,* New York, 1989, Basic Books.

47. Sullivan L: Can we put the brakes on health care costs? *USA Today* 76:26, 1992.

48. Summary of coverage for occupational therapy services under medicare. In Scott S, editor: *Payment for occupational therapy services,* Rockville, Md, 1988, American Occupational Therapy Association.

49. Taylor F: *The principles of scientific management,* New York, 1911, Harper.

50. Upham E: Agriculture for the disabled, *Mod Hosp* 11:74, 1928.

51. Weibe R: *The search for order,* 1877-1920, New York, 1967, Farrar, Strauss & Giroux.

52. Woolley S: Physician, restrain thyself, *Business Week* 2:32, 1993.

53. Words to live by: a reader's guide, *Newsweek* 121:33, 1993.

54. *Workshop on rehabilitation facilities, 1955: department scrapbooks 1955-63,* Archives of the Department of Occupational Therapy, San José State University, San José, Calif.

Occupational Therapy Evaluation and Assessment of Physical Dysfunction

Lorraine Williams Pedretti

ssessment is a process of gathering data, identifying problems, formulating hypotheses, and making decisions for treatment interventions.[11,21] Assessment is carried out using formal and informal screening and evaluation methods including review of the medical record, interview, observation, standardized tests, and nonstandardized tests.[11] In occupational therapy, assessment of occupational performance areas and performance components is the basis for developing treatment objectives and treatment strategies. Treatment is directed to remediation of or compensation for the problems identified in the assessment process.

The terms assessment and evaluation are sometimes used interchangeably. In this chapter, *evaluation* refers to the battery of specific tests of measurable deficits whereas *assessment* refers to a composite picture of the person's functioning based on the results of the evaluation.[23] *Evaluation procedure* refers to one specific method, such as tests or structured observation, used in the evaluation.

EVALUATION AND ASSESSMENT

An initial evaluation takes place before treatment, and reevaluation occurs periodically during the course of occupational therapy intervention.[20] The results of the initial evaluation are used to make an assessment of deficits in performance components, performance areas, and occupational role performance. The assessment is the foundation for selecting treatment objectives and treatment methods.[21] Reevaluation is essential to determine the effectiveness of treatment, to modify treatment to suit the patient's needs, and to revise the assessment. Reevaluation may involve eliminating unattainable goals, modifying goals that were partially or completely achieved, and adding new goals as additional problems are identified or progress is made.

Evaluation and assessment provide the therapist with specific methods of determining his or her own effectiveness as a planner and administrator of treatment. They are the scientific foundation for the decisions in the treatment plan.[21] They provide specific information that can be communicatcd to other members of the rehabilitation team. Furthermore, careful evaluation and assessment can enhance the development of occupational therapy. If evaluation data are collected systematically, they may be used for the development of more standardized evaluation instruments and may contribute to a better understanding of the evaluation and treatment techniques that are suitable and effective in occupational therapy practice.

To be an effective evaluator, the therapist must be knowledgeable about the dysfunction, its causes, course, and prognosis; familiar with a variety of evaluation methods, their uses, and proper administration; and able to select evaluation methods that are suitable to the patient and the dysfunction. Thus an understanding of possible dysfunction in performance areas, performance components, and applicable treatment principles is essential. When performing evaluations the therapist must approach the patient with openness and without preconceived ideas about his or her limitations or personality. The therapist must have good observation skills and be able to enlist the trust of the patient in a short time.[24]

THE ASSESSMENT PROCESS

The assessment process (Fig. 4-1) is initiated with *screening,* which refers to reviewing the patient's record, to determine the need for further evaluation and occupa-

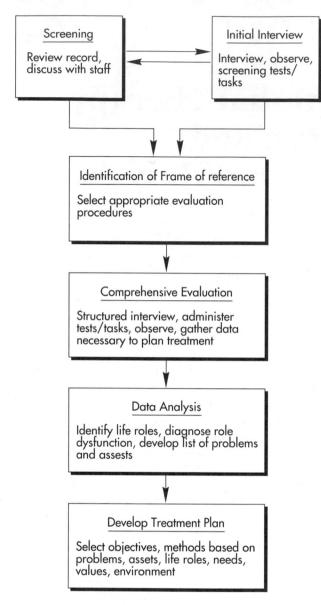

FIG. 4-1   Schematic of assessment process.

tional therapy intervention.[5] Following the screening, an initial evaluation is conducted to determine whether occupational therapy services are needed and the kinds of services required.[20] The occupational therapist may interview the patient, administer selected screening tests, and make observations. The estimated duration of treatment and the need to coordinate treatment with other services may also be determined at this time.[5]

The assessment process continues with identification of an appropriate frame of reference for treatment and the selection of specific evaluation procedures that will yield the information needed as the basis for clinical decision making. Administration of specific tests, clinical observations, structured interviews, standardized tests, performance checklists, and activities and tasks are then used to evaluate specific performance abilities and deficits. Data necessary to plan treatment are obtained and

interpreted.[5] The process continues with an analysis of the results of the evaluation procedures.

An assessment of the individual's occupational roles and role dysfunction is made and a list of problems and assets to be used in planning occupational therapy intervention is made on the basis of this analysis.[20] A treatment plan is then developed, selecting objectives to address problems and selecting suitable methods. It is important that the patient be involved, to the extent possible, throughout the assessment process.

CLINICAL REASONING

During the evaluation and assessment process, problems are identified and intervention strategies are selected based on clinical reasoning and clinical decision making.[21] Clinical reasoning guides decisions about the collection, classification, and analysis of data, and ultimately, determines appropriate goals and methods of treatment.[22] Fleming defined *clinical reasoning* as "the many types of inquiry that an occupational therapist uses to understand patients and their difficulties." She stated that it includes, but is not limited to, hypothetical reasoning and problem solving and refers to the complex processes used when the occupational therapist thinks about the patient, the disability, the circumstances, and the meaning of the disability to the patient.[15]

Clinical reasoning has been the focus of much study in the past several years.[2,15] Mattingly[18] offered a multifaceted concept of clinical reasoning. She described it as "a . . . tacit, . . . imagistic, and . . . phenomenological mode of thinking . . . based on tacit understanding and habitual knowledge gained through experience."[18] Clinical experience results in the development of professional expertise, the kind of knowing that results from doing or action. Such knowledge is difficult to articulate; in a sense it is greater than the knowledge that can be expressed verbally.[18]

Clinical reasoning includes the ability to express theoretical reasons for clinical decisions, but it is more than that. It embodies the tacit knowledge and habitual ways of seeing and doing things and dealing with patients that are based on expertise gained from experience. It is directed to determining appropriate action for the particular patient at a particular time in a specific circumstance. It is not merely the response to a technical question or theoretical hypothesis. In essence it is a process of figuring out how to act and what to do in a specific circumstance involving the patient's well being.[18]

Occupational therapy theory can provide a starting place for clinical reasoning but cannot provide all the answers for the course of action in a particular case. Because each patient is unique and complex, treatment must be individualized and that requires judgment, creativity, and improvisation.[18] Mattingly proposed that clinical reasoning in occupational therapy be primarily directed to the "human world of motives and values and beliefs—a world of human meaning," rather than to a biological world of disease. "Occupational therapists' fundamental task is treating . . . the illness experience," that is, the meaning that the disability has for the individual person.[18]

Occupational therapists teach everyday activities, such as dressing skills and toilet transfers, for the purposes of increasing self-care independence. In the teaching process, they are confronted with the patient's experiences of profound life changes brought about by the disability, the loss of capacities taken for granted, and reorientation to the world as a person with physical and functional limitations. The therapist treats not only the physical dysfunction, but the person who has the dysfunction. The therapist's role is to help the patient confront the limitations, "claim the disability," reclaim a changed body and functioning, and develop a new sense of self with meaning, purpose, and value. Thus the simple application of theoretical constructs to arrive at answers to questions about appropriate intervention strategies is only a part of the clinical reasoning process. The therapist must plan treatment based on the unique meaning of the disability to the particular patient and not just the physical impairments resulting from the disability.[18]

In a pilot study of clinical reasoning it was found that occupational therapists practicing in physical disabilities used six stages of clinical reasoning during the initial assessment. These were (1) obtaining information from the medical record, referral statement, and reports before meeting the patient; (2) selecting assessments based on medical diagnosis, prognosis, and the patient's ability to cooperate and participate in the evaluation; (3) implementing the assessment plan by interacting with the patient and carrying out selected evaluations and tests; (4) defining problems and possible causes; (5) defining treatment objectives based on the problem list in conjunction with the patient; selecting treatment tasks and plans to carry out additional assessment; and (6) evaluating the effectiveness of the assessment plan and the reliability of evaluation results.[22]

In this study therapists used the medical diagnosis to select assessments, to recall standard problem lists for the diagnoses, and to select objectives and methods of treatment.[22] This approach reflects a medical model of clinical reasoning, which focuses on the diagnosis.[13] It is a formula approach that bypasses important considerations about the patient as a person, critical factors in effective treatment planning and treatment outcomes.[18,22] This approach has value as an element of clinical reasoning but it omits the complex needs, unique situation, and meaning of the disability in the patient's life as important considerations for treatment planning. The occupational therapist uses a medical model of reasoning when considering the patient's physical disability but when concerned with individualizing treatment, facilitating independence, and creating a new future, other reasoning strategies are used.[13,14] Fleming[13] proposed

that three types of reasoning are used by occupational therapists. These are (1) procedural reasoning to consider physical problems, (2) interactive reasoning to guide interactions with the patient, and (3) conditional reasoning to consider the patient in his or her personal and social context and future.[14,15] Thus clinical reasoning is a multifaceted process that results in an intervention plan to meet the individual's unique needs not only for remediating physical dysfunction and improving performance but for reclaiming a valued sense of self and a meaningful life.[18]

CONTENT OF THE EVALUATION

The initial occupational therapy evaluation should include an evaluation of the patient's goals, functional abilities, and deficits in occupational performance areas: activities of daily living (ADL), work and productive activities, and play or leisure skills.[3,4,7] Performance components should also be evaluated with particular attention to the sensorimotor component and cognitive integration and cognitive components. Psychosocial skills and psychological components[7] are also evaluated or observed during the initial visits with the patient. The occupational therapist may need to plan remediation for these latter components and for the more obvious sensorimotor deficits or refer the patient to the appropriate service for remediation, depending on the severity of the problems. The occupational therapist should obtain information about the patient's medical, educational, and work histories, family, and cultural background.[3] The patient's environment as a determinant of occupational performance should also be evaluated. The social, cultural, and physical environments are all performance contexts that influence occupational functioning. The disabling and enabling factors of the patient's environments and person-environment relationships require evaluation and consideration in treatment planning.[7,17] This information should guide the therapist in selecting appropriate and meaningful treatment objectives and methods. Structuring treatment on the basis of the patient's needs, values, and sociocultural milieu is critical to eliciting his or her full participation in the treatment process.

METHODS OF EVALUATION
Medical Records

Data gathered from the medical record are an important part of the assessment process. The medical record can provide information on the diagnosis, prognosis, medical history, precautions, current treatment regime, social data, psychologic data, and other rehabilitation therapies. Daily notes from nurses and physicians can give information about current medications and the patient's reactions and responses to the hospital, treatment regime, and persons in the treatment facility.[23] Ideally the occupational therapist should have had the opportunity to study the medical record before seeing the patient to begin specific evaluation. The therapist may have to begin the evaluation, however, without benefit of the information in the medical record, with an interview and some simple screening tests. The information from the medical record serves as a good basis for selecting evaluation procedures and possibly an approach to the patient. It indicates problem areas and helps the therapist focus attention on the relevant factors of the case.[24]

Interview

The initial interview is a valuable step in the evaluation process. During the interview the occupational therapist gathers information on how the patient perceives his or her roles, dysfunction, needs, and goals, and the patient can learn about the role of the occupational therapist and occupational therapy in the rehabilitation program.[24] An important outcome of the initial interview is the development of rapport and trust between therapist and patient.

The initial interview should take place in an environment that is quiet and ensures privacy. The therapist should plan the interview in advance to know what information must be acquired and to prepare some specific questions. The interviewer and patient should set aside a specified period of time for the interview. The first few minutes of the interview may be devoted to getting acquainted and orienting the patient to the occupational therapy clinic or service and to the role and goals of occupational therapy.

The two essential elements for a successful interview are a solid knowledge base and active listening skills. These abilities require study, practice, and preparation. The therapist's knowledge will influence the selection of questions or topics to be covered in the interview. The interview should reflect the therapist's knowledge and cover the areas that are relevant both to occupational therapy and to the construction of a meaningful treatment plan. The interviewer who actively listens demonstrates respect for and a vital interest in the patient.[1] In active listening, the receiver (therapist) tries to understand what the sender (patient) is feeling or the meaning of the message. The therapist then puts that understanding into his or her own words and feeds it back to the patient for verification, for example, by "This is what I believe you mean. . . . Have I understood you correctly?" The therapist does not send a new message, such as an opinion, judgment, advice, or analysis. Rather, the therapist sends back only what he or she thinks the patient meant.[16]

Throughout the interview the therapist should listen to ascertain the patient's attitude toward the dysfunction. The patient should have an opportunity to express what he or she sees as the primary problems and goals for rehabilitation. These may differ substantially from the therapist's judgment and must be given careful consideration when therapist and patient reach the point of setting treatment objectives together. As the interview progresses, there should be an opportunity for the patient to ask questions as well. The therapist must have good listening and observation skills to gather maximum information from the interview.

It probably will be necessary to take notes or record the initial interview. The patient should be advised of this method in advance, understand the reasons why, know the uses to which the material will be put, and be allowed to view or listen to the tape if he or she desires.[23,24]

During the initial phase of the interview the therapist should explain the role of the therapist, the purpose of the interview, and how the information is to be used. As the interview progresses the therapist may seek the desired information by asking appropriate questions and guiding the responses and ensuing discussion so that relevant topics are addressed. The occupational therapist may wish to seek information about the patient's family and friends, community and work roles, educational and work histories, leisure and social interests and activities, and the living situation to which the patient will return. Information about how the patient spends and manages time is important. This can be determined by using a tool such as the daily schedule described below, the activity configuration described by Watanabe,[25] or the Activities Health Assessment described by Cynkin and Robinson.[12] The interview can be concluded with a summary of the major points covered, information gained, estimate of problems and assets, and plans for further occupational therapy evaluation.

The daily schedule

The therapist should interview the patient to get a detailed account of his or her activities for a typical day (or week) before the onset of physical dysfunction. Information that should be elicited is as follows:

Rising hour
Morning activities with hours
Hygiene
Dressing
Breakfast
Work/leisure/home management
Child care
Luncheon
Afternoon activities with hours
Work/leisure/home management
Child care
Rest
Social activities
Dinner
Evening activities with hours
Leisure and social activities
Preparation for retiring
Bedtime

The amount of time spent on each activity should be recorded carefully. During the interview the therapist should be careful not to allow the patient to gloss over or omit any of the daily activities by cuing the patient with appropriate questions.

The therapist might ask, "What time did you get up?", "What was the first thing that you did?", "When did you eat lunch?", "Who fixed it for you?" The review of the daily schedule as it was before the disability may evoke many recollections of family, friends, social, community, vocational, and leisure activities about which the patient may share information freely. At times, this digression from the schedule itself is desirable to elicit a well-rounded picture of the patient's roles and relationships and some ideas of his or her needs, values, and personal goals. In other instances, tangential conversation should be limited or discouraged to focus the patient's attention on the specific daily schedule. If memory or communication disorders make the construction of the daily schedule impossible in the manner described, friends or family members may be consulted for an approximation of the patient's activities pattern.

A second daily schedule of present activities pattern in the treatment facility (or at home if the patient is an outpatient or is treated at home) is then constructed. It is important during this interview to ask the patient who helps him or her with each activity and how much assistance is needed and received. A discussion and comparative analysis of these two schedules between therapist and patient should yield valuable information about the patient's needs, values, satisfaction-dissatisfaction with the activities pattern, primary and secondary goals for change, interests, motivation, interpersonal relationships, and fears. On the basis of this information it becomes possible to set priorities for treatment objectives according to the patient's needs and values rather than to the therapist's priorities. Activities that will be meaningful to the patient in his or her particular environment and social group, which may be appropriate for use in the intervention plan, begin to emerge. Their potential for facilitation of change may be presented, and selection of therapeutic modalities to meet objectives that have been agreed on can be made.

The daily schedule can reveal the patient's concepts of life roles to the occupational therapist. Thus it enables the therapist to view the patient as a functioning human being rather than merely a diagnosis or disability. Treatment can then be based on the individual needs of the patient rather than on standard evaluation and treatment regimes established for a certain disability. Knowing the patient's roles, interests, and activities is most helpful for diagnosing role dysfunction. It is valuable for determining the patient's values and establishing realistic possibilities for resumption of former roles or for structuring new ones.

Observation

Some aspects of the evaluation of the patient will be based on the occupational therapist's observation of the patient during the interview and the evaluation procedures that follow. As treatment begins the occupational therapist will base some of the reevaluation of the patient on observations during treatment. The occupational therapist can gain much information by observing the patient as he or she approaches or is approached. What is the posture, mode of ambulation, and gait pattern? How is he or she dressed? Is there obvious motor dysfunction? Are there apparent musculoskeletal deformities? What is the facial expression, tone of voice, and manner of speech? How are the hands held and used? Are there pain mannerisms, such as protection of an injured part or grimaces and groans?

In addition to these informal observations, which can be made during the first few minutes of the initial contact with the patient, occupational therapists use structured observation to evaluate performance of self-care, home management, mobility, and transferring. Evaluation of these skills is usually carried out by observing the patient perform them in real or simulated environments. The therapist can determine the patient's level of independence, speed, skill, need for special equipment, and the feasibility of further training.

The rapport and trust that develop between the patient and the therapist are based on the communication between them. The communication in the interview and observation phases of the evaluation is critical to all subsequent interactions and thus to the effectiveness of treatment. The patient needs to sense that he or she has been heard and understood by someone who is empathetic and who has the necessary knowledge and skills to facilitate rehabilitation. The therapist needs to project self-confidence and confidence in the profession, setting the tone for all future interaction with the patient, and enhancing the development of the patient's trust in the therapist and in the potential effectiveness of occupational therapy.[24]

Formal Evaluation Procedures

The evaluation of performance is a major responsibility in occupational therapy. Along with the review of records, interview, and observations, the evaluation is carried out through procedures such as tests and measurements in occupational therapy. Relevant and accurate assessment is critical to decision-making for planning treatment, determining school and community living placement, considering admission to and discharge from clinical programs, and other dispositions that may be based on test results. Thus in reporting evaluation data, it is essential that the information be supported by relevant and accurate testing procedures.[9]

Occupational therapists use both standardized and nonstandardized evaluations. It is assumed that standardized tests are superior to nonstandardized tests and that most clinicians would prefer to use standardized tests.[2] Yet there are relatively few standardized evaluation procedures in occupational therapy.[20] Many evaluation procedures in use have unknown reliability and validity. Many are informal instruments developed by occupational therapists to suit the needs of their own practice settings. Still others are adaptations of existing evaluation instruments and are used with patients other than those for whom they were designed. Standardized instruments designed by other professionals for their own disciplines are also used by occupational therapists.[10,27] The development of occupational therapy evaluation instruments that are reliable, valid, and grounded in theory would increase confidence in occupational therapy practice. There is a need to broaden the repertoire of standardized tests used in occupational therapy evaluation and assessment.[9,10,27]

Standardized tests

A standardized evaluation procedure includes instructions for administration and scoring and has statistical evidence of validity and reliability. It also has established norms, which allow the score of the person being evaluated to be compared with those of a norm group.[8,9]

Occupational therapists have been encouraged to use standardized tests to record information obtained from patients. It was proposed that using standardized tests improves the ability to formalize occupational therapy evaluations based on quantitative assessment. Results of the initial evaluation and follow-up evaluations can then be reported in a consistent, objective, and reliable manner. This approach requires that occupational therapists increase their knowledge and skill in testing and thus enhance professional credibility.[26]

Many standardized tests were designed by professionals other than occupational therapists for use in their own disciplines. Occupational therapists are using such tests in the areas of measuring achievement, development, intelligence, manual dexterity, motor skills, personality, sensorimotor function, and vocational skills.[8,10] The *Mental Measurements Yearbook*,[19] *An Annotated Index of Occupational Therapy Evaluation Tools*,[8] *Occupational Performance Assessment*,[11] and *Assessment and Evaluation: An Overview*[23] are excellent sources of information about standardized tests. Current health care journals and psychological abstracts are other sources of information about standardized evaluations that may be relevant to occupational therapy.[9] Although it is desirable to have standardized and objective evaluations in occupational therapy, professional judgment and interpretation are always an important part of the evaluation procedure.[20]

To use standardized tests properly, the occupational therapist needs knowledge and certain skills. The therapist should:

1. be familiar with available tests applicable to the area of practice
2. identify the behavioral dimension measured by the tests
3. be able to interpret information on validity, reliability, and norms
4. understand the theoretical reason for selecting and using the tests
5. be able to administer, score, and interpret standardized tests
6. recognize the need for further evaluation of function
7. integrate and correlate data from all observations and evaluation procedures to develop a treatment plan based on theory
8. recognize the need for reassessment of the patient's performance.[6]

Non-standardized tests

In contrast to standardized tests, a nonstandardized evaluation tool is subjective and has no specific instructions for administration, no criteria for scoring, nor does it provide information on interpreting results of the evaluation.[20] The results and interpretation of nonstandardized tests depend on the clinical skill, experience, judgment, and bias of the evaluator.[9] Some nonstandardized evaluation procedures provide broad criteria for scoring and interpretation but still require the use of considerable subjective professional judgment.[20] The manual muscle test, described in Chapter 9, is an example of such a test. Several other nonstandardized evaluation procedures are described in this text.

SUMMARY

The occupational therapy evaluation of the patient with physical dysfunction includes an examination of medical records, interview, observation, and the administration of specific formal and informal evaluation procedures. The assessment of the patient is based on an analysis of the data gathered from evaluation and is used to identify problems and assets in the patient's life and plan appropriate treatment strategies.

Occupational therapists have developed many informal evaluation procedures that are useful in particular treatment facilities. These include tests, checklists, and rating scales. Many of these have been developed into standardized tests. The need for reliable standardized tests pertinent to occupational therapy continues, however, as occupational therapists have recognized the need to identify and employ discipline-specific evaluation procedures to help establish the scientific base of the profession.

The selection of the appropriate evaluation procedures will depend on the patient's diagnosis, medical history, lifestyle, interests, living situation, needs, values, and environment. Clinical reasoning in the occupational therapy assessment is based on information gathered during the evaluation and used to select appropriate treatment objectives, methods, and progression in the construction of the treatment plan, discussed in the next chapter.[24]

REVIEW QUESTIONS

1. Define *evaluation*.
2. Differentiate evaluation from assessment.
3. List four purposes of occupational therapy evaluation.
4. Which skills must the occupational therapist possess to be an effective evaluator?
5. List and describe the steps in the assessment process.
6. Define and discuss *clinical reasoning*.
7. List and differentiate three types of clinical reasoning.
8. Which specific occupational performance areas and performance components should be evaluated by the occupational therapist when treating patients with physical dysfunction?
9. Describe four methods of evaluation that the occupational therapist may use in the evaluation process.
10. Along with diagnosis and medical data, which other important factors about the patient should be considered by the occupational therapist during the assessment and later in treatment planning?
11. Compare standardized and nonstandardized tests. What are some advantages and disadvantages of each?
12. To use standardized tests, the occupational therapist should have certain skills. List at least five that were identified in the chapter.

REFERENCES

1. Allen C: The performance status examination: paper presented at the American Occupational Therapy Association Annual Conference, San Francisco, October 1976. Cited in Hopkins HL, Smith HD, editors: *Willard and Spackman's occupational therapy,* ed 6, Philadelphia, 1983, JB Lippincott.
2. *American Journal of Occupational Therapy,* Special issue on clinical reasoning, 45(11), 1991.
3. American Occupational Therapy Association: Standards of practice for occupational therapy services for clients with physical disabilities, *Reference manual of the official documents of The American Occupational Therapy Association.* Rockville, Md, 1986, The Association.
4. American Occupational Therapy Association: Uniform occupational therapy evaluation checklist, *Reference manual of the official documents of the American Occupational Therapy Association.* Rockville, Md, 1986, The Association.
5. American Occupational Therapy Association: Uniform terminology system for reporting occupational therapy services, *Reference manual of the official documents of The American Occupational Therapy Association.* Rockville, Md, 1986, The Association.
6. American Occupational Therapy Association: Hierarchy of competencies relating to the use of standardized instruments and evaluation techniques by occupational therapists, *Reference manual of the official documents of the American Occupational Therapy Association,* Rockville, Md, 1989, The Association.
7. American Occupational Therapy Association: Uniform terminology for occupational therapy, third edition, *Am J Occup Ther* 48(11):1047-1054, 1994.
8. Asher, IE: *An annotated index of occupational therapy evaluation tools,* Rockville, Md, 1989, The American Occupational Therapy Association.
9. Atchison B: Selecting appropriate assessments, *Physical disabilities special interest section newsletter* 10:2, American Occupational Therapy Association, 1987.
10. Bowker A: Standardized tests utilized by therapists in the field of physical disabilities, *Physical disabilities special interest section newsletter* 6:4, American Occupational Therapy Association, 1983.
11. Christiansen C: Occupational performance assessment. In Christiansen C, Baum C, editors: *Occupational therapy: overcoming human performance deficits,* Thorofare, NJ, 1991, Slack.
12. Cynkin S, Robinson AM: *Occupational therapy and activities health: toward health through activities,* Boston, 1990, Little, Brown.
13. Fleming MH: Clinical reasoning in medicine compared with clinical reasoning in occupational therapy, *Am J Occup Ther* 45(11):988, 1991.
14. Fleming MH: The therapist with the three-track mind, *Am J Occup Ther* 45(11): 1007, 1991.
15. Fleming MH: Aspects of clinical reasoning in occupational therapy. In Hopkins HL, Smith HD, editors: *Willard and Spackman's occupational therapy,* ed. 8, Philadelphia, 1993, JB Lippincott.
16. Gordon T: PET: *Parent effectiveness training,* New York, 1970, The New American Library.
17. Letts L and associates: Person-environment assessment in occupational therapy, *Am J Occup Ther* 48(7):608, 1994.
18. Mattingly C: What is clinical reasoning? *Am J Occup Ther* 45(11):979, 1991.
19. Mitchell JV, editor: *Mental measurements yearbook,* ed 11, Highland Park, NJ, 1992, Rutgers University.
20. Mosey AC: *Occupational therapy, configuration of a profession,* New York, 1981, Raven Press.
21. Opacich KJ: Assessment and informed decision-making. In Christiansen C and Baum C, editors: *Occupational therapy: overcoming human performance deficits,* Thorofare, NJ, 1991, Slack.
22. Rogers JC, Masagatani G: Clinical reasoning of occupational therapists during the initial assessment of physically disabled patients, *Occup Ther J Res* 4:195, 1982.
23. Smith HD: Assessment and evaluation: an overview. In Hopkins HL, Smith HD, editors: *Willard*

and Spackman's occupational therapy, ed. 8, Philadelphia, 1993, JB Lippincott.

24. Smith HD, Tiffany EG: Assessment and evaluation: an overview. In Hopkins HL, Smith HD, editors: *Willard and Spackman's occupational therapy,* ed 6, Philadelphia, 1983, JB Lippincott.

25. Watanabe S: Activities configuration, 1968 regional institute on the evaluation process, *Final report RSA-123-T-68,* New York, 1968, American Occupational Therapy Association.

26. Watson M: Analysis: standardized testing objective, *Physical disabilities special interest section newsletter* 6:4, American

Occupational Therapy Association, 1983.

27. Watts JH and associates: The assessment of occupational functioning: a screening tool for use in long-term care, *Am J Occup Ther* 40:231, 1986.

Treatment Planning

Lorraine Williams Pedretti

A treatment plan is the design or proposal for a therapeutic program. Pelland[8] described it as "the core of occupational therapy practice." The treatment plan is based on a critical analysis of performance deficits and the unique circumstances of the individual patient. These factors make occupational therapy intervention complex and treatment planning a challenge for therapists. Effective treatment planning is possible if the therapist has made a thorough and careful assessment; reviewed, analyzed, and summarized the assessment data; identified treatment goals and objectives; and selected appropriate treatment methods. Furthermore, the treatment plan should include ongoing reevaluation, data collection, and development of treatment priorities.[2] In short, the treatment plan includes long- and short-term treatment objectives and methods based on identified problems and indicates how the program should progress.

The importance of writing a treatment plan cannot be overstated. Specific objectives must be outlined in an orderly and sequential manner to be clear to the therapist, patient, and other concerned personnel. The treatment plan helps the therapist proceed efficiently and provides a standard for measuring the progress of the patient and the effectiveness of the plan.

Practicing therapists sometimes work intuitively and find it difficult to articulate the rationale for their treatment plans.[2] Such clinicians may be working in a trial and error manner, wasting precious time and money. They may be poorly prepared to defend their course of action to themselves, the patient, or the rehabilitation team. They may lack confidence in their reports about the patients assigned to them. The lack of a stated treatment plan can present problems to other staff members who may have to substitute in the absence of the assigned therapist.

Perhaps one of the most important purposes for writing a treatment plan is that it allows the therapist to analyze the proposed course of action. In so doing, the therapist should ask many questions. Some of these are the following:

1. What is the most appropriate frame of reference or treatment approach on which to base the treatment plan?
2. What are the patient's capabilities and assets?
3. What are the patient's limitations and deficits?
4. What does occupational therapy have to offer this patient?
5. What are the goals of treatment?
6. What are specific long-term and short-term objectives?
7. Are the treatment objectives consistent with the patient's needs and personal aspirations?
8. If objectives are not compatible, how do they need to be modified?
9. Which treatment methods are available to meet these objectives?
10. When should the patient have met the objectives?
11. What standards will be used to determine when the patient has reached an objective?
12. How will the effectiveness of the treatment plan be evaluated?
13. What is the estimated length of treatment?

The treatment plan affirms the therapist's competence and the professionalism of occupational therapy. It can provide a systematic method for gathering research data and documents the purposes and effectiveness of occupational therapy services.

THE TREATMENT PLANNING PROCESS

The occupational therapy treatment planning process (Fig. 5-1) is one of identifying problems and finding their solutions to promote health, well-being, and optimal functioning in persons who are ill or disabled. It is a problem-solving process that has a logical progression.[4] Hopkins[4] described a generic problem-solving process and applied it to treatment planning. The first step is assessment, analysis, and identification of problems. Then prospective solutions are explored and treatment objectives developed. A plan of action, the treatment plan, is designed and implemented. The outcomes of the

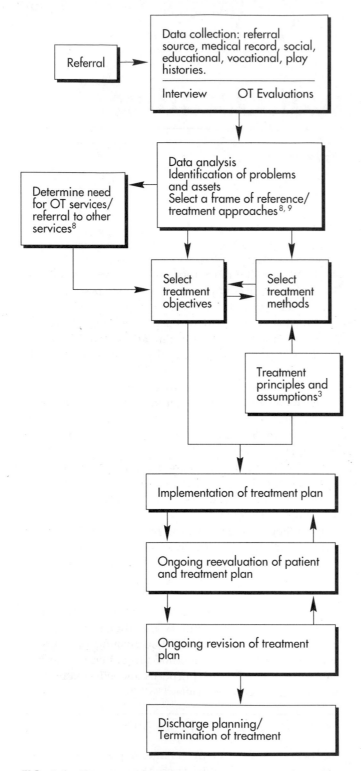

FIG. 5-1   Treatment planning process.

plan are assessed and the plan is modified if necessary. Finally, the treatment is terminated when the plan has been achieved or treatment is no longer feasible.[4]

DATA GATHERING

After the patient is referred for occupational therapy services, the therapist must gather data to develop an ap-

propriate treatment plan. Sources for these data are the referral form; the medical record; social, educational, vocational, and play histories; interview of the patient or family and friends; and the results of evaluation procedures completed by occupational therapy and other services. The details of the assessment process were discussed in Chapter 4.

DATA ANALYSIS AND PROBLEM IDENTIFICATION

After data have been gathered, they are analyzed to identify functions and dysfunctions, and it is determined if occupational therapy can be employed to alleviate the problems.[9] From a careful analysis of all of the data, a list of problems and assets is developed that forms the basis of the treatment plan. Deficits in the performance areas and performance components that may be amenable to occupational therapy intervention should be noted. Limitations that require intervention by other professional services should be communicated through the appropriate referral process. How the patient's assets can be used to enhance progress toward independence should be determined.

SELECTING A FRAME OF REFERENCE OR TREATMENT APPROACH

A treatment plan should be based on one or more of the occupational therapy frames of reference or a specific treatment approach to determine which evaluation procedures, objectives, and methods will be most appropriate for the patient.[8,9] The problem-solving process is influenced by the frame of reference or treatment approach being used. Several approaches are available in treatment today and each has its particular philosophy, body of knowledge, and methods of evaluation and treatment, though there is some overlap. The selection of a frame of reference or treatment approach provides the therapist some guidelines for the clinical reasoning process in treatment planning.[4]

For example, if the therapist is treating a patient with a fractured arm resulting in limited joint motion and muscle weakness from disuse, the biomechanical approach might be selected. Evaluation procedures in this approach focus on joint range of motion measurement and muscle strength testing. Treatment might involve therapeutic exercise and activities. On the other hand, if the patient has hemiplegia, the therapist might choose the neurodevelopmental (Bobath) approach and would evaluate muscle tone and postural mechanisms. Treatment would be directed to normalizing tone through positioning, handling techniques, and special movement patterns, and facilitating a more normal postural mechanism through activities that demand weight shifts and weight bearing. A discussion of the occupational therapy frames of reference is beyond the scope of this text. See Chapter 1 for a discussion of the biomechanical, rehabilitative, and sensorimotor approaches to treatment and the occupational performance model as a frame of reference for treatment planning.

SELECTING AND WRITING TREATMENT GOALS AND OBJECTIVES

Treatment goals and objectives are written to address the problems identified in the occupational therapy assessment. After gathering data, selecting a frame of reference and one or more treatment approaches, some general kinds of treatment methods that would facilitate the patient's rehabilitation may come to mind. For example, following the evaluation, it may be apparent that the patient could benefit from training in activities of daily living (ADL). Having ideas for methods can facilitate the selection and writing of treatment objectives. Writing objectives and selecting treatment methods actually are concurrent and mutually dependent elements of the treatment planning process.

Goals

Goals are general statements that describe global or general changes in function at some time in the future. Goals may also be long-term objectives. For example, a goal might be: *The patient will be independent in self-care.* Because self-care encompasses many activities, it is not possible to achieve this goal without many intervening objectives.

Objectives

Objectives are steps in the process of achieving goals. An example of an objective toward reaching the goal just stated would be: *The patient will transfer to and from the toilet without assistance.* The paragraphs that follow focus on writing objectives.

A treatment objective is a statement of intent describing a proposed change in a patient. The statement clearly conveys the change in function, performance, or behavior that the patient will demonstrate when the treatment procedure or program has been successfully completed. Whenever possible the therapist should select objectives and plan the treatment program in conjunction with the patient. The therapist and patient determine objectives that are attainable by the end of a treatment program so that treatment procedures relevant to those objectives may also be selected. Evaluation of progress is based on achievement of the objectives selected. Objectives should reflect the patient's needs and should be consistent with the general goals stated on the referral and determined by the assessment. The occupational therapy objectives should complement those of other rehabilitation services.

When clearly defined objectives have not been stated, there is no sound basis for selecting appropriate treatment methods, and it is impossible to evaluate the effectiveness of the treatment program. It is important to state objectives to measure the degree to which the patient is able to perform in the desired manner.

Writing Treatment Objectives

The method for writing treatment objectives, described below, is based on models for writing competency-based educational objectives described by Mager[7] and Kemp.[6]

A comprehensive objective conveys an idea of what the patient will be like when the objective has been achieved. The idea conveyed is identical to the one the therapist and the patient have in mind. It succeeds in communicating their intent and describes the terminal behavior of the patient well enough to preclude misinterpretation. A comprehensive treatment objective is a statement of three elements: (1) terminal behavior, (2) conditions, and (3) criterion.

Terminal behavior

Terminal behavior is the physical change(s), behavior or performance skill that the patient is expected to display.[7] The terminal behavior statement is composed of an action verb and the subject or object being acted upon. For example: *To remove the blouse. Remove* is the action verb, and the *blouse* is the object of the action.

Conditions

These are the circumstances required for the performance of terminal behavior. The conditions answer questions such as "Is special equipment needed?", "Are assistive devices necessary?", "Is supervision or assistance necessary?", "Are special environmental arrangements necessary?", and "Are special cues necessary?"[6,7] For example, "If given verbal cues, the patient will remove the blouse" indicates that the patient will be able to remove the blouse only when there is someone present to provide verbal cues. This statement describes a special circumstance that enables adequate performance of the terminal behavior, *to remove the blouse.*

Obviously many treatment objectives are achieved by patients without any special devices, equipment, environmental modification, or human assistance. Therefore the statement of conditions is not necessary in many objectives. It is an optional element and should be used only when some special circumstance is required to enable the performance of the terminal behavior. The treatment methodology and the time frame in which the treatment program is to take place are *not* considered conditions.

Criterion

The criterion is the performance standard or degree of competence the patient is expected to achieve, stated in measurable or observable terms.[6,7] The criterion answers questions such as how much, how often, how well, how accurately, how completely, and how quickly.[6] If it is possible to estimate the patient's potential level of competence, it is important to include a criterion or performance standard in the objective so the therapist can determine the achievement of the stated terminal behavior with certainty. Like conditions, the criterion is an optional element in the treatment objective. While it is desirable to state a performance standard, it is not always necessary or possible. For example, in the objective, *With minimal assistance the patient will transfer to the toilet,* a performance standard is not necessary because the accomplishment of the transfer is evidence of achievement of the desired skill. In this example, *with minimal assistance* is the condition.

Muscle grades, increases in range of joint motion, degree of competence in task performance, and speed of performance are some examples of criteria. While it is sometimes necessary to state the length of the treatment program in an objective to satisfy insurance requirements, length of treatment is *not* a criterion.

Sample Objectives

Here are some sample treatment objectives and an analysis of their elements.

1. *Given assistive devices, the patient will eat independently in 30 minutes.* In this objective the terminal behavior is the statement *the patient will eat.* Here *eat* is the action verb and the object of the action, food, is implicit. The conditions are *given assistive devices.* This statement indicates the special circumstances, in this case devices, that will make eating possible. The performance standards are *independently in 30 minutes.* This statement says that the patient will be able to eat without human assistance and will achieve eating a meal within 30 minutes, a reasonable amount of time for this activity.

2. *The joint range of motion (ROM) of the left elbow will increase.* This objective is a good statement of terminal behavior. It indicates the kind of change in physical function that is expected as a result of the treatment program. Conditions are not necessary because there will be no special circumstances needed for the patient to demonstrate or perform the increased range of motion. The objective does need a criterion, however, because the amount of increase in range of motion is not indicated, making it difficult to measure progress. It can be reworded as follows: *The joint ROM of the left elbow will increase from 0 to 120 degrees to 0 to 135 degrees.* This wording adds the criterion of a 15 degree increase in ROM, which is measurable.

3. *The patient will operate the control systems of the left above-elbow prosthesis without hesitation.* In this objective *operate the control systems* is the terminal behavior. *Operate* is the action verb and *control systems* are the objects of the action. This is the skill that is expected as a result of the prosthetic training program. Conditions are not necessary because the desired goal is for the patient to be able to perform this skill under any circumstances.

Without hesitation is the criterion. It is an observable level of skill indicative of automatic performance.

4. *Given assistive devices, the patient will dress herself in less than 20 minutes.* To *dress herself* is the terminal behavior. Dress is the action verb and the object of the action is *herself.* The availability of assistive devices is a necessary condition for this patient to perform this task and so the statement of conditions, *given assistive devices,* is needed. The criterion or performance standard is stated in terms of speed and indicates that dressing within 20 minutes is a reasonable expectation for this patient and for this task.

5. *Given equipment set-up and assistive devices, the patient will use mobile arm supports to feed himself independently.* The equipment set-up and the availability of assistive devices constitute the conditions for this objective, and the criterion for performance under these circumstances is *independently,* which indicates that once the equipment and devices are provided, the task of eating can be performed without further human assistance.

There are many variables and unknown factors in the performance and functions of persons with physical dysfunction. Therefore the degree to which they can benefit from, participate in, or succeed at rehabilitation programs cannot be predicted with certainty. This fact makes it difficult for therapists always to write comprehensive treatment objectives. The therapist should attempt to write such objectives, however, using past experience with similar patients and knowledge gained during the assessment process to describe desired terminal behavior, conditions, and criteria for each treatment objective. If comprehensive objectives cannot be written, it is recommended that a specific statement of terminal behavior be used until applicable conditions and criteria become apparent. The stated terminal behaviors can then be modified to become comprehensive objectives as treatment progresses.

SELECTING TREATMENT METHODS

When objectives have been selected, the treatment methods to help the patient achieve them are chosen. This is probably one of the most difficult steps in the treatment planning process. The frame of reference, treatment approach, or a treatment principle or assumption that is applied to the cause of an identified problem should underlie the selection of an appropriate treatment method.[3] For example, after peripheral nerve injury and repair when nerve regeneration is progressing, a principle would be that the use of reinnervated muscles will help to maintain or increase their tone and strength. Therefore graded therapeutic activity or exercise may be the method of choice to effect the desired goals. Many other factors will influence the selection of treatment methods. Some of the factors that should be considered in the selection of treatment methods are the following:

1. What is the goal for the patient?
2. What are the precautions or contraindications that affect the occupational therapy program?
3. What is the prognosis for recovery?
4. What were the results for evaluations in occupational therapy and other services?
5. What other treatment is the patient receiving?
6. What are the goals of other treatment programs, and are the occupational therapy goals compatible with them?
7. How much energy does the patient expend in other therapies?
8. What is the state of the patient's general health?
9. What are the patient's interests, vocational skills, and psychologic needs?
10. What is the patient's physical and sociocultural environment?
11. What roles will the patient assume in the community?
12. What kinds of activities or exercises will be most useful and meaningful to the patient?[5]
13. How can treatment be graded to meet the patient's changing needs as progression or regression occurs?
14. What special equipment or adaptations of therapeutic equipment are needed for the patient to perform maximally?

When treatment methods are selected, it should be clear to others reading the treatment plan exactly how the methods will be used to reach specific objectives. Sometimes several methods may be needed to achieve one objective, or the same methods may be used to reach several objectives.

IMPLEMENTING TREATMENT PLAN

When at least one objective and one or more treatment methods have been selected, the treatment plan is implemented. The patient engages in the procedures that have been designed to ameliorate problems and capitalize on assets. A comprehensive treatment plan may evolve over time. For example, while a lengthy evaluation procedure is in progress, such as ADL, the patient may have commenced a program of therapeutic activity to strengthen specific muscle groups. Therefore, as the assessment is being completed, an increasing number of problems may be identified, and additional objectives and methods may be added to the treatment plan.

REEVALUATING THE PATIENT AND THE INITIAL TREATMENT PLAN

Once the treatment plan is implemented, its effectiveness is evaluated on an ongoing basis through continuous observation and reevaluation. The therapist must be an alert observer and ask: (1) Are the objectives suitable to the patient's needs and capabilities? (2) Are the methods most appropriate for fulfilling the treatment objectives? (3) Does the patient relate to the treatment methods and see them as worthwhile and meaningful? (4) Are the treatment objectives realistic, and are they consistent with the patient's personal objectives? In addition to these observations, the therapist may reevaluate physical functions and performance skills with the same evaluation procedures used in the initial assessment. Gains or losses may then be compared to baseline function recorded at the outset. This approach provides objective evidence of change that is required for reimbursement and validates the treatment plan.

Scrutinizing the treatment plan in this way will enable the therapist to modify the plan as needed. The criterion for determining the effectiveness of the plan is the progress of the patient toward the stated objective(s).

REVISING THE TREATMENT PLAN

The information gained from observations and reevaluation of the patient, as outlined above, may necessitate some revision or modification of the initial treatment plan. The patient's progress may be enough to increase duration, complexity, or resistance of the activity, for example. In degenerative diseases in which maintenance of optimal function is often a primary objective, resistance, duration, and complexity of activity may need to be decreased to accommodate the gradual decline of physical resources. The patient's motivation or inability to see the therapeutic program as helpful or meaningful may necessitate change in treatment approaches and methods. The initial plan is continually revised according to the patient's needs and progress. This process of reevaluation, revision, and reimplementation of the treatment plan goes on throughout the course of the therapeutic program.[8,9]

DISCHARGE PLANNING AND TERMINATING TREATMENT

The whole treatment program is directed to preparing the patient to return home or other suitable living arrangement. Discharge planning is actually a continual process that occurs throughout the treatment program. All treatment is directed to preparing the patient to return to the community. Often therapy will continue on a less intensive basis at home or other living environment.

As the treatment program in the primary health care facility progresses, discharge planning should be initiated. This planning is a team effort that involves the patient, the family, and all rehabilitation specialists concerned with the patient's care.

Preparation for discharge includes medical considerations, provision of assistive devices and mobility equipment, planning a home activity or exercise program, and making a home visit to assess architectural barriers in the environment. Discharge planning should include patient education and education and training of caregivers for a smooth transition. Arrangement for home care therapies and referral to appropriate community agencies is another important aspect of discharge planning.[10]

The psychological preparation of the patient and family members is an important aspect of discharge planning. They may not be psychologically prepared for or functionally capable of managing the transition to the new environment. Generalizing learning from the health care facility to the home may be difficult for the patient. The family may not know the patient's capabilities or how best to give assistance. Providing emotional support, training, counseling, and resource information to the patient and the family is helpful in easing the transition. The family needs information about the following: the patient's ADL status and performance expectations; solutions to accessibility problems in the home, work place, and community; information on home modification; how to obtain, use, and care for assistive devices or mobility equipment; and availability of community resources such as emergency care, self-help groups, respite care, and independent living centers.[11] Maintaining a connection with the primary care facility as a resource for information or further treatment can be reassuring and helpful.[1]

Termination of treatment involves a final assessment of the patient that clearly indicates objectives achieved, partially achieved, or not achieved in the treatment program. The discharge summary is written on the basis of these data and indicates expected future performance of the patient. Termination can affirm the success of the treatment program, but termination is not always achieved. Patients may be discharged before objectives of treatment are met and treatment is concluded.[4] The patient may be referred to another facility or to home care where another therapist assumes the continuity of the treatment program. Careful communication between therapists and agencies is necessary to assure a smooth transition and continuity of care.

TREATMENT PLAN MODEL

The treatment plan model (Fig. 5-2) is useful for teaching treatment planning during academic preparation, and it may be modified for clinical use. The student is presented with a hypothetical case study or an actual patient and is directed to complete the treatment plan, using the *treatment planning guide.* (Box 5-1.) If given a hypothetical patient, the student is directed to complete the *evaluation summary* section of the treatment plan according to his or her knowledge of the particular diagnosis and its resultant disability. A sample treatment plan follows. It was completed according to this model.

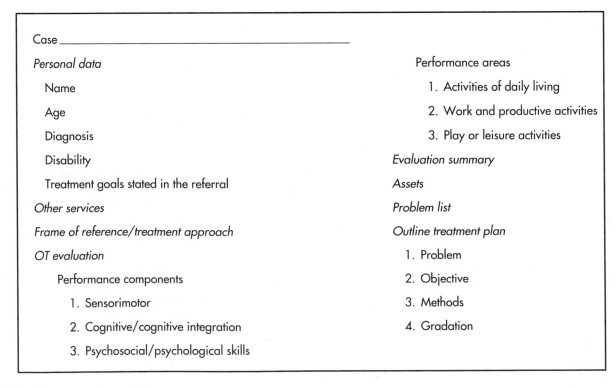

FIG. 5-2 Treatment plan model.

BOX 5-1

TREATMENT PLANNING GUIDE

The treatment planning guide is a reference for filling out a treatment plan for either an actual or a hypothetical patient.

PERSONAL DATA

Fill in the requested information from the medical record or case study.

Name	Disability
Age	Treatment aims stated in the referral
Diagnosis	

OTHER SERVICES

List and describe briefly other services the patient is using.

Physician	Psychology/psychiatry
Nursing	Educational services
Respiratory therapy	Spiritual counseling
Social service	Community social groups/day care
Speech pathology	Home health care services
Physical therapy	Sheltered employment
Vocational counseling	

FRAME OF REFERENCE/ TREATMENT APPROACH

State the frame of reference and treatment approach on which the treatment plan is based. More than one may be necessary.

OT EVALUATION

From the list below, select the performance components and performance areas that should be evaluated. Indicate whether evaluation will be determined by testing or by observation.

Performance components

Sensorimotor
- Muscle strength
- ROM
- Physical endurance
- Standing tolerance
- Walking tolerance
- Sitting balance
- Involuntary movement
- Movement speed
- Level of motor development
- Equilibrium/protective responses
- Coordination/muscle control
- Spasms
- Spasticity
- Stage of motor recovery (stroke patient only)
- Postural reflex mechanism
- Functional movement patterns
- Hand function
- Swallowing/cranial nerve functions
- Sensation—touch, pain, temperature, proprioception, taste, smell

- Body schema
- Motor planning
- Stereognosis
- Visual perception
  - Visual fields
  - Spatial relations
  - Position in space
  - Figure/background
  - Perceptual constancy
  - Visual-motor coordination
  - Depth perception
  - Perception of vertical/horizontal elements
  - Eye movements
- Functional auditory perception

Cognitive/cognitive integration
- Memory
- Judgment
- Safety awareness
- Problem-solving ability
- Motivation
- Sequencing
- Rigidity

BOX 5-1—cont'd

TREATMENT PLANNING GUIDE

Abstract thinking
Functional language skills
    Comprehension of speech/writing
    Ability to express ideas
    Reading
    Writing
Functional mathematical skills
    Mental calculations
    Written calculations
Psychosocial/psychological skills
  Self-identity
  Self-concept
  Coping skills
  Maturity (developmental level)
  Adjustment to disability
  Reality functioning
  Interpersonal skills—dyadic and group interactions

Performance areas
Self-care
  Feeding
  Dressing
  Hygiene
  Transferring
  Community mobility
Work and productive activities
  Work habits and attitudes
  Potential work skills
  Work tolerance
  Home management
  Child care
Play/leisure
  Past and present leisure interests/play activities
  Modes of relaxation

EVALUATION SUMMARY

Summarize findings from tests and observations.

ASSETS

List the assets of the patient and his or her situation that can be used to enhance progress toward maximum independence.

PROBLEM LIST

Identify and list the problems that require occupational therapy intervention.

OBJECTIVES

Write specific treatment objectives in comprehensive form. Each should relate to a specific problem in the problem list and be identified by the corresponding number.

METHODS OF TREATMENT

Describe in detail appropriate treatment methods for the patient.

GRADATION OF TREATMENT

Briefly state how treatment methods will be graded to enhance the patient's progress.

SAMPLE TREATMENT PLAN

The following treatment plan is not a comprehensive plan for the hypothetical patient. Rather, it presents a sampling of parts of a proposed treatment program. The plan deals with four of the problems on the Problem List. The reader is encouraged to add objectives and methods to address additional problems and make the plan a more comprehensive one.

CASE STUDY

Mrs. R. is 49 years old. She has two sons. One is age 26 and married, and the other is age 17. Mrs. R. is divorced. She and her younger son live with her married son, his wife, and their 4-year-old boy. Before the onset of her illness, Mrs. R. lived in an apartment with her younger son.

Mrs. R. had Guillain-Barré syndrome. She has been left with residual weakness of all four extremities. Mrs. R. uses a standard wheelchair for mobility.

Mrs. R. appears thin and frail. She speaks in a weak voice and appears to be passive and discouraged. She feels she cannot accomplish anything. The home situation is poor. Mrs. R. does not communicate with her daughter-in-law, and there are conflicts between the couple and Mrs. R. concerning the management of the teenage son. Mrs. R. feels unable to assert her authority as his mother or to express her needs and feelings. The disability has brought about the loss of her independence and has changed her role in relation to her younger son.

Her daughter-in-law reported that Mrs. R. is dependent for self-care, never attempts to help with homemaking, and isolates herself in her room much of the time. She believes that her mother-in-law is capable of more activity "if only she would try." She says she is willing to allow Mrs. R. to do some of the household work.

Mrs. R. was referred for occupational therapy services as an outpatient for restoration or maintenance of motor functioning and increased independence in ADL.

TREATMENT PLAN

Personal Data
Name: Mrs. R.
Age: 49
Diagnosis: Guillain-Barré syndrome

Disability: Residual weakness, upper and lower extremities
Treatment aims stated in referral: Restoration or maintenance of motor functioning; increased independence in ADL

OTHER SERVICES

Physician: prescription of medication; maintenance of general health; supervision of rehabilitation program
Physical therapy: muscle strengthening; ambulation and transfer training

Social service: individual and family counseling
Community social group: socialization

FRAME OF REFERENCE

Occupational performance

TREATMENT APPROACHES

Biomechanical and rehabilitative

OT EVALUATION

Performance Components
Sensorimotor
 Muscle strength: test
 Passive ROM: test
 Physical endurance: observe, interview
 Walking tolerance: observe, interview
 Movement speed: observe
 Coordination: test, observe
 Functional movement: test, observe
 Sensation (touch, pain, thermal, proprioception): test
Cognitive/cognitive integration
 Judgment: observe

Safety awareness: observe
 Motivation: observe, interview
Psychosocial/psychological skills
 Coping skills: observe
 Adjustment to disability: observe, interview
 Social skills
 Interpersonal relationships: observe

Performance Areas
Self care: observe, interview
Home management: observe, interview

SAMPLE TREATMENT PLAN – cont'd

EVALUATION SUMMARY

Muscle testing revealed that all muscles are the same grades bilaterally: scapula and shoulder muscles are F+ to G (3+ to 4); elbow and forearm muscles are F+ to G (3+ to 4); wrist and hand musculature is graded F+ (3+). Trunk muscles are G (4); all muscles of the hip are G (4); except adductors and external rotators, which are F+ (3+). Knee flexors and extensors are G (4). Ankle plantar flexors and dorsiflexors are F (3), and all foot muscles are F− (3−) to P (2).

All joint motions within normal to functional range. Physical endurance limited to 1 hour of light activity of upper extremities, with some ambulation, before rest. Mrs. R. uses a wheelchair for energy conservation and propels it using both arms and legs. Slight incoordination, evident on fine hand function, caused by muscle weakness.

Sensory modalities of touch, pain, temperature, and proprioception are intact. No cognitive deficits were observed. Mrs. R. is passive and discouraged about her disability. She feels she cannot accomplish anything and tends to stay in her room alone.

Before onset of illness, Mrs. R. lived independently with her 17-year-old son. Since her illness, she and her son have moved in with her 26-year-old son, his wife, and their 4-year-old son. This arrangement has proved less than ideal. There is little communication between Mrs. R. and her daughter-in-law. There are conflicts between the couple and Mrs. R. about the management of her teenage son.

The disability has brought about the loss of Mrs. R.'s independence and has changed her roles as homemaker and mother. She feels unable to assert her authority as mother of her 17-year-old or to express her needs and feelings.

Mrs. R. manages some personal care such as facewashing and hair and teeth care. She needs some assistance with dressing and has difficulty with buttons and zippers. She requires an adaptive toothbrush and needs assistance in toilet transferring and showering. Mrs. R. does not perform any home management tasks but is potentially capable of light activities such as table setting, dusting, and folding clothes. Mrs. R.'s daughter-in-law is willing to allow her mother-in-law some household activities if understanding about their respective roles can be established.

ASSETS

Some functional muscle strength
Good joint mobility
Potential for good living situation

Presence of able-bodied adults who can assist
Potential for some further recovery
Good sensation

PROBLEM LIST

1. Muscle weakness
2. Low physical endurance
3. Limited walking tolerance
4. Mild incoordination
5. Self-care dependence

6. Homemaking dependence
7. Dependent transferring
8. Isolation, apparent depression
9. Reduced social interaction
10. Lack of assertiveness

PROBLEM 1

Muscle weakness

Objective

Muscle strength of shoulder flexors will increase from F+ (3+) to G (4).

Method

Light progressive resistive exercise to shoulder flexion: patient is seated in a regular chair, wearing a weighted cuff one half the weight of her maximum resistance above each elbow. Lifts arms alternately through 10 repetitions and then rests. Repeated using three quarters maximum resistance, then full resistance. Activities: reaching for glasses in overhead cupboard and placing them on the table, replacing glasses in cupboard when dry; rolling out pastry dough on a slightly inclined pastry board; wiping table, counter, and cupboard doors, using a forward push-pull motion; Turkish knotting project with weaving frame set vertically in front of her and tufts of yarn on right and left sides, at hip level.

Gradation

Increase resistance, number of repetitions, and length of time as strength improves.

PROBLEM 1

Muscle weakness

Objective

Strength of wrist flexors and extensors and finger flexors will increase from F + (3 +) to G (4).

Method

Light progressive resistive exercises for wrist flexors and extensors: patient is seated, side to table, with pronated forearm resting on the table and hand extended over edge of table; a hand cuff, with small weights equal to one half of her maximum resistance attached to the palmar surface, is worn on the hand; patient extends the wrist through full range of motion against gravity for 10 repetitions, then rests. Exercise is repeated, using three quarters maximum resistance and then full resistance. The same procedure is used to exercise wrist flexors, except that the forearm is supinated on the table, and the weights are suspended from the dorsal side of the hand cuff. Activities to improve finger flexors: tearing lettuce to make a salad; handwashing panties and hosiery. Progress to kneading soft clay or bread dough.

Gradation

Increase resistance, repetitions, and time.

PROBLEM 5

Self-care dependence

Objective

Given assistive devices, Mrs. R. will be able to dress herself independently within 20 minutes.

Method

Putting on bra: using a back-opening stretch bra, pass bra around waist so that opening is in front and straps are facing up; fasten bra in front at waist level; slide fastened bra around at waist level so that cups are in front; slip arms through straps and work straps up over shoulders; adjust cups and straps. Putting on shirt: place loose fitting blouse on lap with back facing up and neck toward knees; place arms under back of blouse and into arm holes; push sleeves up onto arms past elbows; gather back material up from neck to hem with hands and duck head forward and pass garment over head; work blouse down by shrugging shoulders and pulling into place with hands; use button hook to fasten front opening. Putting on underpants and slacks: sitting on bed or in wheelchair, cross legs, reach down, and place one opening over foot; cross opposite leg, place other opening over foot; uncross legs, work pants up over feet and up under thighs (a dressing stick may be used to pull pants up if leaning forward is difficult); shift hips from side to side and work pants up as far as possible over buttocks; stand, if possible, and pull pants to waist level, then sit and pull zipper up with prefastened zipper pull; use Velcro at waist closure on slacks. Putting on socks: using stretch socks and seated, cross one leg, place sock over toes and work sock up onto foot and over heel; cross other leg and repeat. Putting on shoes: using slip-on shoe with Velcro fasteners, use procedure for socks.

Gradation

Progress to more difficult tasks such as pantyhose, tie shoes, dresses, pullover garments.

PROBLEM 6

Homemaking dependence

Objective

Given assistive devices, Mrs. R. will perform homemaking activities.

Methods

Using a dust mitt, patient dusts furniture surfaces easily reached from wheelchair such as lamp tables and coffee table; sits at sink to wash dishes; practices folding small items of clothing such as panties, nylons, children's underwear, while sitting at kitchen table; have Mrs. R.'s daughter-in-law observe activities at treatment facility; work out an acceptable list of activities and a schedule with both women. Discuss how Mrs. R. could make some contributions to home management routines; ask Mrs. R. to keep activity diary, noting any performance difficulties and successes for review at next visit.

Gradation

Increase number of household responsibilities. Increase time spent on household activities.

SAMPLE TREATMENT PLAN – cont'd

PROBLEM 8
Isolation, depression

Objective
Mrs. R. will reduce time spent alone from 6 waking hours to 3 waking hours.

Method
Establish acceptable graded activity schedule between Mrs. R. and son and daughter-in-law; include homemaking tasks and socialization with family through playing games, watching TV, preparing and eating meals, and conversing; family members encourage Mrs. R. to be with them but to be accepting if she refuses; have Mrs. R. keep activities diary for review; determine how time is spent and discuss how it could be more productive and enjoyable. Initiate avocational activity, such as needlework or tile mosaics, to complete at home; set goals for where and how much activity will be performed.

Gradation
Increase time spent out of own room; include friends, neighbors, family, in household social activities; plan a community outing for shopping or lunch.

REVIEW QUESTIONS

1. Define *treatment plan*.
2. Why write a treatment plan?
3. Why base the treatment plan on a specific frame of reference or treatment approach?
4. List the steps in developing a treatment plan.
5. List, define, and give examples of the three elements of a comprehensive treatment objective.
6. If a comprehensive objective cannot be written, which element would be *most* important to identify first?
7. List six factors to consider when selecting treatment methods.
8. Is it necessary to develop a complete comprehensive treatment plan before treatment can begin?
9. Is it ever necessary to change the initial treatment plan?
10. What criterion is used to evaluate the effectiveness of a treatment plan?
11. How does a therapist know when to modify or change a treatment plan?
12. What are some of the concerns and preparations for termination of treatment?

REFERENCES

1. Baum C: Identification and use of environmental resources. In Christiansen C, Baum C: *Occupational therapy, overcoming human performance deficits,* Thorofare, NJ, 1991, Slack.
2. Christiansen C: Occupational therapy: intervention for life performance. In Christiansen C, Baum C: *Occupational therapy, overcoming human performance deficits,* Thorofare, NJ, 1991, Slack.
3. Day D: A systems diagram for teaching treatment planning, *Am J Occup Ther* 27:239, 1973.
4. Hopkins HL: Problem solving. In Hopkins HL, Smith HD, editors: *Willard and Spackman's occupational therapy,* ed 8, Philadelphia, 1993, JB Lippincott.
5. Hopkins HL and associates: Therapeutic applications of activity. In Hopkins HL, Smith HD, editors: *Willard and Spackman's occupational therapy,* ed 6, Philadelphia, 1983, JB Lippincott.
6. Kemp JE: *The instructional design process,* New York, 1985, Harper & Row.
7. Mager RF: *Preparing instructional objectives,* ed 2 (rev.), Belmont, Calif, 1984, David S. Lake.
8. Pelland MJ: A conceptual model for the instruction and supervision of treatment planning, *Am J Occup Ther* 41:351, 1987.
9. Smith HD: Assessment and evaluation: an overview. In Hopkins HL, Smith HD, editors: *Willard and Spackman's occupational therapy,* ed 8, Philadelphia, 1993, JB Lippincott.
10. Spencer EA: Functional restoration: preliminary concepts and planning. In Hopkins HL, Smith HD, editors: *Willard and Spackman's occupational therapy,* ed 8, Philadelphia, 1993, JB Lippincott.
11. Versluys HP: Family influences. In Hopkins HL, Smith HD, editors: *Willard and Spackman's occupational therapy,* Philadelphia, 1993, JB Lippincott.

Documentation of Occupational Therapy Services

Janet L. Jabri

Documentation of occupational therapy services refers to the written record of all information that is relevant to the patient or client from occupational therapy admission to discharge. The documentation process is initiated immediately upon receipt of the initial referral, and the actual documentation includes confirmation of the referral, initial evaluation, ongoing daily and/or weekly progress notes, periodic interim reassessments, and a discharge summary. Backup documentation, not usually entered into the official medical record, may include evaluation test results, checklists, or patient worksheets. The full record contains pertinent information about the patient's status, progress, and performance.

There is no standard or single method for documenting occupational therapy services within the profession. The types of records and reports to be written may be determined by the treatment facility and by the funding agencies.[4,8] Regardless of the method for documentation, it is critical that all entries be clear, concise, objective, accurate, and complete. Because the documentation is part of a legal record, omissions or errors in the record may cause doubts about the accuracy of the entire record.[3] The occupational therapist is responsible for ensuring that all documentation requirements are met in a timely fashion.

PURPOSES FOR DOCUMENTATION

Documentation is a very important part of occupational therapy practice. Effective documentation of occupational therapy services serves many purposes, including the following:

1. communicating progress to the physician and other health care professionals
2. facilitating continuity of treatment when staff changes occur
3. providing clear, objective data about the patient on which future treatment can be based
4. providing justification for continued treatment for utilization review committees
5. ensuring payment for the service by third party payers
6. complying with the law and aiding in litigation
7. providing a method to ensure patient rights and advocacy
8. interpreting the treatment program to the patient, family and other interested individuals or agencies
9. evaluating the effectiveness of occupational therapy intervention
10. ensuring facility accreditation from organizations such as the Joint Commission for the Accreditation of Healthcare Organizations (JCAHO) or the Commission for Accreditation of Rehabilitation Facilities (CARF)
11. providing data for research and the advancement of the professionalism of occupational therapy
12. facilitating training and student education programs.[3,4,6,8]

RECORDS AND REPORTS
THE OCCUPATIONAL THERAPY FILE

In some facilities the occupational therapy service maintains separate departmental files. This file includes supporting records, notes, and worksheets as well as copies of the reports prepared for the permanent legal record. The supporting data may include tests results such as a muscle test form, treatment observations such as an activities of daily living (ADL) checklist, informal therapy team conference notes, or treatment plan approaches. The supporting data form the basis of the reports that will become part of the permanent legal record.

Maintaining a separate occupational therapy file offers

increased efficiency and other advantages. The record is accessible for convenient review and updating of all data. The permanent legal record is used by many treatment team members and is not always readily available. The occupational therapy record file is readily accessible and provides more detailed information for clinicians who cover in the absence of the primary therapist, ensuring more effective continuity of treatment. Finally, the record is available for review during patient care/family conferences or during any treatment session.

THE PERMANENT LEGAL RECORD

The permanent legal record contains defined information from the entire treatment team. The documents in this record are considered the only official information related to that patient or client. Each facility determines the official contents of this record, which may be based on requirements set by internal systems, licensing agencies, accrediting bodies, and third party payers. This record will be used within the facility by the treatment team for understanding the full patient treatment picture, by utilization reviewers to determine justification for continued treatment, and by quality assurance teams to assess overall patient outcomes and services. These records may also be used by third party payers to determine payment for services, by the court system for legal litigation, and by outside agencies for continued treatment or services after discharge from the facility.

The occupational therapy documents contained in the permanent legal record consist of the doctor's referral, initial evaluation, ongoing progress notes, interim reassessments, and the discharge summary. These records consist of a concise summary of all tests and observations, treatment goals, treatment plans, and progress toward the established goals. In addition, the occupational therapist may be required to provide entries in other sections of the permanent record such as the interdisciplinary care plan or the patient care conference note.

THE RECORDS AND REPORTS PROCESS AND FORMATS
THE REFERRAL

Occupational therapy evaluation and treatment is usually initiated by receipt of a patient/client referral. This referral is generally, but not always, received from the physician and may specify the reason for requesting the referral. When a physician's referral is required, it should include the occupational therapy treatment diagnosis, the onset date of the treatment diagnosis, a request for evaluation and/or other specific treatment orders, the date, and physician's signature.[1]

The first entry into the permanent record may be to document receipt of the referral and the initial plan of action. The response time is established by each facility but is usually within 24 to 48 hours upon receipt of the referral.

Sample of Referral Receipt

11/5/95 Occupational Therapy referral received and full evaluation initiated this date.

INITIAL EVALUATION

The initial evaluation is a three-step process. The first step is to gather general information about the patient to establish a database. The second step is to complete the assessment and establish a baseline of patient performance. The final step is to use the information obtained in steps one and two and apply clinical reasoning skills to draw sound conclusions and establish the treatment goals and plan.

Step 1: Building the General Information Data Base

The therapist begins the initial evaluation process by reviewing data obtained from the permanent record. He or she also interviews referring sources, the patient, and family members, and observes patient performance and behavior to build a general information data base. This data base includes the patient's name, address, important phone numbers, family members, third party payers (both primary and secondary), family, educational and work histories. In addition the data base includes pertinent medical, physical, and mental status information related to specific primary and secondary diagnoses as well as other related prior levels of function information. Information regarding expected treatment outcomes and discharge plans is also pertinent.

This information provides baseline information, and the appropriate data will be integrated into the initial evaluation report. Extraneous information may be kept in the occupational therapy record for reference during the treatment process.

Step 2: Establishing the Performance Baseline

The second step in the initial evaluation involves assessments and tests to establish the performance baseline. Accuracy in administering tests and recording evaluation results is critical. All future assessment reports will compare progress to this baseline, and the degree of improvement may determine the course and amount of treatment approved by physicians and third party payers.

The occupational therapy file should contain detailed results of all evaluations that were completed. These may include the following: (1) range of motion (ROM) measurements; (2) manual muscle testing, sensory testing, and perceptual/cognitive evaluation results; and (3) ADL, functional mobility, home management, vocational, and avocational assessment findings.

Step 3: Establishing the Treatment Plan

The final step involves using the data gathered in the previous two steps to establish a clear plan of action. This process is one of determining the problems impeding function and then applying clinical reasoning skills to determine predictable functional outcomes. The result is a clear set of goals with a plan of treatment to accomplish those goals.

THE INITIAL EVALUATION REPORT

Initial evaluation formats vary greatly from setting to setting. Most facilities have printed forms that the therapist fills out rather than completing a narrative report. There are pros and cons for either format. Forms ensure that information is complete. The subheadings trigger a written response for all evaluation areas. A form's limited space encourages brevity and conciseness. In general, the form saves time and most team members find it faster for gleaning needed information. The form also presents a ready format for computer keyboard input. The form may not meet the specialized documentation needs of all diagnoses, however, or provide sufficient space for important information not covered by the subheadings. The main advantage of the narrative format is its adaptability to the special needs of the individual patient. The narrative format, however, generally takes longer to complete and to read.

The initial evaluation, whether it is a form (Figs. 6-1 and 6-2) or narrative format, can be divided into several distinct sections as follows: (1) general information, which includes patient identifying information, medical history, and prior level of function; (2) clinical evaluation and interpretation; (3) functional status assessment; and (4) the evaluation summary, which includes problem identification, short and long term goals, and the treatment plan.

General Information

The first section consists of basic patient identifying information. It includes the patient's name, medical record or account number, the referring physician, and the referral and evaluation dates. This section details pertinent medical history including a list of primary treatment and any related secondary diagnoses with their onset dates. This section should list any precautions or contraindications that need to be observed during treatment. The patient's prior level of function, prior living situation, and previous vocation and avocational level of function are also noted (Fig. 6-1).

Clinical Evaluation

This section is a synopsis of evaluation results (Fig. 6-2). It is helpful to relay standardized results or use standardized rating scales for easy interpretation by others. Standardized scales also ensure reliable replication of the evaluation process at reassessment and discharge times. The evaluations performed will depend upon the specific diagnosis. For example, a brain injured patient may require a physical assessment (ROM, motor function, and sensory) as well as perceptual and cognitive testing. For a mental disorder such as depression, the assessment may focus primarily on behavior and cognitive parameters.

Functional Status Assessment

This section evaluates the functional performance of the patient. The clinical evaluation results have substantial bearing on these assessments; again a standardized scale is imperative to ensure reliability of results through the treatment process. The scope of this occupational therapy assessment will depend upon the defined roles of the department within the facility. In the sample form (Fig. 6-2) bed mobility, transfers, wheelchair mobility, and daily living skills are assessed. A sample levels-of-assistance scale is provided in Table 6-1.

Evaluation Summary

The evaluation summary is the most important section of the report. In this section the previously recorded information is analyzed and a problem list is developed. The problems listed are those factors that will impede the patient from obtaining maximal independence. It should be noted that this list may include problems that occupational therapy intervention may not directly affect. These problems will influence the treatment approach taken by the occupational therapist. Using this problem list, the occupational therapist must set realistic and functional therapy goals. Writing therapy goals is the most critical portion of the initial evaluation process. The goals are predictions of the patient outcome. The occupational therapist must apply theoretical knowledge and clinical reasoning skills to predict one or more treatment outcomes for the patient. These initial goals are the indicators that will be used to measure the effectiveness of the therapy intervention and the success for the patient.

The goals can be divided into two groups: long-term goals and short-term goals. Long-term goals are the maximal predicted outcomes expected for that patient after the full treatment program has been completed. Short-term goals describe the level of function expected after a predesignated period of treatment intervention, usually 1 week or 1 month. Each goal must reflect a measurable, realistic, and functional outcome for the patient. For example, a long-term goal for a patient currently requiring maximum assistance for eating might read, "The patient will eat independently using an adapted utensil." The short-term goal for the next week might read, "The patient will require moderate assistance for eating using an adapted utensil."

Finally, a treatment plan must be established. The treatment plan lists the treatment interventions that the therapist will use to assist the patient in achieving predetermined goals. This plan includes the treatment frequency and duration. For the previous goal, daily eating retraining and upper extremity functional strengthening for two weeks may be a treatment plan established to achieve increased independence in eating.

The summary section may also include a discharge plan once therapy has been completed and a checkbox to note that goals have been discussed and reflect the goals of the patient and/or family. Finally, if the physician's referral was for an evaluation only or did not spec-

OCCUPATIONAL THERAPY

SANTA CLARA VALLEY MEDICAL CENTER
OCCUPATIONAL THERAPY DEPARTMENT
Page 1 of 2

Service _____ ☐ Inpatient ☐ Outpatient

☐ Initial ☐ Interim ☐ Discharge
(Rating scales on back of form)

INFORMATION

Onset Date: _____ Referral Date: _____ Sex: M F Language: _____
Diagnosis

Medical History:

Precautions/Diet:

Living Situation:

A/Vocational History:

UPPER EXTREMITY

Range of Motion
☐ Refer to range of motion form

Muscle Picture
☐ Refer to muscle test form

Sensation
(Light touch, pain, kinesthesia, other)

Hand Function

Dominance: ☐ Right ☐ Left

	Right			Left		
	Grip	3 point	Lateral	Grip	3 point	Lateral
Initial						
Interim/DC						
Norm						

Splinting:

OTHER MOTOR
(Endurance, head/trunk posture and control, sitting/standing balance, reflexes, LE picture, functional ambulation)

VISUAL PERCEPTUAL SKILLS

VISUAL	Initial	Interim/DC	PERCEPTUAL	Initial	Interim/DC
Visual Attention			Motor planning		
Near Acuity			Graphic praxis		
Distance Acuity			Body scheme		
Pursuits			R/L discrimination		
Saccades			Form		
Ocular Alignment			Size		
Stereopsis			Part/whole		
VisualFields			Figure ground		
Visual Neglect			Position in space		

SCALE: 0 = intact; 1 = impaired; 2 = severely impaired; 3 = unable to perform
COMMENTS:

Wears corrective lenses ☐Y ☐N   Testing not indicated ☐

COGNITION AND BEHAVIOR
(Orientation, initiation, direction following, memory, judgement, organization, problem solving, impulsivity, attention span)

DISPOSITION - White - MEDICAL RECORD   Yellow - O.T. Chart   Therapist's Signature:_____

9502   SCVMC 6628-17

FIG. 6-1 Occupational therapy evaluation form, page 1 of 2. Reprinted with permission, Occupational Therapy Department, Santa Clara Valley Medical Center, San José, Calif.

SANTA CLARA VALLEY MEDICAL CENTER
OCCUPATIONAL THERAPY EVALUATION
Page 2 of 2

Service _____ ☐ Inpatient ☐ Outpatient

☐ Initial   ☐ Interim   ☐ Discharge

(Rating scale on back of form)

OCCUPATIONAL THERAPY

BED MOBILITY

ACTIVITY	Initial	Interim D/C	Goal
Rolling R			
Rolling L			
Bridging			
Scooting			
Long Sit			
Sidelying to Sit			

Bed:
Positioning:

Caregiver Training:

Comments:

TRANSFERS

ACTIVITY	Initial	Interim D/C	Goal
Bed			
Toilet			
Tub/Shower			
Car/Van Seat			
Furniture			

Type: Equipment:
Caregiver Training:

Comments:

WHEELCHAIR

ACTIVITY	Initial	Interim D/C	Goal
Management			
Weight Shift			
Home			
Community			
In/Out of Car			

Type: Weight Shift Type:
Positioning/Cushion:

Caregiver Training:

Comments:

DAILY LIVING SKILLS

ACTIVITY	Initial	Interim D/C	Goal
Eating			
Upper Body Dressing			
Lower Body Dressing			
Hygiene/Grooming			
Bathing			
Toileting			
Kitchen			
Homemaking			
Community			
Communication Tasks			

Equipment:

Home Environment:

A/Vocational/Driving Skills:

Caregiver Training:

Comments:

Problems:

Goals/Recommendation: ☐ Patient/Caregiver participated in goal setting

X _____ / _____ / _____
Frequency / Session Length / Duration of Treatment

_____   _____   _____
Therapist's Signature   Date   Physician's Signature

DISPOSITION - White - MEDICAL RECORD Yellow - O.T. Chart   9502 PAGE 2 of 2   SCVMC 6628-17

FIG. 6-2 Occupational therapy evaluation form, continued, page 2 of 2. Reprinted with permission, Occupational Therapy Department, Santa Clara Valley Medical Center, San José, Calif.

TABLE 6-1 Definitions of Levels of Assistance

LEVEL OF ASSISTANCE	ABBREVIATION	DEFINITION
Independent	Ind.	Patient requires no assistance or cuing in any situation.
		Patient is trusted in all situations 100% of the time to do the task safely.
Supervision	Sup.	The caregiver is not required to provide any hands-on guarding but may need to give verbal cues for safety.
Contact Guard/Standby	Con. Gd./Stby	The caregiver must provide hands-on contact guard or be within arms length for the patient's safety.
Minimum Assistance	Min.	The caregiver provides 25% physical and/or cuing assistance.
Moderate Assistance	Mod.	The caregiver assists the patient with 50% of the task.
		The assistance can be physical and/or cuing.
Maximum Assistance	Max.	The caregiver assists the patient with 75% of the task.
		The assist can be physical and/or cuing.
Dependent	Dep.	Patient is unable to assist in any part of the task. The caregiver performs 100% of the task for the patient physically and/or cognitively.

Adapted from Occupational therapy evaluation form, Occupational Therapy Department, Santa Clara Medical Center, San José, Calif. Reprinted with permission.

ify the treatment intervention now planned, a physician's review of the plan and verifying signature may be necessary.

THE INTERIM ASSESSMENT REPORT

If treatment occurs over an extended time, it may be necessary to complete a full reassessment. The format is often the same as the initial evaluation. The main difference is that this report reflects the differences between the initial evaluation results and the present clinical status. The interim report reflects progress made toward the predicted goals and is a measure of success of the treatment intervention. The new evaluation results may present an opportunity for revising initial goals and treatment timelines. Interim assessments are an important tool for the ongoing utilization review process. It allows the therapist to justify continued treatment intervention by clearly assessing the effectiveness and the efficiency of the treatment that has occurred.

THE DISCHARGE SUMMARY REPORT

At the completion of the treatment regime, it will be necessary to document the status of the patient. The format can be the same as that used for the initial evaluation and interim assessments. This summary is a description of the final status of the patient at the time of discharge from the particular setting. It is important to compare accurately the progress made from the initial assessment to discharge. Some key elements may be added to the discharge summary. These include a statement of which goals were achieved, which goals were not achieved and why, and most important, discharge recommendations. These recommendations should clearly indicate additional interventions and follow-up needed to ensure continued functional improvement or maintenance.

The discharge summary is a key document because it reflects the total progress and all accomplishments achieved for the case. The data can be used for many purposes. Quality assurance committees may use the data to evaluate effectiveness of the treatment. The data may also be used for outcome studies to prove effectiveness for treatment within certain diagnostic categories. In addition, insurance payers may use the report to determine payment for the service, and other service agencies such as outpatient clinics use the data to help establish goals and treatment plans in the new treatment setting.

THE PROGRESS NOTE

Progress notes may be required on a per treatment, daily, or weekly basis. Generally daily notes are very brief and reflect patient response to the treatment, treatment provided, and progress noted. Revision of the treatment plan and goals are not always necessary.

Weekly progress notes are more thorough and should summarize the treatment provided, the treatment frequency, the patient's response to treatment, and progress toward goals or lack of progress with justification. The goals should be updated and the treatment plan revised. The new goals and treatment plan are usually considered short-term goals and reflect the expected outcome for the following week's treatment regime.

Various styles or formats for progress notes are used to ensure consistency of the content of the notes. SOAP notes are one format frequently used. The acronym stands for *subjective* (the patient's view of the problem), *objective* (the clinical findings about the problem), *assessment* (important data from reevaluations), and *plan* (treatment goals and modalities to be used).[8] This method of recording information is based on the system designed by Weed[9] in the Problem Oriented Medical Record.[5,6] Another format for short daily notes states the problem, progress, description of the treatment program, and future plans. Still another possibility is to record the treatment frequency, goal, method, patient's response and progress, and future treatment plan.

Brief Daily Note Sample

Patient actively participated in eating retraining and RUE strengthening program. Patient ate 75% of his meal with adapted utensils and required minimal assistance for cutting meat. Established treatment plan to continue.

Weekly Progress Note Sample

Patient has been seen daily for eating retraining and RUE functional strengthening program. The patient is able to eat 75% of his meal using adapted utensils and with minimal assistance for cutting meat. Previously patient ate 50% of meal and required moderate assist for cutting meat. The patient will eat independently with no assistive devices in one week.

SOAP Note Sample

S.   Patient stated satisfaction with feeding self.
O.   The patient is able to eat 75% of his meal using adapted utensils and with minimal assistance for cutting meat. Previously patient ate 50% of meal and required moderate assistance for cutting meat.
A.   The patient continues to exhibit low endurance for maintaining hand grip and poor strength in elbow flexors strength (fair to fair minus).
P.   Achieve independent eating with no assistive devices in one week via eating retraining and RUE functional strengthening program.

Problem Focus Progress Note Sample

Problem: Assisted eating.
Progress: The patient was able to eat 75% of his meal using adapted utensils and with minimal assistance for cutting meat. Previously patient ate 50% of meal and required moderate assistance for cutting meat.
Program: Eating retraining and RUE functional strengthening program.
Plan: Achieve independent eating with no assistive devices in 1 week.

QUALITY OF DOCUMENTATION CONTENT

The quality of the documentation content is of the utmost importance. Documentation must be well organized, objective, accurate, and must contain only pertinent information. Conciseness and brevity are dictated by time constraints for both the writer and the reader. The therapist must consider who will read the report,[2] which may influence what needs to be reported and how the report will be written. Whether a report is written for other clinicians, insurance payers, or a lay person may determine the medical terminology or medical abbreviations used as well as the amount of detail needed for understanding by the reader.

The content of documentation is legally governed. Laws have been enacted to ensure quality care and cost containment. The written record is the primary means of justifying appropriate treatment by the appropriate clinician in the most cost-effective environment. To preserve the rights of the patient, the record must be factual and include no value judgments that may be prejudicial to the patient.[7,10]

Health records may be used in litigation for settling insurance claims and may be examined by third party payers, fiscal intermediaries, and other utilization review boards.[7,10] The review of the records is governed by principles of ethical practice in relation to confidentiality, and the records are under strict control of the physician or health care agency. No privileged information, verbal or written, can be released without written consent of the patient.[3] In addition, the patient has the right to know what is in the record and can ask for the information. The physician is responsible for providing the information in the manner in which he or she sees fit.

It is important to remember that the legal written record is the only acceptable proof of the treatment intervention. If it is not written it did not happen, in the eyes of outside reviewers, whether it be a third party payer or a jury. The following documentation guidelines help ensure that the therapist meets legal and ethical obligations:

1. Date all entries for accurate sequencing of the treatment.
2. Document missed treatments.
3. Document at the time of treatment so the entry will completely and accurately reflect the treatment session.
4. Document in specific facts rather than in general terms.
5. Do not criticize another health care provider in the written record.
6. Do not change a legal record after the fact without clarifying the time and nature of the change.[7]

REPORTING SYSTEMS
THE PROBLEM ORIENTED MEDICAL RECORD

The Problem Oriented Medical Record (POMR) was devised by Dr. Lawrence L. Weed at Case Western Reserve University.[9] It is based on a computer-compatible model and follows a systematic progression from evaluation to progress reporting. It is a problem-solving model that is readily accepted by occupational therapists and can be implemented in any setting. It offers a method by which evaluation and treatment standards can be documented and enforced.[5]

The POMR encourages an interdisciplinary model in which all health care services integrate information into one document. The data base is composed of physical, social, and demographic information contained in one report. From this data base a problem list is formulated and kept at the front of the record. It serves as an index to all problems and may include anticipated problems.

Each problem is numbered and named, and these designations remain the same for each hospitalization of the patient. All of the treatment plans must be titled and numbered according to the problem list, dated, and signed. For example, by reading all of the notes that refer to problem number 3, the health care worker can learn what each service is contributing to the patient's total rehabilitation at any given time.[5]

All progress notes are dated, numbered, and titled according to the problem to which they refer. All progress notes are recorded together. They are written according to the previously mentioned SOAP outline. Progress notes are written whenever a staff member has relevant information to record. The frequency of entries to the record may reflect policies of the treatment facility, acuteness of the patient's condition, or need for continued evaluation.[5] The record concludes with a problem-oriented discharge summary.

The POMR facilitates communications between health disciplines because all progress notes are intermixed and all personnel are bound by the same criteria for recording. All services are up-to-date on progress in other areas, and treatment can be adjusted accordingly. The patient can be educated about his condition and progress. The POMR allows for adequate documentation required for quality assurance and third party payer requirements.

The accurate documentation of services is an outcome of the treatment process. The POMR offers a recording system that can improve the standards of documentation.[5]

THE OCCUPATIONAL THERAPY SEQUENTIAL CLIENT CARE RECORD

The Occupational Therapy Sequential Client Care Record (OTSCCR) created by Llorens[4] is unique to occupational therapy. Rather than being based on medical or psychological reporting systems, it is organized according to a theoretical framework consistent with the characteristics, objectives, and goals of occupational therapy. As the field of occupational therapy has developed, there has been an increased effort to measure quality of care, achieve autonomy in decision making, be accountable to patients and funding agencies, and assume professional responsibility for services. Llorens described the client care record as the "key document for determining quality and effectiveness of care."[4]

The OTSCCR system combines the theoretical framework of Llorens' Occupational Therapy Developmental Analysis, Evaluation, and Intervention Schedule with the scientific method of the POMR for documenting care in occupational therapy. The OTSCCR includes a data base, information about the evaluation process, problem identification, an occupational therapy plan, progress notes, and a discharge summary. It is based on developmental frame of reference and occupational performance model, and data are recorded and analyzed according to the performance areas and performance components of the occupational performance model.

The OTSCCR documents factual information about the client based on actual behavior. It is designed to span the total time the client is served by occupational therapy from admission to discharge. It is retained by the occupational therapy department for use in preparing reports and communicating with the client and other interested persons or agencies.[4]

AUTOMATED DOCUMENTATION SYSTEMS

With the development of computer technology, there has been a substantial increase in therapy documentation software systems. These systems range from primary documentation formats to integrated systems that not only provide basic documentation but also complete billing processes, provide administrative tracking information, and collate outcome data.

The ultimate advantage in using an automated system lies in the time savings not only in the documentation time but in the time spent on collating data for outcome studies and other required administrative reports. In addition, data handling abilities are far more advanced and accurate than that of manual systems. Disadvantages of automated systems include the following: (1) the difficulty of securing a system that meets all the needs of the program or requests from outside agencies; (2) the cost of sufficient hardware to meet the needs of the facility; and (3) the cost of training as well as staff acceptance of using the system.[6]

SUMMARY

Documentation of occupational therapy services consists of written records and reports that contain pertinent information about the patient's status, progress, and performance. The occupational therapist is responsible for keeping accurate records to document the patient's evaluation results, the identified problems, the treatment goals and plan and the patient's progress toward the established plan.

Documentation is necessary for administrative tasks, reimbursement, communication, quality assurance, educational, and legal purposes. It is essential to justify the necessity and cost of treatment. It also contributes to advancing the validity of occupational therapy.

Occupational therapy documentation includes the referral, evaluation data, initial evaluation, progress notes, interim reassessments, and the discharge summary. Records and reports should reflect clear, concise, accurate, and objective information about the patient. The reader of the documents must be considered when reports are being written to avoid misinterpretation and misunderstanding. Documentation should be well organized and developed according to an agreed-upon system for internal consistency of the record.

REVIEW QUESTIONS

1. What is meant by documentation of occupational therapy services?
2. When is the documentation process initiated?
3. List at least five purposes of documentation.
4. What is the difference in content between the occupational therapy file and the permanent legal record? Which kinds of documents are contained in each?
5. Briefly summarize the content of the initial evaluation report.
6. How is the treatment plan developed?
7. What is contained in an interim assessment report?
8. What is contained in the discharge summary report?
9. List two formats for progress notes.
10. Why is excellent documentation important?
11. Describe the POMR and OTSCCR recording systems.
12. What is the advantage of an automated documentation system?

REFERENCES

1. Allen C, Foto M, Moon-Sperling T, Wilson D: A payer's review of documentation. In Acquaviva J, editor: *Effective documentation for occupational therapy,* Rockville, Md, 1992, American Occupational Therapy Association.
2. Baum CM, Luebben AJ: *Prospective payment systems,* Thorofare, NJ, 1986, Slack.
3. Gleave GJ: Medical records and reports. In Willard HS, Spackman CS, editors: *Occupational therapy,* ed 4, Philadelphia, 1971, JB Lippincott.
4. Llorens LA: *Occupational therapy sequential client care record manual,* Laurel Md, 1982, Ramsco Publishing.
5. Potts LR: The problem oriented record: implications for occupational therapy, *Am J Occup Ther* 26:6(288), 1972.
6. Robertson S: Why we document. In Acquaviva J, editor: *Effective documentation for occupational therapy,* Rockville, Md, 1992, American Occupational Therapy Association.
7. Steich T: Legal implications in documentation: fraud, abuse and confidentiality. In Acquaviva J, editor: *Effective documentation for occupational therapy,* Rockville, Md, 1992, American Occupational Therapy Association.
8. Tiffany EG: Psychiatry and mental health. In Hopkins HL, Smith HD, editors: *Willard and Spackman's occupational therapy,* ed 6, Philadelphia, 1983, JB Lippincott.
9. Weed LL: *Medical records, medical education and patient care,* Chicago, 1971, Year Book Medical Publishers.
10. Welles C: The implications of liability: guidelines for professional practice, *Am J Occup Ther* 23:1(18), 1969.

Motor Learning and Teaching Activities in Occupational Therapy

Lorraine Williams Pedretti, Darcy Ann Umphred

Teaching and learning are the essential elements of the therapeutic process. Learning is the acquisition of skills or information that changes a person's behavior, attitudes, insights, or perceptions.[4] Learning takes place within the person. The therapist, as teacher, can only provide the environment and design and guide the experiences that facilitate learning.[14] The occupational therapist instructs the patient (learner) in the skills that facilitate independence and personal development. Many of the skills that occupational therapists teach are motor skills. Complex cognitive processes may or may not be involved in these activities. The learning necessary for motor execution is referred to as *procedural,* and the learning necessary for highly contextual, categorical, analytical, and cognitive activities is called *declarative.*[10]

Different areas of the brain are involved in the storage and retrieval of the memory for motor procedures and for declarative tasks. For this reason, environments that enhance optimal learning vary according to the type of learning desired.[2,17] Because occupational therapy is so intricately interwoven with motor learning and motor control, a therapist needs to understand the interactions between the various stages of motor learning and the relationship of tasks to environmental sets, reinforcement scheduling, practice environment, and the limitations of the patient.

MOTOR LEARNING AND OCCUPATIONAL THERAPY

Motor learning is the acquisition of motor skills. It is "a set of processes associated with practice or experience leading to relatively permanent changes in the capability for responding."[17] The desired outcome of motor learning is a permanent change in motor behavior or skill as a result of practice and experience. Motor programs are formatted initially to match the context and goal of the activity but in time to generalize to similar tasks but different environments. The ability to retain what is learned is of utmost importance in motor learning.[7] Once learned, encoding for long-term retention and retrieval depend upon the context of the activity, the amount and type of practice performed, the motivation and attention of the learner, and the feedback both from the therapist and from the learner's inherent feedback mechanisms.[15]

Occupational therapy is concerned with the acquisition of relevant life skills, both procedural and declarative. Measurement tools used to evaluate these skills require motor output and are the result of motor programs learned for achieving maximal independence for living. The focus in occupational therapy is on learning specific functional tasks or skills to reach occupational performance goals. Motor learning, on the other hand, focuses more on *how* motor skills are learned, controlled, and retained, with the primary focus on the learner. Thus motor learning and occupational therapy are both concerned with learning motor skills, but one emphasizes results or outcomes and the other emphasizes the learner and the process.

Two core concepts of occupational therapy theory are the use of purposeful activities as treatment modalities and the active participation of the patient in the treatment process.[7] Gliner[3] proposed that purposeful activity could be the common ground between the fields of motor learning and occupational therapy. He proposed an "ecological" or event approach to motor learning in which the environment (object and task) and the performer must be considered as a unit with the "environment providing meaning and support to the performer's actions."[3] In this approach the skill is related to the immediate object or environment, and the focus is on adaptation to the environment. The learner can engage in different skills using different strategies for adaptation. The learner discovers appropriate muscular organizations for the motor skill to be performed. There are many possibilities for performing the same task. The performer discovers the variables and with many trials and practice refines the muscular organization of the task until it is performed in the most efficient way.[3] Since Gliner originally presented his theoretical constructs, motor learning concepts have evolved beyond theory to clinically relevant treatment that can be the focus of research.

In occupational therapy the patient interacts with the environment, and the occupational therapist structures the patient-environment interaction and learning experiences to optimize effectiveness in the acquisition of occupational performance goals. For example, assume a patient needs to learn to sit on a chair while eating his dinner. Selecting which food to eat first and deciding how small to cut the meat and whether to interact with someone else while eating are cognitive tasks and require declarative memory. The tasks of cutting the meat and maintaining the postural mechanism and balance while sitting are procedural. These tasks need to become automatic without much cognitive energy expenditure. Thus the therapist's intervention needs to incorporate the context of the environment (sitting on a hard surface while eating) as well as distracting the patient's attention from the motor strategies needed to sit so that they become automatic. To facilitate carryover into life experiences, the therapist also needs to incorporate both cultural and psychological dimensions appropriate to the patient. The context within which the patient learns and practices a task can dramatically affect the outcome.

THE ACQUISITION OF MOTOR SKILLS

In the treatment process, patients are engaged in instruction and practice to perform motor behaviors beyond their present skill level. Many factors affect motor learning, including the following: (1) arousal of the central nervous system (CNS), (2) attention to the task, (3) motivation of the patient, (4) type of memory needed (auditory, visual, or kinesthetic), (5) level of movement required (simple to complex), (6) practice schedule, (7) type of practice, (8) type and timing of clinician's reinforcement and (9) the environmental context within which the task must be accomplished. Motor skills used in treatment may have been learned before but because of the disability, must be relearned or learned in a different way.

The therapist acts as a teacher and facilitator by providing instructions, giving physical and verbal guidance, providing feedback about faulty performance, suggesting modifications, and providing reinforcement. The therapist must decide which activities are to be mastered, how to structure the therapy session, the order of presentation of treatment tasks, and how to provide practice for the greatest retention of learning.[17] To optimize learning, all of these decisions whenever possible should be made with the patient's input, consent, and cooperation. By empowering the patient the arousal, attention, and motivational components are incorporated into the motor learning environment.

The type of movement required for the task greatly influences the type of practice or practice context selected. The patient is always a critical variable when determining the complexity of the task. The demands on memory, information processing, task organization, and the number of components interacting with the state of the patient's CNS following injury will be the true determinants of the type of practice selected.[17,20,21]

Simple and discrete tasks usually are learned best by introduction of whole learning in which the patient practices the entire task at once. A transfer from bed to chair is considered a simple task and often can be learned as one procedure rather than a series of components such as the following: (1) lock the chair, (2) move weight forward to edge of chair, (3) shift weight over feet, (4) stand up, (5) pivot, and (6) sit down. Teaching six components or procedural programs as part of the transfer may increase the difficulty level proportionately. Intermediate skills and serial tasks often are learned more easily if taught in a progressive-part context. For example, learning a dance might be considered an intermediate skill. It may require walking or stepping to a beat along with a variety of interlimb and intralimb movements while moving on a diagonal and with a partner. If the dance has a fixed sequence, a progressive-part schedule might consist of practicing the first few movements and then adding more steps, always starting from the beginning. Some skills can be learned in a pure-part context. If the skill is cutting food on a plate, whether the individual cuts the meat or the vegetables first does not matter. All types of cutting are required and thus a pure-part learning can be used. To learn a very complex skill, a whole to part to whole sequence generally leads to optimal retention. Knowing the whole while working on component parts helps with long-term retention.

Stages of Motor Learning

The practice schedule (practice versus rest periods or time between practice) selected for therapy should match the patient's stage of motor learning. During the *skill acquisition stage* the patient is getting the idea of the movement. Errors are frequent and performance inefficient and inconsistent. Thus frequent repetition and frequent feedback are necessary. Generally at this stage a mass practice schedule is used. The mass practice is often done on a daily schedule as in a rehabilitation department. As the patient moves to a *skill refinement stage,* both the patient and the therapist should recognize an improvement in performance, a reduction in the number and degree of errors, and an increase in consistency and efficiency of the movement. Often a distributed practice schedule is advised. For example, practice might be 3 times per week, tapering to 2 times or 1 time. This schedule is similar to a home or outpatient program.

When motor learning progresses to the *skill retention*

stage with the patient able to perform movement and achieve functional goals, a random practice schedule is best, empowering the patient to practice at his or her own pace. The objective is to retain the skill and transfer that skill to different settings. In these varied contexts, the patient needs to modify the timing, force, sequencing, balance, postural integrity, and ongoing excitation of all the neurons in the brain stem and the spinal motor neurons (the motor pool) to succeed at the task. This involves motor problem-solving and is a hallmark of motor learning. The more novel the task, the more intensive the mass practice must be. For some activities mass practice leads to better performance and retention, but for other activities distributed or random practice may lead to better retention. Factors such as memory loss, low levels of cognition, and severe emotional distress can influence motor learning and behavior and need to be considered for practice schedule selection.

MEASURES OF LEARNING

The structure and quality of practice and feedback about performance influence transfer.[17] Transfer enables the patient to call upon previous experience to perform new tasks in new situations.[7] In traditional learning models, when a patient practiced a motor skill (such as putting on shoes) and was evaluated as successful during the practice session, it was assumed that the task was learned. But this method of evaluation does not ensure that skills are retained or that they can be generalized to other situations. For example, if the patient learns to put on trousers, can he also put on undershorts? If he can put on trousers in the hospital room, can he also put them on at home? If the instruction takes place on Monday, will he be able to perform the same skill on Thursday without practice during the intervening days?[7,17] To measure learning and skill retention, performance must be assessed again later, not in a practice session but in as realistic a setting as possible.[9,16]

Experts in the field of motor learning studied the effects of practice and feedback on learning and long-term retention. Although the process of skill acquisition by normal humans is not yet fully understood, studies showed that certain factors facilitate learning and enhance long-term retention and generalization of motor tasks.[17] Of great importance are the type of practice, practice context, stages of motor learning, and type and frequency of feedback. No doubt future research will show therapists how to modify the learning environment to enhance the rate and efficiency of motor learning.[7,8,13]

PRACTICE
Random Practice

If several tasks are planned for the treatment session, it is best to present them in random order. For example, the patient may be asked to pick up cones, cubes, buttons, and spheres in random order. The prehension pattern for each is different, requiring the patient to reformulate the solution to the motor problem each time a different object is approached. Practice involves not only repetition of the same motor patterns but also the formulation of plans to solve motor problems.[16] If motor skill acquisition is measured by performance during a random practice session, learning may not appear to be taking place as rapidly as during repetitive or blocked practice. Repeated solving of motor problems has been shown to aid retention more than repetitive practice of the same motor skills.[17]

Blocked Practice

Blocked practice refers to the repeated performance of the same motor skill. For example suppose a patient is asked to pick up a cup from the left and place it on a saucer on the right side of a table. The patient needs to solve the motor problem only once or twice and then repeat the motor skill over and over again. If measured during the practice session performance appears to improve faster with blocked practice. In blocked practice, however, the patient need not attend to the task, once learned, because it no longer requires novel solutions. There are no alternative activities to cause forgetting and reformulation of the solution to the motor problem, a process that enhances long-term learning and retention.[16,17]

In early learning or with confused patients, blocked practice may be necessary. The patient needs to practice the same movements over and over to establish the motor pattern. For example, it may be helpful at the outset to practice with the same open front shirt repeatedly before introducing a jacket or housecoat that requires similar movement patterns.[16]

Practice Contexts

Practicing in different contexts facilitates generalization of learning. Practice conditions affect transfer and retention. Transfer enables an individual to perform similar tasks in a new context by drawing on past experience. Transfer indicates the motor retention stage of motor learning has been reached.[16] For example, the patient who learns to sponge bathe the upper body in the hospital lavatory and can perform the task in her home bathroom has transferred the learning to a new context. Motor skills required to perform the task are applied in the new context although neither motor skills nor environment are identical.

Practice under variable conditions can increase generalization of learning. Dressing training, for example, can alternate between the patient's room and the occupational therapy clinic's ADL area. Various types of clothing requiring similar motor patterns should be used. Undershorts could be alternated with trousers and shirts with cardigan sweaters in dressing practice, for instance. Training should be done in the environment most appropriate to the task and should be as realistic as possible. For example, eating should take place at a table with the appropriate utensils and real food.[16]

Feedback/Reinforcement

Information about whether a movement has been successful in achieving a goal is critical in motor learning.[16,17] If learners do not get the *intrinsic feedback* necessary to rate their motor performance, learning may be poor or nonexistent. In such instances, feedback must be provided by some *extrinsic* source such as the therapist or teacher or a mechanical device such as a biofeedback machine.[17]

Intrinsic Feedback

Intrinsic feedback is information received by the learner as a result of performing the task.[17] It arises from sensory stimulation to tactile receptors, proprioceptors, and visual and vestibular systems while performing the task and after the task is completed (i.e., the results of the action).[16] This feedback may not be brought to conscious awareness, but should be processed within the cortical as well as the cerebellar structures to determine whether the motor patterns selected for task accomplishment were correct or need refinement. For example, a patient putting on a shirt can feel the movements of joints and muscles and the sensation of the shirt on the skin as the task progresses. He can sense whether arms and hands are in the correct position to grasp the edge of a shirt front or push an arm through a sleeve. He can feel the fabric on the arms and trunk so he knows whether a sleeve is pulled up over the shoulder. When the task is completed, he can look in the mirror and see that the shirt is properly adjusted, the buttons are buttoned and the collar is flat. In reality the patient does not notice all these variables but does recognize whether the task is accomplished. If the task has been completed the patient decides whether the quality of the accomplishment was acceptable. If the CNS determines that corrections are appropriate, the plan will be modified the next time the task is practiced. In patients with sensory, perceptual, or cognitive impairments, the capacity for intrinsic feedback may be mildly to severely limited. If intrinsic feedback is not possible or is distorted by sensory or motor dysfunction, extrinsic feedback is needed for motor learning.[16,17]

Extrinsic Feedback

Feedback about performance from an outside source such as a therapist or a mechanical device is called *extrinsic feedback*. It is used to augment intrinsic feedback.[16,17] Extrinsic feedback can provide information about (1) performance and (2) results.

Performance feedback

Verbal feedback about the process or performance provides the patient with information about the movements in achieving a motor skill.[10,16,17] For example, the therapist might say, "You need to raise your arm a little higher" or "You are not holding on to the edge of the shirt tightly enough." This feedback informs the performer of the movement's effectiveness in achieving the goal of putting on a shirt.

Results feedback

The therapist provides feedback about the outcome, product, or results of the motor actions.[10,16,17] The therapist might say, "The shirt is put on correctly; it looks neat and each button is lined up with its buttonhole." Results feedback can also point out faulty performance and facilitate the revision of movement patterns. The therapist could point out that the buttons are not lined up with correct buttonholes or that the body of the shirt is twisted. The patient then can revise his movement plan to correct the faulty performance.[16]

Therapists should use performance feedback more than results feedback during treatment sessions. Performance feedback is directed toward correcting faulty movement patterns. The frequency and level of extrinsic feedback are determined by the task being performed and the stage of learning.[16,17] Feedback should be given more frequently in early stages of learning so that the patient can correct performance errors.[16] Studies have demonstrated that when enough feedback has been provided for the patient to correct important errors in movement, it should be gradually decreased. This declining schedule of feedback actually enhances long-term retention of activities learned in the rehabilitation program because the patient uses inherent feedback to self-correct.[17]

From his studies on the effect of feedback on learning, Schmidt[17] concluded that summary feedback, which is given after a series of trials with no feedback, aided retention more than feedback given after each trial. Performance during practice declined, however. The reason may be that, for the patient to succeed at the task, intrinsic feedback is needed during the trials to correct errors in movement. It is also possible that frequent feedback delays the development of the patient's intrinsic feedback, and intrinsic feedback is a desirable outcome of rehabilitation.

COMPONENTS OF MOTOR CONTROL

Various components interact within the motor control system, including range of motion (ROM), muscle strength, synergy patterns, state of the motor pool, balance, postural integrity, direction, speed, and context of the environment. Each component affects the performance of the entire system. A problem, deficit, or imbalance in one component causes the other aspects of the system to compensate by modifying their function to allow the patient to succeed at the desired task. If musculoskeletal aspects such as ROM, muscle strength, or joint integrity are compromised, the CNS components may accommodate to perform a task. If lack of joint stabilization causes peripheral instability, the CNS may increase the firing rate of motor neurons to muscles that normally provide that stabilization. In that case, a hypertonic muscle or synergy can develop that limits motor function but corrects the instability. During treatment the therapist must decide whether to allow the patient to self-correct using dysfunctional motor components or whether to use extrinsic feedback and a contrived environment so the patient can succeed at the task. Neither automatically leads to better performance or retention of motor learning. The first choice may allow the patient to succeed at the task in a limited environmental context. The second choice may lead to dependency on the therapist for task success unless the therapist relinquishes control of the motor patterns and the patient uses intrinsic feedback to self-correct. Whether the environment is initially contrived or not, for motor learning to be measured it needs to be functionally independent in the context in which the task is performed.

TEACHING ACTIVITIES IN OCCUPATIONAL THERAPY
CHARACTERISTICS OF AN EFFECTIVE TEACHER

The effective teacher is enthusiastic about the learning content and enjoys teaching. The teacher is positive, realistic, accepting, empathetic, and nonjudgmental toward the learners. Consistency in approach and expectations are additional assets to the teacher who is flexible, adaptable, attentive, and able to motivate learners. The effective teacher gives positive and honest reinforcement to learners and observes and analyzes their behaviors to evaluate the outcome of learning. Such characteristics enhance the possibility of moving the learner toward independence and thus to successful treatment outcomes.[4] The effective teacher remains in the teaching role and does not become friend, mother, brother, or confidant to the learner.[14] Thorough knowledge of the skill to be taught and the ability to present it clearly are essential.[4] Poor preparation or uncertainty about the skill cause the patient to lose confidence in the therapist. For the effective teacher also to be a master clinician, additional personality characteristics may be needed. A master clinician dealing with motor learning problems, acts as a guide to the patient. That guide directs the patient through an interaction that is compassionate, bonding, and accepting of the individual as a unique and worthwhile human being. That master constantly empowers the patient to gain control over his or her cognitive, psychosocial, and motor systems to attain occupational independence and a better quality of life.[21]

INDIVIDUAL AND GROUP TREATMENT

The therapist is responsible for planning individual and group instruction. Treatment plans and group protocols, analogous to lesson plans, include problems, goals, teaching methods, and methods to evaluate treatment outcomes. The occupational therapist assumes responsibility for facilitating the achievement of treatment goals.

In group treatment the therapist must understand group structure, group process and function, act as a group leader, and facilitate group roles.

In physical disabilities practice, most treatment is on an individual basis. Group treatment is appropriate, however, when treatment goals are best reached through group interaction, when the therapist is treating two or more patients with similar problems, for cutting costs, and for practice without extensive extrinsic feedback. A therapeutic group may meet to share and resolve problems, explore interests, perform tasks, or participate in common activities.[4,14]

Treatment groups may be formed for conversation, decision making, discovery, or instruction. In an instructional group, the leader teaches or demonstrates a skill that the members all need to learn.[4] The instructional group may be used for skill acquisition and refinement. In physical disabilities practice, group treatment is focused on task performance rather than group process. If the group activity has multiple goals and varied contexts, the skill retention phase of motor learning might be the focus.

Instructional groups may be described as project or parallel groups.[4,14] In a parallel group, members work in the presence of one another with minimal sharing of tasks. Examples are the reality orientation group and hemiplegia exercise group. Members of a project group, however, are involved in a common short-term or long-term task that requires sharing or interaction, either competitive or cooperative. Little interaction may take place other than that necessary for completion of the task.[14] Examples are a cooking group or a ball-toss game.[18] Group patients may be at various stages of motor learning. Altering the task and changing the context requires intrinsic feedback to modify motor plans. This adaptation should enhance future retention and retrieval of motor plans.

Generally the group should include no fewer than 4 nor more than 20. Members' problems and/or characteristics should be compatible. The treatment environment should be appropriate for the activities to be performed. Space should be adequate and comfort of each group member assured. The style of leadership, group format, group roles, and communications should match group treatment goals and learning needs.[4]

THE TEACHING/LEARNING PROCESS

The teaching/learning process is a systematic problem-solving process. It involves four steps as follows: assessment, plan design, instruction, and feedback/evaluation (Fig. 7-1).[9]

Assessment

The teacher or therapist must assess self, learner characteristics, learning needs, learning skills and style, and the situation.[4,9] During the evaluation phase the therapist assesses the patient's cognitive status, perceptual deficits,

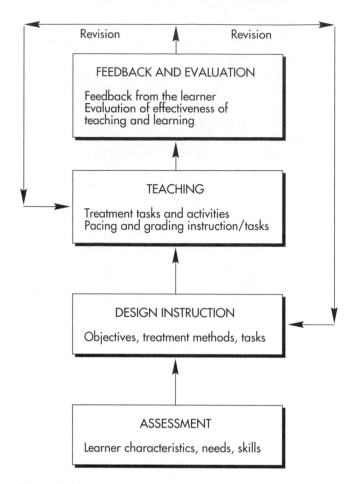

FIG. 7-1 Steps in the teaching-learning process. (Adapted from Kemp, JE: *The instructional design process,* New York, 1985, Harper & Row.)

and physical limitations. Psychosocial readiness is considered as are the patient's attitudes, feelings, and emotional state in relation to the task, the therapist, and the teaching process.[4] This information is essential for estimating the patient's readiness for learning, planning appropriate treatment, and selecting methods of teaching. The interaction of the cognitive, psychosocial and motor systems generates conditions that form a unique individual. A therapist should always evaluate how a change in one system affects the other two. These interactions have become a focus of occupational therapy research.[13]

Readiness for learning implies that the learner possesses the necessary cognitive, perceptual, and physical skills to master the learning task. Because the condition of the brain and nervous system is so important in learning, the therapist must assess CNS functions to select appropriate tasks and teaching methods.[4] Therapists sometimes begin with tasks that are too hard because the patient's cognitive, perceptual, motivational and/or physical capacities have been overestimated.[14]

Teaching Plan Design

The therapist plans treatment or instruction after assessing learner abilities and needs. The therapist writes spe-

cific learning or treatment objectives and plans, instructional tasks and methods to suit the learner. The learning environment is selected and prepared,[4] as determined by the various components of motor learning and the patient's learning stage.[17]

The patient's motivation to perform treatment tasks will have an important effect on participation in the learning process. The learner's perception of the relevance, value, and meaning of the learning task will influence involvement in performance. Motivation may be intrinsic or extrinsic. Intrinsic motivation derives from an internal drive, is self-initiated, and occurs when the learner needs to know something and is ready to learn. External motivation derives from an outside stimulus, such as the therapist encouraging certain actions. Learning through extrinsic motivation takes more effort, concentration, and time than learning that is intrinsically motivated. Much learning is probably driven by a combination of intrinsic and extrinsic motivation.[4]

The patient's age, sex, interests, and cultural group must be considered in selecting relevant treatment activities. If the patient is part of this decision-making process, the selected task will closely match patient goals and enhance motivation. Choosing age-appropriate tasks, considering possible sex-role identification of activities, and assessing the value of activities in the patient's culture help motivate him or her to perform treatment tasks.[14] The importance of cultural consideration cannot be overemphasized and plays a major role in the attainment of functional carry-over into real-life situations.[12] Activities that are relevant to life roles and meaningful in the patient's family or social group ensures greater motivation and participation than activities that seem irrelevant. Relevance is determined by the patient and his or her support systems and not by the therapist. The learner needs to understand why the activity is to be done and how it relates to recovery and resumption of important life activities.[4]

Instruction

The therapist teaches the task or activity in a way that is understandable and meaningful. Repetition may be important, especially for patients with cognitive or perceptual limitations. Patients should be given opportunities for questions and clarification.[4]

It is important for patients to be challenged in task performance and yet to experience some success. Tasks that are too difficult for success are detrimental to motivation. On the other hand, tasks that are too easy do not help the patient move to higher levels of accomplishment. Activities must challenge the patient without being so difficult they cause discouragement. Activities may be graded in the complexity of their physical and cognitive demands as well as in levels of required supervision and assistance.[4]

Tasks should be taught in a relevant environment and activities context. For example, practice in brushing hair is most appropriately done as part of the normal morning hygiene activities in the patient's bathroom rather than in the middle of the afternoon in the occupational therapy clinic.[14]

Pacing and grading instruction

Pacing refers to structuring the instruction and the practice so that the learner can progress at his or her own speed. Once the patient is beyond skill acquisition, practice that extends over time and practice sessions spaced with rests or alternative activities are more effective for retention than long periods of concentrated practice on the same task.[4,17]

Learning should also be graded from simple to complex. In designing the learning experience, the therapist should analyze the activity and break it down into its component steps when appropriate. Simple tasks requiring simple motor plans should be taught as a whole movement activity. For pure-part learning, steps can be taught singly; as each step is mastered, another step is added until the patient masters the whole task.[13,14,17]

One way to grade patient performance is to use backward or forward "chaining" instruction. In backward chaining, the therapist assists through all steps of the activity, then allows the patient to perform the last step independently. Then the patient performs the last two steps, three steps, and so on until he or she can perform the whole activity independently. This method is consistent with whole-part-whole practice. In forward chaining, the patient performs the first step independently and then the therapist helps the patient perform the rest of the steps. The patient then performs the first two steps, then three steps, and so on until he or she can perform the activity independently. Forward chaining is a sequential step approach to motor learning.[6,11,19] Chaining may be helpful for patients with difficulty with sequencing or remembering the steps of the activity.

Active participation and repetition

One of the primary principles of occupational therapy is active patient participation in the treatment process. It is important for the patient to be actively engaged in learning. It is not enough to have an activity described or demonstrated. The patient must perform and learn the activity at a tactile and kinesthetic level to ensure retention.[10,14] Active participation not only enhances learning but enables the patient to control the process, to direct the action.

Repetition of cognitive learning strategies differs from repetition of a motor learning program. Repetitious practice of incorrect actions that do not promote fluid, efficient movement still lead to motor learning, but probably not to success at the functional task. Some researchers believe that incorrect practice makes change more difficult because motor patterns tend to become permanent with repetition.[4]

Feedback/Evaluation

Feedback and reinforcement are closely connected. Confirmation of successful responses encourages the learner to continue learning.[9] The learner also needs feedback so that mistakes will be recognized and performance modified. The kind of feedback depends upon whether the task requires declarative or procedural learning. Declarative learning depends on the neural connections of the limbic and cortical structures. Procedural learning's neural network is more intricately involved with cortical and noncortical motor centers.[10]

Reinforcement may be intrinsically derived from the personal satisfaction of successful performance or may be provided extrinsically by the therapist. Verbal reinforcement in a cognitive task may be direct and very meaningful; yet in a motor task, that external reinforcer may override the intrinsic mechanism and not allow self-correction. Cognitive behavior that is reinforced tends to be repeated. Extrinsic feedback should be realistic, honest, and appropriate to the task. That is, the therapist need not exclaim loudly in superlatives when a shoe has been tied. Rather, a positive statement about how the shoe was tied and will keep the shoe on the foot is more appropriate. Similarly, if the motor performance is not going to reach the goal, offer to repeat the instruction, possibly in a different sensory mode.[14]

Constructive criticism must be thoughtful and tactful, yet honest. It should be nonthreatening to avoid evoking defensiveness. False praise can be just as confusing and insulting as criticism. Constructive suggestions for alternative action should be included with criticism.[4] Considerable reinforcement may be needed in the early stages of learning whether the task is cognitive or motor-based. As tasks are mastered, less reinforcement is necessary.[14,17]

In evaluating the effectiveness of the teaching/learning process the therapist must ask: How did it go? Were treatment objectives achieved? What was the extent or quality of achievement of objectives? Here is an opportunity for the therapist to get feedback from the learner(s). Feedback can be verbal and reflect the learners' affective reactions to a group activity, for example, or it can be behavioral, reflecting performance that was not possible before instruction.[4]

Progress can be evaluated by repeating initial evaluation tests. The results can provide objective evidence of the effectiveness of treatment. A muscle test may show a change in grade of strength, and a self-care reevaluation can reflect a change in the level of independent dressing. For billing and legal documents, the therapist needs to make sure that all measurements are objective and quantifiable. Descriptive or subjective record-keeping often helps the therapist remember behaviors that cannot be measured objectively, but do reflect change in the cognitive, psychosocial, or motor systems. Although that information is important in therapeutic record-keeping, it is not part of professional justification for payment of services. Third party payers are generally concerned with statistics and have little interest in the nuances of CNS change and therapeutic procedures.[20]

INSTRUCTION: THE TEACHING PROCESS

Instruction can be subdivided into four steps (Fig. 7-2). The process must be modified, of course, if the patient is unable to interact with the external world. The following teaching process can serve as a guide for patients who comprehend and interact with the environment.

Preparation: The Preinstruction Phase

After the patient has been evaluated, the therapist selects treatment objectives with the patient. What is the patient to learn to do? How competent should the learner become? How long will it take to achieve each objective? The therapist may also analyze potential treatment activities at this stage, considering the physical and cognitive demands and component steps. Teaching methods (to be discussed in more detail later) are then selected.

The preinstruction process includes preparing the therapy space. Furniture should be arranged, areas cleared, and equipment and materials gathered. Treatment time should not be wasted while the therapist prepares for treatment. When the patient is present, he or she should be positioned comfortably and correctly for the activity.[5]

Demonstration: The Instruction Phase

Once the preparations are complete, instruction begins. The therapist should put the patient at ease and arouse the patient's interest in the activity. Explanation of the purposes and benefits of the activity can help to motivate participation. The therapist then demonstrates the activity. In general, the therapist should explain and demonstrate the activity, one step at a time. Key points are stressed and instruction is given clearly, completely and patiently. Repetition and review are often necessary. The therapist should not present any more than the patient can successfully master at one time. Words should be few and simple. Some patients require tactile and kinesthetic cues or gentle manual guidance along with verbal and demonstrated instruction.[5]

Return Demonstration: Performance Stage

Once the therapist has taught the activity, the patient should perform the skill, demonstrating whether or not the instruction has been grasped. To ask, "Do you understand?" following the demonstration is not enough. The therapist should observe the performance and correct errors as they occur. To reinforce understanding, ask the patient to explain key points as the activity is performed. The therapist should observe until it is clear that the patient is performing the activity correctly.[5]

Follow-up: Supervision

When the patient is performing the activity correctly, the therapist may be able to attend to other patients or duties. Some continuous supervision is necessary, however. The therapist may periodically observe the patient's performance from a distance or may occasionally offer assistance and recheck performance. The therapist gives the patient opportunities to ask questions, corrects faulty performance, and provides realistic, positive, and appropriate feedback. The degree of independent performance may be graded by tapering off coaching and close supervision as the patient masters the skills.[5]

METHODS OF TEACHING

Methods of instruction depend on the patient's cognitive level, perceptual functions, physical status, and motivation. Teaching methods require different levels of perceptual and cognitive function and access one or more sensory systems in transmitting data to the cerebral cortex for information processing and execution of the motor plan. In therapy, methods may be combined. It is important for the method to suit the patient's learning style and level of comprehension.

TEACHING THROUGH THE AUDITORY SYSTEM: VERBAL INSTRUCTION

When using verbal instruction, the therapist speaks an instruction and expects the patient to carry it out. For example, the therapist says, "Brush your hair." Such a command assumes that the patient understands the words spoken, has previous experience with the activity, can retain the memory of the command, can retrieve it from memory, has retained the motor patterns associated with the hairbrush and the act of brushing hair, can plan and execute the motor task associated with the command, and is motivated to brush the hair. Patients with deficits in receptive language, auditory perception, auditory or visual memory, and motor planning (praxis), to name a few, will have considerable difficulty following

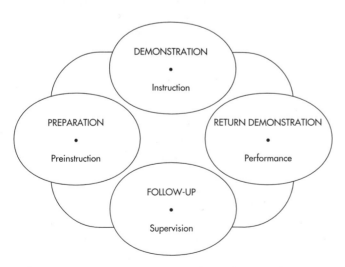

FIG. 7-2   Steps in the instruction phase of the teaching-learning process.

verbal instructions only. Generally, this method is the least effective.

TEACHING THROUGH THE VISUAL AND AUDITORY SYSTEMS: VERBAL INSTRUCTION AND DEMONSTRATION

Demonstrating an activity while giving verbal instruction can enhance learning considerably. Two sensory systems are engaged, the auditory and the visual. The therapist not only describes the steps of the activity but demonstrates them as well. The therapist may brush his or her own hair and ask the patient to imitate what was shown or may ask the patient to perform in parallel, one step at a time. With this method of instruction receptive language skills and auditory memory are not as critical but the ability to imitate motor acts must be intact. Patients with motor planning deficits (apraxia) will not be able to plan movements to imitate the therapist's demonstration. Poor visual or auditory memory may also hamper the learning process when using this method.

TEACHING THROUGH THE SOMATOSENSORY/VESTIBULAR SYSTEMS: TOUCH, PROPRIOCEPTION, AND MOTION

For patients who have deficits in the ability to follow auditory and demonstrated instructions, it may be necessary to augment instruction with input to the somatosensory system. If using tactile, proprioceptive, or movement stimuli to cue the patient, the therapist may choose to use no words or just short simple commands. Some demonstration may also be appropriate. The therapist may say, "Brush your hair" and then may touch the patient's hand and move the hand to the hairbrush. This action alone may be enough to cue the patient to perform the task. If not, the therapist may lift the patient's hand, holding the hairbrush and simulating the movement pattern of hair brushing on the patient's head. In many instances, the feeling of the correct movements and the tactile cue to pick up the brush facilitate the auditory and visual input of the demonstration and enhance learning.

Guiding is a special form of tactile, proprioceptive, and vestibular input. It is based on the work of Felicie Affolter and is described by Bonfils[1] in detail in Chapter 25. The patient is guided through the activity with the close physical contact of the therapist throughout the movement process. Little or no verbal instruction is given. It is performed in contact with a reference of solid support such as a table or counter surface, rather than moving through the air. The purpose of guiding is to give the patient familiar sensory input.

During the guiding process, the patient may take over some of the movement as the brain recognizes it from past experience.[1] As learning takes place, the therapist may decrease the amount of guiding and use less intense sensory input. When guiding, the therapist stands behind the patient and places his or her arms along the surfaces of the patient's arms. The therapist places her hand over the patient's hand and guides it along the surface of the table or vanity to reach the brush. The brush is grasped by the patient's hand, with the therapist's hand over top. The hand is guided back along the vanity surface and to the patient's body. The body may be used as a solid surface of support as the arm is guided toward the head. The therapist then guides the patient's arm through the brushing movements with the head now as the solid support.

The sensorimotor approaches described in Part III, Unit Two of this text all use somatosensory input in their methods of teaching motor skills. The use of tactile and proprioceptive cues is very helpful for patients who are apraxic and cannot imitate movements or have "forgotten" motor patterns associated with common implements such as a hairbrush. The effectiveness of this approach may be limited with patients who have severe tactile and proprioceptive sensory losses or who resist being touched.

SUMMARY

The fields of motor learning and occupational therapy are both concerned with the acquisition and retention of motor skills. It is important to focus on both how the skills are acquired and the end results of performance. Occupational therapy is a teaching process with goals that often incorporate teaching motor skills for independent living. Although the therapist is the instructor and the patient is the learner, the therapist needs to be open to learning from the patient. Learning and retention are influenced by the structure and quality of practice and feedback for both the patient and the clinician. When learning a motor strategy, random practice and summary feedback have been shown to have a positive effect on long-term retention. Blocked practice is useful in the early stages of learning to establish motor patterns and increase performance. Skill acquisition is best measured at some time after practice sessions to evaluate retention because testing skill acquisition during practice sessions does not measure long-term retention.

Instruction and practice should be appropriately paced for the learner and graded in complexity. Backward and forward chaining in instruction are two ways of grading independent performance. Practice is best done in the context most appropriate to the activity. Practice under variable conditions will facilitate ability to generalize learning.

Feedback is necessary to correct faulty motor performance. Feedback may be intrinsic or extrinsic. Intrinsic feedback is sensory information from task performance and outcome. Extrinsic feedback is received from an outside source such as the therapist or a mechanical device. Extrinsic feedback should be realistic, honest, and appropriate. It should enable the patient to revise erroneous motor acts. The frequency of extrinsic feedback should be decreased as performance is mastered. Summary feedback, given after several trials at a task, is more helpful for long-term retention than immediate and frequent feedback. Feedback about how the task is performed helps the patient develop the capacity for intrinsic feedback.

In occupational therapy for physical dysfunction, most treatment is done in individual sessions. Group treatment may be used, however. Groups are usually project or parallel types with the primary focus on task performance rather than group process and depend on the patient's level of cognitive and psychosocial function. The occupational therapist is responsible for planning and executing individual and group treatment. The treatment plan is analogous to an instructional lesson plan and should be developed following the steps in the teaching/learning process: (1) assessment, (2) plan design (3) instruction, and (4) evaluation. The instruction phase can be further broken down into (1) preinstruction/preparation, (2) demonstration/instruction, (3) return demonstration/performance, and (4) follow-up/supervision.

Methods of instruction depend on the patient's physical and cognitive status and motivation. Instruction may use the auditory, visual, and somatosensory systems. Multisystem input often facilitates learning. Teaching methods can be graded to accommodate the learner's cognitive and perceptual abilities.

To achieve the goals of acquiring essential motor skills, the learner must be ready for learning, that is, be prepared and have enough physical and cognitive resources to perform the task. The patient must also be motivated. Task relevance is essential to motivation. The clinician's role includes evaluating the patient, setting goals, and selecting appropriate activities with the patient, providing instruction and feedback, and evaluating treatment outcomes.

REVIEW QUESTIONS

1. What is the result of learning?
2. Define motor learning.
3. What is the difference between procedural and declarative skills?
4. What is the difference in the emphasis on learning motor skills between occupational therapy and motor learning theory?
5. What is meant by the 'ecological' approach to motor learning?
6. What is the difference between whole learning and progressive-part learning? Give an example when each might be used.
7. List and define the stages of motor learning.
8. How is learning measured?
9. What is meant by transfer of learning? How is it measured?
10. Describe two types of practice. What are the advantages and disadvantages of each?
11. What is meant by practice context?
12. Why is feedback/reinforcement important to learning?
13. Describe two types of feedback.
14. List the components of motor control.
15. List at least 8 characteristics of an effective teacher.
16. What are some reasons to use group treatment?
17. List and define the overall steps in the teaching/learning process.
18. What are some of the important factors a therapist must consider about the patient when designing the instructional (treatment) plan?
19. What is meant by pacing or grading instruction?
20. List the steps in the instruction phase of the teaching process.
21. List three main methods of teaching, accessing the sensory systems used as the mode of instruction. Give examples of how you would teach a patient to use a spoon to eat mashed potatoes using each method.

REFERENCES

1. Bonfils K: The Affolter approach. In Pedretti LW: *Occupational therapy practice skills for physical dysfunction*, ed 4, St Louis, 1995, Mosby-Yearbook.
2. Cai Z: The neural mechanism of declarative memory consolidation and retrieval: a hypothesis, *Neuroscience & Biobehavioral Reviews* 14(3):295-304, 1990.
3. Gliner JA: Purposeful activity in motor learning theory: an event approach to motor skill acquisition, *Am J Occup Ther* 39(1):28, 1985.
4. Hames CC, & Joseph DH: *Basic concepts of helping*, ed 2, Norwalk, Conn, 1986, Appleton-Century-Crofts.
5. Hopkins HL, Tiffany EG: Occupational therapy—base in activity. In Hopkins HL, Smith HD editors: *Willard and Spackman's occupational therapy*, ed 7, Philadelphia, 1988, JB Lippincott.
6. Humphrey R, Jewell K: Developmental disabilities. I. Mental retardation. In Hopkins HL, Smith HD, editors: *Willard and Spackman's occupational therapy*, ed 8, Philadelphia, 1993, JB Lippincott.
7. Jarus T: Motor learning and occupational therapy: the organization of practice, *Am J Occup Ther* 48(9):810, 1994.
8. Kaplan M: Motor learning: implications for occupational therapy and neurodevelopmental treatment. *Developmental disabilities: special interest section newsletter* 17(3):1-4, 1994.
9. Kemp JE: *The instructional design process*, New York, 1985, Harper and Row.
10. Kupfermann I: Learning and memory. In Kandel ER, Schwartz JH, Jessell TM: *Principles of neural science*, ed 3, New York, 1991, Elsevier.
11. Levy LL: Section A, Behavioral frame of reference. In Hopkins HL, Smith HD: *Willard and Spackman's occupational therapy*, ed 8, Philadelphia, 1993, JB Lippincott.

12. Llorens L, Umphred D, Burton G, Glogoski-Williams D: Ethnogeriatrics: implications for occupational therapy and physical therapy. *Physical and Occupational Therapy in Geriatrics* 11 (3), 1993.

13. Mathiowetz V, Haugen JB: Motor behavior research: implications for therapeutic approaches to central nervous system dysfunction. *Am J Occup Ther* 48(8):734-745, 1994.

14. Mosey AC: *Activities therapy,* New York, 1973, Raven Press.

15. Newton R: Contemporary issues and theories of motor control: assessement of movement and balance. In Umphred DA: *Neurological rehabilitation,* St Louis, 1995, Mosby-Yearbook.

16. Poole J: Application of motor learning principles in occupational therapy, *Am J Occup Ther* 45(6):530, 1991.

17. Schmidt RA: Motor learning principles for physical therapy. In *Contemporary management of motor control problems, proceedings of the II step conference,* Alexandria, Va, 1991, Foundation for Physical Therapy.

18. Schwartzberg S: Tools of practice, Section 2, Group process. In Hopkins HL, Smith HD, editors: *Willard and Spackman's occupational therapy,* ed 8, Philadelphia, 1993, JB Lippincott.

19. Umphred DA: Classification of treatment techniques based on primary input systems: inherent and contrived feedback/loop systems included. In Umphred DA, editor: *Neurological rehabilitation,* ed 3, St Louis, 1995, Mosby-Yearbook.

20. Umphred DA: Introduction and overview: multiple interactive conceptual models: frameworks for clinical problem solving. In Umphred DA, editor: *Neurological rehabilitation,* ed 3, St Louis, 1995, Mosby-Yearbook.

21. Umphred DA: Limbic complex: influence over motor control and learning. In Umphred DA, editor: *Neurological rehabilitation,* ed 3, St Louis, 1995, Mosby-Yearbook.

PART TWO

Evaluation and Treatment: The Performance Components

CHAPTER 8

Evaluation of Joint Range of Motion

Lorraine Williams Pedretti

Joint measurement is a primary evaluation procedure for physical dysfunctions that could limit joint motion. These dysfunctions include skin contracture caused by adhesions or scar tissue; arthritis, fractures, burns, and hand trauma; displacement of fibrocartilage or presence of other foreign bodies in the joint; bony obstruction or destruction; and soft tissue contractures, such as tendon, muscle, or ligament shortening. Limited range of motion (ROM) also can be secondary to spasticity, muscle weakness, pain, and edema.[8,11]

Range of motion is the arc of motion through which a joint passes. Passive ROM is the arc of motion through which the joint passes when moved by an outside force, such as the therapist. Active ROM is the arc of motion through which the joint passes when moved by the muscles acting on the joint. In normal individuals passive ROM is very slightly greater than active ROM.[9] If passive ROM is significantly more than active ROM at the same joint, it is likely that there is muscle weakness.[11]

ROM measurements help the therapist determine appropriate treatment goals and select appropriate treatment modalities, positioning techniques, and other strategies to reduce limitations. Specific purposes for measuring ROM are to (1) determine limitations that interfere with function or may produce deformity, (2) determine additional range needed to increase functional capacity or reduce deformity, (3) determine the need for splints and assistive devices, (4) measure progress objectively, and (5) record progression or regression.

Formal joint measurement is not necessary for every patient. If joint limitation is not a primary symptom, or the disability is of recent onset, with proper positioning and daily ROM exercises, limited ROM would not be anticipated. In such cases, however, ROM should be observed by using active ROM or by putting all joints through passive ROM. Normal ROM varies from one person to another. Establish norms for each individual by measuring the uninvolved part if possible.[4] Otherwise the therapist uses average ranges listed in the literature. The therapist should check records and interview the patient for the presence of fused joints and other limitations caused by old injuries. Joints should not be forced when resistance is met on passive ROM. Pain may limit ROM and crepitation may be heard on movement in some conditions.

PRINCIPLES AND PROCEDURES IN JOINT MEASUREMENT

Before measuring joint range of motion, the therapist should be familiar with average normal ROMs, joint structure and function, normal end-feels, recommended positioning for self and patient, and bony landmarks related to each joint and joint axes.[4,9] The therapist should be skilled in correct positioning and stabilization for measurements, palpation, alignment and reading of the goniometer, and recording measurements accurately.[9]

VISUAL OBSERVATION

The therapist should observe the joint and adjacent areas.[3] The therapist asks the patient to move the part through the available ROM, if muscle strength is adequate, and observes the movement.[4] The therapist should look for compensatory motions, posture, muscle contours, skin color and condition, skin creases and compare the joint with the noninjured part, if possible.[3] The therapist should then move the part through its range to see and feel how the joint moves and to estimate ROM.

PALPATION

Feeling the bony landmarks and soft tissue around the joint is an essential skill, gained with practice and experience. The pads of the index and middle fingers are used for palpation. The thumb is sometimes used. The therapist's fingernails should not make contact with the patient's skin. The pressure is applied gently but firmly enough to detect underlying muscle, tendon, or bony structures. For joint measurement, the therapist must palpate to locate bony landmarks for placement of the goniometer.[3]

POSITIONING OF THERAPIST AND SUPPORT OF LIMBS

The therapist's position varies, depending on the joints being measured. When fingers or wrist joints are being measured, the therapist may sit next to or opposite the patient. When the larger joints of the upper or lower extremity are being measured, the therapist may stand next to the patient on the side being measured. The patient may be seated or lying down. The therapist needs to employ good body mechanics in posture and in lifting and moving heavy limbs. The therapist should use a broad base of support and stand with the head upright, keeping the back straight. The feet should be shoulder-width apart with the knees slightly flexed. The therapist's stance is in line with the direction of movement. The limb is supported at the level of its center of gravity, approximately where the upper and middle third of the segment meet. The therapist's hands should be in a relaxed grasp that conforms to the contours of the part. Additional support can be given by resting the part on the forearm.[3]

PRECAUTIONS AND CONTRAINDICATIONS

In some instances, measuring joint ROM is contraindicated or should be undertaken with extreme caution. It is contraindicated if there is a joint dislocation or unhealed fracture, immediately following surgery of any soft tissue structures surrounding joints, and in the presence of myositis ossificans.[3]

Joint measurement must always be done carefully. Extreme caution is needed if (1) there is joint inflammation; (2) the patient is taking medication for pain or muscle relaxants; (3) there is osteoporosis, hypermobility, or subluxation of a joint; (4) the patient has hemophilia; (5) there is hematoma; and (6) bony ankylosis is suspected.[3]

END-FEEL

Passive ROM is normally limited by the structure of the joint and surrounding soft tissues. Thus ligaments, the joint capsule, muscle and tendon tension, contact of joint surfaces, and soft tissue approximation may limit the end of a particular range of motion. Each of these structures has a different end-feel as the therapist moves the joint passively through the ROM. End-feel is the resistance to further motion. Practice and sensitivity are required for the therapist to detect different end-feels and to distinguish the normal from the abnormal.[3,9] End-feel is normal when full ROM is achieved and the motion is limited by normal anatomical structures. Abnormal end-feel occurs when the ROM is increased or decreased or when ROM is normal but structures other than normal anatomy stop the ROM.[3]

Normally end-feel is hard, soft, or firm. An example of hard end-feel is bone contacting bone when the elbow is passively extended and the olecranon process contacts the olecranon fossa. Soft end-feel can be detected on knee flexion when there is soft tissue apposition of the posterior aspects of the thigh and calf. A firm end-feel has a firm or springy sensation that has some give as when the ankle is dorsiflexed with the knee in extension and the ROM is limited by tension in the gastrocnemius muscle.[3]

In pathological states, soft end-feel occurs sooner or later in the ROM than is normal or in a joint that normally has a hard or firm end-feel. The end-feel may be "boggy," which could indicate soft tissue edema or synovitis. Firm end-feel occurs sooner or later than is normal or in joints that normally have a soft or hard end-feel. It could indicate muscular, capsular, or ligamentous shortening. Hard end-feel occurs sooner or later in the ROM than is usual and in joints that normally have a soft or firm end-feel. It may be felt in joints with loose bodies, degenerative joint disease, fractures, or dislocations. A bony grating or bony block may be detected. There may be an "empty" end-feel in instances where the end of ROM is not reached because of pain; thus no resistance is felt because the patient may be using protective muscle splinting or there is muscle spasm.[3,9] Normal end-feels for each joint are noted with the directions for joint measurement below.

TWO-JOINT MUSCLES

When measuring the ROM of a joint that is crossed by a two-joint muscle, the ROM of the joint being measured may be affected by the position of the other joint because of passive insufficiency.[3] That is, joint motion is limited by the length of the muscle. A two-joint muscle feels taut when it is at its full length over both joints before it reaches the limits of the normal ROM of both joints.[7] For example, passive finger extension is normally limited when the wrist is in full extension because of the passive insufficiency of the finger flexors that cross the wrist and finger joints. When measuring joints crossed by two-joint muscles, it is necessary to place the joint not being measured in a neutral or relaxed position to place the two-joint muscle on slack. For example, when measuring finger extension, the wrist should be placed in the neutral position to avoid full stretch of the finger flexors over all of the joints they cross. Similarly, when measuring hip flexion, the knee should also be flexed to place the hamstrings in the slackened position.[3]

METHODS OF JOINT MEASUREMENT
THE 180° SYSTEM

In the 180° system of joint measurement, 0° is the starting position for all joint motions. For most motions the anatomical position is the starting position. The body of the measuring instrument, the goniometer, is a semicircle that is superimposed on the body in the plane in which the motion is to occur. The axis of the joint is the axis of the arc of motion. All joint motions begin at 0° and increase toward 180°.[5,9] The 180° system is used later in this chapter to describe procedures for joint measurement.

THE 360° SYSTEM

In the 360° system of joint measurement, movements occurring in the coronal and sagittal planes are related to a full circle. When the body is in the anatomical position, the circle is superimposed on it in the same plane in which the motion is to occur with the joint axis as the pivotal point. "The 0° (360°) position will be overhead and the 180° position will be toward the feet."[5] Thus, for example, shoulder flexion and abduction are movements that proceed toward 0°, and shoulder adduction and extension proceed toward 360°.[5] The average normal ROM for shoulder flexion is 170°. Therefore using the 360° system, the movement would start at 180° and progress toward 0° to 10°. The ROM recorded would be 10°. On the other hand, shoulder extension that has a normal ROM of 60° would begin at 180° and progress toward 360° to 240°, and 240° would be the ROM recorded.[5] The total ROM of extension to flexion would be 240° − 10°, that is, 230°.[5,6]

Some motions cannot be related to the full circle. In these instances a 0° starting position is designated, and the movements are measured as increases from 0°. These motions occur in a horizontal plane around a vertical axis. They are (1) forearm pronation and supination, (2) hip internal and external rotation, (3) wrist radial and ulnar deviation, and (4) thumb palmar and radial abduction (carpometacarpal flexion and extension).[5]

GONIOMETERS

The instrument used for measuring ROM is the goniometer. Goniometers are made of metal or plastic, come in several sizes, and are available from medical and rehabilitation equipment companies.[5,9] The word *goniometer* is derived from the Greek *gonia*, which means angle, and *metron*, which means measure.[9,12] Thus goniometer literally means to measure angles.

The goniometer consists of a stationary (proximal) bar and a movable (distal) bar.[9] The body of the stationary bar is a small protractor (half circle) or a full circle printed with a scale of degrees from 0° to 180° for the half-circle and 0° to 360° for the full-circle goniometer.[4] The movable bar is attached at the center or axis of the protractor and acts as a dial. As the movable bar rotates around the protractor, the dial points to the number of degrees on the scale.

Two scales of figures are printed on the half circle. Each starts at 0° and progresses toward 180° but in opposite directions. Because the starting position in the 180° system is always 0° and increases toward 180°, the outer row of figures is read if the bony segments being measured are end to end, as in elbow flexion. The inner row of figures is read if the bony segments being measured are alongside one another, as in shoulder flexion.

Fig. 8-1 shows five styles of goniometers. The first (Fig. 8-1, *A*) is a full-circle goniometer that has calibrations for both the 360° and the 180° systems printed on its face. This goniometer has longer arms and is convenient for use on the large joints of the body. Fig. 8-1, *B*, shows a half-circle instrument used for the 180° system. This goniometer is radiopaque and could be used during x-ray examinations if necessary. Its dial is notched at two places for accurate motion reading regardless of whether the convexity of the half circle is directed toward or away from the direction of motion. Thus the examiner does not have to reverse the goniometer, obscuring the scale. A special finger goniometer is shown in Fig. 8-1, *D*. Its arms are short and flattened. It is designed to be used over the finger joint surfaces rather than on their lateral

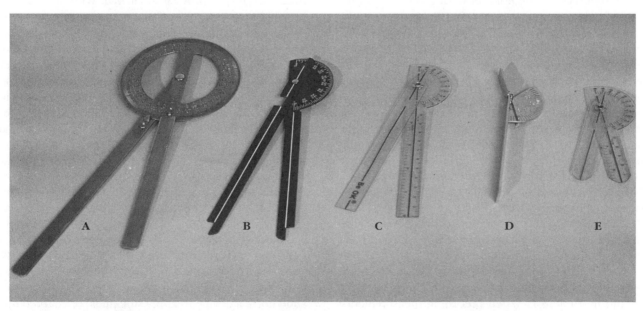

FIG. 8-1 Types of goniometers.

aspects, as is done in most of the larger joint motions. Small plastic goniometers are shown in Fig. 8-1, *C* and *E*. These are inexpensive and easy to carry. The longer one can be used with both large and small joints. The smaller is simply a larger one that has been cut for use as a finger goniometer. The dials of transparent goniometers are marked or notched in two places.

One important feature of the goniometer is the fulcrum. The nut or rivet that acts as the fulcrum must move freely, yet it must be tight enough to remain where it was set when the goniometer is removed following joint measurement.[4] Some goniometers have a locking nut that is tightened just before removing the goniometer for easy, accurate readings.[5]

There are other types of goniometers. Some use fluids with a free-floating bubble that provides the reading after the motion is completed.[5] Others can be attached to a body segment and have dials that register range of motion.[3] A tape measure or metric scale may also be used to measure ROM of some joints by measurement of the distance between two segments. For example, the distance between the center of the tips of two fingers may be measured for finger abduction, and opposition may be evaluated by measuring the distance between the thumb tip and little finger tip.[3]

RECORDING MEASUREMENTS

When using the 180° system, the evaluator should record the number of degrees at the starting position and the number of degrees at the final position after the joint has passed through the maximum possible arc of motion.[9] Normal ROM always starts at 0° and increases toward 180°. When it is not possible to start the motion at 0 degrees because of a limitation of motion, the ROM is recorded by writing the number of degrees at the starting position followed by the number of degreees at the final position.[3] For example, elbow ROM limitations can be noted as follows:

Normal: 0° to 140°

Extension limitation: 15° to 140°

Flexion limitation: 0° to 110°

Flexion and extension limitation: 15° to 110°

Abnormal hyperextension of the elbow may be recorded by indicating the number of degrees of hyperextension below the 0° starting position with a minus sign followed by the 0° position and then the number of degrees at the final position.[9] For example:

Normal: 0° to 140°

Abnormal hyperextension: −20° to 0° to 140°

There are alternate methods of recording ROM. The evaluator is advised to learn and adopt the particular method required by the health care facility.

A sample form for recording ROM measurements is shown in Fig. 8-2. Average normal ROMs are listed on the form and in Table 8-1. When recording measurements,

every space on the form should be filled in. If the joint was not tested, "NT" should be entered in the space.[3]

It should be noted that movements of the shoulder (glenohumeral) joint are accompanied by scapula movement as outlined. Glenohumeral joint motion is highly dependent on scapula mobility, which gives the shoulder its flexibility and wide ranges of motion. Although it is not possible to measure scapula movement with the goniometer, the evaluator should assess scapula mobility by observation of active motion or by passive movement before proceeding with shoulder joint measurements. Scapular ROM is noted as full or restricted.[3] If scapula motion is restricted, as when musculature is in a state of spasticity or contracture, and the shoulder joint is moved into extreme ranges of motion (for example, above 90° of flexion or abduction), glenohumeral joint damage can result.

When joint measurements may be performed in more than one position (for example, as in shoulder internal and external rotation), the evaluator should note on the record in which position the measurement was taken. The examiner should also note any pain or discomfort experienced by the subject, the appearance of protective muscle spasm, whether active or passive ROM was measured, and any deviations from recommended testing procedures or positions.[9]

RESULTS OF EVALUATION AS BASIS FOR TREATMENT PLANNING

Following joint measurement, the therapist should analyze the results in relationship to the patient's life role requirements. The therapist's first concern should be to correct ROMs that are below functional limits. Many ordinary activities of daily living (ADL) do not require full ROM. Functional ROM refers to the amount of joint range necessary to perform essential ADL without the use of special equipment.[8] The first concern of treatment is to try to increase ROMs that are limiting performance of self- and home-maintenance tasks to functional ROM.[8] For example, a severe limitation of elbow flexion affects eating and oral hygiene. Therefore it is important to increase elbow flexion to nearly full ROM for function. Likewise, a severe limitation of forearm pronation affects eating, washing the body, telephoning, child care, and dressing. Because sitting comfortably requires hip ROM of at least 0° to 90°, if hip flexion is limited, a first goal might be to increase it to 90°. Of course, if additional ROM can be gained, the therapist should plan the progression of treatment to increase the ROM to the normal range.

Some ROM limitations may be permanent. In such cases the role of the therapist is to work out methods to compensate for the loss of ROM. Possibilities include assistive devices, such as a long-handled comb, brush, or shoe horn, a device to apply stockings, or adapted meth-

JOINT RANGE MEASUREMENTS

Patient's name _____ Chart no. _____

Date of birth _____ Age _____ Sex _____

Diagnosis _____ Date of onset _____

Disability _____

LEFT				RIGHT		
3	2	1	**SPINE**	1	2	3
			Cervical spine			
			Flexion 0-45			
			Extension 0-45			
			Lateral flexion 0-45			
			Rotation 0-60			
			Thoracic and lumbar spine			
			Flexion 0-80			
			Extension 0-30			
			Lateral flexion 0-40			
			Rotation 0-45			
			SHOULDER			
			Flexion 0 to 170			
			Extension 0 to 60			
			Abduction 0 to 170			
			Horizontal abduction 0-40			
			Horizontal adduction 0-130			
			Internal rotation 0 to 70			
			External rotation 0 to 90			
			ELBOW AND FOREARM			
			Flexion 0 to 135-150			
			Supination 0 to 80-90			
			Pronation 0 to 80-90			
			WRIST			
			Flexion 0 to 80			
			Extension 0 to 70			
			Ulnar deviation 0 to 30			
			Radial deviation 0 to 20			
			THUMB			
			MP flexion 0 to 50			
			IP flexion 0 to 80-90			
			Abduction 0 to 50			
			FINGERS			
			MP flexion 0 to 90			
			MP hyperextension 0 to 15-45			
			PIP flexion 0 to 110			
			DIP flexion 0 to 80			
			Abduction 0 to 25			
			HIP			
			Flexion 0 to 120			
			Extension 0 to 30			
			Abduction 0 to 40			
			Adduction 0 to 35			
			Internal rotation 0 to 45			
			External rotation 0 to 45			
			KNEE			
			Flexion 0 to 135			
			ANKLE AND FOOT			
			Plantar flexion 0 to 50			
			Dorsiflexion 0 to 15			
			Inversion 0 to 35			
			Eversion 0 to 20			

FIG. 8-2 Form for recording joint ROM measurement.

TABLE 8-1   Average Normal ROM (180° Method)

JOINT	ROM	ASSOCIATED GIRDLE MOTION	JOINT	ROM
CERVICAL SPINE			**WRIST**	
Flexion	0° to 45°		Flexion	0° to 80°
Extension	0° to 45°		Extension	0° to 70°
Lateral flexion	0° to 45°		Ulnar deviation (adduction)	0° to 30°
Rotation	0° to 60°		Radial deviation (abduction)	0° to 20°
THORACIC AND LUMBAR SPINE			**THUMB***	
Flexion	0° to 80°		DIP flexion	0° to 80°-90°
Extension	0° to 30°		MP flexion	0° to 50°
Lateral flexion	0° to 40°		Adduction, radial and palmar	0°
Rotation	0° to 45°		Palmar abduction	0° to 50°
			Radial abduction	0° to 50°
SHOULDER			Opposition	
Flexion	0° to 170°	Abduction, lateral tilt, slight elevation, slight upward rotation	**FINGERS***	
Extension	0° to 60°	Depression, adduction, upward tilt	MP flexion	0° to 90°
			MP hyperextension	0° to 15°-45°
Abduction	0° to 170°	Upward rotation, elevation	PIP flexion	0° to 110°
Adduction	0°	Depression, adduction, downward rotation	DIP flexion	0° to 80°
			Abduction	0° to 25°
Horizontal abduction	0° to 40°	Adduction, reduction of lateral tilt	**HIP**	
Horizontal adduction	0° to 130°	Abduction, lateral tilt		
Internal rotation		Abduction, lateral tilt	Flexion	0° to 120° (bent knee)
Arm in abduction	0° to 70°			
Arm in adduction	0° to 60°		Extension	0° to 30°
External rotation		Adduction, reduction of lateral tilt	Abduction	0° to 40°
Arm in abduction	0° to 90°		Adduction	0° to 35°
Arm in adduction	0° to 80°		Internal rotation	0° to 45°
			External rotation	0° to 45°
ELBOW			**KNEE**	
Flexion	0° to 135°-150°			
Extension	0°		Flexion	0° to 135°
FOREARM			**ANKLE AND FOOT**	
Pronation	0° to 80°-90°		Plantar flexion	0° to 50°
Supination	0° to 80°-90°		Dorsiflexion	0° to 15°
			Inversion	0° to 35°
			Eversion	0° to 20°

Data adapted from American Academy of Orthopaedic Surgeons: *Joint motion: method of measuring and recording.* Chicago, 1965, The Association; Esch D, Lepley M: *Evaluation of joint motion: methods of measurement and recording,* Minneapolis, 1974, University of Minnesota Press.
* *DIP,* Distal interphalangeal; *MP,* metacarpophalangeal; *PIP,* proximal interphalangeal.

ods of performing a particular skill. See Chapter 26 for further suggestions of ADL techniques for those with limited ROM.

In many diagnoses, as with burns and arthritis, loss of ROM can be anticipated. The goal of treatment is to prevent joint limitation with splints, positioning, exercise, activity, and application of the principles of joint protection before it occurs.

Limitations of ROM, their causes, and the prognosis for increasing ROM will suggest treatment approaches. Some of the specific methods used to increase ROM are discussed elsewhere in this text. These include passive or active stretching exercise, resistive exercise, strengthening of antagonistic muscle groups, activities that require active motion of the affected joints through the full available ROM, splints, and positioning. To increase ROM

the physician may perform surgery or may manipulate the part while the patient is under anesthesia. The physical therapist may employ manual stretching with heat and massage.[8]

PROCEDURE FOR JOINT MEASUREMENT

Average normal ROM for each joint motion is listed in Table 8-1, in Fig. 8-2, and before each of the following procedures for measurement. The reader should keep in mind that these are averages and that there may be considerable variation in ROM from one individual to another. Normal ROM is affected by age, sex, and other factors such as lifestyle and occupation.[9] Therefore the subject in the illustrations may not always demonstrate the average ROM listed for the particular motion.

The goniometer in the illustrations is shown so that the reader can most easily see its correct positioning. However, the examiner may not always be in the best position for the particular measurement. For the purposes of clear illustration, the examiner is necessarily shown off to one side and may have only one hand on the instrument. Many of the motions require that the examiner be squarely in front of the subject or that the examiner's hands obscure the goniometer. How the examiner holds the goniometer and supports the part being measured are determined by factors such as position of the patient, degree of muscle weakness, presence or absence of joint pain, and whether active or passive ROM is being measured. The examiner and subject should be positioned for the greatest comfort, correct placement of the instrument, and adequate stabilization of the part being tested to effect the desired motion in the correct plane.

General procedure — 180° method of measurement

1. Have subject comfortable and relaxed in appropriate position.
2. Explain and demonstrate to subject what you are going to do, why, and how you expect him or her to cooperate.
3. Uncover joint to be measured.
4. Establish and palpate bony landmarks for the measurement.
5. Stabilize joints proximal to joint being measured.
6. Move part passively through ROM to estimate available ROM and get the feel of joint mobility.[9]
7. Return part to the starting position.[9]
8. At starting position place axis of goniometer over axis of joint. Place stationary bar on proximal or stationary bone and movable bar on distal or moving bone. Avoid goniometer dial going off semicircle by always facing curved side away from direction of motion, unless the goniometer can be read when it moves in either direction.
9. Record number of degrees at starting position and remove goniometer.[9] Do not attempt to hold goniometer in place while moving joint through ROM.
10. Evaluator should hold part securely above and below joint being measured and *gently* move joint through available ROM to determine full passive ROM. *Do not force joints.* Watch for signs of pain and discomfort. Unless otherwise indicated, passive ROM should be measured.
11. Reposition goniometer and record number of degrees at final position.
12. Remove goniometer and gently place part in resting position.
13. Record reading at final position and any notations on the evaluation form.

DIRECTIONS FOR JOINT MEASUREMENT—180° SYSTEM
THE SPINE[1,3,4,9,10]
Cervical Spine

Measurement of motions of the neck are the least accurate, because there are few bony landmarks and much soft tissue overlying bony segments.[4] X-ray is the best means to make an accurate measurement of the specific joints.[10] Approximate estimates of cervical flexion, extension, rotation, and lateral flexion may be made by using the goniometer or by estimating the number of degrees of motion, using a fixed axis and estimating the arc of motion from that point (Figs. 8-3 to 8-10.)[1,4]

Cervical flexion

0° to 45° (Fig. 8-3)

Position of the subject. Sitting or standing erect.

Measurement of motion. The subject is asked to flex the neck so that the chin moves toward the chest. The number of degrees of motion may be estimated, or the examiner may measure the number of inches or centimeters from chin to the sternal notch.[1,3,9] If a goniometer is used, the axis is placed over the angle of the jaw. The examiner grasps the corner of the protractor, which is positioned with the arc upward, and steadies his or her arm by resting it against the subject's shoulder. The arms of the goniometer are aligned with a tongue depressor, which the subject is holding between the teeth. As the subject performs neck flexion, the movable bar of the goniometer is adjusted downward to align with the new position of the tongue depressor.[4,9]

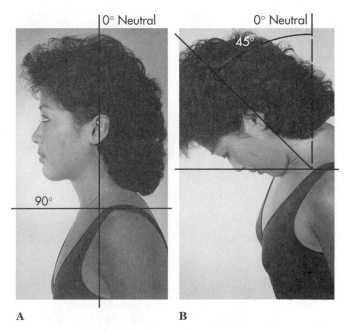

FIG. 8-3 Cervical flexion. **A,** Starting position. **B,** Final position.

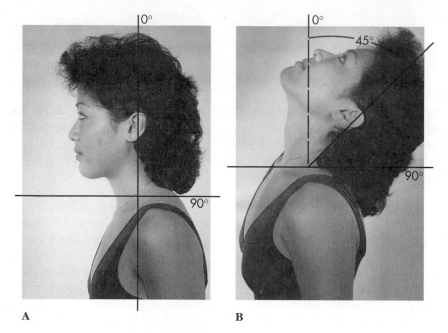

FIG. 8-4 Cervical extension. **A,** Starting position. **B,** Final position.

Cervical extension

0° to 45° (Fig. 8-4)

Position of the subject. Sitting or standing erect.

Measurement of motion. The subject is asked to extend the neck as if to look at the ceiling, so that the back of the head approaches the thoracic spine. The number of degrees of motion can be estimated or the number of inches or centimeters from chin to sternal notch may be measured.[3] If a goniometer is used, the axis is again placed over the angle of the jaw. The examiner grasps the corner of the protractor, which is now positioned with the arc downward, and steadies his or her arm against the subject's shoulder. The movable bar of the goniometer is moved upward to align with the tongue depressor as the subject extends the neck.[4,9]

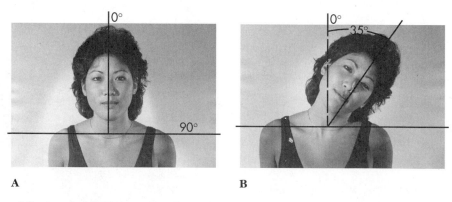

FIG. 8-5 Cervical lateral flexion. **A,** Starting position. **B,** Final position.

Lateral flexion

0° to 45° (Fig. 8-5)

Position of the subject. Sitting or standing erect.

Measurement of motion. The subject is asked to flex the neck laterally without rotation, moving the ear toward the shoulder. The number of degrees of motion may be estimated, or the examiner may measure the number of inches or centimeters between the mastoid process and the acromion process of the shoulder.[1,3] If a goniometer is used, the axis is placed over the spinous process of the seventh cervical vertebra. The stationary bar may be over the shoulder and parallel to the floor so that the motion begins at 90° or it may be aligned with the thoracic vertebra for a starting position of 0°. The movable bar is aligned with the external occipital protuberance.[1,9]

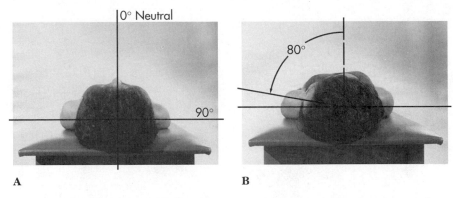

FIG. 8-6 Cervical rotation. **A,** Starting position. **B,** Final position.

Cervical rotation

0° to 60° (Fig. 8-6)

Position of the subject. Lying supine or seated.

Measurement of motion. The subject is asked to rotate the head to right or left without rotating the trunk. The amount of rotation may be estimated in degrees from the neutral position[1] or a tape measure may be used to mea-sure the distance from the tip of the chin to the acromion process of the shoulder. The measure is taken first in the anatomical position and then again after the neck has been rotated.[3] In the lying position, if a goniometer is used, it is set at 90°, and the axis is placed over the vertex of the head. The stationary bar is held steady, parallel to the floor or to the acromion process on the side being tested. The movable bar is aligned with the tip of the nose.[4,9]

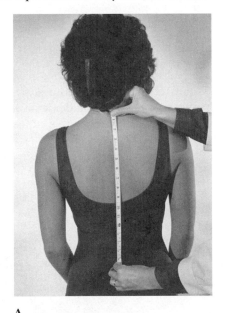

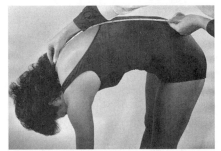

FIG. 8-7 Spine flexion. **A,** Starting position. **B,** Final position.

Thoracic and Lumbar Spine
Flexion

0° to 80° and + 4 inches (Fig. 8-7)

Position of the subject. Standing erect.

Measurement of motion. Four methods of estimating the range of spinal flexion are as follows: (1) measuring the number of degrees of forward flexion of the trunk in relation to the longitudinal axis of the body. The exam-iner must hold the pelvis stable with the hands and any change in the subject's normal lordosis should be ob-served; (2) indicating the level of the fingertips along the front of the subject's leg; (3) measuring the number of inches or centimeters between the subject's fingertips and the floor; and (4) measuring the length of the spine from the seventh cervical vertebra to the first sacral ver-tebra when the subject is erect and again after the subject has flexed the spine (Fig. 8-7).[3,9] The fourth method is probably the most accurate of these clinical methods.[1] In a normal adult there is an average increase of 4 inches (10 cm) in length in forward flexion of the spine.[3] If the subject bends forward at the hips with a straight back, there will be no difference in length.

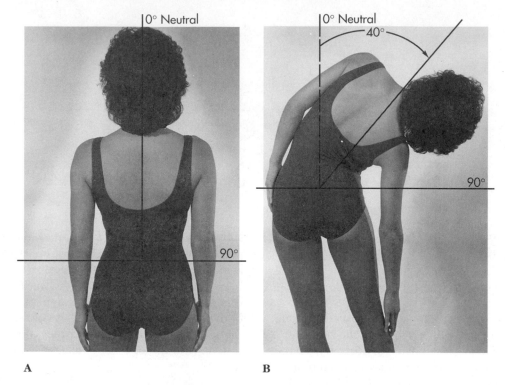

FIG. 8-8   Spine lateral flexion. **A,** Starting position. **B,** Final position.

Lateral flexion

0° to 40° (Fig. 8-8)

Position of the subject. Standing erect.

Method of measurement. Several methods may be used to estimate the range of lateral flexion of the trunk. The steel tape measure may be held in place during the motion and used to estimate the number of degrees of lateral inclination of the trunk compared with the vertical position. Other methods include (1) estimating the position of the spinous process of C7 in relation to the pelvis (Fig. 8-8); (2) measuring the distance of the fingertips from the knee joint in lateral flexion; (3) measuring the distance between the tip of the third finger and the floor;[3] and (4) using a long arm goniometer, placing the axis on S1, the stationary bar perpendicular to the floor, and the movable bar aligned with C7.[1,9]

Extension

0° to 30° (Fig. 8-9)

Position of the subject. Standing erect or lying prone.

Method of measurement. The subject is asked to bend backward while maintaining stability of the pelvis. The examiner stabilizes the pelvis from the anterior when the measurement is taken in the standing position, if necessary. The range of extension is estimated in degrees from the vertical, using the superior iliac crest as the pivotal

point in relation to the spinous process of C7. In the lying postion, a pillow is placed under the abdomen and the hands are placed at shoulder level on the treatment table. The pelvis is stabilized with a strap or by an assistant and the subject extends the elbows to raise the trunk from the table. A perpendicular measurement is taken of the distance between the suprasternal notch and the supporting surface at the end of the ROM.[3]

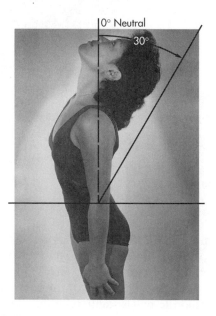

FIG. 8-9   Spine extension.

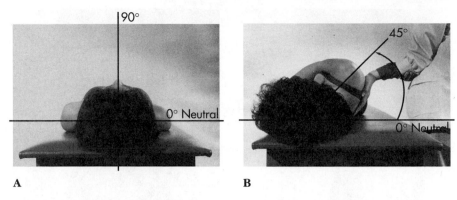

FIG. 8-10 Spine rotation. **A,** Starting position. **B,** Final position.

Rotation

0° to 45° (Fig. 8-10)

Position of the subject. Lying supine or standing.

Method of measurement. The subject is asked to rotate the upper trunk while maintaining neutral position of the pelvis. The examiner may fix the pelvis firmly to maintain the neutral position. This step is especially important if the subject is in the standing position. This motion is recorded in degrees, using the center of the crown of the head as a pivotal point and the arc of motion made by the shoulder as it moves upward or forward.

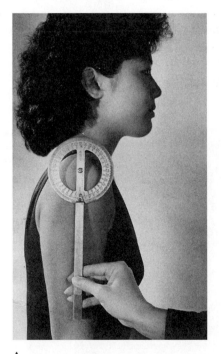

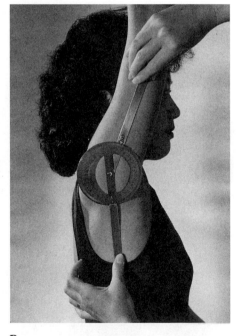

FIG. 8-11 Shoulder flexion. **A,** Starting position. **B,** Final position.

UPPER EXTREMITY[1,2,3,5,9,10]
Shoulder
Flexion

0° to 170° (Fig. 8-11)

Position of the subject. Seated or supine with humerus in neutral rotation.

Position of goniometer. Axis is in the center of humeral head just distal to the acromion process on the lateral aspect of humerus. Stationary bar is parallel to trunk, and movable bar is parallel to humerus. Note that when the shoulder is flexed, the axis point moves upward and backward to the posterior surface of the shoulder. Thus to take the measurement of the final position, the goniometer should be placed on the lateral surface of the shoulder aligned with the imaginary axis through the center of the humeral head, which is just slightly superior to the crease formed by the deltoid mass.

End-feel. Firm.

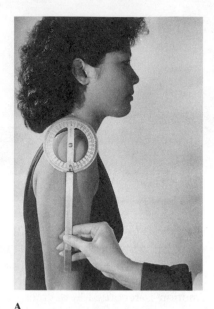
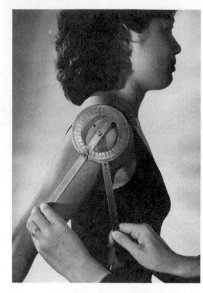

A   **B**

FIG. 8-12 Shoulder extension. **A,** Starting position. **B,** Final position.

Extension

0° to 60° (Fig. 8-12)

Position of the subject. Seated or prone, with no obstruction behind humerus and humerus in neutral rotation.

Position of goniometer. Same as for flexion, but the axis point remains the same for starting and final positions. Movement should be accompanied by slight upward tilt of the scapula. Excessive scapular motion should be avoided.

End-feel. Firm.

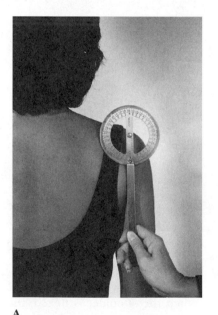
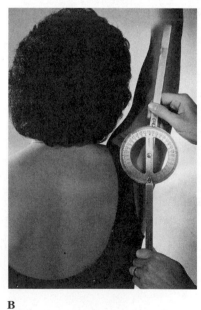

A   **B**

FIG. 8-13 Shoulder abduction. **A,** Starting position. **B,** Final position.

Abduction

0° to 170° (Fig 8-13)

Position of the subject. Seated or lying prone, with humerus in adduction and external rotation. Measure on posterior surface.

Position of goniometer. Axis is on acromion process on posterior surface of shoulder. Stationary bar is parallel to trunk, and movable bar is parallel to humerus.

End-feel. Firm.

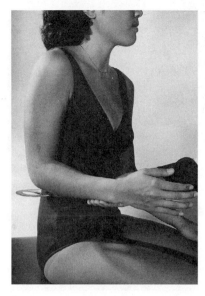
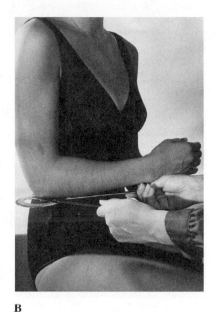

A   **B**

FIG. 8-14   Shoulder internal rotation, shoulder adducted. **A,** Starting position. **B,** Final position.

Internal rotation

0° to 60° (Fig. 8-14)

Position of the subject (used if abduction cannot be achieved).[3] Seated with humerus adducted against

trunk, elbow at 90° and forearm at midposition and perpendicular to body.

Position of goniometer. Axis on olecranon process of elbow and stationary bar and movable bar parallel to forearm.

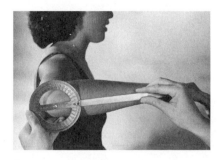
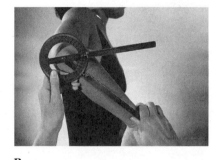

A   **B**

FIG. 8-15   Shoulder internal rotation, shoulder abducted (alternate position). **A,** Starting position. **B,** Final position.

Internal rotation (alternate position)

0° to 70° (Fig. 8-15)

Position of the subject (used if there is no danger of posterior dislocation and abduction is possible).[3] Seated or supine with humerus abducted to 90°, elbow flexed to 90° and forearm in midposition.

Position of goniometer. Axis on olecranon process of elbow and stationary bar and movable bar parallel to forearm.

End-feel. Firm.

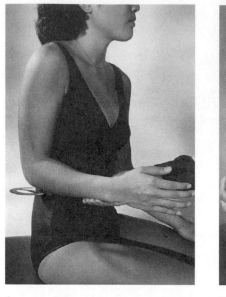
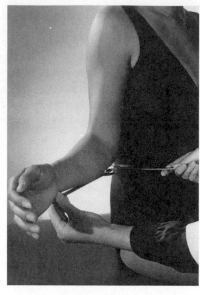

A   **B**

FIG. 8-16   External rotation, shoulder adducted. **A,** Starting position. **B,** Final position.

External rotation

0° to 80° (Fig. 8-16)

Position of the subject (used if abduction is not possible).[3] Seated, humerus adducted, elbow at 90° and forearm in midposition, perpendicular to the body.

Position of goniometer. Axis on olecranon of elbow. Stationary bar and movable bar parallel to forearm.

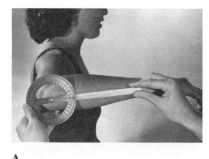
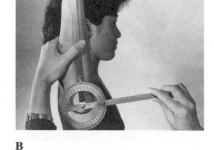

A   **B**

FIG. 8-17   Shoulder external rotation, shoulder abducted (alternate position). **A,** Starting position. **B,** Final position.

External rotation (alternate position)

0° to 90° (Fig. 8-17)

Position of the subject (used if there is no danger of anterior dislocation of the humerus).[3] Seated or supine with humerus abducted to 90°, elbow flexed to 90° and forearm pronated.

Position of goniometer. Axis on olecranon process of elbow and stationary bar and movable bar parallel to forearm.

End-feel. Firm.

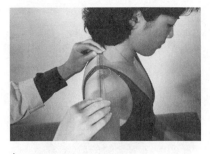
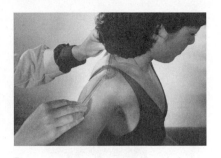

FIG. 8-18   Shoulder horizontal abduction. **A,** Starting position. **B,** Final position.

Horizontal abduction

0° to 40° (Fig. 8-18)

Position of the subject. Seated erect with the shoulder to be tested abducted to 90°, elbow extended and palm facing down. The therapist may support the arm in abduction.

Position of goniometer. The axis is over the acromion process. The stationary bar is parallel over the shoulder toward the neck, and the movable bar is parallel to the humerus on the superior aspect.

End-feel. Firm.

Horizontal adduction

0° to 130° (Fig. 8-19)

Position of subject and goniometer. Same as for horizontal abduction.

End-feel. Firm.

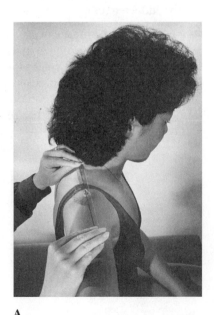
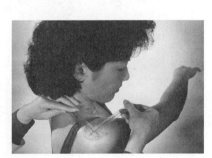

FIG. 8-19   Shoulder horizontal adduction. **A,** Starting position. **B,** Final position.

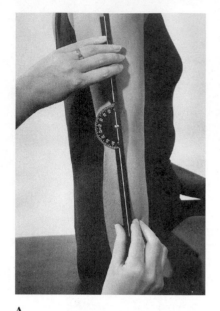
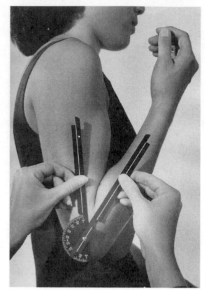

A   **B**

FIG. 8-20   Elbow flexion. **A,** Starting position. **B,** Final position.

Elbow

Extension to flexion

0° to 135°-150° (Fig. 8-20)

Position of the subject. Standing, sitting, or supine with humerus adducted and externally rotated and forearm supinated.

Position of goniometer. Axis is placed over the lateral epicondyle of humerus at end of elbow crease. Stationary bar is parallel to midline of humerus, and movable bar is parallel to radius. After the movement has been com-

pleted, the position of the elbow crease changes in relation to the lateral epicondyle because of the rise of the muscle bulk during the motion. The axis of the goniometer should be repositioned so that it is over, although it will not be directly on, the lateral epicondyle.

End-feel. Hard or firm.

Forearm

Supination

0° to 80° or 90° (Fig. 8-21)

Position of the subject. Seated or standing with humerus adducted, elbow at 90° and forearm in midposition.

Position of goniometer. Axis is at ulnar border of volar aspect of wrist, just proximal to the ulna styloid. Movable bar is resting against the volar aspect of the wrist, and the stationary bar is perpendicular to the floor. After the forearm is supinated, the goniometer should be repositioned so that the movable bar rests squarely across the center of the distal forearm.

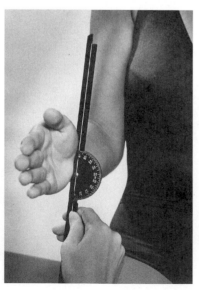
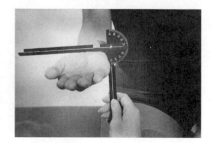

A   **B**

FIG. 8-21   Forearm supination. **A,** Starting position. **B,** Final position.

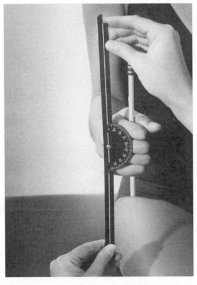

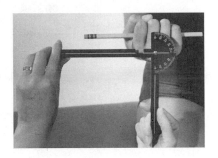

A   B

FIG. 8-22 Forearm supination (alternate method). **A,** Starting position. **B,** Final position.

Supination (alternate method)
0° to 80° or 90° (Fig. 8-22)

Position of the subject. Seated or standing with humerus adducted, elbow at 90° and forearm in midposition. Place pencil in hand so it is held by subject perpendicular to floor.

Position of goniometer. Axis is over the head of third metacarpal, and stationary bar is perpendicular to floor. Movable bar is parallel to pencil.

End-feel. Firm.

Pronation
0° to 80° or 90° (Fig. 8-23)

Position of the subject. Seated or standing with humerus adducted, elbow at 90° and forearm in midposition.

Position of goniometer. Axis is at the ulnar border of the dorsal aspect of the wrist, just proximal to the ulna styloid. The movable bar is resting against the dorsal aspect of the wrist, and the stationary bar is perpendicular to the floor. After the forearm is pronated, reposition the goniometer so that the movable bar rests squarely across the center of the dorsum of the distal forearm.

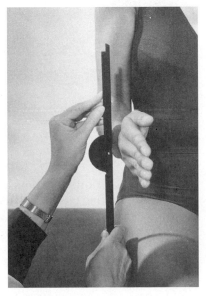

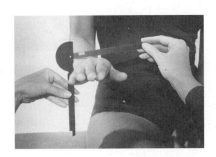

A   B

FIG. 8-23 Forearm pronation. **A,** Starting position. **B,** Final position.

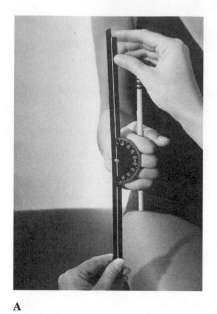
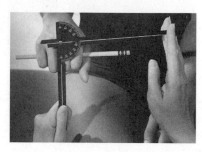

FIG. 8-24 Forearm pronation (alternate method). **A,** Starting position. **B,** Final position.

Pronation (alternate method)

0° to 80° or 90° (Fig. 8-24)

Position of the subject. Seated or standing with humerus adducted, elbow at 90° and forearm in midposition. A pencil is placed in the hand so that it is held perpendicular to the floor.

Position of goniometer. Axis is over the head of the third metacarpal, stationary bar is perpendicular to the floor, and movable bar is parallel to pencil.

End-feel. Hard or firm.

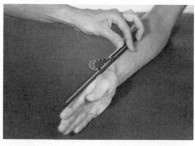
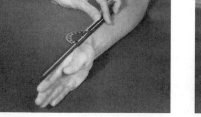

FIG. 8-25 Wrist flexion. **A,** Starting position. **B,** Final position.

Wrist
Flexion

0° to 80° (Fig. 8-25)

Position of subject. Seated with forearm in midposition and hand and forearm resting on table on ulnar border, the fingers are relaxed or extended. This measurement may also be taken with the forearm pronated and resting on a table.

Position of goniometer. If measured with the forearm in midposition the axis is on lateral aspect of wrist just distal to radial styloid in anatomical snuff box. Stationary bar is parallel to radius, and movable bar is parallel to metacarpal of index finger. If measured with the forearm pronated the axis is placed at the wrist just beneath the ulna styloid, the movable bar is aligned with the fifth metacarpal, and the stationary bar with the ulna.

End-feel. Firm.

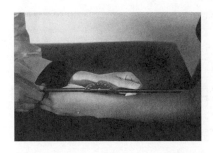
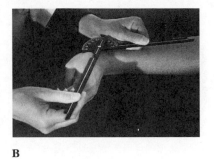

A   B

FIG. 8-26   Wrist extension. **A,** Starting position. **B,** Final position.

Extension

0° to 70° (Fig. 8-26)

Position of subject and goniometer. Same as for wrist

flexion except that the fingers should be flexed.

End-feel. Firm.

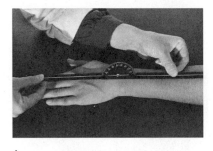
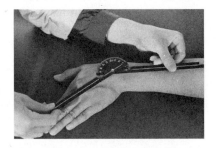

A   B

FIG. 8-27   Wrist ulnar deviation. **A,** Starting position. **B,** Final position.

Ulnar deviation

0° to 30° (Fig. 8-27)

Position of the subject. Seated with forearm pronated, wrist at neutral, fingers relaxed in extension and palm of hand resting flat on table surface.

Position of goniometer. Axis is on dorsum of wrist at base of third metacarpal, over the capitate bone. Stationary bar is parallel to third metacarpal.

End-feel. Firm.

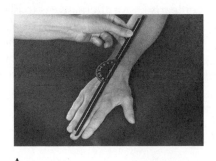
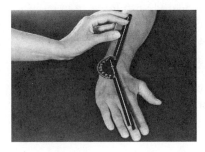

A   B

FIG. 8-28   Wrist radial deviation. **A,** Starting position. **B,** Final position.

Radial deviation

0° to 20° (Fig. 8-28)

Position of subject and goniometer. Same as for ulnar deviation.

End-feel. Hard.

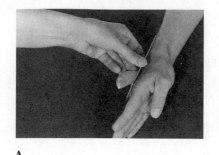
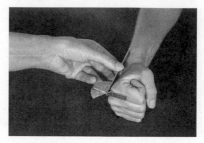

A   **B**

FIG. 8-29   MP flexion. **A,** Starting position. **B,** Final position.

Fingers

Metacarpophalangeal (MP) flexion

0° to 90° (Fig. 8-29)

Position of the subject. Seated with elbow flexed, forearm in midposition, wrist at 0° neutral, and forearm and hand supported on firm surface on ulnar border.

Position of goniometer. Axis is centered on dorsal aspect of the MP joint. Stationary bar is on top of metacarpal, and movable bar is on top of proximal phalanx.

End-feel. Hard or firm.

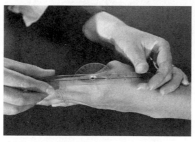

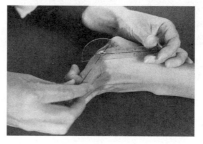

A   **B**

FIG. 8-30   MP hyperextension. **A,** Starting position. **B,** Final position.

MP hyperextension

0° to 15°-45° (Fig. 8-30)

Position of the subject. Seated with forearm in midposition, wrist at 0° neutral, IP joints relaxed or in flexion, and forearm and hand supported on a firm surface on ulnar border.

Position of goniometer. Axis is over lateral aspect of MP joint of index finger. Stationary bar is parallel to metacarpal, and movable bar is parallel to proximal phalanx. Fifth finger MP joint may be measured similarly. ROM of third and fourth fingers can be estimated by comparison. An alternative is to place the goniometer on the volar aspect of the hand. Using the edge of the goniometer, the axis is aligned over the MP joint being measured, the stationary bar is parallel to the metacarpal, and the movable bar parallel to the proximal phalanx.

End-feel. Firm.

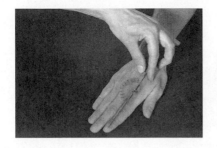

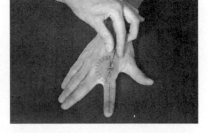

A   B

FIG. 8-31   MP abduction. **A,** Starting position. **B,** Final position.

MP abduction
0° to 25° (Fig. 8-31)

Position of the subject. Seated with forearm pronated, wrist at 0° neutral deviation, fingers straight, resting on a firm surface.

Position of goniometer. Axis is centered over MP joint being measured. Stationary bar is over corresponding metacarpal, and movable bar is over corresponding proximal phalanx.

End-feel. Firm.

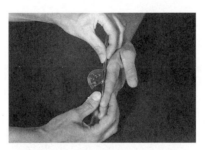

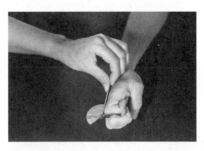

A   B

FIG. 8-32   PIP flexion. **A,** Starting position. **B,** Final position.

Proximal interphalangeal (PIP) flexion
0° to 110° (Fig. 8-32)

Position of the subject. Seated with forearm in midposition, wrist at 0° neutral, and forearm and hand supported on a firm surface on ulnar border.

Position of goniometer. Axis is centered on dorsal surface of PIP joint being measured. Stationary bar is placed over the proximal phalanx, and movable bar is over distal phalanx.

End-feel. Usually hard.

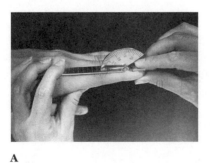

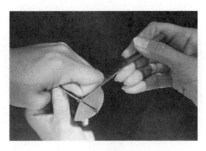

A   B

FIG. 8-33   DIP flexion. **A,** Starting position. **B,** Final position.

Distal interphalangeal (DIP) flexion
0° to 80° (Fig. 8-33)

Position of the subject. Seated with forearm in midposition, wrist at 0° neutral, and forearm and hand supported on the ulnar border on a firm surface.

Position of goniometer. Axis is on dorsal surface of DIP joint. Stationary bar is over middle phalanx, and movable bar is over distal phalanx.

End-feel. Firm.

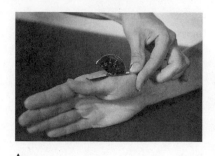
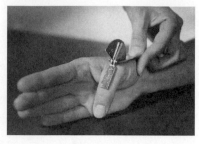

A   **B**

FIG. 8-34   Thumb MP flexion. **A,** Starting position. **B,** Final position.

Thumb
MP flexion

0° to 50° (Fig. 8-34)

Position of the subject. Seated with the elbow flexed, the forearm in 45° of supination, wrist at 0° neutral, supported on a firm surface.

Position of goniometer. Axis is on dorsal surface of MP joint. Stationary bar is over thumb metacarpal, and movable bar is over proximal phalanx.

End-feel. Hard or firm.

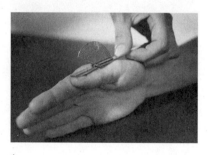
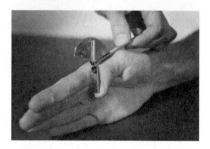

A   **B**

FIG. 8-35   Thumb IP flexion. **A,** Starting position. **B,** Final position.

Interphalangeal (IP) flexion

0° to 80°-90° (Fig. 8-35)

Position of the subject. Same as described for PIP and DIP finger flexion.

Position of goniometer. Axis is on dorsal surface of IP joint. Stationary bar is over proximal phalanx, and movable bar is over distal phalanx.

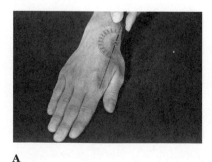
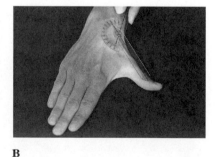

A   **B**

FIG. 8-36   Thumb radial abduction. **A,** Starting position. **B,** Final position.

Radial abduction (carpometacarpal [CMC] extension)

0° to 50° (Fig. 8-36)

Position of the subject. Seated with forearm pronated and hand palm down, resting flat on firm surface.

Position of goniometer. Axis is over CMC joint at base of thumb metacarpal. Stationary bar is parallel to radius, and movable bar is parallel to thumb metacarpal.

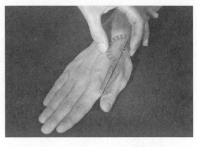
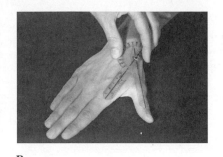

A **B**

FIG. 8-37 Thumb radial abduction (alternate method). **A,** Starting position. **B,** Final position.

Radial abduction (alternate method)
0° to 50° (Fig. 8-37)

Position of subject and goniometer. Subject is positioned same as described in first method. Axis is over the CMC joint at the base of the thumb metacarpal. The sta-

tionary and movable bars are together and parallel to the thumb and the first metacarpals. Neither will be directly over these bones.

End-feel. Firm.

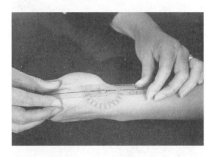
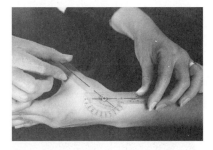

A **B**

FIG. 8-38 Palmar abduction. **A,** Starting position. **B,** Final position.

Palmar abduction (CMC Flexion)
0° to 50° (Fig. 8-38)

Position of the subject. Seated with forearm at 0° midposition, wrist at 0°, and forearm and hand resting on ulnar border. The thumb is rotated so that it is at right angles to the palm of the hand.

Position of goniometer. Axis is at the junction of the thumb and index finger metacarpals. Stationary bar is over radius, and movable bar is parallel to the thumb and index finger metacarpals.

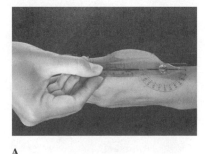
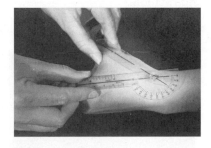

A **B**

FIG. 8-39 Palmar abduction (alternate method). **A,** Starting position. **B,** Final position.

Palmar abduction (alternate method)
0° to 50° (Fig. 8-39)

Position of subject and goniometer. Subject is positioned same as described in first method. Axis is at junc-

tion of the thumb and index finger metacarpals. The stationary and movable bars are lined up together parallel to the thumb and the index finger metacarpals.

End-feel. Firm.

Opposition (Fig. 8-40)

Deficits in opposition may be recorded by measuring distance between centers of the pad of the thumb and pad of fifth finger with a centimeter ruler.

End-feel. Soft or firm.

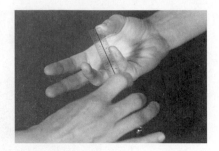

FIG. 8-40   Thumb opposition to fifth finger.

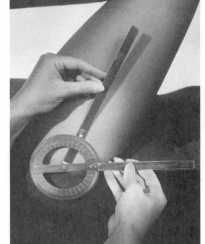

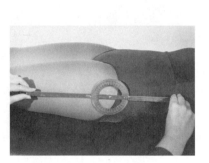

A

B

FIG. 8-41   Hip flexion. **A,** Starting position. **B,** Final position.

LOWER EXTREMITY[3,5,6,9]
Hip
Flexion

0° to 120° (Fig. 8-41)

Position of the subject. Supine lying with hip and knee in 0° neutral extension and rotation.

Position of goniometer. Axis is on lateral aspect of hip over greater trochanter of femur. Stationary bar is centered over the middle of the lateral aspect of the pelvis, and movable bar is parallel to long axis of femur on lateral aspect of thigh. Knee is bent during the motion.

End-feel. Soft.

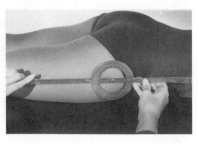

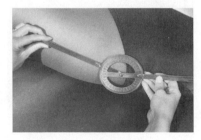

A

B

FIG. 8-42   Hip extension. **A,** Starting position. **B,** Final position.

Extension (hyperextension)

0° to 30° (Fig. 8-42)

Position of the subject. Prone lying with hip and knee at 0° neutral extension and rotation.

Position of goniometer. Same as for hip flexion.

End-feel. Firm.

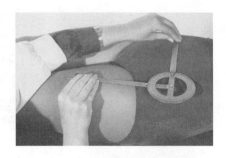
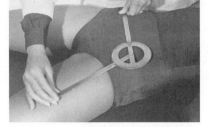

A   B

FIG. 8-43   Hip abduction. **A,** Starting position. **B,** Final position.

Abduction
0° to 40° (Fig. 8-43)

Position of the subject. Supine, lying with legs extended and hip in 0° neutral rotation, pelvis level.

Position of goniometer. Axis is placed on anterior superior iliac spine. Stationary bar is placed on a line be-

tween two anterior superior iliac spines, and movable bar is parallel to longitudinal axis of femur over anterior aspect of thigh. Note that starting position is at 90° for this measurement, and recording of measurement should be adjusted by subtracting 90° from total number of degrees obtained in arc of joint motion.

End-feel. Firm.

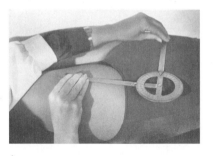
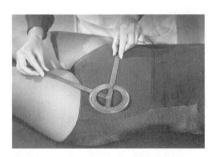

A   B

FIG. 8-44   Hip adduction. **A,** Starting position. **B,** Final position.

Adduction
0° to 35° (Fig. 8-44)

Position of subject and goniometer. Supine, lying with hip and knee of the leg to be tested in extension and

neutral rotation. The leg not being tested should be abducted. The goniometer is positioned the same as for hip abduction.

End-feel. Firm.

Internal rotation
0° to 45° (Fig. 8-45)

Position of the subject. Seated with hip in 0° neutral rotation and hip and knee flexed to 90°. Knee is flexed over the end of the treatment table. A small roll or towel may be placed under the distal end of the femur to maintain it in a horizontal plane. The contralateral hip is abducted, and the foot may be supported on a stool.

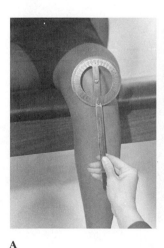
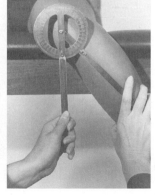

A   B

FIG. 8-45   Hip internal rotation. **A,** Starting position. **B,** Final position.

Position of goniometer. Axis is on center of patella of knee. Stationary and movable bars are parallel to longitudinal axis of tibia on anterior aspect of lower leg. Stationary bar remains in this position, perpendicular to floor, while movable bar follows tibia as hip is rotated.

End-feel. Firm.

External rotation

0° to 45° (Fig. 8-46)

Position of subject and goniometer. Seated with hip in 0° neutral rotation and hip and knee of leg to be tested flexed to 90°. The other leg should be (1) flexed at the knee so that the lower leg is back under the table or (2) flexed at the hip and knee so that the foot is resting on the table. These positions allow the motion to take place without obstruction. The trunk should remain erect during the performance of the motion. The goniometer is positioned as for internal rotation.

End-feel. Firm.

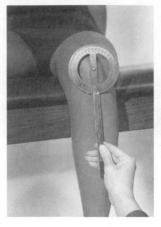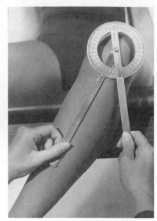

A   B

FIG. 8-46   Hip external rotation. **A,** Starting position. **B,** Final position.

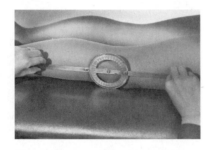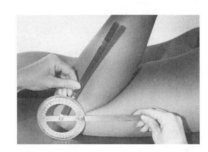

A   B

FIG. 8-47   Knee flexion. **A,** Starting position. **B,** Final position.

Knee
Extension-flexion

0° to 135° (Fig. 8-47)

Position of the subject. Prone lying with knees and hips extended, and hip in 0° neutral rotation.

Position of goniometer. Axis is centered on lateral aspect of knee joint at tibial condyle. Stationary bar is on lateral aspect of thigh parallel to the longitudinal axis of femur. Movable bar is parallel to longitudinal axis of tibia on lateral aspect of leg.

End-feel. Soft.

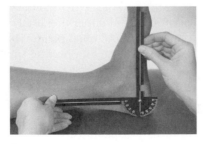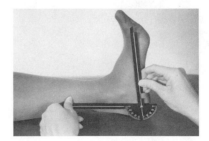

A   B

FIG. 8-48   Ankle dorsiflexion. **A,** Starting position. **B,** Final position.

Ankle
Dorsiflexion

0° to 15° (Fig. 8-48)

Position of the subject. Supine lying or seated with knee flexed at least 30°. Ankle is at 90° neutral position and the foot is in 0° of inversion and eversion.

Position of goniometer. Axis is placed approximately 1.5 cm below medial malleolus.[3] Stationary bar is parallel

to midline of lower leg and movable bar parallel with first metatarsal. (This measurement may also be taken on the lateral side of the foot). Note that measurement begins at 90°, so 90° must be subtracted when recording joint measurement.

End-feel. Firm.

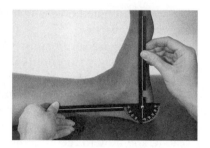
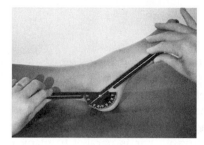

A   **B**

FIG. 8-49 Ankle plantar flexion. **A,** Starting position. **B,** Final position.

Plantar flexion

0° to 50° (Fig. 8-49)

Position of subject and goniometer. Same as for dorsiflexion.

End-feel. Firm or hard.

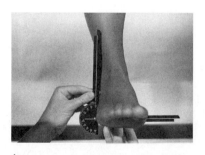
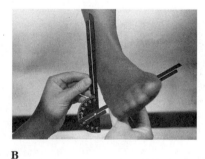

A   **B**

FIG. 8-50 Ankle inversion. **A,** Starting position. **B,** Final position.

Inversion

0° to 35° (Fig. 8-50)

Position of the subject. Supine with the knee and hip extended and in 0° neutral rotation, the ankle in the 90° neutral position and foot over the edge of the table; or sitting with knee flexed to 90°, the leg over the edge of the supporting surface, and ankle in 90° neutral position.

Position of goniometer. Axis is placed at lateral border of foot near heel. Stationary bar is parallel to longitudinal axis of tibia on lateral aspect of leg. Movable bar is parallel to plantar surface of heel.

End-feel. Firm.

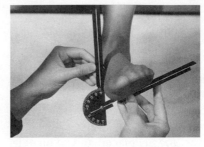

A   B

FIG. 8-51 Ankle eversion. **A,** Starting position. **B,** Final position.

Eversion

0° to 20° (Fig. 8-51, see p. 105)

Position of the subject. Same as for inversion.

Position of goniometer. Axis is on medial border of foot just proximal to metatarsal-phalangeal joint. Stationary bar is parallel to longitudinal aspect of tibia on medial aspect of lower leg. Movable bar is parallel to plantar surface of sole. Note that measurements for inversion and eversion both begin at 90°. Therefore this amount must be subtracted from total when recording measurement.

End-feel. Hard.

SUMMARY

Joint measurement is used to evaluate ROM in persons whose physical dysfunction affects joint mobility. ROM measurements are used in setting treatment goals, selecting treatment methods, and making objective assessments of progress.

The occupational therapist who does joint measurement should know the principles of joint measurement related to inspection, palpation, positioning and stabilization, precautions and contraindications, end-feel, and two-joint muscles. The therapist should also know normal average ROMs, how to use the goniometer, how to read it, and how to record joint ROM measurements.

The procedure for measuring joint ROM involves correct positioning for patient and therapist, exposure of joints to be measured, palpation, appropriate stabilization and handling of parts, and correct placement of the goniometer at the beginning and end of the range of motion.

Directions and illustrations for measuring all of the major joint motions in the neck, trunk, and upper and lower extremities are included in this chapter. The content is designed for the development of the fundamental techniques of joint measurement.

REVIEW QUESTIONS

1. Describe general rules for positioning the goniometer when measuring joint ROM.
2. With which diagnoses would joint measurement be a primary evaluation procedure?
3. List and discuss four purposes of joint measurement.
4. Is formal joint measurement necessary for every patient? If not, how may ROM be evaluated?
5. What is meant by palpation? How is palpation done?
6. In observing joints and joint motions, what should the therapist look for?
7. List at least five precautions or contraindications to joint measurement.
8. What is meant by end-feel? Describe soft, firm, and hard end-feels and name one joint for each.
9. When measuring a joint crossed by a two-joint muscle, how should the joint not being measured be positioned?
10. Describe the steps in the procedure for joint measurement.
11. How is joint ROM measurement recorded on the evaluation form?
12. List the average normal ROM for elbow flexion, shoulder flexion, finger MP flexion, hip flexion, knee flexion, and ankle dorsiflexion.
13. Describe how to read the goniometer when using the 180° system of joint measurement.
14. List three common causes of joint limitation.
15. Define what is meant by functional range of motion.
16. Discuss two approaches to treatment of joint limitation in occupational therapy.
17. List six treatment methods that could be used by occupational and physical therapy to increase ROM.

EXERCISES

1. Measure all of the upper extremity joint motions of a normal subject. Record the findings on the form in Figure 8-2.
2. Repeat the first exercise, but the subject should play the role of someone with several joint limitations.

3. Observe joint motions used in ordinary activities of daily living (self-care, home management). Estimate the functional ranges of motion for the following joint motions: Shoulder flexion, external rotation, internal rotation, abduction; elbow flexion; wrist extension; hip flexion and extension; knee flexion; ankle plantar flexion.

REFERENCES

1. American Academy of Orthopaedic Surgeons: *Joint motion: method of measuring and recording,* Chicago, 1965, The Association.
2. Baruch Center of Physical Medicine: *The technique of goniometry,* Unpublished manuscript.
3. Clarkson HM, Gilewich GB: *Musculoskeletal assessment, Joint range of motion and manual muscle strength,* Baltimore, 1989, Williams & Wilkins.
4. Cole T: Measurement of musculoskeletal function: goniometry. In Kottke FJ, Stillwell GK, Lehmann JF, editors: *Krusen's handbook of physical medicine and rehabilitation,* ed 3, Philadelphia, 1982, WB Saunders.
5. Esch D, Lepley M: *Evaluation of joint motion: methods of measurement and recording,* Minneapolis, 1974, University of Minnesota Press.
6. Hurt SP: Considerations of muscle function and their application to disability evaluation and treatment: joint measurement, Reprinted from *Am J Occup Ther* 1:69, 1947; 2:13, 1948.
7. Kendall FP, McCreary EK: *Muscles, testing and function,* ed 3, Baltimore, 1983, Williams & Wilkins.
8. Killingsworth A: Basic physical disability procedures, San José, Calif, 1987, Maple Press.
9. Norkin CC, White DJ: *Measurement of joint motion: a guide to goniometry,* Philadelphia, 1985, FA Davis.
10. Rancho Los Amigos Hospital: *How to measure range of motion of the upper extremities,* Unpublished manuscript.
11. Smith HD: Assessment and evaluation: an overview. In Hopkins HL, Smith HD, editors: *Willard and Spackman's occupational therapy,* ed 8, Philadelphia, 1993, JB Lippincott.
12. Thomas CL, editor: *Taber's cyclopedic medical dictionary,* ed 13, Philadelphia, 1977, FA Davis.

Evaluation of Muscle Strength

Lorraine Williams Pedretti

Many physical disabilities cause muscle weakness. Loss of strength places slight to substantial limitations on the performance of occupational roles, depending on the degree of weakness and whether the weakness is permanent or temporary. The occupational therapist must assess the weakness and plan treatment that will improve strength or compensate for the loss of strength if it is not expected to improve.

The manual muscle test (MMT) is a means of evaluating muscle strength. It measures the maximal contraction of a muscle or muscle group. The criteria used to measure strength are evidence of muscle contraction, amount of ROM through which the joint passes, and amount of resistance against which the muscle can contract, including gravity as a form of resistance.[6,8] The MMT is used to determine amount of muscle power and to record gains and losses in strength.

CAUSES OF MUSCLE WEAKNESS

Disabilities in which a loss of muscle strength is a primary symptom or direct result of the disease or injury include (1) the lower motor neuron disorders, such as peripheral neuropathies and peripheral nerve injuries, spinal cord injury (because those muscles innervated at the level[s] of the lesion generally have a lower motor neuron paralysis), Guillain-Barré syndrome, and cranial nerve dysfunctions; (2) primary muscle diseases, such as muscular dystrophy and myasthenia gravis; and (3) neurological diseases in which the lower motor neuron is affected, such as in amyotrophic lateral sclerosis or multiple sclerosis. Disabilities in which a loss of muscle strength is caused by disuse or immobilization rather than by a direct effect of the disease process include burns, amputation, hand trauma (unless there is an accompanying nerve injury), arthritis, fractures, and a variety of other orthopedic conditions. Although MMT is not appropriate for upper motor neuron disorders such as stroke or head injury, it may reveal some residual weakness in the final stages of recovery when spasticity and synergy patterns have disappeared and the patient has achieved isolated control of voluntary muscle function. In these instances some assessment of strength can be of value in designing a treatment program. (See Chapter 10 for methods of evaluating motor function of patients with upper motor neuron disorders.)

LIMITATIONS RESULTING FROM MUSCLE WEAKNESS

Muscle weakness can restrict the performance of occupational roles and thus prevent pursuit of self-care as well as vocational, leisure, and social activities. These limitations are assessed through muscle testing combined with performance testing. Given good to normal endurance, the patient with good (G) to normal (N) muscle strength will be able to perform all ordinary activities of daily living (ADL) without undue fatigue.[10] (Ordinary ADL are considered here to be all self-maintenance tasks, mobility, and vocational roles except strenuous labor.) The patient with fair plus (F+) muscle strength usually has low endurance and will fatigue more easily than one with G to N strength. The patient will be able to perform independently many ordinary ADL but may require frequent rest periods, however. The patient with muscle grades of fair (F) will be able to move parts against gravity and perform light tasks requiring little or no resistance.[8,10] Low endurance is an important problem and will limit the amount of activity that can be done. The patient can probably eat finger foods and perform light hygiene if given the time and rest periods needed to reach the goals.[10] If muscle strength in the lower extremities is only F, ambulation will not be possible.[8] Poor (P) strength is considered below functional range, but the patient can perform some ADL with mechanical assistance, and range of motion (ROM) can be maintained independently.[8] Patients with muscle grades of trace (T) and zero (0) are completely dependent and can perform no ADL without externally powered devices. Some activities are possible with special controls on equipment, such as electric wheelchair, electronic communication devices, and hand splints.[10]

PURPOSES FOR EVALUATING MUSCLE STRENGTH

Muscle testing, particularly the evaluation of individual muscles, is essential for diagnosis in some neuromuscular conditions, such as peripheral nerve lesions and spinal cord injury. In peripheral nerve or nerve root lesions the pattern of muscle weakness may help determine which nerve or nerve roots are involved and whether the involvement is partial or complete. Careful evaluation can help determine the level(s) of spinal cord involvement.[9] Therefore muscle testing along with sensory evaluation can be an important diagnostic aid in neuromuscular conditions.

The purposes for evaluating muscle strength are (1) to determine the amount of muscle power available and thus establish a baseline for treatment; (2) to discern how muscle weakness is limiting performance of ADL; (3) to prevent deformities that can result from imbalances of strength; (4) to determine the need for assistive devices as compensatory measures; (5) to aid in the selection of activities within the patient's capabilities; and (6) to evaluate the effectiveness of treatment.[10]

METHODS OF EVALUATION

Muscle strength can be evaluated in several ways. The most precise method is a test of individual muscles, as nearly as that is possible. In this procedure the muscle is carefully isolated through proper positioning, stabilization, and careful control of the movement pattern, and its strength is graded. This type of muscle testing is described by Kendall and McCreary[9] and Cole, Furness, and Twomey.[7] Another and perhaps a more common method of manual muscle testing is to assess the strength of groups of muscles that perform specific motions at each joint. This type of testing was described by Daniels and Worthingham[8] and, for the most part, is the form that is presented later in this chapter. Functional motion tests, functional muscle tests, or screening tests are also used to assess muscle strength. These tests are not as precise as manual muscle testing, and their purpose is to make a general evaluation of muscle strength and to determine areas of weakness and the need for more precise testing. Finally, muscle strength can be observed in the performance of ordinary activities.[8] During an ADL performance evaluation, for example, the therapist can observe for difficulties and movement patterns that may signal weakness, muscle imbalance, poor endurance for activity, and substitutions that are used for function. The performance evaluation should always be part of the assessment of strength.

RESULTS OF EVALUATION AS A BASIS FOR TREATMENT PLANNING

When planning treatment for the maintenance or improvement of strength, the occupational therapist must consider several factors before determining treatment priorities, goals, and modalities. The results of the muscle strength assessment will suggest the progression of a strengthening program. What is the degree of weakness? Is it generalized or specific to one or more muscle groups? Are the muscle grades generally the same throughout, or is there significant disparity in muscle grades? If there is disparity, is there an imbalance of strength between the agonist and antagonist muscle that will require protection of the weaker muscles during treatment and ADL? Where there is substantial imbalance between an agonist and antagonist muscle, treatment goals may be directed toward strengthening the weaker group while maintaining the strength of the stronger group. Muscle imbalance may also suggest the need for orthoses to protect the weaker muscles from overstretching while recovery is in progress. Devices such as the bed footboard to prevent overstretching of the weakened ankle dorsiflexors and the wrist cock-up splint to prevent overstretching of weakened wrist extensors are examples. Muscle grades will suggest the level and type of therapeutic exercise and activity that can help to maintain or improve strength. Is the weakness mild (G range), moderate (F to F+), or severe (P to 0)?[10] Muscles graded F−, for example, could be strengthened by using active assisted exercise or activity against gravity. Muscles graded P likewise will require active exercise in the gravity-decreased plane with little or no resistance to increase strength. Further discussion of appropriate exercise and activity for specific muscle grades appears in Chapter 18.

The endurance of the muscles (how many repetitions of the muscle contraction are possible before fatigue sets in) is an important consideration in treatment planning. Frequently one of the goals of the therapeutic activity program is to increase endurance as well as strength. Because the manual muscle test does not measure endurance, the therapist should assess it by engaging the patient in periods of exercise or activity graded in length to determine the amount of time that the muscle group can be used in sustained activity. There is usually a correlation between strength and endurance. Weaker muscles will tend to have less endurance than stronger ones. When selecting treatment modalities for increasing endurance, the therapist may elect not to tax the muscle to its maximal ability but rather to emphasize repetitive action at less than the maximal contraction to increase endurance and prevent fatigue.[10]

Sensory loss, which often accompanies muscle weakness, complicates the ability of the patient to perform in an activity program. If there is little or no tactile or proprioceptive feedback from motion, the impulse to move is decreased or lost, depending on the severity of the sensory loss. Thus the movement may appear weak and ineffective even when strength is adequate for performance of a specific activity. With some diagnoses, a sensory stimulation program may be indicated to increase the patient's sensory awareness and feedback from the part. In other instances the therapist may elect to help the patient compensate for the sensory loss through visual devices such as mirrors, video playback, and biofeedback, which can be used as adjuncts to the strengthening program.

Another important consideration is the diagnosis and expected course of the disease. Is strength expected to increase, decrease, or remain about the same? If it is expected to increase, what is the expected recovery period? What effect will exercise or activity have on muscle function? Will too much activity delay the progress of the recovery? If muscle power is expected to decrease, how rapid is the progression? Are there factors to be avoided that can accelerate the decrease in strength, such as a vigorous exercise program? If strength is declining, is special equipment practical and necessary? How much muscle power is needed to operate the equipment? How long will the patient be able to operate a device before a decrease in muscle power makes it impracticable?[10]

The therapist should assess the effect of the muscle weakness on the ability to perform ADL, which can be observed during the ADL evaluation. Which tasks are most difficult to perform because of the muscle weakness? How does the patient compensate for the weakness? Which tasks are most important for the patient to be able to perform? Is special equipment necessary or desirable for the performance of some ADL, such as the mobile arm support for independence in eating?[10]

If the patient is involved in a total rehabilitation program and receiving several other health care services, the strengthening and activity programs must be synchronized and well balanced to meet the patient's needs rather than the needs of the professionals, their schedules, and possibly their competition. The occupational therapist needs to be aware of the nature and extent of the programs in which the patient is engaged in physical therapy, recreation therapy, and any other services being received. Ideally the team should plan the exercise or activity program together to determine that the programs complement one another. Questions that may be asked are: What is the patient doing in each of the therapies? How long is each treatment session? Are the goals of all of the therapies similar or complementary, or are they divergent and conflicting? Is the patient being overfatigued in the total program? Are the various treatment sessions in rapid succession, or are they well spaced to meet the patient's need for rest periods?

On the basis of these considerations and of others pertinent to the specific patient, the occupational therapist can select enabling and functional activities designed to maintain or increase strength, improve performance of ADL, and enable the use of special equipment while protecting weak muscles from overstretching and overfatigue.

RELATIONSHIP BETWEEN JOINT ROM AND MUSCLE WEAKNESS

One criterion used to grade muscle strength is the excursion of the joint on which the muscle acts, that is, did the muscle move the joint through complete, partial, or no ROM. Another criterion is the amount of resistance that can be applied to the part once the muscle has moved the joint through the available ROM. In this context ROM is not necessarily the full average normal ROM for the given joint. Rather, it is the ROM available to the individual patient. When measuring joint motion, discussed in Chapter 8, it is the *passive* ROM that is the measure of the range available to the patient. Passive ROM, however, is no indication of muscle strength. When performing muscle testing, the occupational therapist must know what the patient's available passive ROM is in order to assign muscle grades correctly. It is possible that the passive ROM is limited or less than the average for that joint motion but that the muscle strength is normal. Therefore it is necessary for the therapist either to have measured joint ROM or to move the joint passively to assess the available ROM before administering the muscle test. For example, the patient's passive ROM for elbow flexion may be limited to 0° to 110° because of an old fracture. If the patient can flex the elbow joint to 110° and hold against moderate resistance during the muscle test, the grade would be G. In such cases the examiner should record the limitation with the muscle grade, for example, 0-110°/G.[8] Conversely, if the patient's available ROM for elbow flexion was 0° to 140°, and he or she flexed the elbow against gravity through only 110°, the muscle would be graded F −, because the part moved through only partial ROM against gravity. When the therapist determines the patient's available ROM before performing the muscle test, he or she can grade muscle strength on that basis rather than by using the average normal ROM as the standard.

LIMITATIONS OF THE MANUAL MUSCLE TEST

The limitations of the manual muscle test are that it cannot measure muscle endurance (number of times the muscle can contract at its maximum level), muscle coordination (smooth rhythmic interaction of muscle function), or motor performance capabilities of the patient (use of the muscles for functional activities).[7]

The manual muscle test cannot be used accurately with patients who have spasticity caused by upper motor neuron disorders, such as cerebrovascular accident (stroke) or cerebral palsy. In these disorders muscles are often hypertonic; muscle tone and ability to perform movements are influenced by primitive reflexes and the position of the head and body in space. Also, movements tend to occur in gross synergistic patterns that make it impossible for the patient to isolate joint motions, which is demanded in the manual muscle testing procedures.[2,3,6,11]

CONTRAINDICATIONS AND PRECAUTIONS

Assessment of strength using the MMT is contraindicated when there is dislocation or unhealed fracture; after surgery, particularly of musculoskeletal structures; if there is myositis ossificans; and in the presence of pain and inflammation.[6]

Special precautions must be taken when the patient is taking pain medications or muscle relaxants; has osteoporosis; has subluxation or hypermobility of a joint; has hemophilia or cardiovascular disease; has had abdominal surgery or has an abdominal hernia; and when fatigue can exacerbate the patient's condition.[6]

KNOWLEDGE AND SKILL OF THE EXAMINER

Validity of the manual muscle test depends on the examiner's knowledge and skill in using the correct testing procedure. Careful observation of movement, careful and accurate palpation, correct positioning, consistency of procedure, and experience of the examiner are critical factors in accurate testing.[8,9]

To be proficient in manual muscle testing, the examiner must have detailed knowledge about all aspects of muscle function. Joints and joint motions, muscle innervation, origin and insertion of muscles, action of muscles, direction of muscle fibers, angle of pull on the joints, and the role of muscles in fixation and substitution are important considerations. The examiner must be able to locate and palpate the muscles; recognize whether the contour of the muscle is normal, atrophied, or hypertrophied; and detect abnormal movements and positions. Knowledge and experience are necessary to detect substitutions and to interpret strength grades with accuracy.[9]

It is necessary for the examiner to acquire skill and experience in testing and grading muscles of normal persons of both sexes and of all ages. Many factors affect muscle strength. The age, gender and lifestyle of the subject, the muscle size, type and speed of contraction, the effect of previous training for the testing situation, and the joint position during the muscle contraction all can affect muscle strength.[6] Experience can help the examiner differentiate strength grades if these factors are taken into account.[12]

GENERAL PRINCIPLES OF MANUAL MUSCLE TESTING

PREPARATION FOR TESTING

When preparing to administer the muscle test, the examiner should observe contour of the part, comparative symmetry of muscle on both sides, and any apparent hypertrophy or atrophy. During passive ROM the examiner can estimate muscle tone. Is there lesser or greater than normal resistance to passive movement? During active ROM the examiner can observe quality of movement, such as movement speed, smoothness, rhythm, and any abnormal movements such as tremors.[12]

Correct positioning of the subject and the body part is essential to effective and correct evaluation. The subject should be positioned comfortably on a firm surface. Clothing should be arranged or removed so that the examiner can see the muscle or muscles being tested. If the subject cannot be placed in the correct position for the test, the examiner must adapt the test and use clinical judgment in approximating strength grades.[12] In addition to correct positioning, test validity depends on careful stabilization, palpation of the muscles, and observation of movement.[8]

GRAVITY FACTORS INFLUENCING MUSCLE FUNCTION

Gravity is a form of resistance to muscle power. It is used as a grading criterion in tests of the neck, trunk, and extremities, meaning that the muscle grade is based on whether or not a muscle can move the part against gravity.[9] Movements against gravity are in a vertical plane, that is, away from the floor or toward the ceiling and are used with grades F, G, and N. Movements against gravity and resistance are performed in a vertical plane with added manual or mechanical resistance and are used with F+ to N grades. Tests for the weaker muscles (O, T, P, and P+ grades) are often performed in a horizontal plane, that is, parallel to the floor, to reduce the resistance of gravity on the muscle power. This position has been referred to as the gravity-eliminated, gravity-decreased, or gravity-lessened test position.[8,9,12] Gravity eliminated is the common term to designate this position.[12] Because it is not possible completely to eliminate the effect of gravity on muscle function, however, gravity-decreased or gravity-lessened may be more accurate terms. The term gravity-decreased is used in this chapter.[8,9]

In many muscle tests the effect of gravity on the ability to perform the movement must be considered in grading muscle power. It is of lesser importance, however, in tests of the forearm, fingers, and toes because the weight of the part lifted against gravity is insignificant compared with the muscle strength.[8,9] Therefore the examiner may choose to do the tests for F to N in the gravity-decreased plane. In other tests, positioning for movements in the gravity-decreased position or the against-gravity position may not be feasible. For example, in the test for scapula depression, positioning to perform the movement against gravity would require the subject to assume an inverted position. In individual cases, positioning for movement in the correct plane may not be possible because of confinement to bed, generalized weakness, trunk instability, immobilization devices, and medical precautions. In these instances the examiner must adapt the positioning to the patient's needs and modify the grading using clinical judgment.

If tests of the forearm, fingers, and toes are done against gravity rather than in the gravity-decreased plane, the standard definitions of muscle grades can be modified when recording muscle grades. The partial ROM against gravity is graded P, and the full ROM against gravity is graded F.[8] Such modifications in positioning and grading should be noted by the examiner when recording results of the muscle test.

For consistency in procedure and grading, the gravity-decreased positions and against-gravity positions are used in the muscle testing procedures described later, except where the positioning is not feasible or would be awkward or uncomfortable for the subject. Modifications in positioning and grading have been cited with the individual tests.

MUSCLE GRADES

Although the definitions of the muscle grades are standard, the assignment of muscle grades during the manual muscle test depends on clinical judgment, knowledge, and experience of the examiner,[8] especially when determining slight, moderate, or maximal resistance. Age, sex, body type, occupation, and avocations all influence the amount of resistance that a particular subject can take.[8,9] Normal strength for an 8-year-old girl will be considerably less than for a 25-year-old man, for example. Additionally, strength tends to decline with age, and full resistance to the same muscle group will vary considerably from an 80-year-old man to a 25-year-old man.[6,9] Therefore the amount of resistance that can be applied to grade a particular muscle group as N or G varies from one individual to another.[8,9]

The amount of resistance that can be given also varies from one muscle group to another. Muscle strength is relative to the cross-sectional size of the muscle. Larger muscles have greater strength.[6,8] For example, the flexors of the wrist are larger and therefore have more power and can take much more resistance than the abductors of the fingers. The examiner must consider the size and relative power of the muscles and the leverage used when giving resistance.[10] The amount of resistance applied should be modified accordingly. When only one side of the body is involved in the dysfunction causing the muscle weakness, the examiner can establish the standards for strength by testing the unaffected side first.

Because weak muscles fatigue easily, results of muscle testing may not be accurate if the subject is tired. There should be no more than three repetitions of the test movement because fatigue can result in grading errors if the muscle becomes tired as a result of low endurance.[6,7] Pain, swelling, or muscle spasm in the area being tested may also interfere with the testing procedure and accurate grading. Such problems should be noted on the evaluation form.[12] Psychological factors must also be considered in interpreting muscle strength grades. The examiner must assess the motivation, cooperation, and effort put forth by the subject when interpreting strength.[8]

In manual muscle testing, muscles are graded according to the following criteria[8,13]:

Number Grade	Word/Letter Grade	Definition
0	Zero (0)	No muscle contraction can be seen or felt.
1	Trace (T)	Contraction can be felt, but there is no motion.
2 −	Poor minus (P −)	Part moves through incomplete ROM with gravity decreased.
2	Poor (P)	Part moves through complete ROM with gravity decreased.
2 +	Poor plus (P +)	Part moves through incomplete ROM (less than 50%) against gravity or through complete ROM with gravity decreased against slight resistance.[8]
3 −	Fair minus (F −)	Part moves through incomplete ROM (more than 50%) against gravity.[8]
3	Fair (F)	Part moves through complete ROM against gravity.
3 +	Fair plus (F +)	Part moves through complete ROM against gravity and slight resistance.
4	Good (G)	Part moves through complete ROM against gravity and moderate resistance.
5	Normal (N)	Part moves through complete ROM against gravity and full resistance.

The purpose of using plus or minus designations with the muscle grades is to "fine grade" muscle strength. These designations are likely to be used by the experienced examiner. Two examiners testing the same individual may vary up to a half grade in their results, but there should not be a whole grade difference.[12]

SUBSTITUTIONS

The brain "thinks" in terms of movement and not contraction of individual muscles.[8] Thus a muscle or muscle group may attempt to compensate for the function of a weaker muscle to accomplish a movement. These movements are called trick movements or substitutions.[6,9] Substitutions can occur during the manual muscle test. To test muscle strength accurately, it is necessary for the therapist to give careful instructions, to eliminate substitutions in the testing procedure by correct positioning, stabilization, palpation of the muscle being tested, and to ensure careful performance of the test motion without extraneous movements. The correct position of the body should be maintained and movement of the part performed without shifting the body or turning the part to allow substitutions.[6,9] The examiner must palpate contractile tissue (muscle fibers or tendon) to detect tension in the muscle group under examination. It is only through correct palpation that the examiner can be certain that the motion observed is not being performed by substitution.[8]

In the tests that follow, possible substitutions are described at the end of the directions. The examiner should be familiar with these substitutions to detect them and correct the procedure. Detecting substitutions is a skill gained with time and experience.

MUSCLE EXAMINATION

Patient's name _____ Chart no. _____

Date of birth _____ Name of institution _____

Date of onset _____ Attending physician _____ MD

Diagnosis:

LEFT   RIGHT

				Examiner's initials				
				Date				
			NECK	Flexors	Sternocleidomastoid			
				Extensor group				
			TRUNK	Flexors	Rectus abdominis			
				Rt. ext. obl. / Lt. int. obl. Rotators	{ Lt. ext. obl. / Rt. int. obl.			
				Extensors	{ Thoracic group / Lumbar group			
				Pelvic elev.	Quadratus lumb.			
			HIP	Flexors	Iliopsoas			
				Extensors	Gluteus maximus			
				Abductors	Gluteus medius			
				Adductor group				
				External rotator group				
				Internal rotator group				
				Sartorius				
				Tensor fasciae latae				
			KNEE	Flexors	{ Biceps femoris / Inner hamstrings			
				Extensors	Quadriceps			
			ANKLE	Plantar flexors	{ Gastrocnemius / Soleus			
			FOOT	Invertors	{ Tibialis anterior / Tibialis posterior			
				Evertors	{ Peroneus brevis / Peroneus longus			
			TOES	MP flexors	Lumbricales			
				IP flexors (first)	Flex. digit. br.			
				IP flexors (second)	Flex. digit. l.			
				MP extensors	{ Ext. digit. l. / Ext. digit. br.			
			HALLUX	MP flexor	Flex. hall. br.			
				IP flexor	Flex. hall. l.			
				MP extensor	Ext. hall. br.			
				IP extensor	Ext. hall. l.			

Measurements:

Cannot walk   Date   Speech

Stands   Date   Swallowing

Walks unaided   Date   Diaphragm

Walks with apparatus   Date   Intercostals

KEY

5	N	Normal	Complete range of motion against gravity with full resistance.
4	G	Good*	Complete range of motion against gravity with some resistance.
3	F	Fair*	Complete range of motion against gravity.
2	P	Poor*	Complete range of motion with gravity eliminated.
1	T	Trace	Evidence of slight contractility. No joint motion.
0	0	Zero	No evidence of contractility.
S or SS			Spasm or severe spasm.
C or CC			Contracture or severe contracture.

*Muscle spasm or contracture may limit range of motion. A question mark
should be placed after the grading of a movement that is incomplete from
this cause.

FIG. 9-1   Muscle examination. Adapted with the express permission and authority of the
March of Dimes Birth Defects Foundation.

LEFT   RIGHT

				Examiner's initials						
				Date						
			SCAPULA	Abductor	Serratus anterior					
				Elevator	Upper trapezius					
				Depressor	Lower trapezius					
				Adductors	Middle trapezius					
					Rhomboids					
			SHOULDER	Flexor	Anterior deltoid					
				Extensors	Latissimus dorsi					
					Teres major					
				Abductor	Middle deltoid					
				Horiz. abd.	Posterior deltoid					
				Horiz. add.	Pectoralis major					
				External rotator group						
				Internal rotator group						
			ELBOW	Flexors	Biceps brachii					
					Brachioradialis					
				Extensor	Triceps					
			FOREARM	Supinator group						
				Pronator group						
			WRIST	Flexors	Flex. carpi rad.					
					Flex. carpi uln.					
				Extensors	Ext. carpi rad.					
					l. & br.					
					Ext. carpi uln.					
			FINGERS	MP flexors	Lumbricales					
				IP flexors (first)	Flex. digit. sub.					
				IP flexors (second)	Flex. digit. prof.					
				MP extensor	Ext. digit. com.					
				Adductors	Palmar interossei					
				Abductors	Dorsal interossei					
				Abductor digiti quinti						
				Opponens digiti quinti						
			THUMB	MP flexor	Flex. poll. br.					
				IP flexor	Flex. poll. l.					
				MP extensor	Ext. poll. br.					
				IP extensor	Ext. poll. l.					
				Abductors	Abd. poll. br.					
					Abd. poll. l.					
				Adductor pollicis						
				Opponens pollicis						
			FACE							

Additional data:

FIG. 9-1, cont'd Muscle examination.

PROCEDURE FOR MANUAL MUSCLE TESTING

Testing should be performed according to a standard procedure to ensure accuracy and consistency. The tests that follow are divided into steps: (1) position, (2) stabilize, (3) palpate, (4) observe, (5) resist, and (6) grade.

First the subject (S) should be *positioned* for the specific muscle test. The examiner (E) should position himself or herself in relation to S. Then E *stabilizes* the part proximal to the part being tested to eliminate extraneous movements, isolate the muscle group, ensure the correct test motion, and eliminate substitutions. E should then demonstrate or describe the test motion to S and ask S to perform the test motion and return to the starting position. E makes a general observation of the form and quality of movement, looking for substitutions or difficulties that may require adjustments in positioning and stabilization. E then places fingers for *palpation* of one or more of the prime movers, or its tendinous insertion, in the muscle group being tested and asks S to repeat the test motion. E again *observes* the movement for possible substitution and the amount of range completed. When S has moved the part through the available ROM, S is asked to hold the end position. E removes the palpating fingers and uses this hand to *resist* in the opposite direction of the test movement; for example, when elbow flexion is tested, E applies resistance in the direction of extension. E usually must maintain stabilization when resistance is given. These muscle tests use the break test; that is, the resistance is applied after S has reached the end of the available ROM.

Muscles exert different amounts of force at various points in the ROM. In the break test, resistance is applied near the weakest point in the ROM. If the examiner is consistent and always uses the same procedure, however, reliability of the results will not be affected. Functional interpretation of the muscle grade may be not as accurate, however.[8]

S should be allowed to establish a maximal contraction (set the muscles) before the resistance is applied.[8,10] E applies the resistance after preparing S by giving the command to hold. Resistance should be applied gradually in a direction opposite to the line of pull of the muscle or muscle group being tested. The break test should not evoke pain, and resistance should be released immediately if pain or discomfort occurs.[8] Finally, E grades the muscle strength according to the preceding standard definitions of muscle grades. This procedure is used for the tests of strength of grades F and above. Resistance is not applied for tests of muscles from P to 0. Slight resistance is sometimes applied to a muscle that has completed the full ROM in the gravity-decreased plane to determine if the grade is P+. Fig. 9-1 shows a sample form for recording muscle grades.

SEQUENCE OF MUSCLE TESTING[8]

To avoid frequent repositioning of the subject, the tests can be given in the sequence outlined so that they are performed in order of backlying position, facelying position, sidelying position, and finally, sitting position (see Box 9-1).

LIMITATIONS OF INSTRUCTIONS FOR PROCEDURES

The following directions do not include tests for the face, neck, and trunk. Refer to Kendall and McCreary,[9] Clarkson and Gilewich,[6] or Daniels and Worthingham[8] for these tests.

MANUAL MUSCLE TESTING OF THE UPPER EXTREMITY*

Motion

Scapula elevation, neck rotation, and lateral flexion

Muscles[8]	Innervation (Nerve, Nerve Roots)[8,9]
Upper trapezius	Accessory nerve, (Cr. 11), C2,3,4
Levator scapula	Dorsal scapular nerve, C3,4,5

Procedure for Testing Grades Normal (N or 5) to Fair (F or 3)

Position: S is seated erect with arms resting at sides of body. E stands behind S toward the side to be tested.

Stabilize: Chair back can offer stabilization to the trunk, if necessary.

Palpate: The upper trapezius parallel to the cervical vertebrae, near the shoulder-neck curve.[8]

Observe: Elevation of the scapula as S shrugs the shoulder toward the ear, rotates and laterally flexes the neck toward the side being tested at the same time (Fig. 9-2, A).[9]

Resist: With one hand on top of the shoulder toward scapula depression and with the other hand on the side of the head toward derotation and lateral flexion to the opposite side (Fig. 9-2, B).[9]

Procedure for Testing Grades Poor (P or 2), Trace (T or 1), and Zero (0)

Position: S lying prone with the head in midposition. E stands opposite the side being tested.

Stabilize: Weight of the trunk on the supporting surface is adequate stabilization.

Palpate: The upper trapezius as described above while observing S shrug the shoulder being tested. Because of the positioning, the neck rotation and lateral flexion components are omitted for these grades (Fig. 9-2, C).

Grade: According to standard definitions of muscle grades.

Substitutions: Rhomboids and levator scapula can elevate the scapula if the upper trapezius is weak or absent. In the event of substitution, some downward rotation of the acromion would be observed during the movement.[4,10,13]

---

* E refers to examiner or therapist, S is subject or patient. Normal (5) to fair (3) tests are performed so muscle moves part in vertical plane or against gravity. Poor (2) to zero (0) tests move part in horizontal plane or gravity-decreased position.

BOX 9-1

SEQUENCE OF MUSCLE TESTING

Backlying (spine)

Grades N to F

Scapula abduction and upward rotation

Shoulder horizontal adduction

All tests for forearm, wrist, and fingers can be given in the backlying position if necessary

Grades P to O

Shoulder abduction

Elbow flexion

Hip abduction

Hip adduction

Hip external rotation

Hip internal rotation

Foot inversion

Foot eversion

Sidelying

Grades N to F

Hip abduction

Hip adduction

Foot inversion

Foot eversion

Grades P to O

Shoulder flexion

Shoulder extension

Hip flexion

Hip extension

Knee flexion

Knee extension

Ankle plantar flexion

Ankle dorsiflexion

Facelying (prone)

Grades N to F

Scapula depression

Scapula adduction

Scapula adduction and downward rotation

Shoulder extension

Shoulder external rotation

Shoulder internal rotation

Shoulder horizontal abduction

Elbow extension

Hip extension

Knee flexion

Ankle plantar flexion

Grades P to O

Scapula elevation

Scapula depression

Scapula adduction

Sitting

Grades N to F

Scapula elevation

Shoulder flexion

Shoulder abduction

Elbow flexion

All forearm, wrist, finger, and thumb movements

Hip flexion

Hip external rotation

Hip internal rotation

Knee extension

Ankle dorsiflexion with inversion

Grades P to O

All forearm, wrist, finger, and thumb movements

Ankle dorsiflexion with inversion

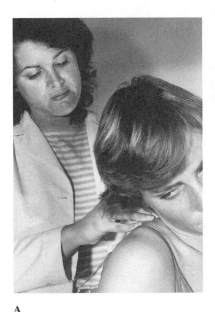
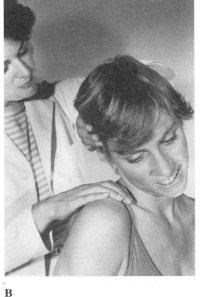
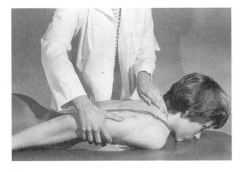

A   **B**   **C**

FIG. 9-2   Scapula elevation. **A,** Palpate and observe. **B,** Resist. **C,** Gravity-decreased position.

Motion

Scapula depression, adduction, and upward rotation

Muscles[1,4]	Innervation[6]
Lower trapezius	Accessory nerve, spinal portion
Middle trapezius	Accessory nerve, spinal portion
Serratus anterior	Long thoracic nerve, C5,6,7

Procedure for Testing Grades N (5) to F (3)

Position: *S* lying prone with arm positioned overhead in approximately 120° to 130° of abduction and resting on the supporting surface. *E* stands next to *S* on the opposite side.[6,8]

Stabilize: Weight of the body is adequate stabilization. This test is given in the gravity-decreased position because it is not feasible to position *S* for the against-gravity movement (head down).

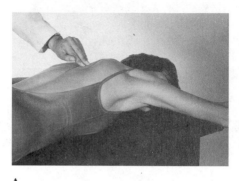
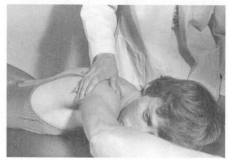
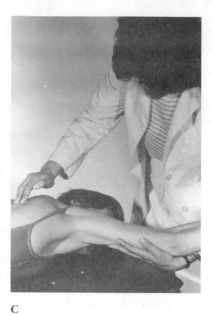

A   B   C

FIG. 9-3   Scapula depression. **A,** Palpate and observe. **B,** Resist. **C,** Test for Grades P to O.

If deltoid is weak, arm may be supported and passively raised by *E* while *S* attempts the motion.[8]

Palpate: The lower trapezius distal to the medial end of the spine of the scapula and parallel to the thoracic vertebrae approximately at the level of the inferior angle of the scapula.[8]

Observe: *S* lift the arm up off the supporting surface. During this movement, there is strong downward fixation of the scapula by the lower trapezius (Fig. 9-3, *A*).[8]

Resist: At the lateral angle of the scapula toward elevation and abduction (Fig. 9-3, *B*).[8] Resistance may be given on the dorsum of the forearm in a downward direction if shoulder and elbow strength are adequate.[9]

Procedure for Testing Grades P (2), T (1), and 0

Position and stabilize: As described for previous test. No stabilization is required unless it is necessary for *E* to support *S*'s arm because of weak posterior deltoid and triceps.

Palpation and observation: Same as described for previous test (Fig. 9-3, *C*).

Grade: According to modified grading criteria. F for full ROM: P if 50% ROM was achieved.[8]

Substitutions: Rhomboids may substitute. Rotation of the inferior angle of the scapula toward the spine is evidence of substitution.[13]

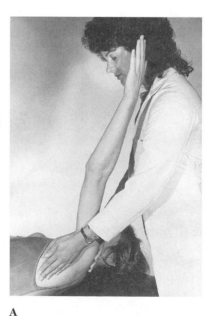
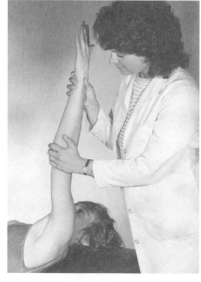
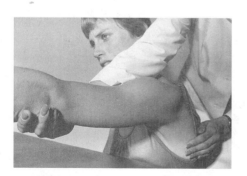

A   B   C

FIG. 9-4   Scapula abduction. **A,** Palpate and observe. **B,** Resist. **C,** Gravity-decreased position.

Motion

Scapula abduction and upward rotation

Muscles[8,9]	Innervation[8,9]
Serratus anterior	Long thoracic nerve, C5,6,7

Procedure for Testing Grades N (5) to F (3)

Position: S lying supine with the shoulder flexed to 90° and slightly abducted, elbow extended or fully flexed.[6,8,9] E stands next to S on the side being tested.
Stabilize: Over the shoulder.
Palpate: The digitations of the origin of the serratus anterior on the ribs, along the midaxillary line and just distal and anterior to the axillary border of the scapula.[8] Note that muscle contraction may be difficult to detect in women and overweight subjects.
Observe: S reach upward as if pushing the arm toward the ceiling, abducting the scapula (Fig. 9-4, A).[8]
Resist: At the distal end of the humerus and push arm directly downward toward scapula adduction (Fig. 9-4, B).[6,8] If there is

shoulder instability, E should support the arm and not apply resistance. In this instance, only a grade of F (3) can be tested.[6]

Procedure for Testing Grades P (2), T (1), and 0

Position: S seated at a high table with the arm resting on it in 90° of shoulder flexion.[8] E supports S's arm slightly above the table surface to eliminate resistance from friction and the weight of the arm.
Stabilize: Over the shoulder to be tested.
Palpate: The digitations of the serratus anterior on the ribs along the midaxillary line just distal and anterior to the axillary border of the scapula.
Observe: For abduction of the scapula as the arm moves forward (Fig. 9-4, C).[8] Weakness of this muscle produces "winging" of the scapula.[7]
Grade: According to standard definitions of muscle grades.
Substitutions: Pectoralis major may pull scapula forward into abduction at its insertion on humerus. E observes for humeral horizontal adduction followed by scapula abduction.[6,10]

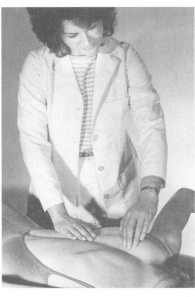 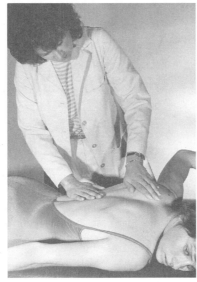 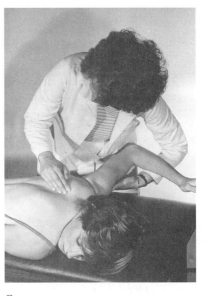

A   B   C

FIG. 9-5   Scapula adduction. **A,** Palpate and observe. **B,** Resist. **C,** Test for Grades P to O.

Motion

Scapula adduction

Muscles[8,9]	Innervation[8]
Middle trapezius	Spinal accessory nerve, C3,4
Rhomboids	Dorsal scapular nerve, C5

Procedure for Testing Grades N (5) to F (3)

Position: Lying prone with the shoulder abducted to 90° and elbow flexed to 90°, humerus resting on the supporting surface. E stands on the side being tested.[8,9]
Stabilize: Weight of the trunk on the supporting surface is usually adequate stabilization or over the midthorax to prevent trunk rotation, if necessary.
Palpate: The middle trapezius between the spine of the scapula and the adjacent vertebrae in alignment with the abducted humerus.
Observe: Movement of the vertebral border of the scapula toward the thoracic vertebrae as the arm is lifted off the supporting surface (Fig. 9-5, A).

Resist: At the vertebral border of the scapula toward abduction (Fig. 9-5, B).[6,8]

Procedure for Testing Grades P (2), T (1), and 0

Position and stabilize: As described for previous test, but E now supports the weight of the arm by cradling under the humerus and forearm.[10] S may also be positioned sitting erect with arm resting on a high table and the shoulder midway between 90° flexion and abduction.[8] E stands behind S in this instance.
Palpate and observe: The middle trapezius. Ask E to bring the shoulders together as if assuming an erect posture. Observe movement of the scapula toward the vertebral column (Fig. 9-5, C).
Grade: According to standard definitions of muscle grades.
Substitutions: Posterior deltoid can act on the humerus and produce scapula adduction. Observe for humeral extension being used to initiate scapula adduction. Rhomboids may substitute but scapula will rotate downward.[6,10,13]

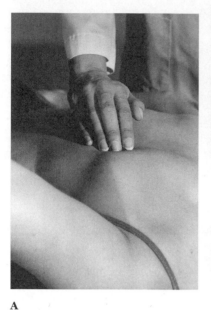
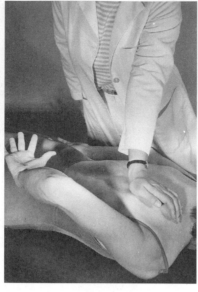
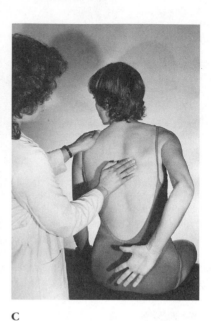

A   **B**   **C**

FIG. 9-6   Scapula adduction and downward rotation. **A,** Palpate and observe. **B,** Resist, **C,** Gravity-decreased position.

Motion

Scapula adduction and downward rotation

Muscles[6,7]	Innervation[6,7]
Rhomboids major and minor	Dorsal scapular nerve, C5
Levator scapula	Dorsal scapular nerve, C3,4,5
Middle trapezius	Spinal accessory nerve, C3,4

Procedure for Testing Grades N (5) to F (3)

Position: *S* lying prone with the head rotated to the opposite side; arm on the side being tested is placed in shoulder adduction and internal rotation with the elbow slightly flexed and the dorsum of the hand resting over the lumbosacral area of back. *E* stands opposite the side being tested.[6,7,8]

Stabilize: Weight of the trunk on the supporting surface offers adequate stabilization.[6,9]

Palpate: Rhomboid muscles between the vertebral border of the scapula and the 2nd to 5th thoracic vertebrae.[8,9] (They may be more easily discerned toward the lower half of the vertebral border of the scapula, because they lie under the trapezius muscle.)

Observe: As *S* raises the hand up off the back.[6] During this motion the anterior aspect of the shoulder must lift from the table surface. Observe scapula adduction and downward rotation while the shoulder joint is in some extension (Fig. 9-6, *A*).[8]

Resist: On the vertebral border of the scapula toward abduction and upward rotation (Fig. 9-6, *B*).

Procedure for Testing Grades P (2), T (1), and 0

Position: *S* sitting erect with the arm positioned behind the back in the same manner described for previous test. *E* stands behind *S* a little opposite the side being tested.[8]

Stabilize: Trunk by placing one hand over the shoulder opposite the one being tested to prevent trunk flexion and rotation.

Palpate: The rhomboids.

Observe: Scapula adduction and downward rotation as *S* lifts the hand away from the back (Fig. 9-6, *C*).

Grade: According to standard definitions of muscle grades.

Substitutions: Middle trapezius, but the movement will not be accompanied by downward rotation. Posterior deltoid acting to perform horizontal abduction or glenohumeral extension can produce scapula adduction through momentum. Scapula adduction would be preceded by extension or abduction of the humerus.[10,13] Pectoralis minor could tip the scapula forward.[6]

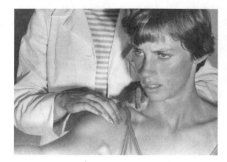
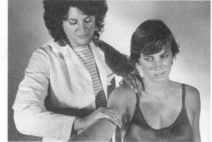
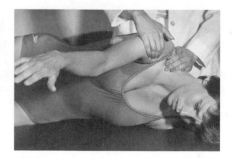

A   **B**   **C**

FIG. 9-7   Shoulder flexion. **A,** Palpate and observe. **B,** Resist. **C,** Gravity-decreased position.

Motion

Shoulder flexion

Muscles[8]	Innervation[8]
Anterior deltoid	Axillary nerve, C5,6
Coracobrachialis	Musculocutaneous nerve, C6,7

Procedure for Testing Grades N (5) to F (3)

Position: *S* seated with the arm relaxed at the side of the body with the hand facing backward. A straightback chair may be used to offer trunk support. *E* stands on the side being tested and slightly behind *S*.[6,8,13]

Stabilize: Over the shoulder being tested, but allow the normal abduction and upward rotation of the scapula that occurs with this movement.[8]

Palpate: The anterior deltoid just below the clavicle on the anterior aspect of the humeral head.[6]

Observe: *S* flex the shoulder joint by raising the arm horizontally to 90° of flexion (parallel to the floor) (Fig. 9-7, *A*).[8]

Resist: At the distal end of the humerus downward toward shoulder extension (Fig. 9-7, *B*).[6,7]

Procedure for Testing Grades P(2), T(1), and 0

Position: *S* in sidelying. Side being tested is superior. If *S* cannot maintain weight of the arm against gravity, it can be supported on a smooth, powdered board placed under it or by *E*. *E* stands behind *S*.[8,13] If the sidelying position is not feasible, *S* may remain seated, and the test procedure described above can be performed with grading modified.[8]

Palpate and observe: Same as described for previous test. The arm is moved forward toward the face to 90° of shoulder flexion (Fig. 9-7, *C*).

Grade: According to standard definitions of muscle grades. If the seated position was used for the tests of grades poor to zero, partial ROM against gravity should be graded poor.[8]

Substitutions: Pectoralis major, clavicular fibers, can perform flexion through partial ROM while performing horizontal adduction. Biceps brachii may flex the shoulder, but the humerus will first be rotated externally for the best mechanical advantage. The upper trapezius will assist flexion by elevating the scapula. Observe for flexion accompanied by horizontal adduction, external rotation, or scapula elevation.[10,13]

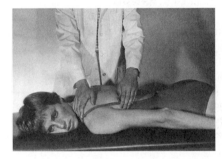
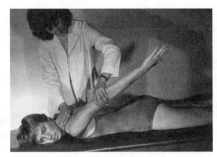
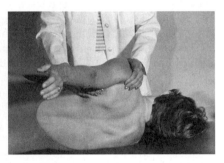

A   **B**   **C**

FIG. 9-8   Shoulder extension. **A,** Palpate and observe. **B,** Resist. **C,** Gravity-decreased position.

Motion

Shoulder extension

Muscles[4,8,9]	Innervation[8]
Latissimus dorsi	Thoracodorsal nerve, C6,7,8
Teres major	Inferior subscapular nerve, C5,6
Posterior deltoid	Axillary nerve, C5,6

Procedure for Testing Grades N (5) to F (3)

Position: *S* prone lying with the shoulder joint adducted and internally rotated so that the palm of the hand is facing up.[6] *E* stands on the opposite side.

Stabilize: Over the scapula on the side being tested.

Palpate: The teres major along the axillary border of the scapula. The latissimus dorsi may be palpated slightly below this point or closer to its origins parallel to the thoracic and lumbar vertebrae.[6,8] The posterior deltoid may be found over the posterior aspect of the humeral head.

Observe: As *S* lifts the arm up off the table extending the shoulder joint (Fig. 9-8, *A*).

Resist: At the distal end of the humerus in a downward and outward direction, toward flexion and slight abduction (Fig. 9-8, *B*).[6,8,9]

Procedure for Testing Grades P(2), T(1), and 0

Position: *S* in the sidelying position; *E* stands behind *S*.

Stabilize: Over the scapula. If *S* cannot maintain the weight of the part against gravity, *E* should support *S*'s arm or place a smooth board between the arm and the trunk. If the sidelying position is not feasible, *S* may remain in the prone lying position and the test may be performed as described for previous test with modified grading.[8]

Palpate: The teres major or latissimus dorsi as described for previous test.

Observe: *S* move the arm backward in a plane parallel to the floor (Fig. 9-8, *C*).

Grade: According to standard definitions of muscle grades. If the test for grades poor to zero was done in the prone lying position, completion of partial ROM should be graded poor.[8]

Substitutions: Scapula adduction will affect some shoulder extension. Observe for flexion of the shoulder or adduction of the scapula preceding extension of the humerus.[10]

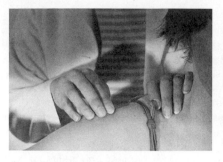 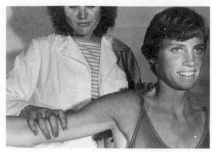 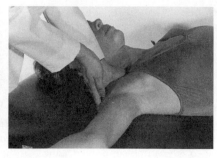

A   B   C

FIG. 9-9 Shoulder abduction. **A,** Palpate and observe. **B,** Resist. **C,** Gravity-decreased position.

Motion

Shoulder abduction

Muscles[8,9]	Innervation[8]
Middle deltoid	Axillary nerve, C5,6
Supraspinatus	Suprascapular nerve, C5

Procedure for Testing Grades N (5) to F (3)

Position: *S* seated with the arms relaxed at sides of body. The elbow on the side to be tested should be slightly flexed and the palms facing toward the body. *E* stands behind *S*.[6]

Stabilize: Over the scapula on the side to be tested.[8,9]

Palpate: The middle deltoid over the middle of the shoulder joint from the acromion to the deltoid tuberosity.[8,9,10] The supraspinatus may be difficult to palpate because it lies under the trapezius muscle, but it may be palpated in the supraspinatus fossa.

Observe: *S* abduct the shoulder to 90°. During the movement *S*'s palm should remain down and *E* should observe that there is no external rotation of the shoulder or elevation of the scapula.[8,9,10] (Fig. 9-9, *A*).

Resist: At the distal end of the humerus as if pushing the arm down toward adduction (Fig. 9-9, *B*).

Procedure for Testing Grades P(2), T (1), and 0

Position: *S* in supine lying with the arm to be tested resting at the side of the body, palm facing in and the elbow slightly flexed. *E* stands in front of the supporting surface toward the side to be tested.

Stabilize: Over the shoulder to be tested.

Palpate and observe: Same as described for previous test. *E* asks *S* to bring the arm out and away from the body, abducting the shoulder to 90° (Fig. 9-9, *C*).

Grade: According to standard definitions of muscle grades.

Substitutions: The long head of the biceps may attempt to substitute. Observe for elbow flexion and external rotation accompanying the movement. The anterior and posterior deltoids can act together to effect abduction. The upper trapezius may attempt to assist. Observe for scapula elevation preceding the movement.[6,10,13]

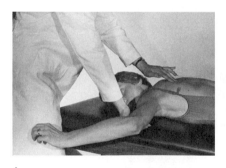 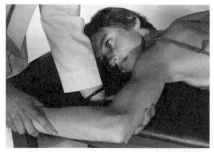 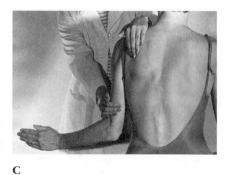

A   B   C

FIG. 9-10 Shoulder external rotation. **A,** Palpate and observe. **B,** Resist. **C,** Gravity-decreased position.

Motion

Shoulder external rotation

Muscles[4,8,9,10]	Innervation[4,8,9]
Infraspinatus	Suprascapular nerve, C5,6
Teres minor	Axillary nerve, C5,6

Procedure for Testing Grades N (5) to F (3)

Position: *S* lying prone with the shoulder abducted to 90° and the humerus in neutral (0°) rotation, elbow flexed to 90°. Forearm is in neutral rotation, hanging over the edge of the table, perpendicular to the floor.[6,7] *E* stands in front of the supporting surface toward the side to be tested.[8,9]

Stabilize: At the distal end of the humerus by placing a hand under the arm on the supporting surface to prevent shoulder abduction.[6,9]

Palpate: The infraspinatus muscle just below the spine of the scapula on the body of the scapula or the teres minor along the axillary border of the scapula.[8]

Observe: Rotation of the humerus so that the back of the hand is moving toward the ceiling (Fig. 9-10, *A*).[6,8,9]

Resist: On the distal end of forearm toward the floor in the direction of internal rotation (Fig. 9-10, *B*).[8,9]

Procedure for Testing Grades P (2), T (1), and 0

Position: *S* seated with arm adducted and in neutral rotation at the shoulder. The elbow is flexed to 90° with the forearm in neutral rotation. *E* stands in front of *S* toward the side to be tested.[6]

Stabilize: Arm against the trunk at the distal end of the humerus to prevent abduction and extension of the shoulder and over the shoulder to be tested.[5,6,13] The hand stabilizing over the shoulder can be used to palpate the infraspinatus simultaneously.

Palpate: The infraspinatus and teres minor as described for previous test.

Observe: Movement of the forearm away from the body by rotating the humerus while maintaining neutral rotation of the forearm (Fig. 9-10, *C*).[13]

Grade: According to standard definitions of muscle grades.

Substitutions: If the elbow is extended and *S* supinates the forearm, the momentum could aid external rotation of the humerus. Scapular adduction can pull the humerus backward and into some external rotation. *E* should observe for scapula adduction and initiation of movement with forearm supination.[10,13]

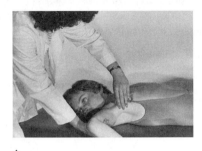
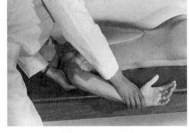
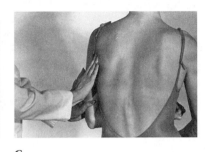

| A | B | C |

FIG. 9-11 Shoulder internal rotation. **A,** Palpate and observe. **B,** Resist. **C,** Gravity-decreased position.

Motion

Shoulder internal rotation

Muscles[8,9,10]	Innervation[4,5,8]
Subscapularis	Subscapular nerve, C5,6
Pectoralis major	Anterior thoracic nerve, C5 through T1
Latissimus dorsi	Thoracodorsal nerve, C6,7,8
Teres major	Subscapular nerve, C5,6

Procedure for Testing Grades N (5) to F (3)

Position: *S* lying prone with the shoulder abducted to 90° and the humerus in neutral rotation, the elbow flexed to 90°. The forearm is perpendicular to the floor. *E* stands on the side to be tested just in front of *S*'s arm.[6,7]

Stabilize: At the distal end of the humerus by placing a hand under the arm and on the supporting surface as for external rotation.[6,8,9]

Palpate: The teres major and latissimus dorsi along the axillary border of the scapula toward the inferior angle.

Observe: Movement of the palm of the hand upward toward the ceiling, internally rotating the humerus (Fig. 9-11, *A*).[8]

Resist: At the distal end of the volar surface of the forearm anteriorly toward external rotation (Fig. 9-11, *B*).[6,8,9]

Procedure for Testing Grades P (2), T (1), and 0

Position: *S* seated with the shoulder adducted and in neutral rotation, elbow flexed to 90° with the forearm in neutral rotation. *E* stands on the side to be tested.[13]

Stabilize: Arm at the distal end of the humerus against the trunk to prevent abduction and extension of the shoulder.

Palpate: The teres major and latissimus dorsi as described for previous test.

Observe: *S* move the palm of the hand toward the chest, internally rotating the humerus (Fig. 9-11, *C*).

Substitutions: If the trunk is rotated, gravity will act on the humerus, rotating it internally. *E* should observe for trunk rotation. If the arm is in extension, pronation of the forearm can substitute.[10,13] Elbow extension or shoulder abduction can be used to substitute.[6]

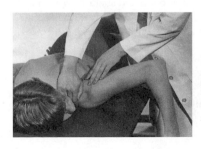
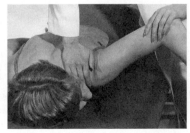
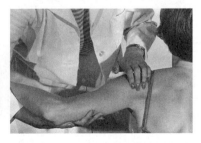

| A | B | C |

FIG. 9-12 Shoulder horizontal abduction. **A,** Palpate and observe. **B,** Resist. **C,** Gravity-decreased position.

Motion

Shoulder horizontal abduction

Muscles[4,8,10]	Innervation[8]
Posterior deltoid	Axillary nerve, C5,6
Infraspinatus	Suprascapular nerve, C5,6

Procedure for Testing Grades N (5) to F (3)

Position: S prone with the shoulder abducted to 90° and in slight external rotation, elbow flexed to 90°, and forearm perpendicular to the floor. E stands on the side being tested.[9,10]

Stabilize: Over the scapula.[8]

Palpate: The posterior deltoid below the spine of the scapula and distally toward the deltoid tuberosity on the posterior aspect of the shoulder.[8]

Observe: Movement of the arm as it is lifted toward the ceiling, horizontally abducting the humerus (Fig. 9-12, *A*).

Resist: Just proximal to the elbow obliquely downward toward adduction and horizontal adduction (Fig. 9-12, *B*).[9]

Procedure for Testing Grades P (2), T (1), and 0

Position: S seated with the arm in 90° abduction, the elbow flexed to 90°, and the palm down, supported on a high table or by E. If a table is used, powder may be sprinkled on the surface to reduce friction.

Palpate: Posterior deltoid as described for previous test.

Observe: As the arm is pulled backward into horizontal abduction (Fig. 9-12, *C*).

Grade: According to standard definitions of muscle grades.

Substitutions: Latissimus dorsi and teres major may assist the movement if the posterior deltoid is very weak. Movement will occur with more shoulder extension rather than at the horizontal level. Scapula adduction may produce slight horizontal abduction of the humerus, but trunk rotation and shoulder retraction would occur.[10,13]

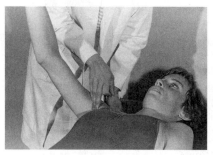 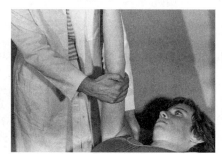 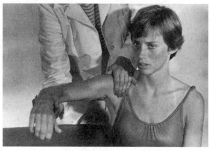

A   B   C

FIG. 9-13   Shoulder horizontal adduction. **A,** Palpate and observe. **B,** Resist. **C,** Gravity-decreased position.

Motion

Shoulder horizontal adduction

Muscles[4,10]	Innervation[4,8]
Pectoralis major	Medial and lateral anterior thoracic nerves, C5,6,7,8, T1
Anterior deltoid	Axillary nerve, C5,6
Coracobrachialis	Musculocutaneous nerve, C6,7

Procedure for Testing Grades N (5) to F (3)

Position: S supine with the shoulder abducted to 90°, elbow flexed or extended. E stands next to S on the side being tested or behind S's head.[4,6,8]

Stabilize: The trunk by placing one hand over the shoulder on the side being tested to prevent trunk rotation and scapula elevation.

Palpate: Over the insertion of the pectoralis major at the anterior aspect of the axilla.

Observe: S move the arm toward the opposite shoulder, horizontally adducting the humerus to a position of 90° of shoulder flexion.[9] If S cannot maintain elbow extension, E may guide the forearm to prevent the hand from hitting S's face (Fig. 9-13, *A*).

Resist: At the distal end of the humerus in an outward direction toward horizontal abduction (Fig. 9-13, *B*).[6,8]

Procedure for Testing Grades P (2), T (1), and 0

Position: S seated next to a high table with the arm supported in 90° of shoulder abduction and slight flexion at the elbow.[4,13] Powder may be sprinkled on the supporting surface to reduce the effect of resistance from friction during the movement, or E may support the arm.

Stabilize: Over the shoulder on the side being tested, using the stabilizing hand simultaneously to palpate the pectoralis major muscle.

Palpate: Pectoralis major as described for previous test.

Observe: S move the arm toward the opposite shoulder, horizontally adducting it in a plane parallel to the floor (Fig. 9-13, *C*).

Substitutions: Muscles may substitute for one another. If the pectoralis major is not functioning, the other muscles will perform the motion, which will be considerably weakened.[10]

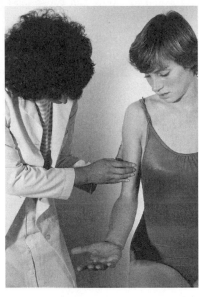
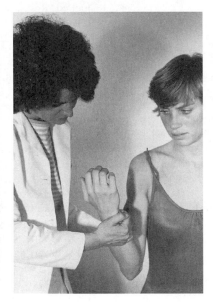
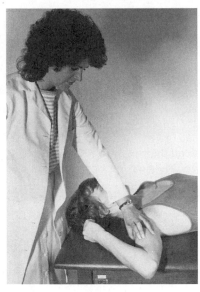

A   B   C

FIG. 9-14 Elbow flexion. **A**, Palpate and observe. **B**, Resist. **C**, Gravity-decreased position.

Motion

Elbow flexion

Muscles[8,9,10]	Innervation[9]
Biceps brachii	Musculocutaneous nerve C5,6
Brachialis	Musculocutaneous nerve C5,6
Brachioradialis	Radial nerve C5,6

Procedure for Testing Grades N (5) to F (3)

Position: S sitting with the arm adducted at the shoulder and extended at the elbow, held against the side of the trunk. The forearm is supinated to test for the biceps, primarily. (Forearm should be positioned in pronation to test for the brachialis, primarily and in midposition to test for brachioradialis).[8] E stands next to S on the side being tested or directly in front of S.

Stabilize: Humerus in adduction.

Palpate: The biceps brachii over the muscle belly on the middle of the anterior aspect of the humerus. Its tendon may be palpated in the middle of the antecubital space.[6,8] (Brachioradialis is palpated over the upper third of the radius on the lateral aspect of the forearm just below the elbow. Brachialis may be palpated lateral to the lower portion of the biceps brachii, if the elbow is flexed and in the pronated position).[10]

Observe: Elbow flexion, movement of the hand toward the face. E should observe for maintenance of forearm in supina-

tion (when testing for biceps) and for relaxed or extended wrist and fingers (Fig. 9-14, *A*).[10]

Resist: At the distal end of the volar aspect of the forearm, pulling downward toward elbow extension (Fig. 9-14, *B*).[6,8,9]

Procedure for Testing Grades P (2), T (1), and 0

Position: S supine with the shoulder abducted to 90° and externally rotated, elbow extended and forearm is supinated. E stands at the head of the table on the side being tested. (S may also be seated, side being tested resting on the treatment table, which is at axillary height, humerus in 90° abduction, elbow extended, and forearm in neutral position.)[6]

Stabilize: The humerus. The stabilizing hand can be used simultaneously for palpation here.

Palpate: The biceps as described for previous test.

Observe: Elbow flexion, movement of the hand toward the shoulder.[8] Watch for maintenance of forearm supination and relaxation of the fingers and wrist (Fig. 9-14, *C*).[10]

Grade: According to standard definitions of muscle grades.

Substitutions: Brachioradialis will substitute for biceps, but the forearm will move to midposition during flexion of the elbow. Wrist and finger flexors may assist elbow flexion, which will be preceded by finger and wrist flexion.[8,10] Pronator teres may assist. Forearm pronation during the movement may be evidence of this substitution.[10]

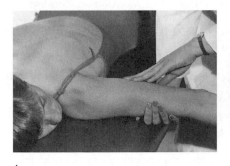
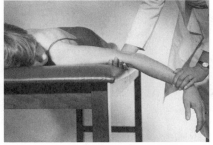
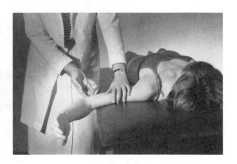

A   B   C

FIG. 9-15 Elbow extension. **A**, Palpate and observe. **B**, Resist. **C**, Gravity-decreased position.

Motion

Elbow extension

Muscles[8,9]	Innervation[8,9]
Triceps	Radial nerve, C7,8
Aconeus	Radial nerve, C7,8

Procedure for Testing Grades N (5) to F (3)

Position: *S* prone with the humerus abducted to 90° and in neutral rotation, elbow flexed to 90°, and the forearm, which is perpendicular to the floor, in neutral rotation. *E* stands next to *S* just behind the arm to be tested.[6,9,13]

Stabilize: The humerus by placing one hand for support under it, between *S*'s arm and the table.[9]

Palpate: The triceps over the middle of the posterior aspect of the humerus or the triceps tendon just proximal to the olecranon process on the dorsal surface of the arm.[6,8,10]

Observe: Extension of the elbow to just less than maximum range. The wrist and fingers remain relaxed (Fig. 9-15, *A*).

Resist: In the same plane as the forearm motion at the distal end of the forearm, pushing toward the floor or elbow flexion. Before resistance is given, be sure that the elbow is not locked. Resistance to a locked elbow can cause joint injury (Fig. 9-15, *B*).[8]

Procedure for Testing Grades P (2), T (1), and 0

Position: *S* supine with the humerus abducted to 90° and in external rotation, elbow fully flexed, and forearm supinated. *E* is standing next to *S* just behind to the arm to be tested.[8] An alternate position is with *S* seated, shoulder abducted to 90° and internally rotated, elbow flexed, and forearm in neutral position, resting on a table or powder board.[6]

Stabilize: The humerus by holding one hand over the middle or distal end of it to prevent shoulder motion.

Palpate: The triceps as described for previous test.

Observe: Extension of the elbow or movement of the hand away from the head (Fig. 9-15, *C*).

Grade: According to standard definitions of muscle grades.

Substitutions: Finger and wrist extensors may substitute for weak elbow extensors. Observe for finger and wrist extension preceding elbow extension. When upright, gravity and eccentric contraction of the biceps will effect elbow extension from the flexed position.[10]

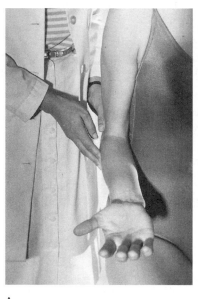 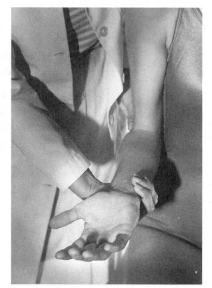 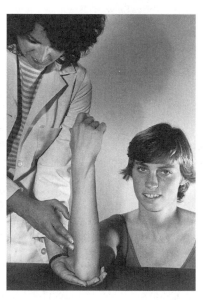

A	**B**	**C**

FIG. 9-16 Forearm supination. **A,** Palpate and observe. **B,** Resist. **C,** Gravity-decreased position.

Motion

Forearm supination

Muscles[4,8,10]	Innervation[8]
Biceps brachii	Musculocutaneous nerve, C5,6
Supinator	Radial nerve, C6

Procedure for Testing Grades N (5) to F (3)

Position: *S* seated with the humerus adducted, the elbow flexed to 90°, and the forearm in full pronation. *E* stands next to *S* on the side to be tested.[6,8]

Stabilize: The humerus just proximal to the elbow.[8,11]

Palpate: Over the supinator muscle on the dorsal-lateral aspect of the forearm, below the head of the radius. The muscle can be best felt when the radial muscle group (extensor carpi radialis and brachioradialis) are pushed up out of the way.[4] *E* may also palpate the biceps on the middle of the anterior surface of the humerus.[6]

Observe: Supination, turning the hand palm up. Because gravity assists the movement, after the 0° neutral position is passed, the therapist may apply slight resistance equal to the weight of the forearm[6] (Fig. 9-16, *A*).

Resist: By grasping around the dorsal aspect of the distal forearm with the fingers and heel of the hand, turning the arm toward pronation (Fig. 9-16, *B*).

Procedure for Testing Grades P (2), T (1), and 0

Position: *S* seated, shoulder flexed to 90° and the upper arm resting on the supporting surface. Elbow flexed to 90° and the forearm in full pronation in a position perpendicular to the floor.[6,13] *E* stands next to *S* on the side to be tested.

Stabilize: The humerus just proximal to the elbow.

Palpate: The supinator or biceps as described for previous test.
Observe: Supination, turning the palm of the hand toward the face (Fig. 9-16, *C*).
Grade: According to standard definitions of muscle grades.
Substitutions: With the elbow flexed, external rotation and horizontal adduction of the humerus will effect forearm supination. With the elbow extended, shoulder external rotation will

place the forearm in supination. The brachioradialis can bring the forearm from full pronation to midposition. Wrist and thumb extensors, assisted by gravity, can initiate supination. *E* should observe for external rotation of the humerus, supination to midline only, and initiation of motion by wrist and thumb extension.[10,13]

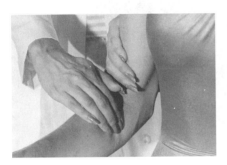

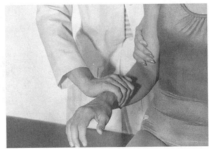

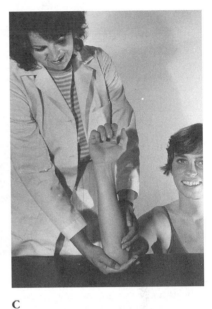

A   B   C

FIG. 9-17   Forearm pronation. **A,** Palpate and observe. **B,** Resist. **C,** Gravity-decreased position.

Motion

Forearm pronation

Muscles[4,10]	Innervation[9]
Pronator teres	Median nerve, C6,7
Pronator quadratus	Median nerve, C8, T1

Procedure for Testing Grades N (5) to F (3)

Position: *S* seated with the humerus adducted, elbow flexed to 90° and the forearm in full supination. *E* stands beside *S* on the side to be tested.[6,8]
Stabilize: The humerus just proximal to the elbow to prevent shoulder abduction.[6,8,9]
Palpate: The pronator teres on the upper part of the volar surface of the forearm, medial to the biceps tendon and diagonally from the medial condyle of the humerus to the lateral border of the radius.[6,8-10]
Observe: Pronation, turning the hand palm down (Fig. 9-17, *A*).[8]
Resist: By grasping over the dorsal aspect of the distal forearm

using the fingers and heel of the hand and turn toward supination (Fig. 9-17, *B*).

Procedure for Testing Grades P (2), T (1), and 0

Position: *S* seated, shoulder flexed to 90°, elbow flexed to 90°, and the forearm in full supination. The upper arm is resting on the supporting surface and the forearm is perpendicular to the floor.[13] *E* stands next to *S* on the side to be tested.
Palpate: Palpate the pronator teres as described for previous test.
Observe: Pronation, turning the palm of the hand away from the face (Fig. 9-17, *C*).
Grade: According to standard definitions of muscle grades.
Substitutions: With the elbow flexed, internal rotation and abduction of the humerus will produce apparent forearm pronation. With the elbow extended, internal rotation can place the forearm in a pronated position. Brachioradialis can bring the fully supinated forearm to midposition. Wrist flexion, aided by gravity, can effect pronation.[6,8,10,13]

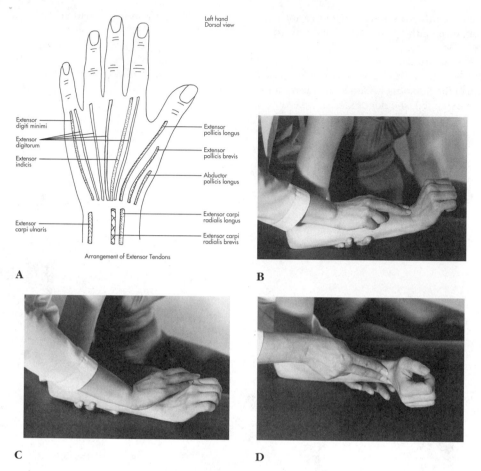

FIG. 9-18 **A,** Arrangement of extensor tendons at wrist. **B,** Wrist extension with radial deviation. Palpate and observe **C,** Resist. **D,** Gravity-decreased position.

Motion

Wrist extension with radial deviation

Muscles[8,9,10]	Innervation[10]
Extensor carpi radiallis longus	Radial nerve, C5,6,7,8
Extensor carpi radialis brevis	Radial nerve, C5,6,7,8
Extensor carpi ulnaris	Radial nerve, C6,7,8

Procedure for Testing Grades N (5) to F (3)

Position: *S* seated or supine with the forearm resting on the supporting surface in pronation, the wrist at neutral, and the fingers and thumb relaxed. *E* sits opposite *S* or next to *S* on the side to be tested.[8,9]

Stabilize: Over the volar aspect of the midforearm to distal forearm.[8,9]

Palpate: The extensor carpi radialis longus and brevis tendons on the dorsal aspect of the wrist at the bases of the 2nd and 3rd metacarpals respectively.[6,8] The tendon of the extensor carpi ulnaris may be palpated at the base of the 5th metacarpal, just distal to the head of the ulna (Fig. 9-18, *A*).[4,8,10]

Observe: Wrist extension and radial deviation, lifting the hand up from the supporting surface and moving it medially (to the radial side) simultaneously. The movement should be performed without finger extension, which could substitute for the wrist motion (Fig. 9-18, *B*).[8,10]

Resist: Over the dorsum of the 2nd and 3rd metacarpals toward flexion and ulnar deviation (Fig. 9-18, *C*).[8,9]

Procedure for Testing Grades P (2), T (1), and 0

Position: As described for previous test, except that the forearm is resting in midposition on its ulnar border.[8,13]

Stabilize: At the ulnar border of the forearm, supporting it slightly above the table surface.[8]

Palpate: Radial wrist extensors as described for previous test.

Observe: Extension of the wrist with movement of the hand away from the body (Fig. 9-18, *D*).

Grade: According to standard definitions of muscle grades.

Substitutions: Wrist extensors can substitute for one another. In the absence of the extensor carpi radialis muscles, the extensor carpi ulnaris will extend the wrist but in an ulnar direction. The combined extension and radial deviation will not be possible. The extensor digitorum communis muscle and the extensor pollicis longus can initiate wrist extension, but finger and/or thumb extension will precede wrist extension.[6,10,13]

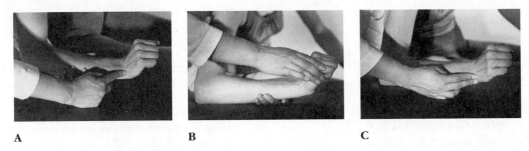

FIG. 9-19 Wrist extension with ulnar deviation. **A,** Palpate and observe. **B,** Resist. **C,** Gravity-decreased position.

Motion
Wrist extension with ulnar deviation

Muscles[8,9,10]	Innervation[9]
Extensor carpi ulnaris	Radial nerve, C6,7,8
Extensor carpi radialis longus	Radial nerve, C5,6,7,8
Extensor carpi radialis brevis	Radial nerve C5,6,7,8

Procedure for Testing Grades N (5) to F (3)
Position: S seated, forearm in pronation, wrist neutral, fingers and thumb relaxed. E sits opposite or next to S on the side to be tested.
Stabilize: Over the volar aspect of the midforearm to distal forearm.[8,9]
Palpate: Extensor carpi ulnaris tendon at the base of the 5th metacarpal, just distal to the ulna styloid, and the extensor carpi radialis longus and brevis tendons at the bases of the 2nd and 3rd metacarpals.
Observe: S bring the hand up from the supporting surface and move it laterally (to the ulnar side) simultaneously. E should observe that the movement is not preceded by thumb or finger extension (Fig. 9-19, *A*).[8,10]
Resist: Over the dorsal-lateral aspect of the 5th metacarpal toward flexion and radial deviation (Fig. 9-19, *B*).[8,9]

Procedure for Testing Grades P (2), T (1), and 0
Position: As described for previous test, except that the forearm is in 45° of pronation.
Stabilize: Arm at the volar aspect of the forearm, supporting it slightly above the supporting surface.[8,9]
Palpate: Extensor tendons as described above.
Observe: S bring the hand away from the body and move it ulnarly at the same time (Fig. 9-19, *C*).
Grade: According to standard definitions of muscle grades.
Substitutions: In the absence of the extensor carpi ulnaris muscle, the extensor carpi radialis longus and brevis muscle can extend the wrist but will do so in a radial direction. The ulnar deviation component of the test motion will not be possible. Long finger and thumb extensors can initiate wrist extension, but the movement will be preceded by finger and/or thumb extension.[6,10,13]

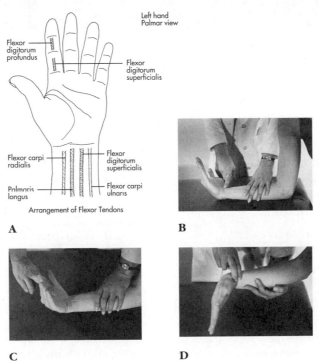

FIG. 9-20 **A,** Arrangement of flexor tendons at wrist. **B,** Wrist flexion with radial deviation. Palpate and observe. **C,** Resist. **D,** Gravity-decreased position.

Motion

Wrist flexion with radial deviation

Muscles[9]	Innervation[5,8,9]
Flexor carpi radialis	Median nerve, C6,7,8
Flexor carpi ulnaris	Ulnar nerve, C8, T1
Palmaris longus	Median nerve, C7,8, T1

Procedure for Testing Grades N (5) to F (3)

Position: S seated or supine with the forearm resting in nearly full supination on the supporting surface, fingers and thumb relaxed.[6,10] E is seated next to S on the side to be tested.
Stabilize: Over the volar aspect of the midforearm.[8,9]
Palpate: Muscle tendons. The flexor carpi radialis tendon can be palpated over the wrist at the base of the second metacarpal bone. The palmaris longus tendon is at the center of the wrist at the base of the 3rd metacarpal, and the flexor carpi ulnaris tendon can be palpated at the ulnar side of the volar aspect of the wrist at the base of the 5th metacarpal (Fig. 9-20, A).[4]
Observe: S bring the hand up from the supporting surface toward the face, deviating the hand toward the radial side simultaneously. E should observe that the fingers remain relaxed during the movement (Fig. 9-20, B).

Resist: In the palm at the radial side of the hand over the 2nd and 3rd metacarpals toward extension and ulnar deviation (Fig. 9-20, C).

Procedure for Testing Grades P (2), T (1), and 0

Position: S seated with the forearm in midposition with the ulnar border of the hand resting on the supporting surface.[8,13] E sits next to S on the side to be tested.
Stabilize: At the ulnar border of the forearm, slightly above the supporting surface.
Palpate: Wrist flexor tendons as described for previous test.
Observe: S move the hand toward the body and in a radial direction, flexing the wrist. Movement should not be initiated with finger flexion (Fig. 9-20, D).
Grade: According to standard definitions of muscle grades.
Substitutions: Wrist flexors can substitute for one another. If flexor carpi radialis is weak or nonfunctioning in this test, flexor carpi ulnaris will produce wrist flexion, but in an ulnar direction, and the radial deviation will not be possible. The finger flexors can assist wrist flexion, but finger flexion will occur before the wrist is flexed. The abductor pollicis longus, with the assistance of gravity, can initiate wrist flexion.[6,10]

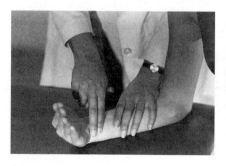
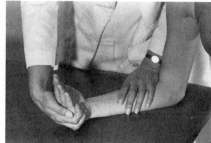
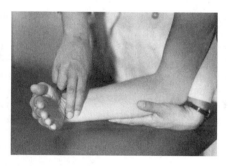

A   B   C

FIG. 9-21 Wrist flexion with ulnar deviation. **A,** Palpate and observe. **B,** Resist. **C,** Gravity-decreased position.

Motion

Wrist flexion with ulnar deviation

Muscles[8]	Innervation[5,8,9]
Flexor carpi ulnaris	Ulnar nerve, C8, T1
Palmaris longus	Median nerve, C7,8, T1
Flexor carpi radialis	Median nerve, C6,7,8

Procedure for Testing Grades N (5) to F (3)

Position: S seated or supine with the forearm resting in nearly full supination on the supporting surface, fingers and thumb relaxed. E is seated opposite or next to S on the side to be tested.[8,9]
Stabilize: Over the volar aspect of the middle of the forearm.[8,9]
Palpate: Flexor tendons on the volar aspect of the wrist, the flexor carpi ulnaris at the base of the 5th metacarpal, the flexor carpi radialis at the base of the 2nd metacarpal, and the palmaris longus at the base of the 3rd metacarpal.[4]
Observe: S bring the hand up off the supporting surface, flexing the wrist and deviating it ulnarly simultaneously (Fig. 9-21, A).

Resist: In the palm of the hand over the hypothenar eminence toward extension and radial deviation (Fig. 9-21, B).[6,9]

Procedure for Testing Grades P (2), T (1), and 0

Position: S seated with the forearm resting in 45° of supination on the ulnar border of the arm and hand.[8,11] E sits opposite S or next to S on the side being tested.
Stabilize: S's arm can be supported slightly above the supporting surface and stabilized at the dorsal-medial aspect of the forearm to prevent elbow and forearm motion.
Palpate: Wrist flexor tendons as described for previous test.
Observe: S bring the hand toward the body, flexing and deviating the wrist ulnarly simultaneously (Fig. 9-21, C).
Grade: According to standard definitions of muscle grades.
Substitutions: Wrist flexors can substitute for one another. If flexor carpi ulnaris is weak or absent, flexor carpi radialis can produce wrist flexion in a radial direction and the ulnar deviation will not be possible. The finger flexors can also assist wrist flexion, but the motion will be preceded by flexion of the fingers.[10,13]

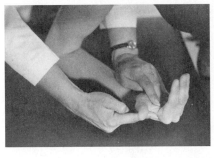
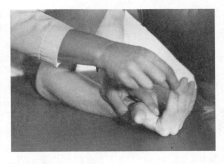
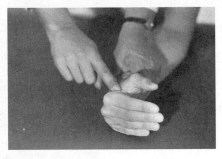

A   **B**   **C**

FIG. 9-22 MP flexion with IP extension. **A,** Palpate and observe. **B,** Resist. **C,** Gravity-decreased position.

Motion

Metacarpophalangeal (MP) flexion with interphalangeal (IP) extension

Muscles[1,4]	Innervation[8]
Lumbricals 1 and 2	Median nerve, C6,7
Lumbricals 3 and 4	Ulnar nerve, C8, T1
Dorsal interossei	Ulnar nerve, C8, T1
Palmar interossei	Ulnar nerve, C8, T1

Procedure for Testing Grades N (5) to F (3)

Position: S seated with forearm in supination, wrist at neutral, resting on the supporting surface.[8] The MP joints are extended and the IP joints are flexed.[13] E sits next to S on the side being tested.

Stabilize: Over the palm to prevent wrist motion.

Palpate: The first dorsal interosseous muscle just medial to the distal aspect of the 2nd metacarpal on the dorsum of the hand. The remainder of these muscles are not easily palpable because of their size and deep location in the hand.[10,13]

Observe: S flex the MP joints and extend the IP joints simultaneously (Fig. 9-22, A).[9]

Resist: Each finger separately by grasping the distal phalanx and pushing downward on the finger into the supporting surface toward MP extension and IP flexion, or apply pressure first against the dorsal surface of the middle and distal phalanges toward flexion, followed by application of pressure to the volar surface of the proximal phalanges toward extension (Fig. 9-22, B)[9]

Procedure for Testing Grades P (2), T (1), and 0

Position: S seated or supine with the forearm and wrist in midposition and resting on the ulnar border on the supporting surface.[8] MP joints are extended and IP joints are flexed. E sits next to S on the side being tested.

Stabilize: The wrist and palm of the hand.

Palpate: As described for previous test.

Observe: S flex the MP joints and extend the IP joints simultaneously (Fig. 9-22, C).

Grade: According to standard definitions of muscle grades.

Substitutions: Flexor digitorum profundus and superficialis may substitute for weak or absent lumbricals. In this case, MP flexion will be preceded by flexion of the distal and proximal interphalangeal joints.[10,13]

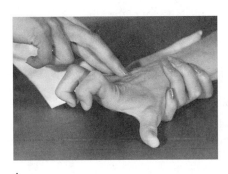
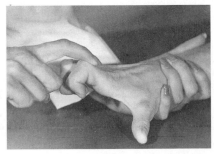
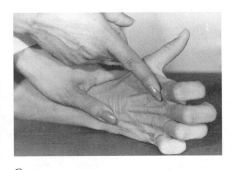

A   **B**   **C**

FIG. 9-23 MP extension. **A,** Palpate and observe. **B,** Resist. **C,** Gravity-decreased position.

Motion

MP extension

Muscles[8,9,10]	Innervation[8]
Extensor digitorum communis	Radial nerve, C6,7,8
Extensor indicis proprius	
Extensor digiti minimi	

Procedure for Testing Grades N (5) to F (3)

Position: S seated with the forearm pronated and the wrist in the neutral position, MP and IP joints partially flexed.[6,8] E sits opposite or next to S on the side to be tested.

Stabilize: The wrist and metacarpals slightly above the supporting surface.[8,9]

Palpate: The extensor digitorum tendons where they course over the dorsum of the hand.[6,8] In some individuals, the extensor digiti minimi tendon can be palpated or visualized just lateral to the extensor digitorum tendon to the 5th finger. The extensor indicis proprius tendon can be palpated or visualized just medial to the extensor digitorum tendon to the first finger.

Observe: *S* raise the fingers away from the supporting surface, extending the MP joints but maintaining the IP joints in some flexion (Fig. 9-23, *A*).

Resist: Each finger individually over the dorsal aspect of the proximal phalanx toward MP flexion (Fig. 9-23, *B*).[8,9]

Procedure for Testing Grades P (2), T (1), and 0

Position: Same as described for previous test, except that *S*'s forearm is in midposition and the hand and forearm are supported on the ulnar border.[8]

Stabilize: Same as described for previous test.
Palpate: Same as described for previous test.
Observe: *S* move the fingers backward, extending the MP joints while keeping the IP joints somewhat flexed (Fig. 9-23, *C*).

Grade: According to standard definitions of muscle grades.
Substitutions: With the wrist stabilized, no substitutions are possible. When the wrist is not stabilized, wrist flexion with tendon action can produce MP extension.[6,10,13]

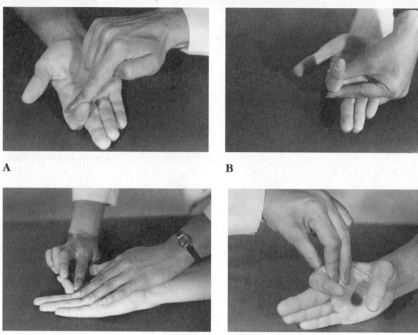

A   **B**   **C**   **D**

FIG. 9-24   PIP flexion. **A,** Palpate and observe. **B,** Position to assist with isolation of PIP joint flexion. **C,** Resist. Therapist checks for substitution by flexor digitorum profundus. **D,** Gravity-decreased position.

Motion

PIP flexion, 2nd through 5th fingers

Muscles[8,9]	Innervation[8,9]
Flexor digitorum superficialis	(FDS) Median nerve, C7,8, T1

Procedure for Testing Grades N (5) to F (3)

Position: *S* seated with the forearm in supination, wrist at neutral, fingers extended, and hand and forearm resting on the dorsal surface.[8] *E* sits opposite or next to *S* on the side being tested.

Stabilize: MP joint and proximal phalanx of the finger being tested.[6,8,9]

Palpate: The FDS tendon on the volar surface of the proximal phalanx. A stabilizing finger may be used to palpate in this instance.[10] The tendon supplying the 4th finger may be palpated over the volar aspect of the wrist between the flexor carpi ulnaris and the palmaris longus tendons, if desired.[4]

Observe: *S* flex the PIP joint while maintaining the DIP joint in extension (Fig. 9-24, *A*). If isolating PIP flexion is difficult, hold all of the fingers not being tested in MP hyperextension and PIP extension by pulling back over the IP joints. This maneuver inactivates the flexor digitorum profundus so that *S* cannot flex the distal joint (Fig. 9-24, *B*).[4,13] Most individuals cannot perform isolated action of the PIP joint of the 5th finger even with this assistance.[10]

Resist: With one finger at the volar aspect of the middle phalanx toward extension.[8,9] If the index finger is used to apply resistance, the middle finger may be used to move the DIP joint to and fro to verify that the flexor digitorum profundus (FDP) is not substituting (Fig. 9-24, *C*).

Procedure for Testing Grades P (2), T (1), and 0

Position: *S* seated with the forearm in midposition and the wrist at neutral, resting on the ulnar border.[13] *E* sits opposite or next to *S* on the side to be tested.

Stabilize: The MP joint and proximal phalanx of the finger.[8,9] If stabilization during the motion is difficult in this position, the forearm may be returned to full supination, because the effect of gravity on the fingers is not significant.

Palpate and observe: The same as described for previous test, except that the movement is performed in a plane parallel to the floor (Fig. 9-24, *D*).

Grade: According to standard definitions of muscle grades. If the test for grades poor and below is done with the forearm in full supination partial ROM against gravity may be graded poor.[8]

Substitutions: The FDP may substitute for the FDS. DIP flexion will precede PIP flexion.[6,10,13] Tendon action of the long finger flexors accompanies wrist extension and can produce an apparent flexion of the fingers through partial ROM.[10,13]

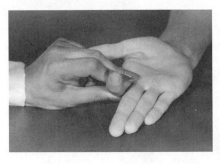 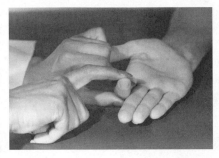 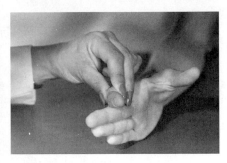

A   B   C

FIG. 9-25   DIP flexion. **A,** Palpate and observe. **B,** Resist. **C,** Gravity-decreased position.

Motion

DIP flexion, 2nd through 5th fingers

Muscles[8]	Innervation[8]
Flexor digitorum profundus	Median and ulnar nerves, C8, T1

Procedure for Testing Grades N (5) to F (3)

Position: S seated with the forearm in supination, the wrist at neutral, and the fingers extended. E sits opposite or next to S on the side being tested.[8]

Stabilize: The wrist at neutral and the PIP joint and middle phalanx of the finger being tested.[13]

Palpate: Use the finger stabilizing the middle phalanx to simultaneously palpate the FDP tendon over the volar surface of the middle phalanx.[8,10]

Observe: S bring the fingertip up away from the supporting surface, flexing the DIP joint (Fig. 9-25, A).

Resist: With one finger at the volar aspect of the distal phalanx toward extension (Fig. 9-25, B).[6,8,9]

Procedure for Testing Grades P (2), T (1), and 0

Position: S seated with the forearm in midposition and with wrist at neutral resting on the ulnar border.[13] S may be positioned with the forearm supinated, if necessary.

Stabilize: Same as described for previous test.

Palpate: The same as described for previous test.

Observe: S flex the DIP joint (Fig. 9-25, C).

Grade: According to standard definitions of muscle grades except that if the test for grades poor and below was done with the forearm in full supination, movement through partial ROM may be graded poor.[8]

Substitutions: None possible during the testing procedure if the wrist is well stabilized, because the FDP is the only muscle that can act to flex the DIP joint when it is isolated. During normal hand function, however, wrist extension with tendon action of the finger flexors can produce partial flexion of the DIP joints.[10,13]

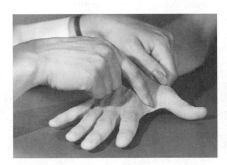

A   B

FIG. 9-26   Finger abduction. **A,** Palpate and observe. **B,** Resist.

Motion

Finger abduction

Muscles[8]	Innervation[8]
Dorsal interossei	Ulnar nerve, C8, T1
Abductor digiti minimi	Ulnar nerve, C8, T1

Procedure for Testing Grades N (5) to F (3)

Position: S seated or supine with the forearm pronated, wrist at neutral, and fingers extended and adducted. E is seated opposite or next to S on the side to be tested.[8]

Stabilize: The wrist and metacarpals slightly above the supporting surface.

Palpate: The 1st dorsal interosseous muscle on the lateral aspect of the second metacarpal or of the abductor digiti minimi on the ulnar border of the 5th metacarpal. The remaining interossei are not palpable.[6,8]

Observe: S spread the fingers apart, abducting them at the MP joints (Fig. 9-26, A).

Resist: The first dorsal interosseous by applying pressure on the radial side of the the proximal phalanx of the 2nd finger in an ulnar direction (Fig. 9-26, B); the 2nd dorsal interosseous on the radial side of the proximal phalanx of the middle finger in an ulnar direction; the 3rd dorsal interosseous on the ulnar side of the proximal phalanx of the middle finger in a radial direction; the 4th dorsal interosseous on the ulnar side of the proximal phalanx of the ring finger in a radial direction: the abductor digiti minimi on the ulnar side of the proximal phalanx of the little finger in a radial direction.[9]

Procedure for Testing Grades P (2), T (1), and 0

The tests for these muscle grades are the same as described for previous test. Because the test motions were not performed against gravity, some judgment of the examiner must be used in grading. For example, partial ROM in gravity-decreased position may be graded poor and full ROM graded fair.[8]

Substitutions: Extensor digitorum communis can assist weak or absent dorsal interossei, but abduction will be accompanied by MP extension.[10,13]

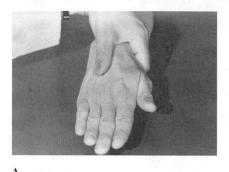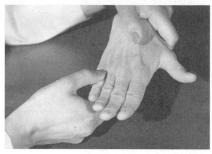

A   **B**

FIG. 9-27   Finger adduction. **A,** Therapist observes movement of fingers into adduction. Palpation of these muscles is not possible. **B,** Resist.

Motion

Finger adduction

Muscles[8,9]	Innervation[8]
Palmar interossei, 1, 2, 3	Ulnar nerve, C8, T1

Procedure for Testing Grades N (5) to F (3)

Position: S seated with forearm pronated, wrist in neutral, and fingers extended and abducted.[8]

Stabilize: The wrist and metacarpals slightly above the supporting surface.

Palpate: Not palpable.

Observe: S adduct the 1st, 4th and 5th fingers toward the middle finger (Fig. 9-27, *A*).

Resist: The index finger at the proximal phalanx by pulling it in a radial direction, the ring finger at the proximal phalanx in an ulnar direction, and the little finger likewise (Fig. 9-27, *B*).[9] These muscles are very small and resistance will have to be modified to accommodate to their comparatively limited power.

Procedure for Testing Grades P (2), T (1), and 0

The test for these muscle grades is the same as described for previous test. The examiner's judgment must be used in determining degree of weakness. Achievement of full ROM may be graded fair and partial ROM graded poor.[8]

Substitutions: Flexor digitorum profundus and superficialis can substitute for weak palmar interossei, but IP flexion will occur with finger adduction.[10,13]

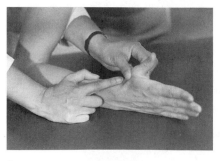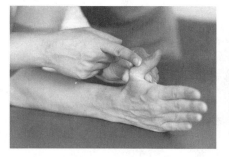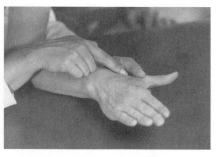

A   **B**   **C**

FIG. 9-28   Thumb MP extension. **A,** Palpate and observe. **B,** Resist. **C,** Gravity-decreased position.

Motion

Thumb MP extension

Muscles[8,9]	Innervation[8,9]
Extensor pollicis brevis	Radial nerve, C6,7,8

Procedure for Testing Grades N (5) to F (3)

Position: S seated or supine, forearm in midposition, wrist at neutral, and hand and forearm resting on the ulnar border.[8] The thumb is flexed into the palm at the MP joint and the IP is extended, but relaxed. E sits opposite or next to S on the side to be tested.

Stabilize: The wrist and the thumb metacarpal.

Palpate: The extensor pollicis brevis (EPB) tendon at the base of the 1st metacarpal on the dorsoradial aspect. It lies just medial to the abductor pollicis longus tendon on the radial side of the anatomical snuff-box, which is the hollow space created between the EPL and EPB tendons when the thumb is fully extended and radially abducted.[4,6]

Observe: S extend the MP joint. The IP joint remains relaxed (Fig. 9-28, *A*). It is difficult for many individuals to isolate this motion.

Resist: On the dorsal surface of the proximal phalanx toward MP flexion (Fig. 9-28, *B*).[8,9]

Procedure for Testing Grades (P), (T), and (0)

Position and stabilize: Positioning and stabilizing are the same as described for previous test, except that the forearm is fully pronated and resting on the volar surface.[13] *E* may stabilize the 1st metacarpal, holding the hand slightly above the supporting surface. The test may also be performed in the same manner as for grades normal to fair, with modification in grading.[8]

Palpate and observe: Palpation is the same as described for previous test. MP extension is performed in a plane parallel to the supporting surface (Fig. 9-28, *C*).

Grade: According to standard definitions of muscle grades. If midposition of forearm was used, partial ROM is graded poor and full ROM is graded fair.[8]

Substitutions: Extensor pollicis longus may substitute for extensor pollicis brevis. IP extension will precede MP extension.[6,10,13]

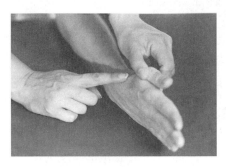 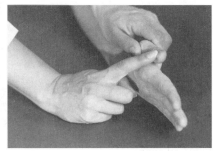 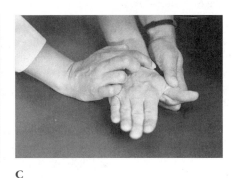

A   B   C

FIG. 9-29 Thumb IP extension. **A,** Palpate and observe. **B,** Resist. **C,** Gravity-decreased position.

Motion

Thumb IP extension

Muscles[8,9,10]	Innervation[8,9]
Extensor pollicis longus	Radial nerve, C6,7,8

Procedure for Testing Grades N (5) to F (3)

Position: S seated or supine, forearm in midposition, wrist at neutral, and hand and forearm resting on the ulnar border.[8] The MP joint of the thumb is extended or slightly flexed, and the IP is flexed fully into the palm. *E* sits opposite or next to S on the side being tested.

Stabilize: The wrist at neutral, 1st metacarpal and the proximal phalanx of the thumb.

Palpate: The extensor pollicis longus tendon on the dorsal surface of the hand medial to the EPB tendon, between the head of the 1st metacarpal and the base of the 2nd on the ulnar side of the anatomical snuff box.[4,8]

Observe: S bring the tip of the thumb up, out of the palm, extending the IP joint (Fig. 9-29, *A*).

Resist: On the dorsal surface of the distal phalanx, down toward IP flexion (Fig. 9-29, *B*).[8,9]

Procedure for Testing Grades P (2), T (1), and 0

Position and stabilize: Positioning and stabilizing are the same as described for previous test, except that the forearm is fully pronated.[13] *E* may stabilize so that *S*'s hand is held slightly above the supporting surface. The test may also be performed in the same position as for grades normal to fair with modification in grading.

Palpate and observe: Palpation is the same as described for previous test. IP extension is performed in the plane of the palm, parallel to the supporting surface (Fig. 9-29, *C*).

Grade: According to standard definitions of muscle grades. If the test was performed with the forearm in midposition, partial ROM is graded poor.[8]

Substitutions: A quick contraction of the flexor pollicis longus followed by rapid release will cause the IP joint to rebound into extension. IP flexion will precede IP extension.[6,10] Abductor pollicis brevis, flexor pollicis brevis, the oblique fibers of the adductor pollicis, and the 1st palmar interossous can extend the IP joint because of their insertions into the extensor expansion of the thumb.[9,13]

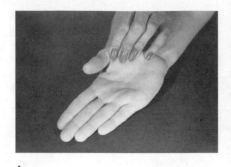
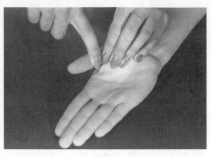

A   **B**

FIG. 9-30   Thumb MP flexion. **A**, Palpate and observe. **B**, Resist.

Motion
Thumb MP flexion

Muscles[8,9]	Innervation[8,9]
Flexor pollicis brevis	Median and ulnar nerves, C6,7,8, T1

Procedure for Testing Grades N (5) to F (3)
Position: S seated or supine, the forearm fully supinated, the wrist in the neutral position, and the thumb in extension and adduction. E is seated next to or opposite S.[6,8,9]
Stabilize: The 1st metacarpal and the wrist.
Palpate: Over the middle of the palmar surface of the thenar eminence just medial to the abductor pollicis brevis muscle.[8] The hand that is used to stabilize may also be used for palpation.
Observe: S flex the MP joint while maintaining extension of the IP joint (Fig. 9-30, A). It may not be possible for some indi-

viduals to isolate flexion to the MP joint. In this instance, both MP and IP flexion may be tested together as a gross test for thumb flexion strength and graded according to the examiner's judgment.
Resist: On the palmar surface of the first phalanx toward MP extension (Fig. 9-30, B).[6,8,9]

Procedure for Testing Grades P (2), T (1), and (0)
Positioning, stabilizing and palpating are the same as described for previous test.
Observe: S flex the MP joint so that the thumb moves over the palm of the hand.
Grade: Full ROM is graded fair; partial ROM is graded poor.[8]
Substitutions: Flexor pollicis longus can substitute for flexor pollicis brevis. In this case, isolated MP flexion will not be possible and MP flexion will be preceded by IP flexion.[6,10,13]

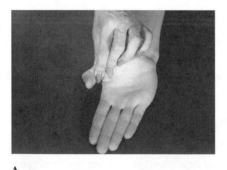
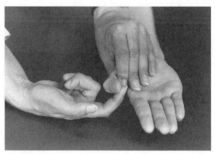

A   **B**

FIG. 9-31   Thumb IP flexion. **A**, Palpate and observe. **B**, Resist.

Motion
Thumb IP flexion

Muscles[8,9,10]	Innervation[8]
Flexor pollicis longus	Median nerve, C7,8, T1

Procedure for Testing Grades N (5) to F (3)
Position: S seated with the forearm fully supinated, wrist in neutral position, and thumb in extension and adduction.[8] E is seated next to or opposite S.
Stabilize: The wrist, 1st metacarpal, and the proximal phalanx of the thumb in extension.[6,8,9]
Palpate: The flexor pollicis longus tendon on the palmar surface of the proximal phalanx. In this instance, the palpating

finger may be the same one used for stabilizing the proximal phalanx.
Observe: S flex the IP joint in the plane of the palm (Fig. 9-31, A).[8]
Resist: On the palmar surface of the distal phalanx, toward IP extension (Fig. 9-31, B).[8,9]

Procedure for Testing Grades P (2), T (1), and 0
The test for these muscle grades is the same as described for previous test. The examiner's judgment must be used in determining degree of weakness. Achievement of full ROM may be graded fair and partial ROM graded poor.[8]
Substitutions: A quick contraction and release of the extensor pollicis longus may cause an apparent flexion of the IP joint. E should observe for IP extension preceding IP flexion.[6,10,13]

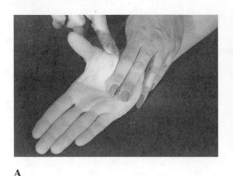
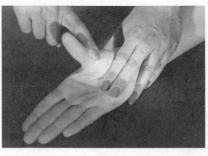
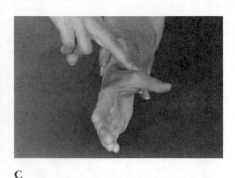

A B C

FIG. 9-32 Thumb palmar abduction. **A,** Palpate and observe. **B,** Resist. **C,** Gravity-decreased position.

Motion
Thumb palmar abduction

Muscles[9,10]	Innervation[9]
Abductor pollicis brevis	Median nerve, C6,7,8, T1

Procedure for Testing Grades Fair (F) to Normal (N)
Position: *S* seated or supine, forearm in supination, wrist at neutral, thumb extended and adducted, and carpometacarpal (CMC) joint rotated so that the thumb is resting in a plane perpendicular to the palm. *E* sits opposite or next to *S* on the side to be tested.[6,8,9]
Stabilize: The metacarpals and wrist.
Palpate: The abductor pollicis brevis muscle on the lateral aspect of the thenar eminence, lateral to the flexor pollicis brevis muscle.[8]
Observe: *S* raise the thumb away from the palm in a plane perpendicular to the palm (Fig. 9-32, *A*).[9]

Resist: At the lateral aspect of the proximal phalanx, downward toward adduction (Fig. 9-32, *B*).[9]

Procedure for Testing Grades P (2), T (1), and 0
Position: As described for previous test, except that the forearm and hand are resting on the ulnar border.[13]
Stabilize: The wrist and metacarpals.
Palpate: The abductor pollicis brevis muscle on the lateral aspect of the thenar eminence.
Observe: *S* move the thumb away from the palm in a plane at right angles to the palm of the hand and parallel to the supporting surface (Fig. 9-32, *C*).
Grade: According to standard definitions of muscle grades.
Substitutions: Abductor pollicis longus can substitute for abductor pollicis brevis. Abduction will take place more in the plane of the palm, however, rather then perpendicular to it.[10,13]

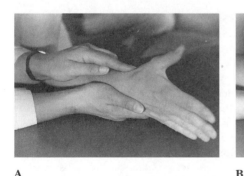
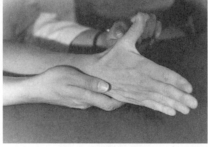
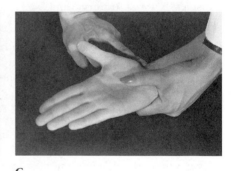

A B C

FIG. 9-33 Thumb radial abduction. **A,** Palpate and observe. **B,** Resist. **C,** Gravity-decreased position.

Motion
Thumb radial abduction

Muscles[9]	Innervation[9]
Abductor pollicis longus	Radial nerve, C6,7,8

Procedure for Testing Grades N (5) to F (3)
Position: *S* seated or supine, forearm in neutral rotation, wrist at neutral, thumb adducted and slightly flexed across the palm. Hand and forearm are resting on the ulnar border.[9] *E* sits opposite or next to *S* on the side being tested.
Stabilize: The wrist and metacarpals of the fingers.[8,9]

Palpate: The abductor pollicis longus tendon on the lateral aspect of the base of the first metacarpal. It is the tendon immediately lateral (radial) to the extensor pollicis brevis tendon.[4,8]
Observe: *S* move the thumb out of the palm of the hand, abducting it in the plane of the palm (Fig. 9-33, *A*).
Resist: At the lateral aspect of the distal end of the 1st metacarpal toward adduction (Fig. 9-33, *B*).[8,9]

Procedure for Testing Grades P (2), T (1), and 0
Position: As described for previous test, except that the forearm is in full supination and the forearm and hand are resting on the dorsal surface.[8]

Stabilize: The wrist and palm of the hand.

Palpate: Same as described for previous test.

Observe: *S* move the thumb out away from the palm of the hand in the plane of the palm, parallel to the supporting surface (Fig. 9-33, *C*).

Grade: According to standard definitions of muscle grades.

Substitutions: Abductor pollicis brevis can substitute for abductor pollicis longus. Abduction will not take place in the plane of the palm, but however, rather in a more ulnarward direction.[10,13]

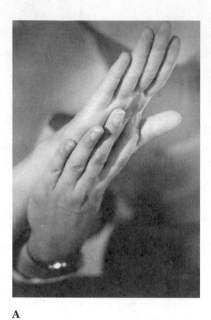
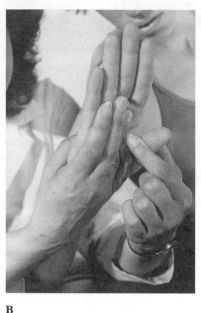
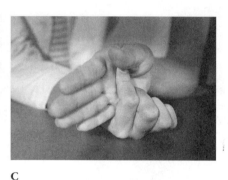

A   **B**   **C**

FIG. 9-34   Thumb adduction. **A,** Palpate and observe. **B,** Resist. **C,** Gravity-decreased position.

Motion

Thumb adduction

Muscles[8,9]	Innervation[8,9]
Adductor pollicis	Ulnar nerve, C8, T1

Procedure for Testing Grades N (5) to F (3)

Position: *S* seated or supine, forearm pronated, wrist at neutral, thumb in palmar abduction.[8,13] *E* is sitting opposite or next to *S* on the side to be tested.

Stabilize: The wrist and metacarpals, supporting the hand slightly above the resting surface.[8]

Palpate: Adductor pollicis on the palmar side of the thumb web space.[10]

Observe: *S* bring the thumb up to touch the palm (Fig. 9-34, *A*).[8] (The palm is turned up in the illustration to show the palpation point.)

Resist: By grasping the proximal phalanx of the thumb near the metacarpal head and pulling downward, toward abduction (Fig. 9-34, *B*).[8]

Procedure for Testing Grades P (2), T (1), and 0

Position: Same as described for previous test, except that the forearm is in midposition and the forearm and hand are resting on the ulnar border.[13]

Stabilize: Over the wrist and palm of the hand.

Palpate: Same as described for previous test.

Observe: *S* bring the thumb in to touch the radial side of the palm of the hand or the 2nd metacarpal (Fig. 9-34, *C*).

Grade: According to standard definitions of muscle grades.

Substitutions: Flexor or extensor pollicis longus muscles may assist weak or absent adductor pollicis. If one substitutes, adduction will be accompanied by thumb flexion or extension preceding adduction.[10,13]

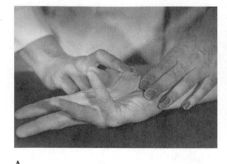
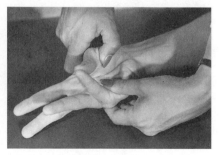

A   **B**

FIG. 9-35   Thumb opposition. **A,** Palpate and observe. **B,** Resist.

Motion

Opposition of the thumb to the 5th finger

Muscles[8,9]	Innervation[8,9]
Opponens pollicis	Median nerve, C6,7,8, T1
Opponens digiti minimi	Ulnar nerve, C8, T1

Procedure for Testing Grades N (5) to F (3)

Position: S seated or supine with forearm in full supination, wrist at neutral, thumb in palmar abduction, and 5th finger extended.[6,8,9] E sits opposite or next to S on the side to be tested.

Stabilize: The forearm and wrist.

Palpate: The opponens pollicis along the radial side of the shaft of the first metacarpal, lateral to the abductor pollicis brevis. The opponens digiti minimi cannot be easily palpated.[8,10]

Observe: S medially rotate the thumb across the palm to touch the thumb pad to the pad of the 5th finger, which flexes and rotates toward the thumb.[6] (Fig. 9-35, A).

Resist: At the distal ends of the 1st and 5th metacarpals toward

derotation of these bones and flattening of the palm of the hand (Fig. 9-35, B).[8]

Procedure for Testing Grades P (2), T (1), and 0

The procedure described for previous test may be used for these grades, if grading is modified to compensate for the movement of the parts against gravity. For example, movement through full ROM would be graded fair and through partial ROM would be graded poor.[8]

Substitutions: Abductor pollicis brevis will assist with opposition by flexing and medially rotating the CMC joint, but the IP joint will extend. The flexor pollicis brevis will flex and medially rotate the CMC joint, but the thumb will not move away from the palm of the hand. The flexor pollicis longus will flex and slightly rotate the CMC joint, but the thumb will not move away from the palm and the IP joint will flex strongly.[10,13] The DIP joints of the thumb and little finger may flex to meet, giving the appearance of full opposition.[6]

MANUAL MUSCLE TESTING OF THE LOWER EXTREMITY

Motion

Hip flexion

Muscles[4,6,8-10]	Innervation[4,8-10]
Psoas major	Lumbar plexus, L1,2,3,4
Iliacus	Femoral nerve, L2,3
Rectus femoris	Femoral nerve, L2,3,4
Tensor fascia latae	Superior gluteal nerve,
Sartorius	Femoral nerve, L2,3,4,5, S1
Pectineus	Femoral nerve, L2,3

Procedure for Testing Grades N (5) to F (3)

Position: S seated with knees flexed over the edge of the table

and feet above the floor. E stands next to S on the side being tested.[6]

Stabilize: The pelvis at the iliac crest on the side being tested. S may hold onto the edge of the table or fold arms across chest.[6,8,9]

Palpate: The psoas and iliacus are difficult to palpate. The rectus femoris may be palpated on the middle anterior aspect of the thigh just lateral to the sartorius muscle.[4,10]

Observe: S lift the leg up from the table flexing the hip through the remainder of the ROM. Observe for internal rotation, external rotation, and abduction accompanying the flexion as signs of substitution or muscle imbalance in this muscle group (Fig. 9-36, A).[6,9]

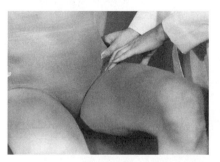

A

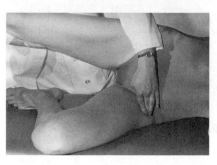

B

C

FIG. 9-36 Hip flexion. **A,** Palpate and observe. **B,** Resist. **C,** Gravity-decreased position.

Resist: Just proximal to the knee on the anterior surface of the thigh, down toward the table into hip extension (Fig. 9-36, *B*).[6,8,9]

Procedure for Testing Grades P (2), T (1), and 0

Position: *S* sidelying. *E* stands behind *S*, supporting the upper leg in neutral rotation and slight abduction, with the knee extended.[8] The lower leg (to be tested) is extended at the hip and knee.

Stabilize: Weight of the trunk may be adequate stabilization, or *E* may stabilize the pelvis.[8]

Palpate: Same as described for previous test.

Observe: *S* bring the lower leg up toward the trunk, flexing the hip and knee (Fig. 9-36, *C*).[8]

Grade: According to standard definitions of muscle grades.

Substitutions: The hip flexors can substitute for one another. If the iliacus and psoas major muscles are weak or absent, hip flexion will be accompanied by other movements: abduction and external rotation (sartorius), abduction and internal rotation (tensor fascia latae), adduction (pectineus).[8,10] If the anterior abdominal muscles do not stabilize the pelvis, it will flex on the thighs; the hip flexors may hold against resistance, but not at maximum ROM.[9]

Motion

Hip extension

Muscles[8,9]	Innervation[8]
Gluteus maximus	Inferior gluteal nerve, L5, S1,2
Semitendinosis	Sciatic nerve, L5, S1,2,3
Semimembranosis	Sciatic nerve, L4,5, S1,2
Biceps femoris (long head)	Sciatic nerve, L5, S1,2,3

Procedure for Testing Grades N (5) to F (3)

Position: *S* lying prone with the hip at neutral and the knee flexed to about 90°. *E* stands next to *S* on the opposite side.[9] Two pillows may be placed under the pelvis to flex the hips.[6]

Stabilize: Over the iliac crest on the side being tested.[8]

Palpate: The gluteus maximus on middle posterior surface of the buttock.[10]

Observe: *S* lift the leg from the supporting surface, extending the hip while keeping the knee flexed to minimize action of the hamstring muscles on the hip joint (Fig. 9-37, *A*).

Resist: At the distal end of the posterior aspect of the thigh, downward, toward flexion (Fig. 9-37, *B*).[8,9]

Procedure for Testing Grades P (2), T (1), and 0

Position: Sidelying. *E* stands in front of *S*, supporting the upper leg in extension and slight abduction.[8] The lower leg (to be tested) is flexed at the hip and knee.

Stabilize: The pelvis over the iliac crest.[8]

Palpate: Same as described for previous test.

Observe: *S* bring the lower leg backward, extending the hip but maintaining flexion of the knee (Fig. 9-37, *C*).

Grade: According to standard definitions of muscle grades.

Substitutions: Elevation of the pelvis and extension of the lumbar spine can produce some hip extension. In supine position, gravity and eccentric contraction of the hip flexors can return the flexed hip to extension.[10] Hip external rotation, abduction, or adduction may be used to substitute.[6]

Motion

Hip abduction

Muscles[8-10]	Innervation[8,9]
Gluteus medius	Superior gluteal nerve, L4,5, S1
Gluteus minimus	Superior gluteal nerve, L4,5, S1
Tensor fascia latae	Superior gluteal nerve, L4,5, S1

Procedure for Testing Grades N (5) to F (3)

Position: *S* sidelying, upper leg (to be tested) has the knee extended and hip extended slightly beyond the neutral position; lower leg is flexed at the hip and knee to provide a wide base of support.[6] *E* stands in front of *S*.[6,8,9]

Stabilize: The pelvis over the iliac crest.[8,9]

Palpate: The gluteus medius on the lateral aspect of the ilium above the greater trochanter of the femur.[8]

Observe: *S* lift the leg upward, abducting the hip (Fig. 9-38, *A*).

Resist: Just proximal to the knee in a downward direction, toward adduction (Fig. 9-38, *B*).[8]

Procedure for Testing Grades P (2), T (1), and 0

Position: *S* lying supine with both legs extended and in neutral rotation. *E* stands next to *S* on the opposite side.[8]

Stabilize: The pelvis at the iliac crest on the side to be tested and the opposite limb at the lateral aspect of the calf.[8]

Palpate: Use the hand stabilizing over the pelvis to palpate the gluteus medius muscle simultaneously by adjusting the position of the hand so that the fingers are touching the lateral aspect of the ilium, above the greater trochanter, as described for previous test.

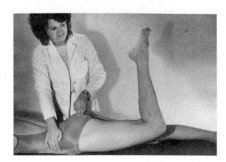
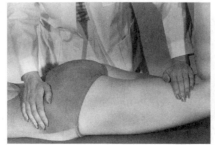
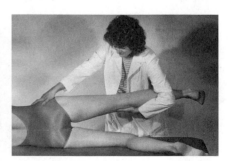

A **B** **C**

FIG. 9-37 Hip extension. **A,** Palpate and observe. **B,** Resist. **C,** Gravity-decreased position.

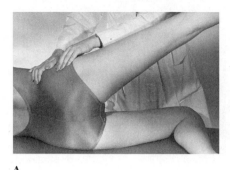
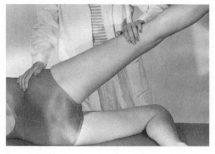
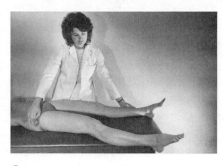

A   B   C

FIG. 9-38 Hip abduction. **A,** Palpate and observe. **B,** Resist. **C,** Gravity-decreased position.

Observe: *S* move the free leg sideward, abducting the hip as far as possible and maintaining neutral rotation during this movement (Fig. 9-38, *C*).[8]
Grade: According to standard definitions of muscle grades.
Substitutions: Lateral muscles of the trunk may contract to bring the pelvis toward the thorax, effecting partial abduction at the hip.[8] If the hip is externally rotated, the hip flexors may assist in abduction.[6,8,10]

Motion

Hip adduction

Muscles[4,8-10]	Innervation[4,8,9]
Adductor magnus	Obturator and sciatic nerve, L2,3,4,5, S1
Adductor brevis	Obturator, L2,3,4
Adductor longus	Obturator, L2,3,4
Gracilis	Obturator, L2,3,4
Pectineus	Femoral and obturator, L2,3,4

Procedure for Testing Grades N (5) to F (3)

Position: *S* sidelying on right for test of right leg or on left side for test of left leg; body in a straight line with legs extended. *E* stands behind *S*. This test may also be done with *S* in the supine position.[6,7,8]
Stabilize: Support *S*'s upper leg in partial abduction while *S* holds on to the supporting surface for stability.[5,8,9]
Palpate: Any of the adductor muscles as follows: adductor magnus at the middle of the medial surface of the thigh; adductor longus at the medial aspect of the groin; gracilis on the medial aspect of the posterior surface of the knee, just anterior to the semitendinosus tendon.[10]
Observe: *S* raise the lower leg up from the supporting surface, keeping the knee extended. Observe that there is no rotation, flexion, or extension of the hip or pelvic tilting (Fig. 9-39, *A*).[9]
Resist: Over the medial aspect of the leg, just proximal to the knee, downward toward abduction or outward if tested in supine. (Fig. 9-39, *B*).[6,8,9]

Procedure for Testing Grades P (2), T (1), and 0

Position: *S* supine; limb to be tested is abducted to 45°. *E* stands next to *S* on the opposite side.
Stabilize: Over the iliac crest on the side to be tested.[8]
Palpate: Same as described for previous test.
Observe: *S* adduct the leg toward midline (Fig. 9-39, *C*).
Grade: According to standard definitions of muscle grades.
Substitutions: Hip flexors may substitute for adductors. *S* will internally rotate the hip and tilt the pelvis backward. Hamstrings may be used to substitute for adduction. *S* will externally rotate the hip and tip the pelvis forward.[9,10]

Motion

Hip external rotation

Muscles[8-10]	Innervation[8,9]
Quadratus femoris	Sacral plexus, L4,5, S1
Piriformis	Sacral plexus, L5, S1,2
Obturator internus	Sacral plexus, L5, S1,2
Obturator externus	Obturator nerve, L3,4
Gemellus superior	Sacral plexus, L5, S1,2
Gemellus inferior	Sacral plexus, L4,5, S1

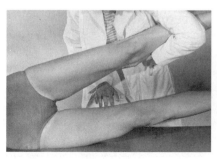
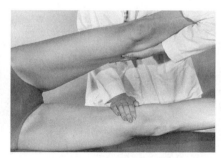
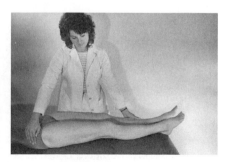

A   B   C

FIG. 9-39 Hip adduction. **A,** Palpate and observe. **B,** Resist. **C,** Gravity-decreased position.

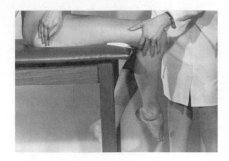
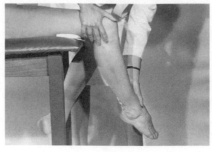
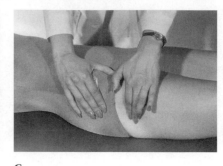

A   B   C

FIG. 9-40   Hip external rotation. **A,** Palpate and observe. **B,** Resist. **C,** Gravity-decreased position.

Procedure for Testing Grades N (5) to F (3)

Position: *S* seated with knees flexed over the edge of the table. A small pad or folded towel is placed under the knee on the side to be tested. *E* stands in front of *S* toward the side to be tested.[8,9]

Stabilize: On the lateral aspect of the knee on the side to be tested. *S* may grasp the edge of the table to stabilize the trunk and pelvis.[8,9]

Palpate: Difficult or impossible to palpate these deep muscles. Action of the external rotators may be detected by palpating deeply posterior to the greater trochanter of the femur.[8]

Observe: *S* rotate the thigh outwardly, moving the foot medially (Fig. 9-40, *A*).

Resist: At the medial aspect of the lower leg, just proximal to the ankle in a lateral direction, toward internal rotation.[6,8,9] Resistance should be given carefully and gradually, because the use of the long lever arm can cause joint injury if sudden forceful resistance is given. Subjects with knee instability should be tested in supine position.[6,8] (Fig. 9-40, *B*).

Procedure for Testing Grades P (2), T (1), and 0

Position: *S* lying supine with hips and knees extended; hip to be tested is internally rotated. *E* is standing next to *S* on the opposite side.[8]

Stabilize: The pelvis on the side to be tested.

Palpate: Action of the external rotators may be detected by palpating deeply posterior to the greater trochanter of the femur.[8]

Observe: *S* roll the thigh outward (laterally). Gravity may assist this motion once *S* has passed the neutral position. *E* may use one hand to palpate and the other to offer slight resistance during the second half of the movement to compensate for the assistance of gravity. If the range can be completed with slight resistance, a grade of poor can be given (Fig. 9-40, *C*).[8]

Grade: According to standard definitions of muscle grades for fair to normal muscles. Muscles are graded poor if ROM in the gravity-decreased position can be achieved against slight resistance during the second half of the ROM. A grade of trace can be assigned if contraction of external rotators can be detected by the deep palpation, described for previous test, when the movement is attemped in the gravity-decreased position.[8]

Substitutions: Gluteus maximus may substitute for the deep external rotators when the hip is in extension. Sartorius may substitute, but external rotation will be accompanied by hip flexion, abduction, and knee flexion.[6,10]

Motion

Hip internal rotation

Muscles[4,8-10]	Innervation[8-10]
Gluteus minimus	Superior gluteal nerve, L4,5, S1
Gluteus medius	Superior gluteal nerve, L4,5, S1
Tensor fascia latae	Superior gluteal nerve, L4,5, S1

Procedure for Testing Grades N (5) to F (3)

Position: *S* seated on a table with the knees flexed over the edge with small pad placed under the knee. *E* stands next to *S* on the side to be tested.[8] (*E* is shown on the opposite side in the illustration so that the palpation and stabilization will be apparent.)

Stabilize: At the medial aspect of the knee. *S* may grasp the edge of the table to stabilize the pelvis and trunk.[8,9]

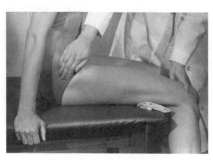
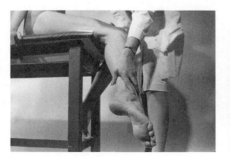
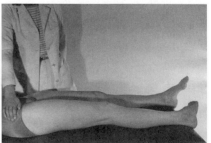

A   B   C

FIG. 9-41   Hip internal rotation. **A,** Palpate and observe. **B,** Resist. **C,** Gravity-decreased rotation.

Palpate: The gluteus medius between the iliac crest and the greater trochanter.[4]

Observe: S rotate the thigh inwardly, moving the foot laterally. E should observe that S does not lift the pelvis on the side being tested (Fig. 9-41, A).[8]

Resist: At the lateral aspect of the lower leg, pushing the leg medially and thus the thigh toward external rotation. The resistance is stressful to the knee joint. Subjects with knee instability should be tested in the supine position described for next test (Fig. 9-41, B).[6,8,9]

Procedure for Testing Grades P (2), T (1), and 0

Position: S supine with hips and knees extended; hip to be tested in external rotation. E stands on the opposite side.[8]

Stabilize: Over the iliac crest on the side to be tested.[8]

Palpate: Same as described for previous test.

Observe: S rotate the thigh inwardly or medially. As in external rotation, gravity may assist the motion once the neutral position is passed, but less than in the test for external rotation (Fig. 9-41, C).

Grade: According to standard definitions of muscle grades.

Substitutions: Hip adduction and knee flexion; trunk medial rotation may also cause some internal rotation of the hip.[6,10]

Motion

Knee flexion

Muscles[4,8-10]	Innervation[4,8,9]
(Hamstrings)	
Biceps femoris	Sciatic nerve, L5, S1,2,3
Semitendinosus	Sciatic nerve, L4,5, S1,2
Semimembranosus	Sciatic nerve, L4,5, S1,2

Procedure for Testing Grades N (5) to F (3)

Position: S lying prone with knees and hips in extension and neutral rotation.[5,6,8,9] E stands next to S on the opposite side, toward the lower end of the supporting surface.[8]

Stabilize: Firmly over the posterior aspect of the thigh, above the tedinous insertion of the knee flexors.[8]

Palpate: For the biceps femoris tendon on the lateral aspect of the posterior surface of the knee as it nears its insertion on the head of the fibula or for the semitendinosus tendon in the middle of the posterior surface of the knee.[4,10] It is the most prominent tendon on the back of the knee.[4]

Observe: S flex the knee to slightly less than 90° (Fig. 9-42, A).[10]

Resist: By grasping S's leg over the posterior aspect of the ankle and pushing downward toward knee extension.[8] Note that not

as much resistance can be applied to knee flexion in this position as when tested with the hip flexed as in sitting (Fig. 9-42, B).[9]

Procedure for Testing Grades P (2), T (1), and 0

Position: S sidelying with knees and hips extended and in neutral rotation. E stands next to S and supports the upper leg in slight abduction to allow testing of the lower leg.[8]

Stabilize: Over the medial aspect of the thigh.

Palpate: The semitendinosus as described for previous test.

Observe: S flex the knee of the lower leg (Fig. 9-42, C).

Grade: According to standard definitions of muscle grades.

Substitutions: Sartorius may substitute or assist the hamstrings, but hip flexion and external rotation will occur simultaneously.[8,10] Gracilis may substitute, causing hip adduction with knee flexion. Gastrocnemius may assist or substitute if strong plantar flexion of the ankle occurs during knee flexion.[8]

Motion

Knee extension

Muscles[8]	Innervation[8]
Quadriceps femoris group	Femoral nerve, L2,3,4
Rectus femoris	
Vastus intermedius	
Vastus medialis	
Vastus lateralis	

Procedure for Testing Grades N (5) to F (3)

Position: S sitting with knees flexed over the edge of the table, feet suspended off the floor. S may lean backward slightly to release tension on the hamstrings and grasp the edge of the table for stability.[8] E stands next to S on the side to be tested.

Stabilize: Thigh by holding hand firmly over it, or place one hand under S's knee to cushion it from the edge of the table. S may grasp the edge of the table.[6,8,9]

Palpate: Any of the muscles in the quadriceps femoris group as follows: rectus femoris on the anterior aspect of the thigh; vastus medialis on the "anteromedial aspect of the lower third of the thigh"; vastus lateralis on the "anterolateral aspect of the lower third of the thigh."[10] Vastus intermedius cannot be palpated.[10]

Observe: S raise the leg toward the ceiling, extending the knee to slightly less than full ROM. Observe for hip movements as evidence of substitutions (Fig. 9-43, A).

Resist: On the anterior surface of the leg, just above the ankle, with downward pressure toward knee flexion.[8,9] S should not be allowed to "lock" the knee joint at the end of the ROM

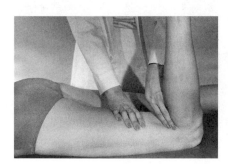
A

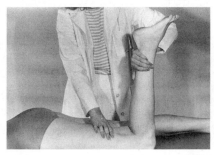
B

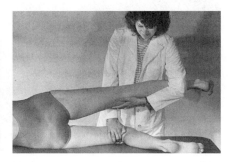
C

FIG. 9-42 Knee-flexion. **A,** Palpate and observe. **B,** Resist. **C,** Gravity-decreased position.

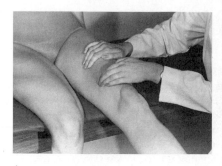
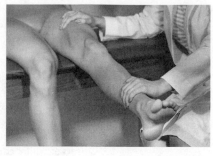
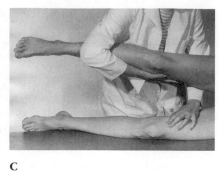

A   **B**   **C**

FIG. 9-43   Knee extension. **A,** Palpate and observe. **B,** Resist. **C,** Gravity-decreased position.

when full extension is achieved.[6,8] Maintenance of a slight amount of knee flexion will prevent this condition. Resistance to a locked knee can cause joint injury (Fig. 9-43, *B*).[8]

Procedure for Testing Grades P (2), T (1), and 0

Position: *S* sidelying on the side to be tested. The lower leg is positioned with the hip extended and the knee flexed to 90°. *E* stands behind *S*.

Stabilize: The upper leg in slight abduction with one hand and with the other over the anterior aspect of the thigh on the leg to be tested.[8]

Palpate: Any of the muscles, as described for previous test, with the same hand used to stabilize *S*'s thigh. Then ask *S* to straighten the leg, extending the knee. Observe for hip movements as signs of substitution (Fig. 9-43, *C*).

Grade: According to standard definitions of muscle grades.

Substitutions: Tensor fascia latae may substitute for or assist weak quadriceps. In this case, hip internal rotation will accompany knee extension.[8,9]

Motion

Ankle plantar flexion

Muscles[4,8-10]	Innervation[9]
Gastrocnemius	Tibial nerve, S1,2
Soleus	Tibial nerve, L5, S1,2
Plantaris	Tibial nerve, L4,5, S1

Procedure for Testing Grades N (5) to F (3)

Position: *S* lying prone with the hips and knees extended and the feet projecting beyond the edge of the table. *E* stands at the lower end of the table facing *S*'s feet.[5,6,9]

Stabilize: Weight of the leg is usually adequate stabilization.

Palpate: The gastrocnemius on the posterior aspect of the calf of the leg, or the soleus, slightly lateral to and beneath the lateral head of the gastrocnemius.[10] The gastrocnemius tendon above the calcaneus may also be palpated.[8]

Observe: *S* pull the heel upward, plantar flexing the ankle. Observe for flexion of the toes and forefoot before movement of the heel as evidence of substitutions (Fig. 9-44, *A*).[9,10]

Resist: On the posterior aspect of the calcaneus as if pulling downward and on the forefoot as if pushing forward. If there is considerable weakness, pressure to the calcaneus may be sufficient (Fig. 9-44, *B*).[9]

Procedure for Testing Grades P(2), T (1), and 0

Position: *S* lying on the side to be tested; hip and knee of the lower limb are extended and the ankle is in midposition. The upper limb may be flexed at the knee to keep it out of the way. *E* stands at the lower end of the table.[8]

Stabilize: Over the posterior aspect of the calf.[8]

Palpate: As described for previous test.

Observe: *S* pull the heel upward, pointing the toes down. Observe for toe flexion, inversion, or eversion of the foot as evidence of substitutions (Fig. 9-44, *C*).

Grade: According to standard definitions of muscle grades.

Substitutions: Flexor digitorum longus and flexor hallucis longus can substitute for plantar flexors, producing toe flexion and flexion of the forefoot, with incomplete movement of the calcaneus. Substitution by the peroneus longus and brevis will cause foot eversion, and substitution by the tibialis posterior will cause foot inversion. Substitution by all three will effect

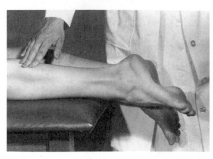
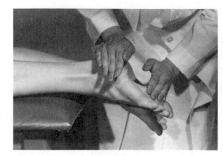
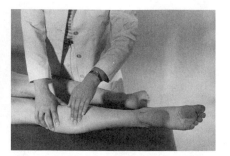

A   **B**   **C**

FIG. 9-44   Ankle plantar flexion. **A,** Palpate and observe. **B,** Resist. **C,** Gravity-decreased position.

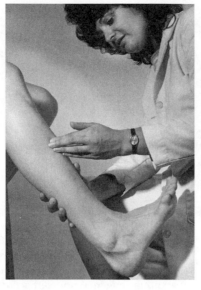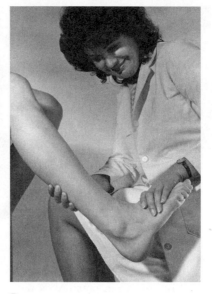

A   B

FIG. 9-45 Ankle dorsiflexion with inversion. **A,** Palpate and observe. **B,** Resist.

plantar flexion of the forefoot, with limited movement of the calcaneus.[8,10]

Motion

Ankle dorsiflexion with inversion

Muscles[7-9]	Innervation[7-9]
Tibialis anterior	Peroneal nerve, L4,5, S1
Peroneus tertius	Deep peroneal nerve, L5, S1

Procedure for Testing Grades N (5) to F (3)

Position: *S* seated with the legs, flexed at the knees, over the edge of the table. *E* sits in front of *S*, slightly to the side to be tested. *S*'s heel can rest in E's lap.[8,9]

Stabilize: The leg just above the ankle.

Palpate: The tibialis anterior tendon on the anterior medial aspect of the ankle.[6,8] Muscle fibers may be palpated on the anterior surface of the leg, just lateral to the tibia.[10]

Observe: *S* pull the forefoot upward and inward, keeping the toes relaxed, dorsiflexing and inverting the foot. Watch for extension of the great toe preceding the ankle motion as a sign of muscle substitution (Fig. 9-45, *A*).[8]

Resist: On the medial dorsal aspect of the foot, toward plantar flexion and eversion (Fig. 9-45, *B*).[8,9]

Procedure for Testing Grades P (2), T (1), and 0

The same position and procedure described for previous test may be used with modified grading. The test may also be performed with *S* in sidelying or supine position.[6,8]

Grade: If the against-gravity position is used in the procedure for grades P to 0, clinical judgment of the examiner must be used to determine muscle grades. Partial ROM against gravity can be graded poor. If the test is performed in the supine position for these grades, standard definitions of muscle grades may be used.[8]

Substitutions: Extensor hallucis longus and extensor digitorum longus may assist or substitute. Movement will be preceded by extension of the great toe or by all of the toes.[6,8,9,10]

Motion

Foot inversion

Muscles[8,9]	Innervation[6,7]
Tibialis posterior	Tibial nerve, L5, S1

Procedure for Testing Grades N (5) to F (3)

Position: *S* lying on the side to be tested, with the hip in neutral rotation, knee extended, and ankle in slight plantar flexion.[8]

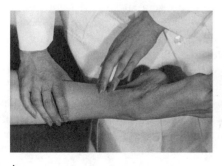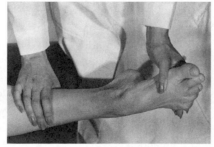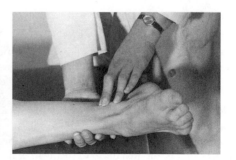

A   B   C

FIG. 9-46 Foot inversion. **A,** Palpate and observe. **B,** Resist. **C,** Gravity-decreased position.

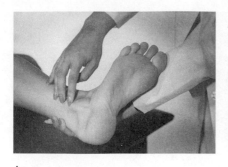
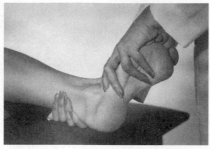
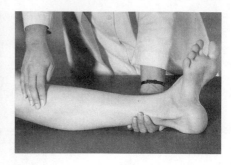

A   B   C

FIG. 9-47   Foot eversion. **A,** Palpate and observe. **B,** Resist. **C,** Gravity-decreased position.

The upper leg may be flexed at the knee to keep it out of the way. *E* stands at the end of the table, facing *S*'s feet.

Stabilize: Leg to be tested above the ankle joint on the dorsal surface of the calf, being careful not to put pressure on the tibialis posterior muscle.[8]

Palpate: The tendon of the tibialis posterior muscle between the medial malleolus and navicular bone or above and just posterior to the medial malleolus.[6,8]

Observe: *S* move the foot upward (medially) and inverting it, keeping the toes relaxed. There normally will be some plantar flexion as well (Fig. 9-46, *A*, see page 145).[8,9]

Resist: On the medial border of the forefoot toward eversion (Fig. 9-46, *B*).[6,8,9]

Procedure for Testing Grades P (2), T (1), and 0

Position: *S* lying supine with the hip extended and in neutral rotation, knee extended, and the ankle in midposition.

Stabilize: Same as described for previous test.

Palpate: Same as described for previous test.

Observe: *S* move the foot inward (medially), inverting it while keeping the toes relaxed (Fig. 9-46, *C*).

Grade: According to standard definitions of muscle grades.

Substitutions: Flexor hallucis longus and flexor digitorum longus can substitute for tibialis posterior. Movement will be accompanied by toe flexion, or toes will flex when resistance is applied.[8-10]

Motion

Foot eversion

Muscles[8,9]	Innervation[8,9]
Peroneus longus	Peroneal nerve, L4,5, S1
Peroneus brevis	
Peroneus tertius	

Procedure for Testing Grades Normal (N) and Fair (F)

Position: *S* sidelying with the lower leg to be tested in hip extension and neutral rotation, knee in extension, and ankle in midposition. The upper leg is flexed at the knee to keep it out of the way.[8,9]

Stabilize: Above the ankle on its medial suface, supporting the foot slightly above the table surface.[8,9]

Palpate: The peroneus longus over the upper half of the lateral aspect of the calf, just distal to the head of the fibula. Its tendon can be palpated on the lateral aspect of the ankle, above and behind the lateral malleolus. Peroneus brevis tendon may be palpated on the lateral border of the foot, proximal to the base

of the 5th metatarsal.[8,10] Its muscle fibers can be found on the lower half of the lateral surface of the leg, over the fibula.[8]

Observe: *S* turn the sole of the foot outward, everting it. (Note that this movement is normally accompanied by some degree of plantar flexion.)[9,10] Observe for dorsiflexion or toe extension as evidence of substitutions (Fig. 9-47, *A*).

Resist: Against the lateral border and the plantar surface of the foot toward inversion and dorsiflexion (Fig. 9-47, *B*).[9]

Procedure for Testing Grades P (2), T (1), and 0

Position: *S* lying supine, hip extended and in neutral rotation.[8] The knee is extended and ankle is in midposition.

Stabilize: The leg under the calf.

Palpate: The same as described for previous test.

Observe: *S* move the foot in a sideward or lateral direction, thus everting it (Fig. 9-47, *C*).

Grade: Grade according to standard definitions of muscle grades.

Substitutions: Peroneus tertius, while everting the foot, also dorsiflexes it. If it is substituting for peroneus longus and peroneus brevis, dorsiflexion will accompany eversion. Extensor digitorum longus can also substitute for the peroneals, and toe extension will precede or accompany eversion.[6,10]

FUNCTIONAL MUSCLE TESTING

The functional muscle test is a useful tool when screening muscles for normal strength.[8,12] It is used by occupational therapists in some health care facilities where specific muscle testing is the responsibility of the physical therapy service. To avoid duplication of services, the occupational therapist may wish to perform a functional muscle test to assess the general strength and motion capabilities of the patient. In dysfunctions in which muscle weakness is not a primary or important symptom, discrete muscle testing may not be needed. Instead, a general estimate of strength is desirable and adequate to plan treatment and measure progress. Sometimes a quick functional muscle test may be performed to identify areas of substantial weakness that deserve discrete testing. Thus the functional muscle test may serve as a screening tool,[6] conserving the examiner's time and the subject's energy.

Various screening tests have been devised. In one, the examiner passively places the part in the position used for the normal test, without considering gravity, and asks the subject to hold the position against resistance. Still another method tests both sides simultaneously while the subject is in the sitting position. If the subject cannot hold against resistance in the screening test, the more thorough manual muscle test should be administered. Observation of the subject performing ordinary ADL can also be used as a screening test of baseline strength for function.[8]

The following functional muscle test should be performed while the subject is comfortably seated in a sturdy chair or wheelchair.

The subject is asked to perform the test motion against gravity or in the gravity-decreased position, if the former is not feasible.

In all of the tests the subject is allowed to complete the test motion before the examiner applies resistance. The resistance is applied at the end of the ROM while the subject maintains the positon and resists the force applied by the examiner. The examiner may make modifications in positioning to suit individual needs. As in the manual muscle tests, the examiner should stabilize proximal parts and attempt to rule out substitutions. The reader should be familiar with joint motions, their prime movers, manual muscle testing, and muscle grades before performing this test.

FUNCTIONAL MUSCLE TEST

Scapular elevation (upper trapezius and levator scapula): S elevates shoulders, and E pushes down on shoulders into depression.

Scapular abduction (serratus anterior): With S's arms positioned in 90° of elbow and shoulder flexion, E pushes at shoulder into scapular adduction.

Scapular adduction (middle trapezius and rhomboids): S extends shoulder and flexes elbow fully, producing scapular adduction. E pushes at shoulder joint into scapular abduction.

Scapular depression (lower trapezius, latissimus dorsi): S extends arm down at side of body as if reaching to floor. E attempts to push arm up at a point just proximal to elbow joint. Muscles act to stabilize scapula and prevent elevation.

Shoulder flexion (anterior deltoid and coracobrachialis): With S's shoulder flexed to 90° and elbow flexed or extended, E pushes down on arm proximal to elbow into extension.

Shoulder extension (latissimus dorsi and teres major): S moves shoulder into full extension. E pushes from behind at a point proximal to elbow into flexion.

Shoulder abduction (middle deltoid and supraspinatus): S abducts shoulder to 90° with elbow flexed or extended. E pushes down on arm just proximal to elbow into adduction.

Shoulder horizontal adduction (pectoralis major, anterior deltoid): S crosses arms in front of chest. E reaches from behind and attempts to pull arms back into horizontal abduction at a point just proximal to elbow.

Shoulder horizontal abduction (posterior deltoid, teres minor, infraspinatus): S moves arms from full horizontal adduction as just described to full horizontal abduction. E pushes forward on arms just proximal to elbow into horizontal adduction.

Shoulder external rotation (infraspinatus and teres minor): S holds arm in 90° of shoulder abduction and 90° of elbow flexion, then externally rotates shoulder through available ROM. E supports or stabilizes upper arm proximal to elbow and pushes from behind at dorsal aspect of wrist into internal rotation.

Shoulder internal rotation (subscapularis, teres major, latissimus dorsi, pectoralis major): S begins with arm as described for external rotation but performs internal rotation. E supports or stabilizes upper arm as before and pulls up into external rotation at volar aspect of wrist.

Elbow flexion (biceps, brachialis): With forearm supinated, S flexes elbow from full extension. E sits opposite subject and stabilizes upper arm against trunk while attempting to pull forearm into extension at volar aspect of wrist.

Elbow extension (triceps): With S's upper arm supported in 90° of abduction (gravity-decreased position) or 160° shoulder flexion (against-gravity position), elbow is extended from full flexion. E pushes forearm into flexion at dorsal aspect of wrist.

Forearm supination (biceps, supinator): Upper arm is stabilized against trunk by S or E. Elbow is flexed to 90°, and forearm is in full pronation. S supinates forearm. E grasps distal forearm and attempts to rotate it into pronation.

Forearm pronation (pronator teres, pronator quadratus): S is positioned as described for forearm supination except that forearm is in full supination. S pronates forearm. E grasps distal forearm and attempts to rotate it into supination.

Wrist flexion (flexor carpi radials, flexor carpi ulnaris, palmaris longus): S's forearm is supported on its dorsal surface on a tabletop or armrest. Hand is moved up from tabletop, using wrist flexion. E is seated next to or opposite S and pushes on palm of hand, giving equal pressure on radial and ulnar sides into wrist extension or down toward tabletop.

Wrist extension (extensor carpi radialis longus and brevis, extensor carpi ulnaris): S's forearm is supported on a tabletop or armrest, resting on its volar surface. Hand is lifted from tabletop, using wrist extension. E sits next to or opposite S and pushes on dorsal aspect of palm, giving equal pressure at radial and ulnar sides into wrist flexion or down toward tabletop.

Finger MP flexion and IP extension (lumbricales and interossei): With forearm and hand supported on tabletop on dorsal surface, E stabilizes palm and S flexes MP joints while maintaining extension of IP joints. E pushes into extension with index finger across proximal phalanges or pushes on tip of each finger into IP flexion and MP extension.

Finger IP flexion (flexors digitorum profundus and sublimis): S is positioned as described for MP flexion. IP joints are flexed while maintaining extension of MP joints. E attempts to pull fingers back into extension by hooking fingertips with those of S.

Finger MP extension (IP joints flexed) (extensor digitorum communis, extensor indicis proprius, extensor digiti minimi): S's forearm and hand are supported on a table surface, resting on ulnar border. Wrist is stabilized by E in 0° neutral position. S moves MP joints from flexion to full extension (hyperextension) while keeping IP joints flexed. E pushes fingers at PIP joints simultaneously into flexion.

Finger abduction (dorsal interossei, abductor digiti minimi): S's forearm is resting on volar surface on a table. E may stabilize wrist in slight extension so that hand is raised slightly off supporting surface. S abducts fingers. E pushes two fingers at a time together at the proximal phalanges into adduction. First, index finger and middle fingers are pushed together, then ring finger and middle fingers, and finally little finger and ring fingers. Resistance is modified to accommodate small muscles.

Finger adduction (palmar interossei): S is positioned as described for finger abduction. Fingers are adducted tightly. E attempts to pull fingers apart one at a time at the proximal phalanges. First, index finger is pulled away from middle finger then ring finger is pulled away from middle finger, and finally little finger is pulled away from ring finger. In normal hand, adducted finger 'snaps' back into adducted position when E pulls it into abduction and lets go quickly. An alternate method is for examiner to place index finger between two of S's fingers. S should adduct against it, thus estimating amount of force or pressure that S is exerting.

Thumb MP and IP flexion (flexor pollicis brevis and flexor pollicis longus): S's forearm should be supported on a firm surface, with elbow flexed at 90° and forearm in 45° supination. Thumb is flexed across palm. E pulls on tip of thumb into extension.

Thumb MP and IP extension (extensor pollicis brevis and extensor pollicis longus): S is positioned as for thumb MP and IP flexion. Thumb is extended away from palm. E pushes on tip of thumb into flexion.

Thumb palmar abduction (abductor pollicis longus and abductor pollicis brevis): S is positioned as described for thumb flexion and extension. Thumb is abducted away from palm in a plane perpendicular to palm. S resists movement at metacarpal head into adduction.

Thumb adduction (adductor pollicis): S is positioned as for all other thumb movements. Thumb is adducted to palm. E attempts to pull thumb into abduction at metacarpal head or proximal phalanx.

Opposition of thumb to 5th finger (opponens pollicis, opponens digiti minimi): S is positioned with elbow flexed to 90° and dorsal surface of forearm and hand resting on a tabletop or armrest. Thumb is opposed to 5th finger, making pad-to-pad contact. E attempts to pull fingers apart, applying force at metacarpal heads of both fingers.

FUNCTIONAL MUSCLE TEST OF THE LOWER EXTREMITIES

All of these tests can be performed with S sitting with legs flexed over edge of supporting surface and feet slightly above floor, except for hip extension test.

Hip flexion (psoas major, iliacus): S flexes hip, bringing leg up from seat; E pushes down on distal aspect of the thigh.

Hip extension (gluteus maximus): S lying prone lifts leg from supporting surface. E pushes down on posterior distal aspect of thigh. Test can be done with knee flexed to 90°.

Hip abduction (gluteus medius): S moves leg to be tested away from other leg. Leg is supported by E from posterior aspect of knee to reduce effect of resistance from friction on supporting surface. E pushes inward at distal lateral aspect of thigh.

Hip adduction (adductor group): E places palm of hand at medial aspect of distal thigh of leg to be tested and asks S to bring legs together, knees touching. E pulls outward on leg.

Hip external rotation (obturators, gemelli, piriformis, quadratus femoris): S moves foot medially by rotating hip externally. E pushes at medial aspect of ankle in lateral direction while stabilizing at lateral aspect of thigh, just above knee.

Hip internal rotation (gluteus minimus): S moves foot laterally by internally rotating hip. E pushes at lateral aspect of ankle in medial direction while stabilizing at medial aspect of thigh, just above knee.

Knee flexion (hamstrings): S flexes knee so that leg is flexed under seat of supporting surface. E pulls forward at posterior aspect of ankle.

Knee extension (quadriceps femoris group): S extends knee, straightening leg in seated position. E pushes downward on anterior distal aspect of ankle. To avoid injury, S should not lock knee but should maintain a slight amount of knee flexion during resistance.[6] E can assist by stabilizing with one hand under knee being tested.

Ankle plantar flexion (gastrocnemius, soleus): S is asked to point foot downward. E places hand on metatarsal heads and pushes upward toward dorsiflexion.

Ankle dorsiflexion with inversion (tibialis anterior): S points foot upward and inward simultaneously. E pushes on medial dorsal aspect of foot in downward and lateral direction.

Foot inversion (tibialis posterior): S turns sole of foot medially while maintaining neutral position between plantar flexion and dorsiflexion of ankle. E pushes on medial border of forefoot in outward direction.

Foot eversion (peroneal group): S turns sole of foot laterally while maintaining neutral position of ankle, as just described. E pushes on lateral border of foot in inward direction.

SUMMARY

Manual muscle testing evaluates the level of strength in a muscle or muscle group. It is a primary evaluation tool for patients with motor unit disorders, and orthopedic conditions. It does not measure muscle endurance or coordination, however, nor can it be used accurately if spasticity is present.

Accurate assessment of muscle strength depends on the knowledge, skill, and experience of the examiner. Although there are standard definitions of muscle grades, clinical judgment is important in accurate evaluation.

Muscle test results are used to plan treatment strategies to increase strength and/or compensate for weakness. Functional muscle tests can be used to assess the general level of strength available for ADL and to screen for patients who need specific manual muscle testing.

REVIEW QUESTIONS

1. List three general classifications of physical dysfunction in which muscle weakness is a primary symptom.
2. Given F+ muscle strength and low endurance, in which kinds of activities can the patient be expected to participate?
3. List at least three purposes for evaluating muscle strength.
4. Discuss five considerations and their implications in treatment planning that are based on the results of the muscle strength evaluation.
5. Define endurance and discuss its correlation with muscle strength.
6. How can muscle weakness be differentiated from joint limitation?
7. If there is joint limitation, can muscle strength be measured accurately? How is strength recorded when available ROM is less than normal?
8. What does the manual muscle test measure?
9. What are the limitations of the manual muscle test?
10. When is the manual muscle test contraindicated?
11. What are the criteria for determining muscle grades?
12. In relation to the floor as a horizontal plane, describe or demonstrate what is meant by the terms "with gravity assisting," "with gravity decreased," "against gravity," and "against gravity and resistance."
13. List five factors that can influence the amount of resistance against which a muscle group can hold.
14. Define the muscle grades: N (5), G (4), F − (3 −), F (3), P (2), P − (2 −), T (1), and zero (0).
15. Define what is meant by substitution.
16. How are substitutions most likely to be ruled out in the muscle testing procedure?
17. List the steps in the muscle testing procedure.
18. Is it always necessary to perform the manual muscle test to determine level of strength? If not, what alternative may be used to make a general assessment of strength? Generally describe the procedure.
19. Describe or demonstrate the muscle testing procedures for testing grades of normal to fair for the following muscle groups: scapula adduction, shoulder flexion, elbow extension, forearm pronation, wrist flexion, opposition, hip extension, knee flexion, and ankle dorsiflexion.
20. List the purposes of functional muscle testing.

REFERENCES

1. Basmajian JF: *Muscles alive,* ed 4, Baltimore, 1978, Williams & Wilkins.
2. Bobath B: *Adult hemiplegia: evaluation and treatment,* ed 2, London, 1978, William Heinemann Medical Books.
3. Brunnstrom S: *Movement therapy in hemiplegia,* New York, 1970, Harper & Row.
4. Brunnstrom S: *Clinical kinesiology,* Philadelphia, 1972, FA Davis.
5. Chusid J: *Correlative neuroanatomy and functional neurology,* ed 19, Los Altos, Calif, 1985, Lange Medical Publications.
6. Clarkson HM, Gilewich GB: *Musculoskeletal assessment,* Baltimore, 1989, Williams and Wilkins.
7. Cole JH, Furness AL, Twomey LT: *Muscles in action,* New York, 1988, Churchill Livingstone.
8. Daniels L, Worthingham C: *Muscle testing,* ed 5, Philadelphia, 1986, WB Saunders.
9. Kendall FP, McCreary EK: *Muscles: testing and function,* ed 2, Baltimore, 1983, Williams & Wilkins.
10. Killingsworth A: *Basic physical disability procedures,* San José, 1987, Maple Press.
11. Landen B, Amizich A: Functional muscle examination and gait analysis, *J Amer Phys Ther Assoc* 43:39, 1963.
12. Pact V, Sirotkin-Roses M, Beatus J: *The muscle testing handbook,* Boston, 1984, Little, Brown.
13. Rancho Los Amigos Hospital, Department of Occupational Therapy: *Guide for muscle testing of the upper extremity,* Downey, Calif, 1978, Professional Staff Association of the Rancho Los Amigos Hospital.

Evaluation of Motor Control

Maureen Forte Undzis, Barbara Zoltan,
Lorraine Williams Pedretti

Motor control is the ability to make dynamic postural adjustments and regulate body and limb movement.[35] Complex neurological systems — that is, the cerebral cortex, basal ganglia, and cerebellum — collaborate to make motor control possible. When a neurological insult occurs, such as stroke or head injury, or there is a disease like multiple sclerosis or Parkinson's, motor control is affected. Functional recovery depends on the amount of damage and the neurological recovery expected.

Motor control is assessed from a functional framework and in its component parts to help the evaluator plan appropriate treatment intervention. Components necessary for motor control include normal postural tone and postural mechanisms, normal muscle tone, selective movement, and coordination.

POSTURAL MECHANISM

Normal postural mechanisms are automatic movements that provide an appropriate level of stability and mobility.[10] These automatic reactions develop in the early years of life and allow for trunk control and mobility, head control, midline orientation of self, weight-bearing and weight-shifting in all directions, dynamic balance, and controlled voluntary limb movement.[6,10]

The components of a normal postural mechanism include normal postural tone and control, integration of primitive reflexes and mass patterns, righting reactions, equilibrium and protective reactions, and selective voluntary movement.[6,10]

In patients who have suffered central nervous system damage (CNS) such as stroke or brain injury, the normal postural mechanism is disrupted. The patient's movements are dominated by abnormal tone and mass pattern,

lacking balance and stability. Movements are slow and uncoordinated. It is imperative that therapists evaluate the extent of damage to the postural mechanism in patients with CNS trauma or disease.

Postural tone is tonus that is present in the postural muscles, high enough to resist gravity, yet low enough to allow movement.[6] It allows us to adjust automatically and continuously to movements.[40] Postural control is the ability of a person to control or regulate specific postural outputs.[29] This control provides the foundation for voluntary selective movements, because normal selective movement cannot be superimposed on abnormal tone.

The following automatic reactions, which are part of the postural mechanism, are important to evaluate in patients with CNS trauma or disease.

RIGHTING REACTIONS

These automatic reactions maintain and restore the normal position of the head in space and its normal relationship with the trunk, as well as the normal alignment of the trunk and limbs. Without effective righting reactions, the patient will have difficulty getting up from the floor, getting out of bed, sitting up, and kneeling.[6]

EQUILIBRIUM REACTIONS

Equilibrium reactions, elicited by stimulation of the labyrinths, maintain and regain balance in all activities.[6,26] They ensure sufficient postural alignment when the body's supporting surface is changed, altering the center of gravity.[26] Without equilibrium reactions, the patient will have difficulty maintaining and recovering balance in all positions and activities.

PROTECTIVE REACTIONS

Protective reactions are associated with equilibrium reactions, and consist of protective extension of the arms and hands which is used to protect the head and face when one is falling.[6,21] Without protective reactions, the

Darcy Ann Umphred is gratefully acknowledged for reviewing and assisting with this chapter.

patient may fall or be reluctant to bear weight on the affected side during normal bilateral activities.

Formal testing of these reactions may be difficult because of the cognitive and physical limitations of the patient or time constraints of the therapist. The therapist can evaluate righting reactions, however, during transfers and ADL. Equilibrium and protective reactions can be observed when the patient shifts farther out of midline than necessary during functional activities.

REFLEXES OR SYNERGISTIC PATTERNS

The symmetrical and asymmetrical tonic neck reflex and tonic labyrinthine reflex may interfere with the patient's abilities as described in the paragraphs that follow.

Asymmetrical Tonic Neck Reflex

The patient with *asymmetrical tonic neck reflex* (ATNR) may have difficulty maintaining the head in midline while moving the eyes toward or past midline.[5] The patient may be unable (1) to extend an arm without turning the head or (2) to flex the arm without turning the head the other way.[5,13] The patient may be unable to move either or both arms to midline, especially when in the supine position, because movement of the arms is dependent on head positioning. This positioning causes asymmetry in the arms. Thus this synergy makes it difficult or impossible to bring an object to the mouth, hold an object in both hands, or grasp an object in front of the body while looking at it.

Symmetrical Tonic Neck Reflex

The patient with *symmetrical tonic neck reflex* (STNR) will be unable to support the body weight on hands and knees, maintain balance in quadruped, and/or crawl normally without fixating the head.[6] The patient will have difficulty moving from lying to sitting because when the head is lifted to initiate the task, increased hip extension resists the movement. As the patient struggles to sit up, increased leg extension may also interfere.[13] The patient will have difficulty with bed-to-wheelchair transferring because as the arms and head are extended to initiate the transfer, one or both legs may show increased flexion, which may cause the patient to slide under the bed. Additionally, the affected leg may actually lift off the floor, causing an inability to bear weight.[13]

Tonic Labyrinthine Reflex

The patient exhibiting poorly integrated *tonic labyrinthine reflex* (TLR) will be severely limited in the ability to move. A few examples of functional limitations are the inability to lift the head in supine, initiate flexion to sit up independently from supine, roll over, or sit in a wheelchair for long periods.[6,13] In attempting to move from a supine to sitting position, the patient will experience domination of extensor tone until halfway up when flexor tone begins to take over. Flexor tone continues until full sitting is reached, resulting in the head falling forward, the spine flexing, and the patient falling forward.[5] Sitting in a wheelchair for extended periods can result in increased extensor tone as the patient hyperextends the head to view the environment. The knee is extended, the foot is pushed forward off the foot plate, and eventually the patient may slip or remain in a half-lying asymmetrical position.[13]

Positive Supporting Reaction

The *positive supporting reaction* is caused by pressure on the ball of the foot. This stimulus elicits extension and internal rotation of the hip, knee extension, ankle plantar flexion, and foot inversion. The patient with a positive supporting reaction will have difficulty placing the heel on the ground for standing, putting the heel down first in walking, and having normal body weight transference in walking.[6,13] The patient will have difficulty getting up from or sitting in a chair and walking down steps because it is not possible to move the joints in weight-bearing because the leg remains stiff in extension. The rigid leg can carry the patient's body weight but is unable to contribute to any balance reactions. All balance reactions, therefore, are compensated with other parts of the body.[5]

Crossed Extension Reflex

The *crossed extension reflex* causes increased extensor tone in one leg when the other leg is flexed. Therefore, if the patient with hemiplegia (who is influenced by this reflex) flexes the unaffected leg for walking, a strong extensor hypertonicity occurs in the affected leg and interferes with the normal pattern of ambulation. By the same token, the patient can bridge (lift buttocks) in bed with the weight supported by both legs; if the unaffected leg is lifted (flexed), however, a total extension pattern occurs in the affected leg, and the bridge cannot be maintained.[5,13]

Grasp Reflex

The patient with a *grasp reflex* will not be able to release objects placed in the hand, even if active finger extension is present.[13]

The reflexes just discussed are rarely seen in isolation because motor behavior is accomplished through the interaction of several reflexes. See Chapter 20 for a table listing these reflexes and reactions.

AUTOMATIC ADAPTATION OF MUSCLES TO CHANGES IN POSTURE

Normal muscles will allow for smooth and well-controlled mobility against the force of gravity. The limb can be placed; that is, it can be moved by the examiner and it will feel light, following the movement actively.[6] Otherwise, the limb will feel heavy and flop down if released by the examiner. The limb may also feel resistive to movement, which indicates that it does not have the ability to combat gravity appropriately for function.

If reflexes or stereotypic patterns are not integrated and righting, equilibrium, and protective reactions are impaired, patients will have difficulty using their limbs for function. They may not be able to place their limbs, stabilize an object or manipulate an object. They may not be able to use their limbs to prevent a fall or maintain their balance.

NORMAL MUSCLE TONE

Normal muscle tone, a component of the normal postural mechanism, is a continuous state of mild contraction, or a state of preparedness.[40] It is dependent on the integrity of peripheral and CNS mechanisms and the properties of muscle. There is a tension between the origin and insertion of a muscle, felt as resistance by the therapist when passively manipulating the limbs. The tension is determined partly by mechanical factors (connective tissue and visoelastic properties of muscle) and the degree of motor unit activity.[16] When passively stretched, the muscle offers a small amount of involuntary resistance. The loss of normal muscle tone will interfere with normal selective movement. Normalizing muscle tone is therefore essential for gaining functional motor control.

Normal muscle tone relies on normal function of the cerebellum, motor cortex, basal ganglia, midbrain, vestibular system, spinal cord functions, neuromuscular system, and a normally functioning stretch reflex.[6] The stretch reflex is mediated by the muscle spindle, a sophisticated sensory receptor continuously reporting sensory information from muscles to the CNS. See Chapter 20 on Neurophysiology for more detail on the muscle spindle and other proprioceptors influencing muscle tone.

Normal muscle tone varies from one individual to another and is dependent on factors such as age, sex, and occupation. There is a range that is considered normal. Normal muscle tone is characterized by the following:

1. effective coactivation (stabilization) at axial and proximal joints.
2. ability to move against gravity and resistance.
3. ability to maintain the position of the limb if it is placed passively by the examiner and then released.[6]
4. balanced tone between agonist and antagonist muscles.
5. ease of ability to shift from stability to mobility and vice versa as needed.
6. ability to use muscles in groups or selectively, if necessary.[19]
7. resilience or slight resistance in response to passive movement.[14]

EVALUATING MUSCLE TONE

Objective evaluation of muscle tone in the patient with CNS dysfunction is difficult because of its continuous fluctuation and relationship to the postural mecha-

nism.[6,23] Stereotypic reflexes and associated reactions will alter postural tone. For example, when lying supine, a patient's level of tone is less than when sitting or standing. The level and distribution of tone caused by modulation over the state of the motor pool changes as the position of the patient's head in space and its relation to the body changes.[6] Therefore tone cannot be evaluated in isolation of postural mechanisms, motor function, synergies present, task specificity, and other variant factors related to motor control.

Abnormal muscle tone is usually described using the following terms: flaccid, hypertonic, and/or rigid. The therapist needs to recognize the differences between these tone states and identify them when clinically examining the patient to use appropriate treatment techniques.

GENERAL GUIDELINES FOR MUSCLE TONE EVALUATION

The steps that follow describe correct procedures for evaluating muscle tone.

1. Record the test position of the patient because body and head position influence muscle tone. Patients' upper extremity muscle tone is evaluated in sitting when possible.
2. Grasp the patient's limb proximal and distal to the joint to be tested and move the joint slowly through its range to determine the free and easy range of motion available. The therapist's hands hold the limb on the lateral aspects to avoid giving tactile stimulation to the muscle belly of the muscle being tested. Note also if the limb feels light or heavy, indicating the ability of the limb to adapt automatically to changes in position against gravity.
3. Clinical examination of abnormal muscle tone involves holding the patient's limb as just described and moving it rapidly through its full range while the patient is relaxed.
4. Remember that the patient's posture (i.e., patient sitting symmetrically weight-bearing vs. slumped or leaning to one side) will affect the results of the tone evaluation. Facilitate the maintenance of symmetrical sitting position for testing, as is feasible.
5. Record findings for various muscle groups or movements (Fig. 10-1).

FLACCIDITY

Flaccidity, or hypotonicity, is a decrease of normal muscle tone. Hypotonicity is usually the result of peripheral nerve injury, a disruption of the reflex arc at the neuron level, cerebellar disease, or frontal lobe damage and is seen temporarily in the shock phase after cerebral or spinal insult (e.g., stroke or spinal cord injury).[32] The muscles feel soft and offer no resistance to passive movement. Usually a wide range of motion (ROM) is possible.[46] If the flaccid limb is moved passively, it will feel

A. Body Handling Skills: key: N = normal, Imp. = Impaired, U = Unable, NT = not tested

	ADM	DC	COMMENTS
Head Control			
Trunk Control			
Sitting Balance			
Standing Balance			
Bed Mobility			
Reach Feet			

B. U.E,. Spasticity: key: 0 = none, Min. = minimal, Mod. = moderate
Sev. = Severe, C = clonus, R = rigidity, F = flaccidity, N.T. = not tested

MUSCLE GROUPS	ADMISSION		DISCHARGE	
	Right	Left	Right	Left
Shoulder abductors				
Shoulder horizontal abductors				
Shoulder extensors				
Shoulder internal rotators				
Elbow flexors				
Elbow extensors				
Forearm supinators				
Forearm pronators				
Wrist flexors				
Wrist extensors				
Thumb flexors				
Finger flexors				
Finger extensors				
Intrinsics				
Other:				

Comments:

FIG. 10-1   Upper extremity muscle tone evaluation, part of Occupational Therapy Stroke Evaluation. (Reproduced with permission from the Occupational Therapy Dept., Rancho Los Amigos Medical Center, Downey, Calif.)

heavy; if moved to a given position and released, the limb will drop because the muscles are unable to resist gravity.[4] Deep tendon reflexes are diminished or absent.[13,19] In stroke or spinal cord injury, flaccidity is usually present initially, then changes to hypertonicity.

HYPERTONICITY

Hypertonicity, also called spasticity, is increased muscle tone. There are various definitions of hypertonicity, one of the most common being an increased or hyperactive stretch reflex causing an increased resistance to passive stretch.[40,44] Hypertonicity can occur when there is a lesion in the premotor cortex, the basal ganglia, or the cerebellum.[10] Damage to upper motor neuron systems results in increased stimulation of the lower motor neurons with a resultant increased alpha motor activity (hypertonicity).[20] Any neurologic condition changing upper motor neuron pathways that directly or indirectly inhibit or facilitate alpha motor neuron activity may result in hypertonicity.[23]

Hypertonicity is characterized by hypertonic muscles,

hyperactive deep tendon reflexes, and clonus.[36] The hypertonicity usually occurs in definite patterns of flexion or extension.[6,27,36] Typically, the patterns of hypertonicity occur in the antigravity muscles of the upper and lower extremities.

Cerebral and spinal hypertonicity differ. Hypertonicity associated with stroke or head injury is often seen in combination with other residual motor deficits such as rigidity and ataxia. It is influenced by position change and labyrinthine and tonic neck reflexes.[23] Spinal cord hypertonicity that is generally seen in patterns of flexion or in flexion/extension is often violent in nature, with severe episodic muscle spasms.[23,41] The degree of hypertonicity in incomplete spinal lesions varies, depending on the degree and direction of remaining supraspinal influences.[41]

Occurrence of Hypertonicity

Hypertonicity is commonly seen in upper motor neuron disorders, such as multiple sclerosis, cerebral palsy, spinal cord injury and disease, cerebral vascular accident (CVA), head injury, and brain tumors or infections.

Factors Influencing Hypertonicity

The postural mechanism influences the degree and patterns of hypertonicity. Therefore the position of the body and head in space and the head in relation to the body influence the state of the motor generators and thus the degree and distribution of abnormal tone.[6] Extrinsic factors that influence the degree of hypertonicity include the presence of contractures, anxiety, fear, environmental temperature extremes, pain, infection, urinary tract obstruction, heterotopic ossification, sensory overload, and emotion.[20,23] Therapeutic intervention should strive to empower the patient to reduce, eliminate, or cope with these extrinsic factors.

Method of Evaluation for Hypertonicity

Hypertonicity fluctuates, making accurate measurement difficult because of the factors described that influence it. Several methods of evaluating hypertonicity have been documented.[6,7,8] Bobath[5,6] proposed that a specific evaluation of hypertonicity is not necessary; rather, assessment of the distribution of abnormal tone should be part of a comprehensive evaluation of the postural mechanism including selective movement. A 5-point ordinal scale for grading the resistance encountered during passive muscle stretching was described by Ashworth as follows: 0 = normal muscle tone; 1 = slight increase in muscle tone, "catch" when limb moved; 2 = more marked increase in muscle tone, but limb easily flexed; 3 = considerable increase in muscle tone; and 4 = limb rigid in flexion or extension.[7] Brunnstrom[8] describes hypertonicity together with synergies (see Chapter 22). Using the criteria that have been suggested for estimating the severity of hypertonicity and being aware of hypertonicity's changing character and the factors that influence muscle tone, the therapist can estimate the degree and pattern of hypertonicity. The ultimate purpose of assessing hypertonicity is to determine how function and/or stability is impaired as a result of this muscle tone problem.

Measuring the Degree of Hypertonicity

Following the general guidelines for muscle tone assessment, the therapist can determine if there is flaccidity, hypertonicity, or rigidity. When hypertonicity is first developing (for example, following the flaccid stage after stroke), it is necessary to move the part more quickly to detect mild stretch reflex activity, a sign of developing hypertonicity.

The following scale is suggested as a guide for estimating the degree of hypertonicity.[24]

Minimal. Palpable stretch reflex (SR) is elicited, but passive movement beyond that point is easily accomplished. If active motion is present, decreased speed of reciprocation will be noted.

Moderate. Visible stretch reflex (SR) is elicited and passive movement beyond the point of SR is difficult and slow. Moderate hypertonicity will influence upright posture.

Severe. Strong visible SR is elicited which halts passive motion. Strong resistance to passive joint motion beyond the point of SR is felt with resultant ROM limitations.

Clonus may also be present. This condition is repetitive muscle contraction in response to a quick stretch.

An alternative evaluation method recommended by Bobath[6] and used by many clinicians assesses muscle tone as part of the evaluation of the postural mechanism. The therapist moves the patient's limbs using specific movement patterns that are to be learned or performed later in treatment. Normally, muscle tone adapts quickly to changes in position. If the limb is placed in a given position and then the therapist's hands are removed, the limb does not fall, and there is no resistance to the movement as the limb is placed. Conversely, if hypertonicity is influencing the passive movement during placing, resistance is felt with movement in a direction opposite to the pattern of hypertonicity; uncontrolled assistance to the passive movement is felt with movement toward the pattern of hypertonicity. Bobath[6] provides an extensive evaluation with the specific movement patterns to be tested.

Often a combination of both of the evaluation methods described will be most useful not only in planning intervention strategies, but in describing the patient's muscle tone picture to physicians and other allied health personnel.

Manual muscle testing is not appropriate for patients who exhibit hypertonicity or rigidity because the relative tone and strength of spastic muscles are not voluntary or selective. They are influenced by the position of the head and body in space, abnormal contraction, deficits in tactile and proprioceptive sensation, and failures in reciprocal innervation.[6]

RIGIDITY

Rigidity is an increase of muscle tone of agonist and antagonist muscles simultaneously. Both groups of muscles contract steadily, resulting in increased resistance to passive movement in any direction and throughout the ROM.[15,32] Rigidity is a sign of involvement of the extrapyramidal pathways in the circuitry of the basal ganglia, diencephalon, and brainstem.[14]

Characteristics of Rigidity

A feeling of constant resistance occurs throughout the ROM when the part is moved passively in any direction. This condition is called plasticity or lead-pipe rigidity because of the similarity to the feeling of bending solder or a lead pipe. In rigidity the deep tendon reflexes are normal or only moderately increased.[15,32] Another type of rigidity is the cogwheel type in which there is a rhythmic give in the resistance throughout the ROM, much like the feeling of turning a cogwheel.[32] It is crucial for the therapist to differentiate between the two types of rigidity in evaluation, documentation, and treatment.

Occurrence of Rigidity

Rigidity occurs as a result of lesions of the extrapyramidal system, such as in Parkinson's disease, some degenerative diseases, encephalitis, tumors,[14] and traumatic brain injury. Cogwheel rigidity occurs in some types of Parkinsonism and also after administration of high doses of reserpine or chlorpromazine and its derivatives. It can also occur after carbon monoxide poisoning.[3] Decerebrate (extension) posturing and decorticate (flexion) posturing can occur with diffuse brain injury or anoxia. Frequently there are lesions of both the pyramidal and the extrapyramidal systems, and rigidity and hypertonicity of muscles may occur together.[15]

Assessing muscle tone is only one component of evaluating motor control. Assessment of actual movement is imperative to determine functional abilities and limitations.

EVALUATING UPPER EXTREMITY MOTOR RECOVERY

Along with tone evaluation, the occupational therapist performs an evaluation of upper extremity movement and control. The therapist identifies where and how much the patient's motor control is dominated by stereotypic patterns of movement and where some isolated movement may be present. The degree to which abnormal tone interferes with selective control is identified. Also, determining in which direction of movement hypertonicity occurs and how it impacts function will assist in determining surgical intervention needs.

Although focusing on upper extremity movement, the therapist must also examine the whole patient, posture, and movement in general. An understanding of how people normally move will enhance the therapist's skills at recognizing the abnormal movements or postures that impact upper extremity function.

Begin examination by noting the patient's overall posture. Is the patient's posture symmetrical with equal weight-bearing on both hips (if sitting) or on both feet (if standing)? Note how the patient moves in general. Is the head aligned or tilted to one side? Is one shoulder elevated? Is the trunk twisted or long on one side, shortened on the other? Abnormalities of these kinds will affect the patient's ability to move the limbs normally. Current therapy focuses heavily on quality movement, achieving as normal functional movement as possible, as well as whether or not a particular function can be accomplished.

Evaluation and treatment often occur together. For example, if asymmetry is noted, the therapist facilitates to correct this condition before going on with testing. In doing so, the therapist still gets valuable information about the patient's ability to respond to tactile input as well as how much abnormal tone and/or movement is present. Once an overall observation is made, the therapist can look more specifically at the amount and type of motor recovery present in the upper extremities.

Testing is usually done with the patient in sitting, but observing upper extremity control in standing may give the therapist a more realistic indication of how much impairment there is, especially if the patient will eventually be ambulatory. Functionally, there are many activities of daily living done standing as well as sitting.

In the 1950s and 1960s Brunnstrom[8] observed progressive changes in motor function and behavior in the motor recovery process from CVA. The various stages of motor function as adapted from Brunnstrom are as follows. The method of testing follows the description.

No motion

No motion can be elicited from the involved upper extremity.

Reflex responses

These movements are limited to generalized or localized reaction to applied stimuli.[24]

Associated reactions

An associated reaction is an abnormal increase in tone in the involved extremity when there is activity that requires excessive effort of the unaffected limbs. The involved extremity will often appear to move, though it is actually a change in tone creating the movement, usually in a synergy pattern. Associated reactions can be tested by resisting motion at a joint in an uninvolved limb or by having the patient squeeze an object with the sound hand. These reactions can also be observed during patient transfers because this activity requires effort.[8]

Mass pattern responses (synergistic)

Voluntary motion is present, but limited to total limb movements in flexion and/or extension, without the ability to isolate individual joint motion or deviate from a stereotyped patterned movement response.[8,24] This response can be evaluated by asking the patient to move at only one joint and observing if motion occurs at more than one joint. With patterned movement, the patient will be unable to move one joint in isolation.

The following is adapted from the Hemiplegic Evaluation Guide from Rancho Los Amigos Medical Center,[24] based on Brunnstrom.[8] It is adapted and presented here with permission as an example of how flexion and extension patterns can be evaluated and described (Fig. 10-2.)

Flexion pattern response

Evaluating the *flexion pattern response* (scapular adduction and elevation, shoulder abduction and external rotation, elbow flexion and forearm supination, wrist flexion, and finger flexion):

III. SENSORY MOTOR ASSESSMENT (continued)

F. Mass Pattern Responses: key: 0 = zero, W = weak, M = moderate, S = strong.
Observe active R.O.M. and effect of head and trunk position on motion.

	ADMISSION		DISCHARGE	
1. FLEXION PATTERN	Right	Left	Right	Left
Shoulder abduction/elevation				
Elbow flexors				

Comments: Note any motion occuring at forearm, wrist and band.

OCCUPATIONAL THERAPY EVALUATION

	ADMISSION		DISCHARGE	
2. EXTENSION PATTERN	Right	Left	Right	Left
Shoulder Adduction/Internal Rotation				
Elbow Extension				

Comments: Note any motions occuring at forearm, wrist and hand.

Key: N = normal, WE = with ease, WD = with difficulty, U = unable, NT = not tested

G. Deviation From Patterns

	ADMISSION		DISCHARGE	
	Right	Left	Right	Left
Shoulder add./Int. rot. with Elbow flexion				
Shoulder abduction with Elbow extension				
Forearm pronation with Elbow flexion				
Forearm supination with Elbow extension				

Comments:

H. Wrist and Hand Recovery: record grasp and pinch measurements

	ADMISSION		DISCHARGE	
	Right	Left	Right	Left
Stable Wrist During Grasp				
Mass Grasp: Notch #				
Mass Release (3 inch cube)				
Lateral Pinch				
Palmar Pinch				
Individual Finger Motions				

Comments:

I. Selective With Pattern Overlay

	ADMISSION		DISCHARGE	
	Right	Left	Right	Left
Integrate prox. to distal control (stack cones)				
Reciprocal total U.E. motion (tether ball)				
Rapid elbow flexion–extension				
Rapid wrist flexion–extension				

Comments:

HAND FUNCTION: (Functional Use Test)

Class #
Involved Side:
Describe highest function:

FIG. 10-2   Upper extremity motor control assessment, part of Occupational Therapy Stroke Evaluation. (Reproduced with permission from the Occupational Therapy Dept., Rancho Los Amigos Medical Center, Downey, Calif.)

1. With the patient seated and the involved arm positioned straight down at the side, ask the patient to attempt to bend the elbow without moving at any other joint.
2. Observe for motion occurring at the other joints.
3. If the patient is unable to isolate elbow movement and shoulder elevation is consistently noted with elbow flexion, the pattern can be described at shoulder and elbow as weak, moderate, or strong as follows:

Shoulder: Weak: Elevates up to 30° in any plane.

Moderate: Elevates between 30° and 60° in any plane.

Strong: Elevates above 60° in any plane.

Elbow: Weak: Flexes up to 60°.

Moderate: Flexes between 60° and 100°.

Strong: Flexes above 100°.

Forearm, wrist, and hand motion can be described separately because the motion can vary.

Extension pattern response

Evaluating the *extension pattern response* (scapular abduction and depression, shoulder adduction and internal rotation, elbow extension, forearm pronation, and wrist and finger flexion or extension):

1. Position the patient in sitting with the shoulder at 90° of abduction and maximal external rotation. The elbow is positioned in maximum flexion. (The arm may be supported in a starting position by the therapist.) Ask the patient to straighten the elbow as far as possible.
2. Observe for motions occurring at other joints. If the patient is unable to isolate elbow movement from shoulder horizontal adduction and/or other components of the extension pattern, the shoulder and elbow patterned motion can be described as follows:

Shoulder: Weak: Contraction of shoulder adductors and internal rotators. May move through partial range of shoulder adduction and internal rotation.

Moderate: Able to go through full ROM in shoulder adduction and internal rotation.

Strong: Takes strong resistance at the end of these ranges.

Elbow: Weak: Contraction of triceps. May go through partial extension range.

Moderate: Able to go through full available range in extension.

Strong: Takes strong resistance at end of extension range.

Forearm, wrist, and hand motion can be described separately because these may vary.

Deviation from pattern

Voluntary control deviates from the synergy though motion is predominantly patterned when functional tasks are attempted. Testing involves asking the patient to perform movements that deviate from the synergies. For example, ask the patient to attempt the following movements and observe for patient's ability to accomplish them.[24]

1. Ask the patient to touch the back of the uninvolved shoulder with the involved hand (shoulder protraction and horizontal adduction with elbow flexion).
2. Ask the patient to touch the therapist's finger held out to the patient's involved side (shoulder abduction with elbow extension).
3. Ask the patient to pick up an object from the therapist's hand, which is four inches above the patient's involved knee (elbow flexion with forearm pronation).
4. Ask the patient to reach out to receive an object in the hand (elbow extension and forearm supination).

From these attempts the therapist can discern whether or not the patient is beginning to deviate from pattern. See Fig. 10-2 for sample recording form.

For the wrist and hand, the therapist can evaluate the following:

Wrist stability. Ask the patient to make a fist and observe for stability of the wrist joint in neutral to 30° of extension.

Individual finger motions. Ask the patient to touch the tip of each finger with the tip of the thumb or perform drumming action with the fingers. Observe for selectivity in movements. If grasp appears voluntarily controlled, it can be measured with a dynamometer, as can pinch if isolated finger motions are observed.

Selective with pattern overlay

Joint movement in the limb is isolated with selective voluntary control occurring in a variety of planes and directions. When the limb is functionally stressed or given increased demands for normal reciprocation, however, synergistic responses may be seen proximally. Selective control will revert to more patterned responses when attempts are made to coordinate and integrate proximal and distal control for functional activities.

Examples of activities to ask the patient to perform are as follows (see Fig. 10-2):

1. Have the patient attempt to cross midline with the involved limb to pick up an object on a table in front of the uninvolved limb. Have patient place it about two feet to the side of the involved limb. Observe for integration of proximal and distal control.[24] If pattern overlay is present, the patient's shoulder may elevate, or the patient may not be able to cross midline.
2. Ask the patient to make a fist with the involved hand and repeatedly hit a tether ball placed at chest level, an arm's length in front.[24] Pattern overlay will be observed if movements are not smooth, if the patient leans to the side to get the arm elevated, or if the shoulder hikes.
3. Ask the patient to perform rapid reciprocal motion. (a) Elbow flexion/extension: Ask patient to flex and extend the involved elbow rapidly. Compare with uninvolved side, if possible, to note abnormalities. (b) Wrist flexion/extension: Ask patient to rapidly flex and extend involved wrist. Again, compare this movement to that of the uninvolved side if possible.[24]

Selective movement

Ability to control movement at each isolated joint and maintain coordinated selectivity is evaluated with the performance of functional activities.

EVALUATING FUNCTIONAL USE OF THE LIMB(S)

The occupational therapist has the challenge of maximizing the patient's ability to return to purposeful and meaningful activities within his or her physical and social environment.[45] The therapist must keep this in mind throughout the process of facilitating upper extremity control. Therefore, evaluating function and functional potential are paramount in helping the patient to actualize functional, realistic goals.

There are many ADL tests to look at the whole picture of functioning. One test, the Functional Test for the Hemiplegic/Paretic Upper Extremity, addresses the patient's ability to use the involved arm for purposeful tasks. It contains tasks ranging from those that involve basic stabilization to more difficult tasks requiring fine motor manipulation and proximal stabilization. Examples of tasks are holding a pouch, stabilizing a jar, wringing a rag, hooking and zipping a zipper, folding a sheet, and putting in a light bulb overhead. This test provides objective documentation of functional improvement and is administered in 30 minutes or less.[47]

Fugl-Meyer and associates developed a quantitative assessment of motor function following stroke, using Brunnstrom methods and by measuring such parameters as range of motion, pain, sensation, and balance. This test is used throughout the world as a reliable and valid research tool. The scores on the Fugl-Meyer Assessment correlate with activities of daily living.[17]

The therapist may also use observational skills during ADL evaluation to determine the functional use and potential for use of the involved upper extremity, taking into consideration the patient's cognition, sensation, and other physical factors. Whatever evaluation method is used, the therapist can then set a functional goal for the upper extremity, for example, that the patient will use the involved upper extremity as a minimal active assist. The following descriptors are suggested[1]:

Minimal stabilizing assist. The patient is able to use the involved upper extremity to stabilize objects being manipulated by the uninvolved extremity. This task is accomplished by the weight of the extremity alone. The extremity can be placed by the uninvolved arm for this stabilization.

Minimal active assist. The patient is able to use the involved arm and hand to assist in accomplishing a single part of an activity, for example, actively holding the arm away from the body for dressing or hygiene activities performed by the uninvolved arm and hand.

Maximal active assist. The patient is able to use the involved arm and hand in all activities that require motor control for pushing or pulling, stabilizing, and gross grasp and release.

Incorporation of the involved upper extremity in all bilateral tasks associated with activities of daily living. The patient is able to use the involved upper extremity to assist the uninvolved or less involved arm in all self-care tasks and light home skills, though extremity still is not normal. May not have adequate ability to assist in activities requiring speed and precise use.

OCCUPATIONAL THERAPY CONSIDERATIONS BASED ON RESULTS OF MOTOR CONTROL EVALUATION

Although the therapist bases treatment on the patient's overall evaluation results, including cognition, vision, perception, sensation, psychological aspects, and occupational needs,[37] motor control evaluation results suggest some directions for treatment. Several approaches to motor control treatment are described in detail in Chapters 21 through 25. The following are some general directions for treatment.

For low tone and limited to no motion in the upper

extremity, the therapist needs to facilitate increased tone necessary for motion that is controlled and selective. Weight-bearing and proprioceptive input facilitates normal tone and control. Caution is needed to avoid encouraging abnormal patterns of movement. Therapeutic activities for improving strength may be appropriate if motion is selective and not patterned. The goals of treatment should be to effect a balance of strength and tone between agonist and antagonist muscles.[9] The arm can be positioned as normally as possible during ADL tasks to provide sensory and proprioceptive feedback. Patient education in proper positioning and joint protection is important to protect the joint structures and prevent trauma.

For hypertonicity in the upper extremity, which usually accompanies synergy or patterned movement, treatment methods that use techniques of inhibition (such as the sensorimotor approaches described in Chapters 21 through 25) may be appropriate, depending on the disability, severity and distribution of the hypertonicity, and concomitant problems. The goal of treatment is to balance the tone for more normal movement. Therefore, inhibition of the spastic muscles and facilitation of the antagonist muscles is necessary, using one of the sensorimotor approaches to treatment.

In some cases hypertonicity is severe enough to require progressive inhibition casting or splinting.[3,33,37,43] Casting provides the necessary circumferential pressure that will prevent soft tissue contractures and maintain the normal length of the muscle for functional ROM.[28,35]

Serial casting is most successful when a contracture has been present for less than 6 months. The cast may be bivalved for skin protection and to allow the therapist to work with the extremity out of the cast. However, many clinicians believe that a non-bivalved cast is more effective and actually causes less skin breakdown.[3] A dropout cast, which can be used as part of the serial casting process, has a cut-out, allowing movement of the joint into the desired direction. For example, for an elbow that has flexor hypertonicity, the dorsal upper arm portion of a long arm cast can be cut out to allow the triceps to be facilitated to extend the arm.

A combination of peripheral nerve blocks and casting or splinting is often used.[3,28] Lidocaine blocks, which are short-blocks, can be administered before casting to alter hypertonicity to a manageable level for easier limb positioning. Phenol blocks that can last up to three months can be used to allow the therapist to increase antagonist control and strength to gain a balance of muscle control.[28,45]

Physical agent modalities such as cold, heat, and neuromuscular electrical stimulation can be used as preparation for or in conjunction with purposeful activity, provided the therapist has the appropriate education and skill to carry them out. These modalities can help inhibit or reduce hypertonicity temporarily to allow the development of antagonistic control and modulation over the state of the motor generators.

Patients with severe hypertonicity accompanied by severe pain may require evaluation of the cause of the pain. Drug therapy and/or other pain management techniques may be part of the treatment approach. The three drugs most commonly used are diazepam, dantrolene, and baclofen.[3,28] Diazepam is a centrally acting, habituating drug, and its sudden discontinuance may cause seizures. Dantrolene is a peripherally acting drug that can cause weakness lasting up to a week and liver damage. Baclofen is a centrally acting drug that is more effective with spinal cord injuries than with cerebral injuries. Its potential side effects are confusion, hallucination, and increased seizures. No matter which drug is used, it is crucial for the occupational therapist to communicate to the medical staff any noted side effects that interfere with the patient's overall function.

Another treatment objective is to teach the patient to manage muscle tone to accomplish essential daily living activities. Positioning and movement in patterns opposite to hypertonic or synergistic patterns are important in developing quality movement that is as close to normal as possible. The patient should be taught how to modulate the abnormal tone or how to instruct others to do so. The patient should also be taught how to incorporate the upper extremities as much as possible into all daily living activities.[18] Activities of daily living, crafts, games, and work activities can be used to teach incorporation of the extremities for a total approach to treatment.[45]

Even when motor control is adequate for some function, sensory and perceptual abilities of the patient may affect the therapist's expectations for functional goal achievement. Perception may alter the patient's abilities, requiring the therapist to lower expected goals.[2]

COORDINATION

Coordination is the ability to produce accurate, controlled movement. Such movement is characterized by smoothness, rhythm, appropriate speed, refinement to the minimum number of muscle groups necessary to produce the desired movement, and appropriate muscle tension, postural tone, and equilibrium.

To effect coordinated movement, all of the elements of the neuromuscular mechanism must be intact. Coordinated movement is dependent on the contraction of the correct agonist muscles with simultaneous relaxation of the correct antagonist muscles together with the contraction of the joint fixator and synergist muscles. In addition, proprioception, body schema, and the ability to judge space accurately and to direct body parts through space with correct timing to the desired target must be intact.[4]

OCCURRENCE OF INCOORDINATION

Coordination of muscle action is under the control of the cerebellum and influenced by the extrapyramidal system. Knowledge of the body schema and body-to-space

relationships is essential to the production of coordinated movement, however. Therefore, many types of lesions can produce disturbances of coordination.[4] Disturbances of movement from causes other than cerebellar lesions can interfere with coordination. Noncerebellar causes include diseases and injuries of muscles and peripheral nerves, lesions of the posterior columns of the spinal cord, and lesions of the frontal and postcentral cerebral cortex. Paralysis of the limbs caused by a peripheral nervous system lesion prevents carrying out tests for coordination even though CNS mechanisms are intact.[32]

Cerebellar dysfunction can cause incoordination that can affect any body region and cause a variety of clinical symptoms. For example, the patient may have postural difficulties that include slouching or leaning positions (bilateral lesions) or spinal curvature (unilateral lesions) and wide-based standing. Eye movements, both voluntary and reflexive, may be affected as well as the resting position of the eye.[46] The following are common signs of cerebellar dysfunction that the therapist may encounter.

Ataxia. Ataxia is the result of a cerebellar lesion. It is seen as delayed initiation of movement responses, errors in range and force of movement, and errors in the rate and regularity of movement. It results in incoordination and irregularity of movement. There is a staggering wide-based gait with reduced or no arm swing. Step length may be uneven, and the patient may have a tendency to fall to the side of the lesion. Ataxia will result in a lack of postural stability with patients tending to fixate to compensate for their instability.[11,22,31]

Adiadochokinesis. This dysfunction is an inability to perform rapidly alternating movements, such as pronation and supination or elbow flexion and extension, and results from lesions of the cerebellum.[14]

Dysmetria. Cerebellar lesions can cause dysmetria, which is an inability to estimate the ROM necessary to reach the target of the movement. It is evident when touching the finger to the nose or an object on a table or in placing limbs in voluntary movement.[14]

Dyssynergia. Literally, dyssynergia is a "decomposition of movement" in which voluntary movements are broken up into their component parts and appear jerky. It results from cerebellar lesions and can cause problems in articulation and phonation.[14]

Tremor. An intention tremor that is associated with cerebellar disease occurs during voluntary movement, is often intensified at the termination of the movement, and is often seen in multiple sclerosis. The patient with intention tremor may have trouble performing tasks that require accuracy and precision of limb placement (for example, drinking from a cup or inserting a key in a lock). A resting tremor occurs as a result of disease of the basal ganglia.[11]

Rebound phenomenon of Holmes. This is a lack of a "check reflex," that is, the inability to stop a motion quickly to avoid striking something. For example, if the patient's arm is flexed against the resistance of the examiner and the resistance is released suddenly and unexpectedly, the patient's hand will hit his or her face or body.[11,14]

Nystagmus. An involuntary movement of the eyeballs in an up-and-down, back-and-forth, or rotating direction is called nystagmus. It interferes with head control and fine adjustments required for balance. Nystagmus can occur as a result of vestibular system, brain stem, or cerebellar lesions.[14]

Dysarthria. Dysarthria is explosive or slurred speech caused by an incoordination of the speech mechanism resulting from cerebellar lesions. The patient's speech may also vary in pitch, appear nasal and tremulous, or both.[11,14]

The following are signs of extrapyramidal disease that produces incoordination.[6,19]

Tremors. Resting tremors, such as the pill-rolling tremor seen in Parkinsonism, result from lesions of the basal ganglia.[14]

Choreiform movements. These are irregular, purposeless, coarse, quick, jerky, and dysrhythmic movements of variable distribution. They may also occur during sleep and result from lesions of the basal ganglia.[14]

Athetoid movements. These are continuous, slow, wormlike, arrhythmic movements that primarily affect the distal portions of the extremities. They occur in the same patterns in the same subject and are not present during sleep. Athetoid movements result from lesions of the basal ganglia.[14]

Spasms. These are involuntary contractions of large groups of muscles of the arm, leg, or neck that result from lesions of the corticospinal tracts or extrapyramidal involvement.[11]

Dystonia. Dystonia results in bizarre twisting movements of the trunk and proximal muscles of the extremities. Torsion spasms and spasmodic torticollis may occur. Dystonic movements tend to involve large portions of the body and produce grotesque posturing with bizarre writhing movements. They are caused by lesions of the basal ganglia.[11]

Ballism. A rare symptom that is produced by continuous, gross, abrupt contractions of the axial and proximal musculature of the extremity. It causes the limb to fly out suddenly, occurs on one side of the body (hemiballism), and is caused by lesions of the opposite subthalamic nucleus.[11,14]

CLINICAL EVALUATION OF COORDINATION

Incoordination consists of errors in rate, rhythm, range, direction, and force of movement.[22] Therefore observation is an important element of the evaluation. The neurologic examination for incoordination may include the nose-finger-nose test, the finger-nose test, the heel-knee test, the knee pat (pronation-supination) test, hand pat and foot pat tests, finger wiggling, and drawing a spiral.[4,32] Such tests can reveal dysmetria, dyssynergia, adiadochokinesis, tremors, and ataxia. Usually these examinations are performed by the neurologist.

OCCUPATIONAL THERAPY EVALUATION OF COORDINATION

Because occupation is the hallmark of occupational therapy, the occupational therapist should seek to translate the clinical evaluation to a functional one. Selected activities and specific performance tests can reveal the effect of incoordination on function, the primary concern of the occupational therapist. The occupational therapist can observe for coordination difficulties during ADL evaluation. The therapist can prepare simulated tasks that require coordinated muscle function, such as writing, placing objects into containers, tossing and catching a bean-bag or ball, or playing a board game.[42] The therapist should observe for irregularity in the rate of movement and sudden corrective movements in an attempt to compensate for incoordination. Thus, movement during the performance of various activities may appear irregular and jerky and overreach the mark.[32] The following general guidelines and questions can be used when evaluating incoordination:

1. Assess the patient's tone and joint mobility.
2. Observe the patient in the sitting position and locate any overdeveloped muscle bulk.
3. Observe for ataxia proximally to distally during functional upper extremity movement. Are movements away from or toward the body more difficult for the patient? Where, within the range of movement, is ataxia most prevalent?
4. Stabilize joints proximally to distally during the functional task and note differences in patient performance as compared with performance without stabilization.
5. Observe for resting or intention tremor in patient. Are the eyes and speech affected?
6. Apply weight cuffs or similar adaptation to the extremity during the functional task to establish if weighting or resistance will be an effective treatment option. Note the amount of resistance provided.

7. Does patient's emotional status affect coordination?
8. How do the patient's ataxia or coordination problems affect function?
9. Perform an occupational history interview, asking about the patient's roles, routines, goals, and environment to determine what functions are important for the patient to be able to perform.

Several standardized tests of motor function and manual dexterity outlined by Smith[42] are available and can be used to evaluate coordination. Some of these include: The Purdue Pegboard,[39] The Minnesota Rate of Manipulation Test,[34] Lincoln-Oseretsky Motor Development Scale,[30] The Pennsylvania Bimanual Work Sample,[38] The Crawford Small Parts Dexterity Test,[12] and the Jebsen-Taylor Hand Function Test.[25]

RESULTS OF EVALUATION AS A BASIS FOR TREATMENT PLANNING

Admittedly, treatment of incoordination is difficult, and several approaches may be used. Incoordination arising from lesions of the corticospinal system may be improved using one of the sensorimotor approaches directed to the normalization of muscle tone and the development of more normal movement patterns. Specific sensory input is used to change muscle tone and evoke adaptive motor responses. Activities graded on the basis of normal motor learning and control may be helpful in attaining proximal stability and then mobility. Therapy directed toward the modulaton of reflexes and synergies and the enhancement of motor control mechanisms, such as the righting and equilibrium reactions, can help to improve coordination. Weight-bearing, joint approximation, placing and holding techniques, and fixed points of stability (tabletop) can be helpful.[10] Begin with small ranges of movement and gradually increase as the patient progresses. Work initially in the plane and direction of movement that are easiest for the patient, and progress toward more difficult areas. Some of the involuntary movements of cerebellar or extrapyramidal origin are difficult to manage or change. Pharmacological agents or surgical intervention may be employed by the physician in an effort to control tremors or other involuntary movements. Therapists have used weights on the extremities and proximal fixation in an effort to help the patient gain an improvement in motor control. These are sometimes helpful but often not practical in day-to-day activities. Methods and devices to compensate for incoordination may be necessary to make ADL safer, more possible, and more satisfying. A thorough occupational history interview is necessary, however, to make appropriate equipment choices and determine adaptive strategies that the patient will carry over to the home environment. Some of these strategies are described in Chapter 26.

SUMMARY

Motor control is the ability to make dynamic postural adjustments and regulate body and limb movement. It is the result of the interaction of complex neurological systems. Evaluation of motor control includes assessment of the postural mechanism, muscle tone, selective movement, and coordination. Automatic reactions as well as stereotypic reflexes and synergistic patterns are evaluated.

The presense of abnormal elements of motor control affect the quality of movement and the ability to perform functional tasks. The occupational therapist evaluates muscle tone, upper extremity recovery, and coordination using tests and observation of movement during performance of functional activities. The results of the motor control evaluation can aid the therapist in selecting the appropriate treatment approach, such as one of the sensorimotor approaches and/or compensatory methods.

REVIEW QUESTIONS

1. What are the components of a normal postural mechanism?
2. Describe equilibrium reactions and the functional implications of their presence in motor behavior.
3. Describe functional difficulties encountered when the asymmetrical tonic neck reflex is present.
4. Describe the automatic adaptation of muscles to changes in posture.
5. Define muscle tone.
6. Describe the characteristics of normal muscle tone.
7. Describe the characteristics of hypotonicity (flaccidity).
8. In which diagnoses does flaccidity usually occur?
9. Describe the characteristics of hypertonicity.
10. In which diagnoses does hypertonicity usually occur?
11. How is rigidity unlike hypertonicity, and how is it like hypertonicity?
12. List five factors that can influence hypertonicity negatively.
13. Why should the evaluation of muscle tone be performed in conjunction with the patient's overall motor function?
14. List the components of and procedure for an upper extremity muscle tone evaluation and a selective movement evaluation.
15. Describe the upper extremity flexion pattern response.
16. How can flexion and extension pattern responses be tested?
17. Define coordination.
18. List several factors on which normal coordination is dependent.
19. Which types of disabilities produce incoordination?
20. How is coordination evaluated?
21. What should the therapist observe when evaluating coordination by means of performance of ordinary activities?

REFERENCES

1. Andric M: Projecting the upper extremity functional level. In Professional Staff Association of Rancho Los Amigos Medical Center: *Stroke rehabilitation: state of the art 1984,* Downey, Calif, 1984, Los Amigos Research and Education Institute.
2. Bernspang B, Viitanen M, Erickson S: Impairments of perceptual and motor functions: their influence on self-care ability 4 - 6 years after a stroke, *The Occup Ther J of Res* 9:27-37, 1989.
3. Berrol S: The treatment of physical disorders following brain injury. In Wood RL, Eames P, editors: *Models of brain injury rehabilitation,* Baltimore, 1989, Johns Hopkins University Press.
4. Bickerstaff ER: *Neurological examination in clinical practice,* ed 3, London, 1973, Blackwell Scientific Publications.
5. Bobath B: *Abnormal postural reflex activity caused by brain lesions,* ed 2, London, 1975, William Heinemann Medical Books.
6. Bobath B: *Adult hemiplegia: evaluation and treatment,* ed 2, London, 1978, William Heineman Medical Books.
7. Bohannon RW, Smith MB: Interrater reliability of a modified Ashworth scale of muscle spasticity, *Phys Ther* 67:206-207, 1987.
8. Brunnstrom S: *Movement therapy in hemiplegia,* New York, 1970, Harper & Row.
9. Carr JH, Shepherd RB: *A motor relearning program for stroke,* ed 2, Rockville, Md, 1987, Aspen.
10. Charness A: Stroke/head injury: a guide to functional outcomes in physical therapy management, Rockville, Md, 1986, Aspen.
11. Chusid J.G.: *Correlative neuroanatomy and functional neurology,* ed 18, Los Altos, Calif, 1982, Lange Medical Publications.
12. Crawford Small Parts Dexterity Test: The Psychological Corporation, 304 East 45th St, New York, N.Y. 10017

13. Davies PM: *Steps to follow: a guide to treatment of adult hemiplegia,* New York, 1985, Springer Verlag.
14. deGroot J: *Correlative neuroanatomy,* ed 21, Norwalk, Conn, 1991, Appleton & Lange.
15. DeMyer W: *Technique of the neurologic examination: a programmed text,* ed 2, New York, 1974, McGraw-Hill.
16. Duncan PW, Badke MB: Determinants of abnormal motor control. In Duncan PW, Badke MB: *Stroke rehabilitation: the recovery of motor control,* Chicago, Ill, 1987, Year Book Publishers.
17. Duncan PW, Badke MB: Measurement of motor performance and functional abilities following stroke. In Duncan PW, Badke MB: *Stroke rehabilitation: the recovery of motor control,* Chicago, Ill, 1987, Year Book Publishers.
18. Eggers O: *Occupational therapy in the treatment of adult hemiplegia,* London, 1984, William Heinemann Medical Books.
19. Farber S: *Neurorehabilitation: a multisensory approach,* Philadelphia, 1982, WB Saunders.
20. Felten DL, Felten SY: A regional and systemic overview of functional neuroanatomy. In Farber S: *Neurorehabilitation: a multisensory approach,* Philadelphia, 1982, WB Saunders.
21. Fiorentino M: *Normal and abnormal development: the influence of primitive reflexes on motor development,* Springfield, Ill, 1972, Charles C Thomas.
22. Ghez C.: The cerebellum. In Kandel ER, Schwartz JH, Jessel TM: *Principles of neural science,* ed 3, New York, 1991, Elsevier.
23. Griffith ER: Spasticity. In Rosenthal M and associates, editors: *Rehabilitation of the head injured adult,* Philadelphia, 1983, FA Davis.
24. Hazboun V: *Occupational therapy evaluation guide for adult hemiplegia,* Downey, Calif, 1991, Los Amigos Research and Education Institute.
25. Jebsen RH and associates: An objective and standardized test

of hand function, *Archives of Physical Medicine and Rehab,* 50(6):311-319, 1969.
26. Jewell MJ: Overview of the structure and function of the central nervous system. In Umphred DA, editor: *Neurological rehabilitation,* ed 2, St Louis, 1990, Mosby-Yearbook.
27. Johnstone M: *Restoration of motor function in the stroke patient,* ed 2, New York, 1983, Churchhill Livingstone.
28. Keenan MA: The orthopedic management of spasticity, *J Head Trauma Rehabil* 2(2):62, 1987.
29. Lee WA: A control systems framework for understanding normal and abnormal posture, *Am J Occup Ther* 439(5):291-301, 1989.
30. Lincoln-Oseretsky Motor Development Scale: C.H. Stoelting Co., 424 N. Hohman Ave., Chicago, IL 60624
31. Marsden CD: The physiological basis of ataxia, *Physiotherapy* 61:326, 1975.
32. Mayo Clinic and Mayo Clinic Foundation: *Clinical examinations in neurology,* ed 5, Philadelphia, 1981, WB Saunders.
33. McPherson JJ and associates: A comparison of dorsal and volar resting hand splints in the reduction of hypertonus, *Am J Occup Ther* 36:664, 1982.
34. Minnesota Rate of Manipulation Test: American Guidance Service, Inc., Publisher's Bldg., Circle Pines, Mn 55014.
35. Newton RA: Motor control. In Umphred DA, editor: *Neurological rehabilitation,* ed 2, St Louis, 1990, Mosby-Yearbook.
36. Okamoto GA: *Physical medicine and rehabilitation,* Philadelphia, 1984, WB Saunders.
37. Pelland MJ: Occupational therapy and stroke rehabilitation. In Kaplan PE, Cerrillo LJ: *Stroke rehabilitation,* Boston, 1986, Butterworth Publishers.
38. Pennsylvania Bi-Manual Work Sample: Educational Test Bureau, American Guidance Service, Inc., Publisher's Bldg., Circle Pines, Mn 55014.

39. Purdue Pegboard: Science Research Associates, Inc., 259 East Erie St., Chicago, Ill 60611.

40. Ryerson S: Hemiplegia resulting from vascular insult or disease. In Umphred DA, editor: *Neurological rehabilitation,* ed 2, St Louis, 1990, Mosby-Yearbook.

41. Schneider F: Traumatic spinal cord injury. In Umphred DA, editor: *Neurological rehabilitation,* ed 2, St Louis, 1990, Mosby-Yearbook.

42. Smith HD: Occupational therapy assessment and treatment. In Hopkins HL, Smith HD: *Willard and Spackman's occupational therapy,* ed 8, Philadelphia, 1993, JB Lippincott.

43. Snook JH: Spasticity reduction splint, *Am J Occup Ther* 33:648,1979.

44. Thilmann AF, Fellows SJ, Garms E: The mechanism of spastic muscle hypertonus, BRN, 114:233-244, 1991.

45. Tomas ES and associates: Nonsurgical management of upper extremity deformities after traumatic brain injury, *Phys Med and Rehabil: State of the Art Reviews,* vol. 7(3), Oct, 1993.

46. Urbscheit NL: Cerebellar dysfunction. In Umphred DA, editor: *Neurological rehabilitation,* St Louis, 1990, Mosby-Yearbook.

47. Wilson DJ, Baker LL, Craddock JA: *Functional test for the hemiplegic/paretic upper extremity,* Downey, Calif, 1984, Los Amigos Research and Education Institute.

Dysphagia: Evaluation and Treatment

Karen L. Nelson

Eating is the most basic activity of daily living (ADL), necessary for survival from birth throughout the life span. Dysphagia is defined as the inability to swallow. Deglutition refers to the normal consumption of solids or liquids. Other components of eating include the ability to reach for food, place it in the mouth, chew it, and swallow it.

The occupational therapist is trained to evaluate and treat all components of eating. These components are motor control; muscle tone and positioning of the trunk, head, and upper and lower extremities; inhibition of primitive reflexes; oral and pharyngeal function; and the treatment of sensory, perceptual, and cognitive dysfunction, which may interfere with the eating process.

This chapter provides the occupational therapist with a foundation for the evaluation and treatment of the adult patient with an acquired dysphagia. Anatomic and developmental dysphagias are beyond the scope of this chapter. Some of the conditions that can result in an acquired dysphagia are cerebral vascular accident (CVA), head injury, brain tumor, anoxia, Guillain-Barré syndrome, multiple sclerosis, amyotrophic lateral sclerosis, Parkinson's disease, myasthenia gravis, poliomyelitis, and quadriplegia.

ANATOMY AND PHYSIOLOGY OF NORMAL SWALLOW

Deglutition, the normal consumption of solids or liquids, is a complex sensorimotor process involving the brain stem, the cortex, six cranial nerves, the first three cervical nerve segments, and 48 pairs of muscles.[13,32,35] A normal swallow requires all these structures to be intact (Fig. 11-1). Therefore the occupational therapist treating the patient with dysphagia must have a thorough understanding of the anatomy and physiology of swallowing (Fig. 11-2, *A* to *E*). The swallowing process can be divided into four stages: (1) oral preparatory phase, (2) oral phase, (3) pharyngeal phase, and (4) esophageal phase[27] (Table 11-1).

ORAL PREPARATORY PHASE

The oral preparatory phase of swallowing begins with the act of looking at and reaching for food.[11] Visual and olfactory information stimulates salivary secretions. Salivation plays an important role as a triggering mechanism for the entire swallowing process.[38] As tactile contact is made with the food, the jaw comes forward to open. The lips close around a glass or utensil to remove the food. The labial musculature forms a seal to prevent any material from leaking out of the oral cavity.

As chewing begins, the mandible moves in a strong, combined rotary and lateral direction. The upper and lower teeth shear and crush the food. The tongue moves laterally to push the food between the teeth. The buccinator muscles of the cheeks contract to act as lateral retainers to prevent food particles from falling into the sulcus between the jaw and cheek.[24] The tongue sweeps through the mouth, gathering food particles and mixing them with saliva to shape a bolus. The tongue carries sensory information of taste, texture, and temperature of the bolus or liquid through the seventh and ninth cranial nerves to the brain stem. The chewing action of the mandible and tongue is repeated rhythmically until a cohesive bolus is formed. The posterior portion of the tongue forms a tight seal with the velum, preventing slippage of the bolus or liquid into the pharynx.[8,12]

When liquids are introduced into the oral cavity, the tongue moves anteriorly, stopping behind the incisors and forming a groove. The shape of this groove along the dorsal surface of the tongue funnels the liquid toward the pharynx.[16]

In preparation for the next stage, the bolus, having been formed into a cohesive mass, is held between the anterior tongue and palate. The tongue cups around the bolus to seal it against the hard palate. The larynx and the pharynx are at rest during this phase of the swallowing process. The airway is open.

I would like to acknowledge Deborah Morawski, OTR, for the time and effort provided to review and contribute to this chapter revision.

TABLE 11-1 Swallowing Process*

STRUCTURE	MUSCLE	MOVEMENT	CRANIAL NERVE	SENSATION
ORAL PREPARATORY STAGE				
Jaw	Pterygoideus medialis	Opens jaw	Trigeminal (V)	Face, temple, mouth, teeth, mucus
	Pterygoideus medialis and lateralis	Protrudes lower jaw; moves jaw laterally		
	Masseter	Closes jaw		
	Digastricus; mylohyoideus; geniohyoidcus	Depresses lower jaw		
Mouth	Orbicularis oris	Compresses and protrudes lips	Facial (VII)	
	Zygomaticus minor	Protrudes upper lip		
	Zygomaticus major	Raises lateral angle of mouth upward and outward (smile)		
	Levator anguli oris	Moves angle of mouth straight upward		
	Risorius	Draws angle of mouth backward (grimace)		
	Depressor labii inferioris	Draws lower lip downward and outward		
	Mentalis	Protrudes lower lip (pouting)		
	Depressor anguli oris	Draws down angles of mouth		
Tongue	Superior longitudinal	Shortens tongue; raises sides and tip of tongue	Facial (VII)→	Taste, anterior two thirds of tongue
	Transverse	Lengthens and narrows tongue	Glossopharyngeal (IX)	Taste, posterior third of tongue
	Vertical	Flattens and broadens tongue	←Hypoglossal (XII)	
	Inferior longitudinal	Shortens tongue		
		Turns tip of tongue downward		
ORAL STAGE				
Tongue	Styloglossus	Elevates and pulls tongue posteriorly	Accessory (XI)	
	Palatoglossus	Elevates and pulls tongue posteriorly; narrows fauces		
	Genioglossus	Depresses, protrudes, and retracts tongue; elevates hyoid	Hypoglossal (XII)	
	Hyoglossus	Depresses and pulls tongue posteriorly		
Soft palate	Tensor veli palatini	Tenses soft palate	←Trigeminal (V)→	Mouth
	Levator veli palatini	Elevates soft palate	←Accessory (XI)	
	Uvulae	Shortens soft palate		
PHARYNGEAL STAGE				
Fauces	Palatoglossus	Narrows fauces	←Vagus (X)→	Membranes of pharynx
	Palatopharyngeus	Elevates larynx and pharynx		
Hyoid	Suprahyoidei	Elevates hyoid anteriorly, posteriorly	←Trigeminal (V)	
	Stylohyoideus			
	Sternothyroideus	Depresses thyroid cartilage	←Cervical segments 1,2,3	
	Omohyoideus	Depresses hyoid		
Pharynx	Salpingopharyngeus	Pharynx elevation	←Glossopharyngeal (IX)	
	Palatopharyngeus	Pharynx elevation		
	Stylopharyngeus	Pharynx and larynx elevation		

* References 13, 14, 24, 26.
Key: ← Movement function
    → Sensory function

TABLE 11-1 Swallowing Process—cont'd

STRUCTURE	MUSCLE	MOVEMENT	CRANIAL NERVE	SENSATION
PHARYNGEAL STAGE				
Pharynx	Constrictor pharyngeus superior	Sequentially constricts the nasopharynx, oropharynx, laryngopharynx	←Vagus (X)→	Membranes of pharynx
	Constrictor pharyngeus medius			
	Constrictor pharyngeus inferior			
	Cricopharyngeus	Relaxes during swallow; prevents air from entering esophagus		
Larynx	Aryepiglotticus	Closes inlet of larynx	←Vagus (X)→	Membranes of larynx
	Thyroepiglotticus			
	Thyroarytenoideus	Closes glottis; shortens vocal cords		
	Arytenoid—oblique, transverse	Adducts arytenoid cartilages		
	Lateral cricoarytenoid	Adducts and rotates arytenoid cartilage		
	Vocalis	Controls tension of vocal cords		
	Postcricoarytenoideus	Widens glottis		
	Cricothyroideus—straight, oblique	Elevates cricoid arch		
ESOPHAGEAL STAGE				
Esophagus	Smooth	Peristaltic wave	←Vagus (X)	

* References 13, 14, 24, 26.
Key: ← Movement function
    → Sensory function

ORAL PHASE

The oral phase of swallowing begins when the tongue moves the bolus toward the back of the mouth.[3] The tongue elevates to squeeze the bolus up against the hard palate. A central groove is formed by the tongue to funnel the food posteriorly. The oral stage of the swallow is voluntary, requiring the person to be alert.[8,27,34] A normal voluntary swallow is necessary to elicit a strong swallow response during the pharyngeal stage that follows. Overall, the oral sequence takes approximately 1 second to complete with thin liquids.

PHARYNGEAL PHASE

The pharyngeal phase of swallowing begins when the bolus passes through the anterior faucial arches and into the pharynx, marking the start of the involuntary component of the swallow. After the swallow response has been triggered, it continues with no pause in bolus movement until the total act is completed. The swallow response is controlled by the medulla oblongata of the brain stem.[35] Within the medulla oblongata, the medullary reticular formation is responsible for screening out all extraneous sensory patterns and for responding only to those patterns that indicate the need to swallow. The reticular formation also assumes control of all motor neurons and related muscles needed to complete the swallow. Higher brain functions such as speech, in addition to the respiratory reflex center, are preempted.[15,35]

When the swallow response is triggered, several physiologic functions occur simultaneously. The velum elevates and retracts, closing the velopharyngeal port to prevent regurgitation of material into the nasal cavity. The entire pharyngeal tube elevates and peristalsis occurs, carrying the bolus into and through both sides of the pharynx to the cricopharyngeal sphincter located at the top of the esophagus.[8] This movement must be rapid and efficient so that respiration is interrupted only briefly.

Concurrently, the larynx elevates beneath the back of the tongue base, protecting the airway. Three actions occur to facilitate closure of the larynx: (1) soft palate elevation and retraction and closure of the nasopharynx; (2) laryngeal displacement anteriorly and superiorly with obliteration of the laryngeal vestibule and closure at the epiglottis and true vocal cords, preventing food from entering the airway; and (3) relaxation and opening of the upper esophageal sphincter.[8,22] As the sphincter relaxes, food passes from the pharynx into the esophagus. If the involuntary swallow response does not occur, neither do these physiologic functions, thus preventing a safe, normal swallow.[23,27]

The entire pharyngeal phase of the swallow takes

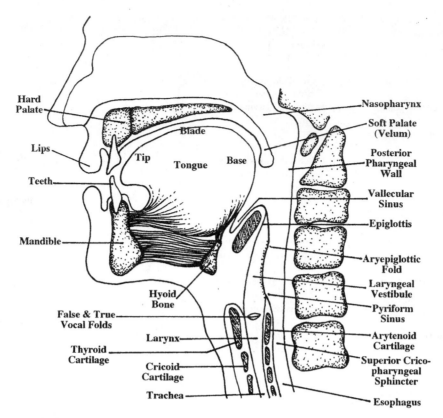

FIG. 11-1   Oral structures, swallowing mechanism at rest. (From René Padilla MS, OTR, Occupational Therapy Department, Creighton University, 1994.)

about 1 second to complete for thin liquids. It is important to note that both voluntary and involuntary components are needed in a normal swallow. Neither mechanism alone is sufficient to produce an immediate, consistent swallow necessary for normal feeding.[27]

ESOPHAGEAL PHASE

The esophageal phase of the swallow starts when the bolus enters the esophagus through the cricopharyngeal juncture. The esophagus is a straight tube, approximately 10 inches in length, which runs from the pharynx to the stomach. The pharynx is separated from the esophagus by the upper esophageal sphincter. The lower esophageal sphincter separates the esophagus from the stomach.[10] The upper third of the esophagus is composed of striated muscle and innervated by the central nervous system. The middle section is made up of striated and smooth muscle and innervated by the enteric nervous system which is visceral. The lower third of the tube is comprised of smooth muscle.[10,22] The food is transported through the esophagus by peristaltic wave contractions. The overall transit time needed for the bolus to reach the stomach varies from 8 to 20 seconds.

EVALUATION

Upon receiving a physician's referral, a thorough dysphagia evaluation must be completed. The occupational therapist needs to review the patient's medical history

and to assess the patient's mental status, physical control of head, trunk, and extremities and oral structures.

MEDICAL CHART REVIEW

Review of the patient's medical chart before the evaluation often reveals important information. The therapist should take note of the patient's diagnosis, pertinent medical history, prescribed medications, and current nutritional status.

The medical diagnosis may help to indicate the cause or type of swallowing problem the patient is experiencing. For example, the presence of a neurological disorder should alert the therapist that dysphagia problems may exist. It is important to learn whether the dysphagia was of sudden or gradual onset. The therapist should seek out information regarding the onset and duration of the patient's swallowing difficulties. The therapist also should note any previous surgeries involving the head, neck, and gastrointestinal tract that affect deglutition.

Particular attention should be paid to reported episodes of pneumonia or aspiration (entry of material into the airway).[27] Aspiration pneumonia is a complication that occurs when food enters or penetrates the lungs. Elevation of the temperature may indicate that a patient is aspirating.

The patient's current nutritional status may be found in the dietary section of the chart or in the nursing progress notes. Consideration should be given to prescribed medications that may alter the patient's alertness, orien-

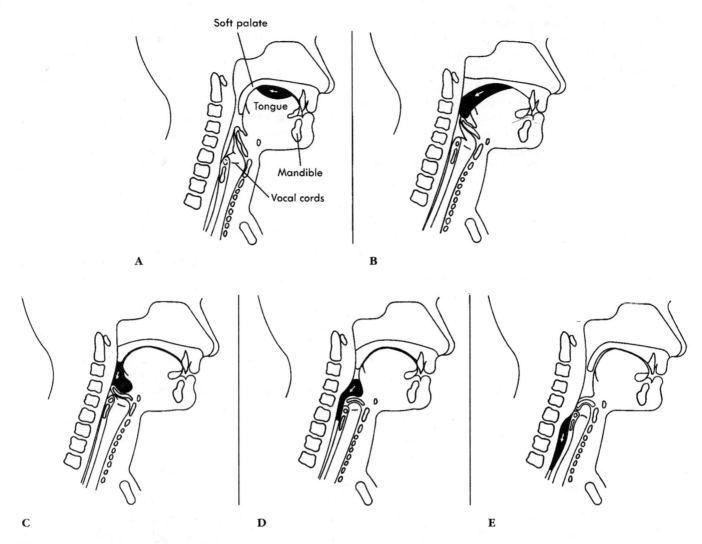

FIG. 11-2 The normal swallow. **A,** Voluntary initiation of swallow. **B,** Swallow response. **C,** Bolus passage through pharynx. **D,** Bolus begins to enter esophagus. **E,** Completion of pharyngeal stage as entire bolus moves into esophagus. (From Logeman J: *Evaluation and treatment of swallowing disorders,* San Diego, 1983, College-Hill Press.)

tation, and muscle control. How the patient is receiving food is important, for example, whether the patient is receiving food orally or through a nasogastric or gastrostomy tube and whether the patient is able to take all nutrients orally or is receiving supplemental tube feedings. The nurses' notes may indicate whether the patient has difficulty managing certain food or liquid consistencies and whether the patient coughs or chokes during eating. The patient's intake and output (I & O) record provides additional information about hydration status.

MENTAL STATUS

It is necessary to assess a patient's ability to participate actively in a feeding evaluation or treatment program. The therapist should establish whether the patient is alert; oriented to name, day, and date; and able to follow simple directions, either verbal or with guidance. The patient who exhibits confusion, dementia, or poor awareness may not be a good candidate for eating, be-

cause chewing and swallowing require voluntary control.[3,4,8]

PHYSICAL STATUS

Head and trunk control are important components for a safe swallow. To evaluate head control, the therapist asks the patient to turn the head from side to side and up and down. Assessment should include the quality of head movement, whether it is smooth and coordinated and whether it is adequate to allow the patient to maintain control with assistance. The therapist also should move the head passively from side to side and up and down to look for stiffness or abnormal muscle tone. Poor head control may indicate decreased strength, decreased or increased muscle tone, or decreased awareness. Head control is important because it develops first; jaw movement follows, and last, quality tongue movement occurs. Head control is also necessary to provide adequate jaw and tongue movement for an optimal swallow response.

In evaluating the patient's trunk control, the therapist observes whether the patient is sitting in midline with equal weight-bearing on both hips. Thus the therapist learns whether the patient can maintain the midline position when provided with postural supports (such as wheelchair trunk supports or a lapboard) and whether a return to midline is possible if loss of balance occurs.

To participate in a feeding training program, the patient must maintain an upright position with head and trunk in midline to provide sufficient alignment of the swallowing structures.[3,7] If the patient has poor head or trunk control, the therapist may assist the patient during evaluation and treatment.

ORAL EVALUATION
Outer Oral Status

The face and mouth are sensitive areas to evaluate. Most adults are cautious about or even threatened by having another person touch their faces. Therefore, as the outer oral structures are evaluated, including the facial musculature and mobility of the cheeks, jaw, and lips, each step of the process should be carefully explained, using terms that are understood by the patient. The therapist also should tell the patient how long he or she will be touching the face, for example, "for a count of three." Working within the patient's visual field, the therapist moves his or her hand(s) slowly toward the patient's face. This allows the patient time to process and acknowledge the approach. If the patient is hypersensitive or resistant to the therapist's touch, the therapist can first guide the patient's hand as needed to evaluate that area.

It is important for the patient to feel comfortable with the therapist's touch during evaluation. If a patient is not comfortable with the face or lips being touched, he or she will certainly be less inclined to allow the therapist's hand inside the mouth.

Sensation

Indications of poor oral sensation are drooling, food on the mouth, or food falling out of the mouth without the patient's awareness. To evaluate the patient's awareness of touch, the vision is occluded and a cotton-tipped swab is used to touch the patient gently with a quick stroke to different areas of the face. The patient is asked to point to where he or she was touched. If pointing is difficult for the patient, the patient is asked to nod "yes" or "no" when touched. The patient with intact sensation responds accurately and quickly.

Ability to sense hot and cold should be evaluated. The therapist may use two test tubes filled with hot and cold water or a laryngeal mirror that is heated and cooled with hot and cold water. The patient is touched on the face or lips in several places and is asked to indicate whether the touch was hot or cold. An aphasic patient may have difficulty answering correctly. In this instance, the therapist has to make an assessment from clinical observations.

Poor sensory awareness affects the patient's ability to move facial musculature appropriately. The patient's self-esteem also may be affected, especially in social situations, if decreased awareness causes the patient to ignore food or liquids remaining on the face or lips.

Musculature

Evaluation of the facial muscles provides the therapist with information regarding the movement, strength, and tone available to the patient for chewing and swallowing.

First the patient's face is observed at rest, and visible asymmetry is noted. If a facial droop is obvious, the therapist should observe whether the muscles feel slack or taut. A *masked* appearance, with little change in facial expression, may also be observed. The therapist should observe whether the patient appears to be frowning or grimacing, with jaw clenched and mouth pulled back. These symptoms may indicate increased or decreased muscle tone. Information obtained through clinical observations should be compared with that seen during actual movement.

To test the facial musculature, the patient is asked to perform the movements listed in Table 11-2. The therapist should note how much assistance the patient requires to perform these movements. As the patient moves through each task, bilateral symmetry is assessed. Asymmetry may indicate weakness or increased tone. Musculature is palpated for abnormal resistance to the movement. Resistance, which feels as if the patient is fighting the movement, is caused by hypertonicity in the antagonist muscle group.

If the patient is able to hold the position at the end of the movement, pressure is applied against the muscle to determine the muscle's strength. The patient with normal strength is able to hold the position throughout the applied resistance. The patient who is able to hold the position briefly against pressure may have adequate strength for chewing and swallowing with assistance. The patient who is unable to move into the testing position independently or with assistance will have difficulty with eating and with facial expression.

Oral reflexes

A patient with a clearly documented neurologic involvement may display primitive oral reflexes that interfere with a dysphagia retraining program. The rooting, bite, and suck-swallow reflexes, normal from 0 to 5 months of age, reappear in adults when higher cortical structures are damaged. The gag, palatal, and cough reflexes, which should be present in adults and act to protect the airway, may be impaired. Specific evaluation techniques can be found in Table 11-3. Persistence of these primitive oral reflexes interferes with the patient's development of isolated motor control needed for chewing and swallowing.

Inner Oral Status

Evaluation of the patient's inner oral status includes an examination of oral structures, tongue musculature, pa-

TABLE 11-2   Outer Oral Motor Evaluation

FUNCTION	INSTRUCTION TO PATIENT	TESTING PROCEDURE*
Facial expression	Lift your eyebrows as high as you can.	Place one finger above each eyebrow. Apply downward pressure.
	Bring your eyebrows toward your nose in a frown.	Place one finger above each eyebrow. Apply pressure outward.
	Wrinkle your nose upwards.	Place one finger on tip of nose and apply downward pressure.
	Suck in your cheeks.	Apply pressure outward against each inside cheek.
Lip control	Smile.	Observe for symmetric movement. Palpate over each cheek.
	Press your lips together tightly, puff out your cheeks.	Place one finger above and one finger below lips. Apply pressure, moving fingers away from each other, check for ability to hold air.
	Pucker your lips as in a kiss.	Apply pressure inwardly against lips (toward teeth).
Jaw control	Open your mouth as far as you can.	Assist patient to maintain head control. Apply pressure from under chin upward and forward.
	Close your mouth tightly. Don't let me open it.	Assist patient to maintain head control. Apply pressure on chin downward.
	Push your bottom teeth forward.	Place two fingers against chin and apply pressure backward.
	Move your jaw from side to side.	Place one finger on left cheek and apply pressure to right.

* Apply resistance only in the absence of abnormal muscle tone.

latal function, and swallowing. By performing the outer oral status evaluation first, the therapist has established a rapport and trust with the patient. Each procedure is first explained to the patient. The therapist works within the patient's visual field and gives the patient time to process the instructions.

It is important to place only a wet finger or tongue blade into the patient's mouth, because the mouth is normally a wet environment and a dry finger or tongue blade is uncomfortable.[11] After a count of three, the therapist removes the finger and allows the patient to swallow the saliva. The therapist should wear latex gloves for protection from infections. Appropriate hand washing techniques are also necessary.

Dentition

Because the adult uses teeth to shear and grind food during bolus formation, the therapist needs to evaluate the condition and quality of the patient's teeth and gums.

For evaluation purposes, the mouth is divided into four quadrants: right upper, right lower, left upper, and left lower. Each quadrant is evaluated separately, and each side separately, that is, right upper side, then right lower side. First the therapist slides a wet fifth finger under the patient's upper lip and moves it back toward the cheek, rubbing the gums three times.[11] The therapist notes whether the patient's gums are bleeding, tender, or inflamed and whether the gums feel spongy or firm. Loose teeth and sensitive or missing teeth are also noted.

TABLE 11-3   Oral Reflexes*

REFLEX	EVALUATION	FUNCTIONAL IMPLICATIONS
Rooting (0-4 months)	*Stimulus:* touch patient on right or left corner of mouth.	Limits isolated motor control of lip muscles.
	Response: patient moves lips in direction of stimulus.	Moves head out of midline altering alignment of swallowing mechanism.
Bite (4-7 months)	*Stimulus:* touch crowns of teeth with unbreakable object.	Prevents normal forward, lateral, and rotary movements of jaw necessary for chewing.
	Response: patient involuntarily clamps teeth shut.	
Suck swallow (0-4 months)	*Stimulus:* introduction of food/liquid.	Prevents development of normal voluntary swallow.
	Response: sucking.	
Tongue thrust (abnormal)	*Stimulus:* introduction of food/liquid.	Inferferes with ability to keep lips and mouth closed.
	Response: tongue comes forward to front of teeth.	Prevents tongue from propelling food to back of mouth in preparation for swallow. Prevents formation of bolus, loss of tongue lateralization.
Gag (0-adult)	*Stimulus:* pressure on back of tongue.	Protects airway (not always present in normal adult). Hypersensitive gag reflex can interfere with chewing, swallowing.
	Response: tongue humping, pharyngeal constriction, grimacing.	
Palatal (0-adult)	*Stimulus:* stroke along faucial arches.	Protects airway, closes off nasal passages, triggers swallow response.
	Response: constriction of faucial arches, elevation of uvula.	

* References 16, 38.

The therapist should take caution to avoid placing his or her finger between the patient's teeth until it has been determined that the patient does not have a bite reflex.

After assessing the gums, the therapist turns over his or her finger, sliding the pad against the inside of the patient's cheek and gently pushing cheek outward to feel the tone of the buccal musculature. He or she notes whether the cheek is firm with an elastic quality, too easy to stretch, or tight without any stretch. Observe the condition of inside of the mouth, checking for bite marks on tongue, cheeks, and lips. Now the therapist should remove the finger from the patient's mouth and allow or assist the patient to swallow saliva. Assist the patient to move the lip and cheek musculature into the normal resting position. This procedure is repeated for each quadrant. The therapist should avoid moving the finger across midline from right to left side of the patient's gums because this practice can be annoying.

If the patient has dentures, the therapist must discern whether the fit is adequate for chewing. Because dentures are held in place and controlled by normal musculature and sensation, changes in these areas, or marked weight loss, affect the patient's ability to use dentures effectively.[14] The dentures should fit over the gums without slipping or sliding during eating or talking. Because the patient needs to wear dentures throughout the dysphagia training period, necessary corrections or repairs should be completed quickly.[38] A dental consultation may be needed to ensure appropriate fit if dentures cannot be held firmly with commercial adhesive creams or powders. Patients who have gum or dental problems require appropriate follow-up and good oral hygiene to participate in a feeding program. Loose dentures or teeth may necessitate changes in food consistencies that the patient may have otherwise managed.

Tongue movement

The tongue is an intricate part of the normal chewing and swallowing process. Controlled tongue movement is necessary for moving and shaping food in the mouth. The tongue propels the food back in preparation for swallowing; therefore a thorough evaluation of the tongue's strength, range of motion, control, and tone are needed.[8,11,39]

The patient is asked to open the mouth, and the therapist, with a flashlight, can assess the appearance of the tongue and note whether the tongue is pink and moist, angry red, or heavily coated white. A heavily coated tongue may decrease the patient's sensations of taste, temperature, and texture and may indicate poor tongue movement.

In examining the shape of the tongue, the therapist notes whether it is flattened out, bunched up, or rounded. Normally the tongue is slightly concave with a groove running down the middle. The position of the tongue is observed. The examiner should determine whether it is (1) at midline, resting just behind the front teeth in the normal position, (2) retracted or pulled back away from the front teeth, or (3) deviated to the right or left side. A retracted tongue indicates an increase of abnormal muscle tone. The patient displaying tongue deviation with protrusion may have muscle weakness on the affected side, causing the tongue to deviate toward the unaffected side because the stronger muscles dominate. The patient also may have abnormal tone, which results in the tongue deviating toward the affected side.

Grasping the tongue gently between the forefinger and thumb, the therapist can pull the tongue slowly forward. A wet gauze square wrapped around the tip of the tongue may help the therapist to grip it.[11] Next, the therapist walks a wet finger along the tongue from front to back, to determine whether the tongue feels hard, firm, or mushy. The right side is compared with the left side of the tongue. An abnormally hard tongue may be due to increased muscle tone.

While continuing to grip the tongue between forefinger and thumb, the therapist can evaluate the patient's range of motion by moving the tongue forward, side to side, and up and down. The tongue with normal range moves freely in all directions without resistance.[11] Moving the tongue through its range, the therapist can simultaneously evaluate tone. As the therapist pulls the tongue forward, he or she determines whether it comes easily or whether resistance feels as if the tongue were pulling back against the movement, indicating increased tone. A tongue that seems to stretch too far beyond the front teeth is indicative of decreased tone. When moving the tongue side to side, it is noted whether it is easier to move in one direction or the other. Increased abnormal tone makes it difficult for the therapist to move the tongue in any direction without feeling resistance against the movement. The amount of assistance required to reduce or increase tone to within normal limits should be noted. Patients who are confused or apraxic may resist this passive motion but not have an actual increase in tone.

To evaluate the tongue's motor control (strength and coordination), the patient is asked to elevate, stick out, and move the tongue laterally (Table 11-4). If the patient has difficulty following verbal directions, the therapist can use a wet tongue blade to guide the patient through the desired movements. The patient is asked to place the tongue against the tongue blade and to keep it there. The therapist then moves the tongue blade slowly, guiding the patient's tongue in the testing direction.[11] Ease of movement, strength of movement, and coordination of movement are assessed for each direction.

Poor muscle strength or abnormal tone decreases the ability of the tongue to sweep the mouth and gather particles to form a cohesive bolus. If the tongue loses even partial control of the bolus, food may fall into the valleculae, the pyriform sinuses, or the airway, possibly leading to aspiration before the actual swallow.[27] The back of the tongue must also elevate quickly and strongly to propel

TABLE 11-4 Inner Oral Motor Evaluation*

FUNCTION	INSTRUCTION TO PATIENT	TESTING PROCEDURE†
TONGUE		
Protrusion	Stick out your tongue.	Apply slight resistance toward the back of the throat with tongue blade after patient exhibits full ROM.
Lateralization	Move your tongue from side to side.	Apply slight resistance in opposite direction of motion with tongue blade.
	Touch your tongue to your inside cheek — right, left; move it up and down.	Using finger on outside of cheek, push against tongue inwardly.
Tipping	Touch your tongue to your upper lip.	With tongue blade between tongue tip and lip, apply downward pressure.
	Open your mouth. Touch your tongue behind your front teeth.	With tongue blade between tongue and teeth, apply downward pressure on tongue.
	Touch your tongue behind your bottom teeth.	With tongue blade between tongue and bottom teeth, apply upward pressure.
Humping	Say "ng"; say "ga."	Observe for humping of tongue against hard palate. Tongue should flow from front to back.
	Run your tongue along the roof of your mouth, front to back.	Observe for symmetry and ease of movement.
SWALLOW		
Hard palate	Open your mouth and hold it open.	Using flashlight, gently examine for sensitivity by walking finger from front to back.
Soft palate	Say "ah" for as long as you can (5 seconds).	Observe for tightening of faucial arches, elevation of uvula. Using laryngeal mirror, stroke juncture of hard and soft palate to elicit palatal reflex. Observe for upward and backward movement of soft palate.
HYOID ELEVATION (BASE OF TONGUE)	Can you swallow for me?	Place finger at base of patient's tongue underneath the chin, and feel for elevation just before movement of the larynx.
LARYNGEAL		
ROM	I am going to move your Adam's apple side to side.	Grasp larynx by placing fingers and thumb along sides. Move larynx gently side to side, evaluate for ease and symmetry of movement.
Elevation	Can you swallow for me?	Place fingers along the larynx; 1st finger at hyoid, 2nd finger at top of larynx, and so on. Feel for quick and smooth elevation of larynx as patient swallows.
COUGH		
Voluntary	Can you cough?	Observe for ease and strength of movement, loudness of cough, swallow after cough.
Reflexive	Take a deep breath.	As patient holds breath, using palm of hand, push downward (toward stomach) on the sternum. Evaluate strength of reaction.

* References 11, 13, 19.
† Apply resistance in absence of abnormal muscle tone.

the bolus past the faucial arch into the pharynx to trigger the swallow response.[11] The therapist must carefully assess the tongue's function. The patient with poor tongue control may not be a candidate for eating. The therapist first has to normalize tone and improve tongue movement before attempting to feed the patient. The correct selection of appropriate foods also facilitates motor control when the patient is ready for eating.

Clinical evaluation of swallowing

Because aspiration is of primary concern in swallowing, the occupational therapist must carefully evaluate the patient's ability to have a safe swallow. Before presenting the patient with material to swallow, the ability of the patient to protect the airway is assessed. The patient needs an intact palatal reflex, elevation of the larynx, and a productive cough. Directions for evaluating all the components of the swallow are described in Table 11-4. The therapist should note the speed and strength of each component. The patient with intact cognitive skills may accurately report to the therapist where and when there is difficulty with the swallow.[27]

The occupational therapist must assimilate all the information from the evaluation process. Clinical judgment plays an important role in the accurate assessment of dysphagia.[3,11] Questions that must be asked are: Is the patient alert enough to follow through with bolus formation and an immediate swallow when presented with food? With assistance, does the patient maintain adequate trunk and head control, normalizing tone and facilitating quality movement? Does the patient display adequate tongue control to form a partially cohesive bolus and to regulate the speed in which the bolus enters into the pharynx? Is the larynx mobile enough to elevate quickly and strongly? Can the patient handle his or her saliva with minimal drooling? Does the patient have a productive cough strong enough to expel any material that may enter the airway? If the answer is yes to all of the above questions, the therapist may evaluate the patient's oral and swallow control with a variety of food consistencies.

The therapist should request an evaluation tray from dietary services consisting of a sample of puréed food such as pudding or applesauce, soft food such as a banana or macaroni and cheese, and ground tuna with mayonnaise or chopped meat with gravy. The tray also should include a thick drink such as nectar blended with one half banana for a 7-ounce drink, a semi-thick drink such as fruit nectar or a yogurt drink, and a thin liquid such as water.[1,9]

Puréed foods are chosen for patients with decreased motor control with chewing difficulties and or with apraxia to minimize the risk of aspiration. Soft foods are easily formed into a bolus and require less chewing than ground meat for patients who have poor oral motor control. Soft foods also stay together in a cohesive bolus. Ground foods allow the therapist to assess a patient's ability to chew, form a cohesive bolus, and move it in the mouth. Thick liquids move more slowly from front to back, giving the patient with a delayed swallow more time to control the liquid until the swallow response is triggered. Thin liquids are the most difficult to control, because they require a normal swallow to prevent aspiration.

For the patient who appears to have some ability to chew, start with puréed and soft foods and introduce solid materials if the patient is doing well.[11,37,38] The following procedures should be completed after each swallow of food or liquid.

1. Using a fork, the therapist places a small amount (1/3 teaspoon) on the middle of the tongue. A fork allows the therapist greater control of food placement in the mouth.[11,27] This procedure is repeated for each substance for two or three bites to check for fatigue.

2. The therapist palpates for the swallow by placing the index finger at the hyoid notch, the second finger at the top of the larynx, and the third finger along the midlarynx. The therapist can feel the strength and smoothness of the swallow.[11] The therapist also can evaluate the oral transit time by noting when food entered the mouth, when tongue movement was initiated, and when the elevation of the hyoid notch was felt, indicating the beginning of the swallow process. The therapist can time the swallow from the time that hyoid movement begins to when laryngeal elevation occurs, indicating triggering of the swallow response.[27] A normal swallow takes only 1 second to complete for thin liquids.

3. The therapist asks the patient to open the mouth to check for remaining food. Common areas in which food is seen are in the lateral sulci, under the tongue, on the base of the tongue, and against the hard palate.[8,27] Food remaining in the mouth indicates decreased or poor oral transit skills. The patient who exhibits oral motor deficits has increasing difficulty with chewing, shaping a bolus, and channeling food backward as harder consistencies of food are introduced.[11]

4. The therapist asks the patient to say "ah." By listening carefully, the therapist can assess the patient's voice quality and classify the sound production as strong, clear, or gurgly.[11,27] A gurgly voice may result from a delayed swallow response, which allows material to collect in the larynx. The therapist asks the patient to take a second "dry" swallow to clear any pooling of material. Asking the patient to say "ah" again enables the therapist to assess whether the voice quality remains gurgly for any length of time after the dry swallow. If the voice is still gurgly, the therapist should be concerned with the possibility that material has penetrated into the larynx, coming into contact with the vocal cords.[27] In this instance, a videofluoroscopy may be considered.

If the patient has significant coughing episodes, particularly before the therapist feels the initiation of the swallow (elevation of hyoid notch) with any consistency, the procedure should not be continued. If the patient has coughing from food with a puréed consistency, the therapist may try a soft food such as a banana if the patient has good anterior to posterior tongue movement.[11]

A neurologically impaired patient with poor sensation may have difficulty with a puréed consistency because it does not stay together as a bolus. The weight of soft foods may adequately trigger the swallow response. If the patient continues to cough even with soft foods, the swallow evaluation should be discontinued. A patient who is having difficulty at this level can be considered appropriate only for a prefeeding treatment program.

A patient who has difficulty handling solid consistencies may or may not have difficulty with liquids. If the patient is having difficulty with chewing, consider starting the evaluation sequence with ice chips, then proceed as follows. To evaluate the patient's swallow with liquids, start with a thickened (thick) nectar, then a pure nectar (semithick), and finally a thin liquid such as water. Small amounts of the liquid are placed with a spoon on the middle of the patient's tongue. The therapist proceeds by following the sequence used with solids. The therapist evaluates the patient's skill at moving material from front to back, the time of oral transit and swallow, and the voice quality after each swallow. Each liquid consistency is assessed for two or three swallows to check for fatigability.

A patient with a poor swallow may aspirate directly or pool liquids in the pyriform sinuses and valleculae which, when full, overflow into the laryngeal vestibule and down into the trachea. If a patient continues to have a gurgly voice after a second dry swallow or to have substantial coughing with any of the liquid consistencies, the evaluation should be discontinued (Fig. 11-3, *A* to *D*).

It is also important to evaluate the patient's ability to alternate between liquids and solids, which occurs naturally during meals. The therapist presents the patient with the type of food bolus easily handled, then the safest type of liquid tolerated. Assess for coughing when changing consistencies.

A patient with a tracheostomy tube in place can be evaluated by the therapist as previously described. The same criteria must be met before assessing the patient's swallow with food or liquids. The therapist must have a thorough understanding of the types of tracheostomy tubes and varied functions.

There are two main types of tracheostomy tubes: fenestrated and nonfenestrated.[17,27,36] A fenestrated tube is designed with an opening in the middle of the tube to allow for increased air flow. A fenestrated tube is frequently used for patients being weaned from a tube because it allows a patient to breathe nasally as he or she relearns a normal breathing pattern. By placing an inner cannula piece into the tracheostomy tube, the fenestrated opening can be closed off. With the inner cannula in place, a trachea button also may be used to allow the patient to talk. A nonfenestrated tube has no opening. A fenestrated tube is preferred when treating a patient with dysphagia.

A tracheostomy tube, fenestrated or nonfenestrated, may also be cuffed or uncuffed. A cuffed tube has a balloonlike cuff surrounding the bottom of the tube.[27] When inflated, the cuff comes into contact with the trachea wall, preventing the aspiration of secretions into the airway. A cuffed tube is used in cases in which aspiration has occurred. The therapist should consult with

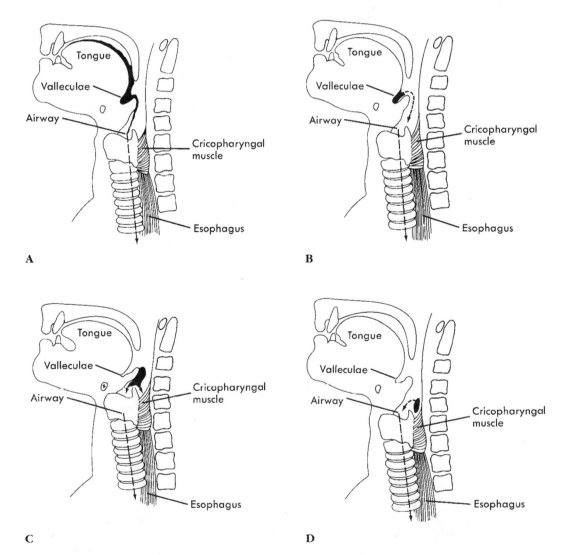

FIG. 11-3 Types of aspiration. **A,** Aspiration before swallow due to reduced tongue control. **B,** Aspiration before swallow due to absent swallow response. **C,** Aspiration during swallow due to reduced laryngeal closure. **D,** Aspiration after swallow due to pooled material in pyriform sinuses overflowing into airway. (From Logeman J: *Evaluation and treatment of swallowing disorders,* San Diego, 1983, College-Hill Press.)

the patient's attending physician to see whether the patient is still at risk of aspirating.

Before presenting the "trached" patient, who has a fenestrated tube, with any materials, the inner cannula is inserted. If the patient has a cuffed tube, present food, and slowly deflate the cuff while suctioning to prevent substances from penetrating the airway. The patient needs to be suctioned orally and through the tracheostomy to ensure that all secretions have been cleared.[8,27] The suctioning procedure can be performed by the nursing staff or a therapist who has been trained and is considered competent.

After presenting food or liquids, the therapist should check for oral transit skills and swallow. Blue food coloring added to food or liquids can aid the therapist in identifying material in the trachea. If the tracheostomy tube is cuffed, the cuff is slowly deflated. The patient is suctioned through the tracheostomy tube to determine whether any material entered the airway. The swallow evaluation should not be continued if material is found in the trachea.[8] The presence of a tracheostomy tube may affect a patient's swallow as secretions are increased and laryngeal mobility is decreased. When evaluation is complete, the patient is thoroughly suctioned. The inner cannula is removed, or the cuff inflated to the level prescribed by the physician.[17,18]

The patient's performance on the swallowing evaluation determines whether he or she is able to participate in a feeding program and at which food and liquid consistencies he or she is able to function efficiently. The therapist must decide which consistency is the safest for the patient. The safest consistency is that which the patient is able to chew, move through the oral cavity, and swallow with the least risk of aspiration.

The indicators of swallowing dysfunction include coughing or throat clearing before, during, or after the swallow; gurgly voice quality; changes in breathing pattern; delayed or absent swallow response; poor cough; and reflux of food after meals.[8,11,27,30] The presence of any swallowing dysfunction can lead to aspiration pneumonia. Acute symptoms of aspiration occurring immediately after the swallow are any change in the patient's color, particularly if the airway is obstructed, gurgly voice, and extreme breathiness or loss of voice.[11,17,18] Over the next 24 hours the therapist and medical staff must observe the patient for other signs of aspiration, such as nasal drip, an increase to profuse drooling of a clear liquid, and temperatures of 100° or greater, which may not have been evident during the clinical examination.[11,21,27] A patient who develops aspiration pneumonia needs to be reevaluated for a change in diet levels or taken off the feeding program, if necessary. An alternative feeding method is required.

Evaluation with videofluoroscopy

An important technique for evaluating a patient's swallow is videofluoroscopy. A videofluoroscopy is a radiographic procedure, using a modified barium swallow recorded on videotape. This technique allows the therapist to see the patient's jaw and tongue movement, to measure the transit times of the oral and pharyngeal stages, and to see the swallow, any residue in the valleculae and the pyriform sinuses, and any aspiration. With a videofluoroscopy, the therapist can determine the cause of any aspiration. A videofluoroscopy also may be used to determine which treatment techniques and the safest diet level may be effective in assisting the patient to achieve a safe swallow.

Aspiration can occur before the swallow because of poor tongue control, pooled material in the valleculae, or a delayed or absent swallow response. Poor laryngeal closure can result in aspiration during the swallow. Aspiration after the swallow is the result of pooled material in the pyriform sinuses overflowing into the trachea. Knowing the reason why a patient is aspirating can aid the occupational therapist in the treatment.[29,30]

A fluoroscopy machine has three components: a fluoroscopy tube, a monitor to view the picture, and an elevation table or platform. A TV videocassette recorder is set up to record the image. Other necessary equipment normally available in a radiology department are lead-lined aprons, lead-lined gloves, and foam positioning wedges.[29] Because the fluoroscopy machine may not lower enough to view a patient seated in a wheelchair, a special plywood seat system or wheelchair platform with a ramp may be required.

A videofluoroscopy is necessary to rule out silent aspiration. Forty percent of dysphagia patients are silent aspirators during the clinical evaluation.[27,28] It is important to rule out the occurrence of aspiration. Other indicators for a videofluoroscopy are difficulties with liquid consistencies and a need to identify specific pharyngeal problems. Some clinicians, however, advocate that all patients should be evaluated by videofluoroscopy regardless of these indicators. Contraindications to performing a videofluoroscopy include rapid progress of the patient, poor level of awareness or poor cognitive status, oral stage problems only, and the physical inability of the patient to undergo the test.

To perform a videofluoroscopy, three people are involved: the radiologist, the occupational therapist, and the person who sets up and runs the video equipment. The patient should be positioned to allow for a lateral view, with the fluoroscopy tube focused on the lips, hard palate, and posterior pharyngeal wall. The lateral view is most frequently used because it allows the therapist to evaluate all four stages of the swallow. This view clearly shows the presence of aspiration. An anteroposterior view also may be needed to evaluate asymmetry in the vocal cords.

During a videofluoroscopy evaluation, the therapist presents the patient with food or liquid to which barium paste or powder has been added.[1,9,29] The therapist mixes or spreads small amounts of paste or powder onto or into each food or liquid consistency. Premixing the consistencies with the barium paste or powder prevents time-consuming interruptions during the actual evaluation.

Food and liquids are presented in the sequence used for the clinical evaluation. Starting with puréed foods, the patient is given 1/3 teaspoon at a time of each consistency and asked to swallow when instructed. Liquids are evaluated separately, beginning with the thickened substance. Small amounts of material are given to reduce the risks of aspiration, if it occurs. An experienced dysphagia therapist may choose to evaluate only foods or liquids that the patient had difficulty with during the clinical examination, rather than to proceed through the entire sequence. The therapist continues to evaluate each consistency until aspiration occurs.

If the patient aspirates during the swallow, allowing material to fall directly into the airway, the therapist should discontinue the evaluation of that consistency. If aspiration occurs before the swallow, secondary to poor tongue control or a delayed swallow reflex, a thicker or denser substance should be tried because it is easier for the patient to control. When evaluating liquids, if the patient aspirates after the swallow because of pooling in the valleculae or pyriform sinuses, the evaluation with that consistency is discontinued.

The solid and liquid consistency that the patient handles without aspiration is selected as the starting point for feeding training. A patient aspirating on puréed or soft foods is not suited to an oral program. The patient who is aspirating thick liquids is not a candidate for liquid intake.

In addition, the videofluoroscopy procedure can be used to observe for fatigue. The patient is asked to take repeated or serial swallows of solids and liquids. The therapist should evaluate the patient's ability to control mixed consistencies of solids and liquids such as soups, and to alternate between solids and liquids. Various compensatory techniques may also be evaluated to determine if the airway can be protected, which may allow the therapist to initiate a feeding program.[29]

A videofluoroscopy is a valuable tool to be used in conjunction with the clinical examination. It can provide the therapist with additional information regarding the patient's difficulties. By identifying silent aspirators, the therapist can feel comfortable with the decisions made in determining a course of treatment. Because videofluoroscopy exposes the patient to radiation, the therapist should exercise good clinical judgment when deciding that videofluoroscopy is needed. The therapist must keep in mind that videofluoroscopy records the patient's performance in an isolated instance and is not a conclusive indicator of the patient's potential ability in a feeding program. If a patient continues to progress without difficulty, a second videofluoroscopy is not necessary. A second videofluoroscopy may be needed, however, to re-evaluate a patient who shows signs of readiness to participate in a feeding program or to determine whether a patient can progress to thin liquids.[11]

When documenting the results of a videofluoroscopy test, foods that were presented, problems that occurred at each stage, and the number of swallows taken to clear the food or liquid are noted. The therapist also should document any facilitation techniques that worked efficiently.[9,29] *This evaluation procedure requires advanced training and should be done only by appropriately trained therapists.*

Evaluation with videoendoscopy. Videoendoscopy (VESS) is a relatively new technique used in evaluation of swallowing. This technique is of value when it is not possible for the patient to participate in a videofluoroscopy or when used as a follow-up evaluation for the patient making rapid progress.[5,37]

The equipment needed for a VESS includes a fiberoptic nasolaryngoscope, video camera, video recorder and television monitor. The therapist first topically anesthetizes one nasal fossa. The therapist then passes a flexible fiberoptic tube through the nasal fossa, positioning the tip just above the palate.[5] The therapist initially examines the swallowing structures. Food and liquids with blue or green food dye added is then introduced as described previously. Bolus formation, tongue movement, swallow, and aspiration, if it occurs, are noted. *This evaluation procedure requires advanced training and should be done only by appropriately trained therapists.*

The results of a thorough evaluation determine the course of treatment to increase a patient's ability to eat. Upon completion of the entire dysphagia evaluation, the therapist should clearly document the patient's major problems, treatment recommendations and plan, and goals. The documentation should be concise and measurable. The treatment plan should include the type of diet needed, the training and facilitation that the patient requires, positioning techniques to be used during feeding, and the type of supervision that must be provided (Fig. 11-4). The treatment recommendations should be communicated to the appropriate nursing and medical staff.

TREATMENT

Because a patient may display more than one problem at each stage of deglutition, the intervention and treatment of dysphagia are multifaceted. The treatment of the patient with dysphagia includes trunk and head positioning and control, hand-to-mouth skills, oral motor skills, and swallowing. Perceptual and cognitive deficits that interfere with eating also are addressed. To treat the patient, the occupational therapist needs to devote 35% to 45% of the patient's total daily treatment time to oral motor and swallowing retraining.[21] A patient with severe problems can require up to 6 months of intense intervention before reaching optimal recovery. In preparing a treatment plan for the patient with acquired dysphagia, the thera-

Dysphagia Evaluation

Pt: _____

Dx: _TBI_____

Onset: _4-13-94_____

Medical hx: _Pt. is a 20 y.o. male who was involved in a single car accident resulting in bihemispheric cerebral damage, brainstem contusion, & subcortical damage to the reticular activating system._

Current nutritional status: _gastrostomy tube, NPO_____

	WNL	Adequate— without assistance	Unable	Comments
Mental status:				
Alert/oriented		c̄ assist		oriented to name, max assist for date
Direction following		c̄ assist		appropriate c̄ guiding
Physical status (symmetry, control, tone):				
Head control		c̄ assist		slight ↑'d tone c̄ head turning
Trunk control		c̄ assist		ataxic, TLR present
Endurance		c̄ assist		fatigues after 30 min.
Respiratory				
Suctioning required	✓			
Tracheostomy	✓			
Outer oral status:				
Facial expressions		c̄ assist		flat affect 2° ↑'d tone to moderate degree
Jaw movement			✓	poor rotary chew, poor jaw glide, pt. uses up & down movt.
Lip movement		c̄ assist		unable to purse & retract, poor lip compression
Sensation		c̄ assist		delayed 2° ↓'d attention
Abnormal reflexes		c̄ assist		suck-swallow present, others absent
Inner oral status (symmetry, control, tone):				
Dentition	✓			good, slightly inflammed gums
Tongue				
Appearance		c̄ assist		slight white coating & mid ℞ tongue laceration
Tone		c̄ assist		↑'d c̄ retraction
Movement: Protrusion		c̄ assist		deviated to ℞
Lateralization		c̄ assist		mild weakness
"ng"→"ga"			✓	poor anterior to posterior
Soft palate/gag reflex:	✓			uvula rises symmetrically
Cough (reflexive/voluntary):	✓			
Swallow:				
Spontaneous	✓			intact
Voluntary	✓			delayed 2° to tone
Laryngeal movement				
Tongue		c̄ assist		requires tone reduction
Elevation		c̄ assist		delayed fatigue factor after serial swallows
Food management:				Overall pt. shows ↓'d cognitive awareness of food in mouth & requires cueing
Puree		c̄ assist		pt. uses suck-swallow
Mechanical soft		c̄ assist		pocketing assist
Chopped/ground		c̄ assist		needed c̄ rotary chew
Regular diet			N/A	
Liquids: Thick		c̄ assist		c̄ straw, 5 sec. delay, Ø cough
Semithick		c̄ assist		c̄ straw, 5 sec. delay, coughing
Thin			N/A	

FIG. 11-4   Dysphagia evaluation.

Dysphagia Evaluation

Major problems:

① ↓'d cognition for attention and awareness of food in mouth s̄ cueing.

② ↑'d jaw & facial tone resulting in poor rotary chew.

③ Poor isolated tongue movements for lateralization, humping.

④ ↑'d laryngeal tone resulting in delayed swallow.

Recommendations/treatment plan:
  (positioning, diet level, environment, techniques)

① Positioning - upright on solid seating surface, slight forward lean.

② Tone reduction techniques for jaw, tongue, & larynx before & during meal.

③ Diet level - pureed & mechanical soft foods, thickened liquids 2x daily c̄ therapist only.

④ Therapeutic feeding in quiet setting.

⑤ No food or liquid in pts. room.

⑥ Monitor patient for signs of aspiration.

⑦ Videofluoroscopy for confirmation.

Long-term goals:

① Independent trunk and head control.

② ↑ attention and awareness of food in mouth to WFL.

③ ↑ isolated motor control of facial expression to WNL.

④ ↑ isolated motor control of jaw, tongue, & larynx to WFL.

⑤ ↑ oral intake for solids from pureed to regular diet.

⑥ ↑ oral intake for liquids from thick to thin.

⑦ Family education.

FIG. 11-4 Continued

pist must identify the symptoms and causes of the patient's deficits.[4,11,14,27,31]

GOALS

The overall goals of occupational therapy in the treatment of dysphagia are as follows[2,3,11,16,27]:

1. to facilitate appropriate positioning during eating
2. to improve motor control at each stage of swallow through normalization of tone and the facilitation of quality movement
3. to maintain an adequate nutritional intake
4. to prevent aspiration
5. to reestablish oral eating to the safest, optimum level

TEAM MANAGEMENT

Because of the complex nature of dysphagia treatment, the development of a team approach facilitates the patient's optimal progress. The dysphagia team should consist of the patient's attending physician, the occupational therapist, the dietitian, the nurse, the physical therapist, the speech-language pathologist, the radiologist, and the patient's family. Each professional contributes expertise toward patient improvement. It is important that all members of the dysphagia team have a thorough working knowledge of treating patients with dysphagia. Interdepartmental in-service is frequently required so that team members have a similar frame of reference.

The occupational therapist's role is to evaluate the patient and to implement the appropriate course of treatment. He or she is also responsible for coordinating the team effort, which includes obtaining physician's orders as needed, communicating with all other team members and staff, family education to ensure proper follow-through, and selecting the appropriate diet. The occupational therapist initiates changes in the patient's program whenever necessary.[4,11,38]

The attending physician's role involves the medical management of the patient's health and safety. The physician oversees all decisions regarding treatment for diet level selection, oral/nonoral feeding procedures, and the progression of treatment as recommended by the team. The physician should reinforce the course of treatment with the patient and the family.[18,21,27,38]

The dietitian is responsible for monitoring the patient's caloric intake. He or she makes recommendations to ensure that the patient receives a balanced nutritional diet in accordance with the medical condition. The dietitian is involved in suggesting types of feeding formulas for the nonoral patient. Diet supplements to augment oral intake may be recommended. In conjunction with the occupational therapist, the dietitian ensures that the proper food and liquid consistencies are served to the patient. Additional in-service training may be necessary for the dietary staff because dysphagia diets vary from traditional medical diets.

The patient's treating physical therapist is involved in muscle reeducation and tone normalization techniques of the trunk, neck, and face. The patient receives treatment in balance, strength, and control. The physical therapist is involved in increasing the patient's pulmonary status for breath support, chest expansion, and cough.[1]

The role of the speech-language pathologist involves the reeducation of the oral and laryngeal musculature used in speaking and voice production. Because these muscles also are used in swallowing, a therapist with dysphagia experience may participate in oral motor and swallowing training during prefeeding and feeding sessions.[21]

The nurse is another key member of the dysphagia team. The nursing staff is responsible for monitoring the patient's medical and nutritional status. The nurse usually is the first to notice changes in the patient's condition, such as an elevated temperature and an increase in secretions indicating swallowing dysfunction. The nurse then informs the physician and occupational therapist of these changes. The patient's oral and fluid intake is recorded in the nursing notes, and the dysphagia team is notified by the nurse when the patient's nutritional status is adequate or inadequate. Supplemental tube feedings that have been ordered by the physician are administered by the nursing staff, which also provides oral hygiene, tracheostomy care, and supervision for appropriate patients during meals.[1,18,27,33]

The patient's family is included as a team member to act as a program supporter. The family frequently underestimates the danger of aspiration; therefore it is important to educate the family and the patient from the first day of evaluation. The family and patient should understand which food consistencies are safe to eat and which foods must be avoided.[2,37]

The roles just described may vary from facility to facility. Designated roles must be clearly defined to ensure a coordinated team approach.

POSITIONING

Proper positioning is essential for treating the dysphagia patient. The patient should be positioned symmetrically with a normal alignment between the head, neck, trunk, and pelvis. To achieve this goal, ideally the patient is seated on a firm surface, such as a chair, with feet flat on the floor, knees at 90° flexion, equal weight-bearing on both ischial tuberosities of the hips, trunk flexed slightly forward (100° hip flexion) with a straight back, both arms placed forward on the table, and head erect in midline with slightly tucked chin.[3,6,14] For the patient who may be bed bound, the same principles apply, equal weight-bearing on both ischial tuberosities for the hips, trunk flexed slightly forward (100° hip flexion) with straight back and both arms placed forward on a bedside table.

Fig. 11-5 *A* and *B* shows two handhold techniques that allow the therapist to assist the patient in maintaining head control. Correct positioning normalizes tone, thereby facilitating quality motor control and function of the facial musculature, jaw and tongue movement, and the swallow process, all of which minimize the potential for aspiration.

A patient who has difficulty moving into the correct position or maintaining the position presents a challenge to the occupational therapist. A more careful analysis of the patient is required to determine the major problem preventing good positioning. Poor positioning may be due to decreased control or balance secondary to hypertonicity or hypotonicity or poor body awareness in space secondary to perceptual dysfunction (Fig. 11-6).[6,11,14] After the cause is identified, the therapist can treat it accordingly. (Specific treatment suggestions can be found later in this chapter.)

To assist in maintaining trunk position, the therapist may consider the use of an adaptive lateral trunk support. Forward trunk support is provided by seating the patient at a table.

ORAL HYGIENE

Oral care by nursing and therapy team members prevents gum disease, the accumulation of secretions, the development of plaque, and the aspiration of food particles that remain after eating. To begin the oral hygiene process, the patient is positioned upright and symmetrically. The patient who is apprehensive or who displays a hy-

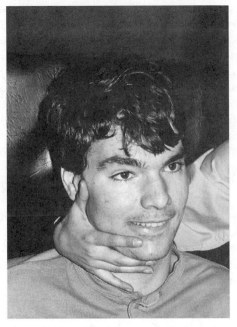

A

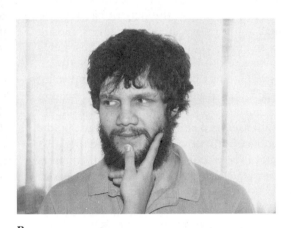

B

FIG. 11-5   Head control. **A,** Side hold position for patients requiring maximum to moderate assistance. **B,** Front hold position for patients requiring minimal assist. (From Meadowbrook Neurological Care Center, San José, Calif, 1988.)

persensitive oral cavity may first require preparation by the therapist. Preparation steps may include firmly stroking outside the patient's mouth or lips with the patient's or therapist's finger. Sensitive gums can also be firmly rubbed, preparing the patient for the toothbrush.

For cleaning purposes, the mouth can be divided into four quadrants. A toothbrush with a small head and soft bristles is used to clean each quadrant, starting with the top teeth and moving from front to back. When brushing the bottom teeth, the therapist brushes from back to

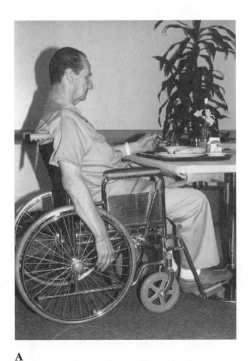

A

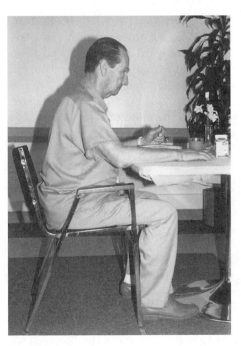

B

FIG. 11-6   Positioning of the patient with dysphagia. **A,** Incorrect positioning. **B,** Correct positioning. (From Meadowbrook Neurological Care Center, San José, Calif, 1988.)

front. Next, holding the toothbrush at a vertical angle, the therapist brushes the inside teeth downward from gums to teeth. Finally, the cutting surfaces of the teeth are brushed. An electric toothbrush is more effective if it can be tolerated by the patient.

After each procedure, the patient is allowed to dispose of secretions. After brushing, the patient is carefully assisted in rinsing the mouth. If the patient can tolerate thin liquids, small amounts of water can be given. Having the patient flex the chin slightly toward the chest helps to prevent the water from being swallowed. The therapist can assist the patient to expel the water by placing one hand on each cheek and, simultaneously, pushing inward on the cheeks while the chin remains slightly tucked. If the patient has no ability to manipulate liquids, a dampened sponge toothette can be used. The therapist and nursing staff also can consider using small amounts of baking soda instead of toothpaste because it is easier to rinse out.[11,14]

Oral hygiene for the nonoral or oral patient can be used as effective sensory stimulation of touch, texture, temperature, and taste. It can be used to facilitate beginning jaw and tongue movement and to encourage an automatic swallow.[11] Lack of oral stimulation over a prolonged time leads to hypersensitivity within the oral cavity. Patients who display poor tongue movement and are eating frequently have food remaining on their teeth or dentures or between the cheek and gum. A patient with decreased sensation is not aware of the remaining food. A thorough cleaning should follow each time the patient eats.

NONORAL FEEDINGS

A patient who is aspirating more than 10% of food or liquid consistencies or whose combined oral and pharyngeal transit time is more than 10 seconds, regardless of positioning or facilitation techniques, is inappropriate for oral eating.[11,27] This patient needs a nonoral nutritional method until he or she is again capable of eating or drinking. Patients who lack the endurance to take in sufficient calories also may require nonoral feedings or supplements.

The two most common procedures for nonoral feedings are the nasogastric tube and the gastrostomy tube.[17,18] A nasogastric tube is passed through the nostril, through the nasopharynx, and down through the pharynx and esophagus to rest in the stomach.[18] The nasogastric (NG) tube is a temporary measure, which should not be used for longer than 3 months.[27]

The advantages of using an NG tube are as follows: (1) it can be inserted and removed nonsurgically, if necessary; (2) it allows the physician to choose between continuous or bolus feedings (a feeding that runs no more than 40 minutes); and (3) it allows the therapist to begin prefeeding and feeding training while the tube is in place. The disadvantages of the NG tube are that (1) it can desensitize the swallow response, (2) that it can in-

terfere with a positioning program (the patient needs to be elevated to 30° during feeding), (3) it can increase aspiration risk, pharyngeal secretions, and nasal reflux, and (4) it can decrease the patient's self-esteem.[20]

Placement of a gastrostomy (G) tube is a minor surgical procedure. The patient receives a local anesthetic, and a small skin incision is made to make an external opening in the abdominal wall. A latex tube is passed through the opening into the stomach. The advantages of using a gastrostomy tube are that (1) it allows the physician to choose between continuous or bolus feedings, (2) it allows the therapist to begin a prefeeding or feeding program while the tube is in place, (3) it carries less risk of reflux and aspiration, (4) it does not irritate or desensitize the swallowing mechanisms, (5) it does not interfere with a positioning program, and (6) it can be removed when the patient no longer requires supplemental feedings or liquids.

The disadvantages of a gastrostomy tube are that the stoma site can become irritated or inflamed and that the tube can be perceived as permanent by the family.[18,20] A gastrostomy tube is the ideal choice for the patient who may require tube feeding or supplemental feedings for longer than 3 months.[27]

A commercially prepared liquid formula that provides complete nutrition usually is used for tube feedings. Many types and brands are available. The physician and dietitian determine which formula is best suited to the patient. The feedings are administered either by a bolus or a continuous method. A bolus feeding takes 20 to 40 minutes to run through either the NG tube or the G tube. It can be gravity-assisted or run through a feeding pump. Bolus feedings can be scheduled at numerous times throughout a 24-hour period. Continuous feedings, which may be better tolerated by the patient, are smaller amounts that are administered continuously by a feeding pump. The feeding pump can be set to regulate the rate that the formula is dripped into the tube. A disadvantage of continuous feedings is that the patient is less mobile, because the pump always accompanies the patient.

While the patient is on a nonoral program, the occupational therapist concentrates efforts on retraining the patient in oral motor control and swallowing. The prefeeding retraining can occur whether the patient is on bolus or on continuous feedings. As a patient begins to eat enough to require an adjustment in the intake amount of formula, however, bolus feedings become the preferred method. A bolus feeding allows the therapist to work with the physician to wean the patient from formula feeding. A bolus feeding can be held back prior to a feeding session, and the number of bolus feedings per day can be decreased as the patient improves. If satisfied by the tube feedings, the patient will not have an appetite and will have decreased motivation to eat.

As the patient improves, oral intake can be increased, and the formula feeding can be used to supplement the patient's caloric intake. An accurate calorie count, determined by recording the percentage of oral intake, assists the physician in decreasing the calories received through the tube feedings as the patient begins to meet nutritional needs orally. If the patient has progressed only enough to handle solids, the NG or G tube can be used to meet the patient's total or partial fluid requirements. Either tube can be removed when the patient is safely able to eat and drink enough to meet caloric and fluid needs.[1,33]

ORAL FEEDINGS

For a patient to be an appropriate candidate for oral feeding, several criteria must be met. The criteria to evaluate a patient's swallow with foods or liquids can be used. To participate in an oral feeding program, a patient must (1) be alert, (2) be able to maintain adequate trunk and head positioning with assistance, (3) have beginning tongue control, (4) manage secretions with minimal drooling, and (5) have a reflexive cough. The therapist needs to identify the food or liquid consistency that is the most appropriate for the patient. The safest consistency with which to initiate the oral program is one that enables the patient to complete the oral and pharyngeal stages combined in less than 10 seconds and to swallow with minimal aspiration (10% or less).[27] The overall goal of an oral feeding program is for the patient to achieve swallowing without any aspiration.

DIET SELECTION

A dysphagia diet must be carefully selected to reflect the needs of the patient. In general, foods chosen for dysphagia diets should (1) be uniform in consistency and texture, (2) provide sufficient density and volume, (3) remain cohesive, (4) provide pleasant taste and temperature, and (5) be easily removed or suctioned when necessary.[11,18] The following foods are contraindicated for dysphagia diets: foods with multiple textures such as vegetable soup and salads; fibrous and stringy vegetables, meats and fruits; crumbly and flaky foods; foods that liquefy such as gelatin and ice cream; and foods with skins and seeds.[9] Garnishes such as lettuce, parsley, and orange wedges also should be avoided because they may be unsafe for the confused patient.

The occupational therapist needs to work closely with the dietitian to develop dysphagia diet levels. Specific dysphagia diets facilitate ordering appropriate foods consistently. Once developed, the medical, nursing, and therapy staff should be educated as to which foods are in each level to ensure the patient's safety. Liquid diet levels also should be established. When requesting a dysphagia diet, the therapist should specify both levels desired, liquid and solid, because a patient may handle each differently.

DIET PROGRESSION

Tables 11-5 through 11-7 list foods in three progressive dysphagia stages.[1,9,33,37] After mastering the stage III or ground food items, the patient may progress to a regular diet. Stage I foods are puréed. This food group is best for patients with little or no jaw or tongue control, a moderately delayed swallow, and a decreased pharyngeal transit, resulting in pooling in the valleculae and pyriform sinuses.[11,27] Puréed foods move more slowly past the faucial arches and into the pharynx, allowing time for the swallow response to trigger. Because puréed foods cannot be formed into an adequate bolus, they offer little opportunity for increasing oral motor control.[11] Stage I foods are best used only to increase the patient's oral intake. The patient should be advanced to the next level as soon as possible.

Stage II items are soft foods that stay together as a cohesive bolus; thus the possibility of particles spilling into the airway is decreased. Stage II foods are best for patients with a beginning rotary chew, enough tongue control with assistance to propel food back toward the pharynx, and a minimally delayed swallow.[11] Mechanical soft foods reduce the risk of aspiration in patients who have both a motor and a sensory loss affecting the start of the swallow response.[3,19] Mechanical soft foods with a density provide increased proprioceptive input throughout the mouth. These foods also stay as a cohesive bolus rather than crumbling and falling uncontrolled into the airway. Because the patient at this diet stage displays improved tongue control, the swallow response is triggered faster as the back of the tongue elevates toward the hard palate. For the patient who is just beginning to chew, mashing the food with a fork enhances the patient's ability to keep it together as a bolus.[11]

Stage III or chopped ground food items require chewing, controlled bolus formation, and a fair swallow. This food group offers a wider variety of consistencies. Meats should be finely cut to facilitate a controlled swallow. Smaller particles are less likely to obstruct the airway and are less of a health risk than large pieces, if minimal aspiration occurs. These foods are safer than items found on a regular diet, yet require work on the part of the patient. Stage III foods work well for patients who have minimal problems with jaw or tongue control and an intact swallow response. The patient who has reached a stage III level needs to be concerned with a delayed swallow only when fatigued.

When a patient is ready to progress to the next diet level, the therapist can adjust the meals by requesting one or two items from the higher group, enabling assessment at the new level. This technique is also appropriate for patients who become fatigued. The patient is thus able to work with the therapist on the harder food item first, then continue the meal with foods that are easier. The therapist also may consider arranging several small meals throughout the day for the patient who fatigues, rather than three traditional meals.

A patient should progress to a regular diet when oral motor control is within functional limits, allowing the patient to chew and form any consistency into a bolus

TABLE 11-5   Dysphagia, Stage I Food Level* (Puréed)

FOOD GROUPS	FOODS ALLOWED	FOODS TO AVOID
Cereals/breads	Cooked refined cereals, cream of wheat/rice, malt-o-meal	All others
Eggs	Custard, puréed egg salad (without onions or celery)	All others
Fruits	Puréed fruit, applesauce	Whole fruits, juicy fruits; all others
Potatoes or substitutes	Mashed (white or sweet) potatoes mixed with thick gravy	All others
Vegetables	Puréed asparagus, beets, carrots, green beans, peas, spinach, squash	All others
Soups	Thickened, strained cream soups — consistency of a puréed vegetable	All others
Meat, fish, poultry, cheese	Puréed meat, pureéed poultry	All others
Fats	Butter, margarine, cream mixed with puréed foods	All others
Deserts	Plain puddings, smooth yogurt without fruit, custard	Any with nuts, coconut, seeds, all others
Sugars/sweets	Honey, sugar, syrup, jelly mixed in with puréed food	All others

* References 29, 33, 37.

and propel it back toward the faucial arches. The patient at this level should be able to swallow any food or liquid consistency with only occasional coughing. Continuing dietary precautions for a patient with a history of dysphagia include avoiding raw vegetables, stringy foods, and foods containing nuts or seeds.[1,9]

Because a patient may exhibit a difference in ability to handle liquids, a progression of liquid levels, separate from the solid levels, should be developed. The liquid progression is divided into three groups: thick, semithick, and thin liquids.[1,9,33] Examples of liquids in these levels are given in Table 11-8.

Thick liquids are made by adding thickening agents such as banana, puréed fruit, yogurt, dissolved gelatin, baby cereal, and cornstarch. A dietitian can provide the occupational therapist with specific recipes. These substances are usually added to the liquids and power-blended for smoothness. The thick drink or soup should stay blended and not be allowed to separate or liquefy. Thick liquids are the appropriate choice for patients with markedly delayed swallow. A thick liquid moves more slowly through the faucial arches, giving some time for the swallow response to trigger. Semithick liquids such as fruit nectars, buttermilk, tomato juice, and yogurt

TABLE 11-6   Dysphagia, Stage II Food Level* (Mechanical Soft)

FOOD GROUPS	FOODS ALLOWED	FOODS TO AVOID
Cereals/Breads	Cooked refined cereals, cream of wheat/rice, malt-o-meal, oatmeal; white, wheat, or rye bread (without crust or seeds); graham crackers, soft French toast without crust	Hard rolls, bread with nuts, seeds, coconut, and fruit. Bread with cracked wheat particles, sweet rolls, waffles, Melba toast, English muffins, popcorn, cereals such as Rice Krispies, corn flakes, puffed rice
Eggs	Custard; boiled, poached, and scrambled eggs; minced egg salad (without onions or celery)	All others
Fruits	Puréed fruit, applesauce, ripe banana and avocado; soft, canned and cooked fruits such as peaches, pears, apricots, pitted plums, stewed prunes, grapefruit, and orange sections (no membrane), baked apple (no skin), cranberry sauce	Fruits with seeds, coarse skins, and fibers, fruits with pits; all raw fruit except those listed as allowed; raisins, grapes, fruit cocktail
Potatoes or substitute	Mashed potatoes (white or sweet), baked potatoes (no skin), soft noodles, spaghetti, and macaroni, finely chopped.	Fried potatoes, potato or corn chips, rice
Vegetables	Cooked or canned artichoke hearts, asparagus tips, beets, carrots, mushrooms, squash, pumpkin, green beans, tomato purée and paste (no skins or seeds)	All other raw, stringy, fried, and dried vegetables; pickles
Soups	Thickened, strained cream soups made with puréed allowed vegetables	All others
Meat, fish, poultry, cheese	Finely ground meat; poultry, tuna (without celery or onions); soft cassaroles, soft sandwiches (without crust); cream or cottage cheese, American cheese	Fish (because of bones); meat, any consistency other than finely ground; bacon; all other cheeses
Fats	Butter, margarine, cream, mayonnaise mixed with food; thick gravy, thick cream sauce	Nuts, olives; all others
Desserts	Plain puddings, custard, tapioca, fruit whip, smooth yogurt, soft cake, cream pie with graham cracker crust	Cookies, cake with nuts, seeds, raisins, dates, coconuts, and fruits not on allowed list; all others
Sugars/sweets	Honey, sugar, syrup, jelly, plain soft milk chocolate bars	Marmalade, coconut; all others

* References 29, 33, 37.

TABLE 11-7 Dysphagia, Stage I Food Level* (Chopped/Ground)

FOOD GROUPS	FOODS ALLOWED	FOODS TO AVOID
Cereals/breads	Cooked cereals, ready-to-eat cereals† such as Rice Krispies, corn flakes, puffed rice; pancakes, French toast, white, wheat, and rye bread (with crust), salt crackers, soda and graham crackers; sweet rolls. English muffins, Melba toast, donuts	Hard rolls, bread with nuts, seeds, coconut, and fruit, coarse cereals such as granola, Grapenuts; popcorn
Eggs	Soft- and hard-boiled, poached, fried, scrambled eggs; egg salad (without onions and celery)	All others
Fruits	Banana, avocado; soft, canned and cooked fruit, ripe fruit	Fruits with seeds, coarse skins and fibers, pits; fruit cocktail
Potatoes or substitutes	Mashed potatoes (white or sweet), creamed potatoes, baked potatoes (without skin), noodles, spaghetti, and macaroni	Fried potatoes, potatoe and corn chips, rice without gravy
Vegetables	Cooked and canned vegetables (without skins, seeds, and stringy fibers)	All raw, stringy, fried, and dried vegetables
Soups	Thickened creamed soups made with puréed or whole allowed vegetables only	All others
Meat, fish, poultry, cheese	Finely diced/minced meat, poultry, tuna (without onions or celery), flaked fish, fish sticks; soft casseroles, sandwiches, and cheeses	Bacon; fish with bones; poultry with skin
Fats	Butter, margarine, cream, mayonnaise, gravy, cream sauces	Nuts; all others
Desserts	Soft cookies, cakes, pies, puddings, custard, yogurt	Cookies, cake with nuts, seeds, coconuts, and fruits not on allowed list; hard pies, crusts/pastries; all others
Sugars/sweets	Honey, sugar, syrup, jelly; plain soft milk chocolate bars	Marmalade, coconut; all others

* References 2, 9, 33, 37.
† Allowed only if thin liquids are appropriate.

drinks are used with patients who have a moderate swallow delay of 3 to 5 seconds.[11,27] Thin liquids, the highest liquid level, require an intact swallow.

PRINCIPLES OF ORAL FEEDING

The therapist should incorporate certain principles into the oral feeding program. First, an important aspect of the oral preparation stage is looking at and reaching for food. Thus the patient must actively participate in the eating process. Food should be presented within the patient's visual field. For the patient with a severe field deficit or unilateral neglect, the therapist needs to assist him or her to scan the plate or tray visually.

When physically possible, the patient should be allowed self-feeding. If the patient does not have a normal hand-to-mouth movement pattern, the therapist must assist the patient to achieve one by guiding the extremity in the correct pattern. Abnormal movement of the upper extremity facilitates abnormal movement in the trunk, head, face, tongue, and pharynx and decreases the patient's functioning.

If the patient is not capable of self-feeding, the therapist can keep the patient actively involved by allowing the patient to choose which food or liquid is preferred for each bite. Food is presented by moving the utensil slowly from the front toward the mouth so that the patient can see the food the entire time. The utensil should not be brought in from the side because the patient will have less preparation time. The patient should be allowed as much control of the situation as possible.

The patient should eat in a normal setting, if possible. For adults, eating is a social activity shared with friends and family. The patient can be redirected if distracted and can use environmental cuing when eating in a dining room with others. Adjustments, such as eating in the dining room but at a separate table, can be made to facilitate patient concentration. The therapist needs to be conscious of how the patient appears to others and help the patient to eat in a normal manner.

The occupational therapist must continually assess the patient's positioning, upper extremity movement, muscle tone, oral control, and swallow. The therapist assists the patient to perform the task correctly and does not allow eating while the patient exhibits an abnormal pattern. If the patient displays poor oral motor skills, the therapist evaluates for food pocketing after every few

TABLE 11-8 Liquids*

THIN LIQUIDS	SEMITHICK LIQUIDS	THICK LIQUIDS
Water	Extra thick milk-shake	Nectar thickened with banana
Coffee, tea	Extra thick eggnog	Nectar with puréed fruit
Decaffeinated coffee	Strained creamed soup	Regular applesauce with juice
Milk	Tomato juice, V-8 juice	Eggnog with baby cereal
Hot chocolate	Plain nectars	Creamed soup thickened with mashed potatoes
All fruit juices	Yogurt and milk blended	
Broth/consommé		
Gelatin dessert		
Ice cream		
Sherbet		

* References 2, 9, 33, 37.

bites. The rate of the patient's intake is monitored. The therapist should determine when too much food is in the mouth and when the patient puts food into the mouth before the previous bite has been cleared. The therapist feels for the swallow with a finger at the hyoid notch if the patient displays abnormal laryngeal tone or a delayed swallow.[11] He or she also assesses voice quality upon completion of the swallow.

The frequency with which the therapist must check each component depends on the skill level and performance of the patient. The more difficulty the patient exhibits, the more frequent the assessment. The therapist may find it necessary to assess after each bite or drink or after a few bites or drinks or after each food item. Use of good observational skills allows the therapist to make the appropriate clinical decision. Specific techniques for evaluation during feeding trials can be found in the swallowing evaluation section of this chapter. After completing the feeding process, the patient should remain in an upright position for 15 to 30 minutes to reduce the risk of refluxing food and of aspirating small food particles that may remain in the throat.[3]

The therapist also must continue to monitor the patient for signs of aspiration while eating and for the development of aspiration pneumonia over time. Although a conservative estimate of aspiration is 10% of material swallowed, measurement is difficult while a patient eats. Patients vary in the amount of aspiration they can tolerate before developing aspiration pneumonia according to age, health, and pulmonary status. The signs of acute and chronic aspiration were outlined previously.

When a patient is participating in oral feedings, careful monitoring of the nutritional status is necessary. The caloric needs are determined by the dietitian and the physician and depend on height, weight, activity level, and medical condition.[27,33] Fluid intake is monitored by having the physician order a calorie count. Each person who supervises or works with the dysphagia patient should record, in percentages, the caloric amount of each item the patient eats or drinks. The dietitian converts the percentages into a daily calorie total. The pa-

tient also should be monitored for physical signs of nutritional deficiency and dehydration. These symptoms are weakness, irritability, decreased alertness, change in eating habits, hunger, thirst, decreased turgor, and changes in amounts or color of urine.[20,38] If a patient is not able to take in the necessary calories (50% of the determined total), supplemental feedings are necessary to make up the difference.[9] The number of supplemental feedings is decided by the physician and the dietitian.

TREATMENT TECHNIQUES FOR THE MANAGEMENT OF DYSPHAGIA

Tables 11-9 through 11-12 provide treatment techniques for the management of dysphagia. They are not intended to be used for all situations. Each patient presents a different clinical picture and may display one deficit or a 0combination of deficits. After careful assessment the therapist must determine the primary cause of the patient's deficits and treat accordingly. The patient must be assessed and treated as a whole person rather than treated as a person with a single deficit.

Treating a patient with dysphagia requires a logical and consistent approach.[11] Abnormal tone, for example, should be normalized before the therapist can expect good motor control. Motor control must be improved before a patient can shape food into a cohesive bolus and achieve an effective swallow. Individualized prefeeding techniques can prepare the patient for eating. The therapist should strive toward facilitating the return of normal eating patterns in each patient.

Continual assessment of treatment by the therapist is essential. The therapist must continually evaluate the patient's response, which should reflect desired change. Therefore the therapist must develop good observational skills.[11] The clinician needs to adapt treatment to performance and progress. For difficult patients, the clinician should seek a consultation with an experienced dysphagia therapist. To develop expertise in dysphagia management, it is recommended that the therapist continue education in this area.

TABLE 11-9 Dysphagic Treatment: Oral Preparatory Stage

STRUCTURE	SYMPTOMS	PROBLEM	PREFEEDING TECHNIQUE	FEEDING TECHNIQUE
Trunk	Leaning to one side	Decreased trunk tone Ataxia	Facilitate trunk strength. Exercise.	Assist patient to hold correct position; assist with head control (Fig. 11-5).
		Increased trunk tone	Have patient clasp hands, lean down, and touch foot, middle, other foot to decrease or normalize tone.	Assist patient to hold correct feeding position; provide with perceptual boundary; consider lateral trunk supports.
		Poor body awareness in space	Patient with hands clasped and arms raised to 90° shoulder flexion moves arms, turning from trunk, side to side.	
	Hips sliding forward out of chair	Increased tone in hip extensors	See above.	Adjust positioning so that patient leans slightly forward at hips, arms forward on table.
		Poor body awareness in space	Provide firm seating surface.	
Head	Inability to hold head in midline	Decreased tone Weakness	Facilitate strength through neck and head exercises, flexion, extension, lateral flexion.	Assist with head control (Fig. 11-5).
	Inability to move head	Increased tone Poor ROM	Tone reduction of head, shoulders, and trunk; facilitate normal movement.	See above.
UE	Spillage of food from utensils	Decreased tone Apraxia Decreased coordination	Facilitate increased tone through weight-bearing, sweeping, or tapping muscle belly of desired muscle.	Guide patient through correct movement pattern; consider adaptive equipment; provide adaptive utensils as needed.
	Inability to self-feed	Increased tone Abnormal movement patterns	Reduce proximal tone from scapula mobilization, weight-bearing through arm.	See above.
Face	Drooling, food spillage from mouth	Decreased lip control	Place a wet tongue blade between patients lips; ask patient to hold tongue blade while therapist tries to pull it out.	Using side handgrip for head control, the therapist approximates lip closure by guiding and assisting with jaw closure.
		Poor lip closure 2° decreased tone, poor sensation	Vibrate lips with back of electric toothbrush down cheek and across lips.	Have patient use a straw when drinking liquids until control improves.
		Apraxia	Lip exercises: movements described in outer oral motor evaluations; patient performs repetitions 2-3 times daily.	Place food to unimpaired side.
			Blow bubbles into glass of liquid with straw.	Use cold food or liquids.
		Decreased sensation	Fan lips so that patient feels drool or wetness on lips or chin to increase awareness.	Teach patient to pat vs. wipe mouth and chin every few bites.
Tongue	Pocketing of food in cheeks or sulci	Poor tongue control for lateralization and/or tipping; decreased tone Poor sensation	Tongue exercises: use movements described in inner oral motor evaluation.	Avoid crumbly foods. Stroke patient's outside cheek where pocketing occurs with index finger back and up toward patient's ear. Instruct patient to check cheek for pocketing.
	Poor bolus formation		Tongue ROM, wrap tip of tongue in wet gauze; gently pull tongue forward, side to side and up and down; move slowly. Pull tongue wrapped in wet gauze forward past front teeth, using index and middle finger to vibrate tongue back and forth sideways to decrease tone and facilitate protrusion.	Avoid crumbly foods. Reduced tone as needed during meal. Double swallow.
	Retracted tongue	Increased tone Retracted jaw	Normalize neck tone. Normalize jaw tone.	Correct positioning (Fig. 11-6).

References 3, 6, 11, 14, 16, 30.
UE, Upper extremities.
2°, Secondary.

TABLE 11-10 Dysphagic Treatment: Oral Stage

STRUCTURE	SYMPTOMS	PROBLEM	PREFEEDING TECHNIQUES	FEEDING TECHNIQUE
Tongue	Slow oral transit Inability to make a "ng-ga" sound	Poor anterior to posterior movement; decreased tone, poor sensation Increased tone	Practice "ng-ga" sounds. Grasping tongue wrapped in gauze, pull it forward past front teeth; use finger or tongue blade to vibrate base of tongue back and forth sideways. Improve tongue ROM (Table 11-9).	Tuck chin towards chest. Position food center, posteriorly. Avoid crumbly foods. Use cold/hot foods vs. warm. Correct positioning. Place index finger at base of tongue under chin. Stroke up and forward.
	Tongue retraction Inability to make a "ng-ga" sound		Grasping tongue wrapped in gauze, pull forward to front teeth; stroke firmly down middle of tongue with edge of tongue blade.	See above.
	Slow oral transit time Inability to channel food back toward pharynx	Inability to form central groove in tongue Apraxia	Facilitate tongue retraction to bring tongue back into normal resting position; vibrate on either side of the frenulum found inside the mouth, under the tongue with finger. Increase jaw control; teach isolated tongue movements (described in Table 11-4).	Correct positioning. Place food away from midline of tongue toward back of mouth. Provide pressure to base of tongue with spoon after food placement.
	Repetitive movement of tongue; food is pushed out front of mouth.	Tongue thrust		
	Food falls off tongue into sulci or food remains on tongue without patient awareness.	Poor sensation	Ice tongue; ice tongue in gauze to prevent ice chips from slipping into the pharynx; brush tongue with toothbrush to stimulate receptors.	Use foods with high density. Alternate presentation of foods—cold, hot during meal.
	Slow oral transmit time; food remains on hard palate; coughing before swallow	Poor tongue elevation; decreased tone	Ask patient to practice k, g, n, d, t sounds. Lightly touch tongue blade or soft toothbrush to roof of mouth at back of tongue, instruct patient to press spot with tongue; resist movement with blade or brush to increase strength. Vibrate tongue at base below chin; provide quick stretch by pushing down on base of tongue.	Correct positioning (Fig. 11-6). With finger under chin at base of tongue, move finger upward and forward to facilitate elevation. Avoid crumbly foods. Double swallow.
	Slow oral transit time. Food remains on back of tongue as patient is unable to elevate tongue to push food to hard palate. Coughing before swallow; retracted tongue	Decreased tone Increased tone Decreased LOA* Weakness Decreased sensation	Tone reduction; grasping tongue with gauze wrapped around tip, pull tongue forward with finger or tongue blade. Vibrate base of tongue right to left. Grasping base of tongue under chin between two fingers, move it back and forth to decrease tone.	Adjust correct positioning by increasing forward flexion at hips, arms forward to decrease tone. Reduce tone as needed; give patient breaks because tone increases with effort. With finger under chin at base of tongue, move finger upward and forward to facilitate elevation.

References 11, 14, 16, 27, 31, 38.
* Level of awareness.

TABLE 11-11 Dysphagia Treatment: Pharyngeal Stage

STRUCTURE	SYMPTOMS	PROBLEM	PREFEEDING TECHNIQUE	FEEDING TECHNIQUE
Soft palate	Tight voice; nasal regurgitation. Air felt through nose or mist seen on mirror when patient says "ah". Decreased tone. Nasal speech	Inadequate soft palate movement; 2° to increased tone, rigidity, decreased tone	Facilitate normal head/neck positioning. Have patient tuck chin into therapist's cupped hand then push into hand as therapist applies resistance. Patient says "ah" afterward. Speed and height of uvula elevation should increase. Follow by thermal application.	Facilitate normal head/neck positioning. With head/neck in midline, have patient tuck chin slightly to decrease rate of food entering into pharynx
	Delayed swallow	Decreased triggering of swallow response	Thermal application: using a laryngeal mirror #00 after being placed in ice water or chips for 10 seconds, touch base of faucial arch. Repeat up to 10 times. Process can be repeated several times a day.	Alternate presentation of food; start very cold substance, then warm. Cold substance can increase sensitivity of faucial arches. Tuck chin slightly forward to prevent bolus entering airway.
Hyoid	Delayed elevation of hyoid bone. Poor tongue elevation	Delayed swallow. Incomplete swallow	Increase tongue humping (Table 11-10) as elevation of tongue and hyoid stimulates triggering of response.	Place index finger under chin at base of tongue and push up forward to facilitate tongue elevation.
	Tongue retraction	Abnormal tongue tone; poor ROM	Tone reduction (Table 11-10).	
Pharynx	Coughing after swallow	Decreased pharyngeal movement. Penetration into laryngeal vestibule	None	If appropriate, alternate presentation of liquid with stage II or stage III solids. Liquid material moves solids through pharynx.
	Coating of pharynx seen on videofluoroscopy. Gurgly voice			Have patient take second dry swallow to clear vallecula. Tilt head to stronger side. Supraglottic swallow
	Seen on videofluoroscopy, AP view. Material residue seen on one side. Weak or hoarse voice	Unilateral pharyngeal movement	None	Compensatory technique for patients with low tone: Have patient turn head toward affected side during swallow to prevent pooling in affected pyriform sinuses. Evaluate technique against its effect on patient positioning and tone in trunk, upper extremities
Larynx	Coughing, choking after swallow	Decreased laryngeal elevation; decreased tone. Weakness	Quick ice up sides of larynx; ask patient to swallow. Assist movement by guiding larynx upward. Vibrate laryngeal musculature from under chin, downward on each side to sternal notch.	Teach patient to clear throat immediately after swallow to move residual. Use supraglottic swallow, Mendelsohn maneuver, effortful swallow.
	Noisy swallow. Audible swallow	Increased tone. Rigidity. Uncoordinated swallow	ROM—place fingers and thumb along both sides of larynx and gently move it back and forth until movement is smooth and easy; tone decreased. Using chipped ice, form pack in washcloth and place around larynx for 5 min	Placing fingers and thumb along both sides of larynx, assist patient with upward elevation before swallow. Double swallow.
Trachea	Continuous coughing before, during, after swallow	Aspiration—before: poor tongue control; during: delayed swallow response; after: decreased pharyngeal movement	Teach patient how to produce a voluntary cough. Ask patient to take a deep breath and cough while breathing out; therapist uses palm of hand to push downward (toward stomach) on the sternum.	Encourage patient to keep coughing; facilitate reflexive cough. Push downward on sternum as patient breathes out. Suction patient if problem in creases.
		Blocked airway	None	Push into patient's sternal notch to assist with cough. Perform Heimlich maneuver. Seek medical assistance.

References 11, 14, 27, 30, 31.

TABLE 11-12 Dysphagia Treatment: Esophageal Stage

STRUCTURE	SYMPTOMS	PROBLEM	PREFEEDING TECHNIQUE	FEEDING TECHNIQUE
Esophagus	Frequent regurgitation of food or liquid and coughing or choking after the swallow: material collecting in a side pocket in esophagus.	Esophageal diverticulum	Requires a medical diagnosis; problem can be seen through traditional barium x-ray study. Surgical correction is needed.	Report symptoms to medical staff. (Therapist cannot treat.)
	Regurgitation of food, coughing, or choking on food after the swallow: inability of food to pass through the pharynx or esophagus	Partial or total obstruction of the pharynx or esophagus	See above.	See above.

References 11, 14, 27, 30, 31.

REVIEW QUESTIONS

1. List the components of dysphagia.
2. List the four stages of swallowing and the characteristics of each.
3. List the physiological functions that occur when the swallow response triggers and explain why these functions are necessary.
4. Why is it necessary to assess a patient's mental status during a dysphagia evaluation?
5. Describe what the therapist should look for when evaluating the trunk and head during the dysphagia evaluation.
6. What information can be gained by the therapist when evaluating the patient's facial motor control?
7. How does poor tongue control contribute to aspiration?
8. Name the components required to protect the airway.
9. What is the safest food sequence to follow for a swallowing evaluation?
10. Describe the finger placement that a therapist can use to feel the strength and smoothness of the swallow.
11. Why should the therapist assess voice quality after a swallow?
12. Will a patient who has difficulty handling solids also have difficulty with liquids?
13. What options does the occupational therapist have when a patient coughs?
14. List the indicators of swallowing dysfunction.
15. List the acute symptoms of aspiration.
16. When is a videofluoroscopy necessary?
17. List the elements in treatment of the dysphagia patient.
18. Describe the position in which a patient should be treated, and give the rationale for this position.
19. What are the indications for placing a patient on a nonoral treatment program?
20. Name five important criteria a patient must meet to participate in an oral feeding program.
21. List the properties of food preferred for diets for patients with dysphagia.
22. Describe the effect that poor hand-to-mouth movements have on the patient's swallow.
23. Why is it important to involve the patient in the eating process?
24. What are the symptoms of nutritional deficiency?
25. Describe two possible treatment techniques used for a patient who displays a masked appearance.
26. Name three treatment techniques the occupational therapist can use for poor rotary jaw movement and increased tone.
27. Describe two ways a therapist can decrease abnormally high tone in the tongue.
28. Describe thermal application as a treatment technique. For which problem is it used?
29. When is use of the 'dry swallow' technique appropriate?
30. How can the therapist facilitate a cough?

REFERENCES

1. Alta Bates Hospital Rehabilitation Services; *Dysphagia evaluation and treatment protocol,* Berkeley, Calif, 1990.
2. American Occupational Therapy Association: *AOTA resource guide: feeding and dysphagia,* Rockville, Md, 1994, The Association.
3. Avery-Smith W.: Management of neurologic disorders: the first feeding session. In Groher M, editor: *Dysphagia: diagnosis and management,* ed 2, Stoneham, Mass, 1992, Butterworth-Heinemann Publishers.
4. Avery-Smith W, Dellaosa D: Approaches to treating dysphagia in patients with brain injury. *Am J Occup Ther* 48:236, 1994.
5. Bastian R: The videoendoscopic swallowing study: an alternative and partner to the videofluoroscopic swallowing study. *Dysphagia* 8:359, 1993.
6. Bobath B: *Adult hemiplegia: evaluation and treatment,* ed 2, London, 1978, William Heinemann Medical Books.
7. Buchholz D, Bosma J, Donner M: Adaption, compensation, and decompensation of the pharyngeal swallow, *Gastrointest Radiol* 10:235, 1985.

8. Cherney L, Pannell J, Cantieri C: Clinical evaluation of dysphagia. In Cherney, L. editor: *Clinical management of dysphagia in adults and children,* Gaithersburg, Md, 1994, Aspen Publishers.

9. Community Hospital Los Gatos-Saratoga, Rehabilitation Services, *Dysphagia protocol,* Los Gatos, Calif, 1992.

10. Conklin JL: Control of esophageal motor function, *Dysphagia* 8:31, 1993.

11. Coombes K: Swallowing dysfunction in hemiplegia and head injury. Course presented by International Clinical Educators, Aug. 24-27, 1986, and Aug. 24-28, 1987, Los Gatos, Calif.

12. Curtis D, Cruess D, Wilgress E: Normal solid bolus swallowing: erect position, *Dysphagia,* 1:63, 1986.

13. Daniels L, Worthington C: *Muscle testing,* ed 5, Philadelphia, 1986, WB Saunders.

14. Davies P: *Steps to follow,* New York, 1985, Springer-Verlag.

15. Donner M, Bosma J, Robertson B: Anatomy and physiology of the pharynx, *Gastrointest Radiol* 10:196, 1985.

16. Farber S: *Neurorehabilitation, a multisensory approach,* Philadelphia, 1982, WB Saunders.

17. Fleming S.: Treatment of mechanical swallowing disorders. In Groher M, editor: *Dysphagia: diagnosis and management,* ed 2, Stoneham, Mass, 1992, Butterworth-Heinemann Publishers.

18. Griggs B: Nursing management of swallowing disorders. In Groher M, editor: *Dysphagia: diagnosis and management,* ed 2, Stoneham, Mass, 1992, Butterworth-Heinemann Publishers.

19. Groher M: Bolus management and aspiration pneumonia with pseudobulbar dysphagia, *Dysphagia* 1:215, 1987.

20. Groher M: Ethical dilemmas in providing nutrition, *Dysphagia* 5:102, 1990.

21. Groher M, Asher I: Establishing a swallowing program. In Groher M, editor: *Dysphagia: diagnosis and management,* Stoneham, Mass, 1984, Butterworth Publishers.

22. Hendrix TR: Coordination of peristalsis in pharynx and esophagus, *Dysphagia* 8:74, 1993.

23. Kahrilas PJ: Pharyngeal structure and function, *Dysphagia* 8:303, 1993.

24. Kendall H, Kendall F, Wadsworth G: *Muscles, testing and function,* Baltimore, Md, 1971, Williams & Wilkins.

25. Lazzara G, Lazarus C, Logeman J: Impact of thermal stimulation on the triggering of the swallow reflex, *Dysphagia* 1:73, 1986.

26. Liebman M: *Neuroanatomy made easy and understandable,* Rockville, Md, 1986, Aspen Publishers.

27. Logemann J: *Evaluation and treatment of swallowing disorders,* San Diego, Calif, 1983, College Hill Press.

28. Logemann J: Treatment for aspiration related to dysphagia: an overview, *Dysphagia* 1:34, 1988.

29. Logemann J: *Manual for the videofluorographic study of swallowing,* ed 2, Austin, Tex, 1993, Pro-Ed. Publishers.

30. Logemann J: Noninvasive approaches to deglutitive aspiration, *Dysphagia* 8:331, 1993.

31. Martin BJW: Treatment of dysphagia in adults. In Cherney L, editor: *Clinical management of dysphagia in adults and children,* Gaithersburg, Md, 1994, Aspen Publishers.

32. Martin RE, Sessler BJ: The role of the cerebral cortex in swallowing, *Dysphagia* 8:195, 1993.

33. Meadowbrook Neurologic Care Center, Rehabilitation Services: *Dysphagia protocol,* 1986, San Jose, Calif, 1986.

34. Miller A: Neurophysiological basis of swallowing, *Dysphagia* 1:91, 1986.

35. Miller AJ: The search for the central swallowing pathway: the quest for clarity, *Dysphagia* 8:185, 1993.

36. Pillsbury H, Buckwalter J: Surgical intervention in dysphagia. In Groher M, editor: *Dysphagia: diagnosis and management,* Stoneham, Mass, 1984, Butterworth Publishers.

37. Rader T, Rende B: Swallowing disorders: what families should know, Tucson, Ariz, 1993, Communication Skill Builders Publishers.

38. Silverman EH, Elfant IL: Dysphagia: an evaluation and treatment program for the adult, *Am J Occup Ther* 33:382, 1979.

39. Stone M, Shawker T: An ultrasound examination of tongue movement during swallowing, *Dysphagia* 1:78, 1986.

Evaluation and Treatment of Visual Deficits

Mary Warren

In order to understand visual perceptual dysfunction following cerebral vascular accident (CVA) and brain injury, it is necessary first to realize that visual perception is a process used by the central nervous system (CNS) to adapt to the environment. Visual perception is not a series of discrete perceptual skills or the function of a single sensory modality, but a process that integrates vision with other sensory input in order to adapt and survive. The activities a person is required to complete in a day will dictate the visual perceptual skill that is needed. Whether or not a patient has a visual perceptual deficit following brain injury will depend on whether the ability to process visual information has been altered so that it prevents completion of a necessary activity of daily living.

ROLE OF VISION IN THE ADAPTATION PROCESS

According to Jean Ayres "the overall function of the brain is to filter, organize and integrate sensory information to make an adaptive response to the environment."[4] The brain receives a variety of sensory information including visual, proprioceptive, tactile, vestibular, and auditory. Vision is used along with information from these other sensory systems to adapt to the environment: to act upon it and to manipulate, mold, and improve it. In adapting to the environment, the brain puts the isolated bits of sensory information it receives together, or integrates them, to form a picture of the environment. This picture, created by sensory input, becomes the context of a situation, and an individual uses this context to make decisions and formulate plans to respond to a situation.

Because sensory input into the CNS is constantly changing, the picture created is dynamic and constantly changing as well. Our decision about how to respond to a situation changes moment by moment with alterations in the sensory context in which we find ourselves.

For example, picture yourself walking on a crowded street at noontime. The sun is shining and people all around you are rushing to complete errands. As you walk down the street you pass by a "street person" huddled against the side of a building. He seems to be highly agitated and is talking furiously to himself and waving his arms. As you pass by, you may think briefly about the social and economic conditions of our times that cause a person to have to live this way. You may feel saddened or angered by his situation but chances are you will not feel personally threatened or in danger. Now picture yourself on the same street, but at midnight. It is dark and instead of a crowd of people rushing about, you are alone. The "street person" is still huddled against the building and he is still in the same agitated state as he was at noontime. This time when you pass by, it is likely that you will walk a little faster and keep a closer eye on this individual; you will feel a greater sense of danger. You will not take time to ponder the conditions of our times but will formulate contingency plans in the event that he comes towards you.[52]

The only differences between these two scenarios are the sensory conditions: the amount of illumination and the number of other people on the street. The street person has not changed; he is no more a threat to you at midnight than he was at noontime. Yet your response to the situation is totally changed by the sensory context of your surroundings.

Successful adaptation to the environment is also dependent on the ability to anticipate information. The key to survival is to stay one step ahead of circumstances whether you are dealing with patients, traffic, or your children. Anticipation enables an individual to plan for situations, and planning allows manipulation of the environment. If we were unable to plan for situations and were only able to react to them once they occurred, we might be able to survive our world but we would not be able to act upon it. Anticipation and planning is driven by the sensory context of our circumstances: "It looks like rain. I'd better take an umbrella" or "It's dark in there. I'd better take a flashlight." How we perceive sensory information determines how we plan our response to each situation.

Given the importance of the sensory context, what role does vision, a basic sensory process, play in the adaptation process? Vision is our most far-reaching sensory system. It is the sensory system that takes us out into our environment; the first to alert us to danger (seeing a threatening storm approach) and the first to alert us to pleasure (seeing your children playing in the yard as you drive up). Because of its far-reaching nature, visual input strongly dominates the construction of the environmental picture we use to adapt. We rely on vision to size up situations. We say to ourselves, "He looks harmless" or "That looks delicious." Our language is peppered with phrases that reflect the importance of vision in decision-making, such as "I'll believe it when I see it," "I'll keep an eye out for it," or "I can see what you mean." Because visual input dominates the construction of sensory context, it plays a very powerful role in the anticipatory process and therefore in our ability to adapt to the environment. It is how we "see" a situation that triggers the planning and decision-making processes.

AN OVERVIEW OF VISUAL PROCESSING WITHIN THE CENTRAL NERVOUS SYSTEM

For vision to be used for adaptation, the raw material of vision (that is, the pattern of light that falls on the retina) must be transformed into images of the environmental surround. Those images must then be conveyed from the occipital cortex to the prefrontal areas of the brain where decision making takes place.[28] The process begins as light enters the eye and passes through the cornea and lens to focus on the retina. The retina then conveys this information over the optic nerve and tract to the lateral geniculate nucleus (LGN) of the thalamus. Because of the crossing of the retinal nasal fibers (of the optic nerve) at the optic chiasm, the LGN receives information from the retinal hemifields of both eyes and integrates information from the two eyes to provide binocular vision.[22,28] After synapsing in the LGN, visual information travels over the geniculocalcarine tracts to the visual cortex. Fig. 12-1 shows these pathways. The visual cortex refines the incoming visual information, sharpening and fine-tuning features such as orientation of line and color to create a general visual image of objects seen by the retina. From the visual cortex, the visual information travels to the prefrontal area of the brain to be used in decision making. Before it can be useful to the prefrontal areas, however, visual information must be combined (integrated) with other incoming sensory information to establish images and relationships between the body and the environmental surround.[28]

To integrate sensory information, visual information travels from the visual cortex towards the prefrontal lobe over two routes: a "northern" or superior route, which takes it through the parietal lobe, and a "southern" or inferior route through the posterior temporal lobe.[27,35] This process is known as parallel-distributed sensory processing (Fig. 12-2). Visual information traveling the southern route through the posterior temporal lobe is processed for visual object information and recognition.[27] The goal of this processing is to identify the object and classify it. Neural processes in the posterior temporal lobe tune into the visual detail of the object and consistency of features by means of information coming in from the macular area of the retina, the area packed with cones and capable of the most acute vision. Processing by the posterior temporal lobe is critical to our ability to tell a can of diet Coke from regular Coke or to distinguish facial features. It is the area of the brain that controls attention to visual detail.

Visual information taking the northern route to the prefrontal lobes travels through the parietal lobe. The parietal lobe is a synthesizer of sensory information, taking bits and pieces of information from all of the sensory modalities and integrating it to create internal sensory maps that are used to orient the body in space.[27] Visual information traveling through the parietal lobe is used to tune the CNS into the presence of the objects surrounding the body and to determine their spatial relationship to the body and to each other. Visual information must be integrated with other sensory information to provide this orientation. Tactual, proprioceptive, kinesthetic, vestibular, and auditory information are needed as well as visual input to assess accurately the relationship between ourselves and the objects that surround us. The map created by information synthesized in the parietal lobe is body-centered and dynamic, changing in shape and content as the body moves through space.[26,28]

The parietal lobe in each hemisphere contains the map for the space on the contralateral side of the body; thus the right hemisphere contains the map for the left side of the body and surrounding space, and the left hemisphere contains the map for the right side of the body and surroundings. The map is not a detailed representation of space but provides a general impression of objects in space on that side of body. The CNS relies on visual information from the peripheral areas of the retinal fields to create and maintain these maps. This area of the brain controls general attention to and awareness of space.[26]

The final destination for visual information traveling through the posterior temporal and parietal lobes is the prefrontal area of the brain where the information is used to make decisions and formulate plans. This area of the brain, along with the premotor cortices and a few other centers, is responsible for planning skilled body movements including eye movements.[28] The frontal eye fields are located in area eight of the prefrontal lobes and are responsible for voluntary visual search of the space on the contralateral side of the body.[8] That is, the frontal eye

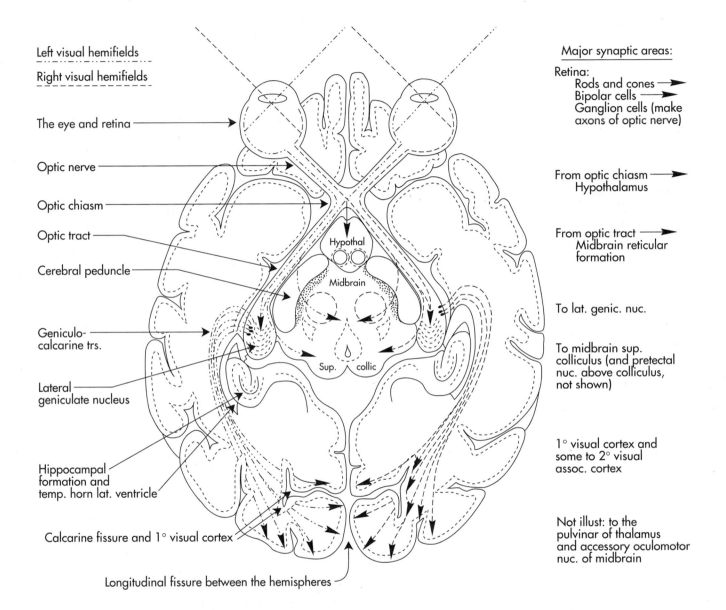

PARALLEL-DISTRIBUTED PROCESSING OF THE VISUAL SYSTEM-I

Schematic inferior view of a horizontal slice of the brain

Left visual hemifields

Right visual hemifields

The eye and retina

Optic nerve

Optic chiasm

Optic tract

Cerebral peduncle

Geniculo-calcarine trs.

Lateral geniculate nucleus

Hippocampal formation and temp. horn lat. ventricle

Calcarine fissure and 1° visual cortex

Longitudinal fissure between the hemispheres

Hypothal

Midbrain

Sup. collic

Major synaptic areas:

Retina:
Rods and cones →
Bipolar cells →
Ganglion cells (make axons of optic nerve)

From optic chiasm →
Hypothalamus

From optic tract →
Midbrain reticular formation

To lat. genic. nuc.

To midbrain sup. colliculus (and pretectal nuc. above colliculus, not shown)

1° visual cortex and some to 2° visual assoc. cortex

Not illust: to the pulvinar of thalamus and accessory oculomotor nuc. of midbrain

The visual system is our most important sense in regard to:

A. Learning, memory, and recall including our ability to see color and fine details as well as the visual surround and global relationships.
B. Communication: use of symbolic language, speaking, and body language.
C. Spatiotemporal orientation in concert with vestibular-proprioceptive systems.
D. Early warning system to pleasure or danger, i.e., vision is our farthest reaching distance receptor and movement detector par excellence.
E. Visual-manual and visual-motor activities.

1°, Primary.

2°, Secondary.

FIG. 12-1 Pathways from retina to LGN to visual cortex. (Drawing courtesy of Josephine C. Moore, PhD., OTR.)

PARALLEL-DISTRIBUTED PROCESSING OF THE VISUAL SYSTEM

Two parallel routes carry visual information from the occipital lobe to the prefrontal lobe and frontal eye field (FEF). Fibers from these two routes distribute to many areas along each route (not illustrated) before terminating in the prefrontal cortex and FEF as illustrated.

(N) = "Northern" or superior route via parietal and frontal lobes.

(S) = "Southern" or inferior route via temporal and frontal lobes.

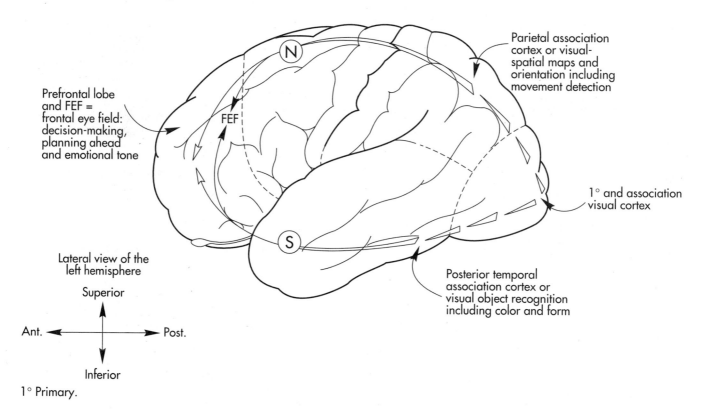

FIG. 12-2 Separate pathways from visual cortex through parietal and posterior temporal lobes to frontal lobe to complete visual processing. (Drawing courtesy of Josephine C. Moore, PhD., OTR.)

fields in the right hemisphere direct visual search toward the left visual space and vice versa. The frontal eye fields conduct visual search based on expectation of where visual information is to be found in the environment; they then direct the eyes to move towards that area. For example, if you were looking for a light switch in a room you would direct your visual search toward the walls because that is where you expect to find a light switch. You would not waste time searching the floor or the ceiling. By directing visual search based on the expected location of crucial visual information, the CNS is able to process visual information very quickly. This arrangement enables us successfully to engage in activities that require rapid visual processing such as driving.

Not all visual information travels over the geniculocalcarine tracts for cortical processing. Many neural pathways leave the optic nerve chiasm and tract and travel to the hypothalamus and brainstem.[24] The brainstem con-

tains several important neural structures involved in visual processing. The superior colliculi, located in the midbrain of the brain stem, are primary brainstem processing centers. The superior colliculi are responsible for reflexive capture of moving visual stimuli appearing in the peripheral visual fields.[24,37] The superior colliculi monitor the peripheral visual field for any unexpected movement. When motion is detected, the colliculi automatically initiate an eye movement toward the direction of the movement. In performing this function, the colliculi serve as an early warning system to prevent the CNS from being caught off guard by events occurring to the side of the individual.[27,34]

The brain stem also contains centers for the control of eye movements. Centers for control of horizontal gaze and vertical gaze are located here as well as those for saccadic eye movements. The nuclei of cranial nerves III, IV, and VI, which control the extraocular muscles of the

TABLE 12-1 Summary of Cortical Hemispheric Functions for Visual Processing and Deficits Secondary to Lesion Site.*

LEFT HEMISPHERE ADVANTAGE		RIGHT HEMISPHERE ADVANTAGE	
More detail-oriented in relation to persons, places, and things		More global or holistic	
Takes in minute details and compares and contrasts these details		Takes a general view of the environment	
Processes visual information sequentially in a systematic item-by-item, serial search strategy		Processes multiple visual inputs simultaneously, grouping them into meaningful categories	
Attends only to right visual fields		Attends globally to both left and right visual fields	
PARIETAL LESION	**POST. TEMP. LESION**	**PARIETAL LESION**	**POST. TEMP. LESION**
Biases attention to detail	Biases attention to global input	Biases attention to detail	Biases attention to global input
Biases brain to right hemisphere advantages	Biases brain to right hemisphere advantages	Biases brain to left hemisphere advantages	Biases brain to left hemisphere advantages
May have right inferior quadrant visual field loss	May have right superior quadrant visual field loss	May have neglect or hemiinattention along with left inferior quadrant visual field loss	May have neglect or hemiinattention along with left superior quadrant visual field loss

* Modified with permission of Josephine C. Moore.

cycs, are also found in the brain stem along with basic visual functions such as the light (pupillary) reflex and the accommodation reflex.[28]

The subcortical areas of the brain are primarily responsible for monitoring the peripheral visual field. A major function of peripheral visual input is to keep the person upright in space.[3] The peripheral system monitors the verticality of structures in the space surrounding you, such as walls, furniture, and buildings, and lines you up with them. If the verticality of these structures is unexpectedly altered, you will have difficulty maintaining an upright posture. For example, when you walk into a fun house, suddenly walls, doors, and floors are on a slant, and you find yourself nauseous and unable to stand upright and walk.

To increase efficiency the hemispheres divide responsibility for some aspects of visual processing. One example can be found in the area of visual attention. Research has shown that the hemispheres differ in how they engage and exercise visual attention. It has been shown that the left hemisphere directs attention towards the right half of the body space, whereas the right hemisphere directs attention towards both the right and left halves of the body space.[19] If a lesion occurs in the left hemisphere, attention may be diminished towards the right visual space, but some attentional capability towards the right side will remain because of the intact right hemisphere. If a lesion occurs in the right hemisphere, however, capability for directing attention towards the left visual space is lost. This asymmetry in the hemispheric direction of visual attention may explain the consistently documented finding that visual inattention or neglect is associated with right hemisphere lesions and rarely observed with left hemisphere lesions.[45]

The hemispheres also differ in the strategy each employs to focus attention. Research has shown that the left hemisphere employs a strict sequential item-by-item

search strategy when scanning the environment.* This strategy gives this hemisphere an advantage in discriminating the subtle differences between objects and a superiority for object identification.[11] Only a limited number of items can be processed at a time, however, and greater mental energy is required to employ the strategy. In contrast, the right hemisphere employs a less spatially selective strategy, processing items by breaking them down into blocks or chunks of information.[32] This enables the right hemisphere simultaneously to process several items and gives it an advantage for identifying configural aspects of objects and processing outlines.[11]

Different areas of the brain have different responsibilities in processing visual information, but all areas must work together for a person to make sense of what is seen and thus use visual information to adapt.[25,28] Millions of long and short fiber tract systems tie the various centers together within and between hemispheres to ensure effective and efficient communication. Like a car in which the fuel-injection system is as critical to performance as the spark plugs, the brain won't run efficiently unless all of its systems are working together. When brain injury or disease occurs, this communication system is disrupted and the organization of visual processing breaks down. Table 12-1 lists effects of various CNS lesions on different aspects of the visual processing system. In reviewing the table, keep in mind that a functional disability in the patient will be observed only in those daily living activities that require the type of visual processing compromised by the lesion. For example, a deficit in the ability to process visual detail caused by a lesion in the left posterior temporal lobe would significantly affect the ability of a proofreader to return to work but might have little effect on a garbage collector's ability to return to work.

---

* References 7, 21, 32, 36, 38, 40.

A HIERARCHICAL MODEL OF VISUAL PERCEPTUAL SKILL

Although while considering individual perceptual skills in this section, remember that the nervous system functions as a unified system: its ability to adapt is a sum of all of its parts working together in unison. Although discrete perceptual skills can be identified, they do not operate independently. Visual perceptual function is organized in a hierarchy of skill levels that interact with and subserve each other.[51] Fig. 12-3 illustrates this hierarchy. Within the hierarchy each skill level is supported by the one that precedes it and cannot properly function without the integration of the lower level skill. As Fig. 12-3 shows the hierarchy consists of visual cognition, visual memory, pattern recognition, visual scanning, visual attention, oculomotor control, visual fields, and visual acuity. The ability to use visual perceptual skill to adapt to the environment is the result of the interaction of all of these skill levels in a unified system.

The highest order visual perception skill in the hierarchy is visual cognition. Visual cognition can be defined as the ability to manipulate visual information mentally and integrate it with other sensory information to gain knowledge and to solve problems, formulate plans, and make decisions. Because visual cognition enables complex visual analysis, it serves as a foundation for all academic endeavors: reading, writing, mathematics, and also many vocations such as artist, engineer, surgeon, architect, and scientist.

Visual cognition, however, cannot occur without the presence of visual memory, the next skill level in the hierarchy. Mental manipulation of visual stimuli requires the ability to create and retain a picture of the object in the mind's eye while the visual analysis is being completed. In addition to being able to store a visual image temporarily in short-term memory, it must also be possible to store the image in long-term memory and then to be able to retrieve it from memory later. For example, to interpret the illusion shown in Fig. 12-4, one must be able to access visual memories of the shape of both a goose and a hawk. Adults or older children can easily resolve this illusion, but most toddlers cannot because they have not yet stored memories of the shapes of these birds.

Before a visual image can be stored in memory there must be recognition of the pattern making up the image. Pattern recognition, which subserves visual memory in the hierarchy, involves identifying the salient features of an object and using these features to distinguish the object from its surroundings.[21] A salient feature is that which distinguishes one object from another. For example, the salient feature that differentiates an *E* from an *F* is the lower horizontal line on the *E*. Pattern recognition comprises two abilities: (1) the ability to identify the configural and holistic aspects of an object: to see its

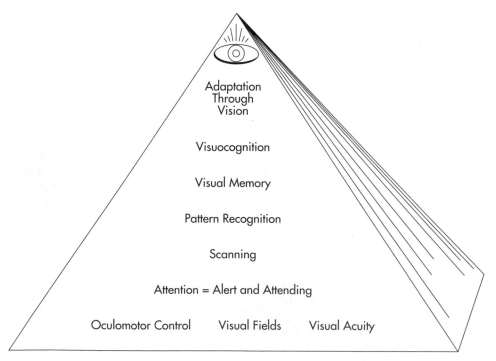

FIG. 12-3 Hierarchy of visual perceptual skill development in central nervous system. (Drawing courtesy of Josephine C. Moore from Warren M: A hierarchical model for evaluation and treatment of visual perceptual dysfunction in adult acquired brain injury. I. Copyright 1993 by the American Occupational Therapy Association, Inc. Reprinted with permission.)

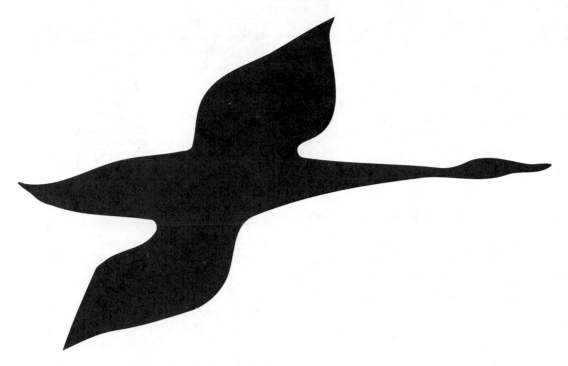

FIG. 12-4 Is this a goose or a hawk? (Visual illusion from Warren M: A hierarchical model for evaluation and treatment of visual perceptual dysfunction in adult acquired brain injury. I. Copyright 1993 by the American Occupational Therapy Association, Inc. Reprinted with permission.)

general shape, contour, and features and (2) the ability to identify specific features of an object such as details of color, shading, and texture.[11] Both aspects of recognition must occur for accurate identification.[7]

Recognition of pattern cannot be accomplished without organized and thorough scanning of the visual scene (the next level in the hierarchy). Visual scanning is accomplished through the use of saccadic eye movements. A saccade is a movement of the eye towards an object of interest in the environment. The purpose of a saccade is to focus the object on the fovea, the area of the retina with the greatest ability to process detail. In scanning a visual array, the eyes selectively focus on the elements that are critical for accurately interpreting the array.[14,30] The most important details are reexamined several times through a series of cyclic saccades to ensure that correct identification is made. Unessential elements in the scene are ignored.[56]

Visual scanning is a motor function and therefore must be driven by a sensory integration process, in this case, visual attention. The saccadic eye movements observed in scanning reflect the engagement of visual attention as it is shifted from object to object. According to Posner and Rafal,[34] shifting of visual attention is accomplished by a three-step cognitive process. The first step is a *disengage* operation in which the eye ceases to focus on the object under study. This step is followed by a *move* operation in which focus is shifted to a new object, and finally by a *compare* operation in which the previous object is compared with the new one for similarities and

differences. The approach taken in trying to locate the face of a friend in a class picture illustrates this three-step process. The eye engages one face, then disengages, moves and fixates on the next face, compares it to the one previously viewed, and so on, systematically continuing this procedure until the desired face is located.

Engagement of visual attention and the other higher level skills in the hierarchy cannot occur unless the brain is receiving clear, concise visual information from the environment. Visual input is provided through three primary sensory components, which form the foundation for all visual processing within the hierarchy. These components are oculomotor control, visual fields, and visual acuity. Oculomotor control ensures that eye movements are completed quickly and accurately. The visual fields register the visual scene and ensure that the CNS receives complete visual information. Visual acuity ensures that the visual information sent to the CNS is accurate. Without these prerequisite sensory components an inadequate image is generated, preventing engagement of higher visual processing.

Brain injury or disease can disrupt visual processing at any skill level in the hierarchy. Because of the unity of the hierarchy, if brain injury disturbs a lower level skill, the skills above it will also be compromised. In this case, it may appear that the patient has a deficit in a higher skill level when the deficit actually has occurred at a much lower level in the hierarchy. For example, a patient who is unable to complete an embedded figures test and appears to have a deficit in the visual cognitive skill of figure/ground perception may, in fact, be experiencing inaccurate pattern recognition caused by an asymmetrical scanning pattern in turn caused by visual inattention compounded by a visual field deficit. Treatment of the higher level skill (figure/ground imperception) will not be successful unless the underlying deficits in visual attention and visual field are addressed first. This effect is similar to that observed in the motor system following brain injury. The high-level problem observed is that the patient cannot use the hand to pick up an object. The underlying deficits are reduced muscle tone and sensation and muscle weakness. Use of the hand for manipulation will be impossible until the deficits in muscle tone, strength, and sensation are addressed in treatment. Effective evaluation and treatment of visual deficits requires an understanding of how brain injury affects the integration of vision at each skill level and how the skill levels interact to enable visual perceptual processing.

EFFECT OF BRAIN INJURY ON VISUAL PERFORMANCE AT EACH SKILL LEVEL

The best way to understand the impact of brain injury on visual performance is to reverse the order of the hierarchy. This section examines how injury disrupts the functioning of each skill level beginning with the foundation skills.

DEFICITS IN OCULOMOTOR CONTROL

Deficits in oculomotor control following brain injury generally result from two types of disruption: either (1) specific cranial nerve lesions occur causing paresis or paralysis of one or more of the extraocular muscles that control eye movements or (2) a disruption of central neural control of the extraocular muscles occurs affecting the coordination of eye movements.[24] In the first case the message to the extraocular muscles through the cranial nerve is blocked; in the second case the message comes through but is scrambled. In both cases the functional result is decreased speed, control, and coordination of eye movements.

Three pairs of cranial nerves (cn) control the extraocular muscles: the oculomotor nerve (cn III), the trochlear nerve (cn IV), and the abducens nerve (cn VI). Between them these nerves are responsible for controlling seven pairs of striated muscles that surround and attach to the two eyeballs. Table 12-2 describes the function of the extraocular muscles controlled by cranial nerves III, IV, and VI.

When a cranial nerve lesion occurs, the muscles controlled by that cranial nerve are weakened or paralyzed. As a result, the eye is unable to move in the direction of the paretic muscles and may even be unable to maintain a central position in the eye socket (i.e., it drifts in or out). Because the eyes must always move together in synergy

TABLE 12-2	Summary of Oculomotor Deficits Associated with Cranial Nerve Lesions	
OCULOMOTOR NERVE 3	**TROCHLEAR NERVE 4**	**ABDUCENS NERVE 6**
Impaired vertical eye movements	Impaired downward and lateral eye movements	Impaired lateral eye movements
Lateral diplopia for near vision tasks	Vertical diplopia for near vision tasks	Lateral diplopia for far vision tasks
Dilation of pupil and impaired accommodation	With bilateral lesion assumes downward head tilt	
Ptosis of eyelid		

and line up evenly to maintain a single visual image, when the movement of one eye is impeded or its position changes and does not match that of the other, the person sees a double image. This condition is known as diplopia or double vision and is the primary functional disruption observed following cranial nerve lesions.[29]

To eliminate the double image, the patient will often assume a head position that avoids the field of action of the paretic muscle. For example, a patient with a left lateral rectus palsy (cn VI) will turn the head towards the left to avoid the need to abduct the eye. A patient with paralysis of the right superior oblique muscle (cn IV) will tilt the head to the right and downward to avoid the action of that muscle.[5] Unless oculomotor function is carefully evaluated, these alterations in head position may be interpreted as resulting from changes in muscle tone in the neck rather than as a functional adaptation purposely assumed to stabilize vision.

Often it is not the cranial nerves that are damaged during brain injury but the neural centers that coordinate their actions. These structures, which were listed earlier, are scattered throughout the brain stem and communicate extensively with cortical, cerebellar, and subcortical areas of the CNS and the spinal cord. During traumatic brain injury, diffuse damage may take place throughout the brain stem, affecting these control centers. If the centers are damaged the person will have difficulty executing eye movements even though the cranial nerves are intact. Disconjugate eye movements may occur causing the person to have difficulty using the eyes together in a coordinated fashion. Dysmetric eye movement, in which the eye undershoots or overshoots a target, may also be observed.[5,24]

These disturbances in ocular motility can create a variety of functional deficits for the patient. The speed and range of eye movement may be diminished, which will reduce the speed at which the patient is able to scan the environment and take in visual information, causing delays in responding to the environment. The patient may have difficulty maintaining a clear image and may experience doubling and blurring of visual images. There may be difficulty focusing at different distances from the body. Depth perception may be diminished. All of these conditions will create significant visual stress for the patient, reducing concentration and endurance for activities. The patient may respond to this increased stress by becoming agitated and uncooperative in therapy sessions and/or complaining of headaches, eye strain, or neck strain.

Because a number of factors can disrupt the control of eye movements, much skill and expertise are needed to make an accurate diagnosis of the oculomotor deficit and design an appropriate treatment intervention. Therapists who provide treatment for this type of dysfunction should do so with the guidance of an optometrist or ophthalmologist who specializes in visual impairment caused by neurological conditions.[17,31]

DEFICITS IN VISUAL ACUITY

Visual acuity is more than just the ability to read a line on the letter chart. In actuality it represents a complex interaction between the optical system (the cornea, lens, and the optic media), which focuses light on the retina, and CNS processing, which transforms that light into visual images.

The first stage of CNS processing begins at the retina. Photoreceptors in the retinal field are programmed to respond to discrete visual stimuli in the environment and activate only when those stimuli are present. For example, a photoreceptor coded for vertical orientation will fire only when a vertical line falls on its receptive field. It is estimated that the retinal field contains nearly one million such discretely coded photoreceptors sending detailed information on the spatial components of objects to the CNS for visual processing. This neural specificity enables the CNS to detect minute differences between patterns and perform precise object identification. Thus we are able to tell a *b* from a *d* and a tangerine from an orange.[10]

For the retina to resolve spatial information, visual images must be focused precisely on the receptors of the retinal field lining the inside of the eye. A defect in the optical system (the cornea or lens or even the length of the eyeball) can cause the images to be poorly focused on the retina.[10]

The three most common optical defects reducing acuity are myopia (nearsightedness), hyperopia (farsightedness), and astigmatism. In myopia the image of an object is focused at a point in front of the retina and is blurred when it reaches the retina. Myopia is corrected by placing a concave lens in front of the eye.[10] In hyperopia the image comes into focus behind the retina causing the image to remain out of focus on the retina.[10] Hyperopia is corrected by placing a convex lens in front of the eye. In astigmatism light is focused differently by two meridians ninety degrees apart. This defect is usually due to a cornea that is not totally spherical but shaped more like a spoon. It results in a blurring of the image because both meridians cannot be focused on the retina; it is corrected by placing a cylindrical lens in front of the eye.[10] Cataracts and corneal opacities, cloudy media, and other conditions can also reduce the quality of the image projected onto the retina.

The health and integrity of the retina also influence the quality of the image sent on to the CNS. The macular area of the retina is particularly critical for identification of visual detail. Unfortunately this structure is also vulnerable to several diseases that destroy its function, including age-related diseases such as macular degeneration and glaucoma, and systemic diseases such as diabetic retinopathy and hypertension. Damage to this area of the retina does not result in blindness but substantially reduces the ability to distinguish visual details such as variations in colors, pattern frequency, and contrast.[15] Accurate identification of patterns and objects becomes difficult because the CNS does not get sufficient information to identify salient features. For example, human faces contain very little differentiation between the facial features. That is, the nose is the same color as the forehead, cheeks, and chin, and eye and hair color are designed to blend with skin tones. Because of the reduced contrast between facial features, persons with macular loss almost universally have difficulty identifying faces even of close friends and family. They must rely on other characteristics such as height, weight, hair color, clothing preferences, and voice to make identification. It is estimated that approximately one in four persons over the age of 80 years has a visual impairment affecting the retina great enough to prevent the individual from reading standard print.[15] This estimate is important to keep in mind because many older patients experiencing CVA or other neurological insult may also have a retinal pathology that adds to their other impairments.

Treatment

The refractive errors found on the physician's evaluation of the optical system can generally be corrected with the use of lenses, medication, or surgery. It is necessary only that the patient be referred to a vision specialist to correct these deficiencies. Other aspects of reduced visual acuity such as reduced ability to see contrast or color cannot be resolved by prescribing a pair of lenses. Treatment in this area requires application of an adaptive approach directed towards changing the environment. Three factors can be manipulated to make the environment more "user friendly" to the person with reduced acuity. These factors are background contrast, illumination, and background pattern.[13]

Contrast. Increasing background contrast is as simple as using a black cup for drinking milk and a white cup for coffee. The key to using contrast effectively is to determine the critical items in the environment needed for orientation or identification and then increase their contrast to surrounding features. For example, if the patient has difficulty walking down stairs because of the reduced contrast between the risers, a line of bright fluorescent tape or paint can be applied to the end of each step to distinguish between them. A carrot may blend into the background of a wood cutting board, but placing the carrot on a white cutting board heightens the definition of the carrot's contours and makes it easier and safer to chop.

Illumination. Increasing the intensity of available light enables objects and environmental features to be seen more readily and reduces the need for high contrast between objects. For example, facial features can be more easily identified if the person's face is fully illuminated. The challenge in providing light is to increase illumination without increasing glare. Halogen and fluorescent lighting provide the best sources of high illumination with minimum glare and are recommended over standard incandescent lighting for both room and reading illumination. In addition to glare, it is also important to minimize shadows. The use of single-bulb or recessed "can" lighting in hallways and rooms should be avoided. Long panels of fluorescent lights should be used instead. If fluorescent lighting cannot be used, 300- to 500-watt torchiere halogen lamps provide excellent illumination with a minimum of shadow. These lamps are relatively inexpensive and can be strategically placed in each room to provide the broadest illumination. For reading, 50-watt halogen desk lamps provide the best illumination.

Pattern. Patterned backgrounds have the effect of camouflaging objects lying on them; anyone who has ever searched for a sewing needle dropped on a patterned rug can attest to this fact. The detrimental effect of pattern on object identification can be minimized by using solid colors for background surfaces such as bedspreads, placemats, dishes, countertops, rugs, towels and furniture coverings. Pattern is also synonymous with clutter in an environment. A patient with difficulty identifying objects will perform better when asked to scan a kitchen shelf with a few orderly items on it than one with dozens of items. The same is true of closets, drawers, sewing baskets, desks, book shelves, counter tops and clinic areas.

VISUAL FIELD DEFICITS

Homonymous hemianopsia (loss of visual field in the corresponding right or left half in each eye) is the most common visual impairment observed following CVA.[58] Although often considered a mild impairment in comparison to the dramatic loss of use of the limbs, a visual field deficit can have an important impact on the ability to adapt to the environment and remain independent. Patients with visual field deficit will experience changes in several areas of performance that affect their ability to correctly and safely complete activities of daily living.

The most significant change occurs in scanning to compensate for the blind portion of the visual field. Instead of spontaneously adopting a wider scanning strategy, turning the head farther to see around the blind field, patients tend to narrow their scope of scanning.[57] They adopt a more protective strategy, turning their heads very little and limiting their scanning to areas immediately adjacent to the body; they concentrate more on sensory input from the tactile, proprioceptive, and vestibular senses.

Although this strategy seems odd following a vision loss, it actually is consistent with how the CNS processes visual information. Research has shown that the brain responds to loss of visual field by exercising perceptual completion.[43] Perceptual completion is a sensory phenomenon in which the brain fills in (perceptually completes) any missing portion of the visual field, thus providing perception of a complete visual scene. The best-known example of the effect of this phenomenon is a person's unawareness of his or her physiologic blind spot. The blind spot comprises five degrees of the visual field; however, the brain fills in this missing visual field and the person operates in total ignorance of the field loss until attempting to change lanes when driving and finding the lane already occupied by another vehicle. Levine[25] reported that persons experiencing field loss are not immediately aware of the absence of vision following onset but only gradually become aware of it through interaction with their environment. Until awareness occurs, the person acts on insufficient and false sensory information and it is likely that mistakes will be observed in activities where full visual field is needed. Thus the person may run into walls or other obstacles when navigating in the environment or may not be able to find items placed within the blind field.

Because of perceptual completion patients do not have the benefit of experiencing a marker indicating a boundary between the seeing and nonseeing field. Instead they experience perception of a complete visual scene in which objects always seem to be appearing, disappearing, and reappearing without warning on the affected side. Uncertainty regarding the accuracy of visual input on the affected side causes the person to adopt a protective strategy, which is more midline and body-centered.[33] This narrowed scope of scanning, however, creates problems in activities in which monitoring of the full visual field is needed, such as driving a car and moving about in a busy environment. In addition to a narrow scope of scanning the speed of scanning decreases, particularly in execution of saccades towards the impaired field. Slow scanning speed compounds any difficulties the patient is experiencing in driving and orienting to the environment.

If the central and particularly the macular portion of the visual field is affected, the person will miss or misidentify detail when viewing objects. Reading presents the greatest challenge and frustration for the patient in this regard.[58] For example, a patient with a left visual field deficit may read the number *8* as a *3* or the word *radish* may be seen as *dish*. Of the two, the reading of numbers is the most difficult; the context of a sentence cues the reader to a misreading, but numbers appear without context. A mistake in reading a number can go unnoticed until a store clerk is given $30.00 for an item that costs $80.00. Patients experiencing these kinds of errors very quickly lose confidence in their ability to pay

bills and manage their checkbook and turn over these very important activities of daily of living to someone else.

Depending on the extent of the visual field loss and the side on which the loss occurs, the patient may experience difficulty guiding the hand in writing and other near vision tasks such as cutting. The top envelope in Fig. 12-5 shows the handwriting of a patient with right visual field loss. In addressing the envelope the patient would lose sight of her hand in her hemianopic field on the right

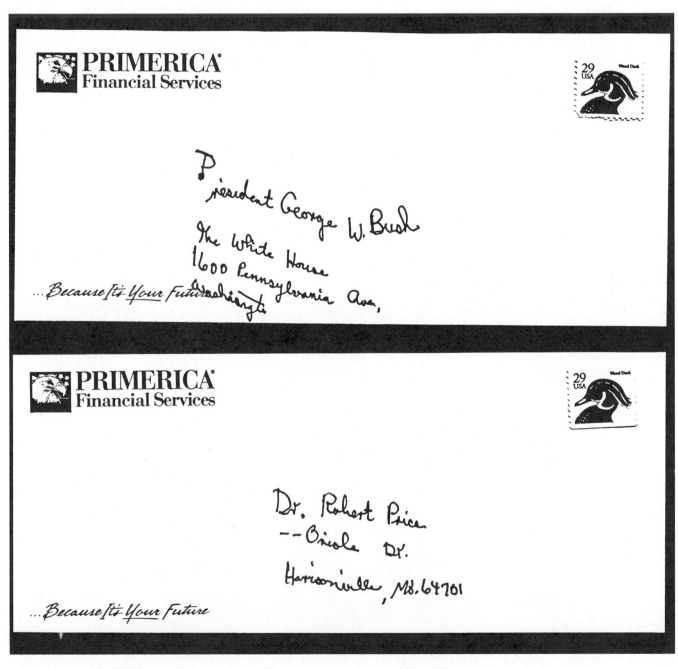

FIG. 12-5   Handwriting completed by patient with right hemianopsia. Upper drawing depicts typical slant as pen moves into hemianopic field. Lower drawing shows improvement after training. (From Warren M: Visuospatial skills: assessment and intervention strategies. In Royeen CB, editor: *AOTA self study series: cognitive rehabilitation,* Rockville, Md, 1994, American Occupational Therapy Association. Reprinted with permission.)

side and subsequently begin to drift downward on that side. The bottom envelope in Fig. 12-5 shows the patient's performance following training.

Evaluation

The most accurate way to measure visual field integrity clinically is through the use of computerized automated perimetry. In automated perimetry a person places the chin on a chin rest and fixates on a central target inside a bowl-shaped device. As the person fixates on the central target, lights are displayed inside the bowl in varying locations and intensities. The person is asked to respond each time a light is seen by pushing a small button. The test is very thorough, presenting lights in over a hundred locations within the field and increasing the intensity of the light in a step threshold sequence if the target is not appreciated the first time. The result is an accurate measurement of the areas of absolute scotoma (total vision loss) and relative scotoma (decreased retinal sensitivity) within the field.

If automated perimetry cannot be obtained, an indication of visual field loss can be achieved using a confrontation test in combination with careful observation of patient performance on daily living activities. In confrontation testing, the examiner sits in front of the patient and has the patient fixate on a centrally placed target (the examiner's nose). The examiner then holds up 1,2,or 5 fingers or a clenched fist separately in each of the four quadrants of the visual field (right upper, right lower, left upper, left lower). The patient indicates how many fingers are seen each time.[23] Clinicians using confrontation testing to quantify field deficit must be careful to correlate their findings with observations of patient performance because confrontation testing alone has been shown to be useful only as a gross indication of deficit.[47] Pertinent observations that may indicate the presence of a visual field deficit include the following: (1) changes in head position when asked to view objects placed in a certain plane, (2) consistently bumping into objects on one side, (3) misplacing objects in one field, and (4) consistent errors in reading.

Treatment

In providing treatment a combination of strategies is used. Remedial strategies focus on increasing the speed and scope of the scanning pattern. The patient must

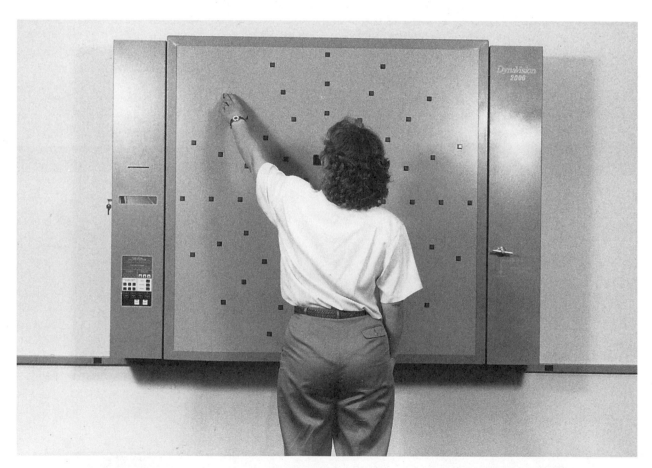

FIG. 12-6   Activity requiring patient to reinforce visual input with tactual feedback. Lights on panel are illuminated one at a time in random patterns. Patient must locate light and press to turn it off. As light is pressed, another light is illuminated. Patient locates as many lights as possible within specified time. (Dynavision 2000, manufactured by Performance Enterprises, Ontario, Canada.)

learn to turn his or her head to compensate for the limitation in field and do so as quickly as possible. Devices such as the Dynavision 2000* unit shown in Fig. 12-6 are extremely effective in teaching patients both speed and scope. Other activities that can be used include ball games in which balls are passed quickly from player to player and balloon batting.

The patient's primary functional limitations will occur as a result of interference from the field deficit in activities that must be completed with vision. Three specific activities that rely on vision are driving, reading, and writing.

Driving is a very complex skill involving the interaction of physical, cognitive, emotional, and visual abilities.[49] A patient's ability safely to resume driving requires a specialized evaluation completed by qualified personnel. From a strictly visual perspective, however, it has been observed that patients with a field deficit experience difficulty primarily in three aspects of driving: (1) changing lanes, (2) merging on and off roadways, and (3) monitoring traffic in multilane situations. The extent to which the patient has difficulty with these maneuvers depends on the severity of the field deficit and the patient's awareness and ability to compensate for the deficit. Speed and scope of scanning are required for compensation. Training should focus on increasing scanning speed and scope and teaching the patient specific strategies to handle the three traffic situations.

The patient's primary complaints in reading will center on difficulty locating and maintaining the correct line of print and accurately identifying words and numbers.[58] Patients with left visual field deficit will experience difficulty returning to the left-hand margin of the reading material to begin a new line of text. Drawing a bold red line down the side of the left margin can provide the patient with a visual cue to use as an anchor to find the left margin.[53] The same technique used on the right margin assists patients with right field loss who are often uncertain when they have reached the end of a line of print. If the patient has difficulty staying on line or moving down to the correct line, a ruler or card can be used under the line of print to keep the patient's place. These techniques can be used when the patient needs to read a recipe or instructions during cooking or to read a bill or financial statement.

Difficulty staying on line when writing is addressed by teaching the patient to monitor the pen tip and maintain visual fixation as the hand moves across the page and into the blind side. Activities that require the patient to trace lines toward the side of the field loss are effective in reestablishing the eye hand lock. Devices that offer feedback, such as a talking pen,* also work well to train the patient to monitor the tip of the pen during handwriting.

Reading, writing, and activities of daily living performance can be enhanced by modifying the visual environment of the patient. Adding color and contrast to the key structures in the environment needed for orientation (for example, door frames and furniture) will assist the patient in locating these structures. Contrast in writing materials can be heightened by using black felt-tip pens and boldly lined paper to assist the patient in monitoring handwriting. The simple addition of more light will often increase reading speed and reduce errors. Reduction of pattern in the environment by cleaning out clutter and using solid colored objects will enhance the patient's ability to locate items.

DEFICITS IN VISUAL ATTENTION, VISUAL SCANNING, PATTERN RECOGNITION, VISUAL MEMORY, AND VISUAL COGNITION
Visual Attention and Scanning

Engagement of visual attention is accomplished through visual scanning. Although these two skills are separated within the hierarchy to assist in understanding them, they cannot be separated in evaluation and treatment of the patient. Any deficit that affects visual attention will be observed through a change in the way the patient scans for visual information.

Visual attention can be divided into two categories: (1) focal or selective visual attention and (2) ambient or peripheral visual attention.[21] Focal attention is used for object recognition and identification. Visual input from the macular area of the retina is used to complete this processing. Focal/selective attention is a highly prized ability in our culture because it enables us accurately to distinguish visual details such as differences between letters and numbers and so contributes greatly to academic achievement. Ambient/peripheral attention is concerned with the detection of events in the environment and their location in space and proximity to the person. It relies on input from the peripheral visual field. To have a fully operational and efficient visual system, these two modes of visual attention must work together. The contribution of each is equally important to perceptual processing. Our culture may prize the contributions of selective attention, but this system could not function efficiently without the perceptual stability provided by peripheral attention.

Research has shown that in normal adults, scanning is consistently completed in an organized, systematic, and efficient pattern.[9,16,34,50] The type of scanning pattern used depends on the demands of the task. In reading, a left-to-right and top-to-bottom rectilinear strategy is used. In scanning an open array (such as a room), a circular left-to-right strategy is generally used with the eye following either a clockwise or counterclockwise pattern.

---

* Dynavision 2000, Performance Enterprises, 76 Major Button's Drive, Markhan, Ontario, Canada L3P 3G7, (905)472-9074.

* Talking Pen, Wayne Engineering, 1825 Willow Road, Northfield, IL, 60093, (312)441-6940.

Studies have shown that disruption in the normal scanning strategy can occur after brain injury. The characteristics of the disruption vary depending on which hemisphere was damaged. Visual scanning deficits associated with right brain injury are characterized by an avoidance in shifting the eye towards the left half of the visual space,[6,12,19] which creates an asymmetrical scanning pattern. Instead of starting the scanning pattern on the left side of a visual array where the majority of adults do, individuals with right brain injuries tend to begin on the right side of the array and stay on the right side. The eyes do not make saccadic movements towards the left, which causes the person to miss both detail and configuration in viewing objects on the left side. As a result, the person may miss some of the visual information needed to make accurate identification and decisions.

The visual inattention associated with right brain injuries is often referred to as visual neglect or unilateral spatial neglect or hemi-inattention.[16*] Although neglect is often used to describe inattention to visual space following either left or right hemisphere lesions, research indicates that the condition occurs only with right brain injuries.[19,45†] The condition of neglect is often confused with the presence of a visual field deficit in the patient. Although both conditions may cause the patient to miss visual information on one side, they are distinctly different conditions and do not have the same effect on the patient's performance. When a visual field deficit occurs, the patient attempts to compensate for the loss by engaging visual attention.[20] The patient directs eye movements towards the side of the vision loss in an attempt to gather visual information from that side. Because of the field deficit, however, the patient may not move the eye far enough to see the needed visual information and so will miss visual input on that side, creating a false impression of hemi-inattention or neglect. In contrast, the patient with true hemi-inattention or neglect has lost the attentional mechanisms in the CNS that drive the search for visual information. No attempt will be made by the inattentive patient to search for information on the left side of the visual space; no eye movements or head turning will be observed toward the left side.[20] The greatest challenge to the therapist comes when the two conditions occur together in the patient. In this case, the patient is missing visual information on the left side because of the field deficit and has no means to compensate for it by directing attention towards the left side. The presence of a visual field deficit exaggerates the inattentive behavior observed in the patient with neglect.[18,54]

Patients with left brain injury often demonstrate a symmetrical decrease in scanning for detail when viewing a visual array.[48] Attention is directed so that the patient broadly scans the visual array for information but does not reexamine aspects of the visual scene to gather additional information. As a result there is a decrease in ability to gather sufficient information to interpret a scene or object accurately, impairing object identification. Left brain injury does not result in hemi-inattention or neglect.

Pattern Recognition

When a patient does not thoroughly and efficiently scan objects, the result will be decreased pattern recognition. Because the right hemisphere directs global attention to the environment, when right brain injury occurs the person's general awareness of the objects that surround him or her in space may be diminished. The patient may not tune into the presence of objects and therefore fail to recognize an object or pattern because he or she does not notice or "see" it.[11,42] Persons with left brain injuries may be aware of objects but have difficulty with identification because it is this hemisphere that directs the focalized item-by-item attentional strategy needed for object recognition and identification.[11,42] Therefore persons with left brain injuries may realize that they are seeing a letter but not be able to distinguish that letter from the one next to it. Any failure in the ability to recognize patterns and objects will diminish the ability to establish an accurate memory of what is seen.

Visual Memory

Visual memory is dependent on accurate pattern recognition. The first step in establishing a visual memory is to construct an accurate sensory model (picture) of the object in the mind's eye.[37,44] Deficits in lower level skills in the hierarchy oculomotor control, acuity, visual field, attention, and/or scanning may cause a critical aspect of an object to be overlooked as the person is viewing it, causing an inaccurate construction of the model. If the model is not accurate, the CNS may not recognize it or may misidentify it, making it difficult for the CNS to establish a visual memory of the object. For example, an individual with a dense left central visual field deficit often misses the first letters of words and as a result may read a word such as *delicious* as *licious*. Whereas *delicious* conjures up a variety of pleasant associations, the word *licious* has no counterpart in memory and so is discarded by the CNS as a nonsense word and not stored in memory. In another example, the same visual field deficit could cause the word *Eight* to be misidentified as *Fight*. These two words, although similar in configuration, cannot be interchanged without greatly altering the context of a sentence. In either case the accuracy of the visual model is compromised, substantially affecting the ability of the nervous system to comprehend and remember it.[16]

---

* Hemi-inattention is considered the more precise term and is preferred to the more vague term of neglect.

† The reason is that the right hemisphere is capable of directing attention towards both right and left sides of the visual space, providing residual visual function with left hemisphere injury.

Fortunately from a treatment standpoint, humans don't store information or learn everything exclusively through the visual channel. It has been hypothesized that models are simultaneously stored in three ways within memory[39]; (1) as a visual representation of the object (for example, color, patterns), (2) as a physical representation of the object (weight, texture, size, shape) and (3) as a verbal representation (the name of the object and definition of its use). The models stored in memory can be retrieved through more than one sensory channel. For example, if I want you to go into the kitchen to get a cup for me, I can tell you to get me a cup (verbal), I can show you a cup and ask you to get me one like it (visual), or I could even put a cup in a bag, ask you to feel its features and get me one just like it (physical). Any one of these three methods would be successful. In real-life daily situations, information about objects is available through several sensory channels. If we don't recognize an object by looking at it, we can pick it up and feel it or we can ask someone to tell us what it is. For this reason, a person with a visual deficit that results in inaccurate pattern recognition can still function fairly well in daily activities for which a variety of sensory information is available. There are three daily living skills that rely almost exclusively on vision for completion, however. These are reading, writing, and driving. Without accurate visual input these skills cannot be performed, limiting activities such as shopping, completing a check or a form, cooking with recipes, and administering medications.

Visual Cognition

Visual cognition represents the highest level of visual skill integration within the nervous system. Although it is the area most often addressed on standard visual perceptual evaluations, it is the area least understood in terms of treatment. Perhaps the reason is that visual cognition is not a separate skill but rather the application of all of the preceding skills in the hierarchy to adaptation to the environment. In other words, visual cognition is the end product of the integration of the foundation skills, visual attention, visual scanning, pattern recognition, and memory. Any deficit in these lower level skills will diminish the ability to apply these skills to adapt cognitively.

Deficits in visual cognition result in difficulties in identifying the spatial properties of objects and mentally manipulating these properties in thought. Many terms are used to describe the deficits that occur in visual cognition, such as spatial agnosia, alexia, disorders of spatial analysis, visual closure and figure/ground perception. These terms, however, do little more than label the deficit; they do not explain why it has occurred. Although labeling deficits provides interesting reading in progress notes and assessment summaries, it does not assist in treatment planning. To treat a deficit, it is necessary to identify what is causing the deficit.

Recent research suggests that one of the most crucial skills enabling visual cognition is the ability to attend selectively to visual information through the focal attention process.[21,34,36] Whereas ambient/peripheral visual processing is instantaneous and largely effortless, selective visual attention relies on serial processing and entails an effortful, stimulus-by-stimulus scanning of the visual array.[7,21] This serial search process becomes increasingly difficult as the number of distracters in the array increases or if the distracters are difficult to discriminate from the target. For example, finding a specific person in a class picture of 100 students is more difficult than finding the person in a class picture of ten, and even more so if the 100 people in the picture are of the same sex and race. Studies of normal populations have shown that this kind of visual processing requires both effort and vigilance and is limited by the global attentional capacity of the person.[36]

Persons with brain injuries demonstrate defined patterns of breakdown in selective attention when completing complex visual tasks. Changes are observed in three areas of selective attention which adversely affect patient performance, as follows: (1) an inability to attend to the critical features and variables between objects, (2) a tendency to restrict scanning to objects on the ipsilateral (sound) side, and (3) an inability to superimpose a structure in scanning an unstructured array.[34,36] These changes cause the person to commit errors in viewing and manipulating complex visual input. For example, in putting together a difficult 500-piece puzzle, a person looks for certain salient features (for example, color, shape) when trying to find a specific puzzle piece. It is also necessary to superimpose some sort of organizational structure on the task, such as deciding to put the border together first, which requires ability to direct attention to both sides of the puzzle. These deficits in the ability to attend selectively to this task greatly affect the ability to complete the puzzle.

Evaluation

Because visual attention and scanning subserve the higher level visual skills of pattern recognition, visual memory and visual cognition, the emphasis in evaluation is on looking at how a patient applies scanning strategies to complete a visual task. Does the patient scan in an organized and efficient manner? Does the patient obtain complete information from scanning? Is the patient able to identify detail correctly? Does the patient's ability to scan decrease as the complexity of the task increases? The answers to these questions indicate whether or not the patient is able to complete the higher level processing skills.

Evaluation is begun by using scanning tests that have a structured array. Letter cancellation and line bisection are two scanning tests shown to be particularly sensitive to the presence of visual inattention.[41,53,55] Letter cancellation involves presentation of several rows of single lower or upper case letters on a page. A designated letter is chosen and the patient is asked to draw a line through that letter each time it appears on the page. Patients with visual inattention secondary to right brain lesions tend to restrict scanning to the right side of the page and subsequently fail to cancel letters on the left side of the page. Patients with inattention secondary to left brain lesions tend to miss letters symmetrically throughout the rows. The deficiency in the scanning pattern is clearly observed in the patient's performance on the page. On a line bisection test, horizontal lines are drawn on a page and the patient is asked to draw a vertical line through the center of each horizontal line.[41] Patients with inattention will tend to displace the vertical line towards their sound side even when cued as to the length of the lines. These tests are simple to administer and yet provide a clear indication of the patient's deficits in scanning.

For the patient with mild inattention, presentation of visual stimuli in a structured lateral array may provide enough of a cue to enable the patient to compensate for the deficit in attention. Therefore it is also useful to present a scanning task with an unstructured array. Albert[2] designed a simple and effective test consisting of numerous short diagonal lines scattered over a page. The patient is asked to place a line through each line that is seen. As with other scanning tests, patients with inattention and right brain injury tend to slash only lines found on the right side of the page. Patients with left brain injuries and inattention show symmetrical omissions. When observing the patient perform the test, it is important to note the type of strategy the patient uses to impose a structure in scanning the random display of lines. Individuals without attentional deficits use either a horizontal lateral strategy, going across the page from left to right, or a vertical lateral strategy, going from top to bottom. Patients with inattention display a random and less organized approach.

A more difficult unstructured scanning test is the star cancellation test of the Behavioral Inattention Test. Wilson, Cockburn and Halligan[55] combined a variety of functional tasks requiring scanning (such as reading a menu and setting a clock) with paper-and-pencil scanning tests into a structured battery called the Behavioral Inattention Test (BIT).* The BIT includes the letter cancellation, line bisection, and slash-the-line tests described previously. The star cancellation test of the BIT consists of a series of large and small stars intermixed with random letters and scattered over a page. The patient is asked to cross out all of the small stars. In completing the test the patient must not only impose a structure for scanning onto an unstructured array but also must attend only to the salient

feature of the target (the size of the star) and ignore large stars and letters. This test has been shown to have a strong correlation to inattention.

The identification of detail required on the letter and star cancellation tests provides an opportunity to observe the patient's ability to attend to visual detail and recognize patterns. Pattern recognition can also be evaluated by asking the patient to complete tasks that require matching, such as matching up two decks of playing cards or sorting items with similar features such as different sized screws and bolts. A computerized evaluation called MATCH* also provides a useful assessment of attention to detail.

The preceding tests are pencil-and-paper tasks presented in a restricted and well defined space. To determine how the patient applies scanning strategy to a broader space, the scanboard test described by Warren[50] can be used. The test consists of a large (24 × 34 inches) board with a series of 10 numbers displayed in an unstructured pattern. The board is placed at eye level and centered at the patient's midline. The patient is asked to scan the board and point out all of the numbers that are seen. The examiner records the pattern the patient follows in identifying the numbers. Research using this test showed that most control subjects without neurological insult (91%) executed either a clockwise or counterclockwise scanning pattern beginning on the left side of the board and proceeding in an organized and systematic fashion until all of the numbers were identified. In contrast only 52% of subjects with neurological insult secondary to CVA demonstrated an organized scanpath.

If the skills of oculomotor function, visual field integrity, visual acuity, visual attention and scanning, and pattern recognition are thoroughly evaluated, it is not necessary to measure visual memory and visual cognition using specific tests. These skills are the product of the integration of the lower level skills in the hierarchy. If the lower level skills are deficient, deficiencies in the higher skills will be observed as well. If the lower level skills are intact, the patient should demonstrate normal execution of these skills.

Instead of formal evaluation of visual memory and visual cognition, the therapist should observe how the patient performs on the tests previously described that measure performance on the skills that contribute to memory and cognition, and then observe how the deficits identified affect the patient's performance of daily living skills requiring complex visual perception. For example, after having identified that a patient has a visual field deficit and an asymmetrical scanning pattern indicative of hemi-inattention, the therapist should observe the patient complete an activity of daily living that involves attending and planning and decision making. The activity

---

* Behavioral Inattention Test, National Rehabilitation Services, 117 North Elm St., P.O. Box 1247, Gaylord, MI 49735, (517)732-3866.

* MATCH computerized test, Life Science Associates, 1 Fenimore Rd., Bayport, NY 11705, (516)472-2111.

may be preparing a meal, sorting and completing laundry, shopping for groceries, measuring the oil level in the car, or completing a job-related task. In observing the patient, the therapist should make special note of how the patient's visual deficit affects ability to process the more complex visual information needed to complete the task. If the patient has difficulty successfully completing the task and the visual deficit appears to be the cause, the therapist should determine if it is possible to improve the patient's performance with treatment of the visual deficit.

Treatment

Deficits in visual attention create asymmetry in scanning and gaps in the visual information sent to the CNS. As a result, the quality of adaptation made by the CNS to the environment decreases because the CNS does not have sufficient or accurate information with which to make decisions. To be successful, treatment must ensure that the patient learns to take in visual information in a consistent, systematic, and organized manner.

Persons with inattention caused by right brain injuries will demonstrate an asymmetrical scanning pattern, restricting scanning to the right half of the visual array. The first step in treatment of this disorder is to teach patients to reorganize their scanning patterns by beginning scanning in the impaired space (or left side) first.[53] Two scanning strategies are taught: a left-to-right rectilinear pattern for reading and a left-to-right circular pattern for scanning an unstructured array. Activities such as solitaire, double solitaire, dominoes, and checkers can help establish the correct scanning strategy.

Persons with left brain injuries do not demonstrate asymmetry in scanning but tend to omit scanning for details in visual arrays. Activities that emphasize conscious attention to detail and careful inspection and comparison of objects should be used. These include any type of matching or sorting activity such as formboards, puzzles, and games such as dominoes.

Because many life skills require orientation to a broad visual space, the treatment activities chosen to facilitate an organized scanning strategy should also require the patient to scan as broad a visual space as possible. The working field should be large enough to require the patient either to turn the head or change body positions to accomplish the task. Many activities and games can be enlarged to require head turning for scanning. For example, formboards can be enlarged to 3 feet by 2 feet size or a tic-tac-toe game can be enlarged.

Any therapeutic activity used to reestablish an organized scanning pattern will be more effective if the patient is required physically to manipulate the objects scanned. Research has shown that a stronger mental representation of a visual image is formed if what is seen is verified by tactual exploration.[4] Whenever possible the treatment should be designed to be interactive. Games such as solitaire or dominoes, or ball games, or activities such as putting together large puzzles are examples of treatment activities with interactive qualities.

Because complex visual processing is dependent on initiation of the stimulus-by-stimulus search strategy of selective visual attention, it is important to include scanning activities that require careful inspection of the detail in visual arrays. Patients should be taught consciously to study objects for their relevant features with emphasis placed on attending to detail in the impaired space. Matching activities that require discrimination of subtle details are especially effective. Many games have these qualities such as solitaire, double solitaire, concentration, connect four, checkers, Scrabble, and dominoes. Large 300- to 500-piece puzzles, word or number searches, crossword puzzles, and needlecrafts such as latchethook also require these skills. Throughout their performance of these tasks, patients should be encouraged to double check their work to make sure that critical details are not missed. Success in regaining selective attention depends on the patient's ability to learn and employ a conscious strategy to compensate for the deficits created by inattention. Insight on the part of the patient into the nature of the visual deficit and how it has affected functional performance is critical to learning compensation successfully.

According to Toglia[46] one of the reasons patients with brain injury do not spontaneously recognize their limitations and the need to compensate is that their concept of their capabilities is based on premorbid experiences, which causes them to overestimate their abilities after injury. Without a realistic understanding of his or her limitations, the patient may be unwilling to employ compensatory strategies. To increase insight, Abreu and Toglia[1] advocate teaching a patient how to monitor and control performance by learning to recognize and correct for errors in performance. This process of error detection is facilitated by giving the patient immediate feedback about the performance and pointing out deficiencies. It can also be facilitated by teaching the patient to use self-monitoring techniques such as activity prediction where the patient predicts how successfully an activity will be performed and identifies the aspects of the activity where errors are likely to occur. The patient then compares actual performance with predicted performance. This technique helps the patient develop anticipatory skills and increase awareness of how the deficit affects functional capabilities.

A final treatment guideline is to practice the skill within context to ensure carry-over of application to daily living activities. The activities given provide a starting place for the therapist to begin reorganizing the strategies needed for successful visual integration. Research has shown, however, that brain-injured patients generally do not spontaneously transfer skills from one learning situation to the next. Toglia[46] suggests that transfer of learning can be facilitated by having the patient apply the learned strategy in different contexts of daily living. For example, the patient can be required to use the strategy of initiating the scanning pattern in the impaired space when selecting clothes from a closet, searching for items in a refrigerator or on a shelf, shopping for groceries, reading, and driving. The more repetition of the strategy under varied circumstances, the more the skill is generalized and transfered to new situations. There is no substitution in therapy for the practice of real-life situations in assisting the patient to develop insight into abilities and compensation for limitations. Some creativity may be needed in scheduling to take the patient out of the clinic, or when that is not possible, in use of clinic space and the environments surrounding the clinic. Cafeterias, gift shops, and office areas within the hospital, streets, fast food restaurants, and shops surrounding the hospital can all be used to expose the patient to more realistic and demanding visual environments. Independent living apartments, simulated work areas, and kitchens within the clinic should also be used regularly in treatment.

SUMMARY

The central nervous system relies on visual information to anticipate and plan adaptation to the environment. Brain injury or disease disrupts the processing of visual information, creating gaps in the visual input sent to the CNS. The quality of the person's adaptation to the environment decreases because the CNS does not have sufficient and/or accurate visual information, to make decisions. Whether or not a person's deficit in visual perceptual processing requires therapeutic intervention depends on the person's lifestyle and whether the visual deficit prevents successful completion of daily living activities.

The framework for evaluation and treatment rests on the concept of a hierarchy of visual perceptual skill levels that interact with and subserve one another. Because of the unity of the hierarchy, a skill function cannot be disrupted at one level without an adverse effect on all perceptual processing. Evaluation must be directed at measuring function at all skill levels with particular emphasis on the foundation skills and visual attention and scanning. Treatment focuses on increasing the accuracy and organization of the sensory input to the system through manipulation of the environment and by providing the patient with strategies to compensate for or minimize the effect of the deficit in daily living activities.

REVIEW QUESTIONS

1. What determines whether a patient has a visual perceptual deficit following brain injury?
2. What is ambient/peripheral vision used for by the CNS?
3. What is the normal scanpath executed by most adults when viewing an unstructured visual array? A structured array?
4. What is the primary compensatory strategy taught to the patient with hemi-inattention?
5. What is the most crucial lower level skill contributing to the ability to complete complex visual processing?
6. What are the three aspects of the environment that can be manipulated to make it more "user friendly" to the person with reduced visual acuity?
7. What changes occur in the scanning pattern following right brain injury?
8. What prevents a patient from automatically compensating for a visual field deficit by turning the head farther to see around the blind field?
9. What kind of protective behaviors do persons adopt following onset of visual field deficit? Why do they adopt these strategies?
10. Describe three treatment strategies for deficits in visual acuity. Give an example of how each could be applied in an activity of daily living.
11. Describe the evaluation for visual field deficits.
12. What are some treatment strategies for teaching the patient to compensate for a visual field deficit?
13. Describe the evaluation for visual scanning.
14. Discuss some treatment strategies for visual scanning and visual inattention.

REFERENCES

1. Abreu BC, Toglia JP: Cognitive rehabilitation: a model for occupational therapy. *Am J Occup Ther* 41:439-448, 1987.
2. Albert ML: A simple test of visual neglect, *Neurology* 23:658-664, 1973.
3. Amblard B, Carblanc A: Role of foveal and peripheral vision information in the maintenance of postural equilibrium in man, *Percept Motor Skill* 51:903-912, 1985.
4. Ayres AJ: *Sensory integration and learning disorders,* Los Angeles, 1972, Western Psychological Services.
5. Baker RS, Epstein AD: Ocular motor abnormalities from head trauma, *Survey of Ophth* 36:245-267, 1991.
6. Belleza T, Rappaport M, Hopkins H, Hall K: Visual scanning and matching dysfunction in brain damaged patients with drawing impairment, *Cortex* 15:19-36, 1979.
7. Bergen JR, Julesz B: Parallel vs serial processing in rapid pattern discrimination, *Nature* 303:696-689, 1983.
8. Bruce CJ, Goldberg M: Physiology of the frontal eye fields, *Trends in Neurosci* 7:436-441,1984.

9. Chedru F, Leblanc M, Lhermitte F: Visual searching in normal and brain damaged subjects, *Cortex* 9:94-111, 1973.

10. Cotman CW, McGaugh JL: *Behavioral neuroscience: an introduction,* New York, 1980, Academic Press.

11. Delis DC, Robertson LC, Balliet R: The breakdown and rehabilitation of visuospatial dysfunction in brain injured patients, *Int Rehabil Med* 5:132-138, 1983.

12. DeRenzi E: *Disorders of space exploration and cognition,* New York, 1982, John Wiley and Sons.

13. Dickman IR: *Making life more livable,* New York, 1985, American Foundation for the Blind.

14. Festinger L: Eye movements and perception. In Bach y Rita P, Collins CC: *The control of eye movements,* New York, 1971, Academic Press.

15. Fletcher D and associates: Low vision rehabilitation: finding capable people behind damaged eyeballs, *Western Journal of Medicine* 154:554-556, 1991.

16. Gianutsos R, Matheson P: The rehabilitation of visual perceptual disorders attributable to brain injury. In Meier MJ, Benton AL, Diller L, editors: *Neuropsychological rehabilitation,* New York, 1987, Guilford Press.

17. Gianutsos R, Ramsey G, Perlin RR: Rehabilitative optometric services for survivors of acquired brain injury, *Arch Phys Med Rehabil* 69:573-578, 1988.

18. Halligan PW, Marshall JC, Wade DT: Do visual field deficits exacerbate visuo-spatial neglect?, *J Neuro Neurosurg Psych* 53:487-491, 1990.

19. Heilman K, Van Den Abel T: Right hemisphere dominance for attention: the mechanism underlying hemispheric asymmetries of inattention (neglect), *Neurology* 30:327-330,1980.

20. Ishiai S, Furukawa T, Tsukagoshi H: Eye fixation patterns in homonymous hemianopia and unilateral spatial neglect, *Neuropsychologia* 25:675-679, 1987.

21. Julesz B: Preconscious and conscious processing in vision. In Chagas C, Gattass R, editors: Pattern recognition mechanisms, experimental brain research, vol 3 (suppl), 1985.

22. Kandel E: Processing of form and movement in the visual system. In Kandel ER, Schwartz JH, editors: *Principles of neural science,* ed 2, New York, 1985, Elsevier.

23. Kanski, JJ: *Clinical ophthalmology,* Toronto, 1984, CV Mosby.

24. Leigh RJ, Zee DS: *Neurology of eye movements,* Philadelphia, 1983, FA Davis.

25. Levine DH: Unawareness of visual and sensorimotor deficits: a hypothesis, *Brain & Cognition* 13:233-281,1990.

26. Mesulam MM: A cortical network for directed attention and unilateral neglect, *Ann Neurology* 10:305-325, 1981.

27. Mishkin M, Ungerleider LG, Macko KA: Object vision and spatial vision: two cortical pathways, *Trends in Neurosci* 6:414-417, 1983.

28. Moore JC: The visual system: in relation to rehabilitation. Workshop sponsored by The Franciscan Health System of Cincinnati, June 18-20, 1993.

29. Neger RE: The evaluation of diplopia in head trauma. *J Head Trauma Rehabil* 4:27-34, 1989.

30. Noton D, Stark L: Scanpaths in eye movements during pattern perception, *Science* 171:308-311, 1971.

31. Padula WV: *A behavioral vision approach for persons with physical disabilities,* Santa Anna, Calif, 1988, Optometric Extension Program Foundation.

32. Palmer T, Tzeng OJL: Cerebral asymmetry in visual attention, *Brain & Cognition* 13:46-58, 1990.

33. Pommerenke K, Markowitsch HJ: Rehabilitation training of homonymous visual field defects in patients with postgeniculate damage of the visual system, *Restorative Neurology, Neuroscience* 1:47-63, 1989.

34. Posner MI, Rafal RD: Cognitive theories of attention and the rehabilitation of attentional deficits. In Meier MJ, Benton AL, Diller L, editors: *Neuropsycho-*

logical rehabilitation, New York, 1987, Guilford Press.

35. Post RB, Leibowitz HW: Two modes of processing visual information: implications for assessing visual impairment, *American Journal Optometry & Physiological Optics* 63:94-96, 1986.

36. Rapesak SZ and associates: Selective attention in hemispatial neglect, *Arch Neurol* 46:178-182, 1989.

37. Ratcliff G, Ross JE: Visual perception and perceptual disorder, *Brit Med Bull* 37:181-186, 1981.

38. Reuter-Lorenz PA, Kinsbourne M: Hemispheric control of spatial attention, *Brain & Cognition* 12:240-266, 1990.

39. Roy EA: Current perspectives on disruptions to limb praxis, *Physical Therapy* 63:1998-2003, 1983.

40. Sagi D, Julesz B: "Where" and "what" in vision, *Science* 228:1217-1219, 1985.

41. Schenkenberg T, Bradford DC, Ajax ET: Line bisection and unilateral visual neglect in patients with neurological impairment, *Neurology* 30:509-517, 1980.

42. Sergent J: Inferences from unilateral brain damage about normal hemispheric functions in visual pattern recognition, *Psychological Bulletin* 96:99-115, 1984.

43. Sergent J: An investigation into perceptual completion in blind areas of the visual field, *Brain* 111:347-373, 1988.

44. Sergent J: The neuropsychology of visual image generation: data, method and theory, *Brain & Cognition* 13:98-129, 1990.

45. Spier PA and associates: Visual neglect during intracarotid amobarbital testing, *Neurology* 40:1600-1606, 1990.

46. Toglia J: Generalization of treatment: a multicontext approach to cognitive perceptual impairment in adults with brain injury. *Am J Occup Ther* 45:505-516, 1991.

47. Trobe JD and associates: Confrontation visual field techniques in the detection of anterior visual pathway lesions, *Ann Neurol* 10:28-34, 1981.

48. Tyler HR: Defective stimulus exploration in aphasic patients, *Neurology* 19:105-112, 1969.

49. van Zomeren AH and associates: Fitness to drive a car after recovery from severe head injury, *Arch Phys Med Rehab* 69:90-96, 1988.

50. Warren M: Identification of visual scanning deficits in adults after cerebrovascular accident, *Am J Occup Ther* 44:391-399, 1990.

51. Warren M: A hierarchical model for evaluation and treatment of visual perceptual dysfunction in adult acquired brain injury. I, II. *Am J Occup Ther* 47:42-66,1993.

52. Warren M: Visuospatial skills: assessment and intervention strategies. In Royeen CB, editor: *AOTA self study series: cognitive rehabilitation*, Rockville, Md, 1994, American Occupational Therapy Association.

53. Weinberg J and associates: Visual scanning training effect on reading-related tasks in acquired right brain damage, *Arch Phys Med Rehab* 60:479-486, 1979.

54. Weintraub S, Mesulam MM: Visual hemispatial inattention: stimulus parameters and exploratory strategies. *J Neuro, Neurosurgery & Psych* 51:1481-1488, 1988.

55. Wilson B, Cockburn J, Halligan P: Development of a behavioral test of visuospatial neglect, *Arch Phys Med Rehab* 68:98-102, 1987.

56. Yarbus AL: Eye movements during perception of complex objects. In Yarbus AL, *Eye movements and vision,* New York, 1967, Plenum Press.

57. Zangemeister WH and associates: Eye head coordination in homonymous hemianopsia, *Journal of Neurology* 226:243-254, 1982.

58. Zihl J: Rehabilitation of visual impairments in patients with brain damage, Unpublished paper, 1993.

Evaluation of Sensation and Treatment of Sensory Dysfunction

Lorraine Williams Pedretti

This chapter is concerned with somatosensory systems of touch (tactile), deep pressure, pain, proprioception, and thermal sensation and the special senses of taste and smell. The specific receptors for these sensory modalities are discussed in Chapter 20. Vision is discussed in Chapter 12.

Sensory information from the environment is received by peripheral receptors and transmitted to the central nervous system via the peripheral and spinal nerves. Almost all sensory information reaching the cerebral cortex is processed through the thalamus. The exception is olfaction, which transmits information directly to the primitive cortex of the medial temporal lobe. Sensory information is used for sensation, control of movement, and maintenance of arousal. While sensation is a conscious experience, not all sensation is perceived (interpreted) before the production of a motor response. For example, the withdrawal of the hand from a hot object is driven by an automatic motor response before the perception that the object is hot occurs.[19]

Diverse sensory systems have in common their ability to extract the same kinds of information from a sensory stimulus. That is, each system carries information about modality (for example, touch, pain, or taste) and the intensity, duration, and location of the stimulus.[19]

SENSATION AND MOTOR PERFORMANCE

The external environment is represented internally through sensation. From this internal representation of the outside world, the information necessary to guide movement is derived.[14] Motor performance in purposeful activity is profoundly dependent on the continuous inflow of sensory information.[14,22] Sensory information is used to manage effective movement and to correct errors in movement through feedback and feedforward mechanisms.[14,21]

FEEDBACK

Sensory feedback about the effectiveness of motor acts is received through the various sensory systems. Sensations derived from the ongoing movement are sent back to the central nervous system (CNS) where a comparison is made between intended action and what is actually happening. When writing, for example, if a wrong word or misspelling occurs, visual and proprioceptive feedback signal that an incorrect motor response has been made. This sensory information is then processed to the central nervous system, and a revision of the motor response is planned and executed. Feedback can be intrinsic, that is, sensations arising from the body during movement, or extrinsic, such as information about effectiveness of motor performance from a therapist or teacher. Feedback control is used primarily to maintain posture and regulate slow movements because feedback processes operate relatively slowly.[14,21]

FEEDFORWARD

Feedforward control is used for rapid movements that are planned in advance. It operates more quickly and controls movement by providing advance information about the act to be performed. This information is used to predict the possibility of movement disturbances and to develop the motor plan.[14] For example, skiing is initiated with feedforward control. It is necessary to anticipate the sensory experience to plan the motor act of descending the ski run. The slope of the ski run, the rate of speed of descent, potential obstacles, and the path to be taken must be considered before the descent is initiated. This anticipation results in assuming a specific posture, setting muscles, initiating the motion, making the

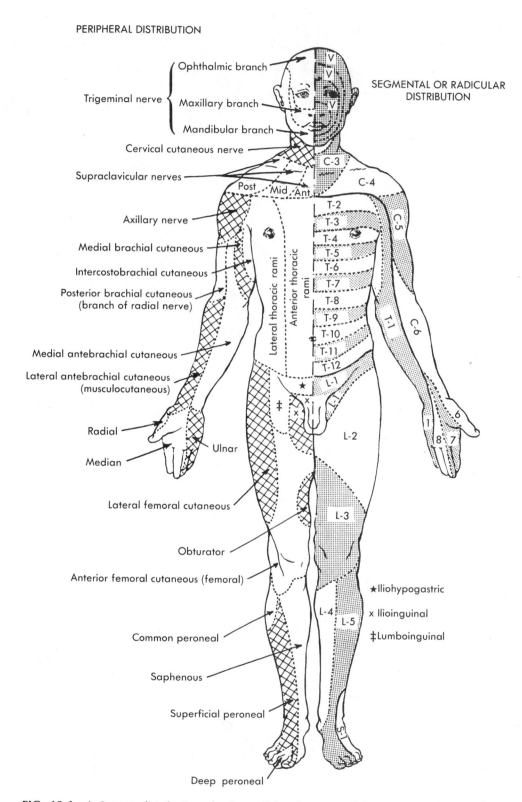

FIG. 13-1   A, Sensory distribution of major peripheral nerves and dermatomes corresponding to spinal cord segments, anterior view. (Reproduced with permission from Chusid JG: *Correlative neuroanatomy and functional neurology,* ed. 19, Copyright Lange Medical Publications, 1985.)

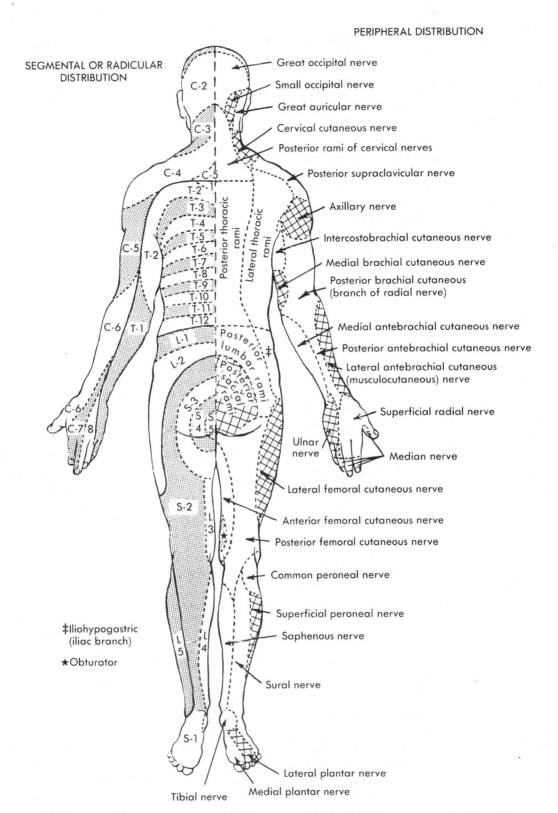

PERIPHERAL DISTRIBUTION

SEGMENTAL OR RADICULAR DISTRIBUTION

Great occipital nerve

Small occipital nerve

Great auricular nerve

Cervical cutaneous nerve

Posterior rami of cervical nerves

Posterior supraclavicular nerve

Axillary nerve

Intercostobrachial cutaneous nerve

Medial brachial cutaneous nerve

Posterior brachial cutaneous (branch of radial nerve)

Medial antebrachial cutaneous nerve

Posterior antebrachial cutaneous nerve

Lateral antebrachial cutaneous (musculocutaneous) nerve

Superficial radial nerve

Ulnar nerve

Median nerve

Lateral femoral cutaneous nerve

Anterior femoral cutaneous nerve

Posterior femoral cutaneous nerve

Common peroneal nerve

Superficial peroneal nerve

Saphenous nerve

Sural nerve

Lateral plantar nerve

Medial plantar nerve

Tibial nerve

‡Iliohypogastric (iliac branch)

★Obturator

FIG. 13-1 B, Sensory distribution, posterior view. (Reproduced with permission from Chusid JG: *Correlative neuroanatomy and functional neurology,* ed. 19. Copyright Lange Medical Publications, 1985.)

appropriate balance responses, and directing movement along a given path toward the destination. As the motor act is being executed, the feedback system operates continuously to correct errors in the intended movement. The feedforward system operates intermittently to anticipate or reevaluate the required action and to plan movement responses.[14,21]

EFFECTS OF SENSORY LOSS ON MOVEMENT

Proprioception and tactile sensation are essential for feedback and feedforward control systems. Patients with impaired sensation have deficits in both feedforward and feedback control. Those with tactile and proprioceptive dysfunction cannot sense position and motion of joints or sense contact with objects, resulting in motor performance deficits. Vision can compensate for the loss of tactile and proprioceptive sensation, but the defects in feedback and feedforward control limit even the patient's ability to use vision effectively. Because the patient cannot sense the resistance of the surface on which the hand is moving or sense the tension in muscles and tendons, jerky movements occur because visual feedback is slow and the errors in direction of movement cannot be corrected in time.[14]

Without sensation the conscious perception of peripheral sensory stimuli is lost, and the affected part(s) may be virtually paralyzed, even when there is adequate recovery of muscle function.[9] Patients with hemiplegia resulting from cerebral vascular accident (CVA) tend not to use the affected hand unless proprioception is intact and two-point discrimination at the fingertip is less than 1 cm apart, indicative of good discriminative sensation. Even slight sensory deficits limit the functional use of the affected hand because there are persistent problems in performing fine motor activities. The highly motivated patient may use visual compensation to engage the affected upper extremity in bilateral activities.[27] Adaptive motor behavior frequently occurs in response to external sensory stimuli, and adequate sensation is essential for effective movement. Therefore it is necessary to understand the patient's sensory status to appreciate fully the causes of the apparent motor dysfunction and to plan appropriate treatment goals and methods.

PRINCIPLES OF SENSORY EVALUATION

Sensation and *sensibility* are terms that refer to the reception, transmission, and interpretation of sensory stimuli. The terms are sometimes used interchangeably, or they may be differentiated.[5,9,18] Callahan defined sensation as the stimuli conveyed to the central interpretive centers by the afferent nerves and sensibility as the ability to perceive or interpret the sensory stimuli.[5] For the purposes of this chapter, the term *sensation* will be used to refer to the ability to identify the sensory modality, its intensity, and location.

Occupational therapists frequently evaluate sensation. It is important for the therapist not only to evaluate the patient's ability to recognize a touch or pinprick stimulus, but also to assess whether sensation is adequate for the performance of activities of daily living.[5] Any patient with CNS or peripheral nervous system (PNS) dysfunction should be routinely evaluated for sensory loss. Patients with CNS dysfunction tend to show loss of many sensory modalities over generalized areas, whereas those with PNS disorders tend to have loss of specific sensory modalities in circumscribed areas. Sensory testing may also be indicated in (1) patients with burns, in whom sensory receptors in the skin are destroyed; (2) patients who have arthritis, in whom joint swelling may cause compression of a peripheral nerve; and (3) patients who sustained traumatic hand injuries, in whom skin, muscles, tendons, ligaments, and nerves may be involved.

Examples of other diagnoses that require sensory testing are peripheral nerve injuries and diseases, spinal cord injuries and diseases, brain injuries and diseases, and fractures. In the latter, sensory testing may help to determine if there is peripheral nerve involvement.

SENSORY SUPPLY TO SPECIFIC AREAS

The sensory distribution of the major peripheral nerves of the body and limbs is shown in Fig. 13-1. When evaluating for peripheral nerve dysfunction, it is important to test the area supplied by the nerve or nerves that are affected. The sensory distribution of the dermatomes that correspond to spinal cord segments is also shown in Fig. 13-1. It is important to test patients with spinal cord injury or disease according to this dermatomal distribution to determine the level or levels of spinal cord lesion and any sparing of spinal cord function.

PURPOSES OF TESTING

By performing a sensory test, the therapist can carefully outline areas of intact, impaired, or absent sensation. This information is sometimes of diagnostic or prognostic value to the physician and provides a baseline for progress. The sensory evaluation can also be used to determine the need to teach the patient how to protect against injury, how to use compensatory techniques (such as visual guidance for movement during activities), and whether a sensory retraining program is feasible. Sensory loss may affect the use of splints and braces, because the patient may be unaware of pressure points during use. Sensory loss may also affect controlled use of a dynamic splint, which requires good sensory feedback for effective operation.

Tests of sensory function do not always accurately predict functional use of the hand. Moberg, cited by Dellon,[9] studied patients with median nerve injury to determine if there was a correlation between results of clinical sensory tests and hand function. He used a series of everyday activities that required several types of grip and

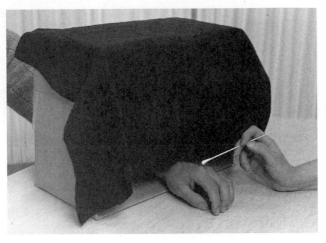
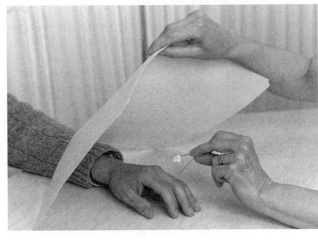

A

B

FIG. 13-2   A, Device for occluding vision during sensory testing: box with cloth drape. **B,** File folder used to occlude vision during sensory testing.

prehension and a test of picking up small objects and placing them in a container (Moberg Picking Up Test) to evaluate hand function. Moberg concluded that tests of touch, pain, temperature, and vibration did not correlate with hand function. There was some correlation between two-point discrimination and hand function.[9] His work is important to occupational therapy because it underscores a primary purpose and principle of occupational therapy practice: to evaluate function or performance. Thus it is important for the occupational therapist not only to evaluate the sensory modalities but to evaluate function as well. The therapist can use one of several hand function tests to observe hand use under simulated conditions. More reliably still, the therapist can observe for spontaneous use of the affected part(s) in bilateral activities of daily living (ADL).

OCCLUDING VISION DURING TESTING

Almost all of the sensory tests described in this chapter require that the patient's vision be occluded so that the test stimuli cannot be seen. Use of a blindfold or keeping the eyes shut are the least desirable methods of occluding vision. A blindfold can be a source of sensory distraction and can be very anxiety-provoking to patients with sensory, perceptual, and balance disturbances.[12] Additionally, it is difficult for many individuals with CNS dysfunction to maintain eye closure because of apraxia and motor impersistence.

There are several alternative methods for occluding vision. As shown later with actual tests, a small screen made by suspending a curtain between two posts is convenient and effective. If such a device cannot be constructed, something similar can be made by folding in the sides of a corrugated box and draping a cloth over one side (Fig. 13-2, *A*), or a file folder can be held over the area being tested (Fig. 13-2, *B*).

TESTS FOR SENSATION

The following tests are based on evaluation tools of clinical neurology and are designed to test gross sensation of adults with CNS or PNS dysfunction.[3,20] The reference list includes additional sensory tests and tests of discrete sensation.[5,9,29] Tests of moving touch, constant touch, vibration sense, and two-point discrimination are described in Chapter 35. Tests for disciminitive tactile perception are described in Chapter 14.

GENERAL PROCEDURE

Testing should take place in a quiet and nondistracting environment. Extraneous noises from the examiner or testing instruments should be minimized. Tests should always be administered to the analogous limb on the normal side if there is unilateral dysfunction, to establish a standard of accuracy for the individual patient and to assure that directions for test administration are comprehended. Parts to be tested should be exposed and positioned comfortably. In some instances it will be necessary for the examiner to support the part manually or with therapy putty, sandbags, or other cushioning material.[5] It is important for the examiner (*E*) to orient the subject (*S*) to the test procedures and to the rationale for administering the tests. The examiner should be sure that the subject understands how to respond. The subject's vision can be occluded by shielding the parts being tested from view.

LIGHT TOUCH AND PRESSURE SENSATION

Tactile sensitivity is critical to performance of all ADL. For example, knowing an object is in the hand or feeling clothes on the body and knowing whether or not they are correctly adjusted is dependent on intact touch sensitivity. Pressure sensation is also important in ADL because it is continuously received in activities such as sitting, pushing drawers and doors, crossing the knees, wearing belts and collars, and a host of other activities that stimulate pressure receptors. It is possible for a patient to have intact pressure sensation if touch is impaired or absent because touch receptors are in the superficial layers of the skin and pressure receptors are in subcutaneous and deeper tissue. Touch sensation is necessary for fine discriminative activities and pressure is a protective sensation because it warns of deep pressure or repetitive pressure that can lead to injury.[5] If touch sensation is impaired, pressure sensation can aid in performance of ADL and substitute for touch feedback in some activities.

Various tools have been used to apply stimuli for the light touch and pressure tests. These include a cotton ball, cotton swab, fingertip, or pencil eraser. All of these objects can provide a gross or cursory evaluation of light touch or pressure sensation. More discrete and accurate testing of cutaneous pressure thresholds of light touch to deep pressure can be performed by using the Semmes-Weinstein Pressure Aesthesiometer* described in Chapter 35.[9,28]

Test for Light Touch Sensation[3,5,15,19]

Purpose: To determine *S*'s ability to recognize and localize light touch stimuli.

Limitations: Patients with receptive aphasia cannot be validly tested.

Materials: A screen or Manila folder to occlude vision. A cotton swab.

Conditions: A nondistracting environment where *S* is seated at a narrow table. The test may also be conducted at the bedside or in a wheelchair. Affected hand and forearm should be supported comfortably on table. *E* sits opposite *S*.

Method: *S*'s hand and forearm are hidden from *S*'s view by placing them under the screen or by *E* holding Manila folder over them. Hand and forearm are touched lightly with a cotton swab at random locations covering area supplied by each peripheral nerve and each dermatome. A few trial stimuli should be administered while *S* is watching to be sure *S* understands procedure and how to respond. Test should be administered on an uninvolved area first to establish a standard. If spasticity is a problem, *E* may support hand on dorsal surface and hold thumb in radial abduction and extension to secure relaxation of fingers for palmar testing (Fig. 13-3 which also shows the screen mentioned earlier).

Responses: After each stimulus, *E* asks if *S* was touched (recognition). *S* responds by nodding or saying "yes" or "no." Screen is lifted or folder is removed after each stimulus, and *S* is asked to point to place where *S* was touched, using unaffected hand if possible. Localization responses are more accurate if *S* is allowed to use vision.[4] If this cannot be done, *S* is asked to describe location, and *E* should select locations that are easy to name (e.g., "knuckle of middle finger").

Scoring: On scoring chart *E* marks a plus (+) for ability to recognize and localize touch stimuli, a minus (−) for ability to

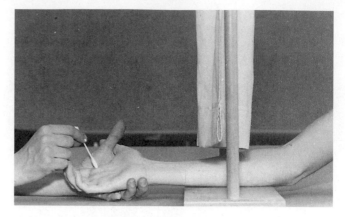

FIG. 13-3   Test for light touch sensation.

recognize only, and a zero (0) for inability to recognize or localize a stimulus (Fig. 13-4).

Interpretation of results: Deviations of ⅗ to 1⅕ inches (1.5 to 3 cm) from the point of application of the stimulus are normal for localization of stimuli, depending on the area of hand or arm touched. Responses should be more accurate on hand than on forearm and more accurate on forearm than on upper arm. Ability to recognize and localize touch indicates intact sensation. Ability to recognize but not localize touch stimuli indicates sensory impairment, and inability to recognize or localize touch stimuli means touch sensation is absent.

Test for Pressure Sensation: Pressure sensitivity may be tested as described for light touch, except that *E* should press hard enough with the cotton swab to dent and blanch the skin. If light touch sensitivity is severely impaired or absent, pressure sensitivity may be intact and may provide important sensory feedback, which can enhance function. Normally pressure stimuli can be localized on the hand from 2.44 to 2.83 mg of pressure[28] (Fig. 13-4).

THERMAL SENSATION

Thermal sensation is another of the protective sensory modalities.[4] The ability to detect temperatures is essential for the prevention of injury in many ADL such as bathing, cooking, and ironing. The ability to detect temperature also contributes to the enjoyment of food and to the detection of uncomfortable environmental temperatures. If the patient lacks accurate thermal discrimination, it will be necessary to teach precautions against injury and to structure ADL to prevent burns. As in the other sensory tests, the results can serve as a baseline for progress, and changes in sensory status may be used to measure recovery or degeneration, depending on the diagnosis.

Techniques such as touching skin with test tubes filled with hot and cold water, immersing the fingers or hand into hot or cold water, or touching small hot or cold compresses to the area being tested have been used in tests for thermal sensation. Another method is the Hot/Cold Discrimination Kit by Rolyan.* This kit includes two

---

*North Coast Medical, 187 Stauffer Blvd, San José, Calif. 95125-1042.

*Smith & Nephew Rolyan, Inc., One Quality Drive, P.O. Box 1005, Germantown, WI 53022.

FORM FOR RECORDING SCORES ON TESTS OF SENSATION

Department of Occupational Therapy

Name_____ Age _____ Sex _____

Diagnosis_____ Disability_____

Date_____

TEST FOR LIGHT TOUCH SENSITIVITY	LEFT	RIGHT
Use a cotton swab and touch random locations on anterior and posterior surfaces. Indicate on diagram: Intact: + Impaired: − Absent: 0	Anterior Posterior	Anterior Posterior

TEST FOR PRESSURE SENSITIVITY	LEFT	RIGHT
Use a cotton swab and press random locations on anterior and posterior surfaces. Indicate on diagram: Intact: + Impaired: − Absent: 0	Anterior Posterior	Anterior Posterior

TEST FOR SUPERFICIAL PAIN	LEFT	RIGHT

Use a large safety pin and touch random locations with sharp and dull ends on anterior and posterior surfaces.
Indicate on diagram:
Sharp:
  Correct response +S
  Sharp reported dull D
  No response −S
Dull:
  Correct response +D
  Dull reported sharp S
  No response −D
	Anterior
	
	Posterior
		Anterior
		
		Posterior

Remarks: _____

FIG. 13-4 Form for recording scores on tests of light touch, pressure, and superficial pain sensation.

metal temperature probes with a thermometer at the head of each, two thermal cups, and a single stem thermometer. One thermal cup is filled with ice and water, and the other is filled with hot tap water. The single thermometer is inserted in the thermal cup. When the desired temperature is reached, the probe is inserted into the thermal cup and allowed to reach the desired testing temperature. The metal probes, which look much like test tubes, are then put in contact with the skin surface to be tested. This kit makes it possible to control temperatures more precisely and to maintain constant temperature stimuli for the duration of the test.

Test for Thermal Sensation[3,7,10,15]

Purpose: To determine S's ability to discriminate between extremes of hot and cold and to detect variations in temperature at four levels.

Limitations: Persons with receptive aphasia cannot be validly tested. It is difficult to control water temperature very accurately, and temperature may change during the administration of the test. The results are subjective and may only detect ability to discriminate gross differences in temperature.

Materials: Four test tubes (3/4-inch or 2-cm diameter) with stoppers. Hot, warm, tepid, and cold water.

Conditions: A nondistracting environment in which S is seated comfortably at a table with both hand and forearm supported on table or alternative positioning described for previous tests.

Method: Subtest I: Two test tubes are used, one filled with cold water (45°F or 7°C) and one with hot water (110°F or 43°C). Extreme temperatures should not be used because they can stimulate the pain receptors. Stoppers are placed in tubes. E touches sides of test tubes to skin surfaces to be tested in random order and at random locations, being sure to cover test area thoroughly (Fig. 13-5).

Subtest II: Four test tubes are used, one filled with cold water, one with tepid water, one with warm water, and one with hot water. E should color code stoppers as follows: yellow: hot, green: warm, orange: tepid, and red: cold. Place stoppers in tubes. E asks S to touch or hold test tubes with affected hand(s) in random order. If S is unable to hold tubes, E may touch each one to S's palm and fingertips.

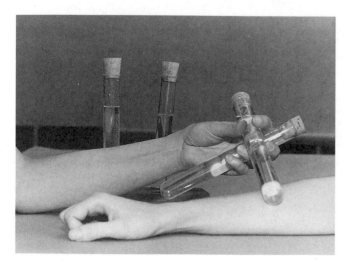

FIG. 13-5   Test for thermal sensation.

Responses: Subtest I: S responds "hot" or "cold" in response to each stimulus. If S is aphasic, E should work out an alternate nonverbal response before beginning tests.

Subtest II: S is asked to arrange test tubes on table from hottest to coldest in order from left to right. E checks correctness of order by color-coded stoppers and/or feeling tubes.

Scoring (Fig. 13-6): Subtest I: E marks a plus (+) if temperature is correctly identified and marks a zero (0) if S cannot distinguish hot from cold. Subtest II is not administered if S cannot succeed at subtest I.

Subtest II: E marks appropriate blanks on form with a check and the appropriate letter to indicate S's responses.

Interpretation of results: Normal adults should be able to complete all items on this test successfully. The normal hand can detect temperatures 1° to 5°C apart.[5]

SUPERFICIAL PAIN SENSATION

Pain is one of the protective sensations that makes possible the detection of potentially harmful stimuli to the skin and subcutaneous tissue.[5] The ability to detect painful stimuli is critical to the avoidance of injury during performance of daily activities and to the prevention of skin breakdown while wearing splints and braces and using wheelchairs, crutches, and other adaptive devices. In normal circumstances, pain sensation warns the individual to move quickly, as when withdrawing a finger from a hot surface, or to adjust the position of clothing, as when an elastic leg band is binding, or to remove an offending article of apparel, as a shoe that is rubbing a blister on the foot. The patient who lacks the ability to detect such painful stimuli is more likely to be injured. If pain sensation is absent or impaired, it is important to teach sensory compensation and safety awareness in the treatment program.

The following test uses a safety pin to apply light pain stimuli. *A new safety pin should be used for each patient; it should be sterilized before testing and discarded after the test.* The examiner should be aware that atrophic skin is particularly susceptible to injury and that a pinprick stimulus, which would not break normal skin, could produce a tiny break in atrophic skin. Skin atrophy occurs after peripheral nerve injury. The interruption of nerve supply interferes with normal tissue nutrition and causes the atrophy.[5] If this possibility is a concern, the end of a straightened paper clip may be used for the test.

Test for superficial pain[3,15,20,22]

Purpose: To make a gross evaluation of superficial pain sensitivity.

Limitations: Persons with receptive aphasia cannot be validly tested. The pulp of fingertips is relatively insensitive to pinprick. Calloused or toughened areas (for example, palms) are normally less sensitive to pinprick than other areas. If S is fearful of a safety pin, the straightened paper clip may be used.

Materials: The screen or a Manila folder to occlude S's vision. A large safety pin or straightened paper clip.

Conditions: A nondistracting environment where S is seated at a narrow table. Affected hand and forearm should be supported comfortably on table. E sits opposite S on other side of table. If it is not possible to position S in this manner, the test may be

FORM FOR RECORDING SCORES ON TESTS OF THERMAL SENSITIVITY

Department of Occupational Therapy

Name_____ Age_____ Sex_____

Diagnosis/Disability_____

Date of Onset_____ Date of Test_____

_____

TEST FOR THERMAL SENSITIVITY

SUBTEST I.

Touch sides of hot and cold test tubes to skin surfaces in random order and at random locations. Record scores on diagrams for tests of arms and hands or list site tested and record scores in columns.

Test site (fill in location tested)   Score (+, 0)

Dates			

Use diagram to record scores on test of arms and hands

SUBTEST II.

	Date	Date	Date
Arrange test tubes in correct order.			
Arrange test tubes in wrong order.			

Indicate arrangement of test tubes by filling in spaces below with H for hot, W for warm, T for tepid, and C for cold.

Date:_____ _____ _____ _____ _____

_____ _____ _____ _____ _____

_____ _____ _____ _____ _____

FIG. 13-6 Form for recording scores on test of thermal sensation.

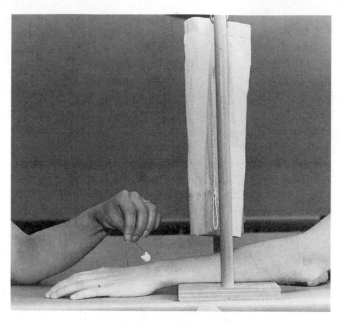

FIG. 13-7   Test for superficial pain sensation.

administered while *S* is in bed or sitting in the wheelchair with arms resting on a lapboard.

Method: The hand and forearm to be tested are hidden from *S*'s view by placing them under the screen or by *E* holding a Manila folder over them. Affected hand and forearm are touched lightly at random locations, using sharp and dull stimuli in random order and at random speed. Each stimulus should be applied with same degree of pressure (Fig. 13-7). It is important to apply stimuli to the area supplied by each peripheral nerve and each dermatome.[5] A few trial stimuli should be conducted with *S* watching to be sure that *S* understands test and knows how to respond. If spasticity is a problem, *E* may support hand on dorsal surface and hold thumb in radial abduction and extension to secure relaxation for palmar testing as shown in Fig. 13-3.

Responses: *S* should be asked to say "sharp" or "dull" in response to each stimulus. If *S* is aphasic or dysarthric, *E* should ask *S* to indicate a response by pointing to appropriate side of an open safety pin in *S*'s view.

Scoring: Callahan[5] recommended the following coding system for responses: *E* marks a plus *S* (+*S*) at stimulus point on scoring chart for a correct response to a sharp stimulus, a minus *S* (−*S*) for no response to a sharp stimulus, and a D if a sharp stimulus is reported as dull; a plus D (+D) for a correct response to a dull stimulus, a minus D (−D) for no response to a dull stimulus, and an *S* if a dull stimulus is reported as sharp.[5] A form for recording results of evaluation is shown in Fig. 13-4.

Interpretation of results: Correct responses to both sharp and dull indicate that potective sensation is intact. Incorrect responses to both sharp and dull are indicative of absent protective sensation. If dull stimuli are reported as sharp, there is hyperanalgesia; if sharp stimuli are reported as dull there is pressure sensation.[5]

OLFACTORY SENSATION (SMELL)

The sense of smell is conveyed by receptors that lie deep in the nasal cavity. Normal individuals can detect thousands of odors and at very low concentrations, making smell discrimination quite extraordinary. The sense of smell is important for detection of noxious and pleasant odors and is associated with the pleasure of taste. It is also connected to neuronal circuits that influence emotional states, and it evokes certain memories. There is great variability of olfactory acuity among normal persons. Olfactory acuity normally declines with age.[11]

Hyposmia is a diminished sense of smell, whereas a loss of the sense of smell is known as *anosmia*. Hyposmia refers to impaired sensation of a general nature. It may occur in patients with cyctic fibrosis of the pancreas, Parkinson's disease, and untreated adrenal insufficiency. Anosmia may be specific or general. Specific anosmia refers to lowered sensitivity to a specific odorant while perception of most other odors remains intact. General anosmia refers to absence of the sense of smell.[11] Anosmia may result from local chronic or acute inflammatory nasal disease or from intracranial lesions that may be the result of cerebral vascular accident, head injury, tumors, and infections. In some disturbances the sense of smell is distorted. There may be perception of odors that do not exist or pleasant odors may be distorted or perceived as noxious. This condition is known as *parosmia*.[3]

Anosmia interferes with function, for example, if the patient has an occupation in which the sense of smell is critical to safety, or for detection of household gas, chemicals, smoke, car exhaust, and noxious environmental odors. The disturbance may interfere with the perception and enjoyment of food odors and taste because decreased sense of smell affects the ability to taste. Therapists may also use olfactory stimulation in the treatment of certain neurological disorders.[13]

Test for Olfactory Sensation

Purpose: To determine if the sense of smell is intact, impaired, or lost and whether the loss is unilateral or bilateral.[3]

Limitations: Persons with receptive aphasia cannot be validly tested. Persons with expressive aphasia who cannot communicate using symbols, such as pictures or words, to indicate responses cannot be validly tested. Test is quite subjective and *E* must rely on *S*'s report.

Materials: Five small opaque or dark-colored bottles containing essences, powders, or crystalline material of familiar and natural odors. Coffee, almond, chocolate, lemon oil, and peppermint are some that are suitable.[3] Vinegar, ammonia, or other irritating chemical odors should not be used in a test of olfaction because they stimulate all receptors of the mucous membranes and tend to be irritating.[10,13] If *S* cannot respond verbally, small cards with the word or a picture for each odor on them will be needed.

Conditions: A nondistracting environment where no strong odors are present with *S* seated or semireclining.

Method: *S* is asked to compress one nostril or this function may be provided by *E*. *S* is then asked to take a breath to demonstrate that the remaining nostril is open. If the substances can be recognized from their appearance, vision is occluded. The cork of the bottle or a cotton swab moistened with essence is held under the open nostril; in the case of solid substances the container may be held under S's nostril. S is asked to take two moderate sniffs. Each of the substances is tried with a short delay between them, and the nostrils are tested alternately using the same and different substances.[3,7,20]

Responses: E asks S if he or she can (1) detect an odor, (2) identify the odor, (3) distinguish if the odors are the same or different to both nostrils.[3,20]

Scoring (Fig. 13-8): E marks a plus (+) on the form if the odor is detected and correctly identified, a minus (−) if an odor is detected and incorrectly identified, and a zero (0) if no odor is detected. Whether or not the same odors are perceived as the same by both nostrils and whether S can differentiate between dissimilar odors presented to each nostril should be noted on the form.

Interpretation of results: Ability to detect and identify odors quickly, ability to detect odor but not identify it, and ability to detect and differentiate odors without identification may all be regarded as normal responses.[3] Distortion of the odor (parosmia) and inability to detect odors (anosmia) are regarded as dysfunctional. If test responses are vague and variable, the results are unreliable, and it is best to postpone the test to a more favorable time.[3]

RECORDING SCORES OF OLFACTORY AND GUSTATORY SENSATION

Name:_____

Age:_____ Diagnosis:_____

Date:_____

Key: + = Can detect and identify odor
      − = Can detect odor, cannot identify odor
      0 = Cannot detect or identify odor
      S = Can detect same odors, both nostrils
      D = Can detect different odors, both nostrils

OLFACTORY SENSATION

	Dates	Left nostril		Right nostril		Comparisons	
Coffee							
Almond							
Chocolate							
Lemon							
Peppermint							

GUSTATORY SENSATION

Key: + = Identifies taste correctly
      − = Cannot identify taste

	Dates			Remarks
Sweet				
Salt				
Sour				
Bitter				

FIG. 13-8   Form for recording scores on olfactory and gustatory sensation.

GUSTATORY SENSATION (TASTE)

Taste receptor cells, located in the taste buds of the tongue, palate, and pharynx, epiglottis, and esophagus, convey taste stimuli to the brain via the facial, glossopharyngeal, and vagus nerves (cranial nerves VII, IX, and X). Generally four basic tastes can be detected: sweet, sour, salty, and bitter. Detection of more complex taste sensations is thought to be due to activation of combinations of receptors for these four basic tastes.[11]

Disturbances of taste may be caused by PNS or CNS lesions.[20] Smokers may demonstrate a decreased sense of taste with aging.[13] Taste is not only basic to the enjoyment of food but is one of the sensory stimuli that triggers salivation and swallowing.[25] Like smell, taste is connected to neural circuits that control emotional states and trigger specific memories.[11] Taste sensation may be of concern to the occupational therapist as part of a comprehensive evaluation of oral-motor mechanisms and for planning feeding training programs.[25]

Test for Gustatory Sensation

Purpose: To determine if the sense of taste is intact, impaired, or absent.

Limitations: The same limitations as cited for the test of olfaction apply here. The most accurate method of administering the test requires that *S* keep the tongue extended.[3,6,25] Therefore *S* must respond by pointing to a word or picture. In instances where *S* has speech but cannot recognize words or pictures, a verbal response should be allowed. If *S* is aphasic, *E* should observe for aversive responses to the sour and bitter stimuli.[25] The appreciation of taste depends on an intact sense of smell.[3,13]

Materials: Sugar or saccharin (sweet), salt or salt substitute (salt), lemon or vinegar (sour), and quinine (bitter) in small containers to test the four basic tastes.[11] Cotton swabs. Response cards with the word for the taste or a picture symbol of the taste on each. A glass, pitcher of water, and a small rinse basin.

Conditions: A nondistracting environment where *S* is seated or semireclining. *E* should sit directly in front of *S*. *S*'s vision should be occluded. The oral cavity should be clean and free of residual food tastes.

Method: *S* is instructed to protrude the tongue, and a small amount of the test substance on the tip of a wet cotton swab is applied to the appropriate place on the tongue: sweet: front/tip of tongue; salt: anterior lateral margins of the tongue; sour: lateral middle margins of tongue; and bitter: posterior tongue margin.[7,11,13] Tastes are presented in that order because the bitter stimulus may evoke an aversive response.[13] If this technique is not effective, rubbing the substance along the side of the protruded tongue should be tried.[3,20] The tongue should be irrigated with plain water between each stimulus.[3,13,15]

Responses: S is instructed to point to a response card before withdrawing the tongue and diffusing the taste to all areas of the tongue.[3,20]

Scoring (Fig. 13-8): *E* should record a plus (+) if the taste is correctly identified and a minus (−) if it cannot be identified.

Interpretation of results: Normal adults should be able to identify all tastes accurately.

POSITION AND MOTION SENSE

Proprioception refers to unconscious information about joint position and motion that arises from receptors in the muscles, joints, ligaments, and bone. The conscious sense of motion may be referred to as *kinesthesia*. Equilibrium (balance) or vestibular sensation is part of proprioception.[1] These senses make it possible to detect joint motion and position of the body or any of its parts. Sensation that is evoked from movement is essential to being able to move effectively. Feedback and feedforward control mechanisms depend on proprioception.[14] These mechanisms provide information about the motion and position of the body and its parts; help in maintaining erect posture, making postural adjustments, and localizing action, the limbs, trunk, and head at any moment. Proprioception, touch, and stereognosis make it possible to write without looking at the pencil, type without looking at the keys, and button clothes behind the back.

The awareness of motion and position is on a subcortical level and normally does not require conscious effort. To test position and motion sense, however, it is necessary to raise the sensation to a conscious level so that the patient can make the appropriate responses. A partial or complete loss of position and motion senses seriously impairs movement, even if muscle function is within normal limits. Therefore it is important for the occupational therapist to know if the patient has the sensory loss so that the motor dysfunction can be more fully understood. The evaluation will help to plan treatment by using compensatory methods or a sensory retraining program.

Test of position and motion sense[3,8,15-17,22]

Purpose: To evaluate *S*'s senses of motion and position.

Limitations: It is very important that *S* comprehend instructions exactly. Thus patients with receptive aphasia may not be validly tested. Movements must be made slowly and carefully enough to be detected. Methods of responding must be well established and understood before beginning the test. The patient's concentration on motion and position is essential.[3]

Materials: For testing hands and forearms, the screen or a Manila folder is used to occlude vision. For testing elbow and shoulder, if space and equipment permit, a screen high and wide enough to conceal *S*'s arm when held overhead or out in front when in a seated position. Curtain on screen should be full, continuous, and attached at top only. If such a screen is not available, an assistant can shield *S*'s vision with a Manila folder.

Conditions: Test should be conducted in privacy in a nondistracting environment. When fingers and wrist are being tested, *S* should be seated at a table with screen in a position to accommodate affected hand and forearm comfortably. *E* should sit opposite *S* on other side of screen and support *S*'s hand for the test. When elbow and shoulder are being tested, *S* should be seated away from table, and curtain screen should be draped over the affected shoulder so that *S* is unable to see the arm. If this position is not feasible, test may be conducted with *S* seated or reclining in bed or seated in a wheelchair.

Responses: To determine appreciation of direction of movement, S should be instructed to respond "up" (away from floor) and "down" (toward floor) or "out" (away from body) and "in" (toward body) as soon as he or she perceives direction of movement. Aphasic subjects may respond by pointing in appropriate direction. If there is one unaffected extremity, as in hemiplegia, S should be asked to imitate, with unaffected extremity, the motion and final position after E has ceased passive movement of the part being tested to evaluate appreciation of motion and position.

Method: Test of fingers: Test positions are index finger flexion, middle finger extension, thumb extension, and little finger flexion, which should be presented in random order. No range of motion should be so extreme as to elicit pain or a stretch reflex. S's hand and forearm should be placed under curtain, resting on dorsal surface. When testing a right hand E should support S's hand with the left palm and hold thumb out of way with the left thumb if necessary. This position should induce relaxation of fingers if S has flexor spasticity. With the right hand E should grasp finger to be tested on each side at distal phalanx to avoid giving pressure cues with E's thumb and index finger. Finger being tested should be separated from others and should be kept from touching palm to avoid cues from contact. Position of E's hands is reversed when testing a left hand (Fig. 13-9).

Test of wrist: Test positions are wrist flexion and extension. The ranges should not be so extreme as to elicit tendon action or a stretch reflex. E's and S's hands are positioned as for testing fingers. E makes a somewhat firmer grasp at sides of S's hand, however, reducing contact between E's palm and back of S's hand.

Test of elbow and shoulder: Starting position for all motions is with S's arm at side, shoulder supported in 20° to 30° of abduction, elbow supported at 90° of flexion, and wrist stabilized at neutral. Test positions are elbow extension, shoulder flexion, shoulder internal rotation, and shoulder flexion-abduction (halfway between 90° of flexion and 90° of abduction). Test positions should be presented in random order. Ranges should not be so extreme as to elicit a stretch reflex or cause pain if there is joint tightness. S should be seated away from table. Curtained screen should be arranged at S's test side. E should

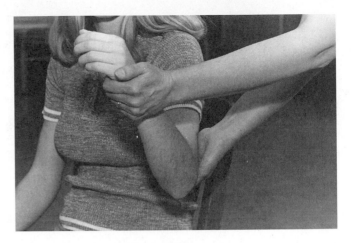

FIG. 13-10 Motion and position sense test of elbow and shoulder.

stand at S's test side and guide limb passively through test positions. When testing a right arm E's right hand should be placed along ulnar border of S's hand and wrist, stabilizing wrist at neutral. E's left hand should be placed on dorsal surface of upper arm just proximal to elbow. Position is reversed when testing left arm. E may carry out all test positions for elbow and shoulder without changing position of hands (Fig. 13-10).

Scoring (Fig. 13-11): Appreciation of direction of movement: E records plus (+) if direction is correctly perceived or zero (0) if direction is not perceived.

Appreciation of position: E records plus (+) if correct response is given, minus (−) if response is delayed or nearly correct, and zero (0) if response is obviously incorrect or no response is given.

Remarks: On the recording form E comments on S's reactions, unusual statements, observations, and individual variations in test procedure adapted for specific dysfunctions.

Interpretation of results: Normal individuals can detect movements of 1 or 2 mm in a joint.[15] A grade of intact was given by Kent[17] if movement could be detected in the first 15° of the ROM. It is possible for normal persons to duplicate the passive motion and position of the part being tested with the analogous uninvolved part quickly and with considerable accuracy.

SENSORY DYSFUNCTION

Sensory disturbances can result from CNS or PNS dysfunction or from cranial nerve disorders. In peripheral and cranial nerve lesions, the sensory disturbance is localized to the area supplied by the affected nerve. Sensory disorders of nerve root origin are localized to the dermatome supplied by the affected nerve root. Sensory dysfunction of CNS origin is more generalized and affects the contralateral side of the body after stroke or head injury, resulting in hemiplegia. Some of the terms associated with sensory disturbances are *anesthesia* (complete loss of sensation); *paresthesia* (abnormal sensation such as tingling or crawling); *hypesthesia* (decreased

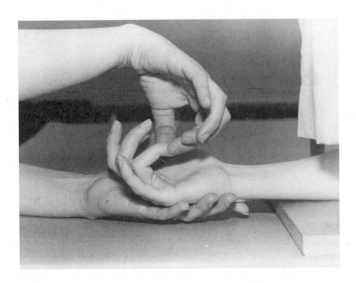

FIG. 13-9 Motion and position sense test of fingers.

FORM FOR RECORDING TESTS OF POSITION/MOTION SENSE

Department of Occupational Therapy

Name_____ Age_____ Sex_____ Onset_____

Diagnosis/disability _____

Date_____

Directions:
  Fingers and Wrist: Grasp part laterally.
  Scoring: Direction of Movement
        + = Intact/correct response
        0 = Absent/incorrect response or no response

      Position Sense
        + = Intact/correct imitation of movement and position
        − = Impaired/delayed response, minor to moderate errors in response
        0 = Absent/significant errors or no response

  Elbow/Shoulder: Starting position for all movements is:
        Shoulder: 20 to 30° of abduction
        Elbow: 90° flexion
        Wrist: Stabilized at neutral
  Scoring: Same as above for fingers and wrist

Test of Motion/Position Sense	Shoulder flexion-abduction	Shoulder internal rotation	Shoulder flexion	Elbow extension	Wrist extension	Wrist flexion	Little finger flexion	Thumb extension	Middle finger extension	Index finger flexion
Appreciation of direction of movement										
Appreciation of position										
Remarks:										

FIG. 13-11   Form for recording the scores on tests of motion/position sense.

sensation); *hyperesthesia* (increased tactile sensitivity); *analgesia* (complete loss of pain sensation); and *hypalgesia* (diminished pain sensation).[6]

Sensory loss may have a profound effect on the patient's ability to function in everyday activities. Therefore it is important to facilitate sensory recovery or reeducation to the extent possible or to teach compensatory techniques and safety precautions.

TREATMENT OF SENSORY DYSFUNCTION

Before treatment of sensory dysfunction can be initiated, a sensory evaluation and an evaluation of functional use of the affected part should be completed. The therapist must have knowledge of the diagnosis, the cause of the sensory dysfunction, the prognosis for return of sensation, and the current progression of recovery. This information may help to determine whether the treatment approach should be remedial, compensatory, or both. The patient who is to begin a sensory reeducation program should be motivated and able to concentrate. Cognitive ability should be adequate to understand the purpose of the training. Motivation to persevere in daily sessions and to make every effort to use the affected part in ADL is important.[4,12]

CENTRAL NERVOUS SYSTEM DYSFUNCTION
Effects of Sensory Loss

Following cerebral vascular accident (CVA) and other CNS disorders such as head injury, sensory loss can be a considerable problem. Sensory loss inhibits movement, even when there is good motor return. The inclination to move is based on sensory input and feedback. Persons with poor sensation have little urge to move. Movement that is attempted may be clumsy or uncoordinated. Sensory loss may contribute to, but is not the only cause of, neglect of the affected extremity so often seen in patients with CVA. The possibility of injury is a serious concern, and the dependence on visual control negates carrying out many activities such as reaching into a purse or pocket to retrieve an item and fastening clothing at the side or back.[12]

Compensatory Treatment

A first concern is safety and ensuring that the patient is not injured by bumping, burning, or becoming snagged in furniture or equipment during performance of ADL. If the loss of sensation is permanent, compensation will facilitate rehabilitation. Examples of compensation are using the less affected hand to perform activities such as cooking, eating, and ironing; using vision to observe motion and location of body parts; testing bath water with the less affected hand or a bath thermometer; and using adaptive devices such as the one-handed cutting board to avoid cutting the affected hand.[26]

The stroke (CVA) patient needs to be made aware of his or her sensory deficits. Safety factors during performance of everyday activities must be continuously brought to the patient's attention and reinforced. To compensate for sensory loss, it may be possible to train the patient to check the position of the limbs by looking at them. Patients must be evaluated for safety awareness and trained to consider safety in hazardous activities. The patient who wishes to return to home management should demonstrate good judgment, safety awareness, and the ability to use visual compensation for sensory loss.[23] Frequent repetition of instructions and cuing by the therapist are often necessary. Cognitive disturbances such as poor memory, perseveration, poor judgment, and inability to see cause-and-effect relationships make it difficult for some patients to learn and attend effectively to compensatory techniques. In such instances, supervision is required.

Remedial Treatment

Sensory bombardment involving as many of the senses as possible has been found to be useful for sensory retraining in some CVA patients. During regular therapeutic activities and handling, the therapist can touch or stroke the affected parts, encourage the patient to observe the movement and touch stimulation. Weight-bearing on legs, arms, and trunk increases proprioceptive feedback.[26]

Eggers[12] advocates integrating sensory retraining with motor retraining, with the Bobath approach as the basis for treatment (see Chapter 24). She described a sensory retraining program that focuses primarily on tactile and kinesthetic reeducation. A prerequisite to sensory retraining is for the therapist to normalize the patient's muscle tone and to find the optimal position for the sensory reeducation activities. The therapist must find ways to stimulate sensation without increasing spasticity. Sufficient time must be allowed for the patient to make responses because many patients exhibit delayed processing of sensory information. Other deficits such as hemianopsia, aphasia, and visual perceptual deficits must be considered when retraining for tactile-kinesthetic functions. Repetition and variation of sensory stimuli are necessary with CNS patients if they are to relearn sensation.[12]

A graded treatment program for sensory deficits is described by Eggers.[12] Initially the patient is allowed to see and hear an object as it is being felt, for the benefit of intersensory facilitation; then vision is occluded during the tactile exploration; and finally, a pad is placed on the table top so that both auditory and visual clues are eliminated and the patient relies on tactile-kinesthetic input alone. The program for tactile-kinesthetic reeducation begins with gross discrimination of objects that are very dissimilar, for example, smooth and rough textures or round and square shapes. Next the patient is asked to estimate quantities (such as number of marbles in a box) through touch. Then the patient must discriminate between large and small objects hidden in sand, progressing to discriminate between two- and three-dimensional objects. Finally, the patient is required to pick a specific small object from among several objects. The reader is referred to the original source for a detailed description of specific training activities.[12]

PERIPHERAL NERVOUS SYSTEM DYSFUNCTION
Treatment of Hypersensitivity

Heightened, uncomfortable, or irritable responses to nonnoxious stimuli often occur after peripheral nerve injury.[2,24] Treatment of hypersensitivity or *dysesthesia* is best done early and should precede a sensory reeducation program provided that there are no open wounds or infection.[24] Many patients with hypersensitivity tend to protect sensitive areas and avoid using the affected part in bilateral ADL. The therapist must reassure the patient that touching hypersensitive areas is beneficial.[2] Desensitization is most often done in hand rehabilitation and burn rehabilitation, which require advanced education and experience. It is beyond the scope of this chapter to outline specific details of desensitization programs. Following is a summary of those discussed by Barber[2] and Schutt and Opitz.[24]

Desensitization includes massage, tapping, or rolling with different textures over hypersensitive areas. Treatment begins at the patient's level of tolerance, then textures are graded to coarser and rougher with increases in force, duration and frequency of application. Vibration and immersion in materials such as soft styrofoam balls, rice, beans, popcorn, buckshot, and plastic squares are also used. This method of treatment is based on increasing the pain threshold of the nerve.[2,24]

Compensatory Treatment

A compensatory approach for patients with PNS dysfunction is similar to that described previously for patients with CNS dysfunction. The patient must be made aware of the specific sensory deficits and taught safety awareness for ADL. It may be necessary to avoid use of the affected limb during bilateral activities that are potentially hazardous.

Callahan[4] proposed the following guidelines for patients with PNS dysfunction who lack protective sensation:

1. Avoid exposure of the involved area to heat, cold, and sharp objects.
2. When gripping a tool or object, be conscious of not applying more force than necessary.
3. Beware that the smaller the handle, the less distribution of pressure over gripping surfaces. Avoid small handles by building up the handle or using a different tool whenever possible.
4. Avoid tasks that require use of one tool for long periods of time, especially if the hand is unable to adapt by changing the manner of grip.
5. Change tools frequently at work to rest tissue areas.
6. Observe the skin for signs of stress (that is, redness, edema, and warmth), and from excessive force or repetitive pressure, and rest the hand if these signs occur.
7. If blisters, lacerations, or other wounds occur, treat them with the utmost care to avoid further injury to the skin and possible infection.
8. To keep skin soft and pliant, follow a daily routine of skin care, including soaking and oil massage to lock in moisture.[4]

The patient with PNS dysfunction may be more capable of learning and attending to the compensatory techniques than the patient with CNS dysfunction. The reason is that perceptual and cognitive skills are intact in patients with PNS dysfunction.

Remedial Treatment

Following nerve injury repair and recovery, the neural impulses received in the sensory cortex from sensory stimulation of the injured hand are altered. The new pattern of neural impulses may be so different as to preclude correct interpretation of the stimulus. Thus although sensory information is received, it cannot be interpreted correctly. The purpose of sensory reeducation is to assist the patient to reinterpret the sensory impulses reaching his or her consciousness. The patient's potential for functional recovery following nerve repair will be enhanced by a sensory reeducation program.[9]

Dellon[9] described a sensory reeducation program that is divided into early and late phases, and progression of the program is based on the recovery process. The nerve recovery is determined by giving specific sensory tests. In the early phase of the program, the focus is on reeducating moving touch, constant touch, pressure, and touch localization. For moving touch, a pencil eraser or fingertip is used to move up and down the area being treated. First, the patient observes the stimulus. Next vision is occluded as the patient concentrates on the stimulus, then opens the eyes to verify what is happening. The patient verbalizes what is being felt, for example, "I feel a soft object moving down the palm of my hand." A similar procedure is followed for constant touch. A pencil eraser is used to press down on one place on the finger or palm in an area where constant touch is recovered. The patient is encouraged to practice these reeducation techniques four times a day for at least 5 minutes each but is directed not to stimulate one hand with the other because this action would send two sets of sensory stimuli to the brain.[4,9]

Late-phase sensory reeducation is initiated as soon as moving and constant touch are perceived at the fingertips and there is good localization, which is often 6 to 8 months after nerve repair at the wrist. The goal in this phase is to facilitate the recovery of tactile gnosis. The exercises involve a series of tactile discrimination tasks, which begin with identification of large objects that are substantially different from one another and progress to objects with more subtle differences. Familiar household objects are used at the outset. The process is to grasp the object while looking at it, then to occlude the vision and concentrate on the perception, and, finally, to look again at the object for reinforcement. The next set of objects are those that differ in texture and then objects that are smaller and require more discrete discrimination. Manipulation of the training objects also contributes to motor recovery. Ultimately, the therapist can incorporate activities that simulate those of the patient's occupational roles.[4,9]

Wynn Parry[29] described a sensory retraining program for patients with PNS injuries affecting the hand. The rationale underlying the technique is that the patient can learn to "lay down a new code" in the CNS. It has been shown that in nerve regeneration following traumatic lesions, there is a marked disturbance of cortical representation of sensory nerve fibers in the hand. The training program works best with patients who are cooperative, well motivated, and need to use their sensation for everyday activities.[29]

The training program begins when the patient has sensation in the fingers, about 6 to 8 months after a nerve suture at the wrist, with the use of large wood blocks of different shapes. The patient's vision is occluded, and a block is placed in the affected hand. The patient is asked to feel it, describe its shape, and compare its weight with a block placed in the unaffected hand. If an incorrect response is given, the patient is allowed to look at the blocks and repeat the manipulation, integrating visual and tactile information. The patient then compares the sensory experience with that of the normal hand. The procedure continues until various shaped blocks have been mastered. Then blocks are used with textures such as sandpaper or velvet on some surfaces. The patient is asked to differentiate textured surfaces from wood surfaces.[29]

In the next phase of training the patient is asked to identify several textures such as sheepskin, leather, silk, canvas, rubber, plastic, wool, carpet, and sandpaper, all presented with the vision occluded. Finally common objects are used in training, and the patient is asked to identify them without the aid of vision. If there are incorrect responses for texture and object identification, the patient is allowed to perform the manipulations while looking at the training objects and to relate what is felt to what is seen. Objects are graded from large to small. Training sessions may be varied by burying objects in a bowl of sand and asking the patient to retrieve a specific object, using a formboard in which to place specific forms, or identifying wooden letters for spelling out words. Training is done in two to four 10-minute sessions a day.[29]

To train touch localization, Wynn Parry[29] recommended the following procedure. Vision is occluded and the therapist touches several places on the volar surface of the hand. The patient is asked to locate each stimulus with the index finger of the unaffected hand. If the response is incorrect, the patient is directed to look at the place where the hand was touched and to relate where the touch was felt to where the stimulus was actually applied.[29]

To evaluate effectiveness of retraining, reevaluation is done at 1 month, 3 months, and 6 months after the initial examination. Criteria used to evaluate treatment effectiveness are time to recognize objects, time to recognize textures, and time for correct localization. To avoid a training effect, the objects and some textures used in testing are different from those used in the training program.[29]

Turner[26] described a sensory reeducation program for patients with peripheral nerve lesions. Retraining is initiated when there is return of protective sensation (deep pressure and pinprick) and touch perception. The retraining activities consist of having the patient identify objects, shapes, and textures with the vision occluded. If the response is incorrect, the patient is allowed to look at the object and compare its sensation in the normal hand to allow the integration of tactile sensation and vision. Activities that may be helpful include using textured dominoes or checkers, handling cut-out shapes, and finding large to small common objects hidden in rice or lentils. Training with these objects is carried out three or four times a day for 3/4 of an hour. The training periods are alternated with periods of general bilateral activity such as pottery, bread-kneading, weaving, and macramé. The patient is encouraged to use the affected hand in bilateral activities and to compare the feelings of the tools and materials in the affected hand with those in the unaffected hand.[26]

A program of sensory reeducation following nerve injury was described by La Croix and Helman.[18] The purpose of the program is to help the patient correctly interpret different sensory impulses. A series of graded stimuli is used in treatment such as constant pressure, movement, light touch, and vibration. The least stressful stimuli are presented first. The patient does the training exercises several times a day for short periods. The exercises are done on the unaffected side and then on the affected side, first with the aid of vision and then with vision occluded. Areas of hypersensitivity are noted. Sensory stimulation such as stroking, deep pressure, rubbing, and maintained touch with different textures and shapes, are used to reduce hypersensitivity.[18]

Sensory reeducation for PNS disorders focuses on applying graded stimuli according to the progression of nerve recovery. Sensory stimuli such as touch localization, moving touch, and constant touch are followed by exercises for tactile discrimination of shape, size, texture, and object identification. Intermodal reinforcement through visual, auditory, and tactile senses is an important part of the reeducation program.

SUMMARY

Exteroceptive receptors convey sensory information from the environment to the brain by way of peripheral and spinal nerves and the spinal cord. Almost all sensory stimuli are processed through the thalamus before reaching the cerebral cortex. Sensation presents the external environment to the brain and provides information necessary to guide purposeful and effective movement responses. Motor performance is dependent on sensory input, and significant motor deficits can result from dysfunction of sensory systems. Movement is guided by sensory feedback and feedforward control systems. Defects in sensation disrupt these systems.

Sensory testing should be part of the comprehensive occupational therapy evaluation of patients with upper and lower motor neuron disorders. It helps the therapist to understand the complexity of the patient's motor dysfunction. Paralyzed muscles are not the sole cause of faulty or absent use of affected limbs. Rather, a sensory disturbance can be the primary or complementary cause of motor paralysis and movement disorders.

This chapter presented clinical screening tests for the senses of touch, pressure, superficial pain, thermal sensation, proprioception, smell, and taste. It provided information on setting up, administering, scoring, and interpreting results of these tests.

REVIEW QUESTIONS

1. Why is sensory evaluation necessary and important to occupational therapy?
2. What types of disabilities should be routinely given sensory evaluation?
3. Describe how light touch sensitivity is evaluated.
4. If the patient recognizes that he or she was touched but cannot localize the stimulus, what grade would be given on the test for light touch?
5. What are the alternatives for responses in the position sense test?
6. Why is it important to grasp the fingers and wrist laterally during the test for position sense?
7. What are some methods for occluding the patient's vision? What are the alternatives to blindfolding or asking the patient to keep eyes closed?
8. Describe two methods for testing thermal sensation.
9. How are olfactory and gustatory sensations related?
10. What is the functional significance of olfactory sensation?
11. Discuss two approaches to the treatment of sensory dysfunction and the purposes of each.
12. Describe the general principles for treatment of hypersensitivity.
13. With which disabilities is desensitization most likely to be used?
14. Describe one approach to sensory reeducation for the patient with CNS dysfunction and one for the patient with PNS dysfunction.
15. What is the neurophysiological principle on which sensory education for PNS dysfunction is based?

REFERENCES

1. Ayres AJ: *Sensory integration and learning disorders,* Los Angeles, 1972, Western Psychological Services.
2. Barber LM: Desensitization of the traumatized hand. In Hunter JM and associates, editors: *Rehabilitation of the hand,* St Louis, 1990, CV Mosby.
3. Bickerstaff ER, Spillane JA: *Neurological examination in clinical practice,* ed 5, London, 1989, Blackwell Scientific Publications.
4. Callahan AD: Methods of compensation and reeducation for sensory dysfunction. In Hunter JM and associates, editors: *Rehabilitation of the hand,* ed 3, St Louis, 1990, CV Mosby.
5. Callahan AD: Sensibility testing: clinical methods. In Hunter JM et al, editors: *Rehabilitation of the hand,* ed 3, St Louis, 1990, CV Mosby.
6. Chusid JG: *Correlative neuroanatomy and functional neurology,* ed 19, Los Altos, Calif, 1985, Lange Medical Publications.
7. deGroot, J: *Correlative neuroanatomy,* Norwalk, Conn, 1991, Appleton & Lange.
8. De Jong R: *The neurologic examination,* New York, 1958, Paul B Hoeber.
9. Dellon AL: *Evaluation of sensibility and re-education of sensation in the hand,* Baltimore, 1981, Williams & Wilkins.
10. De Myer W: *Technique of the neurologic examination: a programmed text,* ed 2, New York, 1974, McGraw-Hill.
11. Dodd J, Castellucci VF: Smell and taste: the chemical senses. In Kandel ER, Schwartz JH, Jessel TM: *Principles of Neural Science,* New York, 1991, Elsevier Science Publishing.
12. Eggers O: *Occupational therapy in the treatment of adult hemiplegia,* Rockville, Md, 1984, Aspen Systems.
13. Farber SD: *Neurorehabilitation, a multisensory approach,* Philadelphia, 1982, WB Saunders.
14. Ghez C: The control of movement. In Kandel ER, Schwartz JH, Jessel TM: *Principles of neural science,* New York, 1991, Elsevier Science Publishing.
15. Gilroy J, Meyer JS: *Medical neurology,* London, 1969, Macmillian.
16. Head H and associates: *Studies in neurology,* London, 1920, Oxford University Press.
17. Kent BE: Sensory-motor testing: the upper limb of adult patients with hemiplegia, *Phys Ther J Am Phys Ther Assoc* 45:550, 1965.
18. La Croix E, Helman J: Upper extremity orthopedics. In Logigian MK, editor: *Adult rehabilitation: a team approach for therapists,* Boston, 1982, Little, Brown.
19. Martin JH: Coding and processing sensory information. In Kandel ER, Schwartz JH, Jessel TM: *Principles of Neural Science,* New York, 1991, Elsevier Science Publishing.
20. Mayo Clinic and Mayo Foundation: *Clinical examinations in neurology,* Philadelphia, 1981, WB Saunders.
21. Montgomery PC: Perceptual issues in motor control. In *Contemporary management of motor control problems: proceedings of the II Step Conference,* Alexandria, Va, 1991, Foundation for Physical Therapy.
22. Occupational Therapy Department, Rancho Los Amigos Hospital: *Upper extremity sensory evaluation: a manual for occupational therapists,* Downey, Calif, 1985.
23. Ruskin A: Understanding stroke and its treatment. In Ruskin A, editor: *Current therapy in physiatry,* Philadelphia, 1984, WB Saunders.
24. Schutt AH, Opitz JL: Hand rehabilitation. In Goodgold J: *Rehabilitation Medicine,* St Louis, 1988, CV Mosby.
25. Silverman EH, Elfant IL: Dysphagia: an evaluation and treatment program for the adult, *Am J Occup Ther* 33:382, 1979.
26. Turner A: *The practice of occupational therapy,* ed 2, New York, 1987, Churchill Livingstone.
27. Waters RL, Wilson DJ, Gowland C: Rehabilitation of the upper extremity after stroke. In Hunter JM and associates, editors: *Rehabilitation of the hand,* St Louis, 1990, CV Mosby.
28. Werner JL, Omer GE: Evaluating cutaneous pressure sensation of the hand, *Am J Occup Ther* 24:347, 1970.
29. Wynn Parry CB: *Rehabilitation of the hand,* London, 1981, Butterworths.

Evaluation and Treatment of Perceptual and Perceptual Motor Deficits

Lorraine Williams Pedretti, Barbara Zoltan, Carol J. Wheatley

Perception is the mechanism by which the brain interprets sensory information received from the environment. The perceived information is then further processed by the various cognitive functions (described in Chapter 15), and the individual may choose to respond by a verbal expression or motor act. Deficits in the motor response system include the apraxias. In early development tactile, proprioceptive, vestibular, and visual perception provide an innate sense of the body scheme, which is basic to all motor function.[4,27,44]

This chapter describes higher level tactile discriminative sensation, body scheme, and praxis. Suggestions for standardized and functional testing are provided. General approaches to treatment are reviewed and suggestions for specific treatment tasks are presented.

GENERAL PRINCIPLES OF EVALUATION

Occupational therapists usually evaluate perception and activities of daily living (ADL) performance separately and attempt to determine the underlying neurobehavioral causes of performance deficits by correlating the results of the separate evaluations.[3] Zoltan, Siev, and Frieshtat,[44] for example, presented several methods of testing perceptual dysfunction but did not address how deficits affect functional performance.[3] Arnadottir[3] recommends the use of ADL to evaluate neurobehavioral dysfunctions and their impact on performance of tasks essential to functional independence. She maintains that it is preferable for occupational therapists to assess neurobehavioral deficits directly from the ADL evaluation rather than doing separate tests and attempting to correlate their results. She developed the Arnadottir OT-ADL Neurobehavioral Evaluation (A-ONE), which provides information on neurobehavioral impairments and deficits in functional performance by evaluating ADL skills.[3] The reader is referred to the original source for more information on this perspective and a detailed description of the A-ONE instrument.[3]

The optimal test battery includes perceptual tests that require a verbal response, motor response, or have flexible response requirements of either mode. With a variety of such tests, the therapist can gather information to discriminate between a deficit in the reception of information or in the verbal or motor output, which, in turn, influences the treatment approach. Observations of performance and analysis of the perceptual-motor demands of functional activities further complement standardized evaluation tools and enable the relating of test results to functional performance.

Before perceptual evaluation, the therapist must have evaluated sensory and motor functions. The therapist should also be aware of language deficits and the patient's general level of alertness and responsiveness.

The patient's age and premorbid status should be considered in the interpretation of performance in perceptual testing. For example, the majority of patients who have sustained a cerebral vascular accident (CVA) are elderly. Numerous changes in visual, auditory, perceptual, and cognitive functions are associated with the natural aging process.[16] Similarly, a young traumatically injured patient may have a history of learning disabilities before a head injury. To interpret test results accurately and establish realistic treatment goals, the therapist should have a clear picture of the patient's premorbid status. If the patient is unable to supply the necessary information, family, friends, and educators should be consulted.

APPROACHES TO TREATMENT

Occupational therapists have used perceptual retraining since the 1950s. They have focused on teaching specific perceptual skills and incorporating perceptual retraining into functional tasks such as ADL. Occupational therapists use perceptual training because performance of functional activities is assumed to be dependent upon perceptual skills as well as motor skills. It is assumed that perceptual deficits affect functional performance adversely, and remediation of or compensation for perceptual deficits is assumed to improve functional performance.[32] Neistadt,[32] in her critical analysis of approaches to treatment for perceptual deficits, described two general classifications of approaches: the adaptive and the remedial. Adaptive approaches provide training in daily living behaviors to facilitate adaptation to the environment for maximal functioning of the patient. In contrast, the remedial approaches seek to cause some change in CNS functions.[32] The effectiveness of the various approaches to the remediation of perceptual deficits has not been well documented and requires scientific investigation, however.[32]

A therapist may use one approach or a combination of approaches in the treatment of perceptual deficits. Many specific activities are suggested for treatment of perceptual deficits in occupational therapy literature but guidelines and protocols for the use of such activities are lacking.[44] For measuring effectiveness of treatment, criteria are needed for successful performance, task grading, objective methods of evaluating performance, and guidelines for task modification.[31] In the absence of such objective criteria the occupational therapist relies on empirical methods to measure and report improvement. The relationship between perceptual deficits and functional performance has been demonstrated in several studies.[5,26,37,40,42]

Treatment of perceptual problems can be difficult and complex. The best results are obtained when the treatment is consistent and done on a daily basis. Zoltan and associates[44] described four approaches used for perceptual training of the hemiplegic patient. The sensory-integrative approach, the neurodevelopmental (Bobath) approach, and the transfer of training approach are classified as remedial. The functional approach is considered adaptive.[32]

REMEDIAL APPROACHES

The sensory-integrative approach is based on neurophysiologic and developmental principles and was described by A. Jean Ayres as a treatment approach for children with sensory-integrative dysfunction.[4,32] It assumes that controlled sensory input can elicit specific motor responses. Thus the sensory-integrative functions of the brain can be influenced by selected activities that provide the necessary input and evoke the desired motor responses. This approach may be impractical for adults because it takes much treatment time to be effective. It is also likely that the adult's CNS does not have the same capacity for learning as the child's because it is thought to have less plasticity. Some therapists report using modifications and selected techniques from this approach with adults with some success.[44]

In the neurodevelopmental (Bobath) approach, perceptual retraining is integral to the handling techniques and feedback about correct movement during the motor retraining program. The experience of the sensation of normal movement and feedback about correct performance enhance the retraining of perceptual functions. Bilateral activities used in the motor retraining program stimulate total body awareness and help to remediate problems of unilateral neglect and homonymous hemianopsia. Weight-bearing activities, an important part of the motor retraining program, enhance proprioception.[44]

The transfer of training approach assumes that practice in a particular perceptual task carries over to performance of similar tasks or practical activities requiring the same perceptual skills. For example, practice in reproducing pegboard designs for spatial relations training could carry over to dressing skills that require spatial judgment (such as matching blouse to body and discriminating between right and left shoes). This approach is common in the treatment of perceptual problems in occupational therapy clinics. Conflicting reports of its effectiveness exist, and further research is needed to determine its benefits.[44]

ADAPTIVE APPROACH

The functional approach is characterized by the repetitive practice of particular tasks that help the patient become more independent in the performance of ADL. This approach is probably the most common one in dealing with perceptual problems. The therapist does not do specific perceptual training. Rather, the patient is made aware of the problem and taught to adapt to or compensate for it. For example, if the patient has trouble dressing because of a body scheme deficit, the therapist may set up a regular dressing pattern and routine and provide cues with repetitive practice. With these adaptations, the patient may learn to dress. Adaptation of environment, methods, or materials is another way to compensate for a perceptual deficit. For example, if the patient is distractible because of visual or auditory figure/ground deficits, the therapist may arrange for treatment in a quiet and uncluttered room to minimize distractions and create the best environment for learning. If the patient has dressing apraxia colored tabs can be sewn into clothing to provide cues for top and bottom, inside and outside.[44]

METHODS OF EVALUATION AND TREATMENT

Stereognosis and graphesthesia are tactile discriminative skills of the parietal lobes. They require a higher level of synthesis than the basic tactile sensory functions of light touch and pressure described in Chapter 13.

STEREOGNOSIS

Stereognosis is the perceptual skill that enables an individual to identify common objects and geometric shapes through tactile perception without the aid of vision. It results from the integration of the senses of touch, pressure, position, motion, texture, weight, and temperature and is dependent on intact parietal cortical function.[20]

Stereognosis is essential to daily living because the ability to "see with the hands" is critical to many daily activities. It is the skill that makes it possible to reach into a pocket or purse and find keys and to reach into a dark room and find the light switch. Stereognosis, along with proprioception, enables the use of all hand tools and performance of hand activities without the need to concentrate visually on the implements being used. Examples are knitting while watching television, sawing wood while focusing on the wood rather than the saw, and using a fork while conversing. A deficit in this perceptual function is called *astereognosis*. Patients who have astereognosis but retain much of their motor function, must visually monitor their hands' activities. Thus they become very slow and purposeful in their movements and tend to be generally less active.

Test for Stereognosis[7,13,22,24]

Purpose: To evaluate a patient's ability to identify common objects and perceive their tactile properties.

Materials: A means to occlude the patient's vision such as a curtain or folder as described in Chapter 13. Typical objects that could be used for identification include a pencil, fountain pen, sunglasses, key, nail, large safety pin, metal teaspoon, quarter, and small leather coin purse. Any common objects may be used, but it is important to consider the patient's social and ethnic background to ensure that he or she has had previous experience with the objects. Three-dimensional geometric shapes (square, sphere, pyramid, etc.) can also be used to test shape and form perception.

Conditions: The test should be conducted in privacy in an environment with minimal distractions. The patient should be seated at a table in a position that accommodates the affected hand and forearm comfortably. The therapist should sit opposite the patient. If the patient is unable to manipulate test objects because of motor weakness, the therapist should assist him or her to manipulate them in as near normal a manner as possible.

Method: The patient's vision is occluded. The patient's hand is resting on dorsal surface on table. Objects are presented in random order. Manipulation of objects is allowed and encouraged. The therapist assists with the manipulation of items if the patient's hand function is impaired.

Responses: The patient should be asked to name the object, or if unable, to describe its properties. Aphasic patients may view a duplicate set of test objects after each trial and point to a choice.

Scoring: A form similar to the one in Fig. 14-1 may be used to score the patient's responses. The therapist marks plus (+) if object is identified quickly and correctly and minus (−) if there is a long delay before identification of object or if the patient can describe only properties (for example, size, texture, material, and shape) of object. The therapist marks a zero (0) if the patient cannot identify object or describe its properties.

Test for Graphesthesia

An additional test of discriminative sensation that measures parietal lobe function is the test for graphesthesia, the ability to recognize numbers, letters, or forms written on the skin.[10,20,33] The loss of this ability is called agraphesthesia. To test graphesthesia, vision is occluded and letters, numbers, or geometric forms are traced on the fingertips or palm with a dull-pointed pencil or similar instrument. The subject tells the examiner which symbol was written.[33] If the patient is aphasic, pictures of the symbols may be used for the patient to indicate a response after each test stimulus.

Treatment of Astereognosis

A graded treatment program for sensory deficits is described by Eggers.[15] Initially the patient is allowed to see and hear an object as it is being felt for the benefit of intersensory facilitation; then vision is occluded during the tactile exploration; and finally, a pad is placed on the table top so that both auditory and visual clues are eliminated and the patient relies on tactile-kinesthetic input alone. The program for tactile-kinesthetic reeducation begins with gross discrimination of objects that are very dissimilar, for example, smooth and rough textures or round and square shapes. Next the patient is asked to estimate quantities (such as number of marbles in a box) through touch. Then the patient must discriminate between large and small objects hidden in sand and progresses to discriminate between two- and three-dimensional objects. Finally the patient is required to pick a specific small object from among several objects. The reader is referred to the original source for a detailed description of specific training activities.[15]

Farber described a treatment approach to retrain for stereognosis in adults and children with CNS dysfunction.[17] First the patient is allowed to examine the training object visually as it is rotated by the therapist. The patient is then allowed to handle the object in the less affected hand while observing the hand. In the next step, the patient is allowed to manipulate the object with both hands while looking. Then the object is placed in the affected hand to be manipulated while the patient looks at it. The patient may place the hand in a mirror-lined, three-sided box during these manipulations to increase visual input. This sequence is then repeated with the vision occluded. Once several objects can be identified consistently, two of the objects may be hidden in a tub of sand or rice. The patient is then asked to reach into the tub and retrieve a specific object. If the sensation of the sand or rice is overstimulating or disturbing, the objects can be placed in a bag.[17]

Vinograd, Taylor, and Grossman[38] described a similar

FORM FOR RECORDING TEST OF STEREOGNOSIS

Department of Occupational Therapy

Name _____ Age _____ Sex _____ Onset _____

Diagnosis/disability _____

Date _____

TEST OF STEREOGNOSIS

COMMON OBJECTS	+ − 0	DESCRIPTION
Pencil		
Fountain pen		
Sunglasses		
Key		
Nail		
Safety pin		
Teaspoon		
Quarter		
Leather coin purse		

Remarks:

FIG. 14-1   Form for recording test of stereognosis.

program. They included objects for discrimination of shape, size, weight, and texture as well as common objects in the training, however. Wooden blocks were included for shape recognition, sandbags and cotton bags for weight recognition, and different grades of sandpaper and smooth leather for texture discrimination.[38]

The effect of intensive stereognostic training on spastic, cerebral, and palsied adults was studied by Ferreri,[18] with some favorable results for improving stereognosis. Training sessions were held for 20 minutes, three to four times a week for a period of 5 weeks. The training program consisted of comparing two different objects or forms using the uninvolved hand, then the involved hand. The subjects were assisted with manipulation of the objects if there was motor paralysis. The examiner talked about the qualities of the objects or forms and emphasized the hand and finger positions. A particular training item was used for each session until five consecutive correct responses were given in the testing portion of the session before a new training item was introduced.[18]

BODY SCHEME

An individual's body scheme is a postural model related to how one perceives the position of the body and the relationship of the body parts.[23] It includes (1) knowledge of body construction, its anatomic elements, and spatial relationships; (2) the ability to visualize the body in movement and its parts in different positional relationships; (3) the ability to differentiate between right and left; and (4) the ability to recognize body health and disease.[4,44] An individual's body scheme is considered the foundation for future skills in the perception of environmental space.[45] Body scheme disorders are associated with parietal lobe damage and can include somatognosia, unilateral neglect, impaired right/left discrimination, and finger agnosia.[1,11,14,29,44]

Tests for Body Scheme Disorders

Asomatognosia refers to a loss of body scheme[23] and is usually evaluated by having the patient point to body parts on command and/or by imitation.[27,35,44,45] In addi-

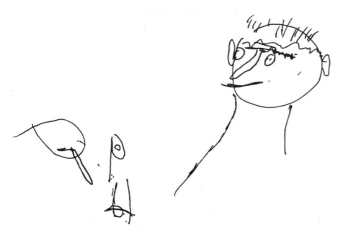

FIG. 14-2 Example of impaired body scheme. Drawing on left is patient's first attempt to draw a face. Therapist asked patient to try again. Second effort is drawing on right.

tion, many clinicians use the draw-a-person test and body and face puzzles.[27,44,45] The clinician, however, must rule out constructional apraxia as the cause of poor performance for these latter tests. An impairment in body scheme is illustrated in Figure 14-2.

Right/left discrimination deficits can occur in extrapersonal space and/or intrapersonal space. The most basic testing of right/left discrimination abilities is to have the patient point to a body part, specifying the right or left side, on self, or on a more advanced level, identify right and left body parts on the examiner.[8]

Unilateral inattention or neglect refers to the inability to integrate perceptions from the left side of the body or the left side of space. Left neglect is more prevalent than neglect or inattention to the right side.[39] Figure 14-3 il-

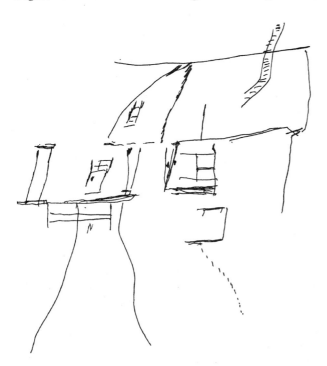

FIG. 14-3 Example of two-dimensional constructional apraxia and inattention of left side in patient's drawing of house. Patient was retired architect.

lustrates evidence of left neglect. Tactile inattention refers to a decreased sensitivity to sensory input to one side of the body.[34] The patient may exhibit an inattention deficit with or without associated visual and sensory impairments, i.e., homonymous hemianopsia. Unilateral neglect is often evaluated through table top tasks such as body or face puzzles, scanning worksheets, or the draw-a-person test.[45] The Benton Visual Retention Test includes an analysis of left- versus right-sided errors.[36] Before using these tests, however, visual field deficits and/or ocular-motor impairment must be ruled out as causes of poor performance. The most effective evaluation of unilateral neglect as it relates to a body scheme disorder is direct observation during dressing and other ADL. See Chapter 12 for a discussion of visual deficits and their evaluation.

The patient with finger agnosia has difficulty naming fingers on command or identifying which finger has been touched.[30] The evaluation of finger agnosia is accomplished through finger localization, naming on command, or having the patient imitate finger movements made by the therapist.[27,35]

Treatment of Body Scheme Disorders

The treatment of body scheme disorders can include the sensory-integrative, transfer of training, functional, or neurodevelopmental approach, or a combination of these. Using the transfer of training approach, the therapist may touch the patient's body parts and have him or her identify them as they are touched. Practice in assembling human figure puzzles and quizzing the patient on body parts are other methods in this approach.[44]

For a remedial approach, unilateral body neglect can be treated by applying sensory input (rubbing patient's arm or leg) before dressing, observing precautions to prevent increased spasticity. The therapist may also engage the patient in activities that focus attention on the neglected side. Examples are placing work materials on the affected side and approaching the patient from the affected side for treatment or conversation. Conversely, using an adaptive or compensatory approach, the therapist may place food, utensils, and work materials on the unaffected side and give all instructions from that side. Repetitive practice and cuing may also be effective. Bilateral weight-bearing with handling techniques of the neurodevelopmental approach can be used to facilitate total body awareness.[44]

PRAXIS

Praxis is the ability to plan and perform purposeful movement. An impairment in the ability to perform purposeful movement, with no loss of motor power, sensation, or coordination and with normal comprehension, is called apraxia.[23] Types of apraxias include ideational, ideomotor, constructional, oral, and dressing apraxia. Because the distinction between ideational and ideomotor apraxia is often difficult, some authors recommend simply using the term apraxia[25] or applying more descriptive terms such as apraxia of symbolic actions or apraxia of utilization of objects.[12]

Any one or a combination of the apraxias can be seen in an individual patient. Because all aspects of ADL require the effective planning and carrying out of skilled purposeful movement, the apraxic patient is faced with a frustrating and devastating residual deficit of brain injury.

Tests of Ideational and Ideomotor Apraxia

Ideomotor apraxia is an inability to carry out a motor act on command, but the patient is able to perform the act automatically. The patient may be able to describe the intended motion verbally, but is unable to execute the motor act at will. Observations of the patient in activity performance is critical to the identification of this deficit. Ideational apraxia is an inability to form the concept of the movement and inability to execute the act in response to a commend or automatically.[23]

Full test batteries of ideational and ideomotor apraxia have been developed.[9,21] Each of these evaluations differentiates praxis abilities with certain body parts (i.e., buccal-facial, unilateral limb, bilateral limb, and total body movements) and by level of concreteness (i.e., on command, imitation, object usage, and nonrepresentational movements). Box 14-1 describes a sample praxis evaluation developed at Santa Clara Valley Medical Center.[45] This screening evaluation is used as an indicator for the need of a more complete praxis evaluation.

Treatment of Ideomotor and Ideational Apraxia

Treatment of ideational and ideomotor apraxia is difficult. Short, clear, concise, and concrete instructions are necessary, because this apraxia is usually the result of a dominant hemisphere lesion; often aphasia is present as well. The task should be broken down into its component steps, and each step should be taught separately. Verbal and demonstrated instructions may be ineffective, and it can be helpful to guide the patient through the correct movements, giving tactile and proprioceptive input to the instruction while also giving brief verbal instruction. After the patient has performed each step of the task separately, the therapist can begin to combine the steps, grading to the complete task.[44] An example of a complete task is hair combing. The therapist can break the task into steps: lift comb; bring comb to hair; move comb across top of head, down left side, down right side, down back; and replace comb on table. Much repetition is necessary to be effective.

Tests of Constructional Apraxia

Constructional apraxia is a deficit in the ability to copy, draw, or construct a design, whether on command or spontaneously.[23] It is the inability to organize or assemble parts into a whole, as in putting together block designs (three-dimensional) or drawings (two-dimensional). This perceptual motor impairment is commonly seen in persons with severe head injury or CVA and is related to a dysfunction of the parietal lobes. Constructional apraxia causes significant dysfunction in ADL that require constructional ability, such as dressing, following instructions for assembling a toy, and stacking a dishwasher. Research has demonstrated its strong correlation with body scheme, dressing, daily living skills, and the ability to use objects purposefully.[5,26,37,42] Figure 14-3, which shows evidence of left neglect, also demonstrates constructional apraxia.

Traditional tests of constructional praxis are the Test of Visual-Motor Skills,[19] the copy administration of the Benton Visual Retention Test[36] and the Rey Complex Figure.[25] The Three-Dimensional Block Construction[6] evaluates three-dimensional constructional praxis. Nonstandardized tests that may be used are drawing, constructing matchstick designs, assembling block designs, or building a structure to match a model. In daily living, tasks such as dressing or table setting require constructional skills. To perform such tasks successfully, there must be integration of visual perception, motor planning, and motor execution.[6,21,31,41,44] A wide variety of tasks is used to evaluate praxis, and test administration differs from one to another.[16] Several studies have gathered data on constructional praxis of unimpaired subjects for use as normative reference for patients with CVA and traumatic brain injury (TBI).[16,31] In a study of constructional praxis in the well elderly, Fall[16] demonstrated that results are influenced by the type of test administration. Subjects tended to score higher on tests that used three-dimensional models as guides for construction than on those that used photographs or drawings. The implications of this finding for occupational therapists are that (1) the type of test administration affects scores, and (2) in teaching patients with construction apraxia, models or demonstration of desired performance will produce better results than the photographs or drawings.[16]

Treatment of Constructional Apraxia

Using a transfer of training approach, the patient may practice simple copying and constructional tasks. Guidance, demonstration, and three-dimensional models may be necessary. The use of landmarks in simple designs may be helpful. Tasks can be graded in complexity (e.g., number of pieces to assemble). The patient can draw on a clay board or in sand rather than on paper to get additional proprioceptive input.[44]

Dressing Apraxia

Dressing apraxia, the inability to plan and perform the motor acts necessary to dress oneself, has been linked with problems of body scheme, spatial orientation, and constructional apraxia.[28,40] Clinically, the patient may have difficulty initiating dressing or may make errors in orientation by putting the clothes on the wrong side of the body, upside down, or inside out.[2]

Treatment of Dressing Apraxia

The therapist teaches a set pattern for dressing and gives cues that help the patient distinguish right from left or

BOX 14-1

PRAXIS (MOTOR PLANNING)

PROCEDURE

The examiner sits directly in front of the patient. The examiner asks the patient to demonstrate or copy actions in the following sequence. First the examiner asks the patient to demonstrate each verbal command listed below. If the patient is unable to perform the action, the examiner demonstrates the action and asks the patient to imitate it. After all items are completed to command and imitation, items 1 through 5 are repeated with the examiner asking the patient to use the real object.

TIME

10 seconds for each item (the examiner times the patient from the start of the gesture to the end of the gesture).

DIRECTIONS

"I AM GOING TO ASK YOU TO TRY SOME DIFFERENT ACTIONS. IN SOME OF THEM, I WILL ASK YOU TO DEMONSTRATE OR COPY MY MOVEMENTS, AND IN SOME I WILL ASK YOU TO USE OBJECTS."

To command
1. "SHOW ME HOW YOU BLOW OUT A MATCH."
2. "SHOW ME HOW YOU DRINK A GLASS OF WATER."
3. "SHOW ME HOW YOU BRUSH YOUR TEETH WITH A TOOTHBRUSH."
4. "SHOW ME HOW YOU CUT PAPER WITH SCISSORS."
5. "SHOW ME HOW YOU THROW A BALL."
6. "SHOW ME HOW YOU SALUTE."
7. "SHOW ME HOW YOU WASH YOUR HANDS."
8. "SHOW ME HOW YOU ACT LIKE A BOXER."

To imitations
The examiner carries out the actions for each test item stating "I AM BLOWING OUT A MATCH, NOW YOU SHOW ME HOW YOU . . .

With the object
The examiner presents the real object for items 1 to 5 and states, "SHOW ME HOW YOU . . . "

Note: During this portion of the test, the examiner should ensure the patient's safe handling of the objects. For bilateral tasks (command 4), the examiner may assist by holding the paper.

Observe for
1. Type of apraxia indicated:
   a. Blowing out match (buccal-facial)
   b. Drinking from glass (buccal-facial, unilateral limb kinetic)
   c. Brushing teeth (buccal-facial, unilateral limb kinetic)
   d. Cutting with scissors (unilateral limb kinetic)
   e. Throwing a ball (unilateral or bilateral limb kinetic)
   f. Saluting (cultural, unilateral limb kinetic)
   g. Washing hands (bilateral limb kinetic)
   h. Boxing (bilateral limb kinetic)
2. Use of body part as the object (BPO)
3. Performance in the correct place of movement (PLM)
4. Which body parts the patient uses to carry out verbal/imitation commands
5. Which movements are easier toward or away from the body
6. Differences in performance: unilateral vs. bilateral, objects vs. no object, verbal vs. imitation

Scale
Rate each item separately:
3 = Unable to perform; unable to attempt response
2 = Severely impaired; poor approximation of accurate response, uses trial and error and response is greater than allotted time
1 = Impaired; able to approximate accurate response for majority of the task, quality or response is compromised or response is greater than allotted time
0 = Intact; response is accurate and within allotted time

Adapted from Zoltan B and associates: *Perceptual motor evaluation for head injured and other neurologically impaired adults*, rev ed, San José, Calif, 1987, Santa Clara Valley Medical Center.

front from back. A helpful method is to have the patient position the garment the same way each time, such as a shirt with the buttons face up and pants with the zipper face up. Labels can be used as cues to differentiate the front from the back of the garment. The garment may be color-coded with small buttons or ribbons for front and back or right and left side.[44]

GENERAL PRINCIPLES OF TREATMENT OF APRAXIA

Understanding the underlying mechanisms and identifying the point of breakdown in a particular action or task is crucial to the effective treatment of apraxia.[28] Activity analysis will identify not only that a patient is unable to put on his shirt but also when and how performance breaks down.[43] Several treatment approaches have proved successful for the treatment of the patient with apraxia. The remedial or transfer of training approach is widely used for constructional apraxia. A functional or adaptive approach combined with the neurodevelopmental approach is effective for the patient with dressing apraxia. Although there may be occasions when a single approach is indicated, more often a combination of techniques or approaches is most effective.[5]

SUMMARY

Perceptual motor deficits affect the patient's overall function. Problems vary in intensity and diversity, depending on the patient's diagnosis and area of brain damage. A systematic comprehensive evaluation of perceptual motor functions is crucial to facilitating achievement of the highest functional potential. The information provided in this chapter is meant to be an overview of the key deficit areas and their clinical evaluation. The reader should seek additional resources for other specific evaluation techniques and procedures.

REVIEW QUESTIONS

1. Why are stereognosis and graphesthesia considered higher aspects of sensory function?
2. How would you adapt a stereognosis test for a patient with aphasia?
3. What are some suggestions for retraining for stereognosis?
4. Which should be evaluated first, praxis or body scheme? Why?
5. List and define the four potential areas of a body scheme disorder.
6. Define apraxia.
7. List four types of apraxia and tell how each can affect ability to perform daily living skills.
8. How is constructional apraxia evaluated?
9. Describe four approaches to treatment of perceptual deficits and give one example of a treatment activity for each.
10. Why is the sensory-integrative approach considered impractical for adult patients?

REFERENCES

1. Anderson E, Choy E: Parietal lobe syndromes in hemiplegia: a program for treatment, *Am J Occup Ther* 24(1):13, 1970.
2. Archibald YM, Wepman JM: Language disturbance and non-verbal cognitive performance in eight patients following injury to the right hemisphere, *Brain* 91:117, 1968.
3. Arnadottir G: *The brain and behavior: assessing cortical dysfunction through activities of daily living,* St Louis, 1990, CV Mosby.
4. Ayres AJ: *Sensory integration and learning disorders,* Los Angeles, 1972, Western Psychological Services.
5. Baum B, Hall K: Relationship between constructional praxis and dressing in the head injured adult, *Am J Occup Ther* 35:438, 1981.
6. Benton AL, Fogel ML: Three-dimensional constructional praxis: a clinical test, *Arch Neurol* 7:347, 1962.
7. Benton AL, Schultz LM: Observations of tactile form perception (stereognosis) in pre-school children, *J Clin Psychol* 5:359, 1949.
8. Boone P, Landes B: Right-left discrimination in hemiplegic patients, *Arch Phys Med Rehabil* 49:533, 1968.
9. Brown J: *Aphasia, apraxia, agnosia,* Springfield, Ill, 1972, Thomas Publishers.
10. Chusid JG: *Correlative neuroanatomy and functional neurology,* ed 19, Los Altos, Calif, 1985, Lange Medical Publications.
11. Critchley M: *The parietal lobes,* London, 1953, Edward Arnold.
12. Dee HL: Visuoconstructive and visuoreceptive deficit in patients with unilateral cerebral lesions, *Neuropsychologia* 8:305, 1970.
13. DeJong R: *The neurologic examination,* New York, 1958, Paul B. Hoeber.
14. DeRenzi E, Scotti G: Autotopagnosia: fiction or reality, *Arch Neurol* 23: 221, 1970.
15. Eggers O: Occupational therapy in the treatment of adult hemiplegia, Rockville, Md, 1984, Aspen Systems.
16. Fall CC: Comparing ways of measuring constructional praxis in the well elderly, *Am J Occup Ther* 41:500, 1987.
17. Farber SD: *Neurorehabiliation, a multisensory approach,* Philadelphia, 1982, WB Saunders.
18. Ferreri JA: Intensive stereognostic training, *Am J Occup Ther* 16:141, 1962.
19. Gardner MF: *The test of visual-motor skills (TVMS),* Burlingame, Calif, 1992, Psychological and Educational Publications.
20. Gilroy J, Meyer JS: *Medical neurology,* London, 1969, Macmillan.

21. Goodglass H, Kaplan E: *Assessment of aphasia and related disorders,* ed 2, Philadelphia, 1972, Thomas Publishers.
22. Head H and associates: *Studies in neurology,* London, 1920, Oxford University Press.
23. Hécaen H, Albert ML: *Human neuropsychology,* New York, 1978, John Wiley and Sons.
24. Kent BE: Sensory-motor testing: the upper limb of adult patients with hemiplegia, *Phy Ther J Am Phys Ther Assoc* 45:550, 1965.
25. Lezak MD: *Neuropsychological assessment,* ed 2, New York, 1983, Oxford University Press.
26. Lorenze EJ, Cancro R: Dysfunction in visual perception with hemiplegia: its relationship to activities of daily living, *Arch Phys Med Rehabil* 43:514, 1962.
27. MacDonald J: An investigation of body scheme in adults with cerebral vascular accident, *Am J Occup Ther* 14:72, 1960.
28. Miller N: Dyspraxia and its management, Rockville, Md, 1986, Aspen Publishers.
29. Mountcastle VB: The view from within: pathways to the study of perception, *Johns Hopkins Med J,* 136:109, 1975.
30. Neistadt ME: Occupational therapy for adults with perceptual deficits, *Am J Occup Ther* 42:434, 1988.
31. Neistadt ME: Normal adult performance on constructional praxis training tasks, *Am J Occup Ther* 43: 448, 1989.
32. Neistadt ME: A critical analysis of occupational therapy approaches for perceptual deficits in adults with brain injury, *Am J Occup Ther* 44:299, 1990.
33. Occupational Therapy Department, Rancho Los Amigos Hospital: *Upper extremity sensory evaluation: a manual for occupational therapists,* Downey, Calif, 1985.
34. Okkema K: *Cognition and perception in the stroke patient: a guide to functional outcomes in occupational therapy,* Gaithersburg, Md, 1993, Aspen Publishers.
35. Sauget J, Benton AL, Hécaen H: Disturbances of the body scheme in relation to language impairment and hemispheric locus of lesion, *J Neuro Neurosurg Psych* 34:496, 1971.
36. Sivan AB: *The Benton visual retention test,* San Antonio, Tex, 1992, The Psychological Corporation.
37. Titus MND and associates: Correlation of perceptual performance and activities of daily living in stroke patients, *Am J Occup Ther* 45:410, 1991.
38. Vinograd A, Taylor E, Grossman S: Sensory retraining of the hemiplegic hand, *Am J Occup Ther* 16: 246, 1962.
39. Walsh K: *Neuropsychology: a clinical approach,* Edinburgh, Scotland, 1987, Churchill Livingstone.
40. Warren M: Relationship of constructional apraxia and body scheme disorders to dressing performance in adult CVA, *Am J Occup Ther* 35:431, 1981.
41. Warrington E, James M, Kinsborne M: Drawing ability in relation to laterality of lesion, *Brain* 89:53, 1966.
42. Williams N: Correlations between copying ability and dressing activities in hemiplegia, *Am J Phys Med* 46:1332, 1967.
43. Zoltan B: Remediation of visual, perceptual and perceptual motor deficits. In M Rosenthal, editor: *Rehabilitation of the adult and child with traumatic brain injury,* ed 2, Philadelphia, 1989, FA Davis.
44. Zoltan B, Siev E, Freishtat B: *Perceptual and cognitive dysfunction in the adult stroke patient,* ed 2, Thorofare, NJ, 1986, Charles B Slack.
45. Zoltan B and associates: *Perceptual motor evaluation for head injured and other neurologically impaired adults,* rev ed, San José, Calif, 1987, Santa Clara Valley Medical Center.

C H A P T E R   1 5

Evaluation and Treatment of Cognitive Dysfunction

Carol J. Wheatley

Cognitive deficits are perhaps the most devastating residual problems following a cerebral vascular accident (CVA), traumatic brain injury (TBI), or acquired disease resulting in brain damage. Cognition involves the skills of understanding and knowing, the ability to judge and make decisions, and an overall general environmental awareness.[18] Cognitive processing spans a wide continuum. It can involve multiple sensory input from external sources or can be carried on with only intrinsic material. Cognition allows individuals to use and process the information perceived to think and act.

Metacognition, described as "knowing about knowing,"[25] is the ability to know and monitor the individual characteristics of cognitive skills. It is considered the bridge that links together all the various aspects of cognition, and enables a person to choose memory strategies, problem-solving approaches, and reasoning methods that are uniquely beneficial to the completion of a cognitive activity.[46]

The identification and clinical evaluation of discrete cognitive deficits is challenging and complex. Deficit areas are rarely seen in isolation, and the interpretation of a patient's behavior is difficult at best. There are, however, several categories of cognitive deficits that can and should be identified and treated by the occupational therapist along with other allied health professionals. These areas include attention, memory, initiation, planning and organization, mental flexibility, abstraction, insight, problem solving, and calculation abilities. The material in this chapter outlines relevant theoretical principles, and describes additional factors that influence cognitive function, and provides evaluation and treatment applications for these deficit areas.

PRINCIPLES OF COGNITIVE EVALUATION

Therapists should follow established guidelines in evaluating cognitive abilities. The following three guidelines[79] are particularly important:

1. Identify the components of the particular skill to be evaluated that are relatively intact vs. those that are impaired.
2. Observe the patient in a number of settings and activities at different times during the day. Position changes (lying, sitting) can also affect performance, as well as somatic factors (hunger, pain).
3. Using standardized tests and functional activities, establish functional baseline measures. Consider the frequency and severity of the problem. These tests and activities can be used at regular intervals to measure progress.

Several test batteries are available that screen a range of cognitive skills, including the following: the Middlesex Elderly Assessment of Mental State,[29] the Cognitive Assessment of Minnesota,[56] and the Neurobehavioral Cognitive Status Screening Examination.[33] The Arnadottir OT-ADL Neurobehavioral Evaluation (A-ONE) provides an analysis of functional activities to determine cognitive skill deficit areas.[7] The Cognitive Rehabilitation Workbook provides a pre/post test, as well as treatment exercises, for community living skills such as constructing a schedule and reading a map.[23]

THEORETICAL PRINCIPLES OF COGNITIVE EVALUATION

Several theoretical principles should be incorporated into the administration and interpretation of the clinical cognitive evaluation.

Cognition and Other Deficits

Cognition should always be considered in relation to other potential deficit areas. The quality of cognitive processes and skills depends on the integrity of the patient's sensory, language, visual, and perceptual systems. For example, the patient may be unable to attend to and concentrate on a particular task mainly because of an underlying deficit in visual scanning. This interrelationship makes it crucial that the occupational therapist administer the sensory, visual, and perceptual evaluations before initiating cognitive testing.

Team Approach to Evaluation

Discussion of the occupational therapy evaluation results with the other members of the team increases the therapist's understanding of the patient's capacity. The occupational therapy approach to cognitive skills tends to emphasize the processing of visual, tactile, and spatial information, which are largely mediated by the right hemisphere of the brain. Consultation with the speech pathologist concerning the patient's auditory, language, and linguistic/cognitive abilities is essential because these skills are processed mostly by the left brain hemisphere. Physical therapists can provide observations on the patient's visual perceptual functioning during gross motor and ambulation tasks. The psychologist or neuropsychologist can provide information regarding the individual's intellectual range with an overview of the relative strengths and weakness of the various skills. In addition, the family can provide the team with a description of the patient's functioning before the onset of the disability. Without prior knowledge of all these areas, interpretation of the occupational therapy cognitive evaluation may be inaccurate and invalid. The therapist should always look at the total picture when interpreting patient behavior, and frequently, the conclusions are the result of much team discussion.[43,63] The team may also include the physician, therapeutic recreation specialist, and other disciplines, depending on the goals of the facility.

Testing Environment

The testing environment influences the results of the cognitive evaluation. The concept of environment includes not only the physical features and time of day, but the amount of structure and feedback provided by the examiner as well. For example, the patient's ability to attend to tasks may be very different early in the morning while lying in bed compared with taking a structured test while in a wheelchair with cuing provided by the examiner. The patient's behavior in the foreign environment of the hospital or rehabilitation facility may be quite different from performance in the familiar home setting. Controversy among health team members about the patient's cognitive status often occurs when, in fact, discrepancies are merely the result of environmental differences in the administration and nature of testing. Instead of being alarmed by these differences in test results, the more constructive approach is to analyze and use the information in designing the most effective remediation plan.

Optimal Test Battery

The optimal test battery involves a selection of tests, standardized and normed for the population, as well as a variety of functional activities, for example, homemaking. Therapists need standardized tests to provide objective, quantifiable data, to measure the extent of the deficit compared to an established norm, to document progress, and to enable discharge planning. In addition, the common terminology, concepts, and testing conditions of standardized tests facilitate communication between practitioners. Functional activities provide opportunities to observe the practical implications of the deficits revealed by the standardized tests, known as ecological validity,[31,39] and allows the therapist better to predict the person's functioning in the home environment.

Therapist's Approach

When introducing a cognitive test to a patient, the therapist should avoid a condescending attitude or a too bright, false positive manner. No matter what the level of functioning, the patient still deserves to be approached on an age-appropriate level. It is important not to offer choices when there actually aren't any, such as "Would you like to do some tests today?" Instead, offer choices between tests: "Would you prefer to perform coordination tests or cognitive tests?" while acknowledging that all of the tests must be completed eventually. Don't ask for cooperation as a personal favor ("I would like you to . . .") or imply that the test is a joint effort ("Let's do some testing today!"). Instead, recognize each person's responsibility, by such phrases as "Here are some geometric shapes, and your job is . . . ." It is also important that the therapist does not provide cues as to the patient's right or wrong responses: as an alternative, randomly reward the patient's effort throughout the test by such comments as: "Good job", or "You put a lot of effort into that test."[35]

Test Administration

It is vital that the therapist adhere to the instructions that accompany standardized tests, or the results of the tests are invalidated. It is possible, however, to test beyond the limits of a standardized assessment tool by following the rules as given, but once completed, exploring various modifications and, importantly, documenting the adaptations and results.[35] Frequently the therapist develops a repertoire of management strategies to support the optimum functioning of the patient, but because the strategies are seldom documented, they must be rediscovered (or sometimes not) by other therapists who are working with that individual.

Cognition and Aging

The final principle of cognitive evaluation relates to the elderly patient with brain damage. In the normal aging process, linguistic skills of reading and writing, general intellectual capacity, arithmetic, and immediate memory remain relatively stable. The older adult, however, tends to process information more slowly, is less mentally flexible, and has more difficulty with abstract concepts and learning large amounts of material.[15] In addition, research indicates that the elderly are more easily distracted than younger individuals.[20] It is therefore crucial that, before testing the elderly patient with brain damage, the therapist have a clear picture of the patient's premorbid cognitive functioning. This information can usually be provided by the patient's family and friends.

An area of growing concern to geriatric therapists is the patient with Alzheimer dementia.[47] Seven levels of cognitive decline have been identified, based on the patient's cognitive status and functioning in everyday tasks.[52] The goal of therapeutic intervention is to maximize the patient's functioning, increase safety, minimize confusion, develop behavioral management strategies, and serve as a resource to families.[8,21,28]

APPROACHES TO TREATMENT

The treatment of cognitive deficits should follow the same principles outlined previously. Various treatment approaches proposed in occupational therapy literature include the following:

- The *adaptive* approach focuses on the skills that are relatively intact, to develop compensatory methods for deficit areas. Treatment activities are functional, real-life tasks.[44,45]
- The *remedial,* or transfer of training, approach uses practice with activities designed to target the deficit areas. Typically, table top pencil-and-paper tasks are used, involving skills that have been found to be deficient by formal testing.[79]
- The *process* approach emphasizes the therapist's need to continuously adapt the treatment to the patient's changing status and the changing environment. Treatment guides the patient through the sequence of detection, discrimination and analysis, and hypothesis generation while performing therapeutic activities.[1,2]
- The *multicontext treatment* approach uses factors external to the patient (environmental context, nature of the task, and criteria of learning) as well as internal factors (metacognition, processing strategies, and the characteristics of the learner). A particular strategy is targeted and practiced in multiple environments to increase the likelihood of transfer, with a variety of tasks and movement demands.[67]
- *Applied behavioral analysis* has been used to retrain for functional skills, using the behavioral approaches of shaping, fading, and reinforcement.[27]

- *Sensory-integration* theory has been applied to adults with brain damage,[9,79] as has the *cognitive disability* theory developed for patients with psychiatric diseases.[3,4] The reader is also referred to Chapter 12 for details regarding the use of the *hierarchical* model of visual processing with recommendations for treatment.

Therapists may choose to follow a certain treatment philosophy or may adopt a more eclectic approach, blending treatment models based on the response of the patient.

A treatment task can be analyzed and modified in several ways to increase a patient's performance.[65] This process, commonly referred to as providing structure, does not provide information regarding the specific types of cuing or feedback the therapist found valuable. A treatment activity can be graded by changing the task parameters, which include the environment, familiarity with the task, directions for completing the task, number of items, spatial arrangement of items, and response rate required.

Examples of task grading are the treatment of an inattentive patient in a quiet, uncluttered environment and the treatment of the patient with poor memory in the same environment every day. Various environmental cues can be established in the person's work area to stimulate recall.

Cues are provided via systematic interpersonal interaction with the therapist or others and modified according to the patient's response. Cues can direct a patient's attention to a particular aspect of a task, guide problem solving, and facilitate recall. Examples of cues are repetition ("Try again"), analysis ("What do these objects have in common?"), and direction of attention ("Look here on your left").[68] Whenever possible, the patient should be involved in the development of the cuing system, because the patient will select those cues that are most meaningful.

The therapist must always be aware that the ultimate goal of treatment is the internalization of cues or reduction of need for environmental cuing for successful performance.[79]

The following eight-step model provides a framework for the approach of treatment:

1. Select a task or strategy
2. Obtain a baseline measure.
3. Set goals with the client.
4. Choose and teach strategies.
5. Practice strategies.
6. Obtain a post practice measure.
7. Develop transfer and generalization strategies for real-life situations.
8. Practice transfer and generalization.[30]

The aging process affects an individual's cognitive abilities, although treatment has been shown to improve performance.[10] It is important for the therapist to keep this fact in mind when treating the elderly patient with brain damage. Repetition and practice are important, as are limiting distractions and extraneous information.[5,53] In addition, the therapist should always allow enough time for the patient to respond and use appropriate sensory cuing whenever possible. Several resources offer a variety of treatment tasks and ideas.[19,23,69,79]

COMPUTERS IN COGNITIVE RETRAINING

Computers for cognitive rehabilitation were once thought to hold great promise as an independent treatment modality, but expectations have lessened in recent years.[54] Currently computers are viewed as a valuable tool for rehabilitation, because they provide a means by which to practice cognitive skills that are taught by the therapist.[30] Documented research studies are beginning to support the efficacy of computers to augment a multifaceted cognitive rehabilitation program.[34,39] For successful application, the therapist must keep up with state-of-the-art software and critically analyze what is currently available.

Before the clinician selects a computer system, the available software for that particular system should be explored.[38] Available software includes games, educational programs, and software specifically designed for cognitive rehabilitation.[30] Specific programs can be purchased for remediation of deficits in arithmetic, attention and concentration, concept formation, nonverbal memory, reasoning, association, categorization, cause and effect, problem solving, organization, generalization, level of abstraction, judgment of safety, spatial orientation, sequencing, and verbal memory.

An additional consideration in computer-assisted cognitive rehabilitation is the input device. Patients with brain damage may require a mouse, inverted trackball, oversized joystick, light pen, or touch screen to compensate for specific motor deficits. These and other adaptive input devices may also require additional custom adaptations by the occupational therapist.[30,40]

Computers have enabled the development of a number of electronic devices that can be used in compensation for cognitive and memory impairments.[48] These include alarm watches, pocket computerized data storage units, electronic pillboxes, and telephones with phone number memory features.

For additional information on computer resources for individuals with disabilities and specific software used to treat these and other related areas, the reader is referred to Chapter 28 and references 22, 30, 32, 34, and 41.

EVALUATION AND TREATMENT OF SPECIFIC DEFICIT AREAS

Just as cognitive function is interdependent with basic sensory input, specific cognitive skills are also interdependent. For example, an individual cannot display effective problem-solving skills if he or she cannot attend to or remember a particular task. Therefore, a specific progression of testing should be followed that reflects a hierarchy of cognitive skills. Following is the recommended sequence of testing.

ORIENTATION AND ATTENTION

Orientation refers to an individual's ongoing awareness of the situation, the environment, and the passage of time. Immediately following any traumatic injury, a person must develop an awareness of the events that preceded the accident and those occurring since that time. Following a CVA, the individual frequently is disoriented initially, and as the mental state clears, orientation to surroundings increases. A TBI can result in a period of coma, the length of which is indicative of the severity of injury. See also Chapters 41 and 42 on cerebral vascular accidents and traumatic head injury for further discussion.

An unimpaired person is typically oriented to person (Who am I?), to place (Where am I?), and to time (What year, month, day, or time of day is it?). Orientation is related to an individual's memory capacity, because a person must be able to remember past occurrences to place current events in their proper perspective. Following a severe TBI or CVA, a person may initially be confused regarding identity, which indicates a *disorientation to person.* This deficit is more global than an inability to speak one's name, which may occur in the case of aphasia (difficulty with the verbal expression of any message). The patient may also confuse the identities of other individuals, such as thinking that the therapist is a family member. *Orientation to place* refers to an individual's knowledge of the fact that he or she is in a hospital, for example, or the name of the immediate town, city, and state. Difficulty in monitoring the passage of time can result in *time disorientation.* Patients often have difficulty beyond simply remembering the date; they may confuse the sequence of events in time. For example, a patient may report that a certain family member visited the previous day, when that person actually may have visited a week earlier. As with all aspects of cognition, discussion with other team members is critical to ensure a comprehensive understanding of the patient's deficit.

Topographical orientation describes an individual's awareness of his or her position in relationship to the environment: the room, building, town, for example. Functional examples of this disorder are noted when a patient becomes confused while attempting to leave a room, locate another therapy department, or travel to the cafeteria. These individuals frequently perform better in the familiar environment of the home and community, but deficits may still be apparent.

Attention is an active process that allows the individual to focus on the environmental information and sensations that are relevant at a particular time. Attention involves the simultaneous engagement of alertness, selectivity, sustained effort, flexibility, and mental tracking.[64] A patient must be alert and awake and able to select a relevant focus of interest. The patient must be able to maintain focus for as long as needed, yet be able to shift focus if another event of interest or importance occurs. In addition, the person must ignore information if it is not relevant and must be able to track multiple sequences of information simultaneously. Because these skills underlie all aspects of cognitive functioning, they are frequently affected by TBI or CVA, and deficits may hinder all higher skill levels. For example, a patient who is unable to attend to a task for more than a few seconds cannot take in all the necessary information to perform a higher level reasoning task.

The two types of information processing relevant to attention are *automatic* and *controlled processing.*[77] Automatic processing is used by the individual at a subcortical level, whereas controlled processing is used when new information is being considered. Two disorders, focused attentional deficit and divided attentional deficits, are related to these two types of information processing. A focused attentional deficit occurs when an automatic response is replaced by a controlled response. An example of this deficit familiar to many clinicians is the patient with a CVA concentrating on trying to walk. A divided attentional deficit, on the other hand, occurs when the function of controlled processing is inadequate for the individual to process all the information required for task completion. This deficit results in the patient becoming "overloaded." The patient typically responds by reverting to focused attention. For example, if the patient with a CVA is asked a question while ambulating, he or she will frequently stop walking to engage in conversation.

Concentration requires sustained focused attention, also referred to as *vigilance.* Patients may be highly distractible or very sensitive to events in their immediate environment, which pulls their focus away from the task at hand. It is important to note which types of stimuli (e.g., visual, auditory, tactile, gustatory), appear to distract the patient easily. A low stimulus environment or "quiet room" is frequently available in various areas of the hospital or rehabilitation center. This room is designed for minimal visual stimuli and insulation from nearby noise and activity. Some individuals have the opposite problem on the continuum. That is, they can become very deeply focused on a given stimulus or activity and have difficulty maintaining a general awareness of events occurring around them. Each extreme is undesirable; an unimpaired individual is able to focus, sustain a low-level of awareness of peripheral events, and disengage, then reengage concentration as needed.

Evaluation of Orientation and Attention

Orientation to person, time, and place can be assessed informally by asking the patient basic questions about his or her identity, the date, time of day, season of the year, and the name of the hospital, city, and state. Because patients' levels of orientation can vary, it is best to ask these questions several times to determine the consistency of the patient's awareness. Topographical orientation can be assessed by observing a patient travel from one site to another or by asking the patient to draw a floorplan of his or her room, therapy area, or home, verifying the latter with the family. Orientation questions and route-finding are also included as part of the Rivermead Behavioural Memory Test.[75]

Examples of standardized tests of attention include the Knox Cube Test[61] and Trail Making Test.[6] The reader is referred to references 35 and 79 for additional information on these and other standardized tests of attention. The occupational therapist's evaluation of attention should include structured clinical observation and activity analysis during functional tasks.

Treatment of Orientation and Attention

Orientation. Efforts should be made by all staff and family who come into contact with the patient to reestablish orientation as frequently as possible. External aids such as calendars, bulletin boards, and "orientation boards" with pertinent information (for example, the name of the facility, the date, season, and current events) are often used in rehabilitation centers. An orientation group can be scheduled to meet at the start of each day to review the day's upcoming events and previous day's happenings.[37]

Attention. The initial goal of treatment is to identify the optimal environment that enables the patient to attend for the longest time. As attention and concentration improve, the therapist can increase the duration as well as the complexity of the activity. Finally, the patient should be gradually weaned from the low-stimulus environment as tolerance increases. Formalized attention-training models are available.[13,48,60]

MEMORY

Memory is a dynamic continuation of the attentional process that includes the factor of time. As an individual is able to maintain focus on a task, the information becomes stored in the memory process. Memory requires environmental input, central nervous system (CNS) change, maintenance of that change, and related behavioral or informational output.[24] The memory process is summarized in Fig. 15-1. Breakdown of the memory process can occur at any level. If a patient is unable to attend, the information may never enter the system. Some patients are able to process information in short-term or working memory, but never encode the material into long-term storage. Others can store the information, but have a deficit in the retrieval process. Patients with memory deficits, who need to expend additional effort to learn new material, may also have difficulty forgetting information when it is no longer needed. It is critical that the therapist be well prepared when planning to teach new information to a patient, to avoid the necessity to

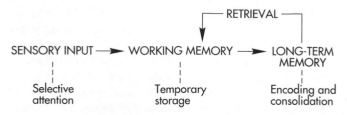

FIG. 15-1   The memory process.

force the person to unlearn, then relearn new information or procedures.

The ability to recite or reproduce information is generally taken as an indication of recall and is referred to as *declarative memory*. Often tests require a person to repeat a word list or draw a set of geometric designs, or a therapist may quiz a patient about events occurring earlier in the day. Declarative memory is subdivided into two categories. *Episodic memory* refers to an individual's personal history and lifetime of experiences. *Semantic memory* describes the general fund of knowledge shared by groups of people, such as language and rules of social behavior. This type of memory is generally less affected following injury.[30]

Some patients may have a considerable deficit in declarative memory, but their *procedural memory,* memory for a skill or series of actions,[30] may be less impaired. For example, a person may be unable to tell a therapist the steps in making a sandwich and cup of coffee, but may be able to perform the activity relatively correctly. It is this skill that enables a patient to learn new self-care techniques despite severe memory deficits on standardized memory tests. This phenomenon underscores the need for integration between test performance and observations made during functional activities.

Everyday memory refers to a person's ability to remember information pertinent to daily life,[76] for example, learning the names and faces of the doctors, nurses, and therapy staff who work regularly with the patient in the hospital or rehabilitation facility. Learning a schedule of appointments or the locations of various departments may be difficult and further complicated by frequent changes; therefore the hospital escort staff often assume this responsibility for the patient. Everyday memory also includes the ability to keep track of daily events in their proper sequence. *Prospective memory* refers to the ability to remember events that are set to occur at some future time, such as an appointment scheduled for later in the day.[76]

A person with memory deficits may tend to *confabulate*,[70] or to fill in the gaps in memory with imaginary material.[70] The person is not aware of adding erroneous information to the factual data and so can become very confused regarding past events. Some memory-deficit patients may deliberately try to "fake it" to cover their embarrassment at the extent of their memory loss, but this practice is not generally considered confabulation.

Just as for any individual, activities or topics of interest or of personal relevance to the patient tend to elicit the best performance. As a result, the family may minimize the deficit: "He can remember if he wants to." It is important to reinforce to the family that, although the impairment may be less with certain types of material, the deficit remains.

Evaluation of Memory Functions

Standardized tests for the evaluation of visual memory include the Benton Visual Retention Test,[58] the Rey Complex Figure,[35] and selected subtests of the Test of Visual Perceptual Skills (TVPS).[26] The Learning Efficiency Test[71] provides comparison of auditory vs. visual recall. The Rivermead Behavioural Memory Test[75] is an evaluation of everyday memory skills. The Contextual Memory Test[68] provides information on the awareness of the deficits and use of strategies.

Questionnaires such as the Subjective Memory Questionnaire[12] can also be valuable, and can be filled out by both the patient and a family member to determine the patient's level of awareness of his or her memory deficits.

Tests can be used to determine where the breakdown in the process occurs. For example, a patient may be unable to remember information in a free recall trial (with minimal or no cues), but may score high on a recognition task of the same information. This pattern suggests that the information was adequately stored in the system, but the patient has a deficit in retrieval. Treatment should then focus on the development of retrieval strategies.

Treatment of Memory Deficits

The occupational therapist, in concert with the psychologist, speech/language pathologist, and other team members, can explore the patient's optimal learning style.[50,73] Because flexibility in adapting to various teaching approaches is often lost or diminished following cognitive deficits, it becomes the responsibility of the therapist to present new information in the most efficient way for the patient. The therapist can identify a patient's learning style by observing the response to instructions (verbal, written, demonstrated, and diagrammatic) for standardized tests and functional activities, as well as by analyzing the data obtained from standardized memory tests. As characteristics of optimal teaching methods become apparent, this information can be communicated to the team, the patient's family, and to the patient, who can learn to request that new information be provided in the most effective manner.

Memory strategies can be divided into two groups: (1) internal, referring to techniques carried out via mental effort by the patient; and (2) external, referring to methods used by the therapist or cues in the environment to trigger an individual's recall. Examples of external cues are verbal reminders from the therapist, signs, cue cards, notebooks, written instructions, and electronic memory aids such as alarm watches and computer data storage units.[48,76] Internal mnemonic strategies include rehearsal, chunking, association, and imagery.[48,74]

The selection of mnemonic strategies can be based upon the characteristics of the learner. For example, a patient who has limited attention and concentration may not be able to use internal mnemonics, but may profit from strategically placed environmental cues. The goal of therapy is to progress from the use of external cues designed by the therapist to internal and external cues established and maintained by the patient independently. A group approach, empowering patients to guide the treatment process, has also been shown to be effective.[49]

The concepts of generalization and transfer are also critical to the learning of new skills. *Transfer of learning* refers to the application of information learned in one situation to another similar situation. *Generalization* refers to the ability to apply knowledge and skills learned to a variety of similar but novel situations.[48] Degrees of transfer can range from near to very far, based on analysis of task characteristics.[66] Individuals with cognitive deficits frequently have difficulty with transfer of learning and may be unable to generalize skills to novel situations. Transfer of new skills must be built into treatment planning, because the patient may not be able to perform such transfers independently. The concept of *domain-specific learning* is based on the assumption that global memory improvement is not likely to be achieved, but the patient is able to learn specific skills relative to a particular situation, and can continue to apply these skills in that environment.[57] An example is the patient who is taught one-handed cooking skills in the occupational therapy department kitchen, but is unable to generalize those skills to the kitchen at home. This patient may be better served if the instruction is provided in the home environment. Job coaching, a type of supported employment, is also based on this premise. The skills needed for the job are taught on the job site rather than being taught in advance training in a setting other than the job site.[72]

EXECUTIVE FUNCTIONS

Deficits in executive skills are generally the result of damage to the frontal lobes of the brain. The patient may demonstrate apathy, indifference, or decreased spontaneity. The patient may also exhibit a slowness of response or absence of initiative unless specifically instructed to perform the task.

Components of executive functioning include goal formation, planning, carrying out the plan, and effective performance.[35] An example of deficits in goal formation is the patient who doesn't think of anything to do, but may respond well to an established routine. On occasion the structured schedule of a hospital or rehabilitation facility may mask deficits in this area, which then become very apparent once the person is discharged to the home where there is less of a routine. Some patients may be

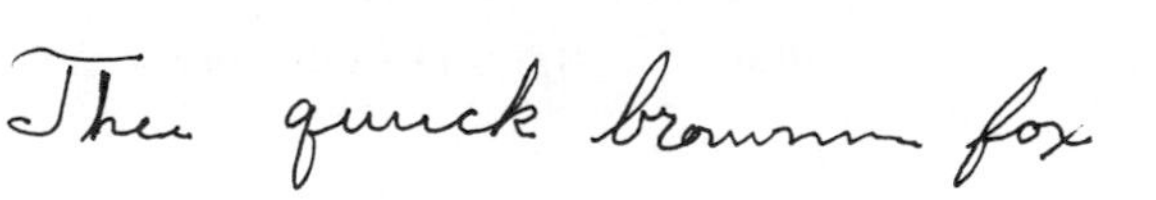

FIG. 15-2 Example of writing perseveration.

able to verbalize an intended goal and plan a course of action, but may be unable to carry it out. These patients often seem far more capable than their behavior actually demonstrates.

When trying to carry out the plan, a patient may demonstrate poor mental flexibility, resulting in perseverative or stimulus-bound behavior. *Perseveration,* which refers to the continuation or repetition of an action beyond its purpose, can be seen in motor acts, verbalizations, or thought processes. The patient can be referred to as having difficulty changing mental set. Fig. 15-2 provides an illustration of writing perseveration. An example of *stimulus-bound behavior* is the patient who impulsively begins the task before instructed or is unable to draw attention away from a task when necessary.

Effective performance requires that the patient continually monitor and adjust performance throughout the execution of the task. Some patients demonstrate an inability to perceive their errors, while others may recognize the error but make no effort to correct it.

Evaluation of Executive Functions

Family members are frequently the best source of information about the patient's executive functioning. A standardized means of observing of these skills is the Profile of Executive Control System (PRO-EX).[59] The therapist should also evaluate these skills through close clinical observation. A homemaking evaluation that involves planning and simultaneously preparing a variety of dishes for a meal may be useful. Perseverative or stimulus-bound behavior should be noted, both as related to a specific environment and to particular tasks.

The therapist must remember, however, that similar behaviors may be related to other clinical deficits such as poor comprehension or apraxia, or may be a sign of depression. Ongoing close observation, evaluation, and consultation with other team members increase the likelihood of correct interpretation and management of patient behavior.

Treatment of Executive Functions

The patient's level of awareness of the executive deficits will determine the treatment approach. A patient with relatively good metacognitive skills, one who can recognize, comprehend, and appreciate the implications of inactivity, may be responsive to self-monitoring strategies or environmental cues. A more severely impaired individual, one who cannot acknowledge or tends to devalue the deficit, may require supervision by another individual. A family member or significant other may be trained to set up a daily routine, provide the verbal prompts needed, and maintain the system of environmental cues established.

REASONING AND PROBLEM-SOLVING SKILLS

Abstract thinking enables a person to see relationships between objects, events, or ideas, to discriminate relevant from irrelevant detail, and to recognize absurdities.[35] These cognitive deficits and resultant behaviors create difficulty in transfer of knowledge to new situations and problem solving.[79] Patients with frontal lobe damage will often lose this ability and think only in the most concrete, literal manner. This literal thinking is often paired with mental inflexibility as described above.

The following is an example of concrete thinking. A patient is asked the interview question: "What brought you to this hospital?", to which the person responded: "My parent's car." The patient is interpreting the question literally, rather than understanding it as a reference to the accident that resulted in brain injury.

Mental processes can also be divided into *convergent thinking,* which enables a person to arrive at a central idea, and *divergent thinking,* which is aimed at generating alternatives.[78] The process of grocery shopping provides an example of both types of thinking. An individual knows that milk, eggs, and butter are needed and by convergent thinking identifies them as dairy products. Then divergent thinking is used to arrive at a list of stores which carry these items.

Problem solving is a complex process involving many cognitive skills. It requires attention, memory, planning and organization and the ability to reason and make judgments. Various types of reasoning can be used in the problem solving process. *Deductive reasoning,* refers to the ability to arrive at conclusions. For example, a patient notices that items grasped in the affected right hand tend to drop to the floor and concludes that the hand is not reliable for grasping and holding. *Inductive reasoning,* enables a person to draw generalizations from specific experiences. For example, after a period of consistent right hand impairments, the patient realizes that the ability to return to a previous occupation involving bilateral manual skills is now questionable.[14,78] The patient must be able to process complex information in order to plan new strategies and to evaluate established strategies.[16]

Evaluation of Reasoning and Problem Solving

Abstract conceptual thinking can be evaluated in a number of ways. The Test of Nonverbal Intelligence (TONI),[17] the Space Visualization subtest of the Employee Aptitude Series,[55] and the Minnesota Paper Formboard Test[36] all assess complex spatial reasoning skills. Object sorting tasks[62] can be useful, particularly for patients whose linguistic skills are limited.

Treatment of Reasoning and Problem-Solving Deficits

The steps that comprise the problem-solving process are as follows:

1. Define the problem.
2. Develop possible solutions.
3. Choose the best solution.
4. Execute the solution.
5. Evaluate the outcome.

This sequence can be taught to the patient, with instructions to use the steps when a problem is encountered in therapy or functional tasks.[14,78] In this manner, the therapist assists the patient in transferring this technique to a variety of situations.

DECREASED INSIGHT AND AWARENESS

Most therapists are familiar with the patient with brain damage who falls out of bed trying to walk to the bathroom despite paralysis. This behavior and others are the result of a lack of awareness or blatant denial of the limitations related to brain damage. This limited insight results in impulsive and unsafe behavior. The patient with this deficit is unable to monitor, correct, and regulate the quality of his or her behavior.[79] A patient's insight frequently increases as the body scheme is modified in response to changes imposed by the disability, which is a long and complex process.

Memory deficits may also complicate the patient's awareness of the frequency with which a problem occurs. For example, the patient who acknowledges difficulty recalling a nurse's name only 2 or 3 times a day may consider the memory problem minimal, although the incidence is actually closer to 12 to 15 times a day. Sometimes the use of a frequency checksheet, recorded by the patient under the supervision of the therapist, may help the person more fully understand the severity of the problem.

An individual may have *anosognosia,* a total inability to recognize deficits that exceeds conscious denial.[51] A team approach is needed to distinguish between neurological and psychological types of awareness deficits.[11] An example is a patient (with intact basic perceptual and language abilities) who cannot recognize her own handwriting on a task performed earlier in the day and accuses the therapist of falsifying the work. This patient may not be responsive to the most carefully designed awareness training program and may be unable to live independently without supervision.

Still other patients are able to recognize and discuss their inappropriate behavior, but may continue to be unable to control it. This trait is referred to as *disinhibited behavior;* the person is unable to exert the usual level of inhibition that prevents acting on impulses. A person may laugh, cry or express other emotions that have no relationship to the actual emotional context of the situation. Other patients may respond with the correct category of emotion, such as laughing at a humorous situation, but the extent and forcefulness of their laughter may be inappropriately exaggerated.

Evaluation of Awareness

Assessment of these disorders is made by behavioral observation and interviews with the family. Subjective questionnaires[12] can be completed by both the patient and a family member, and the results compared and discussed with both parties.

Treatment of Awareness Deficits

Awareness can be further addressed in treatment using the following approaches.[66] Self-estimation can be encouraged by asking questions requiring patient prediction of performance on a certain task. Role reversal can be used between the therapist and patient. Self-questioning during an activity and self-evaluation following completion of the task can also be important tools for increasing awareness.

Behavioral management strategies can be developed to impose restrictions on patient behavior. Specific, direct feedback regarding the inappropriateness of the behavior should be given to the patient. If the person's level of insight and control warrants, internal strategies can be taught, such as "time out", when the person voluntarily leaves the situation. If this approach fails, external controls may be used, and a staff person may escort the patient to a quiet area until behavioral control is once again established. It is critical that the staff person remain calm, because a strong emotional response from staff can further exacerbate the situation.

A group approach can also be useful in providing feedback from peers.[37] Videotaping can provide a visual record of behavior that can be discussed with the patient.

DYSCALCULIA

A deficit in the ability to perform simple calculations can have important implications for an individual's independent functioning in the community. Various types of calculation disorders have been identified.[42] A patient may have difficulty reading (*alexia*) or writing (*agraphia*) the numbers, and consultation should be sought with the speech/language pathologist on the team. *Spatial dys-*

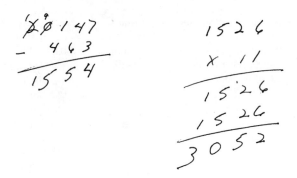

FIG. 15-3 Examples of spatial dyscalculia.

calculia refers to a deficit in the spatial arrangement of the numbers (Fig 15-3). The term *anarithmetria* is applied to the patient who is unable to perform calculations but does not demonstrate deficits in reading and writing numbers or spatially arranging the numbers in the calculation, and premorbidly had satisfactory educational background and academic skills.

Assessment should include number recognition and simple to complex mathematical problems, as well as functionally oriented items such as calculating change, recognition of coins, and budgeting. The Cognitive Rehabilitation Workbook[23] includes everyday calculation tasks, providing pretest and posttest measures and training exercises.

SUMMARY

This chapter has presented basic, underlying principles of cognitive evaluation and treatment, as well as specific deficit evaluation through structured clinical observation, activity analysis, and standardized testing. In addition, general guidelines for treatment application have been provided. The field of cognitive dysfunction is complex and requires that the therapist develop astute observational skills and attain knowledge and understanding of underlying principles of evaluation and treatment techniques. The reader is encouraged to seek additional sources and experiences as needed to refine therapeutic skill in dealing with patients with cognitive dysfunction.

REVIEW QUESTIONS

1. Discuss the difference between cognition and metacognition.
2. List the areas of cognition that the occupational therapist should evaluate.
3. What are the major underlying principles of cognitive evaluation that the therapist must consider?
4. Describe and compare the various theoretical approaches to treatment.
5. What is environmental feedback, or cuing?
6. What are the implications of a deficit in attention and concentration for an individual's functioning in everyday activities?
7. Describe the memory process.
8. How can a therapist choose a memory strategy for a particular patient?

9. What are some behavioral manifestations of poor initiation?
10. What behaviors does the patient with poor mental flexibility and abstraction display?
11. What are the five major stages of problem solving?
12. What tasks should a functional test of dyscalculia include?

REFERENCES

1. Abreu BC, Hinojosa J: The process approach for cognitive perceptual and postural control dysfunction for adults with brain injuries. In Katz N: *Cognitive rehabilitation: models for intervention in occupational therapy*, Boston, 1992, Andover Medical Publishers.
2. Abreu BC, Toglia JP: Cognitive rehabilitation: an occupational therapy model, *Am J Occup Ther* 41:439, 1987.
3. Allen CK: Cognitive disabilities. In Katz N: *Cognitive rehabilitation: models for intervention in occupational therapy*, Boston, 1992, Andover Medical Publishers.
4. Allen CK, Earhart CA, Blue T: *Occupational therapy treatment goals for the physically and cognitively disabled*, Rockville, Md, 1992, The American Occupational Therapy Association.
5. Arenberg D, Robertson-Tchabo E: Learning and aging. In Birren J, Schaie K, editors: *Handbook of the psychology of aging*, New York, 1977, Von Reinhold.
6. *Army individual test battery: manual of directions and scoring*, Washington, DC, 1944, War Department, Adjutant General's Office.
7. Arnadottir G: *The brain and behavior: assessing cortical dysfunction through activities of daily living*. St Louis, 1990, CV Mosby.
8. Aronson MK: Caring for the dementia patient. In Aronson MK, editor: *Understanding Alzheimer's disease*, New York, 1988, Charles Scribner's Sons.
9. Ayres AJ: *Sensory integration and learning disorders*, Los Angeles, 1980, Western Psychological Services.
10. Ball K, Sekuler R: Improving visual perception in older observers, *J Gerontol* 41:176, 1986.
11. Barco PP and associates: Training awareness and compensation in postacute head injury rehabilitation. In Kreutzer JS, Wehman PH: *Cognitive rehabilitation for persons with traumatic brain injury*, Baltimore, 1991, Paul H Brookes Publishing.
12. Bennett-Levy J, Powell G: The subjective memory questionnaire (SMQ): an investigation into the self-reporting of "real life" memory skills, *Br J Soc Clin Psychol* 19:177, 1980.
13. Ben-Yishay Y, Piasetsky EB, Rattock J: A systematic method for ameliorating disorders in basic attention. In Meier MJ, Benton AL, Diller L, editors: *Neuropsychological rehabilitation*, New York, 1980, Guilford Press.
14. Beyer BK: *Practical strategies for the teaching of thinking*, Boston, 1987, Allyn & Bacon.
15. Birren J, Schaie KW, editors: *Handbook of the psychology of aging*, ed 2, New York, 1985, Von Reinhold.
16. Bolger J: Cognitive retraining: a developmental approach, *Clin Neuropsychol* 4:66, 1982.
17. Brown L, Sherbenou RJ, Johnsen SK: *The test of nonverbal intelligence (TONI)*, Austin, Tex, 1982, Pro-Ed.
18. Craine JF: Principles of cognitive rehabilitation. In Trexler LE: *Cognitive rehabilitation: conceptualization and intervention*, New York, 1982, Plenum Press.
19. Craine JF, Gudeman HE: *The rehabilitation of brain functions: principles, procedures and techniques of neurotraining*, Springfield, Ill, 1981, Charles C Thomas Publishers.
20. Crook T: Psychometric assessment in the elderly. In Raskin A, Jawick L: *Psychiatric symptoms and cognitive loss in the elderly*, New York, 1979, Hemisphere Publishing.
21. Davis CM: The role of the physical and occupational therapist in caring for the victim of Alzheimer's disease. In Taira ED: *Therapeutic interventions for the person with dementia*, New York, 1986, The Hayworth Press.
22. DLM Teaching Resources: *Apple computer resources in special education and rehabilitation*, Allen, Tex, 1988, DLM Teaching Resources.
23. Doughtery PM, Radomski MV: *The cognitive rehabilitation workbook*, Rockville, Md, 1987, Aspen Publishers.
24. Filskov S, Boll T: *Handbook of clinical neuropsychology*, New York, 1981, John Wiley & Sons.
25. Flavell JH: *Cognitive development*, Englewood Cliffs, NJ, 1985, Prentice Hall.
26. Gardner MF: *The test of visual perceptual skills (TVPS)*, Burlingame, Calif, 1992, Psychological and Educational Publications.
27. Giles GM: A neurofunctional approach to rehabilitation following severe brain injury. In Katz N: *Cognitive rehabilitation: models for intervention in occupational therapy*, Boston, 1992, Andover Medical Publishers.
28. Glickstein JK: *Therapeutic interventions in Alzheimer's disease*, Rockville, Md, 1988, Aspen Publishers.
29. Golding E: *The Middlesex elderly assessment of mental state*, Thames, England, 1989, Thames Valley Testing.
30. Harrell M and associates: *Cognitive rehabilitation of memory: a practical guide*, Gaithersburg, Md, 1992, Aspen Publishers.
31. Hart T, Hayden ME: The ecological validity of neuropsychological assessment and remediation. In Uzzell BP, Gross Y: *Clinical neuropsychology of intervention*, Boston, 1986, Martinus Nijhoff Publishing.
32. IBM National Support Center for Persons with Disabilities, P.O. Box 2150, Atlanta, Ga. 30055.
33. Kiernan RJ and associates: The neurobehavioral cognitive status examination: a brief but differentiated approach to cognitive assessment. *Ann Int Med* 481-485, 1987.

34. Levin W: Computer applications in cognitive rehabilitation. In Kreutzer JS, Wehman PH: *Cognitive rehabilitation for persons with traumatic brain injury,* Baltimore, 1991, Paul H Brookes Publishing.

35. Lezak MD: *Neuropsychological assessment,* New York, 1983, Oxford University Press.

36. Likert R, Quasha WH: *The revised Minnesota paper formboard test,* New York, 1970, Psychological Corporation.

37. Lundgren CC, Persechino EL: Cognitive group: a treatment program for head injured adults, *Am J Occup Ther* 40:397, 1986.

38. Lynch W: Microcomputer technology in the rehabilitation of brain disorders: advances in clinical rehabilitation, New York, 1988, Springer Publishing.

39. Lynch WJ: Ecological validity of cognitive rehabilitation software, *J Head Trauma Rehabil* 7:36, 1992.

40. Mann WC, Lane JP: *Assistive technology for persons with disabilities: the role of occupational therapy,* Rockville, Md, 1991, The American Occupational Therapy Association.

41. Matthews CG, Harley JP, Malec JF: Guidelines for computer-assisted neuropsychological rehabilitation and cognitive remediation, *Clin Neuropsychol* 5:3, 1991.

42. McCarthy RA, Warrington EK: *Cognitive neuropsychology: a clinical introduction,* San Diego, 1990, Academic Press.

43. Morse PA, Morse AR: Functional living skills: promoting the interaction between neuropsychology and occupational therapy, *J Head Trauma Rehabil* 3:33, 1988.

44. Neistadt ME: Occupational therapy for adults with perceptual deficits, *Am J Occup Ther* 42:434, 1988.

45. Neistadt ME: A critical analysis of occupational therapy approaches for perceptual deficits in adults with brain injury, *Am J Occup Ther* 44:299, 1990.

46. Nelson TO, Narens L: Why investigate metacognition? In Metcalfe J, Shimamura AP, editors: *Metacognition: knowing about knowing,* Cambridge, Mass, 1994, The MIT Press.

47. Oakley F: *Understanding the ABC's of Alzheimer's disease: a guide for caregivers,* Rockville, Md, 1993, American Occupational Therapy Association.

48. Parente R, Anderson-Parente J: *Retraining memory: techniques and applications,* Houston, 1991, CSY Publishing.

49. Parente R, Stapleton M: An empowerment model of memory training, *Appl Cog Psychol* 7:585, 1993.

50. Parente R, Stapleton MC, Wheatley CJ: Practical strategies for vocational reentry after traumatic brain injury, *J Head Trauma Rehabil* 6:35, 1991.

51. Prigatano GP: *Neuropsychological rehabilitation after brain injury,* Baltimore, 1986, The Johns Hopkins University Press.

52. Reisberg B and associates: The global deterioration scale for assessment of primary degenerative dementia, *Am J Psychiatry* 139:1136, 1982.

53. Riege WH and associates: Decision speed and bias after unilateral stroke, *Cortex* 18:345, 1982.

54. Ross FL: The use of computers in occupational therapy for visual-scanning training, *Am J Occup Ther* 46:314, 1992.

55. Ruch FL, Ruch M: *Employee aptitude survey,* San Diego, 1963, Educational & Industrial Testing Service.

56. Rustad RA and associates: *The cognitive assessment of Minnesota.* Tucson, Ariz, 1993, Therapy Skill Builders.

57. Schacter DL, Glisky EL: Memory remediation: restoration, alleviation, and the acquisition of domain-specific knowledge. In Uzzell BP, Gross Y, editors: *Clinical neuropsychology of intervention,* Boston, 1986, Martinus Nijihoff Publishing.

58. Sivan AB: *The Benton visual retention test,* San Antonio, Tex, 1992, The Psychological Corporation.

59. Sohlberg MM: *The profile of executive control system (PRO-EX),* Puyallup, Wash, 1992, Association for Neuropsychological Research & Development.

60. Sohlberg MM, Mateer CA: *Attention process training,* Puyallup, Wash, 1986, Association for Neuropsychological Research & Development.

61. Stone MH, Wright BD: *Knox's cube test,* Wood Dale, Ill, 1980, Stoelting.

62. Strauss AA, Werner H: Disorders of conceptual thinking in the brain injured child, *J Nerv and Ment Dis* 96:153, 1942.

63. Tankle, RS: Application of neuropsychological test results to interdisciplinary cognitive rehabilitation with head injured adults, *J Head Trauma Rehabil* 3:24, 1988.

64. Toglia, J: Attention and memory. In Royeen CB, editor: *AOTA self study series: cognitive rehabilitation,* Rockville, Md, 1993, The American Occupational Therapy Association.

65. Toglia JP: Visual perception of objects: an approach to assessment and treatment, *Am J Occup Ther* 43:587, 1989.

66. Toglia JP: Generalization of treatment: a multicontext approach to cognitive perceptual impairment in adults with brain injury, *Am J Occup Ther* 45:505, 1991.

67. Toglia JP: A dynamic interactional approach to cognitive rehabilitation. In Katz N: *Cognitive rehabilitation: models for intervention in occupational therapy,* Boston, 1992, Andover Medical Publishers.

68. Toglia JP: *The contextual memory test manual,* Tucson, Ariz, 1993, Therapy Skill Builders.

69. Toglia JP, Golisz K: *Cognitive rehabilitation: group games and activities,* Tucson, Ariz, 1990, Therapy Skill Builders.

70. Walsh K: *Neuropsychology: a clinical approach,* Edinburgh, Scotland, 1987, Churchill Livingstone.

71. Webster RE: *The learning efficiency test,* ed 2, Novato, Calif, 1992, Academic Therapy Publications.

72. Wehman PH: Cognitive rehabilitation in the workplace. In
Kreutzer JS, Wehman PH: *Cognitive rehabilitation for persons
with traumatic brain injury: a
functional approach,* Baltimore,
Md, 1991, Paul H Brookes Publishing.
73. Wheatley CJ, Rein JJ: Intervention in traumatic head injury:
learning style assessment. In
Hertfelder S, Gwin C, editors:
*Work in progress: occupational
therapy in work programs,*
Rockville, Md, 1989, The American Occupational Therapy Association.
74. Wilson BA: *Rehabilitation of
memory,* New York, 1987, The
Guilford Press.

75. Wilson B, Cockburn J, Baddeley
A: *The Rivermead behavioural
memory test,* Suffolk, England,
1985, Thames Valley Test.
76. Wilson BA, Moffat N, editors:
*Clinical management of mem-
ory problems,* Rockville, Md,
1984, Aspen Publishers.
77. Wood RL: Management of attention disorders following brain
injury. In Wilson BA, Moffat N:
*Clinical management of mem-
ory problems,* Rockville, Md,
1984, Aspen Publishers.
78. Ylvisaker M and associates:
Topics in cognitive rehabilitation therapy. In Ylvisaker M,
Gobble EM: *Community re-
entry for head injured adults,*
Boston, 1987, Little, Brown.

79. Zoltan B, Siev E, Frieshtat B: *The
adult stroke patient: a manual
for evaluation and treatment of
perceptual and cognitive dysfunction,* rev ed 2, Thorofare,
New Jersey, 1986, Charles B
Slack.

SUGGESTED READING

1. Royeen CB, editor: *AOTA Self
Study Series: Cognitive Rehabilitation,* Rockville, Md, 1993, The
American Occupational Therapy Association.

CHAPTER   16

The Social and Psychological Experience of Having a Disability: Implications for Occupational Therapists

Elizabeth J. Yerxa

I was quite literally separated from the earth, for while I spent my time in an iron lung, in a bed, or in a wheelchair, my feet almost never touched the ground.

But more important, I believe, was being separated from so many of the elemental routines that occupy people . . . I felt no longer connected with the familiar roles I had known in family, work, sports. My place in the culture was gone.

Arnold Beisser[2]

Many years ago I met "Jeff," a patient undergoing rehabilitation at a large hospital in which I worked as an occupational therapist. My encounter with Jeff created a turning point in my thinking about people with disability and influenced the direction of my entire subsequent career.

One day Jeff wheeled into my office. I could see that he was very excited about something. "Betty, if you have a minute, I want to show you something," he exclaimed, his eyes bright with anticipation.

"Sure, Jeff," I replied. "What is it?" He handed me a manuscript. As I examined it I realized that it was a scholarly paper. It was titled something like this: "The Social Status of People with Disabilities as a Maligned Minority Group." Because it was the early 1960s, Jeff's paper conveyed a new idea to me.

"I've written it for a sociology class I'm taking at

UCLA. I thought you might like to read it." His tone of voice conveyed both a question and a hope.

"I'd love to read it," I replied, full of curiosity by now. "Could I borrow it for a few days?" He nodded, left his paper, and told me he'd return by the end of the week.

I took Jeff's paper home that night and read it with increasing interest. He proposed and supported, with many references, the idea that people with disabilities were treated as second-class citizens in American society and were the recipients of pervasive prejudice that limited their life opportunities. I saw images in my mind of events that had occurred at our rehabilitation center, events that had bothered me. For example, I remembered patients being talked about as though they were invisible in conferences at which they were present. I saw patients segregated from professional staff members into separate eating areas and rest rooms clearly labeled "patients" vs. "staff." References to some patients were in terms of "uncooperative" or "has not accepted his or her disability." Such labels were the "kiss of death," because these patients were discharged as soon as possible, often in an atmosphere of contempt and hostility.

With these pictures racing through my mind and the increasing conviction that Jeff was onto something important, I showed his paper to a colleague the next day.

"Take a look at this," I exclaimed. My coworker quickly scanned Jeff's paper. Then she turned to me with a slight smile and tone of incredulity, as though I'd been taken in: "Betty, remember this. Jeff has brain damage!"

Both Jeff's paper and the rejection of his experiences

I am indebted to Carol Stein for helpful suggestions that strengthened this work, to the Occupational Therapy Department at the University of Southern California for their support in preparing the manuscript, and to Marian Karsjens who processed the words so competently.

by this professional colleague created a new impetus for me to explore what it is like to have a disability. I hoped that such a quest would enable me to do a better job as an occupational therapist.

QUESTIONS

This chapter will explore several questions that are central to occupational therapists who work with people who have disabilities. These queries permeate our practice regardless of the technology we employ, the theories that guide us, or the particular type of disability with which the patient must live. The four major themes of this chapter are as follows: (1) Through what pair of glasses do occupational therapists view the recipients of their services? (2) What is it like to have a disability? (3) What, if anything, does our society need to do for people with disabilities? and the bottom-line question (4) How can occupational therapists help improve life opportunities for people with disabilities?

THE PAIR OF GLASSES THROUGH WHICH OCCUPATIONAL THERAPISTS VIEW THEIR PATIENTS

Before examining these important questions, let me identify some of my assumptions. The first assumption is that all professionals, including occupational therapists, wear a particular pair of glasses through which we view the people who receive our services. These glasses are constructed of the beliefs, values, and traditions of the profession and are transmitted via education including clinical socialization.[25] I assume that the lenses worn by occupational therapists are different from those worn by physicians and other medical personnel, even though occupational therapists often practice within a medical or rehabilitation milieu.[60]

Table 16-1 summarizes key values and beliefs of occupational therapists, derived from our history and literature. Occupational therapists' values seem to center upon a humanistic concern for the individual who may have a chronic, severe, and lifelong disability and who will never be cured.[60] The occupational therapists' lenses see the essential humanity of each person, including the need to maximize his or her capacity or capability. Rather than eradicating disease, occupational therapists identify and strengthen the healthy aspects or potentials of the person. Self-directedness and self-responsibility of the person are emphasized rather than compliance or adherence to orders. A generalist, integrated view of the person as one who interacts with his or her environment guides occupational therapy practice rather than a specialist, reductive perspective. This integration is required by our emphasis on patients' daily life activities and their engagement in the occupations expected by their culture. In occupational therapy, therapeutic relationships are based upon a model of mutual cooperation[47] with the

TABLE 16-1	Traditional Values Supporting Practice of Occupational Therapy and Practice of Medicine	
OCCUPATIONAL THERAPY	**MEDICINE**
Essential humanity of patient-agent; obligation to seek life satisfaction for people with severe disability	Freedom from threat of death; responsibility limited to illness
Goal to maintain and enhance health; support healthy aspects of patient-agent	Goal to eradicate disease, pathology; confer the sick role
Self-directedness and responsibility of patient-agent	Patient compliance to orders; moral authority
Generalist, integrated view of patient-agent	Specialist, reductionist emphasis on organ systems
Therapeutic relationship of mutual cooperation with patient-agent; shared authority	Therapeutic relationship of activity of physician, passivity of patient; aesculapian and sapiental authority of physician
Patient-agent acts on environment rather than behavior determined by it	Patient behavior determined by environment and body machine
Faith in patient-agent's potential	Faith in science and healer's competence and charismatic authority
Patient-agent productivity and participation	Patient relieved of all responsibilities except getting well
Play, leisure activities as essential components of balanced life	Recovery from illness, freedom from disease as major concern
Understand subjective perspectives of patient-agent	Emphasis on objectivity, analysis, observation, and diagnosis

Modified from Yerxa EJ: Audacious values: The energy source for occupational therapy practice. In Kielhofner G, editor: *Health through occupation*, Philadelphia, 1983, FA Davis. Reproduced with permission.

patient rather than a model of active therapist, passive patient. The patient is viewed as an agent or actor with goals, interests, and motives and not as one whose behavior is determined by physical laws. The occupational therapist seems to possess faith in the patient's potential ability, which is actualized by engagement in activity.

Therapeutic intervention emphasizes the recipient's productivity and participation rather than relief from responsibility. Occupational therapists seek to facilitate a balance among work, rest, play, and sleep in the patient's daily life rather than only recovery from illness. Finally, the occupational therapist seeks to understand the patient's experience and point of view instead of relying solely upon observation as the only credible source of information. The patient's view is essential to our understanding of people's motivation to engage in the activities of daily life.

By way of contrast, in their classic work, Siegler and Osmond[48] identified important values supporting the traditional practice of medicine. They constitute the glasses through which physicians have historically viewed their patients. These values are based on Aesculapian authority, conferred by society, which defines the physician-patient relationship. The physician has the power to confer the sick role upon the patient. This role requires that the patient admit to being ill, submit to treatment, and curtail his or her usual activities while being exempted from normal responsibilities. The patient's job is to get well by complying with orders.

A physician's authority ends when the illness ends. It does not deal with the state of impairment in which the person recovers from the illness but still has a disability.

The values supporting the traditional practice and science of medicine include freeing the patient from the threat of death; eradicating disease while conferring the sick role; expecting patient compliance; employing a specialist approach in order to possess superior, precise knowledge; promoting a physician-patient relationship in which the physician is active and the patient is passive; perceiving the patient as more or less of a body machine determined by physical laws; placing faith in natural science and the competence of the physician-healer; relieving the patient of everyday responsibilities; focusing on recovery from illness rather than engagement in daily activities; and relying upon an objective, observable assessment of the patient's symptoms to produce a diagnosis and to indicate a course of treatment, which usually employs technology such as drugs or surgery.

Throughout this chapter I will assume that occupational therapists focus on improving the life opportunities for people who often do not recover, but must live with the impact of having a chronic condition. According to the American Occupational Therapy Association, the majority of occupational therapists work with people who have chronic and often severe disabling conditions.[1] Thus, although we may provide services in a medical milieu, occupational therapists view the patient in a different way from the traditional medical perspective of diagnosis, cure, and recovery and we follow a different thought process.

I also assume that our concern for people's capacity to engage in their rounds of daily life activities means that our scope of practice includes not only the hospital but the patient's home and community. Thus occupational therapists practice both within and outside of the medical milieu, often helping patients to become agents. In this sense occupational therapy practice bridges the sometimes alien world of acute medical care with the familiar world of home, family, and culture.

WHAT IS IT LIKE TO HAVE A DISABILITY?

Bickenbach,[5] a philosopher, suggested that society has not yet answered in a satisfactory manner, the "straightforward" and "childishly simple" query, "What does it mean to have a disability?" As with the contrasting glasses worn by physicians and occupational therapists, the answer depends upon one's perception or point of view.

WORLD HEALTH ORGANIZATION (WHO) CLASSIFICATION

In 1980 the World Health Organization,[57] to assess the effectiveness of health care systems, adopted a classification of the outcomes of the physical event of a disability (Definition column of Table 16-2). This classification is used internationally to provide consistent terminology, formulate research questions, and influence public policy.

Impairment means an abnormality of a physiological structure or deviation from a biomedical norm.[5] For example, a fracture-dislocation of the cervical vertebra at the level of C5, 6 is an impairment.

A *disability* is a limitation resulting from the impairment. It may be an inability to perform any activity considered normal or required for some recognized social role or occupation.[5] For example, inability to dress oneself because of the loss of hand function caused by the impairment of the cervical fracture with resultant spinal cord injury constitutes a disability.

A *handicap* is any resulting social disadvantage for an individual that limits the fulfillment of a normal role or occupation.[5] For example, for a person with quadriplegia, the lack of accessibility to a job site caused by architectural or social barriers constitutes a handicap.

Table 16-2 presents the WHO classification as three models of disability. I have expanded these to include the columns labeled "Problem" and "Power" to include some important implications of the separate perspectives. Each of the three classifications — impairment, disability, and handicap — represents a different view of what it is like to have a disability.[5] Because impairment emphasizes pathological structures it reflects the traditional biomedical model of disability. In this view the problem of having a disability resides in the body, which needs to be cured or modified in some way (for example, through surgery or technology). The power to accomplish a solution to the problem therefore rests in the medical profession by virtue of its superior knowledge and authority.

A disability presents a contrasting economic model. The problem resides in those who are unable to contribute to society by fulfilling an occupational or social role as a result of their limitations. The beginning of the rehabilitation movement in the United States was marked by

TABLE 16-2	Three Models of Disability		
DEFINITION	**MODEL**	**PROBLEM**	**POWER**
Impairment	Biomedical	Body	Medicine
Disability	Economic	Individual's contribution to economy	Marketplace/ State
Handicap	Sociopolitical	Social environment	Self-advocacy

Modified from Bickenbach JE: *Physical disability and social policy,* Toronto, 1993, University of Toronto Press.

efforts to restore people with disabilities to gainful employment so that they would contribute to the economic well-being of the country rather than depleting its resources.[5] The power in this model rests in the marketplace or state, which assesses the value of the individual according to his or her capacity to be a productive contributor to society. The state may intervene by providing vocational rehabilitation services to increase productivity.

The handicap model adopts a sociopolitical pair of glasses. In this view the problem does not reside in the body or in the individual's ability to contribute to society's productivity; rather, it resides in the social environment in which the person with a disability goes about daily life. Thus to have a handicap means to experience a social disadvantage or injustice because of social stigma, prejudice, or other environmental constraints.[5] The power and solution, therefore, rest in self-advocacy in which people with disability work to bring about social change to achieve equality of opportunity and justice. An example of such self-advocacy is the political organization by and for people with disability to influence legislation designed to remove barriers to their full participation in society.[44]

Each of these models represents a different perception of what it means to have a disability. According to Bickenbach,[5] none is complete or integrated but rather each model represents only a partial and selective viewpoint. He urges society to develop an integrated, comprehensive model of disability rather than focusing on these partial and conflicting views.

NEED FOR AN INTEGRATED MODEL

The biomedical and economic models necessarily emphasize what is wrong with the person who has a disability as seen by an outside observer (the physician or potential employer). In contrast, the sociopolitical model emphasizes what is wrong with the social environment as seen by the person who has the disability, and in this sense provides an insider's view. Occupational therapists who work with individuals who have lifelong disabilities need an integrating model of what it means to have a disability, one that reflects our ethical values and seeks to understand both the outsider's and insider's view of disability. Although we often provide our services in a medically oriented environment, we know that occupational therapy cannot be limited to concern with the body but must also focus on people's ability to connect with the daily routines of their culture[2] in their own physical and social environments.

One of the insights of the occupational behavior frame of reference,[41] the model of human occupation,[22] and the newly emerging discipline of occupational science[62] is recognition of the complexity of the people served by occupational therapists. In these conceptual frameworks a person is viewed as a multileveled, open system interacting with his or her environment. Thus *all* people, with or without disabilities, have biological, psychological, sociocultural, and spiritual or transcendental levels of existence, open to a multitude of inputs from the outside world.

In the sciences, each level also represents a pair of glasses through which outsiders may perceive a human being. Many respected and powerful academic disciplines tend to focus on only one level, ignoring the others or reducing them to lower levels. For example, medical knowledge, emanating from the natural sciences, may focus primarily on the microbiological level, emphasizing the integrity of body structures. Conversely, sociologists may focus on the level of society and culture. While these are legitimate disciplines, their partial views may fail to address significant aspects of human life, and their tools for helping people may be limited or even distortive. In the realm of people with disability, medicine emphasizes impairment whereas sociology emphasizes handicap.

Because of occupational therapy's values and its emphasis upon what people want and need to do in daily life, many of our theorists seek to integrate and address all of these levels as well as the environments in which people actually live. Although different levels present valid perspectives, they require integration to provide a complete picture, supplemented by (1) the insider's experiences of daily life (that is, experiences of the person with the disability) and (2) the characteristics of the environment.

Occupational therapy's scientists and practitioners need to develop new approaches to augment the strengths and potential of people beyond current models and integrating perspectives. The remainder of this chapter describes a systems view of what it is like to have a disability, emphasizing the complexity and uniqueness of interactions between the individual and the environment.

SOCIAL ATTITUDES TOWARD PEOPLE WITH DISABILITIES

Occupational therapy students at Boston University participated in a class designed to provide a first-person experience of architectural barriers. Students spent most of the day in wheelchairs going about their daily routines as students, visiting classrooms, libraries, and cafeterias. At the end of the day they returned to the classroom for discussion.

Although the students discovered architectural barriers, many were much more impressed with the behaviors of able-bodied people they encountered. Students were the recipients of stares, averted eye contact, obvious social discomfort, and conversations directed to their wheelchair pushers rather than to them. (Most people didn't know these students were able-bodied.) One student put it this way: "I couldn't wait until 4:00 PM when I could get out of that damned wheelchair. What must it be like for people who really have a disability and cannot walk away?"

Outsiders' Views

How society views people with disability, an outsider's view, is sometimes categorized as social attitude. Wright,[58] a social psychologist, has studied society's reactions to people with disabilities for many years. She used the term "spread" to describe how the presence of a disability or atypical physique serves as a stimulus to create other inferred characteristics, assumptions, or expectations about the person who has a disability. For example, a person who is blind may be shouted at as though lack of vision means impaired hearing as well, or a person with cerebral palsy may be assumed to be mentally retarded.

One extreme manifestation of spread is the belief that an individual's life must be a tragedy because of having a disability. This attitude may be expressed in such statements as, "I would rather be dead than have multiple sclerosis." This life sentence to a tragic existence denies that life satisfaction and happiness may ever be obtained in the presence of a disabling condition. It is particularly of ethical concern today when genetic counseling and euthanasia may provide a socially acceptable means by which people with disability may be eliminated.[51] If life is seen as tragic or not worth living, it is a fairly easy step to argue that it is better for everyone if people with disability cease to exist.

Goffman's classic work[19] used the term "stigma" to describe the social discrediting process that reduces the life chances of people with disability or other differences. An obvious impairment is translated into "something bad about the moral status of the signifier." The individual with stigma is seen as not quite human and society tends to impute a wide range of imperfections on the basis of the original stimulus (impairment) and at the same time project some positive (but undesired) attributes such as heroism or a sixth sense.

Stigma often is a societal reaction to fear of the unknown. Despite mainstreaming in education and the removal of many environmental barriers, the general public has little social contact with people who have disabilities and does not know what to expect of them in daily life. As a result, people with disabilities are often categorized as different from other people. This treatment may be complicated by the just-world hypothesis[26]: If the world is just and having a disability is a tragedy, then the person or the family must have done something morally reprehensible to be the recipients of such a fate. Such thinking leads easily into stigmatization and social distancing. Liachowitz[27] argued that, historically, people who were physically different were often the recipients of philanthropy that inadvertently reinforced negative beliefs of helplessness and dependency by society at large. One current example is the approach used in telethons or other fund-raising ventures in which people with disabilities may be portrayed as victims, reinforcing negative attitudes and stigma. In contrast, some network television programs and commercials include people with disabilities as regular participants in daily life, as workers or family members.

Echoing the WHO classification of handicap, Wright[58] posited that outside observers may attribute the behavior of people with disability to their disability rather than their environmental situation, which is often the real culprit. For example, a child's inattentiveness may be accounted for in terms of presumed hyperactivity or mental retardation, disregarding possible environmental contributions to the observed behavior. Thus people with disabilities may be blamed for being unemployed, for example, when, in fact, environmental factors such as employer attitudes, transportation and architectural barriers, community unemployment levels, or family obstacles are the cause rather than personal attributes. Dawes,[12] a research psychologist, pointed out that, in general, people are likely to attribute their own failures to environmental conditions but attribute other people's failures to personality factors. This observation seems to describe how society views people with disability except that failures are blamed on the disability.

Attitudes are often reflected in research approaches. Twenty-five years ago, I conducted a small study comparing the self-esteem of children with and without disability. I expected to find lower self-esteem in the children with disability, but did not. I know now that my expectation was based upon an erroneous assumption that to have a disability meant to have a more negative self-concept. My previous view was recently echoed by another researcher's perspective.[18] Having found that the self-esteem of college students with disabilities was similar to that of nondisabled students, the authors asked, "Why then do people with disabilities have positive self-images?" This question reflects an unstated assumption that such people *should* have negative self-images. This study also was based on the unstated assumption that disability is such a powerful, salient stimulus that it overrides every other aspect of the person and his or her environment, a questionable assumption to say the least. When reading research about people with disabilities, it is useful to determine what assumptions are embedded in the study and what sort of attitudes they reflect.

Siller,[49] a social psychologist, has studied attitudes toward people with disability for twenty years. In a wide-ranging review of the research extant he concluded, "Any inclination to consider disability outside of the larger social context and as something that resides only in the disabled person is destructively wrong."

Cultural Influences

Edgerton,[15] an anthropologist, discussed social reactions to disability within the context of the social rules of culture. "Rules are a . . . shared understanding of how people ought to behave and what should be done if someone behaves in a way that conflicts with that understanding."

Cultural rules influence the treatment of people with

disabilities. Societies differ in the extent to which they relieve their sick members of responsibility. Often when someone is sick the rules are different. For example, the Chinese in Taiwan are more willing than those in America to exempt people who are sick from their responsibilities. In some societies people with severe mental retardation may receive almost total exemption from responsibility to follow the rules, while in others (Northern Salteaux Indians, for example) such people could be burned alive as children. Some societies do not indulge their ill members. For example, it is inexcusable for married females to be sick among the Sarakatsani shepherds of Greece, and anyone too ill to travel was left to die in the Siriond culture of the tropical forests of Bolivia.

Many impairments are culturally recognized and named as brief periods during which the temporarily ill person is expected to behave in ways that would normally be prohibited. Culture also dictates great differences in people's responses to pain. For example, Jews and Italians are encouraged to respond to pain as an expression of their feelings and emotions, whereas other cultures disapprove of such expression.[15] Culture and its rules create profound differences in both the expectations and opportunities for people with disabilities.

Attitudes of Rehabilitation Workers

Many people with disabilities encounter the health care system, but what is known about the attitudes of those providing services? Siller[49] described an array of studies about rehabilitation personnel. First he observed that certain conditions have less appeal to medical students than others. Patients who are elderly, have mental retardation, are dying, or have a chronic disability seem to have less appeal than the patients who are seen as most like the medical students or are perceived as more capable of being helped.

Expectancies of the teacher influence the performance of students, the so-called Pygmalion effect. For example, higher expectations are correlated with better school performance. Several studies in rehabilitation settings support this effect for professionals (who have higher status) and their patients (who have lower status). For example, a correlation was found between the expectations of houseparents and the performance of institutionalized adolescents. Siller[49] concluded that such findings about expectations probably can be generalized to all disability conditions and all rehabilitation professions. Lower expectations may lead to lower performance and higher expectations produce better performance.

Having relatives with a particular type of disability and knowing more about a certain disability are correlated with a professional's preference to work in that area.[49] In another study, counselors who rated people with disability similarly to people without disability were judged by their superiors as more effective than counselors who rated the two groups differently.[49]

Siller[49] observed that medical personnel, particularly physicians, may see themselves as healers. They often have been trained within an acute medical care frame of reference in which passivity on the part of the patient is encouraged or insisted upon. Some rehabilitation professionals may need to emphasize the negative aspects of disability to reassure themselves of the importance of their services. Siller concluded, "One cannot overly stress the crucial importance for those with chronic disabling conditions to be self-sufficient and active in their own behalf."[49]

What sort of attitudes are displayed by occupational therapy students? Lyons[28] studied the attitudes of Australian students. He found that the attitudes of freshmen occupational therapy students did not differ significantly from those of business majors. The occupational therapy students' attitudes did not vary with the years of undergraduate education completed. However, those students who had valued social role contact with people with disabilities (a friend, family, or coworker rather than patient) had significantly more positive attitudes than those without such contact. He recommended that educational programs in occupational therapy facilitate such valued social role contact. In another study of social distance, Lyons[29] found that undergraduate occupational therapy students most preferred to work with people who had less visible types of disabilities and least preferred to work with those with disorders of the mind, namely people with cerebral palsy, mental retardation, mental illness, or alcoholism or those with a criminal record.

Other studies of occupational therapists[3,17] yielded conflicting results, some finding more positive attitudes than those reported by Lyons. Westbrook and Adamson[54] concluded that "occupational therapy students tend to underestimate the normalcy of lives that handicapped people are managing to live in a relatively prejudiced society."

Vash,[52] a psychologist who also has a disability, recounted a rehabilitation conference held in 1974. A psychiatrist addressed the audience, alternately standing up and sitting in a wheelchair, all the while challenging listeners to deny that their perceptions of his competence fluctuated as he stood and sat, over and over. She reported that much discussion followed and that virtually all in attendance acknowledged that their views of his competence *had* changed; the psychiatrist appeared more credible and more worthy of attention when he stood. The experience was emotionally draining for many because it forced them to confront the prejudice they had denied or ignored previously. A wheelchair can be a powerful social symbol conveying devaluation of the person in it.

Vash[52] introduced her work on the psychology of disability with this bit of wisdom:

Some dangers inhere in even acknowledging the validity of the concept "the psychology of disability," since, in the past, it has led to unhelpful exaggerations of the perceived differences between people with disabilities and those without. The fact is, human beings are more alike than different, regardless of variances in their physical bodies, sensory capacities, or intellectual abilities.

How Different Are People with Disabilities?

What is actually known about the similarities and differences between people with and people without disabilities? Siller[49] reported mixed results. He inferred that,

"As soon as one departs from the direct fact of disability, evidence can be provided to demonstrate that persons with disabilities do or do not have different developmental tracks, social skills and percepts, defensive orientations, empathetic potential, etc. Much of the data suggest that if the disabled* do present themselves as "different" this is often a secondary consequence of the social climate rather than inherent disability-specific phenomena.

Weinberg[53] reported that a group of people with disability showed no differences in life satisfaction, frustration, or happiness compared to a group without disabilities. The only difference found was on ratings of the difficulty of life. People with disabilities judged their lives to be more difficult and more likely to remain so. She reported another study in which people with chronic, but not fatal health problems not only seemed to be quite happy but derived some happiness from their ability to cope with their difficulty. She concluded that "we need to question the assumption that physical limitations are directly related to happiness. Instead, it may be that many people with disabilities find happiness despite their disabilities, even though the able-bodied public would not always expect this."[53]

Studies in Sweden showed that among community based people who had had strokes, life satisfaction was not correlated with the degree of physical impairment. Rather it was related to people's ability to achieve their own valued goals.[4]

Another longitudinal study found that, although adolescent girls with cerebral palsy scored significantly lower on physical, social, and personal self-esteem, as adults they no longer scored significantly differently from other able-bodied groups.[31] The authors speculated that their subjects' changed self-esteem might have been due to a greater choice of environments in which to interact, better social relationships, and/or a wider range of experiences in education, work, and commerce.

A study of adolescents with disabilities (cerebral palsy, orofacial clefts, and spina bifida) found that the subjects' self-evaluations of global self-worth did not differ from those of an able-bodied comparison group. Speaking to occupational therapists, the authors concluded that "clinicians should not assume that adolescents with physical disabilities will have problems in self-esteem."[23]

Social attitudes toward people with disability are often stigmatizing and devaluing, increasing the degree of handicap and decreasing life opportunities. Such attitudes may be found among professional rehabilitation workers including occupational therapists. Positive attitudes are associated with valued social role contact as friends, family, or coworkers. Much research supports the finding that people with disabilities are more like nondisabled peers than different from them in life satisfaction, happiness, and self-esteem. Apparently when we know only that a person has an impairment or disability, we cannot assume anything about his or her social or psychological status.

INSIDERS' VIEWS OF HAVING A DISABILITY

How do people with disabilities define themselves? A growing body of literature provides us with the insiders' viewpoint of what it is like to have a disability.

Zola,[63] a sociologist who has a disability, observed that, at its worst, society denigrates, stigmatizes, and distances itself from people with chronic conditions. He experienced little encouragement to integrate his "disabled self into the rest of his life" because this integration would be interpreted as "giving up the struggle to be normal." In letting his disability surface as a real, not necessarily bad part of himself, he was able to shed his superstrong, "I-can-do-it-myself" attitudes and be more demanding of what he needed. Only recently did he come to believe that he had the right to ask for or demand certain accommodations. He currently refuses to accept speaking engagements unless they are held in a fully accessible facility (not only for him as the speaker but for the audience as well).

Vash[52] reported that, at the age of 19, about 3 years after the onset of poliomyelitis, she was rejected for service by the state-funded vocational rehabilitation program. The reason given was that she refused to abandon her "unrealistic" goal of becoming a psychologist for the practical goal of becoming a secretary. She has subsequently had a productive career as a psychologist, professor, and writer who still can't type.

In one of her books, Vash[52] described the impact of disability from her unique insider/outsider perspective as a person with a disability and as a psychologist. She observed that an individual's reactions to having a disability are influenced not only by the type of disability but also by its severity and stability as well as the person's sex, inner resources, temperament, self-image, family support, income, technology, and even government funding trends.

The *stage of life* when disablement occurs influences a person's reaction because it affects the way the person is perceived and the developmental tasks that might be interrupted. The person who is born with a disability or acquires a disability in infancy or childhood may experience isolation or separation from the mainstream in family life, play, and education. A person who acquires a

---

*"Disabled" is Siller's terminology.

disability later in life may face different issues, such as the need to change vocations, find a marital partner, or remain a part of his or her culture via the routines of daily life.[2,52]

In terms of *functions* impaired, Vash[52] believed that different disabilities (such as blindness or paralysis) generate different reactions because each creates different problems or challenges. She observed, however, that the insider-outsider perspective also applies to people with disability. Thus, the person with the disability may feel that his or her condition is not as difficult as that of others; for example, a person who is blind may feel that it would be worse to be deaf. Reactions are also tempered by the impact of the disability on the valued skills and capacities the person has lost. For example, a person who loves music more than the visual arts may have a stronger reaction to loss of hearing than a visual person with the opposite pattern. (Note the use of the word "may" throughout this paragraph, indicating that reactions are individualized and unpredictable.)

The *severity* of disability does not have a direct, one-to-one relationship with the person's reaction to it. Vash[52] stated, "One person can assimilate total paralysis with fair equanimity, while another is devastated by the loss of a finger."

The *visibility* or lack thereof of impairment may influence a person's reactions to his or her disability because of social reactions.[52] For example, invisible disabilities such as pain may create difficulties because other people expect the person to perform in impossible ways. One woman with arthritis indicated that it was easier for her to go grocery shopping when she wore her hand splints because then her disability was visible and people would carry her packages for her without her having to ask.

The *stability* of the disability or the extent to which it changes over time may influence reactions.[52] In some progressive disabilities the individual faces uncertainty as to the degree of limitations as well as, in some cases, a hastened death. Reactions to such disabilities are shaped by these realities and by what the affected people tell themselves about their projected futures. When neither hope for containment nor cure is substantiated the person may experience a new round of disappointment, fear, or anger.

Pain tends to usurp consciousness whenever it is present. As Vash[52] observed, "It is hard to be jolly, creative or maybe even civil when you hurt—but some [people] can learn to do so." Reactions to pain are highly individualized and influenced by culture.[15]

In discussing all of these reactions, Vash[52] observed that they depend, not only on the disability but on the *people* who become disabled. She observed that we need to ask, "What remaining resources do they have for developing effective and gratifying lifestyles?" This question seems particularly important for occupational therapists because of our concern for what people *can* do and how their own occupations influence their health and quality of life. Vash raised other questions relevant to occupational therapists: ". . . what activities and behavior patterns are interrupted by disablement, and how central are these to their happiness? What is the spiritual or philosophical base of their lives?"

Gender influences a person's reactions. Certain societal expectations that people fulfill their social and sexual roles and live up to social ideals may influence men's and women's reactions differently. For example, the need for women to be "physically perfect specimens"[52] or to carry the major responsibility for managing the home and caring for children may create a different impact for women.

Vash[52] gave great importance to the *activities* affected by disablement. In fact she stated that "The impact of disablement is largely contingent on the extent to which it interferes with what you are doing." It is not only actual activities that influence a person's reactions but also the potential ones, held as goals for the future.

Interests, values, and goals influence a person's reaction to disablement. The individual with a limited range of interests may react more negatively to a disability that prevents their expression while an individual with a wide range of interests and goals may adapt more readily. Vash[52] observed that people may not be aware of their interests, values, and goals and therefore may not be conscious of those that have the potential to lead to satisfaction after acquiring a disability. She emphasized the importance of interests: "The more varied this potential, the more protected is the individual from frustration and dejection over being disabled."*

Vash[52] proposed that the *resources* the individual possesses for coping with and enjoying life are assets that may counterbalance the devastation of loss of function. Some of these, such as social skills and persistence, may be developed to a level enabling paid employment whereas others, such as artistic talent or leisure skills, may contribute to a more satisfying life.

Vash[52] is one of the few authors who emphasized the importance of *spiritual and philosophical beliefs* to a person's reactions to disablement. She separated spirituality from religiosity with the observation that people who acknowledge a spiritual dimension of life and who have a philosophy of life into which disablement can be integrated in a meaningful, non-destructive way may be better able to deal with having a disability. Specific religious beliefs may or may not be helpful. The person who views having a disability as punishment for past sins will respond differently from one who views it as a test or opportunity for spiritual development.

Finally, Vash[52] acknowledged the importance of the person's *environment* in influencing his or her reactions to having a disability. Immediate environmental qualities such as family support and acceptance, income, commu-

---

*"Being disabled" is Vash's terminology.

nity resources, and loyal friends are powerful contributors. The institutional environment if one is hospitalized also has a profound effect, especially the attitudes and behaviors of the staff members. The culture and its support or lack thereof for resolving functional problems or protecting the civil rights of people with disabilities is another significant influence.

Vash[52] provided a broad and complex picture of people's reactions to having a disability. In her portrayal of the impact of impairment and disability on the biological, psychological, social, and spiritual levels of the human, she recognized the need to discover resources at all of these levels and stressed the importance of the person's interaction with his or her environment, especially in being able to do something, to act. Vash's work supported both occupational therapy's values and its open systems view of human beings.

A growing body of literature provides insight into the experiences of having a disability.[2,14,35,55] These works provide occupational therapists with a much needed insider's view.

Beisser[2] had just completed medical school at age 23 when he acquired poliomyelitis, which left him totally paralyzed and unable to breathe without a respirator. He spent one year in the hospital occupying the same room. Later, he was able to articulate his experiences with a clarity and sensitivity that enable us almost to share them. Some of his experiences in the hospital are noteworthy.

He frequently felt that those who attended to his body were more the owners of it than he was. Although he was often cold because his paralysis prevented his muscles from generating heat, the nurse doubted his judgment. She would feel his leg and say, "Oh, it's all right, you're not cold." These experiences happened over and over. Beisser[2] observed "They thought they knew how *I* felt better than I did. I was not even acknowledged as a separate person." Although enraged by his imposed powerlessness, he learned that you "cannot get mad in hospitals" because "angry patients come last" (have their needs attended to last). He compared his experience of hospitalization to being a prisoner of war except that, although he depended upon his captor's feelings and behaviors for his self-esteem, he could never become one of them no matter how hard he tried to be a good patient.

Depersonalization was common. Some of the employees upon whom he depended made it clear that it was just a job to them. In one hospital, the first hour of the nurses' shift was spent deciding about coffee breaks. Patient needs were secondary. Sometimes workers even left him in midair in a lift to go on a coffee break. "One of the worst times was at 'change of shift' . . . because then there was absolutely no chance of getting anyone to help even if the problem was urgent." Beisser[2] observed, "To me, what they did or did not do was not 'just a job' but a matter of survival, of both my physical body and my sense of myself as a person."

Fortunately, sometimes he had other sorts of helpers who helped willingly with interest and compassion, whose primary goal was the comfort of patients. When one of them came to a ward of patients, the room brightened and the patients' fears and tensions lessened considerably.

Beisser[2] discussed his reactions to acquiring a disability. First he had to give up the "old and obsolete, preparing the ground for something new." Then he had to find something positive, available for a new commitment. The first step in giving up the old was a grieving process, which involved a gradual reduction in the energy invested in what had been lost. He described traversing through stages of denial (he hadn't really lost anything of value), blaming (whose fault is this?), bargaining (with physicians, God, and universe) that if he did X he would get back what he had lost. When he discovered that there was no one to blame or bargain with or rage against, despair and depression appeared. Although this stage is supposed to lead to acceptance, Beisser[2] asked, "Acceptance of what?" Why would a person accept the loss of something valued unless there was something new of value to take its place? There had to be a positive replacement. In his case he had to find a new way of being, involving his old enthusiasms. The first was sports, then people in his life, and finally work, but these discoveries took a long time.

Although he couldn't become a surgeon, he did become a psychiatrist; although he could no longer play tennis, he could become an enthusiastic sports fan (later he wrote a book about sports). The stages of acceptance, which needed to occur simultaneously with grief, were the following: "Rejection of unfamiliar options; looking for something new; a grudging acceptance of something new; behaving 'as if' you accept it; discovering some of the same satisfaction in the new that you had with the obsolete."

Another insider's view is provided by Robert Murphy,[35] a professor of anthropology who developed a progressive spinal cord tumor that moved from "a little muscle spasm in 1972 to quadriplegia in 1986," the year he wrote this book.

Murphy[35] described his initial reaction to having a disability: "But what depressed me above all else was the realization that I had lost my freedom, that I was to be an occasional prisoner of hospitals for some time to come, that my future was under the control of the medical establishment." This feeling was like falling into a vast web, a trap from which he might never escape.

His view of hospitalization was similar to Beisser's. He described the key rules for a sick person as (1) don't complain! and (2) maintain a cheery exterior. Doctors and nurses appreciate patients who can follow these rules.

The hospital patient must conform to the routine imposed by the establishment. For example, he spent five weeks on one ward where he was bathed at 5:30 every morning because the day shift nurses were too busy to do it. The chain of authority from physicians on down creates a bureaucratic structure that breeds and feeds on impersonality.[35] The totality (social isolation) of such institutions is greater in long-term care facilities such as mental hospitals and rehabilitation centers. A closed-off, total institution generally attempts to erase prior identity and make the person assume a new one, imposed by authority. The hospital requires that the inmates think of themselves primarily as patients, a condition of "conformity and subservience."

In relation to his social world, Murphy[35] experienced an increase in social isolation because some of his friends avoided him and he often encountered physical barriers in his environment. He was surprised to discover that in attending meetings of organizations of people with disabilities, more attention was often paid to the opinions of outside experts who were able-bodied than to his views (in spite of his having a disability and being a professor of anthropology). He observed that people with disability fit into a mold of liminality (invisibility); as their bodies are impaired, so is their social standing. "Their persons are regarded as contaminated; eyes are averted and people take care not to approach wheelchairs too closely."[35] One of his colleagues viewed wheelchairs as portable seclusion huts or isolation chambers. Even so, Murphy[35] expressed a sense of wonder that so many people with disability manage to break out into the world.

A great deal of Murphy's book[35] recounts his struggle for autonomy. Because of changes in his physical condition he decided to have his wife, Yolanda, do the driving. Later he realized that this change was a mistake because it resulted in the loss of his sense of mastery and power. Driving an automobile meant not only mobility but spontaneity and free will. Having to rely on other people and the planning necessary to go anywhere because of his increasing paralysis "invaded my entire assessment of time." He observed that not only he but all people with paraplegia and quadriplegia have problems of planning their activities and often have to conform to the time tables of family members, aides, and service providers.

A major contributor to his sense of mastery was his work as a professor, which he continued as long as possible. But even with his status as an internationally recognized anthropologist and researcher, hospital personnel often saw him as an anomaly. A social worker asked him, "What *was* your occupation?" even though he was working full time and doing research in areas related to medical expertise. Their mindset seemed unable to place him in the mainstream of society. Murphy[35] concluded that people with disability must make extra efforts to establish themselves as autonomous, worthy individuals. His book ended with this observation: "But the essence of the well-lived life is the defiance of negativity, inertia and death. Life has a liturgy which must be constantly celebrated and renewed; it is a feast whose sacrament is consummated in the paralytic's breaking out from his prison of flesh and bone, and in his quest for autonomy."

Williams' autobiography[55] provides a glimpse into the experiences of a woman diagnosed as having autism. It provides a rich portrait of one person's experience of growing up in an alien world. When she was a child, her mother and brother often sided together to put her down. "To them, I was a nut, a retard, a spastic. I threw mentals and couldn't act normal." She sought safety in hanging on to an insular little world in which communication via objects was comfortable but any physical contact with people was anxiety-ridden. "I felt that all touching was pain, and I was frightened" (at the prospect of hugging or being hugged).

Fortunately, her father was sensitive to her needs. "He simply sat within my presence, letting me show him how I felt in the only way I could—via objects. . . . I eventually had the courage to show him some of the secret pictures I'd drawn and the poems I'd written."[55]

Her existence became one of her own construction as she tried to resist intrusion from the outside world of fragments and incoherence. For example, although she could read novels fluently she was unable to understand what books were about. The meaning got lost in "the jumble of trivial words."[55] Concentration was difficult, especially for imposed tasks. Unless the activity was one she had chosen, she would drift off no matter how hard she tried. "Anything I tried to learn, unless it was something I sought and taught myself, closed me out and became hard to comprehend, just like any other intrusion from 'the world.'"

At the end of this odyssey, often similar to that of being on a strange planet, Williams[55] recounted those experiences which had been helpful: "Allowing me my privacy and space was the most beneficial thing I ever got. As much as many of the things I did were dangerous and as much as people could sense my isolation, this isolation was not from being left to my own devices. It stemmed from the isolation of my inner world, and only the unthreatening nature of privacy and space would inspire the courage to explore the world and get out of my world under glass step by step." Williams' book conveys the experiential basis of her behavior, which often might otherwise appear bizarre and incomprehensible to an outside observer. It also offers support for the importance of choices, a safe space for exploration, and intrinsic motivation for engagement in activities.

Dubus,[14] an accomplished novelist, acquired a severe disability when he was hit by an automobile after he had stopped to help a couple whose car had broken down on a busy highway. He was suddenly transformed into a "disabled man" with one leg amputated and the other so badly shattered that he needed to use a wheelchair as a permanent mode of transportation. He gradually moved from initial despair toward surrender and acceptance. Along the way he told of changes in how he perceived his environment.

The world is a different place when seen from a wheelchair. . . . It's a landscape made up of obstacles and traps.

How to get a glass of water the nurse has put out of reach? How to get in and out of a car? How to shave, how to shower? How to reach the dials on the stove? What do you do if your car breaks down? How do you ask for things without making every request a statement of disability?

His solution to the last question was, "I say things like 'I wonder if there's any cheese?' or 'Does anyone want hot chocolate?'"[14]

Like Murphy[35] and Beisser,[2] Dubus[14] experienced a profound change in his sense of time. Everything took him three times as long to do as it had previously. As a result time seemed to move "three times as fast as the action that once used a third of it." Dubus' experiences underline his need to develop extraordinary new skills to manage his space, time, and social relationships as a person with a disability.

These articulate people help us understand the experience of having a disability from an insider's point of view. Increasing amount of literature provides new insights into such experiences including encounters with social stigma, reactions to the medical system, and need to have a supportive environment. Of particular relevance to occupational therapists are their quests for autonomy and a sense of mastery over their daily lives, needs to discover substitute interests for those lost, the essential strength of their unique resources and their embeddedness in the mainstream of humanity. Reading these and other[20,24,39] original sources may provide occupational therapists with new understanding of how to make their services better fit the needs of people as identified by the people themselves. They cast light on how people adapt to the challenges of their environments in the presence of a disabling condition by discovering, enhancing, and using their strengths and resources. This process can be profoundly affected by occupational therapy.

WHAT, IF ANYTHING, DOES SOCIETY NEED TO DO FOR PEOPLE WITH DISABILITIES?

This section will explore the social context of having a disability. The first issue will be that of current trends in terminology followed by changes in health care affecting the life opportunities for people with disability. Finally, some current social policies regarding the civil rights of people with disability and attempts to reduce social handicapping[5] will be presented.

TERMINOLOGY

The language used to communicate ideas about people with disabilities is important because it conveys images about them that may or may not diminish their status as human beings. For example, in the jargon of the medical environment people may be called quads, paras, CPs or that stroke down the hall. This categorization leads easily to viewing individuals as categories (stereotypy) and also as being "engulfed"[5] by their impairments. Additionally,

referring to such people as the disabled or a disabled person seems to make the disability swallow up their entire identity, leaving them outside the mainstream of humanity. How then might one talk about them in a spirit of dignity?

Many years ago, Vash[52] edited a chapter I had written for one of her books. In the margin she wrote, "Why not refer to '*people* with disabilities' rather than 'the disabled'?" This was her way of emphasizing that each individual was a person first with all of the uniqueness *and* the similarity to everyone else that personhood conveys. I have used that terminology throughout this chapter with the intention that *disability* be defined in the broadest sense to include any condition (internal or external) that may interfere with the accomplishment of goals and intentions. *People with disabilities* is increasingly being used by other writers in this field.[5,52,58]

Another issue is that of what to call the recipient of occupational therapy: patient, client, or even patient/client. In a medical setting, *patient* may convey both a sense of ethical responsibility[42] toward as well as a state of passivity and dependence[35] of people receiving care. *Client*, on the other hand, conveys an economic relationship[46] as does *consumer*. What these latter terms may gain in autonomy they seem to lose in beneficence. Therefore, I suggest that the term "patient-agent" be used in a medical setting, to convey both the ethical responsibility of care givers as well as the goal of enabling patients to become agents (an agent is one who acts, who has power, and is capable of producing an effect).

In a community or nonmedical setting it may be appropriate to use terms such as "students" (in an educational program) or the more generic "service recipient." I prefer the latter term because it conveys the important point that occupational therapy is a service and not a commodity to be consumed. Service conveys benefits, help, and usefulness rather than a business relationship (client) in which the buyer may need to beware because the goal of the provider is to maximize his or her profits.

The WHO terminology of impairment, disability and handicap[57] may also be useful in separating the biomedical, economic, and social perspectives of disability. It is used widely in the international community. Whatever terminology is selected needs to be chosen with care and thoughtfulness to assure that it conveys respect, dignity, and a sense of ethical responsibility toward those who receive occupational therapy.

CHANGES IN HEALTH CARE

Changes in the health care system are emanating from the increased population of people with chronic conditions as well as the increased knowledge and activism of those receiving care, especially long-term care such as rehabilitation. These changes will certainly affect the way society provides opportunities for people with disability.

Robinson,[43] a British social scientist who has written about the experience of having multiple sclerosis, urged that major changes be made in the organization of rehabilitative care. Such changes are needed to attain the patient's active and involved commitment to the process of rehabilitation, to achieve a good quality of life, and to restore viable social functioning.

Because rehabilitation is often based on a model of acute medical care, he recommended that the traditional goals of short-term, acute medical care be radically changed to those appropriate to the rehabilitation of people with long-term disabilities. The aim of rehabilitation would thus change from that of cure to alleviation, its focus on handicap rather than impairment,[5] and its style from technique-centered to patient-centered. He recommended that the physician's role change from controller to coordinator and that therapists change from medical agents (carrying out medical orders) to autonomous contractors (who can deal with the long-term complex relationships among impairment, disability, and handicap).[43]

The patient's role would change from that of passive complier with preset goals to active definer of rehabilitation goals. The site of service provision would change from the hospital to the community.[43]

Interestingly, Robinson[43] observed that of the health professions involved in rehabilitation, occupational therapists were most likely to adapt to these needed changes because of their traditional involvement with long-term impairments and "the very adaptability and diversity of occupational therapy, centered around ideas of occupation and activity." As more and more people live with disabilities in an increasingly complex environment,[61] such changes in rehabilitation will be urgently needed to improve the life opportunities of people with disabilities and assure that they can achieve their goals and purposes in their real-life environments.

LEGISLATION

Legislation is another way for society to improve life by decreasing the handicap of people with disabilities. After decades of work by people with disabilities and their advocates, the *Rehabilitation Act of 1973* was passed as a first step toward full recognition of the rights of such people. It prohibited discrimination on the basis of disability in all federally funded programs and activities and required that federal contractors use affirmative action in hiring and promoting qualified people with disabilities.[5]

In 1990, the *Americans with Disabilities Act*[56] was passed, reflecting further progress in achieving civil rights. At the time the Act was passed, of the estimated 43 million people with disabilities residing in the USA, 67% were unemployed. The Act consists of 5 sections (titles) designed to prevent discrimination by employers and businesses on the basis of physical and/or mental disability. It broadens the scope of the *Rehabilitation Act of 1973* to prohibit discrimination by all businesses (not just federally funded ones). It prohibits discrimination on the basis of physical and/or mental disability. Dis-

ability is defined as an impairment that substantially limits a major life activity such as caring for oneself, performing manual tasks, walking, learning, and working.[56] Major provisions include prohibition of discrimination in employment of those with disabilities who are qualified to perform the job, with or without accommodations at the work site; accessibility to all state and local government services without discrimination to individuals with disabilities; and accessibility to public goods and services (for example, restaurants and inns, hospitals, universities, zoos, amusement parks, and homeless shelters). Such accessibility may be achieved through removal of architectural barriers and/or by changes in company policies and practices. Telephone systems must make public accommodations more accessible to hearing-impaired and speech-impaired persons. Finally, the Act prohibits retaliation or coercion against people who seek the rights granted by the *Americans with Disabilities Act*.

Any legislation is only as effective as its enforcement. According to public television,[30] complying with the Act has not resulted in the huge expenditure predicted by many business owners. But although progress is being made, many medium-sized and smaller businesses are still not in compliance, as is true of many universities. As a result, more people with disabilities are filing lawsuits to achieve their rights by bringing about needed changes in their social and physical environments. Occupational therapists may help achieve the goals of the Act by serving as both advocates and sources of information for people with disabilities about their rights.

PUBLIC POLICY

A final point about society's responsibility to people with disability concerns public policy. Bickenbach's entire book[5] deals with the issue of how the decisions made by social entities such as governments affect the lives of individuals with disabilities. He pointed out that such policies ultimately affect almost everyone, because those without a disability are really TABs (temporarily able-bodied). Their status may change because of aging, acute conditions such as fractures, or pregnancy.

Bickenbach[5] concluded that policies ought to promote the goals of respect for, social participation of, and accommodation for people with disabilities. He viewed disablement as a condition of social, structural inequality. He then raised the question of what equality might mean, asking "Equality of what?" For example, it might be defined as equality of respect, antidiscrimination, opportunity, or equality of result (such as political and economic power). After exploring each of these ideas he concluded that equality of capability proves the most just and encompassing goal.

Equality of capability seems relevant to occupational therapy and is reminiscent of Reilly's goal[41] of reduction of incapacity as central to occupational therapy practice. Capability in Bickenbach's view[5] is a "set of functionings, over which a person has a choice, so that the set of a person's capabilities constitute his or her actual freedom of choice over alternative lives he or she can lead.'' The value of this freedom is in its positivity, range of options, and functionings (things people can do or become, have a realistic choice about). For example, equality of capability for a man with blindness might mean a world in which he could rise in the morning, help get the children off to school, bid his wife goodbye, and proceed along the street to his daily work without dog, cane, or guide (if he so desired), proceeding with assurance, knowing that he is a member of the public for whom the streets are maintained with the help of his taxes, and that he shares a world in which he also has a right to live.[5] Equality of capability respects people as agents and emphasizes not what they do choose but what they can and might choose.

In answer to the question of society's responsibilities to people with disability, several directions are now apparent. The words used to refer to people with disabilities need to be chosen carefully so that they convey dignity and reflect individual personhood rather than stereotypy. Changes are needed in the health care system so that a model of long-term commitment to improving life opportunities for people with disabilities takes the place of the current paradigm of acute medical care, leading to more autonomy for both patient-agents and the occupational therapists who serve them. Legislation to protect the civil rights of people with disability needs to be passed, widely publicized, and enforced so that handicap is no longer a social barrier. People with disabilities need to know about their rights to participate fully in life. Finally, society needs to understand and support the goal of equality of capability so that people with disability can enjoy their agency and have full participation in the routines of their culture, to the degree that they so desire.

HOW MAY OCCUPATIONAL THERAPISTS HELP IMPROVE THE LIFE OPPORTUNITIES OF PEOPLE WITH DISABILITIES?
MIND/BODY SPLIT

Several years ago a patient in a large rehabilitation center attempted suicide. The administrators tried to transfer him to a psychiatric facility. That hospital would not accept him because he had a spinal cord injury, however. This incident emphasizes the mind/body split in categorization that forces whole people into medically defined, diagnostic boxes. It is often assumed that a person with a physical disability has a physical impairment that can be fixed via technology and therapy. If such a person displays psychosocial problems, these are viewed as adjustment or behavioral deficits requiring counseling or psychotherapy. Because occupational therapists are educated to provide services both for people diagnosed as

physically disabled or psychiatrically disabled, they might similarly dichotomize their patients and approach those with physical impairments by providing technical solutions including devices and physical modalities. If these patients display emotional reactions such as depression, the occupational therapists might supplement their techniques with counseling or talk therapy. But note that the patient-agent is fragmented and the approach is "doing to" by a professional to a patient. The majority of people seen by occupational therapists have lifelong conditions that cannot be cured,[1] so the fixing is only partially successful and the cost of what is neglected may be high in loss of the patient-agent's autonomy and future quality of life.

OCCUPATION AS THERAPY

In contrast, the occupational therapist might employ occupation as therapy, engaging the recipient of services in self-initiated, self-directed, purposeful (to the patient-agent) activity. Here I do not mean only self-care but rather the whole gamut of playful, creative, and productive human activity that is recognized as meaningful by both that individual and his or her culture. Such occupation helps to put the patient-agent back together again because it is neither exclusively physical nor mental but as Reilly[40] said, is energized by mind and will. The use of occupation, performed by the recipient of occupational therapy services, has several implications relevant to the social and psychological experience of having a disability. First, it enables the expression of the unique pattern of interests possessed by each individual. Pursuing old interests and developing new ones are vital ingredients in enabling people to adapt to their environments in the presence of disabling conditions.[2,32,52,55] The reification of interests through occupation also is a way of tapping into the intrinsic motivation[7] that will energize the person, not only for the short term but for life in the real world of home and community.

Engagement in occupation involves the whole human being in the development of skill, which he or she will possess as a resource. Occupation requires such subroutines as planning, problem solving, application of work habits, knowing and following rules, and identifying and correcting mistakes, all of which contribute to the ability of the eye, hand, and mind[6] to function cooperatively in producing an effect on the environment.

Occupation, because it enables the actor to produce an effect, contributes to a sense of mastery. The need to achieve mastery, efficacy, and autonomy is identified by many authors with disabilities as an important contributor to the quality of their lives and their sense of well-being.[2,35,52] Humans possess an innate need to exercise control over their environments, a need that seems to be rarely recognized in the traditional medical milieu and therefore compounds the impact of the disability. Instead of learned helplessness[45] in which people see themselves as the victims of overwhelming forces in their environments, the ability to do[52] something the person really wants to do contributes to a sense of efficacy. Dawes[12] wrote that self-esteem frequently results from achievement and effort rather than being their precursor. He also cited research supporting the idea that mild depression is often alleviated by simply encouraging and enabling people to engage in the activities they enjoy. Engagement in occupation may contribute to self-esteem and mitigate depressive emotions.

Occupation as therapy enables people to learn those skills they need to fulfill their social roles.[41] For example, Beisser[2] needed to learn how to pursue his interest in sports in a new way (writing a book) and how to work as a physician (as a psychiatrist rather than a surgeon). These are examples of how occupations enabled him to be reconnected with his culture and to find his place in society.

The use of occupation as therapy demands a systems perspective of the recipient, not one limited to impairment, disability, or handicap alone. Occupation involves all levels of the human system (biological, psychological, sociocultural, and spiritual) in interaction with that person's real environment. The activity is the integrator of these levels, producing an output such as competence or skill.

The occupational therapist has a significant, complex, and sensitive part to play in the use of occupation as therapy. He or she creates an environment in which the patient-agent can make an adaptive response. This role requires setting the stage at the right level of challenge for each individual, neither too difficult nor too easy. It also requires suggesting activities consonant with the individual's interests and which may need to be adapted so that the person can perform them. One of my colleagues had a serious traumatic head injury when her children were still young. Her occupational therapist helped her learn how to resume her responsibilities as a mother by doing a task analysis of subroutines. She broke these occupations into small, achievable units, which when accomplished, were synthesized to enable my colleague to achieve the global skills of child care. The ability to resume her role of mother was a powerful contributor to her sense of competence and the reuniting of her family.

Using occupation as therapy requires discovering the resources each individual possesses. This process is grounded in an optimistic view of human nature[40] in which *all* persons are seen as having resources that can be reclaimed,[34] regardless of the degree of impairment. Much of the literature[5,49,52,59] supports the validity of viewing people with disability, not according to what is wrong but to what is right about them. For example, psychologists Wright and Fletcher[59] claimed that a professional preoccupation with the negative leads rehabilitation workers to underestimate people's abilities. They recommended that more attention be given in assessment procedures to the environments in which the patient-agent will live (school, work place, community, etc.). They also urged that evaluators pay as much atten-

tion to describing the strengths and resources of the individual (and his or her environments) as exposing deficiencies and problems.

A study by Burnett and Yerxa[9] of the self-identified needs of community-based people with disabilities demonstrated many unmet needs. Our subjects reported lower confidence levels than a sample of people without disabilities in performing problem-solving, social, recreational, school, vocational, and home skills as well as in community mobility. Basic activities of daily living was the only area of similar confidence. Many of these people had received previous hospital-based rehabilitation services including occupational therapy, yet pervasive needs for the skills required to live in the community persisted. As a result, a new program was established by the authors at a community college. It is directed by Burnett,[8] an occupational therapist. The program includes not only skill development for independent living in the community but training in self-advocacy (to reduce or eliminate handicap).

The use of occupation as therapy reveals the occupational therapist's role as coach (a term suggested by Mary Reilly). Rather than doing to or for the patient, the occupational therapist's role is to foster the patient-agent's adaptive response, often by making it possible for him or her to use strengths and capabilities or develop new ones. This approach takes sensitivity, skill, and an understanding of intrinsic motivation[7] far beyond that required for the "laying on of hands." Just as an athlete needs coaching to achieve the highest level of performance, the recipients of our services need coaching from occupational therapists to reach a level of competence that enables them to achieve their goals in their own environments. This is the process by which patients may be transmuted to agents. We need to study and learn much more about this process, a process that is consonant with needed changes in the health care system.[43]

Finally, the use of occupation as therapy requires that patient-agents learn how to organize their lives to reduce the interference of the disability. This aspect requires a knowledge of how people may organize their time, space, resources, and daily routines to achieve their goals. Almost all of the people who wrote about their experiences of having a disability mentioned problems and frustrations with time, space, and daily routines.[14,35,39] Such organization is becoming more overwhelming as society increases in technological complexity. Some patient-agents may never have learned how to plan and might need help in identifying their goals. This possibility is especially likely if, instead, they have learned helplessness. Occupational therapists with a knowledge of organization can help them organize their lives for maximum satisfaction and participation, contributing to their equality of capability.[5]

MOURNING AND VALUE CHANGES

Wright[58] discussed the common experience of people who acquire a disability as feelings of shame and inferior-ity (caused by the disability) along with avoidance of being identified as a person with a disability. She urged that care givers conceptualize acceptance of disability in a new way. Rather than resignation or preference of one's state over another, she recommended the goal of acceptance of one's disability as nondevaluating. The disability may still be seen as inconvenient and limiting, requiring work to improve certain facets of life, but the person will not feel debased nor need to hide out in shame. Almost all of the people whose experiences were described earlier talked at length about the devaluation they experienced.[35,52,55,63]

The crisis of suddenly having a disability may produce a gamut of emotions and thoughts including disbelief and denial, anger, panic, self-devaluation, and guilt fluctuating with hope and encouragement, feelings of being comforted, relief, and exaltation. These rapidly occurring cycles are highly individual and may become less acute as the person begins to acknowledge reality.[58]

How might health care workers help people through such crises toward nondevaluating acceptance of loss? Wright[58] suggested that what is required is changes in people's value system. These changes include "(1) enlarging the scope of values, (2) subordinating physique relative to other values, (3) containing disability effects, and (4) transforming comparative-status values into asset values." Note that these changes apply both to the person with disability and outsiders, such as occupational therapists and the patient-agent's family members. These value changes are discussed in the paragraphs that follow.

In enlarging the scope of values, the person with a disability may initially be preoccupied with loss, going through a period of mourning. Wright[58] viewed this process as unique to the individual in length and depth. She observed that care givers may overestimate the degree of depression as outsiders, while the insider, because his or her life depends upon it, may have a strong need to cope and to discover and hold onto hope and positive aspects of the situation. Some forces that may keep the person in a mourning state are as follows: (1) a need to hold onto the preferred state that was, (2) the need for time to absorb the changes, and (3) perceptual emphasis on the difference of disability rather than commonalities and continuity with the past. In contrast, the scope of values may be enlarged by the following: (1) comparison of one's state with other states (death or having other disabilities); (2) arousal of dominant values such as awakened pride or the need to deal with the problems at hand; (3) the satiation factor whereby the emotions devoted to mourning are worn out, the person feels wrung out and becomes ready for something new; and finally (4) involvement in the necessities of daily living.

Mourning may not always be protracted or intense but it needs to be recognized as a healing period during which the wound is first anesthetized and then closed gradually with some scarring. Wright[58] observed that as depression lifts, the sheer necessities of living contribute to needed changes in values. Bodily needs prod the per-

son with paraplegia, for example, to try to move or sit up, representing a "here and now" challenge. Mastering the activities of daily living helps enlarge the scope of values, although as Wright observed, "Mastering ADL is surely not sufficient for enjoying a new lease on life." Seeing films of other patient-agents who can manage the ordinary affairs of daily life may also provide valuable support for the person who recently acquired a disability.[58] The occupational therapist's regulated optimism regarding the patient-agent's potential may contribute to a sense of the possible.

As mourning subsides after time for its expression and the opportunity to engage in activity, physique may still hold a potent value. Value changes may eventually override this potency through a shift in emphasis from appearance to personality or capability, reducing the effects of spread.

Containing disability effects involves an increased understanding that, although a physical impairment is a fact that may affect aspects of life, it does not affect all of life nor are all of its effects necessarily negative. Instead, "It involves certain limitations in certain situations. The source of limitation is due to barriers imposed by society and not only to personal incapacity."[58]

Finally, transforming comparative-status values into asset values is an important shift. Status values or judgments of the worthiness of a person can be replaced by asset values. Asset values are attributes that, rather than being competitive or judgmental, are seen as useful or intrinsically worthwhile. For example, being able to get around in one's community while using a wheelchair may constitute an asset value without comparison to how other people do it or even how the person with the disability used to do it. Occupational therapists who enable people to achieve their personal goals by discovering and using their strengths and resources may help people with disability to enlarge their scope of values so that physique is less important than what one can do and be[52] and so that new possibilities are discovered as asset values.

Although psychologists such as Wright[52] and Siller[49] emphasize adjustment to disability, I prefer the broader concept of adaptation with a disability.[33] This goal suggests that the disability or handicap constitutes only one class of challenges among many others with which all human beings must deal to achieve a goodness of fit with their environments. Adaptation places the person with disability within the mainstream of humanity and acknowledges his or her resources gained by evolution. It places proper attention on the social barriers of handicap rather than putting the entire responsibility on the person with disability.

OCCUPATIONAL THERAPIST/ PATIENT-AGENT RELATIONSHIP

Occupational therapists are said to value a model of mutual cooperation[47,60] as the ideal relationship with the patient-agent. This collaborative relationship is different in style and substance from the traditional physician-patient relation in which the professional is active and the patient is passive. What are some characteristics of the occupational therapist/patient-agent relationship?

Peloquin[36] urged that occupational therapists be not only competent but caring. She observed that the profit-drivenness of health care provision often treats patients as mere customers and results in a budgeting of caring actions. Many patients complain about the impersonality and overreliance on technical methods they experience in the hospital or clinic. The system values competence over caring because of three social trends: "(1) emphasis on rational fixing of health care problems, (2) overreliance on methods and protocols, and (3) a health care system driven by business, efficiency, and profits."[36] She challenged occupational therapists to recognize the extent to which such social forces shape the manner in which they relate to patients.

In contrast, Peloquin[36] observed that occupational therapists can be both competent and caring. This goal may be accomplished by getting to know each patient as a person, gaining more power in the system (in order to change it), tempering that power with care, seeking to understand patients' feelings about their illnesses, and rather than acting as authoritarian parents or technicians, to provide patients with opportunities for control over their own lives. These recommendations seem congruent with valuing mutual cooperation in planning and implementing occupational therapy. For example, if the occupational therapist elicits the patient's interests and goals, he or she must get to know each patient as an individual. Providing opportunities for control and self-direction are congruent with the ultimate goal of independent living in the community, whereas expecting compliance with professional orders may seem more efficient but may subvert the learning of habits of independence and self-sufficiency.

Schlaff,[44] an occupational therapist, proposed that occupational therapists help to redefine disability. This redefinition would include working for changes in social attitudes and practices so that society would recognize the dignity and worth of people with disabilities, granting their rights to self-definition and self-direction. The occupational therapist would strive to work in an independent living paradigm as a consultant, helper, and advocate rather than as a diagnostician or a prescriber and manager of treatment. "The consumer is or becomes self-directed, and both the consumer and occupational therapist work to remove community barriers and disincentives [for economic independence]."[44]

Wright's perspective[58] of the client as comanager in rehabilitation echoes the valuing of mutual cooperation by occupational therapy. She observed that if the goal of rehabilitation is independence and self-directedness, it must be nurtured during rehabilitation. She proposed that comanagement could result in increased self-esteem, intrinsic motivation, and better potential for learning be-cause the patient-agent is actively involved. Besides, health care professionals need the knowledge that only the patient-agent can provide to recommend the best course of action. Vash[52] obviously knew herself better than her vocational counselor did when she decided to become a psychologist rather than a secretary. If mutual cooperation is actualized by comanagement, what impediments might get in its way?

Wright[58] observed that the helping relationship itself might get in the way because it conveys subservience and less power for the person being helped, reinforcing the view that the expert has the answers (or should have). The patient-agent might expect and want the professional to take complete charge. In some circumstances, such as acute illness, this approach is necessary and commendable. The shifting of responsibility to the therapist, however, can interfere substantially with the goals of rehabilitation and occupational therapy, especially those of eventual unsupervised and independent living. Wright[58] therefore asserted that "It is essential that the client be brought into a directorship role as soon as feasible."

Wright[58] also acknowledged that helpers may have needs that interfere with comanagement. They might need to assert themselves, display their knowledge, gain power, or achieve satisfaction in an authoritative role. She also cited the increasing pressure for efficiency and cost containment in the system as a stumbling block, because comanagement may require more time and effort than professional prescriptions. Her advice was, "Don't get stuck with the problem; move on to the solution" to prod constructive thinking. For example, why not employ more people with disabilities to work in occupational therapy departments to pave the way for real participation on the part of patient-agents?

Some other suggestions for comanagement are as follows: (1) that patient-agents be given more active roles and responsibilities in the day-to-day activities of the hospital, such as administrative problem-solving; (2) that planning the rehabilitation program be a joint effort of patient-agents and staff; (3) that patient-agents be encouraged to make decisions and evaluate options (at every stage of the therapeutic process); and finally (4) that professionals be given training in encouraging participants to become comanagers.[58] I would add that patient-agents, too, may need training in how to be comanagers and that occupational therapy with its emphasis on self-directed occupations is a likely learning laboratory for the development of such skills.

Wright[58] cited research that supported the long-term effects of comanagement. A group of 100 patients with severe disabilities underwent rehabilitation in a hospital that encouraged their maximum involvement and participation. One year after discharge their status was compared with a control group who had completed a conventional rehabilitation program at the same hospital. The experimental group showed a greater degree of sustained improvement in self-care and ambulation and a lower mortality rate.[58]

Wright[58] concluded with the conviction that, whenever feasible, comanagement on the part of the client should be promoted. This belief should be supported by showing that one likes the patient-agent, being friendly and caring, and showing concern about the patient-agent's welfare. Basic civilities such as introducing oneself and addressing the recipient of services by name are also important. The professional person needs "to question at all times whether the client is at the helm" or whether the person is being "paternalistically directed."[58] This last test is especially important for occupational therapists who may work in an environment in which professional authoritarianism is the norm.

The therapeutic relationship of mutual cooperation and comanagement also extends to the occupational therapist/parent interaction when providing services to a child with a disability. Parents need to learn the skills of relating to a wide range of professionals to obtain needed services, often in an atmosphere that fosters an uneven distribution of power. They deal with the diagnosis of a life-long disability in highly individual ways, attempting a resolution between professionally provided definitions and their everyday experiences of living with a child who is not a clinical category but a real person who has both resources and problems.[50]

Wright[58] viewed the parent as a key participant in the rehabilitation process. Parents offer knowledge about their child, and their cooperation is essential. They also may need help and support in accepting the child's disability as nondevaluating and in learning to cope with the challenges awaiting them.

She cited three characteristics of a constructive professional-parent relationship: (1) parents need to feel that the professional is not working against them and that together they are seeking solutions; (2) they need to believe that the professional likes their child and sees him or her as a special individual; and (3) they need to feel that the professional appreciates their struggle to do the best they can for their child, that though they may have shortcomings they also have strengths and ideas.[58]

Wright[58] proposed that rather than an exaggerated valuing of independence, the goal of balancing independence, dependence, and interdependence is more helpful. Finding this balance is a necessity in all human relationships and it is likely to ensure the proper emphasis on warmth, love, and caring, which every child needs. Independence often means choice and "calling the shots" while still depending upon others for some things. For example, a person might be independent in hiring or firing an attendant for some personal care but dependent in requiring a person to perform such services.

There are many ways to achieve the balance among independence, dependence, and interdependence. For example, the balance might be enhanced by (1) opportu-

nities for parents to observe other children with the same disability as that of their own child, (2) parent discussion groups including brainstorming for problem solving, (3) special techniques that make life easier at home, (4) creating opportunities for specific experiences such as play and leisure activities, (5) the judicious use of reading material to impart factual information and constructive attitudes, and (6) providing the child with the opportunity to assume increasing responsibility for his or her own self-help behavior and activities involving other people[58] (such as doing chores at home).

Occupational therapists can contribute to achieving this balance by working in partnership with the families of children who have disabilities.[16] For example, they can assist family members in setting aside space and time for play, leisure, and social activities in the home as well as personal time and space for the primary care giver who is often the mother.[16] (Housework, child care, lack of financial resources, and fatigue often make such time out essential.) Other ways occupational therapists can help are by (1) reducing environmental barriers to the child's participation in daily life; (2) identifying the child's strengths and resources (reducing negative spread); (3) enlarging the child's scope of activities by providing the necessary time, patience, and opportunity for learning; and (4) helping the family organize its time and resources to avoid frustrations and fatigue and to ensure participation in satisfying family activities.

A study of mothers of children with cerebral palsy[10] uncovered frustration (1) that their input was sometimes disregarded by professionals and (2) at the high rate of turnover of therapists and resulting lack of continuity in the care of their children. These mothers viewed occupational therapists as agents of change, sources of information, and sources of support. Recommendations for occupational therapists working with such children included the following: developing active, respectful listening skills; establishing a priority on therapist continuity; increasing mothers' trust and confidence; providing expressions of optimism; and enabling children to receive as much therapy as possible.

The patient-agent/occupational therapist relationship is both complex and sensitive. It emphasizes the full participation of the service recipient and the model of mutual cooperation in identifying goals. It provides a safe space for growth and the learning of skills, as well as the discovery and nurturing of the patient-agent's resources for adaptation and competence.

NEW MODELS OF PRACTICE

The literature provides several examples of new models of occupational therapy practice with patient-agents who have physical disabilities. These examples have been selected because they appear congruent both with the values of the profession and with the experiences of people with disabilities; they foster positive attitudes and emphasize the strengths and resources of the individual (such as adaptive capacities) and employ occupation as therapy.

Montgomery[34] described the occupational therapy hospital-based clinic as a resource reclamation center. The occupational therapist discovers and augments the patient's potential strengths, which have developed over the three time spans of evolution, development, and learning. As these resources are enhanced through activity, the patient-agent is helped to resume daily living in the real world of home and community, not as a disabled person but as a person who is part of the mainstream of humanity with the same needs and resources as anyone else.

Burke,[7] in a classic article, explored the complex issue of intrinsic motivation that cuts across all dimensions of occupational therapy practice. Her paper provides useful information for how occupational therapists may coach patient-agents to engage in occupations and become self-directed origins rather than pawns. It speaks to creating a just-right challenge from the environment so that patient-agents may make their own adaptive response.

Several models of occupational therapy practice are devoted to the development of independent living skills for community living. Pendleton[37] found that occupational therapists working in rehabilitation centers frequently placed much more emphasis on technical goals (such as range of motion and muscle strengthening) than upon the skills needed for independent living. She urged occupational therapists to devote more time and energy to preparing patient-agents for the capacity to function in their own communities.

The independent living movement[13] arose to increase the self-direction and achieve the civil rights of people with disabilities. It is based on the idea that people with disabilities are the best judges of their own needs. It emphasizes the goals of not only self-care but mobility, employment, accessible living arrangements, out-of-home activity (to enlarge the environment), and consumer assertiveness. This movement appears compatible with the goals and values of occupational therapy in its pursuit of equality of capability, enabling people to manage their own environments including their time, space, and energy. In some respects it addresses the shortcomings of the medical and rehabilitation system, which may foster paternalistic dependency upon professionals. For example, one of its goals is to enable people with disability to take risks. "Without the possibility of failure, the disabled person* lacks true independence and the ultimate mark of humanity, the right to choose for good or evil."[13]

Some models of occupational therapy practice reflect this emphasis upon autonomy, choice, and the skills needed to increase people's capacity for daily living. Several models are based in community settings such as schools and independent living centers rather than in

hospitals. Community-based occupational therapy practice is likely to become more common in the 21st century because of the high cost of hospital care and the need for long-term services for those with chronic conditions.

Cole (now Cole-Spencer),[11] an anthropologist and occupational therapist, described a program for teaching independent living skills. She observed that such skills need to include planning and management and the skills for self-direction rather than task-oriented behavioral capabilities (such as basic self-care). Some skills her program emphasized were as follows: (1) communicating effectively to have one's needs met, (2) identifying and using resources, (3) identifying and comparing choices, (4) making decisions and setting priorities, (5) committing oneself to long-term goals and persisting until they are attained, (6) developing sequential plans so that efforts produce a cumulative effect and outcome, (7) assessing risks and developing judgment about risk taking, (8) managing crises such as medical or financial emergencies, and (9) solving problems. Note that these skills are needed by every human being and are not limited to people with disabilities. (They are even useful for students studying occupational therapy!) Such skills are also developed through engagement in self-directed activity rather than doing to or for the recipients of service.

Burnett (now Burnett-Beaulieu)[8] developed a nontraditional occupational therapy program for community college students with disabilities. The goals of the program are similar to those described by Cole[11] with a primary emphasis upon enabling students with disabilities to function successfully in their roles as college students. She reported that this program often serves as a bridge between medical rehabilitation and life in the mainstream. It includes three levels of skills: (1) self-care, home management, and community mobility; (2) social-recreational, cognitive, and classroom skills; and (3) consumer rights skills. Burnett-Beaulieu[8] posited that these skills can be grouped into a hierarchy with level 1 being basic to the achievement of the other two levels.

Another occupational therapy program was developed by Jackson[21] and colleagues. It was designed for adolescents with developmental disabilities. The Options program is provided at a nonmainstreamed high school campus. Its goal is to enable students to make a successful transition from school to community living through exploring and broadening their choices about employment, living arrangements, and social activities. It focuses not only upon the skills and resources of the students but also on the characteristics of their environments. Parents and family members are included as advocates. An important feature of the program is learning employment skills in supported work environments.

These programs may stimulate occupational therapists to think about and develop new models of community-based practice as a needed alternative to traditional

---

*"The disabled person" is De Jong's terminology.

hospital-based practice. This alternative is urged by revolutionary changes in the health care system,[43] the needs and experiences of people with disability,[35,52,63] and the values and traditions of occupational therapy.[60] We need many more such models to achieve our potential contribution as a profession, to improve life opportunities for people with disabilities, and to influence public attitudes toward people with disabilities in a positive way by emphasizing the skills of such people and their similarities rather than differences as human beings.

TABLE 16-3 Model of Occupational Therapy			
DEFINITION	**MODEL**	**PROBLEM**	**POWER**
Capability	Occupational Therapy	Discover/nurture potential for agency	Human system acting on the environment with a repertoire of skills

SUMMARY

This chapter explored important questions about the social and psychological experiences of having a disability and what implications they hold for occupational therapy practice. I have suggested that the experiences of people with disabilities are important resources for occupational therapists in enabling us to broaden our vision and potential contribution to the quality of life for the recipients of our services. In widening our scope I have suggested the need for a systems view of each individual as one who interacts with a unique environment by engaging in a unique pattern of occupations, dictated by both culture and unique interests.

When Reilly[40] proposed her great hypothesis that humans could influence the state of their own health through the use of hands, mind, and will, she was not only conveying the essence of occupational therapy but perhaps also a much needed new view of health. Occupational therapists work primarily with people with chronic conditions who will never get well. Therefore we need to help society redefine health, not as the absence of impairment or organ pathology but as the possession of a repertoire of skills[38] that enable a person to achieve his or her valued goals. Thus people with irremediable impairments can still look forward to a healthy life.

Returning to Bickenbach's[5] three models of disability (Table 16-2), we can now add a fourth model, that of occupational therapy (Table 16-3). In this model the problem is the need to discover and nurture the individual's potential for agency. The definition is human capability, which emphasizes people's abilities to do what they want and need to do and their opportunities to make choices. Although it may be threatened or diminished by impairment, disability, and/or handicap, capability is the desired outcome of the physical event of a disability. The power rests in the human system itself, which acts on the environment through occupation, possessing a repertoire of skills. This model of occupational therapy assumes that people have or can develop the strengths and resources to achieve their own goals by engagement in occupations. It integrates people with disability into their own environments and welcomes them into the mainstream of society. The model of occupational therapy provides new hope for attaining equality of capability[5] and influencing health.[40]

REVIEW QUESTIONS

1. Compare and contrast the values of occupational therapy with those of traditional medicine.
2. How do these differences in values translate into different, complementary goals for each profession?
3. Define and provide a clinical example of *impairment, disability,* and *handicap* as formulated by the World Health Organization.
4. Describe a systems view of human beings and apply it to occupational therapy for people with physical disabilities.
5. What did Wright mean by *spread?*
6. Define *stigma* as described by Goffman.
7. Why is it essential for occupational therapists and other health professionals to consider the environment and social context of the person with a disability?
8. What did Vash perceive as a danger in referring to the psychology of disability?
9. What type of interpersonal contact did Lyons associate with more positive attitudes toward people with disabilities among occupational therapy students?
10. To what extent is it valid to predict that a person with a disability will have low self-esteem?
11. Provide two examples of how society might demonstrate devaluation of people with disabilities.
12. How do a person's interests, values, and goals influence his or her reactions to acquiring a disability?
13. Describe Beisser's perspective on acceptance of having a disability.
14. What did Murphy mean by *liminality?*
15. Which aspects of Murphy's daily life contributed to his sense of autonomy and which diminished it?
16. How did Dubus' sense of time change after he acquired a disability?
17. What needs that could be met by occupational therapy were revealed in the autobiographies of people with disabilities?

18. Justify the use of the term "people with disabilities" rather than "the disabled."
19. What does the term "patient-agent" convey about the recipient of occupational therapy?
20. What new setting did Robinson predict would become the site of service provision?
21. Name two provisions of the *Americans With Disabilities Act.*
22. Give one example of how a person with a disability might attain equality of capability.
23. What is meant by employing occupation as therapy?
24. Name three possible outcomes of the use of occupation with patient-agents who have physical disabilities.
25. Describe how an optimistic view of human nature influences occupational therapy practice.
26. What unmet needs for community living skills were identified in Burnett and Yerxa's study?
27. How did Wright consider acceptance of one's disability?
28. Differentiate between the terms "adjustment to disability" and "adaptation with disability."
29. Describe the mutual cooperation model of the patient-agent/occupational therapy relationship.
30. List three characteristics of a constructive parent-professional relationship.
31. How might occupational therapists help patient-agents learn to comanage their rehabilitation?
32. Name two goals of the independent living movement.
33. Give three reasons why occupational therapy needs new models of practice.
34. Discuss a new view of health as it applies to people with chronic conditions.

EXERCISES

1. Please read the following description: "James, an adolescent of fourteen, has spastic cerebral palsy, frequently relates to his siblings and peers aggressively, is two years below grade level in reading and arithmetic, and has parents who are rarely present at home."[59] *Stop here.* What is your impression of James?

   Now add this: "James does an outstanding job on his paper route, likes to write poetry and fantasy stories, has a close relationship with his uncle and aunt who live nearby, and is making steady progress in physical therapy." What is your impression of James?

   Relate this exercise to how occupational therapists assess or evaluate their patient-agents.

2. Think of an actual situation involving yourself and a person receiving occupational therapy. Then, in your mind's eye, imagine that a particular person of high status substitutes for the actual person. Would your behavior toward the person change? Would you treat a dignitary or colleague the same way? What if the person had been kept waiting without explanation or examined in front of a group of visitors without consent? Or mechanically set up to do a boring, repetitious, senseless activity? Would a very important person be treated that way? Discuss this exercise as it relates to human dignity and the occupational therapist/patient-agent relationship.

REFERENCES

1. American Occupational Therapy Association: *Summary report: 1990 member data survey,* Rockville, Md, The Association.
2. Beisser A: *Flying without wings: personal reflections on being disabled,* New York, 1989, Doubleday.
3. Benham P: Attitudes of occupational therapy personnel toward persons with disabilities, *Am J Occup Ther* 42:305, 1988.
4. Bernspång B: *Consequences of stroke: aspects of impairments, disabilities and life satisfaction with special emphasis on perception and occupational therapy,* Umeå, Sweden, 1987, Umeå University Printing Office.
5. Bickenbach JE: *Physical disability and social policy,* Toronto, 1993, University of Toronto Press.
6. Bruner JS: Eye, hand, and mind. In Bruner JS, editor: *Beyond the information given: studies in the psychology of knowing,* New York, 1973, WW Norton.
7. Burke JP: A clinical perspective on motivation: pawn versus origin, *Am J Occup Ther* 31:254, 1977.
8. Burnett SE: *Seven modules for independent living skills instruction for physically disabled college students,* Santa Monica Calif. 1982, Disabled Students Center, Santa Monica College.
9. Burnett SE, Yerxa EJ: Community based and college based needs assessment of physically disabled persons, *Am J Occup Ther* 34:201, 1980.
10. Case-Smith J, Nastro MA: The effect of occupational therapy intervention on mothers of children with cerebral palsy, *Am J Occup Ther* 47:811, 1993.
11. Cole JA: Skills training. In Crewe NM, Zola IK, editors: *Independent living for physically disabled people: developing, implementing and evaluating self-help rehabilitation programs,* San Francisco, 1983, Jossey-Bass.
12. Dawes RM: *House of cards: psychology and psychotherapy built on myth,* New York, 1994, The Free Press.
13. De Jong G: Defining and implementing the independent living concept. In Crewe NM, Zola IK, editors: *Independent living for physically disabled people: developing, implementing and evaluating self-help rehabilitation programs,* San Francisco, 1983, Jossey-Bass.
14. Dubus A: *Broken vessels,* Boston, 1991, David R Godine.
15. Edgerton RB: *Rules, exceptions and social order,* Berkeley, 1985, University of California Press.
16. Esdaile SA: A focus on mothers, their children with special needs and other caregivers, *Aus Occup Ther J* 41:3, 1994.

17. Estes J, Deyer C, Hansen R, Russell J: Influences of occupational therapy curricula on students' attitudes toward persons with disabilities, *Am J Occup Ther* 45:156, 1991.

18. Fichten CS, Robillard K, Judd D, Amsel R: College students with physical disabilities: myths and realities. In Eisenberg MG, Glueckauf RL, editors: *Empirical approaches to the psychosocial aspects of disability,* New York, 1991, Springer.

19. Goffman E: *Stigma: notes on the management of spoiled identity,* Englewood Cliffs, NJ, 1963, Prentice-Hall.

20. Hodgins E: Whatever became of the healing art? *Ann New York Acad of Sci* 164:838, 1964.

21. Jackson J: En route to adulthood: a high school transition program for adolescents with disabilities. In Johnson JA, Yerxa EJ, editors: *Occupational science: the foundation for new models of practice,* New York, 1990, Haworth Press.

22. Kielhofner G: *A model of human occupation: theory and application,* Baltimore, 1985, Williams & Wilkins.

23. King GA, Shultz KS, Gilpin M, Cathers T: Self-evaluation and self-concept of adolescents with physical disabilities, *Am J Occup Ther* 47:132, 1993.

24. Kisor H: *What's that pig outdoors? a memoir of deafness,* New York, 1990, Penguin.

25. Konner M: *Becoming a doctor: a journey of initiation in medical school,* New York, 1987, Viking.

26. Lerner MJ, Miller DT: Just world research and the attribution process: looking back and ahead, *Psychol Bull* 85:1030, 1978.

27. Liachowitz CH: *Disability as a social construct: legislative roots,* Philadelphia, 1988, University of Pennsylvania.

28. Lyons M: Enabling or disabling? students' attitudes toward persons with disabilities, *Am J Occup Ther* 45:3, 1991.

29. Lyons M, Hayes R: Student perceptions of persons with psychiatric and other disorders, *Am J Occup Ther* 47:541, 1993.

30. The MacNeil/Lehrer NewsHour, Public Broadcasting System, April 4, 1994.

31. Magill-Evans JE, Restall G: Self-esteem of persons with cerebral palsy: from adolescence to adulthood, *Am J Occup Ther* 45:819, 1991.

32. Matsutsuyu JS: The interest checklist, *Am J Occup Ther* 23:323, 1969.

33. McCuaig M, Frank G: The able self: adaptive patterns and choices in independent living for a person with cerebral palsy, *Am J Occup Ther* 45:224, 1991.

34. Montgomery MA: Resources of adaptation for daily living: a classification with therapeutic implications for occupational therapy, *Occup Ther in Health Care* 1:9, 1984.

35. Murphy RF: *The body silent,* New York, 1990, WW Norton.

36. Peloquin SM: The patient-therapist relationship: beliefs that shape care, *Am J Occup Ther* 47:935, 1993.

37. Pendleton HM: Occupational therapists' current use of independent living skills training for adult inpatients who are physically disabled, *Occup Ther in Health Care* 6:93, 1989.

38. Pörn I: Health and adaptedness, *Theoretical Medicine,* in press.

39. Puller LB: *Fortunate son: the autobiography of Lewis B Puller, Jr,* New York, 1991, Grove Weidenfeld.

40. Reilly M: Occupational therapy can be one of the great ideas of 20th century medicine, *Am J Occup Ther* 16:300, 1962.

41. Reilly M: The educational process, *Am J Occup Ther* 23:299, 1969.

42. Reilly M: The importance of the client versus patient issue for occupational therapy, *Am J Occup Ther* 38:404, 1984.

43. Robinson I: The rehabilitation of patients with long term physical impairments: the social context of professional roles, *Clin Rehab* 2:339, 1988.

44. Schlaff C: Health policy from dependency to self-advocacy: redefining disability, *Am J Occup Ther* 47:943, 1993.

45. Seligman MEP: *Helplessness,* New York, 1975, WH Freeman.

46. Sharrott GW, Yerxa EJ: Promises to keep: implications of the referent "patient" versus "client" for those served by occupational therapy, *Am J Occup Ther* 39:401, 1985.

47. Shortell SM: Occupational prestige differences within the medical and allied health professions, *Soc Sci Med* 8:1, 1974.

48. Siegler M, Osmond H: *Models of madness, models of medicine,* New York, 1975, Macmillan.

49. Siller J: The measurement of attitudes toward physically disabled persons. In Herman CP, Zanna MP, Higgins ET: editors: *Ontario symposium on personality and social psychology,* Vol 3, *Physical appearance, stigma and social behavior,* Hillsdale, NJ, 1986, Lawrence Erlbaum.

50. Thomas D: *The experience of handicap,* New York, 1982, Methuen.

51. Turner C: Death of Canada "right to die" advocate triggers new debate, *Los Angeles Times,* April 8, 1994, A5.

52. Vash CL: *The psychology of disability, Springer series on rehabilitation,* vol 1, New York, 1981, Springer.

53. Weinberg N: Another perspective: attitudes of people with disabilities. In Yuker E, editor: *Attitudes toward persons with disabilities,* New York, 1988, Springer.

54. Westbrook M, Adamson B: Knowledge and attitudes: aspects of occupational therapy students' perceptions of the handicapped, *Aus Occup Ther J* 36:120, 1989.

55. Williams D: *Nobody nowhere: the extraordinary autobiography of an autistic,* New York, 1992, Avon.

56. Williams MR, Russell ML: *ADA handbook: employment and construction issues affecting your business,* Chicago, 1993, Dearborn Financial Pub.

57. World Health Organization: *International classification of impairments, disabilities and handicaps: a manual of classification relating to the consequences of disease,* Geneva, 1980, WHO.

58. Wright B: *Physical disability: a psychosocial approach,* ed 2, New York, 1983, Harper & Row.
59. Wright B, Fletcher BL: Uncovering hidden resources: a challenge in assessment, *Prof Psychol* 13:229, 1982.
60. Yerxa EJ: Audacious values: the energy source for occupational therapy practice. In Kielhofner G, editor: *Health through occupation,* Philadelphia, 1983, FA Davis.
61. Yerxa EJ: Dreams, dilemmas and decisions for occupational therapy practice in a new millenium: an American perspective, *Am J Occup Ther* 48:586, 1994.
62. Yerxa EJ, Clark F, Frank G, and associates: An introduction to occupational science, a foundation for occupational therapy in the 21st century, *Occup Ther in Health Care* 6:1, 1989.
63. Zola, IK: *Missing pieces: a chronicle of living with disability,* Philadelphia, 1982, Temple University Press.

Issues of Sexuality with Physical Dysfunction

Gordon Umphred Burton

The question of why the occupational therapist should be concerned with issues of sensuality or sexuality when dealing with a client often arises. The answer is that sensuality and sexuality are aspects of everyone's activities of daily living (ADL) and directly relate to the quality of each person's life. Thus it is in the domain of occupational therapy. Occupational therapists work with clients in all of the following areas related to sensuality and sexuality (see Box 17-1).

Each of these factors is involved in the sexuality and sensuality of the client. Any physical limitations may make the client question whether there is a chance of being able to make love or have sex. By becoming disabled the client has experienced an assault upon the commonly held roles and practices of the able-bodied population.[4,35] The disabled individual is often incorrectly seen as asexual, an object of pity, and as being unattractive.[26] This image alone would be disabling for anyone, even in the absence of physical disability. Being perceived as unattractive and possibly unlovable is devastating. It could lead to the concept that the disabled individual will never be intimate either emotionally or physically with anyone. This perception may result in total despair for the client and all of his or her significant others.

Charlifue and associates[5] and Kettl and associates[24] found that females with acquired spinal cord injuries reported feeling less than half as attractive after they had become disabled even though spinal cord injury is a disability in which there usually is not an observable physical change in body appearance. Yet there was a major decrease in self-perceived attractiveness shown in these studies. Males have been found to feel demasculinated by the advent of a disability and may feel their male role is threatened.[34]

These examples provide a glimpse into some of the feelings and perceptions that may affect the sensuality and sexuality of the client. These perceptions must be assessed and treated by the occupational therapist to accomplish true rehabilitation of the person with an acquired disability and the habilitation of a person with a congenital disability. In this chapter issues relating to sexuality and sensuality will be examined.

FRAMES OF REFERENCE

Occupational therapy is a holistic practice that attempts to integrate a person's physical being with his or her emotional and psychological being to attain a higher quality of life through the use of purposeful activities. Three frames of reference are explored in relation to how sexuality may fit into each.

THE DEVELOPMENTAL FRAME OF REFERENCE

In the developmental frame of reference it is proposed that development is horizontal, simultaneously occurring in psychosocial, physical, neurophysiological, and cognitive growth and sociocultural skills. At the same time the individual develops chronologically, further maturing earlier development and skills. In this frame of reference physical, physiological, or environmental insufficiencies can develop and can interrupt the growth and development process. Integration of the senses starts before birth and develops into an organization of body schema and body awareness, which not only aids in acquisition of skills but also the feeling of sensuality and sexuality.

Disability can damage either the development of sensuality or encumber already formed perceptions of sensuality.[31] Because physical expression of affection, sensuality, and sexuality may be impaired, the individual may feel an incompetence for self-expression; the result may be isolation and a feeling of inadequacy affecting normal psychosocial development.

THE MODEL OF HUMAN OCCUPATION

The model of human occupation[25] considers the subsystems of volition, habituation, performance, and environment. The concept of volition includes personal causa-

BOX 17-1

- quality of life
- role delineation
- positioning
- cultural aspects
- impulse control
- energy conservation
- muscle weakness
- hypertonicity/hypotonicity

- appreciation of body
- psychosocial issues
- range of motion
- joint protection
- motor control
- cognition
- increased or decreased sensation

tion, values, and interests. If disabled persons have been taught that the disabled are not sensual and sexual and that the disabled cannot attract others to love them physically and emotionally, they will tend not to develop interests of a sexual and sensual nature easily.

Roles and habits are elements in the concept of habituation. Roles are images a person holds of the self that serve as a source of identity. Roles coupled with habits (images of behavior guiding normal routines) form the basis for action. These roles are ways that the person thinks about how he or she should act in life. If the person has been taught that the role of the disabled is asexual and not sensual, this belief will influence the way the person carries out the habits of everyday life. This asexual role may interfere with normal dating, marital life, or procreation. Sensuality may be impaired because of lack of normal sensation and/or growing up frequently experiencing clinical medical touch.

The performance subsection in the model of human occupation is "a collection of images and biological structures and processes which are organized into skills and used in the production of purposeful behavior."[25] Skill is the organization of all systems and abilities necessary to perform purposeful activities. In the case of the disabled it is obvious that some skills may be impaired but that sex is often not thought of as a skill. It *is* a purposeful activity, however, both in intimate relationships and in the role of procreation.

The last component is that of the environment. Braces, splints, wheelchairs, and mobility devices affect the everyday environment of persons with physical disability in a negative way by inhibiting easy access to society, self-actualization, and possibilities for employment. These barriers limit the potential for developing social and intimate relationships.

OCCUPATIONAL PERFORMANCE

The occupational performance model examines three performance areas and five performance components. The three areas of performance are ADL, work and productive activities, and play or leisure. Each of these areas has elements that either communicate or require aspects of sensuality and sexuality. Self-care forces the individual to relate in a sensual way to the body; if self-care is inadequate, the individual may be shunned by others.

Another performance area is play or leisure. Through play the child develops roles and interactive skills, which allows development of deep and intimate relationships in the future. If during play children are taught that the disabled do not get married, have children, or relate to their bodies in a sensual manner this training will affect how they relate to significant others in the future.

Education is an area of performance that is both formal and informal. At school the child learns from peers as well as in the classroom. Although sex education may be taught formally at school, it is through interaction with friends and parents that attitudes and values are shaped. Many disabled children do not have the opportunity to interact with peers who have information regarding sexual issues because of lack of free play or because the disabled child does not have a close enough relationship with a nondisabled child. This situation was especially common when disabled children were kept in special classrooms isolated from the able-bodied children. In addition, parents may be hesitant to inform the child about sexuality or cannot conceive that their child would want or need to know about it.

During work, sexuality is not usually a major issue, but sensuality is always an expression of how the person feels about self, which will operate in relationships at work. If the client is seen as removed or isolated in the work place, it will be difficult to develop relationships.

It is during leisure time that sensuality and sexuality come together to help create a meaningful relationship. Leisure time is used to capitalize on the social and work relationships that can develop into a meaningful intimate relationship. Most sexual expression takes place during leisure time.

The components of occupational performance are the sensorimotor, psychosocial/psychological, and cognitive/cognitive integrative functions. Sensorimotor function is important to the development of sensuality and sexuality in that the processing of sensory information is one of the chief bases and reinforcers for the sexual act.

One of the objects of therapy is to allow the client to feel good about the self and with the body. The motor component of performance can be seen in the physical expression of sexuality. The client needs to know how to perform sexually despite specific physical limitations and how to communicate sexual needs to others.

The psychosocial/psychological component is a consideration for all people, but the disabled may need to be more assertive than the able-bodied population because they more frequently require assistance from others. People with disabilities may need to ask to have doors opened, clothes put on or taken off, or their bodies positioned. Thus they need to learn how to request help or support in a way that is acceptable to the helper and to themselves.

REACTIONS TO SEXUAL ASPECTS OF DISABILITY

Sexuality or sensuality can be an expression of confidence, validation of the self, and one's perceived lovability. When a person becomes disabled or is born with a disability, he or she may feel less positive about self and feel less lovable.[34] Sex can represent how the person is dealing with his or her world. If the person feels inadequate as a sexual, sensual, and lovable human being, there is little chance that he or she will also feel motivated to pursue other avenues of life and vice versa. When a person feels bad about the self, coping with life's problems is difficult. Because sexuality is often used as a barometer of how one feels about oneself, it is often productive for the therapist to help the client feel as positive as possible about the physical and other qualities of the self. A good sexual attitude aids motivation for all aspects of therapy.

The person's perceived self is seldom what is real. Most individuals feel that they have imperfections that everyone else sees, such as a large nose, big thighs, too much hair, or too much or too little height or weight. The therapist must try to help the client adjust self-perceptions to an extent that allows the client to function within the normal parameters of life. The goal is to increase self-esteem and enable the client to feel lovable. Feeling lovable engenders a sense of self-worth, some degree of attractiveness, sexuality, and being capable of intimacy. All of these factors work together to accomplish a realistic balance in a person's life (Fig. 17-1).

Sexuality has been found to be a predictor of marital satisfaction, adjustment to physical disability, and success of vocational training. In society people are often judged by physical attractiveness.[35] In western civilization physical intimacy is closely associated with love, so if a client perceives self as incapable of expressing sensuality or sexuality, the individual may feel incapable of loving and being loved. Without the capability of loving and being loved, the individual may feel isolated and valueless. It is the therapist's role to attempt to prevent feel-

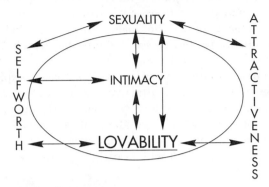

SEXUALITY AND DISABILITY

FIG. 17-1   Sexuality and disability.

ings of worthlessness and hopelessness and to attempt to encourage self-worth and productivity.[14,35]

One of the first questions that comes up when a person acquires a major injury or disability is whether or not sex is still possible. This question quickly gets buried in coping with adjustment to hospital life and activities that make up the daily routine, but it is not forgotten. A common complaint made about medical staff by people with disabilities is that the staff never dealt with nor let the disabled person deal with the topic of sexuality. People with disabilities feel that if their sensuality and sexuality is negated, a significant percentage of their person is being negated. This lack of acceptance results in the loss of feeling treated as a whole person.

Males who are newly disabled report that they feel demasculinated.[34] This problem may take many forms. Lifting weights may no longer be possible. They may not feel as capable of fighting as they once did. Sports and sporting events may not be as accessible as before. Now the person is looking up at others from a wheelchair and may be feeling dependent in getting needs met. It has been found that in both males and females increased dependence by one partner will result in a decrease in the person's sex life,[12] perhaps because the able-bodied partner is less inclined to be aroused by a partner whose body he or she just toileted or bathed. The therapist needs to be sensitive to the possiblity of these perceptions and help the client deal appropriately with the feelings they evoke. Conversations regarding sexuality may be situations in which these feelings can be discussed.

Another possible reaction to the feelings of dependency and demasculinization[34] may be trying to flirt to prove masculinity. Flirting with a female or a male therapist, depending on the client's sexual orientation, may be attempted by the client. The therapist should be alert to the issues the client is working on to prevent doing further damage to the client's sense of self. At the same time, harassment or exploitation of either the therapist or the client must not be allowed.

Females experience many of the same feelings but may interpret and react to them in a different way. Disabled women report feeling unattractive and not desirable because society puts so much emphasis on beauty. This fact may lead to despair if a woman feels that she cannot achieve some of her major goals in life. Thus the female client may flirt to see if she is still perceived as attractive.

Discussion of the topic of sexuality is a way to explore feelings of dependency, attractiveness, and unattractiveness. Communication must be established regarding the feelings of sexual role changes. If clients' perceived roles are threatened, the effects may be pervasive throughout life and should be dealt with as early as possible in treatment.

Clients often ask therapists about sexual aspects related to their disabilities because the therapist deals with other intimate issues such as self-care and personal hygiene. The trust built up in the relationship facilitates this communication. Because the therapist deals with activities such as bathing, dressing, or toileting, the client may feel safe asking questions regarding sex. The therapist should be prepared with information and resources, which does not mean that the therapist must know everything. It certainly does not mean that the occupational therapist should be a sex counselor. In some cases the therapist may be the only appropriate professional to solve specific problems such as correct sexual positioning (to be discussed later). The therapist has an obligation to help the client get the information needed.

VALUES CLARIFICATION

Sexual values of the significant other, the client, and the therapist must be examined for the therapist to interact with the client in the most effective and positive manner in regard to sexual matters.[11,35] Unless the therapist is aware of the thoughts and feelings of all of the individuals involved, the therapist may make incorrect assumptions with devastating results.[8] One of the most direct ways of gaining information is through administration of a sexual history.[8,37] The object of a sexual history is to learn how the individual thinks and feels about sex and bodily functions as well as to discover the needs of those concerned.[8,28] According to some researchers, many disabled individuals had a sexual dysfunction before they became physically disabled, which may be determined during the taking of the sexual history.[29]

Sexual History

The therapist should create an environment that will allow for confidentiality, comfort, and self-expression. In early intervention the therapist should ask about the client's concerns regarding the following: contraception, safe sex, homosexuality, masturbation, sexual health, aging, menopause, or physical changes in the body.

The following are some questions that could be asked. All questions should not be asked at the same time nor would all questions be asked of every client.

- How did you first find out about sexuality?
- In what situation did you first learn about heterosexuality and homosexuality?
- Who furnished you with information about sexuality when you were young?
- Were you ready for the information when you first heard about sexuality?
- Is sexuality important to you at this point in your life?
- How would you describe your sexual activities at this point in your life?
- How do you feel that sexuality expresses your feelings and meets your needs and those of others?
- If you could change aspects of your current sexual situation, what would you change and how would you change them?
- What concerns do you have about birth control, disease control, and your sexual safety?
- What physical, medical, or drug-related concerns do you have relating to your sexuality?
- Have you ever been pressured, threatened, or forced into a sexual situation?
- Which sexual practices have you engaged in in the past (oral, anal, genital, etc.)?
- Which sexual activities have you engaged in that you think are considered "kinky"?
- How important do you think sexuality will be in your future?
- Are there questions or concerns that you have regarding this interview?

After taking the sexual history the therapist may be able to ascertain whether there is guilt connected with the sex act, body parts, or sexual alternatives (such as masturbation, oral sex, sexual positions, or sexual devices). The therapist will be helped by this information because some clients report feelings of guilt or fear in relation to having sex after a heart attack or a stroke (fear that sex may cause a stroke or guilt at supposedly causing the first episode). Another fear is that the presence of catheters, adaptive equipment, and/or scars will not be accepted by the partner. Often performance is an issue. "Can the disabled person do it?" is the question asked by the able-bodied and the disabled alike.

The therapist can furnish the necessary information regarding sexuality by (1) directing the client to other professionals, (2) providing magazines and books, (3) showing movies, or (4) suggesting role models. The therapist must remember that the client's values and preconceived notions are probably being assaulted; the therapist should be tactful. Personal care such as toileting, hygiene (care during menstruation), for example, bathing and birth control are all issues that evoke values regarding sex and body image.

Self-care issues are not usually emphasized enough during acute illness and rehabilitation. Discussing such issues once or twice is not enough. The situation (environment) in which these issues are discussed also needs to be considered. A personal conversation cannot take place in a crowded treatment room, during a rushed and impersonal treatment session, or with a therapist with whom there is no ongoing relationship. The latter is a problem in health care facilities where therapists are frequently rotated or work on a per diem basis. The therapist must create the environment that will allow personal discussions to take place.

Discussion of feelings will also help the client explore the new body or adapt to ongoing degeneration of the body if there is a progressive disability. These conversations may take place while other therapeutic activities are in progress so that billing insurers for time is not an issue.

DEVELOPMENT OF SENSUALITY AND SEXUALITY

How does sexuality develop? The development of a sense of sensuality and sexuality begins before birth. The fetus responds to stimuli within the first eight weeks after conception. As development progresses after birth, a major focus in the child's life becomes the craving and demand for sensation and the accompanying relief of anxiety that accompanies the sensory input.[37] The sensation of touch is interpreted as pleasurable or unpleasurable. Pleasurable sensation is comforting, and the child attempts to prolong the input as can be observed in a baby that cries when nursing is ended.

If on a regular basis satisfaction is not derived from an interaction that should lead to comfort or release of stress and pain, a feeling of anxiety develops. Eventually the child develops distrust and may withdraw from interactions with others. If pleasure in interactions is developed, the ability to maintain the warmth of being close and being nourished is translated into trust, lovability, and bonding with the caretaker.[37] It is here that a sense of intimacy is initiated. Thus trust, intimacy, sensuality, lovability, and later sexuality appear to have a basis in sensory organization.

As a toddler or preschooler (1½ to 4 years) the child will put anything in the mouth and craves oral and tactile sensory input. The child develops the ability to stimulate and satisfy the self and its ego, and sensuality starts to be refined. The ability to explore the immediate world using the hands and mouth as well as other parts of the body allows the child to develop communication, self-gratification, and a feeling of competence. This feeling of competence is derived from the effective use of the body to feel good and accomplish tasks. At this point of development, body parts and body processes are named and the child perceives the body as good. Simultaneously, intimacy between the self and another person is refined, as are sex roles.[13]

Between this early phase in development and adult-

hood, these roles are tested and retested. The child develops improved motor skills to obtain positive sensory input. Children normally start exploring their own bodies as well as the bodies of others at this stage. They explore their genitals when their diapers are being changed and in the bathtub.[13,37] They show interest in looking at nude people. They explore the differences between males and females and may ask about genitals, breasts, and how babies are made. They often like the sensation of being nude and may display their genitals. Ownership of the body and what is done to it is starting to develop at this point. Toileting activities for self and others are usually seen as very interesting. Often "dirty" words for body parts and body functions occur at this stage.[23] In general the child is in an exploratory stage and little or no shame and anxiety will be attached to these activities.

Young school-age children (5-9 years) engage in most of the previously mentioned activities with greater sophistication but also develop other interests in this area. They often think of relations, especially sexual relations between opposite sex partners, as being negative and unacceptable. They talk with friends about sex and sexual matters. They want privacy when toileting, "play doctor" with others, and may compare genitals with peer-age friends. Body changes and sexual tension are heightened and the child may have fantasies of marrying one of the parents.[23] Their sense of ownership of their bodies should be well developed, and they start to feel more control over their bodies and lives. These feelings of adaquacy and self-acceptance are based on how well the person perceives that the previous tasks were accomplished.

This early development of sensuality and sexuality sets the foundation for later perceptions of the body and sense of self. It is important to remember aspects of normal development when working with children who have a disability so that the therapist may encourage age-appropriate activities. When working with adults of all ages, it is important to remember this development and that some of the activities engaged in may stimulate memories of these past events. Some activities may be perceived as a form of infantilism or may bring up unresolved issues for the client or the therapist. This fact is especially true of activities of daily living such as dressing, toileting, hygiene, and general self-care.

SEXUAL ABUSE OF CHILDREN

The life of a child is an evolving barrage of experiences that helps mold and direct the future of this sensitive, unique being. Many experiences, positive and negative, can lead to growth and learning, which, in turn, helps the child mature into a well-adjusted, caring adult member of society. One kind of experience that is deleterious to the growth and adjustment of a child toward adulthood is sexual abuse.[14] Although most adults wish to closet this concept because of the emotional nature of the issue, the problem cannot be ignored. The helplessness of a normal child toward advances from a larger, stronger, more authoritative adult who may be a caregiver is well documented. The inability to run away, to yell, to tell about the experience, or to ward off unwanted touching because of a dysfunctional motor system places the disabled child at a higher risk for sexual abuse than able-bodied children.[1]

The development of normal sensuality and sexuality may be disrupted as a result of sexual abuse and attitudes the child develops toward his or her disabled body.[1] In order to evolve from a giggling child toward a mature sensual adult, the child needs normal relationships, normal experiences, and when matured and ready, normal sensual and sexual interactions with a significant other.

Therapists must increase their awareness of what constitutes sexual abuse. Children with disabilities have long been forced to undress and be examined or treated as part of their care. This treatment is sometimes necessary, but the wishes and dignity of the person should be respected at all times. A college student with an upper extremity amputation related a story that when she was 16 years old, and physically mature, she was instructed to undress down to the waist and walk in front of an assembly of male doctors and medical students to be examined in a pediatric prosthetic clinic. She was humiliated and ashamed and believed that this incident happened only because of her disability. This experience increased a hatred of her disability and her body and made her more self-conscious. Such callous disregard of a client's feelings is a form of abuse and cannot be tolerated in any clinical situation. A child of any age should not be forced to endure the abuse of humiliation.

The many obstacles encountered by the disabled should not interfere with the expression of sensuous and sexual needs that everyone has. As an informed professional, each therapist can help the adult client eliminate unnecessary obstacles that may linger. The therapist can help the client remove and overcome anxieties as well as appreciate each individual's uniqueness.

ATTITUDINAL CONCERNS FROM CHILD TO ADULT

During an interview with an adult who had cerebral palsy the person stated that therapy was either so painful or so clinical that she disassociated herself from sensations in her body during and after therapy. Later in life this reaction became a problem when she was married. She stated that it took seven years of marriage before she could enjoy the sensations of being touched by her husband. She also stated that it was a revolutionary concept for her to realize that a vibrator could be used to give sexual pleasure rather than to activate muscles in therapy.

The therapy session should help the client develop a sense of personal ownership of the body.* This goal is often neglected in working with adults but is especially neglected by health professionals when working with children. If the therapist does not ask permission to touch a client, it could imply that the client does not have the right to control being touched by others. The therapist should guard against communication of this notion to the client. A person who believes that he or she does not have the right to say NO! to being touched, who cannot physically resist unwanted advances and may not even be able to communicate that abuse has taken place, makes a good victim.[1] The effects can be seen in adults. When one client was asked why tone increased in her lower extremities when she was touched, her response was, "I was sexually abused by my father in the name of therapy, and therapy and sexual abuse are synonymous at this point." It was no wonder that she had been resistant to reentering therapy!

Another way of helping clients take charge of their bodies is through naming body parts and body processes. Once the body parts and processes are named, using correct terminology rather than slang, there is the possibility for the client to communicate and to relate in an appropriate manner.[1,7,32,37] The use of the proper terms has the effect of viewing the body in a more positive way, because slang tends to be used to identify negative images.[37]

Children often think that bad things happen only to bad people and consequently may believe that being disabled is punishment for being bad. The adult client who has lost cognitive abilities may be thinking at a childlike level or may hold such beliefs. This concept can be cultural in nature but should be dealt with early to make sure that it does not enter the client's self-perception and hurt his or her body image. To develop the concept that the body (in the case of congenital disabilities) or the "new" body (in the case of acquired disabilities) is acceptable and good may be one of the goals of therapy.[1,7,32,37,41] The client has a better chance of seeing the body in an acceptable way and may approach therapy more favorably. This attitude can be encouraged by pointing out a particularly positive feature about the client's body and mentioning this regularly. The feature could be the hair or eyes or a smile but should be an aspect of the client that can be seen and commented upon by others as well.[9] Commenting on how good the body feels when it is relaxed or how good the sun feels on the body helps the client recognize that the body can be a positive source of pleasure.

Another message from early life that can affect the adult client is the concept that the disabled are asexual and will never have sexual needs or partners.[1,3,7,32,37] While it may be difficult to deal with this concept directly, the therapist may mention to the client that he or she knows of persons with disabilities who are married

---

* References 1,3,7,27,32,37.

and/or have children. In this way the therapist is communicating that there is the possibility that usual sex roles can be continued or fulfilled in the future. If this possibility is not presented, the client may think that all the movies, books, and television programs that deal with normal adult interactions don't apply to the disabled. Such attitudes can promote poor socialization and alienation of the disabled population from the able-bodied population.

ADULT SEXUALITY

Adaptive devices such as braces, wheelchairs, and communication aids can be a detriment to one's perceived attractiveness and sexuality. It may be hard to perceive the self as sexual when there is an indwelling catheter or braces are worn. By discussing the effect of these devices on social interaction, the client can get some ideas about how to handle situations when they arise.[1,29,32,41]

Discussing positioning to reduce pain or spasticity or to enable the client to more comfortably engage in sexual relations will help the client deal with problems before they occur.[8,27,32] Sexual hygiene may be considered as an activity of daily living and so is in the domain of occupational therapy.

The client may feel that his or her masculinity or femininity is threatened by the disability[34] and try to assert sexuality through jokes, flirting, or "passes" at the therapist. It is important for the therapist to realize that the client is seeking confirmation of his or her sexuality. The therapist's response is very important. If the therapist rejects or ridicules the client, the client may be very hesitant to attempt such confirmation of personal attractiveness in future situations that are more socially appropriate. If the therapist rejects the client, the client may deduce that if someone who is familiar with disabled persons is rejecting, there is little chance that anyone unfamiliar with them could accept him or her as lovable. The therapist should not be surprised by such advances and should deal with the situation in a professional manner. Setting personal boundaries appropriate to the client-therapist relationship, while accepting the personhood and needs of the client, is important.

Because it is estimated that up to ten percent of the population is homosexual, the therapist may expect sexual advances from clients of the same sex. It is important to be equally professional in such instances. All of the therapist's interactions should be directed toward creating an environment that promotes the client's self-esteem, positive sexuality, and adjustment to disability.

One way to help the client to discuss intimate matters is asking the client how she will perform a breast self-examination with her disability. A male may be asked how he will perform a self-examination of the testicles. If the treatment facility does not have information about these examinations, they are available from the local Planned Parenthood Association. Each of these activities

falls into the domain of health maintenance and may not have been discussed by others. This interaction will set the stage for discussion of other personal matters, impress upon the client the necessity for concern about personal health, and reaffirm the client's sexual identity.

SEXUAL ABUSE OF ADULTS

Sexual abuse of adults is often not thought of as an area that relates to clients or the disabled but there is sufficient evidence that abuse is a considerable problem.[1] Some people who have disabilities have reported being approached by pimps representing prostitution rings that specialize in providing disabled people for their customers. It appears that there are some persons who are attracted by the idea of having sex with someone who is physically disabled and are willing to pay for this service. Clients should be made aware of the possibility of this type of exploitation. Some clients have reported that medical staff took inappropriate liberties with them and that aides on whom they depended demanded sexual favors. Clients can and should report such assaults to Adult Protective Services. The therapist must also report cases of suspected sexual abuse. The client may be concerned that if abuse is reported, he or she may not be able to get another aide or that, during the time that an aide is being hired, essential assistance will not be available. These are major concerns for a person who is dependent on others for care and these concerns should be respected.

As a general rule therapists do not suspect other care givers, medical staff, aides, transportation assistants, or volunteers, but the therapist should be alert to signs of possible abuse even from these sources.[36] It is a fact of life that some individuals prey on and victimize disabled adults and children and are drawn to the health fields with this motive.[1] The therapist should watch for potential signs of abuse such as the following: 1) clients usually being upset after interacting with a specific person; 2) care givers taking clients off alone for no apparent reason; 3) excessive touching in a sensual manner by care givers; 4) the client's being agitated when around a specific individual; and 5) the client being overly compliant with a specific individual.

Many professional schools do not train the health care workers on the subject of sexuality and disability.[16] Inservice training can be arranged to help the staff be aware of the sexual needs of the disabled.[24,15] Books, articles, video tapes, and training packets are available for professional education.[3,10,11] Unless the staff is educated about the significance of sexuality and related issues, they may have negative feelings about dealing with these matters.[3]

THE EFFECTS OF THE PHYSICAL SYMPTOMS OF DYSFUNCTION

Specific symptoms that may create problems for the disabled persons and their partners and suggestions for

TABLE 17-1   Conditions and Possible Effects on Sexual Functioning

	SYMPTOM															
DIAGNOSES	Anxiety/Fear	Contractures	Cultural Barriers	Decreased Libido	Depression	Impotence	Incontinence	Limited ROM	Loss of Mobility	Loss of Sensation	Low Endurance	Medication	Paralysis/Spasticity	Poor Body Image	Tremor	Catheter/Ostomy
Amputations	x	x	x		x				x	x				x		
Arthritis	x	x	x	x	x			x	x		x	x		x		
Burns	x	x	x		x			x	x	x	x		x	x		
Cardiac	x		x	x	x	x*			x		x	x		x		
Cerebral Palsy	x	x	x		x		x	x	x	x	x		x	x	x	x
CVA	x	x	x	x	x	x	x	x	x	x	x	x	x	x	x	x
Diabetes	x		x	x	x	x			x	x	x			x	x	
Hand Injury	x	x	x		x			x	x	x			x	x		
Head Injury	x	x	x	x+	x	x	x	x	x	x	x	x	x	x	x	x
Musculoskeletal	x	x	x		x		x	x	x	x	x	x	x	x	x	
Spinal Cord Injury	x	x	x		x	x	x	x	x	x	x	x	x	x	x	x

x, Possible involvement; *, Fear or medication as possible causes; +, Increased or decreased

their management are outlined below and summarized in Table 17-1.

Hypertonia

Hypertonia can increase when the muscles are stretched. To avoid quick stretching of muscles involved in a movement pattern, motion should be performed slowly. It is advisable to incorporate rotation into the movement to break up the spasticity. Slow rocking can be used to inhibit the hypertonic musculature. Gentle shaking and/or slow stroking (massage) can also be inhibitory. Heat or cold can also be used to inhibit tone. Clients with hypertonia may need to discuss options for different positions in which to have sexual intercourse. Alternate ways of dealing with personal hygiene (toileting, inserting tampons, gynecological examinations, and birth control) may need to be explored in relation to hypertonicity.

Flaccidity

With low tone (hypotonia) the client may need physical support using pillows or towels or even bolsters to prop up body parts, allowing for endurance and protecting the body from over stretching and fatigue. Sexual positions that allow support of the joints involved need to be explored as well as the client's and partner's attitudes about the positions.

Low Endurance

Low endurance can create problems during sex because the individual may not be able to tolerate prolonged activity. Some techniques for dealing with these problems are work simplification, timing of sex when there is the most energy, and assuming positions in which sexual performance takes less energy.

Loss of Mobility and Contractures

By definition this symptom does not allow for many movement patterns, and positions for sex will be limited due to the limitations of range of motion. Activity analysis must be done in order to find the positions that will allow for sexual activity. This system often requires creative problem-solving on the part of the client, the partner, and the responsible professional counselor.

Joint Degeneration

Conditions such as arthritis can cause pain, damage to the joints, and contractures. Joint damage can be lessened by avoiding stress and repetitive weight bearing on the joints. Activity analysis is needed to reduce joint stress and excessive weight-bearing on the joints. It is necessary to find a position, such as the one represented in Figure 17-2, which takes weight and stress off the knees or hips. This position should not be carried out so it puts undue stress on the back, however. It may not be acceptable for the client if there is limited hip abduction, in which case a sidelying position may be more acceptable. If hip abduction is limited, positions such as those shown in Figures 17-2, 17-5, and 17-9 should be avoided.

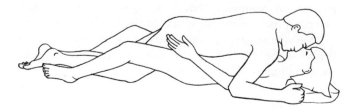

FIG. 17-2 This position places pressure on female's bladder and requires hip abduction but little energy expenditure for her.

Pain

Pain limits the enjoyment of sexual activities.[20] There is usually a time of day that pain is diminished and that energy is at its highest. Sexual activities can be scheduled for such times. Some time after taking medication most people find that pain will be diminished and that sexual activity can be pursued. Communication between partners is especially important when pain is involved. The unaffected partner may feel that his or her needs are not being considered, perhaps because the partner does not understand the strong negative effect of pain, cannot see a physical problem, and may believe that the person with the pain is just not interested. A referral to a counselor who understands the effects of pain may help work out emotional aspects of this problem. The occupational therapist may help the client think of acceptable ways of meeting the partner's sexual needs while not causing pain. Masturbation and mutual masturbation with sexual fantasy are possible ways of meeting sexual needs in these circumstances. In this way the partners are interacting and neither person is feeling isolated.

Loss of Sensation

The loss of sensation can affect the sexual relationship in several ways. The lack of erogenous sensation in the affected area can block proper warning that an area is being abraded (in the case of the vagina not being sufficiently lubricated) or damaged (bladder or even bones if the partner is on top and being too forceful). Lack of sensation can signify a disruption of reflex loop responsible for sensation and reflexogenic erections in the male or lubrication in the female. Either of these issues can be dealt with but they must first be noted. Information on skin care, erections, and lubrication are discussed later in this chapter.

Aging and Sexuality

With aging, changes take place that can affect sexuality. Menopause and the resulting hormonal changes may cause vaginal atrophy and slowed reactions to sexual stimulation. In the male greater stimulation may be needed to develop and maintain an erection, and reaction time between erections may be greater. Partners need to be informed of ways to increase stimulation and to realize that it is quality and not quantity of sexual activity that is important in the relationship. The client should be made aware of the maturing process and its normal effect on sexuality so that the disability is not blamed for all of the problems. It is important not to add dysfunction unrelated to the disability. Following are sexual changes that result from normal aging (see Box 17-2).

Isolation

The environment is composed of objects, persons, and events. In all activities there is a person/environment interaction. Some of the objects with which disabled persons interact are wheelchairs, braces, canes, crutches, and splints. These objects are all hard, cold, and angular. They communicate a hard exterior and a fragile interior and may convey the notion that there is no softness, that it is not safe to hug, and that a person in a wheelchair or in braces or on crutches may get hurt or toppled if touched. Thus the disabled person may grow up feeling isolated by the appliances or, as one client expressed it, "in a plastic bubble." People may relate to the objects around the client in a nonsensual manner, creating events that may reinforce lack of sensuousness and isolation in the client. Often clients feel isolated and different from the "normal" population. This pheonomenon is seen with greater frequency in clients who have been out

---

BOX 17-2

FEMALE

1. Vaginal lubrication decreases and is delayed
2. Size and elasticity of the vagina decreases
3. Size of the uterus decreases
4. Thickness of the vaginal wall decreases
5. Reaction of muscle tone decreases
6. Vaginal itching increases
7. Chance of infection increases
8. Orgasm decreases in length

MALE

1. Strength of orgasm decreases
2. Spontaneous erection decreases (needs extra stimulation)
3. Length of time needed before ejaculation increases
4. Length of time needed before second act increases
5. Size and firmness of the testes decrease
6. Sperm count and quantity of seminal fluid decreases
7. Hardness of erection decreases
8. Decreased steroids may result in decreased muscle strength and drive

of the health care facility for a period of time. Even in the relatively acute phase of the disability, the therapist and the client may role play how to deal with a new partner or how to explain equipment used, such as a catheter. This approach may help ease the client's fears and make him or her feel more comfortable with such issues. At the same time the therapist is communicating the message to the client that sex may be a possibility in the future. It should be pointed out to the client that there has never been a time in human history that disabled people did not exist in society. Thus disabled persons are a part of society and it is not "abnormal" to be disabled. All who live long enough will become disabled to a greater or lesser extent at some time.

Medication

The side effects of medication may cause impotence or delayed sexual response and other problems. Side effects of medication should be discussed with the physician and the pharmacist to see if medications can be altered or changed. If they cannot, acknowledging that the problem is organic may be helpful to the client. Diuretics and antihypertensives may cause impotence, decreased libido, and/or loss of orgasm. Tranquilizers and antidepressants may contribute to decreased libido and even impotence in some individuals.

Performance Anxiety

At times of great emotional stress the male may find that the reflexogenic erection may be inhibited. This problem may lead to increased anxiety in relation to sexuality and create a cycle of dysfunctional inhibition. Taking the focus off of erection and genital intercourse and focusing upon sensuality and making each other feel good is helpful. A massage is one possibility that will allow for more normal physiological reactions. If this approach does not work, a trained counselor may be needed to help deal with this problem, if it has been determined that is not organic in nature.

Skin Care

The person with a disability should be informed that positioning modifications may be needed to allow for better protection of the skin to prevent skin breakdown and to increase pleasure. If a sexual position causes repeated rubbing on the skin, this friction may cause abrasions and result in damage. The therapist and client can discuss methods to prevent the friction through an alternative position, for example. Pressure on bony prominences or a partner exerting pressure in a specific area may also cause problems with skin irritation and must be avoided.

Lubrication

Stimulation of natural lubrication in females is very important but may be overlooked in a woman with paralysis because she may not be able to feel the stimulation and lack of natural lubrication. There should be stimulation to cause reflexive lubrication even when the woman does not feel it. Without proper lubrication, damage may occur without awareness of the problem. If needed, artificial water-based lubricants (such as K-Y Jelly) should be introduced. The individual should also be warned that only water-based lubricants are appropriate because petroleum-based lubricants may cause irritation and will attack latex condoms, causing condom failure. It should be remembered that in heterosexual sex, the female is more likely to be infected with HIV than the male in any given encounter. So condom failure is a major concern.

Erection

To the male the ability to achieve an erection is seen as one of the most significant signs of his masculinity.[34] If awareness of sensory stimulation to the penis is blocked by the sensory loss associated with the paralysis and the male does not try to stimulate a reflexogenic erection, he may believe that he is impotent. This belief may not be true, and the client may go through much anguish needlessly. The client should be encouraged to explore his body. Rubbing the penis, the thighs, or the anus, may be effective to evoke a reflexogenic erection. Even rubbing the big toe has been reported by some men with quadriplegia to stimulate an erection. If the reflex loop is broken, it may not be possible to achieve an erection and alternative methods may need to be explored. The first of these may be forms of sex that do not require an erect penis such as using a vibrator, oral, or digital sex. If the client feels that penile intercourse is the only acceptable alternative there are some possibilities. Injections of hormones that stimulate erections may be used but this practice may lead to problems if the client does not have good judgment, hand dexterity, or has adverse reactions. Use of a vacuum tube is sometimes effective and is one of the less invasive techniques.[37] Surgical implants can be used but may have drawbacks such as infection and skin breakdown. An excellent discussion of these alternatives can be found in the journal, *Sexuality and Disability*, Vol. 12, No. 1, 1994.

Birth Control

There are many issues that the disabled must be aware of regarding birth control.[6,18,27,32] One is the fact that most disabling conditions do not impair fertility (especially for females). This makes it important for the client to be aware of birth control issues and complications of the use of birth control. Condoms require good use of the hands; although an applicator can be adapted in some cases, someone with good hand dexterity must assemble the device beforehand. Diaphragms are not very feasible for people who have poor hand function unless the partner does have hand function and both parties feel comfortable to place the diaphragm as an aspect of foreplay. The contraceptive sponge requires good use of hands. Using "the pill" may increase the risk of thrombosis especially when there is impaired mobility or paralysis. If the client has decreased sensation, the IUD may result in increased complications from bleeding, cramping, puncturing of the uterus, or infection. Use of spermicides requires good control of the hands or the assistance of the partner who has normal hand function. In using any method of birth control, the client must always be concerned with decreasing the chance of infection and using safe sex.

Adaptive Aids

There may be a need to make use of adaptive aids, especially if the client lacks hand function. One aid may be a vibrator for foreplay or masturbation.[16] There are special vibrators adapted for males and females.[8,27,32] Pillows can be used for positioning and other devices can be used for clients who have special needs. The therapist must prepare the client for the concept of using sexual aids before suggesting the option to the client. For example, the therapist can suggest that the client explore, in private, the sensation that the vibrator produces in the lower extremities; the client may discover the possible use of the vibrator or will at least be more open to the idea of using a vibrator as a sexual aid when told how it can be used.

Safe Sex

The issue of safe sex has increased considerably since the advent of AIDS. Safe sex is important also in order to protect against all forms of sexually transmitted diseases (STDs).[18] Clients need to be reassured that this issue is important for them for several reasons. If there is a sensory impairment in and around the genital area the person may not be aware of the infection, which can lead to considerable harm. Having any genital infection allows for an easy entrance for other STDs. The disabled person must be informed of the increased risk for HIV and STDs so that he or she will be extra cautious and thus empowered.

Hygiene Concerns

Catheter care should be addressed, especially when hand function is impaired. Questions may be raised regarding how or if one can have sex when a person has an indwelling catheter. Sex is possible for both males and females but some precautions should be taken. If at any time the catheter becomes chinked or closed off (which will definitely happen in the case of a catheterized male having vaginal intercourse), pressure should not be placed upon the bladder. The length of time of the restriction of flow of urine should be kept as short as possible (not much over 30 minutes), and the bladder should be fully voided before sexual activity. Damage to the bladder and kidneys could result if these precautions are not followed. As a preventive measure the client should not drink fluids at least two hours before sex to avoid the bladder filling during this time. Sexual positions that avoid pressure on the bladder should be used (see Figs. 17-3 to 17-10). Many of the same positions may be used if the client uses a stoma appliance.

It is not uncommon for a person with an impairment of bowel or bladder function to have an occasional episode of incontinence during sexual activities. If the client

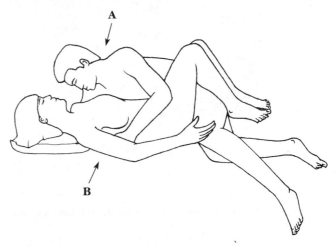

FIG. 17-3 Vaginal entry of *B* requires no hip abduction, and hip flexion tightness would not impede performance. Energy requirements for both parties is minimal. Bladder pressure, catheter safety, and stoma appliance safety should not be an issue in this position for *B*. This position may be recommended if *B* has back pain or is paralyzed, especially if roll is used to support lumbar spine.

and the therapist discuss this possibility and how to deal with it, some of the client's awkwardness may be averted when it occurs. This form of role playing can also be used to go over other scenarios such as "you are heading to the bedroom with a new partner. How will you explain your catheter and appliances to the person?" These may

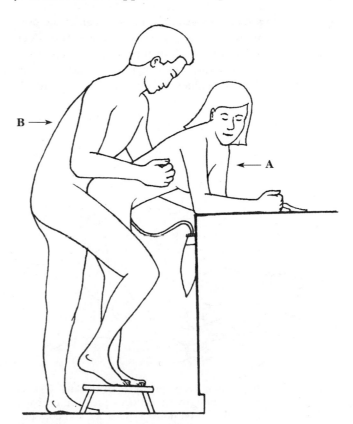

FIG. 17-4 Partner *A* needs little hip abduction but good strength. Partner *B* may find decreased strain on his back. Hip, knee, or ankle joint degeneration would preclude this position for either partner.

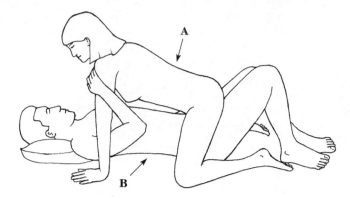

FIG. 17-5 Person *A* must have hip abduction, balance, and endurance but pressure is off of bladder and stoma. If catheter is used it would be unrestricted. Back pain may be avoided by keeping trunk vertical. Person *B*'s hip flexors could be contracted. If low back pain is a problem legs should be flexed and roll placed under low back. If stoma appliance is used this position would avoid interference. If low endurance is a problem this position can be used effectively for *B*.

be awkward conversations for the therapist and the client but it is usually easier to deal with these issues beforehand than waiting for the potential embarassment of the event.

Pregnancy, Delivery, and Child Care

Complications may arise resulting from pregnancy that may affect function and mobility of the client. Before becoming pregnant the women should consider the possibility of respiratory or kidney complications. The effect of the increased weight on transfers, an increased possibility of dysreflexia (autonomic hyperreflexia), and the need for increased bladder and/or bowel care are all

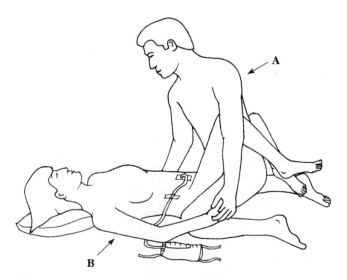

FIG. 17-6 This position keeps pressure off bladder, lessens chance of tubing becoming bent, reduces pressure on back (especially if small roll is used under low back), and does not require *B* to use much energy. Legs do not need to be as high as is shown but if hip flexors are contracted this position may be comfortable.

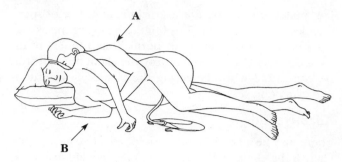

FIG. 17-7 Partner *B* need not expend much energy in this position. Both partners may avoid swayback in this position. Either person may have hemiparesis. Person *B* will not need hip abduction, and pressure on stoma bag may be avoided.

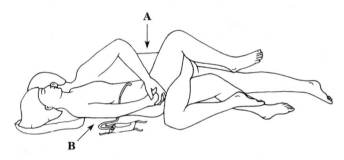

FIG. 17-8 This position can be used if either partner has hemiparesis. If low endurance is a problem this position can be used. Person *A* may avoid swayback in this position.

aspects that should be considered when pregnancy is contemplated.[40] Labor and delivery may present some special problems such as a lack of awareness of the beginning of labor contractions. Induction of labor may be contraindicated if a person has a spinal cord injury at T-6 or above, and the medical staff may not be trained to deal with the possible respiratory problems or dysreflexia that can result. After delivery the disabled parent may need to have modifications made to the wheelchair or consultations may be needed to achieve an optimal level of function for the client in the parenting role.[18]

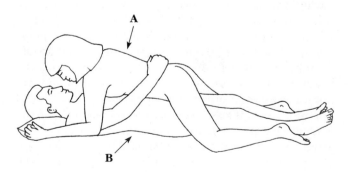

FIG. 17-9 Partner *B* can be paralyzed or have limited ROM. His back may need roll for support and he must be concerned with pressure on his bladder.

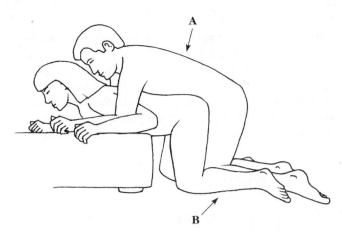

FIG. 17-10   Rear vaginal entry of *B,* who does not need much energy because of support and little or no abduction of hips. Flexion tightness of hips does not affect performance. Due to weight on *B*'s knees, hips, and back as well as inevitable repetitive movement at hips, this would not be a good position for individuals with back, hip, or knee joint degeneration.

EMOTIONAL FACTORS AND METHODS OF EDUCATION

The following techniques or approaches have been effectively used to deal with the emotional apects of some sexual problems of the disabled persons.

Repeat Information

Just mentioning sexual issues once is not enough. Most people, whether they are disabled or not, need to hear information more than once. This fact is especially true for people who are in crisis or who are in the process of adjustment. Too much information, or more information than is asked for, should not be offered at one time. The recipient may become overwhelmed. The therapist should not assume that the client understands all of the information and should have the client ask questions, paraphrase what has been said, or ask questions to see if the information is comprehended.

Discovery of the "New" Body

With any disability the client has suffered an alteration of the perception of the body. In effect the client has a new body and must find altered ways of moving, interpreting sensations, and performing activities of daily living. A large part of the therapeutic experience is to help the client discover how to use this new body as effectively as possible and optimally to process sensory information. The therapist can facilitate this exploration of the new body by creating situations that will encourage awareness of the body through the input of sensation and function.[29] This awareness can be accomplished through exercises that encourage exploration of the body by the client or both the client and his or her sexual partner. Exercises such as gentle tapping or rubbing of a specific area can be developed to see if there is sensation or if the

stimulation causes a change in tone. It should be noted that many people with a disability, such as paralysis, report that they have experienced nongenital orgasms[24] by stimulating other new erogenous areas, often in the area just above where sensation starts to appear. Suggestions for how to use this sensation or change in tone in ADL may be given by the therapist, or the therapist may ask the client to think of ways this change in tone could be used, such as triggering reflex leg extension to assist with putting on pants. This discussion will stimulate problem solving in the client and lead to the client's empowerment.

PLISSIT

This acronym stands for *p*ermission, *l*imited *i*nformation, *s*pecific *s*uggestions, and *i*ntensive *t*herapy. It is a progressive approach to guide the therapist to help the client deal with sexual information.[2] Permission refers to allowing the client to feel new feelings and experiment with new thoughts or ideas regarding sexual functioning. Limited information refers to explaining what effect the disability may have upon sexual functioning. At this point an explanation with great detail is not usually necessary. The next level of information is providing Specific Suggestions. It may be in the therapist's domain to give specific suggestions on how to deal with specific problems that relate to the disability, such as positioning. This level is the highest the average therapist should attempt without education and training because an extensive counseling background is needed to help the client undergo intensive therapy. Intensive therapy should be reserved for the rare client who has an abnormal coping pattern in dealing with sexuality.

Communication

During all aspects of the rehabilitation process the client will need to work on communication with the therapist and staff, as well as with his or her sexual partner. The therapist can facilitate this process by simply giving permission to the client to discuss feelings and techniques that relate to problems, especially in the area of sexuality. The client may need to learn how accurately to communicate sexual needs, desires, and position options to a partner either verbally or nonverbally to have a mutually satisfactory sexual relationship.[24] Each client will have unique problems or issues in this area that may be related to the nature of the disability. An example is a client with Parkinson's disease in whom the lack of facial expression impedes the nonverbal communication of intimacy. The client can be taught verbally to communicate to a partner feelings that were previously conveyed with a smile.

Activity Analysis

To assess the positioning needs of the client, the therapist must analyze the components of the activity. This analysis entails looking at the physical, psychological, social, cultural, and cognitive components of the client's functioning. The activity analysis should be implemented using an objective and professional perspective. The therapist must realize that the sex act itself, if there is one, is only a small fraction of the act of making love and should be treated as just one more activity of daily living that must be analyzed and needs professional assistance. The therapist must also remember that not all partners had sex on a daily, weekly, or even yearly basis before the onset of the disability. The therapist's values and biases should not be imposed on the client, especially if the partners are of the same sex, if there are multiple partners, if masturbation was or is the preferred method of releasing sexual tension, and if the client never had a need for the release of sexual tension.

Sex Education

Some clients may be in need of sex education if they didn't have the information before the disability. Some clients may not have been informed because of the disability, or they may be misinformed about sexual practices.[1] Research has shown that people with hearing impairments have substantially less information regarding sex than do those without hearing impairments.[39] If the occupational therapist is not the one to educate the client or the significant other, he or she should anticipate this need and have knowledge of the resources available for the client to acquire information. It is advisable to avoid pushing only books regarding sexuality and the disabled. Such books are useful but their focus on the disability can be discouraging to some. Books written for the able-bodied such as *The Hite Report on Male Sexuality*,[22] and *The Hite Report*,[21] or *How to Satisfy a Woman Every Time*[19] may be useful. These books not only will give the client an understanding of sex but also will allow the client a chance to see that he or she is normal, while minimizing the focus on the disability. The use of the excellent books available for the disabled such as *Choices: A Guide to Sexual Counseling with the Physically Disabled*,[32] *Reproductive Issues for Persons with Physical Disabilities*,[18] *The Sensuous Wheeler*,[33] *Sexuality and the Person with Traumatic Brain Injury*,[17] *Sex and Back Pain*,[20] and *Enabling Romance*[27] should not be negated, however.

Harassment of Staff

Previously it was stated that clients may have trouble dealing with their feelings regarding attractiveness and that the staff should not overreact or reject the client. At the same time the therapist should *never* permit a client to harass him or her sexually.[30,38] It is harassment when the therapist feels threatened, intimidated, or treated as a sexual object. Sexual harassment is not only damaging to staff morale but to the client as well if it is allowed.[17] Direct feedback should be given explaining that the therapist feels offended and that this behavior is inappropriate and must cease. All of the staff should be informed and develop and implement a plan to modify the client's behavior if it persists.

SUMMARY

Occupational therapists are concerned with the sexuality of their clients because it is related to self-esteem, influences adjustment to disability, and because sexual functioning is an activity of daily living. As with other activities of daily living, a physical dysfunction may necessitate some change in methods of performance. Education, counseling, and activity analysis can be used to solve many common sexual problems confronted by persons with physical dysfunction.

Occupational therapists may provide information and referrals to clients who are concerned with sexual issues. Trained therapists may fulfill counseling roles. Issues of sexual development, sexual abuse, and values need to be considered in sex education and counseling. Through activity analysis and problem solving, the physical symptoms of the disability that affect sexual functioning can usually be managed. A wide variety of sexual practices, sexual expression, and expression of sensuality are possible. The client needs the opportunity to explore his or her needs and acceptable options to meet those needs. The occupational therapist is one of the members of the rehabilitation team who has something to offer in rehabilitating the client in the area of sexuality and sensualty.

REVIEW QUESTIONS

1. List at least five areas related to sensuality or sexuality that are usually the concerns of the occupational therapist.
2. What are some common attitudes of the able-bodied population about sexuality of persons with physical dysfunction?
3. How do these attitudes affect the disabled person's perception of self and attitudes toward his or her own sexuality?
4. How is sexuality related to self-esteem and a sense of attractiveness?
5. Describe some typical questions for sexual history-taking. How can these questions be used to clarify values about sexuality?
6. Describe the stages of sexual development and some positive and negative influences on it.
7. Why is a child with a physical dysfunction more vulnerable to sexual abuse?
8. What are some attitudes about sexuality that may be carried over from childhood to adult life?
9. How do mobility aids and assistive devices impact sexual functioning? How can this situation be managed?
10. What are some signs of potential sexual abuse of adults?

11. What are some suggestions for dealing with the following physical symptoms during sexual activity: hypertonia, low endurance, joint degeneration, and loss of sensation.

12. List some medications that may cause sexual dysfunction.

13. Discuss some issues and precautions relative to birth control for the woman with a physical disability.

14. How is a catheter managed during sexual activity?

15. What are some potential problems in pregnancy, delivery, and child care?

16. Discuss some techniques for educating a person about sexual issues.

17. How should sexual harassment of staff members by clients be handled?

REFERENCES

1. Andrews AB, Veronen LJ: Sexual assault and people with disabilities, *Journal of Social Work and Human Sexuality* 8(2):137-159, 1993.

2. Annon JS: *The behavioral treatment of sexual problems,* Vols. 1, 2, Honolulu, 1974, Enabling Systems.

3. Boyle PS: Training in sexuality and disability: preparing social workers to provide services to individuals with disabilities, *Journal of Social Work and Human Sexuality* 8(2):45-62, 1993.

4. Braithwaite DO: From majority to minority: an analysis of cultural change from able-bodied to disabled, *International Journal of Intercultural Relations* 14:465-483, 1990.

5. Charlifue SW, Gerhart KA, Menter RR and associates: Sexual issues of women with spinal cord injuries, *Paraplegia* 30(3):192-199, 1992.

6. Cole SS, Cole TM: Sexuality, disability, and reproductive issues for persons with disabilities. In Haseltine FP, Cole SS, Gray DB, editors. *Reproductive issues for persons with physical disabilities,* Baltimore, 1993, Paul H Brooks.

7. Cole SS, Cole TM: Sexuality, disability, and reproductive issues through the life span, *Sexuality and Disability* 11(3):189-205, 1993.

8. Cole TM.: Gathering a sex history from a physically disabled adult, *Sexuality and Disability* 9(1):29-37, 1991.

9. Corbett K, Klein S, Bregante JL: The role of sexuality and sex equality in the education of disabled women, *Peabody Journal of Education* 64(4):198-211, 1987.

10. Cornelius DA, Chipouras S, Makas E, Daniels SM: *Who cares? a handbook on sex education and counseling services for disabled people,* Baltimore, 1982, University Park Press.

11. Ducharme S, Gill KM: (1991). Sexual values, training, and professional roles, *J Head Trauma Rehabil* 5(2):38-45, 1991.

12. Edwards DF, Baum CM:. Caregivers burden across stages of dementia, *Occupational Therapy Practice* 2(1):17-31, 1990.

13. Fitz-Gerald M, Fitz-Gerald DR: Involvement in sex education, *Volta-Review* 89(5):96-110, 1987.

14. Froehlich J: Occupational therapy interventions with survivors of sexual abuse, *Occupational Therapy in Health Care* vol 8 (2 & 3): 1-25,1992.

15. Gender AR: An overview of the nurse's role in dealing with sexuality, *Sexuality and Disability* 10(2):71-70,1992.

16. Goldstein H, Runyon C: An occupational therapy education module to increase sensitivity about geriatric sexuality, *Physical and Occupational Therapy in Geriatrics* 11(2):57, 1993.

17. Griffith ER, Lemberg S: *Sexuality and the person with traumatic brain injury: a guide for families,* Philadelphia, 1993, FA Davis.

18. Haseltine FP, Cole SS, Gray DB: *Reproductive issues for persons with physical disabilities,* Baltimore,1993, Paul H Brooks.

19. Hayden N: *How to satisfy a woman every time,* New York, 1982, Bibli O'Phile.

20. Hebert L: *Sex and back pain,* Bloomington, Minn, 1987, Educational Opportunities (800) 654-8357.

21. Hite S: *The Hite report,* New York, 1976, Macmillan.

22. Hite S: *The Hite report on male sexuality,* New York, 1981, Knopf.

23. Johnson TC: Understanding the sexual behaviors of young children, *SIECUS Report,* Aug/Sept, 1991.

24. Kettl P, Zarefoss S, Jacoby K and associates: Female sexuality after spinal cord injury, *Sexuality and Disability* 9(4):287-295, 1991.

25. Kielhofner G: *A model of human occupation,* Baltimore, 1985, Williams & Wilkins.

26. Krause JS, Crewe NM: Chronological age, time since injury, and time of measurment: effect on adjustment after spinal cord injury, *Arch Phys Med Rehabil* 72:91-100, 1991.

27. Kroll K, Klein EL: *Enabling romance,* New York, 1992, Harmony Books.

28. Lefebvre KA: Sexual assessment planning, *J Head Trauma Rehabil* 5(2):25-30,1990.

29. Lemon MA: Sexual counseling and spinal cord injury, *Sexuality and Disability* 11(1):73-97, 1993.

30. McComas J, Hebert C, Giacomin C and associates: Experiences of students and practicing physical therapists with inappropriate patient sexual behavior, *Phys Ther* 73(11):762-769, 1993.

31. Miller BR, Sieg KW, Ludwig FM and associates: *Six perspectives on theory for the practice of occupational therapy,* Rockville, Md, 1988, Aspen.

32. Neistadt ME, Freda M: *Choices: a guide to sex counseling with physically disabled adults,* Malabar, Fl, 1987, Krieger.

33. Rabin BJ: *The sensuous wheeler,* Long Beach, 1980, Barry J Rabin.

34. Romeo AJ, Wanlass R, Arenas S: A profile of psychosexual functioning in males following spinal cord injury, *Sexuality and Disability* 11(4):269-276,1993.

35. Sandowski C: Responding to the sexual concerns of persons with disabilities, *Journal of Social Work and Human Sexuality* 8(2):29-43,1993.
36. Scott R: Sexual misconduct, *PT Magazine of Physical Therapy* 1(10):78, 1993.
37. Smith M: Pediatric sexuality: promoting normal sexual development in children, *Nurse Practitioner* 18(8):37-44,1993.
38. Stockard S: Caring for the sexually aggressive patient: you don't have to blush and bear it, *Nursing* 21(11):72-73,1991.
39. Swartz DB: A comparative study of sex knowledge among hearing and deaf college freshmen, *Sexuality and Disability* 11(2):129-136,1993.
40. Verduyn WH: Spinal cord injured women, pregnancy, and delivery, *Sexuality and Disability* 11(3):29-43,1993.
41. Zani B: Male and female patterns in the discovery of sexuality during adolescence, *Journal of Adolescence* 14:163-178,1991.

SUGGESTED READINGS

Gregory MF: *Sexual adjustment: a guide for the spinal cord injured,* Bloomington, Illinois, 1993, Accent On Living.

Kempton W, Caparulo F: *Sex education for persons with disabilities that hinder learning: a teachers guide,* Santa Barbara, 1989, James Stanfield.
Leyson JF: *Sexual rehabilitation of the spinal-cord-injured patient,* Totowa, 1991, Humana Press.
Rabin BJ: *The sensuous wheeler,* Long Beach, 1980, Barry J. Rabin.
Resources for people with disabilities and chronic conditions, (ed 2), Lexington 1993, Resources for Rehabilitation Inc.
Sandowski C: *Sexual concern when illness or disability strikes,* Springfield, 1989, Charles C. Thomas.
Shortridge J, Steele-Clapp L, Lamin J: Sexuality and disability: A SIECUS annotated bibliography of available print materials, *Sexuality and Disability* 11(2):159-179, 1993.
Sobsey D and associates, editors: *Disability, sexuality, & abuse,* Baltimore, 1991, Paul H Brooks.

ADDITIONAL LEARNING MATERIALS: AGENCIES

American Association of Sex Education Counselors and Therapists
435 N. Michigan Avenue, Suite 1717, Chicago, IL 60611
(312) 644-0828

Association for Sexual Adjustment in Disability
P.O. Box 3579, Downey, CA 90292

Coalition on Sexuality and Disability
122 East Twenty-third Street, New York, NY 10010
(212) 242-3900

Sex Information and Education Council of the United States (SIECUS)
130 West Forty-second Street, Suite 2500, New York, NY 10036
(212) 819-9770

Sexuality and Disability Training Center
University of Michigan Medical Center
Department of Physical Medicine and Rehabilitation
1500 E. Medical Center Drive, Ann Arbor, MI 48109
(313) 936-7067

The Task Force on Sexuality and Disability of the American Congress of Rehabilitation Medicine
5700 Old Orchard Road, Skokie, IL 60077
(708) 966-0095

Evaluation and Treatment: Performance Areas and Performance Components

Therapeutic Modalities

Lorraine Williams Pedretti, Ingrid E. Wade

Traditionally, occupational therapy was associated with the use of arts and crafts as primary therapeutic modalities. In the 1954 (2nd) edition of *Principles of Occupational Therapy* by Helen Willard and Clare Spackman, Spackman stated, "In occupational therapy, exercise of the muscles or motion of the joints is obtained by having the patient himself use the disabled part in the course of some constructive procedure, such as woodworking. Occupational therapy may not be indicated for some patients until they are capable of sustained active motion for brief periods."[37] She stated that the physical therapist uses physical agent modalities* and exercise whereas the occupational therapist uses complementary purposeful activity. She advocated that treatment be coordinated and said it was usually beneficial for occupational therapy to follow physical therapy.[37]

Arts and crafts are still in use as treatment methods and constitute an effective and substantial portion of many occupational therapy programs.[13] But occupational therapy is not restricted to the use of arts and crafts, and the scope of its treatment methods has changed and broadened considerably over the years.

Today occupational therapists are qualified and competent in the use of a wide variety of therapeutic modalities.[1] Their competence is derived from entry level through graduate education, specialty certification, continuing education, and work experience. Indeed, the scope of practice is broad and addresses the continuum of treatment from acute care through advanced rehabilitation. Therefore occupational therapy offers comprehensive services and challenges the skills of the occupational therapy practitioner.

In the context of this chapter, modality includes both media and methods as defined by Reed.[32] A medium is the means by which a therapeutic effect is transmitted. For example, a vestibular ball is a medium. Methods are the steps, sequence, or approach used to activate the therapeutic effect of a medium such as the movements used with the vestibular ball to effect the desired motor responses.[32]

Modalities used in professional practice are influenced by many factors. Reed identified eight factors that influence the selection and discarding of media and methods in occupational therapy. They are as follows: (1) cultural practices, (2) social acceptance or nonacceptance, (3) economics of health care, (4) political factors, (5) available technology, (6) influences of a given theoretical model, (7) historical influences, and (8) research.[32] The evolution of treatment modalities in physical disabilities practice was reviewed in Chapter 2.

In addition to arts, crafts, and other purposeful activities, therapists have become increasingly skillful in applications of therapeutic exercise, physical agent modalities, and the facilitation and inhibition techniques associated with the sensorimotor approaches to treatment, all of which traditionally belonged to the field of physical therapy. These modalities are used by some occupational therapists because they enhance the development of the individual's ability to perform purposeful activities, a primary aim of occupational therapy.

This chapter presents the theory and principles of purposeful activity, enabling activities, and the adjunctive modalities of therapeutic exercise and physical agents.

PURPOSEFUL ACTIVITY

One of the first principles of occupational therapy, stated by Dunton in 1918, is that there must be some useful end to occupation for it to be effective in the treatment of mental and physical disability.[39] This principle implies that the activity or occupation has a purpose and that purposeful activity has an autonomous or inherent goal beyond the motor function required to perform the task.[7] An individual engaged in purposeful activity focuses attention on the goal rather than the processes required to reach the goal.[2,5] Conversely, nonpurposeful activity has been defined as activity in which there is no inherent goal other than the motor function used to perform the

---

* The term *modality* was defined for purposes of the AOTA policy statement "according to *Webster's New World Dictionary,* 2nd College Edition, [as] the employment of or method of employment of, a therapeutic agent"[1]

activity.[39] Attention of the performer is likely to be focused on the activity process or movements rather than a goal. By this definition adjunctive methods such as therapeutic exercise and enabling activities such as moving cones and stacking blocks cannot be considered purposeful activity. This statement does not imply, however, that such media do not have a place in the treatment continuum.

Purposeful activity is the cornerstone of occupational therapy, and its primary treatment modality.[39,41] In its position paper on purposeful activity, the AOTA defined the term as ". . . goal-directed behaviors or tasks that comprise occupations. An activity is purposeful if the individual is an active, voluntary participant and if the activity is directed toward a goal that the individual considers meaningful."[5] The uniqueness of occupational therapy lies in its emphasis on the extensive use of purposeful activity. This emphasis gives occupational therapy the theoretical foundation for its broad application to psychosocial, physical and developmental dysfunction as well as to health maintenance.[2]

Purposeful activity has both inherent and therapeutic goals. For example, sawing wood may have the inherent goal of securing parts for construction of a bookshelf, whereas the therapeutic objectives may be to strengthen shoulder and elbow musculature. The conscious effort of the patient is focused on the ultimate outcome of the movement and not on the movement itself.[7] The patient directs and is in control of the movement. As the patient becomes absorbed in the performance of the activity, it is assumed that the affected parts are used more naturally and with less fatigue.[38] It has been demonstrated that concentration on motion has a detrimental effect on that motion and that muscles controlled by conscious attention and focused effort fatigue rapidly. Therefore it is more sound to focus attention on the activity and its inherent goal than on the muscles or motions being used to accomplish the activity.[7]

Studies have shown the efficacy of purposeful activity. The results of a study by Steinbeck[39] supported the assumption that patients performing purposeful activity are motivated to perform for a longer period than when they are performing nonpurposeful activity. A study of motivation for product-oriented versus non-product-oriented activity by Thibodeaux and Ludwig[41] indicated the need to determine the patient's level of interest in the process and the product and his or her liking of the activity in treatment planning. Rocker and Nelson[34] found that not being allowed to keep an activity product can elicit hostile feelings in normal subjects. Yoder, Nelson, and Smith[44] studied the effects of added-purpose versus rote exercise in female nursing home residents; the added-purpose exercise resulted in significantly more movement repetitions than rote exercise.[44] These studies suggest that goal-directed, purposeful activity increases motivation for participation in sustained activity. In developing a treatment plan, the inherent goals of the activity, the patient's level of interest in the activity, and the meaning of the activity and activity product are important considerations in the ultimate effectiveness of the media and methods selected for treatment.

Purposeful activities are used or adapted for use to meet one or more of the following therapeutic objectives: (1) to develop or maintain strength, endurance, work tolerance, range of motion (ROM), and coordination; (2) to practice and use voluntary, automatic movement in goal directed tasks; (3) to provide for purposeful use of and general exercise to affected parts; (4) to explore vocational potential or train in work skills; (5) to improve sensation, perception, and cognition; (6) to improve socialization skills and enhance emotional growth and development, and (7) to increase independence in occupational role performance. In this text arts, crafts, games, sports, leisure, self-care, home management, mobility, and work-related activities are considered purposeful activities. Several of these activities are treated elsewhere in this text. This section focuses on theory and general principles for selecting and applying purposeful activities as therapeutic media.

THEORY OF ACTIVITY

Occupational therapy was founded on the concept that human beings have an "occupational nature"; that is, it is natural for humans to be engaged in activity, and the process of being occupied contributes to the health and well-being of the organism.[7,11,17] Activity is valuable for the maintenance of health in the healthy person and for the restoration of health after illness and disability. By engaging in relevant, meaningful, and purposeful activity, change is possible and dysfunction is reversible.[11] The occupational therapist acts as facilitator of the change process.[10] Therefore physical dysfunction can be ameliorated when the patient participates in goal-directed (purposeful) activity.[7]

The value of purposeful activity lies in the patient's mental and physical involvement. The activity provides the exercise needed to help develop the use of affected parts and also provides an opportunity to meet emotional, social, and personal gratification needs.[7,38] Cynkin and Robinson[11] pointed out that, for the attainment of optimal function and health, the human being must be consciously involved in problem solving and creative activity, processes that are linked with the use of the hands. Virtually all occupational performance tasks involve the hands.[11]

The activities that form the pattern of one's life, that are performed routinely and automatically, are taken for granted until some dysfunction disrupts their performance. Occupational therapy is founded on the notion that dysfunction can be modified, altered, or reversed toward function through engagement in activities of real life.[11]

Cynkin and Robinson[11] make several assumptions about activities that are summarized as follows:

1. A wide variety of activities is important to the individual. Activities fulfill many of a person's needs and wants, and they are essential to physical and psychosocial growth and development and the attainment of mastery and competence.
2. Activities are socioculturally regulated by the values and beliefs of the culture that defines acceptable behavior for groups of people in the culture. Whether a society is rigid or flexible in its interpretation of acceptable behaviors for various groups, at some point deviations in behavior or activities patterns are deemed unacceptable.
3. Activities-related behavior can change from dysfunctional toward more functional. Persons can change and desire change.
4. Change in activities-related behavior takes place through motor, cognitive, and social learning.[11]

ACTIVITY CONFIGURATION

Selecting appropriate and meaningful activities for the patient should begin with obtaining and analyzing the individual's activity configuration.[41] This model (Fig. 18-1), adapted from Cynkin,[10] includes information about the patient's values, educational history, work history, leisure interests and activities, and vocational interests and plans. It concludes with a daily schedule, a list of life roles, an analysis of the activity balance, and an assessment of developmental tasks. If the person is an outpatient in an advanced rehabilitation program, a daily schedule for the present can be compared with a schedule reflecting activity before the injury or illness. If the patient is acutely ill or in the early stages of rehabilitation, a daily schedule reflecting activity before the injury or illness should be made. This information may be obtained from interviews with the patient and close friends and family members.

Requirements of funding sources and budget regulations may not permit the occupational therapist to spend time with a patient for the sole purpose of this lengthy interview. It is possible to obtain much of this information gradually during regular treatment sessions rather than all at once or through a formal interview.

ACTIVITY ANALYSIS

A careful activity analysis is essential to the selection of appropriate treatment activities. It should yield information about various activities as intervention strategies for physical dysfunction and health maintenance. Activities can be analyzed from three perspectives: the field of action, the actor, and the activity. The *field of action* involves the objects and environment relevant to the performance of the activity and the explicit and implicit rules for performance of the activity in the environment. The *actor* is the person performing the activity. An actor-based analysis examines the performance components required of that person, the relevance of the activity to the person, and relevant sociocultural norms. An analysis

from the *activity* perspective examines intrinsic properties and characteristics and the activity's relationship to the real world, that is "where it fits into socioculturally designed activities patterns and configurations."[11]

Principles of Activity Analysis

If activities are to be used as the core of occupational therapy, their usefulness as therapeutic modalities must be defined, analyzed, and classified.[10] Activities selected for therapeutic purposes should (1) be goal-directed; (2) have some meaning to the patient to meet individual needs in relation to social roles; (3) require the mental or physical participation of the patient; (4) be designed to prevent or reverse dysfunction; (5) develop skills to enhance performance in life roles; (6) relate to the patient's interests; (7) be adaptable, gradable, and age appropriate; and (8) be selected through knowledge and professional judgment of the occupational therapist in concert with the patient.[15]

Biomechanical approach

The biomechanical approach to treatment is likely to be used in lower motor neuron and orthopedic dysfunctions. Improvement of strength, ROM, and muscle endurance are the goals of occupational therapy for such dysfunctions. Thus the emphasis of activity analysis is on muscles, joints, and motor patterns required to perform the activity. An activity should be analyzed in the circumstances under which it is to be performed. Steps of the activity must be identified and broken down into the motions required to perform each step. Range of motion, degree of muscle strength, and type of muscle contraction to perform each step should be identified. The activity analysis model at the end of this chapter is based on the biomechanical approach.

Sensorimotor approaches

Sensorimotor approaches to treatment are likely to be used for upper motor neuron disorders such as cerebral palsy, stroke, and head injury. Activity analysis for these dysfunctions should focus on the movement patterns required in the particular treatment approach. The therapist must also consider the effect of the activity on balance, posture, muscle tone, and the facilitation or inhibition of abnormal reflexes and movements. For example, if using the proprioceptive neuromuscular facilitation (PNF) approach, it is important to incorporate PNF patterns in the activity or to select activities that naturally use these patterns. For the neurodevelopmental (Bobath) approach, postures and movements that inhibit abnormal reflexes and tone are important. These and other sensorimotor approaches and their applications to activity are discussed in Chapters 21 through 25.

Analysis of the perceptual and cognitive requirements of the activity is particularly important for patients with upper motor neuron disorders because these functions are often disturbed. It is important for the therapist to

Patient's Name_____ Age_____ Sex_____

Life Stage_____

Educational History

1. Highest educational level achieved
2. Location and type of schools (public, private, parochial)
3. Subjects of greatest interest
4. Subjects of least interest
5. Average grades achieved
6. Likes/dislikes about school
7. Leisure interests during school years
8. Social groups to which subject belonged
9. Educational level of parents, siblings
10. Future educational plans
11. Career aspirations

Work History

1. Most recent work/job performed
2. Previous jobs
3. Special job training (past, present)
4. Likes and dislikes about jobs, past and present
5. Most preferred jobs (real or imagined)
6. Preferences for working alone or with others
7. Works alone or with others
8. Socializes with co-workers (on the job, off the job)
9. Job supervisor
10. Type of supervision received (close, distant)
11. Most effective/desirable type of supervision
12. Plans for future work or job changes

Leisure Interests and Activities

1. Interest in sports, games, hobbies (specify)
2. Participation in sports, games, hobbies (when, how long)
3. Other leisure interests that would be pursued given adequate time
4. Are leisure skills considered important to life? Why or why not?

Values and Cultural Influences

1. Cultural group with which the patient identifies
2. Describe cultural customs which are important (e.g., celebrations, holiday festivals, foods, religious practices, garments, family traditions).
3. Health practices unique to this culture. Special beliefs about health and illness. Respective roles of ill and well members of family. If raised in another country, attitudes toward health care system in United States. Experiences with U.S. health care system.
4. Describe things (concrete and abstract) that are most valued (e.g., cars, jewels, toys, pictures, family traditions, honesty, integrity, fairness). Why are they valuable?

Daily Schedule

Construct a daily schedule for a typical weekday and typical weekend day in the patient's life. Give details for hour-by-hour activities.

Life Roles

List all occupational roles of the patient (e.g., worker, father, brother, sportsman, gardener).

Life Balance

Approximate percent of time spent by the patient in each of the performance areas of self-maintenance, home and child management, work, and play/leisure.

Life Tasks

Review the patient's life stage and adaptive tasks in progress during this stage. Consider how these tasks influence the use of time and choice of activities.

(Adapted from Cynkin: *Occupational therapy: toward health through activities*, Boston, 1979, Little, Brown.)

FIG. 18-1 Activity configuration/daily schedule. Outline for interview.

select activities that not only meet the requirements for motor performance but that also can be performed with some success.

Adapting and Grading Activity
Adapting activity

It may be necessary to adapt activities to suit the special needs of the patient or the environment. An activity may need to be performed in a special way to accommodate the patient's residual abilities, for example, eating with one hand using a special splint with a utensil holder. An activity may need to be adapted to the positioning of the patient or to the environment, for instance, by setting up a special reading stand and providing prism glasses to enable a patient to read while supine in bed. The problem-solving ability, the creativity, and the ingenuity of occupational therapists in making adaptations are some of their unique skills.

The therapist should remember that for adaptations to be effective, the patient must be able to use them in a comfortable position. The patient must understand the need and purpose of the activity and the adaptations and be willing to perform the activity with the simple modifications. Peculiar and complicated adaptations that require frequent adjustment and modification should be avoided.[38]

Grading activity

Grading an activity means pacing it appropriately and modifying it for the patient's maximal performance. If movement patterns or degree of resistance cannot be obtained when the activity is performed in the usual manner, simple modifications may be made. Changes are usually accepted by the patient if they are not complex and do not require motions that are strained and unnatural. The novice is cautioned that the value of the activity may be diminished if it is designed to be performed with artificial movements or excessive resistance. Such methods discourage participation and interfere with the development of coordination.[19,38] They also require that the patient focus on movements rather than on the goal of the activity, which reduces satisfaction and defeats the primary purpose of purposeful activity as described earlier.

There are many ways in which activities may be graded to suit the patient's needs and the treatment objectives. Activities can be graded for increasing strength; ROM; endurance and tolerance; coordination; and perceptual, cognitive, and social skills.

Strength. Strength may be graded by increasing resistance. Methods include (1) changing the plane of movement from gravity-decreased to against-gravity and by adding weights to the equipment or to the patient, (2) using tools of increasing weight, (3) grading the texture of the materials from soft to hard or fine to rough, or (4) changing to another more or less resistive activity.

For example, a wrap sandbag attached to the wrist increases resistance to arm movements during macramé. A pulley-and-weight system can be attached to an inclined-plane sanding board to increase resistance to the biceps when the sanding block is pulled downward. Springs may be used to increase resistance on a block printing press. When grasp strength is inadequate, grasp mitts may be used to fasten the hand to a tool or equipment handle to assist grip strength and allow arm motion.

Range of motion (ROM). Activities for increasing or maintaining joint ROM may be graded by positioning materials and equipment to demand greater reach or excursion of joints or by adapting equipment with lengthened handles to facilitate active stretching.

An example of a simple adaptation is positioning a large checkerboard in a vertical position to achieve the desired range of shoulder flexion while playing the game (Fig. 18-2). Positioning an object, such as a mosaic tile project, at increasing or decreasing distances from the patient changes the range needed to reach the materials. Tool handles may be increased in size by using a larger dowel or by padding the handle with foam rubber to accommodate limited ROM or to facilitate grasp.

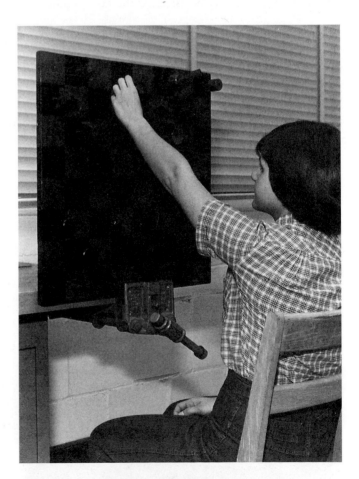

FIG. 18-2   Checkerboard is positioned vertically to increase ROM of shoulder flexion while playing game.

Endurance and tolerance. Endurance may be graded by moving from light to heavy work and increasing the duration of the work period. Standing and walking tolerance may be graded by increasing the time spent standing to work, perhaps at first at a stand-up table (Fig. 18-3), and increasing the time and distance spent in activities requiring walking, perhaps including home management and workshop activities.

Coordination. Coordination and muscle control may be graded by decreasing the gross resistive movements and increasing the fine controlled movements required. An example is progressing from sawing wood with a cross-cut saw to using a coping saw to using a jeweler's saw. Dexterity and speed of movement may be graded by practice at increasing speeds once movement patterns have been mastered through coordination training and neuromuscular education.

Perceptual, cognitive, and social skills. In grading cognitive skills the treatment program can begin with simple one- or two-step activities that require little judgment, decision making, or problem solving and progress to activities with several steps that require some judgment or problem-solving processes. A patient in a lunch preparation group may be assigned the task of buttering

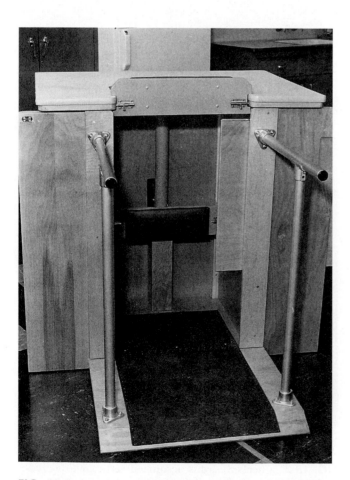

FIG. 18-3 Stand-up table with sliding door, padded knee support, and backrest.

bread that has already been lined up on the work surface. This task could be graded to lining up the bread, then buttering it and placing a slice of lunch meat on it, and, ultimately, to making sandwiches.

Similarly, for grading social interaction the treatment program may be initiated with an activity that demands interaction only with the therapist. The patient can progress to activities requiring dyadic interaction with another patient and, ultimately, to small group activities. The therapist can facilitate the patient's progression from the role of observer to that of participant and then to leader. Concomitantly, the therapist decreases his or her supervision, guidance, and assistance to facilitate more independent functioning in the patient.

SELECTION OF ACTIVITY

In the treatment of physical dysfunction, activities are usually selected for their potential to improve sensorimotor and psychosocial components. Activities selected for improvement of physical performance should provide desired exercise or purposeful use of affected parts. They should enable the patient to transfer the motion, strength, and coordination gained in adjunctive and enabling modalities to useful, normal daily activities. If activities are to be used for physical restoration, they must have certain characteristics, as follows:

1. Activities should provide action rather than position of involved joints and muscles; that is, they should allow alternate contraction and relaxation of the muscles being exercised and allow the joints to course through their available ROM.
2. Activities should provide repetition of motion. That is, activities should allow for a controllable number of repetitions of movement patterns sufficient to be of benefit to the patient.
3. Activities should allow for one or more kinds of grading, such as for resistance, range, coordination, endurance, or complexity.[15,38]

The type of exercise that is needed must be considered. Active and resistive exercises are most often used in the performance of purposeful activity.[38] Requirements for passive and active assisted exercise are harder (although not impossible) to apply to purposeful activities. Other important considerations in the selection of activity are as follows: (1) the objects and environment required to perform the activity; (2) safety factors; (3) preparation and completion time; (4) complexity; (5) type of instruction and supervision required; (6) structure and controls in the activity; (7) learning requirements; (8) independence, decision making, and problem solving required; (9) social interaction potential; (10) communication skills required, and (11) potential gratification to the person.

It is assumed that if the therapist selects an activity in which the patient has an interest, the patient will experience enough satisfaction to sustain performance of the activity. This satisfaction is an important characteristic of intrinsic motivation. Thus it is believed that purposeful activity provides intrinsic motivation to sustain perform-ance.[39] Therapy must be individualized for each patient by means of evaluative tools such as the interest check-list, activity configuration, occupational history, inter-view, and activity analysis.[41]

ENABLING ACTIVITIES

The term enabling activity is used in this text to designate a wide variety of simulations created by occupational therapists to meet an intermediate need in treatment. Enabling activities are considered nonpurposeful be-cause they generally do not have an inherent goal, though they may engage the mental and physical partici-pation of the patient.

The purposes of enabling activities are to practice specific motor patterns, to train in perceptual and cogni-tive skills, and to practice sensorimotor skills necessary for function in home and community.

A common enabling activity used by occupational therapists is use of the inclined sanding board for exer-cise (Fig. 18-4). It was probably derived from the activity of woodworking. There is no end product, it simulates sanding wood on an inclined plane, and is used to exer-cise muscles of the elbow and shoulder. Moving a series of cones from one side of a table top to the other or stacking cones (Fig. 18-5) are other such activities. This activity may be used to train gross coordination and a combined (out of synergy) movement pattern in the Brunnstrom approach, discussed in Chapter 22. Puzzles and other table top perceptual and cognitive training

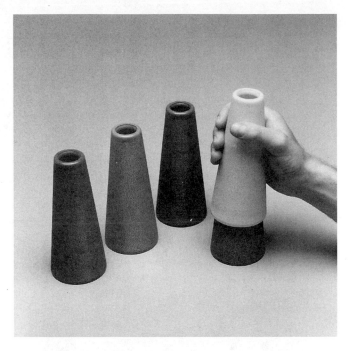

FIG. 18-5   Stacking cones are used to train coordination or specific movement patterns such as reaching and grasping. (Photograph courtesy of North Coast Medical, Inc, San José, Calif.)

media are used to train in visual perceptual functions, motor planning skills, memory, sequencing and problem solving among others (Fig. 18-6). Clothing fastener boards and household hardware boards provide practice in manipulation of everyday objects before the patient is confronted with the real task (Fig. 18-7). At a higher level of technological sophistication, commercial work simu-

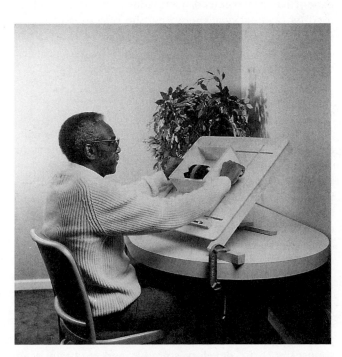

FIG. 18-4   Inclined-plane sanding board simulates sanding wood on an inclined plane and is used to exercise elbow and shoulder musculature. (Reprinted with permission, S&S World-wide, adaptAbility, 1995.)

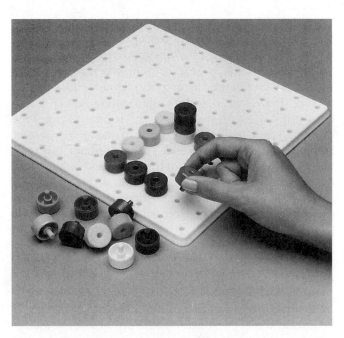

FIG. 18-6   Form, color, pattern and sequencing skills can be practiced with pegboards and puzzles. (Photograph courtesy of North Coast Medical, Inc, San José, Calif.)

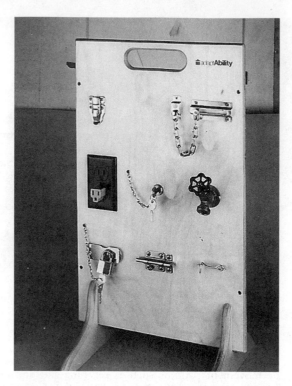

FIG. 18-7 Boards built with household fasteners can be used to practice management of common hardware in the home. (Reprinted with permission, S&S Worldwide, adaptAbility, 1995.)

lators (discussed in Chapter 30) and computer programs to train in cognitive skills are examples of enabling modalities.

Indeed, *many enabling modalities in occupational therapy practice facilitate perceptual, cognitive, and motor learning. Such activities may be appropriate for the skill acquisition stage of learning when the patient is getting the idea of the movement and practicing problem solving. Practice should be daily or frequent and feedback given often so that errors are decreased and skills refined to prepare for performance of real-life purposeful activity.* These activities should be used judiciously, and their place in the sequence of treatment and motor learning should be well planned. They are often used along with adjunctive modalities and purposeful activities as part of a comprehensive treatment program.

ADJUNCTIVE MODALITIES

Adjunctive modalities are preliminary to the use of purposeful activity. They are meant to prepare the patient for occupational performance. Examples are exercise, orthotics, sensory stimulation, and physical agent modalities.[29] In this section, therapeutic exercise and physical agent modalities are presented.

THERAPEUTIC EXERCISE

Early in the history of occupational therapy the psychological effects of purposeful activity were considered primary in the treatment of persons with physical dysfunction.[17] It was later recognized that physical benefits accrued from the performance of activity, and kinesiological considerations were applied in the selection of appropriate therapeutic activities. To apply kinesiologic considerations to purposeful activity, it was necessary to understand the principles of therapeutic exercise.

As treatment methods evolved, occupational therapists began to use therapeutic exercise alone to prepare patients for purposeful activity and to expedite treatment in a health care system constrained by budget and time. The use of therapeutic exercise as a modality raised considerable controversy.[14] The treatment of patients in acute stages of illness and disability imposed new demands and role responsibilities on occupational therapists. Short treatment sessions in acute care, the extent of the patient's physical incapacities, and shortened length of stay in hospital and rehabilitation facilities caused occupational therapists to expand the range of modalities used in treatment.

It was feared that if occupational therapists used exercise or other preparatory modalities, purposeful activity would be forgotten. Exercise and activity were seen as mutually exclusive, yet the principles of exercise had been applied to purposeful activity from early in the history of occupational therapy. Exercise (preparation) and activity (application) are complementary to one another in the treatment continuum, and both should be used in a single treatment plan. If only pure exercise is used the patient has not received occupational therapy.[14] When used by occupational therapists, the purposes of therapeutic exercise should be to remediate sensorimotor dysfunction, augment purposeful activity, and prepare the patient for doing tasks in performance areas.

Definition

Therapeutic exercise is any body movement or muscle contraction to prevent or correct a physical impairment, improve musculoskeletal function, and maintain a state of well-being.[9,20] Specific exercise protocols are used to achieve specific goals. A wide variety of exercise options is available; each should be tailored to meet the goals of treatment and the specific capacities and precautions relative to the patient's physical condition. Exercise can be used to increase ROM and flexibility, strength, coordination, endurance, and cardiovascular fitness.[20]

Purposes

The general purposes of therapeutic exercise are as follows: (1) to develop awareness of normal movement patterns and improve voluntary, automatic movement responses; (2) to develop strength and endurance in patterns of movement that are acceptable and necessary and do not produce deformity; (3) to improve coordination, regardless of strength; (4) to increase power of specific isolated muscles or muscle groups; (5) to aid in overcoming ROM deficits; (6) to increase strength of muscles that will power hand splints, mobile arm supports, and other devices; (7) to increase work tolerance and physical endurance through increased strength; and (8) to prevent or eliminate contractures developing as a result of imbalanced muscle power by strengthening the antagonistic muscles.[31]

Prerequisites for Use

For therapeutic exercise to be effective, the patient must meet certain criteria. Therapeutic exercise is most effective in the treatment of orthopedic disorders (such as fractures and arthritis) and lower motor neuron disorders that produce weakness and flaccidity. Examples of the latter are peripheral nerve injuries and diseases, poliomyelitis, Guillain-Barré syndrome, infectious neuronitis, and spinal cord injuries and diseases.

Therapeutic exercise is contraindicated for patients who have poor general health or inflamed joints or who have had recent surgery.[30] It may not be useful where there is severely limited joint ROM as the result of well established, permanent contractures. As defined and described here, it cannot be used effectively with those who have spasticity and lack voluntary control of isolated motion or those who cannot control dyskinetic movement. The latter conditions are likely to occur in upper motor neuron disorders, which are more amenable to exercise regimes of the sensorimotor approaches to treatment (see Chapters 21-25).

The candidate for therapeutic exercise must be (1) medically able to participate in the exercise regimen, (2) able to understand the directions for the exercise and its purposes, and (3) interested and motivated to perform the exercise. The patient must have available motor pathways and the potential for recovery or improvement of strength, ROM, coordination, or movement patterns, as applicable. It is important that some sensory feedback is available to the patient; that is, sensation must be at least partially intact so the patient can perceive motion and position of the exercised part and sense superficial and deep pain. Muscles and tendons must be intact, stable, and free to move. Joints must be able to move through an effective ROM for those types of exercise that use joint motion. The patient should be relatively free of pain during motion and should be able to perform isolated, coordinated movement. If there is any dyskinetic movement, the patient should be able to control it so the exercise procedure can be performed as prescribed.[30]

Types of Exercise
Exercise to increase muscle strength

Active-assisted, active and resistive isotonic and isometric exercises are used to increase strength. After partial or complete denervation of muscle and during inactivity or disuse, muscle strength decreases. When strength is inadequate, substitution patterns or "trick" movements are likely to develop.[43] A substitution is the attempt to achieve a functional goal by using muscle groups and patterns of motion not ordinarily used because of loss or weakness of the muscles normally used to perform the movements. An example is using shoulder abduction to achieve a hand-to-mouth movement if elbow flexors cannot perform against gravity (Fig. 18-8). When muscle loss is permanent, some substitution patterns may be desirable as a compensatory measure to improve performance of functional activities. Many are not desirable, however, and it is often the aim of therapeutic exercise to prevent or correct substitution patterns.[43]

A muscle must contract at or near its maximal capacity and for enough repetitions and time to increase strength. Strengthening programs generally are based on having the muscle contract against a large resistance for a few repetitions. Strengthening exercises are not effective if the contraction is insufficient.[9,21]

Excess strengthening, however, may result in muscle fatigue, pain, and temporary reduction of strength. If a muscle is overworked, it becomes fatigued and is not able to contract. The type of exercise must suit the muscle grade and the patient's fatigue tolerance level. Fatigue level varies from individual to individual, and the threshold for muscle fatigue decreases in pathological states.[21] Many patients may not be sensitive to fatigue or may push themselves beyond tolerance in the belief that this approach hastens recovery. Therefore the therapist must carefully assess the patient's muscle power and capacity for exercise. The therapist must also supervise the patient closely and observe for signs of fatigue. These signs may be slowed performance, distraction, perspiration, increase in rate of respiration, performance of exercise pattern through a decreased ROM, and inability to complete the prescribed number of repetitions.

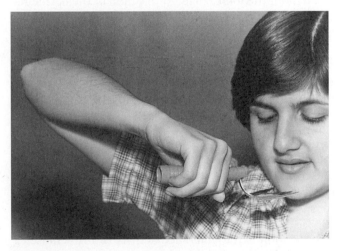

FIG. 18-8 Shoulder abduction is used to compensate for weak elbow flexion.

Exercise to increase muscle endurance

Endurance is the ability of the muscle to work for prolonged periods and resist fatigue. Although a high-load, low-repetition regime is effective for muscle strengthening, a low-load and high-repetition exercise program is more effective for building endurance.[9,12] Having determined the patient's maximum capacity for a strengthening program, the therapist can reduce the maximum resistance load and increase the number of repetitions to adapt the strengthening program to build endurance. This approach is used to build endurance in specific muscles or muscle groups. The strength versus endurance training may be seen on a continuum. Resistance and number of repetitions can be modulated so that gains in both strength and endurance accrue.[9]

Exercise for physical conditioning and cardiovascular fitness

Exercise to improve general physical endurance and cardiovascular fitness uses large muscle groups in sustained, rhythmic aerobic exercise or activity. Examples are swimming, walking, bicycling, jogging, and some games and sports. This type of exercise is often used in cardiac rehabilitation programs in which the parameters of the patient's physical capacities and tolerance for exercise should be well defined and medically supervised. To improve cardiovascular fitness, exercise should be done 3 to 5 days per week at 60 to 90 percent of maximum heart rate or 50 to 85 percent of maximum oxygen uptake. Fifteen to 60 minutes of exercise of rhythmic activities using large muscle groups is desirable.[9]

Exercise for ROM and joint flexibility

Active and passive ROM exercises are used to maintain joint motion and flexibility. Active exercise is done by the performer. Passive exercise is done by an outside force such as the therapist or a device such as the continuous passive motion machine, a mechanical device that can be preset to provide continuous passive motion throughout the joint range. Application of the device requires caution and careful monitoring to prevent mishaps and possible deleterious effects.[9]

Stretching or forced exercise is necessary to increase range of motion. Some type of force is applied to the part when soft tissue (muscles, tendons, ligaments) is at or near its available length. The use of a low-resistance stretch of sustained duration is preferred to high resistance and repetitive quick bouncing movements. The former method is less likely to produce tissue-tearing, trauma, and activation of stretch reflexes in hypertonic muscles. The use of thermal agents or neuromuscular facilitation techniques may enhance static stretching.[9]

Exercise to improve coordination

Coordination is the combined activity of many muscles into smooth patterns and sequences of motion. Coordination is an automatic response monitored primarily through proprioceptive sensory feedback. Kottke differentiated between neuromuscular control and coordination.[19] He defined control as "the conscious activation of an individual muscle or the conscious initiation of a preprogrammed engram." Control involves conscious attention to and guidance of an activity.

An *engram* is a preprogrammed pattern of muscular activity as it is represented in the central nervous system (CNS). An engram is formed only if there are many repetitions of a specific motion or activity. With repetition, conscious effort of the patient is decreased and the motion becomes more and more automatic. Ultimately, the motion can be carried out with little conscious attention. When an engram is excited, the same pattern of movement is produced automatically.

Procedures for the development of neuromuscular control and neuromuscular coordination are briefly outlined later under Exercise Classification. The reader is referred to the original source for a full discussion of the neurophysiologic mechanisms underlying these exercises. Neuromuscular education or control training involves teaching the patient to control individual muscles or motions through conscious attention. Coordination training is used to develop preprogrammed multimuscular patterns or engrams.[19]

Types of Muscle Contraction Used in Therapeutic Exercise[16,21]

Isometric or static contraction. During an isometric contraction there is no joint motion, and the muscle length remains the same. The muscle is set (contracted) or a muscle and its antagonist are contracted at a point in the ROM to stabilize a joint. This action may be without resistance or against some outside resistance, such as the therapist's hand or a fixed object. An example of isometric exercise of triceps against resistance is pressing down against a table top with the ulnar border of the forearm while the elbow remains at 90° flexion.

Isotonic or concentric contraction. During an isotonic contraction there is joint motion and the muscle shortens. This contraction may be done with or without resistance. Isotonic contractions may be performed in positions with gravity decreased or against gravity, according to the patient's muscle grade and the goal of the exercise. An isotonic contraction of the biceps is used when lifting a fork to the mouth for eating.

Eccentric contraction. When muscles contract eccentrically, the tension in the muscle increases or remains constant while the muscle lengthens. This contraction may be done with or without resistance. An example of an eccentric contraction performed without resistance is the slow lowering of the arm to the table. The biceps is contracting eccentrically in this instance. An example of eccentric contraction against resistance is the controlled return of a pail of sand lifted from the ground. Here, the biceps is contracting eccentrically to control the rate and coordination of the elbow extension in setting the pail on the ground.

Exercise Classification

The type of exercise selected depends on muscle grade, muscle endurance, joint mobility, diagnosis and physical condition, treatment goals, position of the patient, and desirable plane of movement.

Isotonic resistive exercise

Resistive exercise uses isotonic muscle contraction against a specific amount of weight to move the load through a certain ROM.[9,16,21] It is also possible to use eccentric contraction against resistance. Resistive exercise is primarily for increasing strength of fair plus to normal muscles but may also be helpful for producing relaxation of the antagonists to the contracting muscles. This latter purpose can be useful if increased range is desired for stretching or relaxing hypertonic antagonists.

The patient performs muscle contraction against resistance and moves the part through the available ROM. The resistance applied should be the maximum against which the muscle is capable of contracting. Resistance may be applied manually or by weights, springs, elastic bands, sandbags, or special exercise devices. It is graded by progressively increasing the amount of resistance (Fig. 18-9).[9,16,21] The number of repetitions that are possible will depend on the patient's general physical endurance and the endurance of the specific muscle.

There are a variety of strength training programs, most based on the principle stated above: that to increase strength, the muscle must contract against its maximal

resistance. The number of repetitions, rest intervals, frequency of training, and speed of movement vary with the particular approach and with the patient's ability to accommodate to the exercise regime.[9]

One specialized type of resistive exercise is the DeLorme method of progressive resistive exercise (PRE).[12,36] PRE is based on the overload principle: that muscles perform more efficiently if given a warm-up period and must be taxed beyond usual daily activity to improve in performance and strength.[12]

During the exercise procedure small loads are used initially and increased gradually after each set of 10 repetitions. The muscle is thus warmed up to prepare to exert its maximal power for the final 10 repetitions. The exercise procedure consists of three sets of 10 repetitions each, with resistance applied as follows: (1) first set, 10 repetitions at 50% of maximal resistance; (2) second set, 10 repetitions at 75% of maximal resistance; and (3) third set, 10 repetitions at maximal resistance.[9,12,36] The load must be sufficient so that the patient can perform 10 repetitions. As strength improves, resistance is increased so that 10 repetitions can always be performed.[9] The patient is instructed to inhale during the shortening contraction and exhale during the relaxation or eccentric contraction.[12,36]

An example of a PRE is a triceps, capable of 12 pounds maximal resistance, extending the elbow, first against 6 pounds, then against 9 pounds, and the final 10 repetitions against 12 pounds. Maximal resistance, the amount of resistance the muscle can lift through the ROM 10 times, is determined by contracting the muscle and moving the part through the full ROM against progressively increasing loads for sets of 10 repetitions until the maximal load that can be lifted 10 times is reached.

At the beginning of the treatment program it is often difficult for the therapist to determine the patient's maximal resistance. Reasons may be that the patient (1) may not know how to exert maximal effort, (2) may be reluctant to exercise strenuously for fear of pain or reinjury, (3) may be unwilling or unable to endure discomfort, and (4) may have difficulty with timing of exercises.

The experience of the therapist and trial and error aid in determining maximal resistance. The therapist should estimate the amount of resistance the patient can take based on the muscle test results and then add or subtract resistance (weight or tension) until the patient can perform the sets of repetitions adequately.

The exercises should be performed once daily four or five times weekly, and rest periods of 2 to 4 minutes should be allowed between each set of 10 repetitions. Modifications of the exercise procedure may be made to suit individual needs. Some possibilities are 10 repetitions at 25% of maximal resistance, 10 repetitions at 50%, 10 repetitions at 75%, and 10 repetitions at maximal resistance. Another possibility is 5 repetitions at 50% and 10 repetitions at maximal resistance. Still another possibility is to omit the second set of exercises. Adjustments

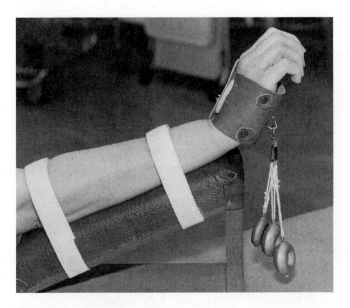

FIG. 18-9 Resistive exercise to wrist extensors, using forearm stabilizer and handcuff to compensate for inadequate grasp.

in the first two sets of exercises may be made to suit the capacity of the individual.[12]

Another approach is the Oxford technique, essentially a reverse of the DeLorme method. The exercise sequence begins with 100% resistance and decreases to 75% and then to 50% on subsequent sets of 10 repetitions each.[12,36] The greatest gains may be made in the early weeks of the treatment program, with smaller increases occurring at a slower pace in the subsequent weeks or months. During performance of the exercise, the therapist should be aware of the following: (1) joint alignment of the exercise device; (2) proper fit and adjustment of the device; (3) ruling out substitute movements; and (4) clear instruction of speed, ROM, and proper breathing.[12,31]

Application to activity. Many purposeful activities lend themselves well to resistive exercise. For instance, leather lacing can offer slight resistance to the anterior deltoid if the lace is pulled in an upward direction. Sanding with a weighted sandblock can offer substantial resistance to the anterior deltoid and triceps if done on an inclined-plane sanding board. Activities such as sawing and hammering offer resistance to upper extremity musculature. Kneading dough and forming clay objects offer resistance to muscles of the hands.

Isotonic active exercise

Isotonic muscle contraction is used in active exercise. Eccentric contraction may also be used. Active exercise is done when the patient moves the joint through its available ROM against no outside resistance.

Active motion through the complete ROM with gravity decreased or against gravity may be used for poor to fair muscles for the purpose of improving strength with the added benefit of maintaining ROM. It may be used with higher muscle grades for the maintenance of strength and ROM when resistance is contraindicated. Active exercise is *not* used to increase ROM because this purpose requires added force not present in active exercise.

In active exercise the patient moves the part through the complete ROM independently. If the exercise is performed in a gravity-decreased plane a powdered surface, skateboard, deltoid aid, or free-moving suspension sling may be used to reduce the resistance produced by friction. It is graded by changing to resistive exercise as strength improves.[16,21]

Application to activity. Activities that offer little or no resistance can be used as active exercise. A needlework activity performed in the gravity-decreased plane can provide active exercise to the wrist extensors or elbow extensors. When a grade of fair or 3 is reached, the wrist can be moved against gravity in an activity such as picking up and placing tiles for a mosaic tile project.

Active-assisted exercise

In active-assisted exercise, isotonic muscle contraction is used. The patient moves the joint through partial ROM, and the range is completed by the therapist (Fig. 18-10) or a mechanical device. Mechanical assistance may be supplied by slings, pulleys, weights, springs, or elastic bands (Fig. 18-11).[36] The goal of active-assisted exercise

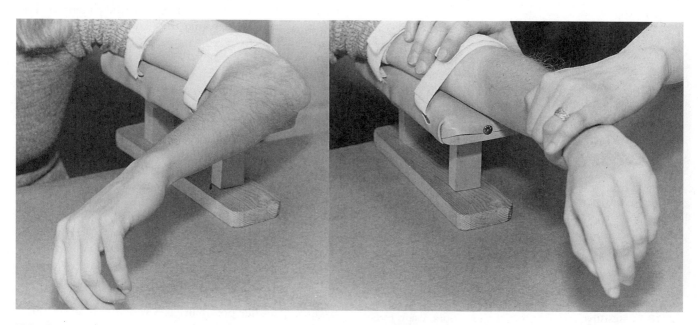

FIG. 18-10 **A,** Patient actively extends elbow from full flexion toward extension in gravity-decreased plane to degree possible. **B,** Therapist assists patient to complete ROM.

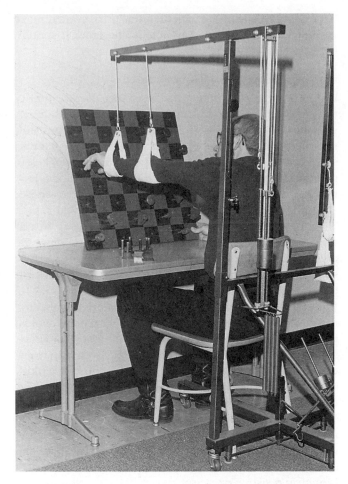

FIG. 18-11   Active-assisted exercise with deltoid aid assisting shoulder in reaching activity.

is to increase strength of trace, poor minus, and fair minus muscles while maintaining ROM. In the case of trace muscles the patient may contract the muscle, and the therapist completes the entire ROM. This exercise is graded by decreasing the amount of assistance until the patient can perform active exercises.[16,21]

Application to activity. If assistance is required to complete the movement, an activity must be structured so that assistance can be offered by the therapist, the patient's other arm or leg, or a mechanical device. Various bilateral activities lend themselves well to active-assisted exercise. Bilateral sanding, bilateral sponge wiping, using a sweeper, and sawing are some examples. In bilateral activities, the unaffected arm or leg can perform the major share of the work and the affected arm or leg can assist to the extent possible.

Passive exercise

In passive exercise there is *no* muscle contraction. Therefore it is of no use for increasing strength. It is not useful to increase ROM because no force is applied to the joint. The purpose of passive exercise is to maintain

ROM, thereby preventing contractures and adhesions and deformity.

To achieve this goal, the exercise should be performed for at least three repetitions, twice daily.[20] It is used when absent or minimal muscle strength (grades 0 to T) precludes the active motion or when active exercise is contraindicated because of the patient's physical condition. During the exercise procedure the joint or joints to be exercised are moved through their normal ranges manually by the therapist or patient or mechanically by an external device such as a pulley or counterbalance sling. The joint proximal to the joint being exercised should be stabilized during the exercise procedure[16] (Fig. 18-12).

Application to activity. It is often possible to include a passive limb in a bilateral activity if the contralateral limb is unaffected. Several of the activities described previously for active-assisted exercise can be used for passive exercise as well.

Passive stretch. For passive stretching, the therapist moves the joint through the available ROM and holds momentarily, applying a gentle but firm force or stretch at the end of the ROM. There should be no residual pain when the stretching is discontinued. Passive stretch or forced exercise is to increase ROM. It is used when there is a loss of joint ROM and stretching is not contraindicated.

If muscle grades are adequate, the patient can move the part actively through the available ROM, and the therapist can take it a little farther, thus forcing or stretching the soft tissue structures around the joint.

Passive stretching requires a good understanding of joint anatomy and muscle function. It should be carried out cautiously under good medical supervision and with medical approval. Muscles to be stretched should be in a relaxed state.[21] The therapist should never force muscles when pain is present unless ordered by the physician to

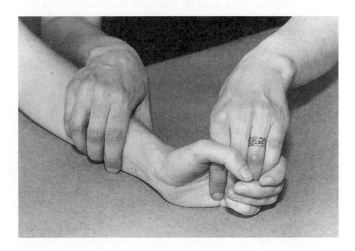

FIG. 18-12   Therapist is performing passive exercise of wrist.

work through pain. Gentle, firm stretching held for a few seconds is more effective and less hazardous than quick, short stretching. The parts around the area being stretched should be stabilized, and compensatory movements should be prevented. Incorrect stretching procedures can produce muscle tearing, joint fracture, and inflammatory edema.[20]

Application to activity. Passive stretching may be incorporated into an activity if an unaffected part guides the movement of the affected part and forces it slightly beyond the available ROM. One example is the passive stretch of wrist flexors during a block printing activity if the block is pressed down with the open hand while the patient is standing.

Active stretch. The purpose of active stretch is the same as for passive stretch, that is, to increase joint ROM. In active stretching, the patient uses the force of the agonist muscle to increase the length of the antagonist. It requires good to normal strength of the antagonist, good coordination, and motivation of the patient. For example, forceful contraction of the triceps to stretch the biceps muscle can be performed. Because the exercise may produce discomfort, there is a natural tendency for the patient to avoid the stretching component of the movement. Therefore supervision and frequent evaluation of its effectiveness is necessary.

Application to activity. Many activities can be used to incorporate active stretching. Slowly sawing wood, for example, requires a forceful contraction of the triceps with a concomitant stretch of the biceps.

Isometric exercise without resistance

Isometric exercise uses isometric contractions of a specific muscle or muscle group. In isometric exercises a muscle or group of muscles is actively contracted and relaxed without producing motion of the joint that it ordinarily mobilizes.

The purpose of isometric exercise without resistance is to maintain muscle strength when active motion is not possible or is contraindicated. It may be used with any muscle grade above trace. It is especially useful for patients in casts, after surgery, and with arthritis or burns.[9]

The patient is taught to set or contract the muscles voluntarily and to hold the contraction for 5 or 6 seconds. The therapist's fingers may be placed distal to the joint on which the muscles act. Without offering resistance, the therapist's fingers provide a kinesthetic image of resistance and help the patient learn to set the muscle. If passive motion is allowed, the therapist may move the joint to the desired point in the ROM and ask the patient to hold the position.

Isometric exercise affects the cardiovascular system, which may be a contraindication for some patients. It may cause a rapid and sudden increase in blood pressure, depending on age of the patient, intensity of contraction, and muscle mass being contracted. Therefore it should be used with caution.[9]

Isometric exercise with resistance

Isometric exercise with applied resistance uses isometric muscle contraction performed against some outside resistance. Its purpose is to increase muscle strength of muscles graded fair+ or 3+ to normal or 5. The patient sets the muscle or muscle group while resistance is applied and holds the contraction for 5 or 6 seconds. Isometric exercises should be performed for one exercise session per day, 5 days a week. Besides manual resistance, the patient may hold a weight or resist against a solid surface, depending on the muscle group being exercised. A small weight held in the hand while the wrist is stabilized at neutral requires isometric contractions of the wrist flexors and extensors.

Exercise is graded by increasing the amount of outside resistance or the degree of force the patient holds against. A tension gauge should be used to monitor accurately the amount of resistance applied. Isometric exercises are effective for increasing strength and also endurance but generally isotonic exercise is the method of choice for these purposes. Isometric exercise has several specific applications, as in arthritis, when joint motion may be contraindicated but muscle strength must be increased or maintained.[16,31] The cardiovascular precautions stated previously are particularly important with isometric resistive exercise.

Application to activity. Any activity that requires holding, or static posture incorporates isometric exercise. Holding tool handles or holding the arm in elevation while painting are examples. This type of exercise, if contraction is sustained, can be very fatiguing.

Exercise for neuromuscular control

It may be desirable to teach control of individual prime movers when they are so weak that they cannot be used normally. The purpose of the exercise is to improve muscle strength and muscle coordination to normal motor patterns. To achieve these ends, the person must learn precise control of the muscle, an essential step in the development of optimal coordination for persons with neuromuscular disease.

To participate successfully in this type of exercise the patient must be able to learn and follow instructions, cooperate, and concentrate on the muscular retraining. Before beginning, the patient should be comfortable and securely supported. The exercises should be carried out in a nondistracting environment. It is important that the patient be alert, calm, and rested. There should be an adequate pain-free arc of motion of the joint on which the muscle acts and good proprioception. Visual and tactile sensory feedback may be used to compensate or substitute for limited proprioception, but the coordination achieved will never be as great as when proprioception is intact.

Procedure. The patient's awareness of the desired motion and the muscles that effect it is first increased by passive motion to stimulate the proprioceptive stretch reflex. This passive movement may be repeated several times. The patient's awareness may be enhanced if the therapist also demonstrates the desired movement and if the movement is performed by the analogous unaffected part. The skin over the muscle belly and tendon insertion may be stimulated to enhance the effect of the stretch reflex. Stroking and tapping over the muscle belly may also be used to facilitate muscle action.[19]

The therapist should explain the location and function of the muscle, its origin and insertion, line of pull, and action on the joint. The therapist should then demonstrate the motion and instruct the patient to think of the pull of the muscle from insertion to origin. The skin over the muscle insertion can be stroked in the direction of the pull while the patient concentrates on the sensation of the motion during the passive movement performed by the therapist.

The exercise sequence then begins with instructing the patient to think about the motion while the therapist carries it out passively and strokes the skin over the insertion in the direction of the motion. The patient is then instructed to assist by contracting the muscle while the therapist performs passive motion and stimulates the skin as before. Next the patient moves the part through the ROM with assistance and cutaneous stimulation while the therapist emphasizes contraction of the prime mover only. Finally the patient carries out the movement independently, using the prime mover.

Coordination exercises must be initiated against minimal resistance if activity is to be isolated to prime movers. If the muscle is very weak (trace to poor), the procedure may be carried out entirely in an active-assisted manner so that the muscle contracts against no resistance and can function without activating synergists.

Progression from one step to the next depends on successful performance of the step without substitutions. Each step is carried out three to five times per training session for each muscle to be exercised, depending on the patient's exercise tolerance.

Exercise for training coordination

The goal of coordination training is to develop the ability to perform multimuscular motor patterns that are faster, more precise, and stronger than those performed when only control of individual muscles is used. The development of coordination depends on repetition. Initially in training, the movement must be simple and slow so the patient can be consciously aware of the activity and its components. Good coordination does not develop until repeated practice results in a well-developed activity pattern that no longer requires conscious effort and attention.

Procedure. Training should take place in an environment in which the patient can concentrate. The exercise is divided into components that the patient can perform correctly. Kottke[19] calls this approach desynthesis. It is important to keep the effort low by reducing speed and resistance to prevent the spread of excitation to muscles that are not part of the desired movement pattern.

When the motor pattern is divided into units that the patient can perform successfully, each unit is trained by practicing it under voluntary control as described previously for training of control. The therapist instructs the patient in the desired movement and uses sensory stimulation and passive movement. The patient must observe and voluntarily modify the motion. Slow practice is imperative to make this monitoring possible. The therapist must offer enough assistance to ensure precise movement and patient concentration on the sensations produced by the movements. With concentration on movement, fatigue occurs rapidly, and the patient should be given frequent short rests. As the patient masters the components of the pattern and performs them precisely and independently, the exercise sequence is graded to subtasks or several components that are practiced repetitively. As the subtasks are perfected, they are chained progressively until the movement pattern can be performed.

The exercise can be graded for speed, force, or complexity, but the therapist must be aware that the increased effort put forth by the patient may result in incoordinated movement. Therefore the grading must remain within the patient's capacity to perform the precise movement pattern. It is important that the motor pattern not be performed incorrectly to avoid the development of faulty engrams.

If central nervous system (CNS) impulses irradiate to muscles not involved in the movement pattern, incoordinated motion results. Constant repetition of an incoordinated pattern reinforces it, resulting in a persistent incoordination. Factors that increase incoordination are fear, poor balance, too much resistance, pain, fatigue, strong emotions, and prolonged inactivity.[19]

Application to activity. Occupational therapy can be used to develop coordination, strength, and endurance. Activities in occupational therapy have the advantage of engaging the patient's attention and interest. Activities should be structured to enable the patient to use the precise movement pattern and to work at speeds consistent with the maintenance of precision.

Occupational therapists, often in conjunction with physical therapists, may initiate coordination training with neuromuscular education and progress to repetitious activities requiring desired coordinated movement patterns. Examples of enabling activities that demand repetitious patterns of nonresistive movement are placing small blocks, marbles, cones, paper cups, or pegs. These activities can later be translated to more purposeful activities such as leather lacing, mosaic tile work, needlecrafts, and repetitive household tasks such as wiping, sweeping, and dusting.

PHYSICAL AGENT MODALITIES

The introduction of physical agent modalities (PAMs) into occupational therapy practice generated considerable discussion and controversy.[40,42] The use of such modalities was initiated by occupational therapists specializing in hand rehabilitation in which inclusion of physical agents in a comprehensive treatment program became necessary and expedient.[33,35] After much study and discussion, AOTA issued an official statement on the use of PAMs by occupational therapists. It stated that occupational therapists may use PAMs as adjuncts to or preparation for performance of purposeful activity. Further, it stipulated that the practitioner must have documented evidence of the theoretical background and technical skills to apply the modality and integrate it into an occupational therapy intervention plan.[3]

Subsequently AOTA published a position paper on physical agent modalities.[4] In this paper the official statement was reiterated, physical agents were defined, and their use as adjuncts to or preparation for purposeful activity was elaborated. It also stated that "the exclusive use of physical agent modalities as a treatment method during a treatment session without application to a functional outcome is not considered occupational therapy."[4] Further, it stated that use of PAMs is not considered entry-level practice: rather, they require appropriate postprofessional education to ensure competence of the occupational therapy practitioner.[4]

Physical agent modalities are used before, or during functional activities to enhance the effects of treatment. The purpose of this section is to introduce the reader to the basic techniques and when and why they might be applied. Examples of the treatment of upper extremity injuries are presented because modalities are most commonly used in occupational therapy for treatment of hand injuries and diseases. The use of the techniques described are not limited to the treatment of hands, however.

Thermal Modalities

In a clinical setting heat is used to increase motion, decrease joint stiffness, relieve muscle spasms, increase blood flow, decrease pain, and aid in the reabsorption of exudates and edema in a chronic condition.[22] Collagen fibers have an elastic component, and when stretched will return to their original length. Applying heat before a prolonged stretch, as in dynamic splinting, allows the permanent elongation of these fibers. The blood flow maintains a person's core temperature at 98.6°F. To attain maximum benefits from heat, tissue temperature must be raised to 105 to 113°F. Precautions must be taken with temperatures above this range to prevent tissue destruction.

Contraindications to the use of heat include acute conditions, sensory losses, impaired vascular structures, malignancies, and application to the very young or very old. The use of heat may substantially enhance the effects of splinting and therapeutic activities that attempt to increase range of motion and functional abilities.

Conduction. Conduction is the transfer of heat from one object to another through direct contact. Paraffin and hot packs provide heat by conduction. Paraffin is stored in a tub that maintains a temperature between 125° and 130°F. An insulating layer of paraffin is applied to the extremity by having the client repeatedly dip the hand into the tub until a thick layer is applied (Fig. 18-13). The hand is then wrapped in a plastic bag and towel for 10 to 20 minutes.[22] This technique has an excellent conforming characteristic, so it is ideal for use on the hands and digits. Partial hand coverage is possible. The paraffin transfers its heat to the hand and the bag and towel act as an insulator against dissipation of heat to the air.

Care must be taken to protect insensate parts from burns. Paraffin should not be applied when moderate to severe edema is present to avoid excessive vasodilation. It cannot be used if open wounds are present. Paraffin can be used in the clinic or incorporated into a home program. The tubs are small, and the technique is safe and easy to use in the home. It is an excellent adjunct to a home program of dynamic splinting, exercises, or general ADL. It may be used in the clinic before therapeutic exercises and functional activities.

Hot packs contain either a silicate gel or a bentonite clay wrapped in a cotton bag and submerged in a hydrocollator, a water tank that maintains the temperature of the packs at 160°-175°F.[22] Because tissue damage may

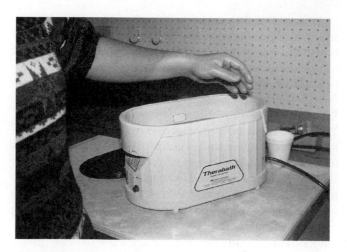

FIG. 18-13 Client's hand is dipped in warm paraffin to prepare hand for performance of therapeutic activities.

occur at these temperatures, the packs are separated from the skin by layers of towels. As with paraffin, precautions should be taken when applying to insensate skin or tissue that has sustained vascular damage. Hot packs are commonly used for myofascial pain, before soft tissue mobilization, and before any activities aimed at elongating contracted tissue.[8] For a client with a hand injury, the packs may be applied to the extrinsic musculature to decrease muscle tone caused by guarding, without heating the hand also. Unless contraindicated, hot packs can be used (with precautions) when open wounds are present.

Convection. Convection supplies heat to the tissues by fluid motion around the tissues. Examples of convection are whirlpool and Fluidotherapy. Whirlpool is more common for wound management than for heat application. Fluidotherapy involves a machine that agitates finely ground corn husk particles, by blowing warm air through them (Fig.18-14). This device is similar to the whirlpool, but corn particles are used instead of water. The temperature is thermostatically maintained, with the therapeutic range being up to 125°F. Studies have shown this technique to be excellent for raising tissue tempera-

ture in the hands and feet.[8] An additional benefit is its effect on desensitization. The agitator can be adjusted to decrease or increase the flow of the corn particles, thus controlling the amount of stimulation to the skin. An extremity can be heated generally, and therefore this technique is effective as a warmup before exercises, dexterity tasks, functional activities, and work simulation tasks.

Conversion. *Conversion* occurs when heat is generated internally by friction, for example, by means of ultrasound. The sound waves penetrate the tissues, causing vibration of the molecules, and the resulting friction generates heat. The energy of sound waves is thus converted to heat energy. The sound waves are applied with a transducer, which glides across the skin in slow continuous motions (Fig. 18-15). Gel is used to improve the transmission of the sound to the tissues. Ultrasound is considered a deep heating agent. At 1 MHz (1 million cycles per second), it can heat tissues to a depth of 5 cm. The previous methods produce heating to 1 cm.[26] Many therapeutic ultrasound machines provide a 3 MHz option for treatment of more superficial structures, with the corresponding heating depth reduced to 3 cm. Ultrasound at frequencies higher than recommended standards can destroy tissue. In addition, precautions must be taken to avoid growth plates in the bones of children, an unprotected spinal cord, and freshly repaired structures such as tendons and nerves. Because of its ability to heat deeper tissues, ultrasound is excellent in treating problems associated with joint contractures, scarring with its associated adhesions, and muscle spasms. When applying the ultrasound, it is beneficial to apply a stretch to the tissues while they are being heated, followed by activities, excercises, and splints to maintain the stretch.

Ultrasound may also be used in a nonthermal application in which the ultrasound waves are used to drive

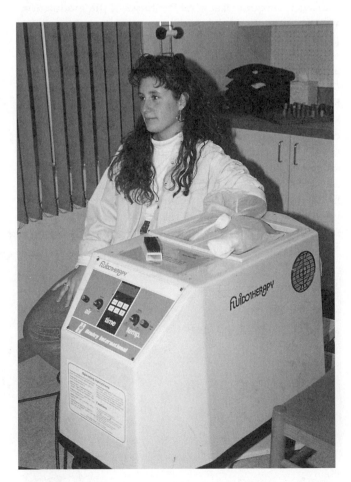

FIG. 18-14 Fluidotherapy uses fine corn particles agitated by warm air to supply heat to tissues.

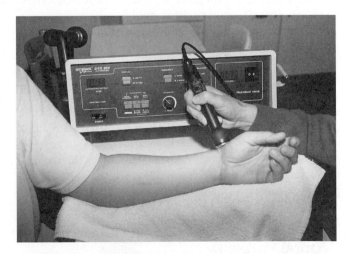

FIG. 18-15 Ultrasound modality converts sound to heat to generate heat internally by friction. It facilitates stretching tissues while they are being heated and is often used before performance of purposeful activities.

antiinflammatory medications into tissues. This process is called *phonophoresis*. Ultrasound is thought to increase membrane permeability for greater symptom relief, and may also be used following corticosteroidal injections.

Cryotherapy, the use of cold in therapy, is often used in the treatment of edema, pain, and inflammation. The cold produces a vasoconstriction, which decreases the amount of blood flow into the injured tissue. Cold decreases muscle spasms by decreasing the amount of firing from the afferent muscle spindles. Cryotherapy is contraindicated for clients with cold intolerance or vascular repairs. The use of cryotherapy may be incorporated into clinical treatment; however, it is particularly useful in a home program.

Cold packs can be applied in a number of ways. There are many commercial packs, ranging in size and cost. An alternative to purchasing a cold pack is to use a bag of frozen vegetables, or a reusable slush bag can be made by combining crushed ice and alcohol in a plastic bag. Ice packs should be covered with a moist towel to prevent tissue injury. The benefit of commercial packs is that they are easy to use, especially if the client is to use them frequently during the day. When clients are working, it is recommended that they keep cold packs at home and at their work, to increase the ease of use. The optimum temperature for storing a cold pack is 45°F.

Other forms of cryotherapy include ice massage and cooling machines. Ice massage is used when the area to be cooled is small and very specific, for example, inflammation of a tendon specifically at its insertion or origin. The procedure entails using a large piece of ice (water frozen in a paper cup) and massaging the area with circular motions until skin is numb, usually 4 to 5 minutes. Cooling devices, which circulate cold water through tubes in a pack, are available through vendors. These devices maintain their cold temperatures for a long time, but they are expensive to rent or purchase. They are very effective at reducing edema immediately after surgery or injury during the inflammatory phase of wound healing.

Contrast baths combine the use of heat and cold. The physical response is alternating vasoconstriction and vasodilation of the blood vessels. The client is asked to submerge the arm, for example, alternating between two tubs of water. One contains cold water (59° to 68°F), and the other contains warm water (96° to 105°F). The purpose is to increase collateral circulation, which effectively reduces pain and edema. As with the use of cold packs, contrast baths are a beneficial addition to a home therapy program. This technique is contraindicated for clients with vascular disorders or injuries.

Electrical Modalities

Electrical modalities are used by an occupational therapist to decrease pain, decrease edema, increase motion, and reeducate muscles to increase a client's functional abilities. Many techniques are available; those most commonly used are presented here. Electrical modalities should *not* be used on clients with pacemakers or cardiac conditions.

Transcutaneous electrical nerve stimulation (TENS) employs electrical current to decrease pain. Pain is classified in three categories: physical, physiological, and psychological. When trauma occurs, an individual responds to the initial pain by guarding the painful body part. This guarding may result in muscle spasms and fatigue of the muscle fibers, especially after prolonged guarding. The supply of blood and oxygen to the affected area is decreased and resultant soft tissue and joint dysfunction occurs.[25] These reactions magnify and compound the problems associated with the initial pain response. The therapist's goal after an acute injury is to prevent this cycle. In the case of chronic pain, the goal is to stop the cycle that has been established. TENS is an effective technique for controlling pain without the side effects of medications. Pain medications are frequently used in conjunction with TENS, which often reduces the duration of their use. TENS is safe to use, and clients can be educated in independent home use.

TENS provides a constant electrical stimulation with a modulated current and is directed to the peripheral nerves through electrode placement (Fig.18-16). The therapist can control several attributes of the modulation waveform such as the frequency, amplitude, and the pulse width. When TENS is applied at a low-frequency setting, endogenous opiates are released. Endorphines are naturally occurring substances that reduce the sensation of pain. The effects of high-frequency TENS are based on the gate control theory originally explained by Melzack and Wall in 1965. This theory describes how the electrical current from TENS, applied to the peripheral nerves, blocks the perception of pain in the brain. Nociceptors (pain receptors) transmit information to the central nervous system through the A delta and C fibers. A fibers transmit information about pressure and touch. It is thought that TENS stimulates the A fibers, effectively saturating the gate to pain perception, and the transmis-

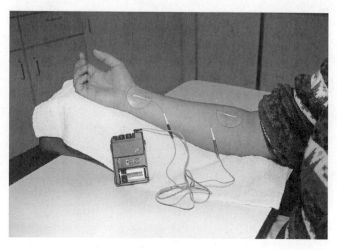

FIG. 18-16 TENS is an electrical device used to control pain.

sion of pain signals via the A delta and C fibers are blocked at the level of the spinal cord.[25]

TENS can be applied for acute or chronic pain. TENS is frequently used postsurgically when it is mandatory that motion be initiated within 72 hours. Examples are tenolysis and capsulotomy surgeries, or after fractures when it is important to maintain tendon gliding through the injured area. TENS can be especially helpful with clients who have a low threshold to pain, making exercising easier. TENS is also useful in treating clients with reflex sympathetic dystrophy because continued active motion is crucial.

TENS can be used to decrease pain from an inflammatory condition, such as tendonitis or a nerve impingement, however it is mandatory that the client be educated in tendon/nerve protection and rest, with a proper home program of symptom management, positioning, and ADL/work modification. Without the sensation of pain, it is possible for the client to overdo and stress the inflamed tissues. It is recommended that other techniques be tried first to decrease pain for these clients. TENS also is used for treating trigger points, with direct electrode application to the trigger point to decrease its irritability.[27]

Neuromuscular electrical stimulation (NMES) provides a continuous interrupted current. It is applied through an electrode to the motor point of innervated muscles to provide a muscle contraction. The current is interrupted to enable the muscle to relax between contractions, and the durations of the on and off times can be adjusted by the therapist. Adjustments can also be made to control the rate of the increase in current (ramp) and the intensity of the contraction.

NMES is used to increase range of motion, facilitate muscle contractions, and strengthen muscles.[28] It may be used postsurgically to provide a stronger contraction for increased tendon gliding, for example, after a tenolysis. It may also be used later in the tendon repair protocol, once the tendon has healed sufficiently to tolerate stress, usually at a minimum of 6 weeks. NMES may be used to strengthen a muscle that has become weakened because of disuse. During the reinnervation phase following a nerve injury, this technique may be used to help stimulate and strengthen a newly innervated muscle. Care must be taken not to overfatigue the muscle. FES can be applied during a dexterity or functional activity, which allows the muscle to be retrained in the purpose of its contraction. As with TENS, NMES may be incorporated into a home program with proper client education and follow-through.

Other techniques that use an electrical current include high-voltage galvanic stimulation (HVGS) and interferential electrical stimulation. These techniques are applied to treat pain and edema.[28] Electrical stimulation may be applied in conjunction with ultrasound through a single transducer to provide heat simultaneously with current. This approach is beneficial in treating trigger points and myofascial pain. Iontophoresis uses a current to drive ionized medication into inflamed tissue and scar tissue. The technique uses an electrode filled with the medication of choice. The transfer of the medicine is caused by applying an electric field that repels the ions into the tissues.

Sample Treatment Plan

The following treatment plan demonstrates how physical agent modalities can be incorporated into the treatment of an individual after a flexor tendon repair. For the complete tendon repair treatment protocol, the reader is referred to the suggested readings at the end of the chapter.

Day 3 to 1 week after surgery: Occupational therapy is initiated. The client is started on an early mobilization program using a modified Kleinert (dorsal blocking) splint and treatment protocol. In addition to wound care, splinting, and exercises, the client is instructed to elevate and apply cold packs to assist in decreasing edema. Cold packs are recommended 6 to 8 times per day for a duration of 10 minutes every application.

If pain is limiting the amount of motion the client is able to achieve within the dorsal blocking splint, a TENS unit may be applied. The unit can usually be discontinued by the end of the first week, once the inflammatory phase of wound healing is complete.

1 to 4 weeks after surgery: The client continues with the just described program. Once the sutures are removed (at approximately 10 days), contrast baths can be initiated in the clinical setting to assist in decreasing edema while also cleansing the wound and hand. Care must be taken to maintain the hand in a protected position while the splint is off and the hand submerged in the baths. Contrast baths can be followed by scar management, protective passive extension, and passive flexion exercises before the splint is reapplied.

4 to 8 weeks: Fluidotherapy or paraffin can begin at this time, providing the digits are taped into flexion to maintain a protected position. If the client continues to have considerable edema, Fluidotherapy is preferred because it is less heat intensive. Fluidotherapy (or paraffin) can be followed by protected passive extension, passive flexion, gentle active flexion, and active extension exercises. Functional activities or resistance to the repaired tendon continue to be contraindicated.

At 6 weeks postsurgically, dynamic extension splinting can begin if full extension has not yet been achieved. A paraffin unit can be incorporated into the home program to heat the tissues (tendons and scar tissue) before splint application to increase scar extensibility. It is recommended that cold packs continue on a regular basis (usually 4 to 6 times per day).

8 to 10 weeks: NMES can begin at this time if full tendon excursion has not been achieved. It is crucial that initially the amplitude be set lower in order to protect the repair by not applying too much force to the repair site. NMES should be followed by active motion, strengthening, and dexterity tasks requiring minimal to moderate resistance as the tendon heals.

Ultrasound can begin for treatment of tendon scar adhesions and decreased tendon gliding. Ultrasound can be used before FES, active exercises, splinting, dexterity activities, strengthening, or a combination of these.

10 to 12 weeks: The client can begin a progressive work conditioning program. The tissues can be heated before exercise with Fluidotherapy, paraffin, or ultrasound, depending on which limitations the client continues to demonstrate. If the digit(s) demonstrates motion within normal limits, then Fluidotherapy can be used for a more general heating of all soft tissues. If the digit continues to lack full motion and tendon pull-through, paraffin and ultrasound (or a combination of the two) can be used before the work conditioning program.

Edema may continue for many months. Therefore a program consistently using cold packs is recommended. These can be especially beneficial once the client returns to work and use of the injured hand increases.

SELECTING APPROPRIATE MODALITIES IN THE CONTINUUM OF CARE

Many years ago treatment roles and responsibilities were more specifically delineated, and occupational therapists treated patients only after they were capable, at least to some degree, of performing purposeful activity.[14] Evolution of treatment methods, trends in health care (see Chapters 2 and 3) and medical technology have significantly altered the role of the respective therapists and expanded the repertoire of treatment modalities that therapists are competent to practice, however.

Patients are now referred to occupational therapy long before they are capable of performing purposeful activity. Therapists are treating patients in the very acute stages of illness and disability. Treatment is directed toward preparing the patient for the time when purposeful activity is possible. This approach may mean the occupational therapist applies a positioning splint to a patient immediately after hand surgery considering how the hand will be used later in treatment and in real life. It means the therapist may use sensory stimulation on the comatose patient because arousal and a return to interacting with persons and objects in the environment will make performance of purposeful activity possible in the future. It means the therapist may apply paraffin to decrease joint stiffness and increase mobility of finger joints before performance of a macramé project.

The unique perspective of the occupational therapist is seeing the potential for performance and using modalities that lead incrementally to performance. The need to employ procedures that maximize purposeful activity are also the concerns of the occupational therapist.[6]

Dutton[14] outlined guidelines for use of both activity and exercise in the same treatment program using the biomechanical and sensorimotor frames of reference. She proposed that exercise is a preparation phase and purposeful activity is the application stage in treatment. Within the biomechanical frame of reference, she stated that movements more easily achieved through exercise are isolated, rhythmical, linear, and reciprocal movements. Also, exercise is more appropriate for increasing range of motion and using excessive resistance for strengthening. Conversely, purposeful activity is more appropriate for coordinated, arrhythmical, diagonal and asymmetrical movements, maintaining range of motion, and increasing endurance.[14]

Further, Dutton stated that the patient's sensorimotor

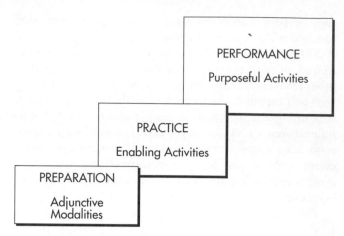

FIG. 18-17 Building blocks of occupational performance: preparation, practice, performance.

and cognitive status need to be considered when the occupational therapist is selecting modalities within the sensorimotor approaches to treatment. If the patient is functioning at a primitive level, using handling techniques ensures quality movement. These techniques are appropriate if the patient is (1) unable to control muscle tone, (2) dependent on tracking the therapist's normal movements, (3) resistant to weight shifts, (4) dependent on conscious monitoring of somatic feedback, and (5) capable of learning only a few movements. As the patient progresses in recovery, handling techniques are decreased and purposeful activity is gradually added to the treatment regime. The advanced patient can control muscle tone, initiate normal movement, perform weight shifts, monitor somatic feedback, and practice motor planning.[14]

Purposeful activity is not appropriate for every phase of treatment. Occupational therapists have developed expertise in handling techniques, facilitation/inhibition, splinting, positioning, massage, exercise, sensory stimulation, physical agent modalities, and other nonpurposeful modalities that meet the needs of the acutely ill or seriously impaired patient. These skills will not be abandoned in favor of a return to the exclusive use of purposeful activity and can be integrated into a comprehensive treatment program that includes purposeful activity if used by competent practitioners[14] (Fig. 18-17).

SUMMARY

Occupational therapists use purposeful activity, therapeutic exercise, enabling activities, and adjunctive modalities in the continuum of treatment, and may use them simultaneously. They apply principles of therapeutic exercise to purposeful activity regularly and use physical agent modalities preceding purposeful activity. In many treatment facilities, the physical therapist is responsible for application of physical agent modalities and the formal therapeutic exercise regime. The occupational therapist provides more general exercise and helps the patient apply newly gained strength, range of motion, and coordination during performance of purposeful activities. The respective therapists' roles may not be sharply defined, with each sharing in exercise and activity aspects of the treatment program according to their expertise, interests, and the roles and responsibilities assigned by the treatment facility.

Purposeful activity is the core of occupational therapy practice. Its value lies in its health giving and remedial nature. The selection of appropriate therapeutic activities is based on the patient's activity configuration and on careful activity analysis. Appropriate therapeutic activity is individualized and designed to be meaningful and interesting to the patient while meeting therapeutic objectives.

Therapeutic activity may be adapted to meet special needs of the patient or the environment. It may be graded for physical, perceptual, cognitive, and social purposes to keep the patient functioning at maximal potential at any point in the treatment program. The uniqueness of occupational therapy lies in its extensive use of goal-directed purposeful activities as treatment modalities.

REVIEW QUESTIONS

1. Define *therapeutic exercise.*
2. What is meant by substitution patterns? Why do they occur?
3. What demand must be made on a muscle for its strength to increase?
4. What happens to a muscle that is fatigued?
5. List four signs of fatigue from excess exercise.
6. List at least four purposes of therapeutic exercise.
7. With which types of disabilities would you use therapeutic exercise? For which disabilities is it less useful? Why?
8. List four precautions or contraindications to therapeutic exercise, and explain why each can preclude the use of therapeutic exercise.
9. What type of exercise should be used if muscle grades are fair+ to good? Why?
10. If a patient has joint pain and inflammation with good muscle strength, what type of exercise should be used? Why?
11. How is passive stretching different from passive exercise?
12. Which physical agent modalities might be used in conjunction with stretching exercise?
13. Describe the procedure and precautions for passive stretching.
14. When beginning PRE, how is the patient's maximal resistance determined?
15. Describe the procedure for PRE to strengthen fair+ wrist extensors.
16. Describe the steps in coordination exercises.
17. List four objectives of therapeutic activities.
18. List at least five requirements ac-tivities need to meet if they are to be used for therapeutic purposes.
19. How can activities be adapted to meet specific therapeutic objectives and allow for grading the therapeutic program?
20. List four ways in which activities can be graded.
21. What three criteria must an activity meet to be useful for exercise purposes?
22. How can the application of physical agent modalities enhance the patient's performance of activities?
23. Name and discuss at least five factors that should be considered in the selection of activities.
24. Can therapeutic activity, therapeutic exercise, and physical agent modalities be used simultaneously in a treatment program? When is each most appropriate? Discuss their integration and elaborate treatment possibilities for the case study presented in the chapter.
25. What is the physiological effect of the application of heat to soft tissue? When might heat be used in occupational therapy?
26. Describe fluidotherapy and its use as a precursor to functional activities.
27. What is the physiological effect of ultrasound? What are some precautions in its use?
28. What is the purpose of contrast baths?
29. List and describe three electrical modalities and discuss their use as preparatory modalities for functional activity.
30. Select one of the following activities and complete an activity analysis according to the model provided in Appendix A: sawing wood, placing mosaic tiles, pulling leather lacing, rolling out dough.

REFERENCES

1. American Occupational Therapy Association: Association policy, occupational therapists and modalities, (Representative Assembly, April, 1983), *Am J Occup Ther* 37(12):816, 1983.
2. American Occupational Therapy Association: Position paper on purposeful activities, *Am J Occup Ther* 37:805, 1983.
3. American Occupational Therapy Association: Official: AOTA statement on physical agent modalities, *Am J Occup Ther,* 45(12):1075, 1991.
4. American Occupational Therapy Association: Position paper: physical agent modalities, *Am J Occup Ther* 46(12):1090, 1992.
5. American Occupational Therapy Association: Position paper: purposeful activity, *Am J Occup Ther* 47(12):1081-1082, 1993.
6. Ayres AJ: Basic concepts of clinical practice in physical disabilities, *Am J Occup Ther* 12(8): 300-302, 1958.
7. Ayres AJ: Occupational therapy for motor disorders resulting from impairment of the central nervous system, *Rehabil Lit* 21:302, 1960.
8. Cannon NM, Mullins PT: *Manual on management of specific hand problems,* Pittsburgh, 1984, American Rehabilitation Educational Network.
9. Ciccone CD, Alexander J: Physiology and therapeutics of exer-

cise. In Goodgold J, editor: *Rehabilitation medicine,* St Louis, 1988, CV Mosby.

10. Cynkin S: *Occupational therapy: toward health through activities,* Boston, 1979, Little, Brown.

11. Cynkin C, Robinson AM: *Occupational therapy and activities health: toward health through activities,* Boston, 1990, Little, Brown.

12. De Lateur BJ, Lehmann J: Therapeutic exercise to develop strength and endurance. In Kottke FJ, Stillwell GK, Lehmann JF, editors: *Krusen's handbook of physical medicine and rehabilitation,* ed 4, Philadelphia, 1990, WB Saunders.

13. Drake M: *Crafts in therapy and rehabilitation,* Thorofare, NJ, 1992, Slack.

14. Dutton R: Guidelines for using both activity and exercise, *Am J Occup Ther,* 43(9):573-580, 1989.

15. Hopkins HL, Smith HD, Tiffany EG: The activity process. In Hopkins HL, Smith HD, editors: *Willard and Spackman's occupational therapy,* ed 7, Philadelphia, 1988, JB Lippincott.

16. Huddleston OL: *Therapeutic exercises,* Philadelphia, 1961, FA Davis.

17. Kielhofner G: A heritage of activity: development of theory, *Am J Occup Ther* 36:723, 1982.

18. Killingsworth A: Activity module for OCTH 120, functional kinesiology, San José State University, Calif, 1989, unpublished.

19. Kottke FJ: Therapeutic exercises to develop neuromuscular coordination. In Kottke FJ, Stillwell GK, Lehmann JF, editors: *Krusen's handbook of physical medicine and rehabilitation,* ed 4, Philadelphia, 1990, WB Saunders.

20. Kottke FJ: Therapeutic exercise to maintain mobility. In Kottke FJ, Stillwell GK, Lehmann JF, editors: *Krusen's handbook of physical medicine and rehabilitation,* ed 4, Philadelphia, 1990, WB Saunders.

21. Kraus H: *Therapeutic exercise,* Springfield, Ill, 1963, Charles C Thomas.

22. Lehmann JF: *Therapeutic heat and cold,* ed 3, Baltimore, 1982, Williams & Wilkins.

23. Llorens L: *Activity analysis for sensory integration (CPM) dysfunction,* 1978, Unpublished.

24. Llorens LA: Activity analysis: agreement among factors in a sensory processing model, *Am J Occup Ther* 40:103, 1986.

25. Mannheimer JS, Lampe GN: *Clinical transcutaneous electrical nerve stimulation,* Philadelphia, 1984, FA Davis.

26. Michlovitz SL: *Thermal agents in rehabilitation,* ed 2, Philadelphia, 1990, FA Davis.

27. Moran CA, Saunders SR, Tribuzi SM: Myofascial pain in the upper extremity. In Hunter JM and associates, editors: *Rehabilitation of the hand,* ed 3, St Louis, 1990, CV Mosby.

28. Mullins PT: Use of therapeutic modalities in upper extremity rehabilitation. In Hunter JM and associates, editors: *Rehabilitation of the hand,* ed 3, St Louis, 1990, CV Mosby.

29. Pedretti LW, Smith RO, Hammel J and associates: Use of adjunctive modalities in occupational therapy, *Am J Occup Ther* 46(12):1075-1081.

30. Rancho Los Amigos Hospital: *Muscle reeducation,* Downey, Calif, 1963, Rancho Los Amigos Hospital, Unpublished.

31. Rancho Los Amigos Hospital: *Progressive resistive and static exercise: principles and techniques,* Downey, Calif, Rancho Los Amigos Hospital, Unpublished.

32. Reed KL: Tools of practice: heritage or baggage? *Am J Occup Ther* 40:597, 1986.

33. Reynolds C: OTs and PAMs: A physical therapist's perspective, *OT Week* 8(37):17, Bethesda, Md, 1994, American Occupational Therapy Association.

34. Rocker JD, Nelson DL: Affective responses to keeping and not keeping an activity product, *Am J Occup Ther* 41:152, 1987.

35. Rose H: Physical agent modalities: OT's contribution, *OT Week* 8(37):16-17, Bethesda, Md, 1994, American Occupational Therapy Association.

36. Schram DA: Resistance exercise. In Basmajian JV, editor: *Therapeutic exercise,* ed 4, Baltimore, 1984, Williams & Wilkins.

37. Spackman CS: Occupational therapy for patients with physical disabilities. In Willard HS, Spackman CS: *Principles of occupational therapy,* Philadelphia, 1954, JB Lippincott.

38. Spackman CS: Occupational therapy for the restoration of physical function. In Willard HS, Spackman CS, editors: *Occupational therapy,* ed 4, Philadelphia, 1971, JB Lippincott.

39. Steinbeck TM: Purposeful activity and performance. *Am J Occup Ther* 40:529, 1986.

40. Taylor E, Humphrey R: Survey of physical agent modality use, *Am J Occup Ther* 45(10):924-931, 1991.

41. Thibodeaux CS, Ludwig FM: Intrinsic motivation in product-oriented and non-product oriented activities, *Am J Occup Ther* 42:169, 1988.

42. West WL, Weimer RB: The issue is: should the representative assembly have voted as it did, when it did, on occupational therapist's use of physical agent modalities?, *Am J Occup Ther* 45(12):1143-1147, 1991.

43. Wynn-Parry CB: Vicarious motions. In Basmajian JV, editor: *Therapeutic exercise,* ed 3, Baltimore, 1982, Williams & Wilkins.

44. Yoder RM, Nelson DL, Smith DA: Added-purpose versus rote exercise in female nursing home residents, *Am J Occup Ther* 43(9):581-586, 1989.

SUGGESTED READINGS

Cooney WP, Lin GT, Kai-Nan A: Improved tendon excursion following flexor tendon repair, J Hand Ther 2:(2),1989.

Strickland JW: Biologic rationale, clinical application, and results of early motion following flexor tendon repair, J Hand Ther 2(2), 1989.

APPENDIX A ACTIVITY ANALYSIS MODEL

The activity analysis offers the reader one systematic approach for looking at the therapeutic potential of activities. This model includes some factors that must be considered about the performer, the field of action, and the activity in the selection of purposeful, therapeutic activity. In it, just two steps of a multistep activity are analyzed for the sake of space and simplicity. The reader is encouraged to complete the motor analysis by considering movements of the shoulder, forearm, and wrist that accompany the pinch and release pattern analyzed.

I. Preliminary Information
1. Name of activity: Pinch pottery
2. Components of the task
   a. Roll some clay into a ball, 3 to 4 inches in diameter.
   b. Place the ball centered on the work table in front of the performer.
   c. Make a hole in the center of the ball with the right or left thumb (Fig. 18-18, *A*).
   d. With the thumb and first two fingers of both hands, pinch around and around the hole from base to top of the ball.
      1. Pinch by pressing thumb against index and middle fingers.
      2. Release pinch by extending thumb and index and middle fingers slightly.
   e. Continue pinching in this way, gradually spreading the walls of the clay until a small bowl of the desired size is formed.
3. Steps of activity being analyzed
   a. Pinch
   b. Release
4. Equipment and supplies necessary
   a. Ball of soft ceramic clay
   b. Wooden table 30 to 32 inches high or a wooden work surface fastened to a table with C clamps
   c. Chair at the work table
   d. Sponge and bowl of water
   e. Ceramic smoothing tool
5. Environment or field of action:[10,11] Occupational therapy

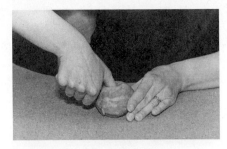

A

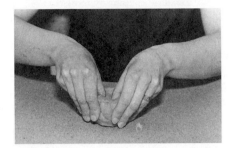

B

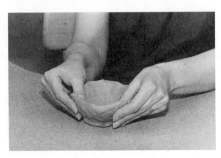

C

FIG. 18-18 A, Opening pinch pot with thumb. **B,** Walls of pot are gradually spread with pinching motion of fingers. **C,** Pinching continues in circular direction until desired size of pot is reached.

workshop or craft activity room. Sink and damp storage area should be available in the work area. There should be ample room around the work table so that the performer is not crowded and can move freely between the table and the sink and damp storage closet. Lighting should be adequate for clear visualization of clay object and work area.
6. Position of the performer in relation to the work surface/equipment: The performer is seated in the chair at the table,

at a comfortable distance for reaching and manipulating the clay and tools. The clay is centered in front of the performer and the tool, sponge, and water bowl are to the right and near the top of the work area.
7. Starting position of the performer: Sitting erect with feet flat on the floor; shoulders are slightly abducted and in slight internal rotation, bringing both hands to the center work surface; elbows are flexed to about 90°; forearms are pronated about 45°; wrists are slightly extended and in ulnar deviation, thumbs are opposed to index and middle fingers, ready to pinch the posterior surface of the opened clay ball (Fig. 18-18, *B*).
8. Movement pattern used to perform the steps under analysis: Flexion of the MP and IP joints of index and middle fingers; opposition and flexion of the thumb (pinch) followed by extension of the MP and IP joints index and middle fingers and extension and palmar abduction of the thumb (release). Repeat pattern around ball of clay until a small bowl of desired size and thickness are formed (Fig. 18-18, *C*).

II. Motor Analysis[18]
1. Joint and muscle activity: List the joint motions for all movements used during performance of the activity. For each indicate amount of ROM used (minimal, moderate, or full), muscle group used to perform the motion, strength required (minimal [P+ to F], moderate [F+ to G], full [G+ to N]), and type of muscle contraction (isotonic, isometric, eccentric). (See Box 18-1.)
2. Grading: Grade this activity for one or more of the following factors:
   a. ROM: Cannot be graded for ROM.
   b. Strength: Grade for strength by increasing the consistency of the clay.

BOX 18-1   MOTIONS FOR PINCH

JT. MOTION	ROM	M. GROUP	STRENGTH	TYPE OF M. CONTRACTION
INDEX AND MIDDLE FINGERS				
MP flexion	Minimal	FDP, FDS lumbricales	Moderate	Isotonic
PIP flexion	Minimal	FDP, FDS	Moderate	Isotonic
DIP flexion	Minimal	FDP	Moderate	Isotonic
Finger adduction	Maximal	Palmar interossei	Moderate	Isometric
THUMB				
Opposition	Full	Opponens pollicis, FPL, FPB	Moderate	Isotonic
MOTIONS FOR RELEASE INDEX AND MIDDLE FINGERS				
MP extension	Minimal	EDC, EIP	Minimal	Isotonic
PIP and DIP extension	Minimal	EDC, EIP	Minimal	Isotonic
Finger adduction	Maximal	Palmar interossei	Moderate	Isometric
THUMB				
Radial abduction	Moderate	APL, APB	Minimal	Isotonic
MP, IP extension	Full	EPL, EPB	Minimal	Isotonic

Adapted from A. Killingsworth, OT120 Activity Module, SJSU.

c. Endurance: Grade for sitting tolerance by increasing the length of activity sessions. Grade for sitting balance by decreasing sitting support.

d. Coordination: Requires fine coordination as performed; grade coordination by adding scored or painted designs to surface; grade to sculpture of small clay figures.

3. Criteria for activity as exercise
   a. Action of joints: Movement localized to flexion and extension of MP and IP joints of index and middle fingers; CMC, MP, and IP joint of thumb.
   b. Repetition of motion: The pinch and release sequence is repeated until the bowl has reached the desired height and thickness.

c. Gradable: The activity is gradable for strength and endurance.

III. Sensory Analysis[23,24]
   1. Check the sensory stimuli received by the person performing the activity. Include any sensory experience obtained from position, motion, materials, or equipment. Describe how sensation is received. (See Box 18-2.)

IV. Cognitive Analysis:[24] Check all that apply and justify your answer. (See Box 18-3.)

BOX 18-2

SENSORY MODALITY		HOW RECEIVED
Tactile	X	Touching clay and tools
Proprioceptive (joint motion and position sense)	X	Awareness of joint position and motion during pinch/release
Vestibular (balance, sense of body, head motion)	X	Maintenance of posture in chair while performing activity
Visual	X	Seeing clay object, environment
Olfactory (smell)	X	Smelling a slight odor of damp clay
Pain	0	
Thermal (temperature)	X	Hands sensing coldness of clay
Pressure	X	Fingertips and thumb tips pressing against walls of clay bowl
Auditory (hearing)	0	
Other		

BOX 18-3

COGNITIVE SKILL		JUSTIFICATION
Memory	X	Remembers instructions
Sequencing (steps in order)	X	Performs steps in order
Problem-solving skills	X	Knows what to do if clay is too wet or too dry, if walls of bowl are too thin or too thick
Following instructions Verbal	X	Able to comprehend and follow verbal and demonstrated instructions
Demonstrated	X	Same
Written	0	
Concentration/attention required	X	Moderate: focuses on bowl and knows when its walls are thin enough and high enough.

V. Safety Factors: What are the potential hazards of this activity? Describe safety precautions necessary for this activity.

There are few hazards in this activity. Ingesting clay or using smoothing tool inappropriately are possible. Also, sitting balance must be adequate to maintain upright posture to perform the activity. Precautions must be taken as follows: (1) Adequate supervision should be provided to ensure appropriate use of clay and tool and (2) the task should be performed from a wheelchair with supports if sitting balance is impaired.

VI. Interpersonal Aspects of Activity[3]
1. Solitary activity: May be done alone.
2. Potential for dyadic interaction: May be done in parallel with one other person but does not require interaction.
3. Potential for group interaction: May be done in a group but does not require interaction.

VII. Psychological/Psychosocial Factors
1. Symbolism in performer's culture:[10] May be seen as more feminine than masculine in mainstream American culture; may be associated with the artistic, liberal, naturalist groups of people in American society.
2. Symbolic meaning of activity to performer: May be seen as leisure skill rather than work: may be regarded as child's play by some persons.
3. Feelings/reactions evoked in performer during performance of activity:[24] The soft, moist, pliable and plastic properties of the clay may evoke soothing feelings in many persons. Others may regard it as messy or dirty. Potential for personal gratification is good because attractive end product is easy to achieve; activity is creative, individualistic, and useful.

VIII. Therapeutic Use of Activity
1. List the autonomous goal of the activity: To make a small clay bowl.
2. List possible therapeutic objective(s) for the activity
   a. To increase pinch strength
   b. To improve coordination of opposition
   c. To increase sitting tolerance

Orthotics

Julie Belkin, Carroll B. English, Carole Adler,
Lorraine Williams Pedretti

Section 1 Hand splinting: Principles, practice, and decision making

Julie Belkin, Carroll B. English

The human hand may be viewed as the brain's most important instrument with which to explore and master the world. It is the only body part that can substitute for other senses. We read with the hand if we suffer loss of vision; we communicate with the hand in the absence of speech or hearing. Our hands give us expression and console us. Even before birth, the fetus is seen to use the thumb as a pacifier. We first explore our hands and explore with our hands as infants. The wonder of the human hand is the precision with which it functions and the extremes of abuse it tolerates. We can and do take our hands for granted because they seem to function effortlessly, that is, until we experience some level of impairment or dysfunction.

The hand does not function independently of the whole human organism. It is connected to the brain via a complex tangle of nerves and is dependent on precise synaptic connections. The hand does not function independently of the upper extremity; stability and control of the shoulder, the elbow, and the wrist are needed to position the hand in space. Dysfunction anywhere from the brain to the fingertips may cause impaired function.

Humans gain independence largely through the control they exercise on their environment, because of the superiority of the human hand and the brain. The skills to tie a knot, open a necklace clasp, wield a hammer, or throw a ball are all unique to the human hand. That we can close a necklace with our vision occluded is testament to the sensibility of the hand. That we can wield a hammer and drive a nail through wood is testament to the integrity of the skin and the strength of the muscles that power the hand. That we can speak volumes with a sweep of our hands or a caressing touch is testament to the aesthetics of the hand. It is a remarkable instrument indeed.

Occupational therapists deal with the human being as a whole, not as just a hand, a toe, or a shoulder. When you change any part, you affect much more. In dealing with the human hand, you will discover how even the smallest impairment may affect function. Loss of placement of the hand may mean an inability to achieve a hand-to-mouth pattern, making independent feeding impossible. Pain anywhere in the hand can affect not only function, but a person's mood and disposition as well. Pain and fear can and do accompany injury, and when our independence or our livelihood is threatened by hand dysfunction, the outcomes are often dramatic. The hand is perhaps most valued only when it ceases to function and we must pay it attention.

Little else so readily calls attention to the hand as a splint. You may not receive comments on a new ring or a recent manicure, but put a splint on your hand and all will take notice. A splint is one of the most important

The authors wish to express their gratitude to North Coast Medical and in particular to Sheila, Jenny, and Susan for their assistance with the graphics for this chapter. We also wish to thank those therapists, students, and patients who have taught us so much over the years.

therapeutic tools therapists can use to minimize or correct impairment and to restore or augment function. The decision to provide or to fabricate a splint requires an in-depth understanding of the pathological condition you wish to affect and of the many splinting choices available.

This chapter serves as an introduction to those anatomical and biomechanical principles necessary to understanding the basic concepts and models of splinting. This chapter (1) briefly reviews the anatomy of the hand and its relationship to principles of splinting; (2) introduces the biomechanics involved in splint design and fabrication; (3) discusses the variety and types of materials available to the therapist for splint fabrication; (4) introduces a decision tree to be used in splint design and decision making; and (5) suggests applications of splinting for some of the more common diagnoses.

ROLE OF THE OCCUPATIONAL THERAPIST

The education an occupational therapist receives in the analysis of activity and the assessment of human occupation and function leads naturally into the use of splinting as one therapeutic tool in the treatment regime. Splints for the hand and upper extremity are most commonly fabricated by occupational therapists, but the occupational therapist also may be called upon to design and fabricate splints for the lower extremity and even for the back or spine. The basic principles of splinting apply, no matter the part being splinted.

Whether a splint is used to protect, prevent, assist, or resist motion, in some way it affects function. Though many other health care professionals participate in the treatment of persons with hand impairment, it is the occupational therapist whose education is most directly related to the discipline of hand rehabilitation. It is because of the hand's contribution to human occupation that the occupational therapist is most often involved in hand therapy and in splint fabrication. Involvement of the occupational therapist in all phases of splint fabrication is recommended, from the initial assessment of need, through the design phase, the fabrication, and the training and follow-up necessary to ensure proper use and fit of the splint.

It is important to focus on restoration of function through every phase of treatment. To do so requires an understanding of the anatomy and biomechanics of the normal, unimpaired hand and the impaired hand. Many excellent texts describe both hand anatomy and biomechanics in extensive detail and should be included in the library of any occupational therapist treating the hand. This chapter reviews the anatomy and biomechanics of the hand that are most pertinent to splinting. The lists of references and suggested readings at the end of this chapter provide several excellent selections for further study.

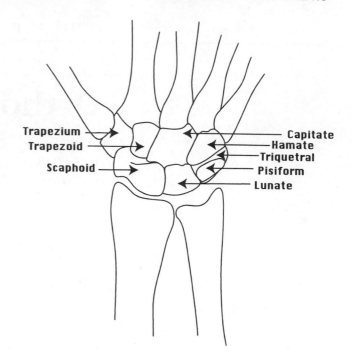

FIG. 19-1 Skeletal structures of the wrist, dorsal view.

One reference of note is the Splint Classification System (SCS),[1] published by The American Society of Hand Therapists (ASHT).* The SCS describes splint nomenclature based on the functional requirement of a splint as well as on the anatomy affected. This nomenclature is quite inclusive of the broad variety of upper extremity splints fabricated by occupational therapists and is suggested for study.

ANATOMICAL STRUCTURES OF THE HAND
Wrist

The hand and wrist are composed of an arrangement of twenty-seven bones that contribute to the mobility and adaptability of the hand. The wrist comprises eight carpal bones arranged in two rows. Each of the carpal bones is cuboid in shape with six surfaces: four articular surfaces and two that receive the attachment of ligaments. The carpal bones form the concave transverse arch and, with the configuration of the distal radius, contribute substantially to the conformability of the hand.[11] The distal ulna does not articulate with any carpal bone, and its contribution to wrist stability is through the attachments of the ulnar collateral ligament, which places a check on radial deviation (Fig. 19-1).

The wrist complex allows for a greater arc of motion than any other joint complex except the ankle. This mobility is due to a unique skeletal configuration and an involved ligamentous system. All motion at the wrist is

* American Society of Hand Therapists, 401 N. Michigan Ave., Chicago, IL 60611-6267.

component motion occurring in more than one anatomical plane; there are no pure or isolated motions. This concept is key in any treatment directed at or across the wrist. Extension occurs with a degree of radial deviation and supination, whereas flexion includes both ulnar deviation and pronation. The wrist cannot be viewed as distinct or separate from the hand. The distal carpal row, including the trapezium, trapezoid, capitate, and hamate, articulates firmly with the metacarpals, and motion is produced across these articulations by muscles that cross the carpals and attach onto the metacarpals. The proximal carpal row, the scaphoid, lunate, and triquetrum, articulates distally with the distal carpal row and proximally with the radius and the triangular cartilage. Gliding motions occur between the carpal rows during flexion, extension, and deviation, with excessive motion checked by the carpal ligaments.

Placement of the hand for functional tasks is reliant on the stability, mobility and precision of placement permitted by the wrist complex. Any mechanism of injury or disease that alters this complex system is translated into some level of dysfunction. Even the simplest splint that crosses the wrist will in some way alter the functional abilities of the hand. Splint designs that attempt to augment or substitute for wrist motion are likely to limit component motions or be too complex to fabricate or wear.

The therapist seeking to position the wrist for function should passively position the wrist in varying degrees of motion while having the patient perform a variety of prehension tasks to determine the optimal wrist position. When static positioning of the wrist is required, the optimal degree of flexion or extension and ulnar or radial deviation will vary with the task and with the patient's preference.

Wrist tenodesis

A concept basic to hand function is that of wrist tenodesis. Tenodesis is the reciprocal motion of the wrist and fingers that occurs during active or passive wrist flexion and extension. Tenodesis is the action of wrist extension producing finger flexion and wrist flexion producing finger extension. It is due to the lack of change in length of the long finger muscles during wrist flexion or extension (Fig. 19-2). Because the extrinsic finger muscle-tendon units have a fixed resting length, and because they cross multiple joints before inserting onto the phalanges, they can affect the position of several joints without any contraction or length change required of the muscles. This concept is crucial to understanding how passive positioning of the wrist affects the resting position of the digits. In the nerve-injured hand, tenodesis is often harnessed by splints to provide function. The spinal cord–injured patient with sparing of a wrist extensor (C6, 7 level) gains considerable function from a tenodesis splint. In dynamic splinting, the effect that tenodesis has

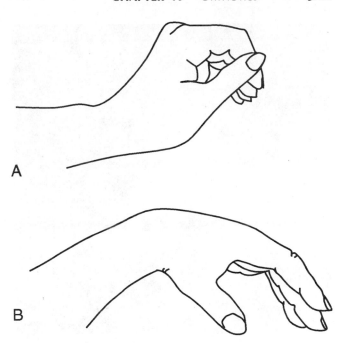

FIG. 19-2 Tenodesis. **A,** Active wrist extension results in passive finger flexion. **B,** Active wrist flexion results in passive finger extension.

on tendon length will in part dictate the wrist position that will optimize forces directed at the digits.

Metacarpal Joints

The metacarpals articulate with the carpal bones proximally and with the phalanges distally. The carpal articulations contribute to the central stability of the second and third metacarpals and to the mobility of the first, fourth, and fifth metacarpals. The first metacarpal, the thumb, articulates with the saddle-shaped trapezium and will be considered separately. The fourth and fifth metacarpals both articulate with the concave distal surface of the hamate; they are highly mobile joints that contribute to the flexible arches of the hand. The second fits into the central ridge of the trapezoid and the third articulates firmly with the facets of the capitate. These articulations form the immobile central segment of the hand around which the other metacarpals rotate.

The distal transverse arch of the hand lies obliquely across the metacarpal heads. This obliquity is critical to the hand's ability to adapt its shape to objects. The hand does not form a cylinder as it closes, but instead assumes the position of a cone. In fisting, the ulnar two digits of the hand contact the palm first and the radial two digits follow. This cascade of the fingers is a direct result of the oblique angle formed at the metacarpal heads. This concept becomes most important in splinting when determining the distal trim lines for a wrist support where full MCP flexion is desired. The splint in Fig. 19-3, *A,* is improperly trimmed distal to the MCP creases. Distal trim

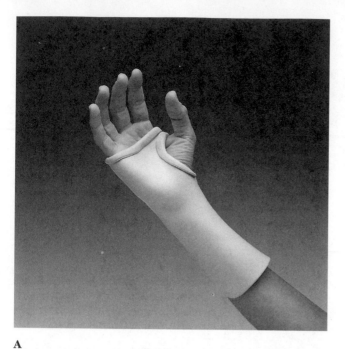

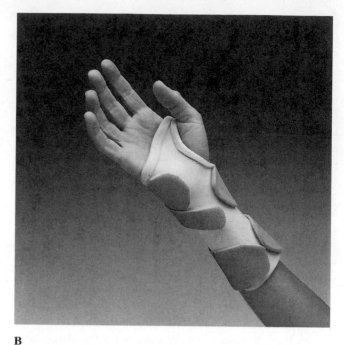

A

B

FIG. 19-3 **A,** Trim lines of splint extend distal to MP creases and limit finger flexion.
B, Splint's distal trim lines fall proximal to MP creases and permit full finger flexion.

lines should be established proximal to the MCP creases as in Fig. 19-3, *B*.

MCP joints

The distal heads of the metacarpals articulate with the proximal phalanges to form the metacarpophalangeal (MCP) joints. Active motion is possible along an axis of flexion and extension and along an axis of abduction and adduction. Additionally, a small degree of conjunct rotation is present at the MCP joints. These axes of motion allow for expansion or spreading of the hand and contribute to the ability of the hand to conform to different shapes and sizes of objects. Attempt to hold a softball without abducting your fingers and the importance of this motion becomes readily apparent. A splint with trim lines along the ulnar border of the hand that extend too far distally, limits both flexion and abduction of the fourth and fifth digits. As a result, the hand will have a limited ability to grasp large objects and function will be restricted (Fig. 19-4, *A*). Distal trim lines that fall proximal to the MCP creases will allow for full MCP flexion (Fig. 19-4, *B*).

Thumb

The articulation of the the base of the first metacarpal with the trapezium forms a highly mobile joint, often compared to the shape of a saddle. The base of the first metacarpal is concave in the anteroposterior plane and convex in the lateral plane. This surface is met by reciprocal surfaces on the trapezium. This configuration allows for a wide arc of motion, with the thumb able to

rotate not only for pad-to-pad opposition but also for full extension and abduction to move away from the palm.[10] One must consider the functional importance of both motions. That is, a thumb posted in permanent opposition may make grasp possible but release of objects impossible. This concept is crucial to the understanding of splints that augment the tenodesis action of the hand by posting the thumb in opposition to the index and long fingers. With such splints, the therapist must carefully consider the degree of abduction and opposition in which the thumb is posted, to maximize both grasp and release.

IP Joints

The proximal interphalangeal (PIP) joints and distal interphalangeal (DIP) joints are true hinge joints with motion in only one plane. This limitation of motion ensures greater stability in these joints, which contributes to their ability to resist palmar and lateral stresses and so impart strength and precision to functional tasks.

Forearm Rotation

A word concerning forearm rotation, or supination and pronation, is necessary because of the importance of these motions to function and to the fitting of splints. Forearm rotation occurs at the elbow as well as at the distal forearm, resulting not only in multiple axes of motion but in a shifting of the positions of the distal ulna and radius. This shifting alters the architecture of the forearm. During pronation the ulnar styloid moves laterally as the radial styloid travels medially. During supination the

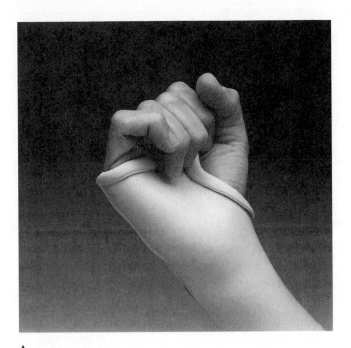

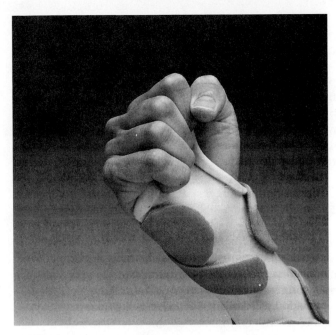

A   B

FIG. 19-4 **A,** Fourth and fifth digits are prevented from full flexion. **B,** Full finger flexion is possible with proper trim lines.

opposite occurs, with the ulnar styloid moving medially. This movement results in a displacement of the styloids, which in turn alters the architecture of the forearm in supination as compared with pronation.

The best way to appreciate this phenomenon is to place your left hand on your right ulnar styloid with your forearm in full pronation. Feel the ulnar styloid displace palmarward as you rotate into supination. Now repeat this motion with your left hand grasped lightly around your proximal forearm, just distal to the elbow crease. Note the rotation and repositioning of the proximal ulna and radius.

To see how this motion will affect the trim lines of a splint, place your right forearm in supination and gently place your left index finger along the radial border of your forearm, with your left thumb along the ulnar border. Hold your finger and thumb in this position as you pronate your right forearm. You will note that your left index finger is now positioned on the dorsum of your forearm, although it started on the volar surface. This rotation and repositioning of the proximal ulna and radius affects the trim lines and fit of splints. Splints are generally used for function with the forearm in pronation, but they are easier to fabricate with the forearm in supination. If the patient does not pronate the forearm just before the splint is cool, for the correct trim lines to be established along the midforearm, the trim line will be high on the radial border and low on the ulnar border.

You may conduct one final experiment to realize the importance of forearm position on hand function. Place a coin of any size on a table top and holding your forearm in neutral (thumb straight up), attempt to pick up the coin. It becomes rapidly apparent that the ability to position the hand for function in great part relies on the more proximal joints of the forearm.

LIGAMENTS OF THE WRIST AND HAND
WRIST

The ligamentous structures of the hand act as checkreins for the hand and wrist, limiting extremes of motion and providing stability. The complex motions of the wrist are dependent in large part on the ligaments that restrain them rather than on the contact surfaces between the carpals and metacarpals. We will briefly consider three groups of ligaments at the wrist, disruption of which results in important functional limitations.

The palmar ligaments are the radioscaphocapitate contributing support to the scaphoid, the radiolunate supporting the lunate, and the radioscapholunate, which connects the scapholunate articulation with the palmar surface of the distal radius. The stability and mobility of the thumb and radial carpus are dependent on the integrity of these ligaments. Disruption of these ligaments results not only in instability and pain at the wrist but in significant dysfunction of the thumb. Splinting is frequently indicated as the treatment of choice to supply stability for pain reduction.

Dorsal stability is provided by the radial and ulnar collateral ligaments. These capsular ligaments, along with the radiocarpal and dorsal carpal ligaments, provide carpal stability while permitting range of motion.

The triangular fibrocartilage complex (TFCC) includes

the ligaments and the cartilaginous structures that suspend the distal radius from the distal ulna and the distal carpus. Modern techniques of arthroscopic evaluation have contributed to greater understanding of this complex and its contribution to wrist stability and to hand function. Tears or strains in this complex are evidenced by pain and weakness with resultant loss of function in resistive tasks. TFCC tears are becoming a more frequent diagnosis, with splinting ordered for support and pain relief.

MCP JOINTS

The MCP joints include a complex structure consisting of a joint capsule, collateral ligaments, and an anterior fibrocartilage or volar plate. The capsule covers the head of the metacarpal and is reinforced by the collateral ligaments. The collateral ligaments run in a dorsal-lateral to palmar-lateral direction, from the head of the metacarpals to the head of the proximal phalanges. The collateral ligaments are configured to allow side-to-side motion when the MCP is in extension and to tighten as the MCP is flexed. The volar plate is attached to the base of the proximal phalanx and loosely attached to the base of the neck of the metacarpal through the joint capsule. This configuration allows for sliding of the plate proximally during MCP flexion. The plate returns to its lengthened state with the MCP in extension and acts as a checkrein to volar displacement of the MCP joint when it is extended.

There is a strong tendency for secondary shortening of the lax collateral ligaments, as well as contraction and adherence of the volar plate when the MCPs are immobilized in extension, resulting in limited MCP flexion and loss of functional grasp patterns. The commonly accepted resting position splint, which places the MCP joints at 60° to 70° of flexion while maintaining PIP and DIP extension, is designed specifically to prevent shortening and maintain the joints in midrange for optimal function. An important consideration here is to ensure that the mobile fourth and fifth digits are positioned in the splint to accommodate their additional degree of mobility by allowing somewhat greater flexion at their MCP joints (Fig. 19-5).

PIP JOINTS

The PIP joint has capsular and ligamentous structures that provide stability and allow for mobility in one plane only. Collateral ligaments on each side of the joint run in a dorsal to palmar direction, inserting into the fibrocartilage plate of the PIP. These ligaments and plate are lax with the PIP joint in flexion and taut with it in extension. The PIP joint is made all the more complex by the inclusion of the extensor mechanism passing through the capsule dorsally and contributing slips to the system of ligaments affecting this joint. The potential for disruption of the extensor mechanism is high. Many of the most commonly fabricated finger splints are used to correct

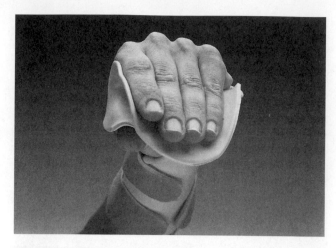

FIG. 19-5 Oblique angle of transverse arch at MCPs must be accommodated to ensure maintenance of more mobile fourth and fifth digits.

the PIP deformities known as boutonniere (Fig. 19-6, *A*) and swan neck deformities (Fig. 19-6, *B*).

DIP JOINTS

The DIP joint has a capsule and ligament similar to the PIP joint but with less structural strength to the terminal insertions of its palmar plate and collateral ligaments. As the structures get smaller, they lose integrity and strength. It is no wonder that one of the most frequent

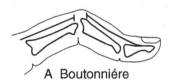

A Boutonniére

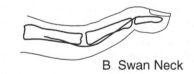

B Swan Neck

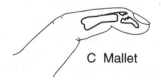

C Mallet

FIG. 19-6 **A**, Boutonniere deformity characterized by PIP joint flexion and DIP joint hypertension. **B**, Swan neck deformity with PIP joint hyperextension and DIP joint flexion. **C**, Mallet deformity with DIP joint flexion and loss of active extension.

injuries to the digits is the disruption of the terminal end of the extensor tendon, resulting in a mallet or "baseball" finger (Fig. 19-6, *C*).

MUSCLES AND TENDONS OF THE FOREARM, WRIST, AND HAND

The important concept to remember when assessing the hand for a splint is that of helping to restore balance, when necessary. Two groups of muscles, which must be balanced, act on the wrist and hand: (1) the extrinsics that arise from the elbow and the proximal half of the midforearm and (2) the intrinsics with origins and insertions entirely in the hand. The extrinsics include both a flexor and extensor group acting on the wrist and on the digits. The intrinsics include the lumbricals, the dorsal and palmar interossei, and the thenar and hypothenar groups.

Smooth coordinated motions of the hand are dependent on a well-integrated balance between and within these two muscle groups. Many of the contractures occupational therapists are called on to correct with splinting are caused by neurologic dysfunction (central or peripheral), which results in imbalance of muscle tone and/or innervation.

NERVE SUPPLY

In discussing the nerve supply to the hand, it is important to mention the continuity of the brachial plexus, from its origins in the spinal cord to its terminal innervations in the hand. Injuries or compressions occurring anywhere along this continuum may result in motor or sensory dysfunction. When splinting the upper extremity, you should understand the pathways of the nerves supplying the upper extremity and the potential sites for entrapment. You must also be aware of sites where the nerves are superficial in the upper extremity, to avoid applying pressure that may cause or add to dysfunction. These sites include the ulnar nerve at the elbow and in the Guyon canal in the palm, the radial nerve at the elbow and in the thenar snuff box, and the digital nerves along the medial and lateral borders of the digits (Fig. 19-7).

Three peripheral nerves supply the motor and sensory function to the hand (Fig. 19-8). The radial nerve is the primary motor supplier to the extensor/supinator muscles. The sensory fibers of the radial nerve supply the dorsum and radial border of the hand. The median nerve provides motor supply to the flexor/pronator group, including most of the long flexors and the muscles of the thenar eminence. The sensory distribution of the median nerve is functionally the most important because it includes the palmar surface of the thumb, index, and long fingers and the radial half of the ring finger. The ulnar nerve supplies most of the intrinsics, the hypothenar muscles, the ulnarmost profundi and the adductor pollicis brevis. The sensory supply of the ulnar nerve includes

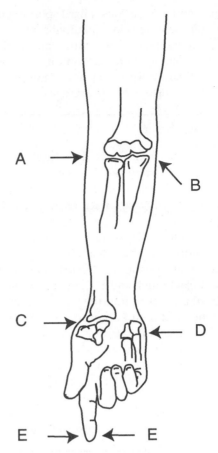

FIG. 19-7 Potential sites for nerve compression from improperly fit splints. **A,** Radial nerve. **B,** Ulnar nerve. **C,** Radial digital nerve in anatomical snuffbox. **D,** Ulnar nerve in Guyon canal. **E,** Digital nerves.

the palmar surface of the ulnar half of the ring finger, the little finger, and the ulnar half of the palm.

Nerve dysfunction is perhaps the most challenging diagnosis the splint maker will encounter. The resultant muscle imbalance leads to (1) dysfunctional posturing of the hand, (2) muscle atrophy that reduces the natural padding of the hand, and (3) lost sensibility that impairs

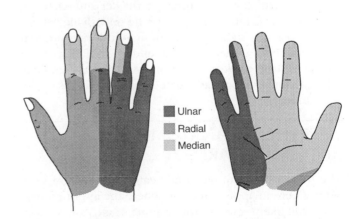

FIG. 19-8 Sensory distribution in hand. Median nerve distribution includes most of prehensile surface of palm.

function and can be hazardous if hard splinting materials are applied to desensate skin. Splinting is directed at prevention of joint and soft tissue contractures and at restoration of functional positioning. Splinting cannot restore sensibility, and care must be taken to minimize limiting sensory feedback further by covering sensate surfaces.

BLOOD SUPPLY

Blood supply to the hand is carried by the radial and ulnar arteries. The ulnar artery lies just lateral to the flexor carpi ulnaris tendon, where it divides into a large branch that forms the superficial arterial arch and a small branch that forms the lesser part of the deep palmar arch. The ulnar artery is vulnerable to trauma where it passes between the pisiform and the hamate (the canal of Guyon). The radial artery divides at the proximal wrist crease into a small superficial branch and a larger deep radial branch. The superficial arterial arch further divides into common digital branches and then into proper digital branches.

Venous drainage of the hand is accomplished by two sets of veins: a superficial and a deep group. It is the superficial venous system with which therapists are most likely to be concerned, as it lies superficially in the dorsum of the hand. Disruption of this superficial system may result in extensive fluid edema in the dorsum of the hand, which demands the therapist's attention.

SKIN

The mobility of the hand is directly related to the type and condition of the skin. If you have ever put on a ring that is slightly too small, only to be unable to remove it, you have experienced the redundancy of the skin on the dorsum of your hand. The skin on the dorsum of the hand is loosely anchored to underlying structures and moves easily to allow flexion and extension of the digits. The ring "problem" occurs because of a greater degree of elasticity in the dorsal skin when it is pulled distally as opposed to when it is pulled proximally. Consider this fact when contemplating the use of finger casts.

The palmar skin, by contrast, is thicker and relatively inelastic. It is firmly connected to the underlying palmar aponeurosis for stability and protection during prehension activities. Furthermore, the underlying fascia of the palmar skin is thicker and protects the nerve endings while acting to supply adequate moisture and oils to the skin surface.

SUPERFICIAL ANATOMY AND LANDMARKS

The therapist venturing to fabricate a splint must consider where to apply force and where the application of force will likely cause further trauma. Hands are remarkable for their deftness and power, given the size of the digits and the lack of protective fascia in the hand. There are bony landmarks over which no hand withstands pressure or shearing forces. The prominent ulnar styloid, the distal head of the radius at the ulnar snuffbox, and the thumb carpometacarpal joint are common sites for pressure. A truism that will always hold in splinting is that *padding adds pressure.* The softest padding added to a too tight splint will only add pressure. When splinting over bony prominences, make a "bubble" over the prominence to relieve pressure. (Make a bubble by applying a mound of padding or therapy putty to the bony prominence itself, before splinting. Later, remove the mound and a bubble will remain in the splint.) When splinting over bony areas where a bubble is not practical, place padding on the bony prominence before applying the warm splint material to build the padding into the splint, where it can help to distribute the forces. Do not add padding to distribute forces after a splint is made.

PREHENSION AND GRASP PATTERNS

A major function of the human hand is to manipulate objects to accomplish a goal. The ability of the human hand to assume a myriad of positions and to apply only the precise amount of pressure necessary to hold an object is owed to the mobility and stability supplied by the skeleton, to the power of the muscles, and to the remarkable degree of sensory feedback from the nerves. This sensory feedback is used to assess the size, shape, texture, and weight of an object. The brain then determines which type of prehension to use. The feedback used in the grasping and lifting of an object is dependent both on the brain interpreting correctly what is seen and on the hand responding appropriately. Once an object is in the hand, further adaptation in prehension will occur if the initial visual assessment was faulty.

Splints can maximize functional prehension. In achieving this goal, the therapist must be aware of what a splint can and cannot do; a splint can stabilize an unstable part, it can position a thumb in opposition, and it can even assist or substitute for lost motion. The splint maker must beware, however, in attempting to do any of the aforementioned, a splint may also limit mobility at uninvolved joints, reduce sensory feedback, add bulk to the hand, and transfer stresses to unsplinted joints proximal or distal to the part being splinted.

The prehension patterns the hand is able to achieve are as exhaustive as the objects that are available to grasp or pinch. Classifications of normal prehension have been attempted by many, and excellent works by Napier and Flatt[7] are presented in the Reference and Suggested Readings sections for further study of the subject. It is possible to reduce the many patterns to two basic classifications, prehension and grasp, from which other patterns may be derived. First, *prehension* is defined as a position of the hand that allows for finger and thumb contact and facilitates manipulation of objects. Second, *grasp* is defined as a position of the hand that facilitates

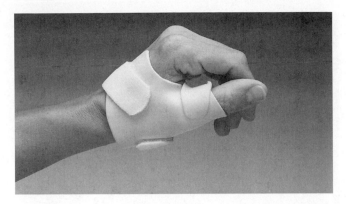

FIG. 19-9 A, Lateral prehension or key pinch in short opponens splint that positions thumb in lateral opposition to index finger.

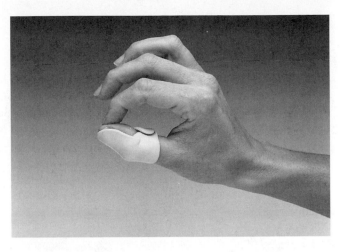

FIG. 19-11 Tip prehension with thumb and index finger in thumb IP blocker that secures IP joint in slight flexion to assist tip prehension.

contact of an object against the palm and the palmar surface of the partially flexed digits.

The thumb is involved in all but one type of grip, that of hook grasp. The position of thumb abduction and rotation is constant in all prehensile actions and remains unchanged despite the size or shape of the object held.[7] The component of carpometacarpal (CMC) and MCP rotation is crucial to precision handling and cannot be overstressed in its importance in splinting to achieve function. This rotation allows for full contact of the thumb in pad-to-pad prehension.

Lateral prehension (Fig. 19-9). The pad of the thumb is positioned to contact the radial side of the index middle or distal phalanx. Most commonly, this pattern is the pattern of prehension used in holding a pen or eating utensil and in holding and turning a key. The most common splint used to simulate this prehension pattern is the short or long opponens splint.

Palmar prehension (Fig. 19-10). This pattern is also called three-jaw chuck pinch. The thumb is positioned in opposition to the index and long fingers. The important component of motion in this pattern is thumb rotation, which allows for pad-to-pad opposition. This prehension pattern is used in lifting objects from a flat surface, in holding small objects, and in tying a shoe or bow. The short and long opponens splints may also be fabricated to position the thumb in palmar prehension.

Tip prehension (Fig. 19-11). In this pattern the IP joint of the thumb and the DIP and PIP joints of the finger are flexed to facilitate tip-to-tip prehension. These motions are necessary to pick up a pin, a nail, or a coin. This prehension pattern is one for which it is difficult to substitute, because it is rarely a static holding posture and is used primarily for manipulation of objects. Once a pin is in the hand, the pattern of prehension will revert to a palmar prehension to provide more skin surface area to retain a small object. The most appropriate splint application to facilitate this prehension pattern is the thumb hyperextension block used to correct arthritic deformities at the IP joint.

Cylindrical grasp (Fig. 19-12). Cylindrical grasp, the most common static grasp pattern, is used to stabilize objects against the palm and the fingers, with the thumb acting as an opposing force. This pattern is assumed when grasping a hammer, pot handle, tumbler or the handhold on a walker or crutch. Splinting offers little to restore this grasp directly, though positioning the wrist in extension offers greater stability to the hand as it assumes this grasp pattern. A dorsal wrist stabilizer offers stability while minimizing palm coverage.

Spherical grasp (Fig. 19-13). Also called ball grasp, this pattern is the one the hand assumes when holding a round object such as a ball or apple. It differs from cylin-

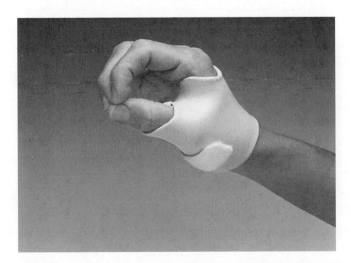

FIG. 19-10 Palmar prehension or 3-jaw chuck pinch in short opponens splint that positions thumb in opposition to index and long fingers.

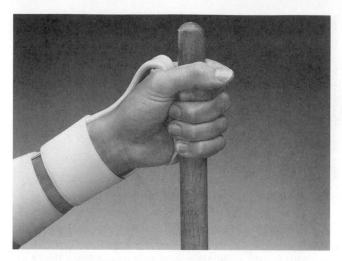

FIG. 19-12   Cylindrical grasp in dorsal splint, which stabilizes wrist to increase grip force and minimizes palm covering.

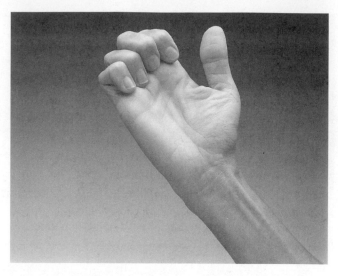

FIG. 19-14   Hook grasp does not involve thumb. Grasp pattern is seen in median and ulnar neuropathy; splinting is aimed at correcting rather than augmenting grasp.

drical grasp primarily in the positioning of the fourth and fifth digits. In cylindrical grasp, the ulnar two metacarpals are supported in greater extension. In spherical grasp, the ulnar two digits assume a more flexed attitude allowing for the cupping of the palm. In splinting, to facilitate or support this pattern of grasp, the wrist-stabilizing splint must be proximal to the distal palmar crease and contoured to allow for the obliquity at the fourth and fifth metacarpal heads.

Hook grasp (Fig. 19-14). This pattern is the only prehension pattern that does not include the thumb to supply opposition. The MCP joints of the fingers are held in extension to slight hyperextension, and the DIP and PIP

joints are held in flexion. This is the attitude the hand assumes when holding the handle of a shopping bag, a pail, or a briefcase. This posture is a dysfunctional one often seen in the nerve-injured hand, and splinting is more commonly directed at correcting this posture than at facilitating it.

Intrinsic plus grasp (Fig. 19-15). This grasp pattern is characterized by the positioning of all the MCPs of the fingers in flexion, the DIP and PIPs in full extension, and the thumb aligned in opposition to the third and fourth fingers. This grasp pattern is used in grasping and holding large flat objects such as books or plates. Intrinsic plus grasp is often lost in the presence of median and/or ulnar nerve dysfunction, and a figure-of-eight or dynamic MCP flexion splint may be used as substitutes.

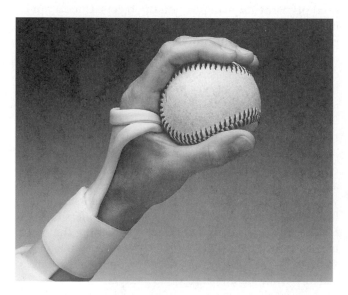

FIG. 19-13   Spherical grasp in dorsal splint. Splint stabilizes wrist to increase grip force and permits metacarpal mobility required for spherical grasp.

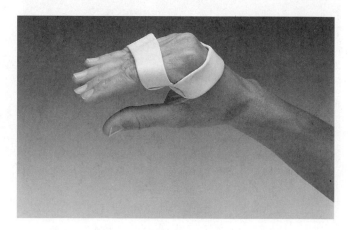

FIG. 19-15   Figure-of-eight splint substitutes for loss of intrinsic function with median and ulnar neuropathy.

MECHANICS OF THE HAND AND PRINCIPLES OF SPLINTING

McCollough and Sarrafian[9] have stated that the three basic motor functions of the upper limb are "prehension and release, transfer of objects in space, and manipulation of objects within the grasp."[9] These functions are dependent on the complex mechanics of the motors that power the limb. These functions are also dependent on the internal and external feedback to which the brain responds when adapting the limb to environmental demands. The task of restoring any one of these basic functions through the application of a splint is complex and relies on an understanding of the mechanics of the hand and the mechanics involved in splinting.

Mechanics deals with the application of force. In the hand, the force required for producing motion is supplied by muscles. The force is then transmitted by the tendons to the bones and joints, with control supplied by the skin and pulp of the fingers and palm.[8] How the application of a splint affects the transmission of force to produce motion depends on (1) the relationship between the axis of rotation of joints and anatomic planes and (2) the forces imposed on the hand.

AXIS OF MOTION

Hollister and Giurintano[8] define *axis of motion* as a stable line that does not move when the bones of a joint move in relation to each other[8] (Fig. 19-16, *A, B*). This stable line is illustrated by Fig. 19-16, *B*, which shows a tire perfectly balanced around its axis of motion. When a tire is perfectly balanced, it does not wobble; it has pure motion around a single point.

If the axis of motion of a joint is aligned in a pure anatomical plane, motion will occur in only one plane. The PIP joint is an example of a single-axis joint in alignment with an anatomical plane. It moves only in the plane of flexion and extension.

Many of the joints of the extremities have more than one axis of motion, however, and these axes deviate from alignment in one plane of motion. For example, the wrist complex has two axes of motion: flexion/extension and radial/ulnar deviation. A joint with multiple axes has conjunct motions in addition to the primary motions described by the joint. These conjunct motions allow for circumduction of the wrist. You may perform an easy exercise to see how these conjunct motions come into play at the wrist. Place your forearm in pronation, relax your fingers and then actively extend your wrist. Note the tendency for the hand to deviate radially and the forearm to supinate slightly; radial deviation and supination are conjunct motions. Likewise, flexion of the wrist produces conjunct motions of ulnar deviation and a tendency toward increased forearm pronation.

The implications for splinting with hinges or coils

A

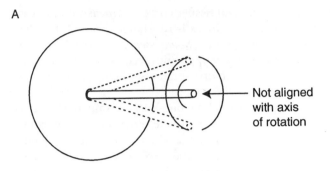

B

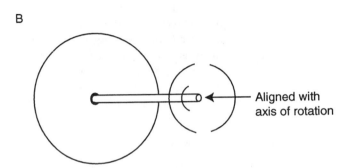

FIG. 19-16 A, Tire not balanced around axis of motion wobbles. If splint hinge is not properly aligned with joint axis of motion, wobble is seen as binding of joint. **B,** Proper alignment of axis of motion in tire results in smooth rotation without wobble. In hinge, proper alignment with joint axis results in smooth, unimpeded motion.

across joints that have conjunct motions are important. The dynamic splint with a hinge or coil has a single axis. If it is placed next to a single-axis joint such as a PIP joint, it can and should be properly aligned with the joint or there will be binding that will limit motion. If it is placed next to a joint with multiple axes and conjunct motions, there will always be some binding or friction, no matter how well aligned, because the hinge or coil cannot allow for or reproduce the conjunct motions available in the unsplinted joint.

FORCE

A thorough discussion of force is beyond the scope of this chapter. It is important to understand certain principles, however, to apply them correctly in splinting. An understanding of the forces applied by levers and the stresses that occur between opposing surfaces can help explain what happens as forces are applied within the body by muscles and externally by splints.

Definitions

The use of the term *force,* as it relates to splinting, describes the effect materials and dynamic components have upon bone and tissue. Force is a measure of stress, friction, or torque. *Stress* is resistance to any force that strains or deforms tissue. *Shear stress* occurs when force is applied to tissues in opposing directions. Pinching skin between the surface of a splint and the underlying bony structures causes shear stress.

Friction occurs when one surface impedes or prevents motion of another surface. Friction is produced in the stiff or contracted joint when soft tissue restriction prevents gliding of the bones. Splints may contribute to friction if they are misaligned in relation to a joint axis. For example, a hinged splint that is not properly aligned with the axis of rotation will limit motion by producing friction as the joint attempts to move.

Torque is the result of the application of force when that force results in rotation of a lever around an axis. The amount of torque created when the lever moves is dependent on the force used and the length of the lever employed. In the body, muscles are the levers that create torque when they act to move a joint. Externally, splints may act as levers to apply the force necessary to move a bone around its axis. The measure of torque is given by the formula:

Torque = (amount of) Force × (length of) Lever arm

Internally, the length of the lever arm is measured as the perpendicular distance from the axis of the joint to the tendon. Externally, the length of the lever arm is measured as the estimated distance from the joint axis to the attachment of force. In splinting, this force is applied through a cuff attached to a line or a static or resilient strap.

Given an equal amount of resistance or load, a 2-foot lever will require half as much force to create motion around an axis as will a 1-foot lever. The important principle for splint makers is as follows: the greater the distance between the attachment of the cuff or strap to the joint axis, the less force required to achieve motion, but the smaller the degree of motion achieved.

Clinically, torque can be dangerous if the splint maker does not consider how splint dimensions and configurations affect the application of force. In splinting, the length of the lever arm is the distance from the joint axis to the point of applied force. For example, if the splint is a finger cast, the length of the cast acts as the lever arm. If the splint includes an outrigger with a finger cuff, as shown in Fig. 19-17, the lever arm is the distance from the cuff to the point of attachment on the outrigger, as indicated in line M.

Rotational and Translational Forces

In addition to being aware of the forces that cause pressure and shear forces, the splint maker must be aware of rotational and translational forces. Although they are involved in all splinting, rotational and translational forces can be most readily seen in dynamic splinting. To understand these forces, it is first necessary to understand the

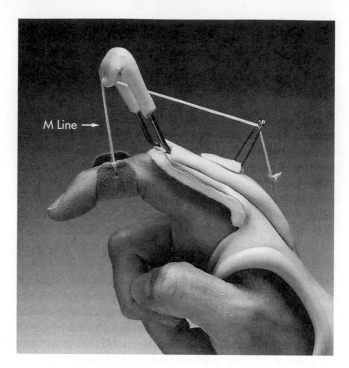

FIG. 19-17   Lever arm of this splint varies with the outrigger line.

concept of angle of approach. The angle of approach is the angle that the line of traction makes as it meets the part being splinted. For example, in the outrigger splint in Fig. 19-18, *A,* the angle of approach between the nylon line and the phalanx is 90°.

The rotational force is the force that makes the joint rotate around its axis and move in a desired direction. For instance, the rotational force in the splint in Fig. 19-18, *A,* is moving the joint into extension. Traction applied at a 90° angle of approach ensures that all the force is going into making the joint rotate around its axis, which in this case is joint extension. If the traction is applied at any

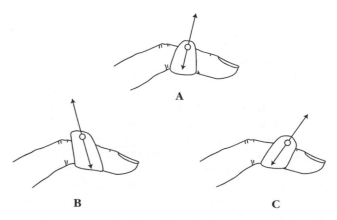

FIG. 19-18   **A,** Angle of approach is 90° to middle phalanx, ensuring force is not dissipated when pulling PIP joint into extension. **B,** Angle of approach less than 90° to axis of middle phalanx compresses joint. **C,** Angle of approach greater than 90° to axis of middle phalanx distracts joint.

angle other than 90°, however, translational force comes into play. It translates some of the rotational force away from producing joint extension and directs the force into joint compression or joint distraction (Fig. 19-18, *B* and 19-18, *C*). The more the angle of approach deviates from 90°, the greater is the amount of translational force. Depending on the type of splint and the condition of the joint, the joint compression or distraction may lead to mere discomfort or to actual joint damage. Translational force also is undesirable because it undermines the effectiveness of the splint.[6]

The challenge in splinting with an outrigger is to position the splint so there is a 90° angle of approach. In the outrigger in Fig. 19-17, as long as the finger does not move, the 90° angle will remain. As soon as the finger moves, however, the 90° angle changes. Few available outriggers allow for this automatic readjustment in position. Therefore, it is very important to adjust the outrigger as the contracture lessens so that at least the initial 90° angle remains.

In summary, splints always apply forces to the part being splinted. If these forces are not understood, the splint will at best be ineffective, and at worst it will cause harm.

APPLICATION OF FORCE THROUGH SPLINTING
Implications of Application of Force

Whether static or dynamic, all splints apply force, which means that they apply some degree of stress on the structures they contact. It is important to minimize or distribute that stress, or the splint will not be tolerated. Excessive stress can cause damage to both superficial and deep structures of the hand and upper extremity. The unimpaired hand tolerates a wide range of stresses by adaptation when possible and by avoidance when not. The impaired hand may lack the protective responses necessary to reposition itself away from the stresses applied by objects or by splints. The classic case is the person with a recently applied cast who experiences rubbing that will result in ulceration if it is not relieved. This is common in cognitively impaired patients who are unable to remove splints left on too long by inattentive caregivers.

Pressure causes ischemia (localized anemia caused by obstruction of blood supply to tissues), and pressure increases when splints are contoured too sharply, when they do not conform uniformly, or when they do not cover a broad enough area of soft tissue. Splints that migrate or move on the hand because of insufficient strapping or contouring, may actually apply pressure in areas that the splint was designed to relieve.

There are techniques for avoiding pressure areas and shear forces in a dynamic splint, particularly where traction is applied to mobilize a finger joint. First, it is important to stabilize the joint(s) proximal to the finger joint being splinted. For instance, to mobilize a PIP joint with an outrigger and cuff, the MCP joint must be held se-

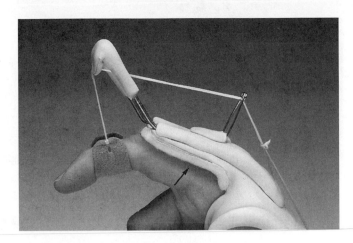

FIG. 19-19   Felt padding distributes pressure over bony dorsal phalanx.

curely so that no movement occurs to cause the splint to produce pressure points elsewhere on the hand or digits. Care must be taken in the contouring of the splint around the proximal phalanx to distribute pressure and prevent motion that could cause shearing over the dorsum of the finger. In this case, padding may be necessary to help distribute pressure over the small and thinly padded phalanx (Fig. 19-19).

Amount of Force to Apply

How much force can be safely applied? The splint maker must apply sufficient force to create motion but not so much to cause ischemia. There are no absolute rules about the amount of force that can be applied to a restricted joint to produce motion. Much depends on the degree of the contracture, how long the restriction has existed, the age of the patient, and the location of the restriction. This leaves the therapist with several options when choosing which force and how much force to apply.

For example, the application of external force in dynamic splints is generally through the addition of rubber bands (or elastic) or springs. Neither option is ideal and both require careful selection and frequent adjustment. The amount of force supplied by rubber bands and springs is dependent on both their thickness and their length. The thickness of the band or spring determines its potential force, while the length of the band or spring (or the number of coils in the spring) determines the range of motion through which the force can be applied. When using either bands or springs, it is desirable to use the optimal force (that is, the greatest tolerable force over the longest wearing time) that does not produce ischemia. To do so, use the midrange of the bands or springs rather than their end ranges, which are either too slack or too strong. A gauge is available to measure the applied force of elastic, which should generally be between 100 and 300 grams. As will be discussed in greater detail in the final section of the chapter, force that can be

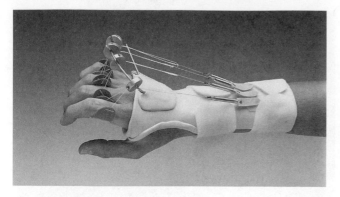

FIG. 19-20   Forearm based four-digit outrigger with dynamic extension assist supplied by springs.

tolerated for longer periods is more likely to result in tissue lengthening.

SPLINT CLASSIFICATIONS

A *dynamic splint* includes a resilient component (elastic, rubber band, or spring), which the patient moves. Dynamic splints are designed to increase passive motion, to augment active motion by assisting a joint through its range, or to substitute for lost motion. Dynamic splints generally include a static base on which to attach the movable, resilient components (Fig. 19-20).

A *static splint* has no resilient components and immobilizes a joint or part. Static splints are fabricated to rest or protect, to reduce pain, or to prevent muscle shortening or contracture. An example of a static splint is a resting pan splint that maintains the hand in a functional or resting position (Fig. 19-21).

A *serial static splint* achieves a slow, progressive increase in range of motion by repeated remolding; each remolding positions the joint at its end range of motion. The serial static splint has no movable, resilient components such as rubber bands or springs; it uses static forces along with remolding and repositioning to achieve its goal. A cylindrical cast designed to reduce a PIP joint flexion contracture through frequent removal and re-

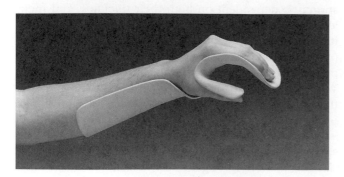

FIG. 19-21   Single-surface static resting splint positions hand in 20° to 30° wrist extension, 45° to 60° MCP flexion, and 15° to 30° PIP and DIP flexion.

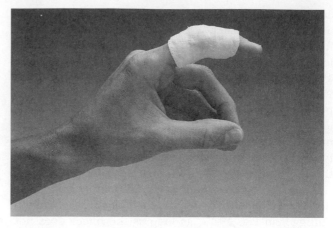

FIG. 19-22   Cylindrical plaster cast to be remade in series of casts to reduce flexion contracture at PIP joint.

casting is a classic example of a serial static splint (Fig. 19-22).

Static progressive splints include a static mechanism that adjusts the amount or angle of traction acting upon a part. Frequently this mechanism is a turnbuckle, cloth strap, nylon line, or a buckle. The static progressive splint is distinguished from the dynamic splint by its lack of a movable, resilient force. It is distinguished from a serial static splint in that its adjustment mechanism is built in, so it does not need to be remolded (Fig. 19-23).

TO SPLINT OR NOT TO SPLINT— AND WHEN TO SPLINT?

Before deciding which splint to make for a particular problem, the therapist must determine if the patient is a good candidate for wearing a splint. There are several issues to examine in this regard.

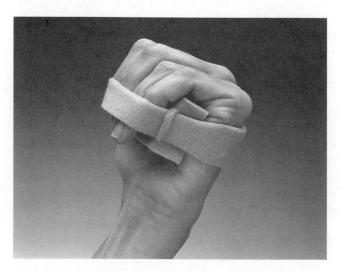

FIG. 19-23   Static progressive web strap adjusts with Velcro closure. Patient may be taught to adjust strap as tolerance permits.

COMPLIANCE ISSUES

First, the therapist must consider whether the patient is likely to comply with the splinting program. The splint may have a negative impact on the patient's ability to be independent in self-care or to function at work. The patient may refuse to wear the splint because of cultural norms; for example, some cultures are very sensitive about calling attention to the hands with anything unattractive. In addition, some patients may be extremely sensitive about their appearance and refuse to wear the splint, even though their cultural values are not offended.

Compliance with a splinting program may be poor because the patient's general motivation to get better is low. On the other hand, some patients may be so highly motivated that they will overdo the splinting program and cause themselves damage. Finally, it is important to consider the patient's cognitive and perceptual ability to follow a splinting program, especially if there is no responsible caretaker.

ABILITY TO DON AND DOFF THE SPLINT ON SCHEDULE

Even if there are no issues of compliance, there may be problems with the patient's donning and doffing (putting on and removing) the splint. For example, the patient may have no one at home to assist in donning and doffing a difficult splint. Or, the hospitalized patient may not have a nursing staff that can follow the wearing schedule or that can apply the splint correctly.

SKIN TOLERANCE AND HYPERSENSITIVITY

The therapist must assess the skin condition of the patient before deciding to splint. If the patient suffers from brain or spinal cord damage, he/she may be diaphoretic and produce excessive perspiration, which can lead to rapid skin maceration. Some patients may be intolerant of any pressure because of extremely thin and fragile skin. Finally, the patient may be hypersensitive because of sensory dysfunction and not tolerate any splinting.

WEARING SCHEDULE

If none of these issues prevents the patient from being a candidate for splinting, the therapist must decide on the best wearing schedule for the splint. Generally, night time is the optimal time for the patient to wear a static splint designed to change range of motion. It is also the time when patients need resting splints to prevent them from sleeping in positions that damage the hand. During the daytime, the patient may wear a dynamic splint or a splint designed to assist function. It is often best to minimize splinting during the day, however, so that the patient can use his hand as normally as possible. Finally, some splints are made purely for exercise and are only worn at specific times for that purpose.

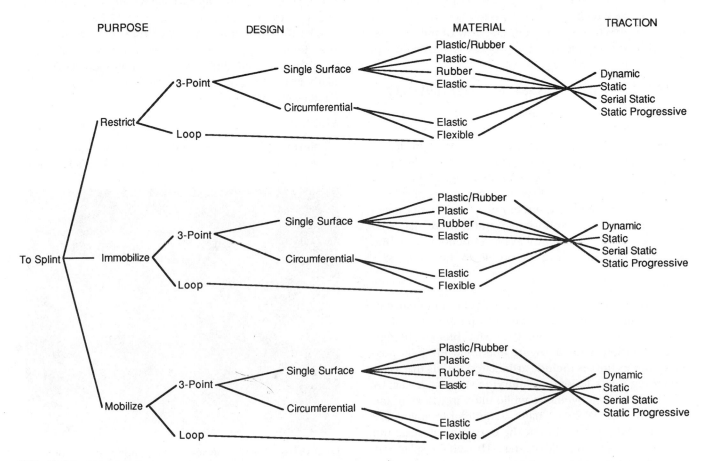

FIG. 19-24 Decision tree.

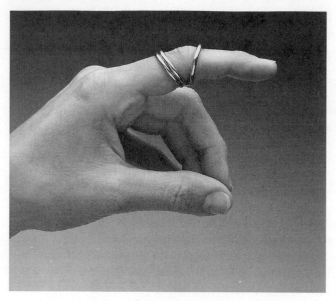

A

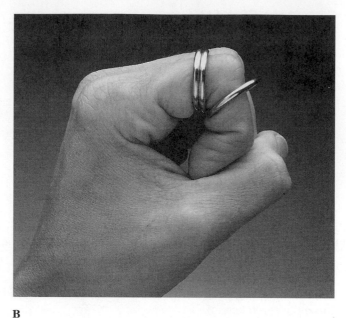

B

FIG. 19-25 Murphy ring splints. **A,** To limit PIP joint hyperextension. **B,** To allow full IP joint flexion.

FRAMEWORK FOR DECISION MAKING

The remainder of the chapter structures the discussion of splints by answering a series of questions. These questions follow the decision-making process you might follow to decide which splint to make and how to make it. A decision tree is used to illustrate the flow of this process. The full decision tree for this process is shown in Fig. 19-24 (see Fig. 19-24 on p. 333).

WHAT IS THE PURPOSE OF THE SPLINT?

Though nomenclatures may vary, the categories presented in the splint classification system (SCS) serve to describe splints in functional rather than in design terms.[1] That is, the SCS describes three overriding purposes of splints: restrictive, immobilizing, and mobilizing. The publication also lists many functions of splints, each of which are placed under one of the three categories, as seen below. Splints may fulfill more than one function or purpose, however, depending on the method of fabrication and the problems they address.

Restrictive Splints

Restrictive splints limit a specific aspect of joint range of motion, but do not completely stop joint motion. One example is the splint in Fig. 19-25 that blocks PIP joint hyperextension while allowing unlimited PIP joint flexion. Other examples include articulated splints that assist in aligning joints following injury or surgical repair, by blocking lateral movement while allowing flexion and extension (Fig. 19-26). Finally, semiflexible splints are available that limit motion at the extremes of range but allow motion in the middle of range. Though the splint may be restrictive, the goal or function of the splint may vary.

Immobilizing Splints

Immobilizing splints may be fit for several reasons including protection to prevent further injury, rest to reduce inflammation or pain, and positioning to facilitate proper healing following surgical repairs. The classic example is the resting pan splint (Fig. 19-21) that serves two of the three functions. A resting splint fit for a patient following a cerebral vascular accident (CVA) positions the wrist and digits to prevent contractures (particularly at the MCP joints) and can protect the desensate hand against damage.

Mobilizing Splints

Mobilizing splints are designed to increase limited range of motion or to restore or augment a patient's function.

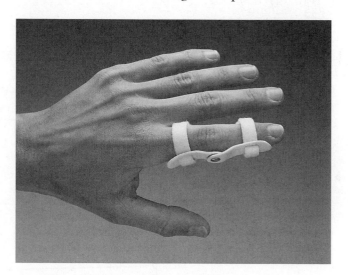

FIG. 19-26 Splint provides lateral support at PIP joint but hinge allows free flexion and extension.

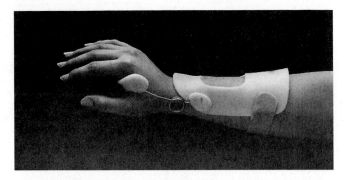

FIG. 19-27 Spring coil splint substitutes for absent wrist extension in radial nerve injury.

The functions of a mobilizing splint may be to assist a weak muscle or substitute for motion lost because of nerve injury or muscle dysfunction (Fig. 19-27). The splint may attempt to balance the pull of spastic muscles unopposed by normal muscle power. In this case, the splint may be preventing deformity as well as assisting function. A splint may resist a weak muscle to improve its strength, or to facilitate tendon gliding after tendon surgery. Frequently, a mobilizing splint is used to increase the range of motion of a contracted joint.

WHICH OF THE DESIGN OPTIONS IS INDICATED?

After you have decided on the purpose of the splint, the next decision relates to its design. Each of the types of splints described earlier (static dynamic, serial static, and static progressive) may be fabricated from one of two design options: (1) three-point or loop or (2) single-surface or circumferential.

Three-Point or Loop Design

All splints are designed to provide some degree of force. That force may be distributed as a continuous loop with equal and opposing forces wrapping around two or more joints (Fig. 19-28). This splint design is called a coaptation splint. On the other hand, the force may be applied through three points of pressure (Fig. 19-29). Although the loop design is generally used only on finger IP joints and for some postoperative splints, versions of the three-point design are used in all other splints.

Loop splints are most frequently used to reduce DIP and PIP joint extension contractures. An extension contracture exists when a joint will not move passively from an extended position into more flexion. This loop design is effective because, unlike a three point splint, it does not block the palmar surface of the joint as it moves into increasing flexion.

Three-point finger splints that incorporate springs, spring wire, or elastics are often used to correct DIP and PIP joint flexion contractures. A flexion contracture exists when a joint will not move passively out of a closed position into extension. These designs include

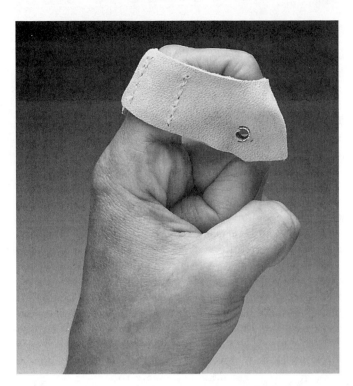

FIG. 19-28 Loop strap designed to increase PIP and DIP joint flexion provides equal force on all surfaces of digit.

two points of pressure, one proximal to the joint and one distal, and the third or central opposing force acting directly over, or close to the joint as in Fig. 19-29. In a three-point finger splint, the force of the central point is equal to the sum of the two forces of the correcting points. This fact is clinically important because tissue tolerance under this central point may be insufficient and may react with pain and inflammation. This problem is seen frequently at the PIP joint. It is important to distribute the pressure over that joint with contoured surfaces that are as broad as possible, and to adjust the spring or elastic force and the wearing time to tolerance.

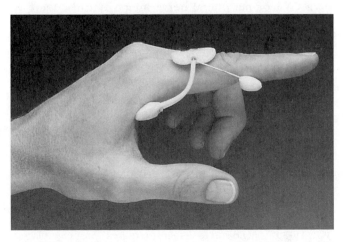

FIG. 19-29 Three-point pressure splint with spring wire reduces PIP joint flexion contractures of 35° or less.

The finger-based three-point splint just described is a unique design, as it does not adhere to the 90° rule. That is, when applied to a joint with a flexion contracture, the angle of approach of the line of traction is never 90°. The more severe the contracture, the more translational force is present; therefore, it is less effective and more uncomfortable than an outrigger or a splint that fully conforms, both of which follow the 90° rule. It is recommended that this design be fitted only in the presence of IP joint flexion contractures of 35° or less. For finger contractures in excess of 35°, a hand or forearm-based outrigger splint is recommended because it can be positioned to apply force at a 90° angle of attack. Alternatively, a conforming, serial static splint can be used, as described in the section on traction.

Single-Surface or Circumferential Design

If a three-point design is chosen, the next decision is whether to use a circumferential or single-surface design for the splint. Single-surface splints are fabricated to cover only one surface, either the palmar or dorsal surface of a limb or the ulnar or radial half of the hand or forearm. Straps are added to create the three points of pressure necessary to secure the splint (Fig. 19-30). Circumferential splints wrap around a part, covering all surfaces with equal amounts of pressure (Fig. 19-31). Straps are used solely to close the splint or to create an overlap. This design option is based on the principle that increasing curves in a material increases its rigidity, while decreasing curves reduces its rigidity. Thus, a thinner ($\frac{1}{16}$ or $\frac{1}{12}$ inch) or highly perforated material can be used for circumferential splints because all the curves add sufficient rigidity, while a thicker ($\frac{1}{8}$ inch) and less perforated material must be used for single-surface splints, which have few curves.

Indications for design choices

Indications for single surface splinting. Single surface splinting is effective for supporting joints surrounded by weak or flaccid muscles, such as following a CVA or peripheral nerve injury. Because there is little or no active motion available, there is no need for the extra control given by circumferential splinting. A single-surface splint is also effective as the base for at-

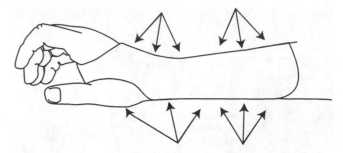

FIG. 19-31 Circumferential splints create multiple 3-point pressure systems to secure splints and ensure immobilization.

taching outriggers in dynamic splinting and for postoperative splints where the fabrication of a circumferential splint may damage repaired structures. The availability of lighter weight plastic and plastic and rubber-like thermoplastics ($\frac{3}{32}$ and $\frac{1}{16}$ inch thicknesses) also offers greater flexibility in the fabrication of hand and forearm-based positioning splints such as cock-up and thumb spica splints.

Indications for circumferential splinting. Circumferential splinting is effective for immobilizing a joint around which there is pain, such as carpal tunnel or tenosynovitis (Fig. 19-32). Because the circumferential design gives comfortable, complete control, it is particularly helpful when the patient has active motion and will be wearing the splint during activity, when shear forces can be a problem. This comfortable, complete control also makes a circumferential design useful for splints that remodel scar and reduce contractures.

Circumferential designs may be useful to support or immobilize unstable joints, because of the even pressure distribution provided by the design. The circumferential design also lends itself to the addition of outriggers. Finally, because of the memory of the elastic materials from which circumferential splints are usually made, se-

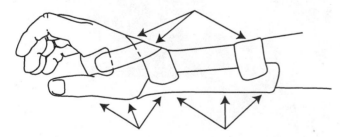

FIG. 19-30 Single-surface splint requires properly placed straps to create 3-point pressure systems to secure splint and ensure proper force for immobilization.

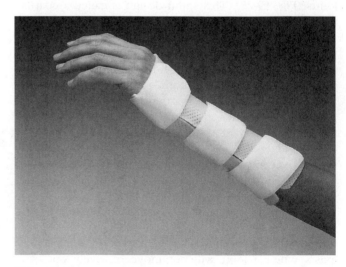

FIG. 19-32 Circumferential gauntlet design.

rial static splinting can be accomplished without having to use new material at each remolding.

Fabrication techniques

The fabrication process for single surface and circumferential splints differs significantly. They do have a starting point in common, and that is the pattern from which the splint will be made. Starting with a paper pattern is recommended, particularly for the beginning splint maker. One very basic rule of splinting is to *get the pattern right before you start working with plastic.*

Fabrication techniques for single-surface splinting.

1. Except for the fingers, ⅛ inch thick material is recommended to obtain sufficient rigidity to hold the joint firmly in position. The broad contours of single-surface splints require thicker materials to provide sufficient support.
2. Trim lines should fall midline along the arm or leg. If the trim lines are left too high, making the trough too deep for the part, the straps will bridge the part and sit up on the edge of the splint, where they are ineffective. The most effective way to secure a splint in place on the forearm is to apply pressure through the splint onto the soft tissue of the forearm muscle bellies. If the forearm trim lines angle below the muscle bellies, the splint will no longer be secured on the muscle bellies (Fig. 19-33).
3. Strapping is critical to secure the splinted part in the splint and to diminish both shear forces and the possibility of pressure areas developing. The splint may require several straps, and wide or crossed straps are suggested to obtain the necessary control. Because the forearm is cone-shaped, straps placed straight across the forearm will contact the skin effectively only on their proximal surface (Fig. 19-34). To have the forearm straps apply effective and well-distributed pressure, place them at an angle.

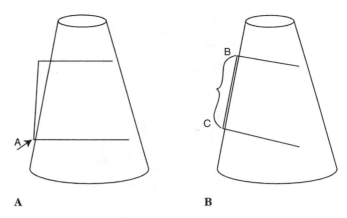

FIG. 19-34 Forearm is cone shaped, gradually widening from wrist to elbow. **A,** Strap placed straight across broader proximal forearm contacts skin only at point **A** and does not secure splint. **B,** Strap placed at angle applies even pressure along line **B C** to secure splint.

4. Conform the splint firmly where there is soft tissue and relieve the pressure, where necessary, over bony prominences (Fig. 19-35).
5. Roll or flare the edges of material wherever a part will move over that edge. Rolled edges are smoother and they distribute pressure over a broader area than a cut edge.
6. A forearm-based splint should extend approximately two thirds of the length of the forearm, as measured from the wrist proximally. A good rule to remember is to bend the patient's elbow fully and mark where the forearm and the biceps muscle meet. The splint should be trimmed ¼ inch below this point to avoid limiting elbow flexion and to prevent the splint from being pushed distally when the elbow is flexed (Fig. 19-36).
7. Most important, to avoid ischemia and shear forces, check the fit of the splint regularly, explain proper procedures to your patients or their care givers, and be prepared to make adjustments.

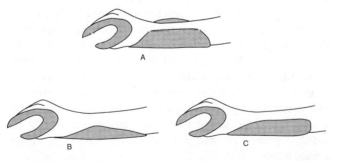

FIG. 19-33 Forearm trim lines. **A,** Trim lines are too high, extending above forearm. Straps will bridge arm and be ineffective. **B,** Trim lines are too low and do not ensure sufficient purchase on forearm. Straps cannot substitute for too low trim lines without applying excessive pressure. **C,** Midline trim lines ensure straps properly secure splint on arm and hand.

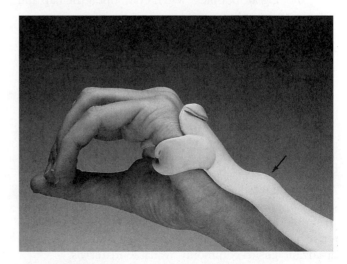

FIG. 19-35 Relief "bubbled" over the ulnar styloid.

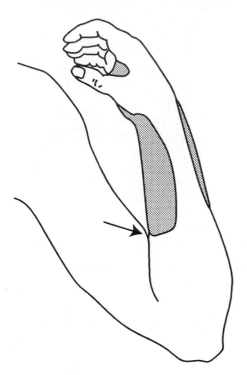

FIG. 19-36 Length of forearm based splint is checked by flexing elbow and noting where biceps meets forearm. Splint is trimmed ¼ to ½ inch distal to point of contact.

Fabrication techniques for circumferential splints.

1. Use a thin or highly perforated elastic material or flexible rubber material that has some memory. For hand and forearm-based splints, thin elastic materials (⅟₁₆, ⅟₁₂ or ³⁄₃₂ inch) provide sufficient strength because of the rigidity provided by the curves of the splint. For splints covering larger areas, a highly perforated ⅛ inch material is recommended.

2. Wrap the material all the way around the part being splinted. The most common technique is to pinch the remaining material together to form a flap. Gently tug on the flap to conform the material, removing air bubbles. When cool, open the flap and trim the splint.

3. Finger splints may have a slight gap with straps attached, or they may be sealed closed and slipped on and off. For all other splints, the opening may be a gap of about 1 inch where small straps are used to secure the opening. Splint donning and doffing is easily accomplished because of the extensive perforation or thinness of the materials being used.

WHICH MATERIAL IS MOST APPROPRIATE FOR THIS SPLINT DESIGN?

After you have decided on the splint's purpose and design, you must choose the appropriate material for constructing the splint. This section will discuss the characteristics, application for splinting, and advantages and disadvantages of commonly available materials.

It is not possible within the scope of this chapter to discuss the characteristics of each material available today. There are, however, some terms in general use that describe handling and molding characteristics. The successful fabrication and application of a splint depend in large part on choosing the most appropriate material, based on a knowledge of the characteristics of each material. Each characteristic can be either an advantage or disadvantage, depending on the type of splint being made. The following is a brief description of material categories and the characteristics of materials within each category. Most of the common suppliers of thermoplastics offer a chart that positions their materials according to these terms.

Categories of Splint Materials

There are four primary categories of thermoplastic materials based on the chemicals or polymers in their formula: plastic, plastic and rubber-like, rubber-like, and elastic. Though it may not be true of every material available, each category of materials has some common characteristics. A fifth category to be considered is flexible splinting materials used in the fabrication of semiflexible splints.

Plastic. Plastic materials tend to have high degrees of conformability and rigidity while having low resistance to stretch. The main advantage of plastics is the light amount of handling required to get a maximum degree of fit. Their disadvantage is that they do not tolerate heavy handling or frequent remolding, because they will stretch and thin.

Rubber-like. The rubber-like materials tend to have a high resistance to stretch but a low degree of conformability. Their main advantage is that they tolerate aggressive handling and frequent remolding. Their disadvantage is that they actually require more aggressive handling during the molding process because of their low degree of drape and their tendency to return to a flat shape when pressure is removed.

Plastic and rubber-like. The plastic and rubber-like materials tend to have characteristics from both ends of the thermoplastic continuum, without any important disadvantages. By every measure, they have a midrange amount of rigidity: less stretch than the plastics but more than the rubber-like materials. They require somewhat more handling than the plastics, but less than the rubber-like materials, while giving greater levels of conformability. The plastic and rubber-like materials tend to be highly versatile for use in the broadest variety of splint applications.

Elastic. The fourth category of materials is the elastics. The handling characteristics of the elastic materials are substantially different from the other materials because they conform by being stretched rather than by having the draping characteristic of materials with plastic in them. Most elastics have a low resistance to stretch and conform easily when stretched. The material properties of the elastics allow for them to be manufactured in thin, highly perforated sheets that are ideal for lightweight circumferential splints.

Flexible. Flexible materials such as cotton duck, neoprene, knit elastics, and plastic-impregnated materials may be used alone or in combination with metal or plastic stays to fabricate semiflexible splints. These materials allow for fabrication of splints that permit partial motion around a joint, yet still limit or protect the part. Semiflexible splints are sometimes used to assist patients with chronic pain in returning to functional activity. Semiflexible splints are also used for geriatric patients and patients with arthritis who often cannot tolerate rigid splints.

Characteristics of Splint Materials

Several materials are available in each of the categories of thermoplastic materials just described. Each of the materials has some handling characteristics that apply when the materials are warm and pliable and some that apply when they are cold or molded. The following is a list of the most common characteristics and how they contribute to the choice of a material for a specific application.

Resistance to stretch. Resistance to stretch describes the extent to which a material resists pulling or stretching. The greater the resistance, the greater the degree of control the splint maker will have over the material. Materials that resist stretch tend to hold their shape and thickness while warm and can be handled more aggressively without thinning. The more resistive materials are recommended for large splints and for splints made for persons who are unable to cooperate in the fabrication process. In contrast, the less resistance to stretch a material has, the more the material is likely to thin during the fabrication process and the more delicately one must handle it. The advantage of stretch is seen in the greater degree of conformability obtained with less effort on the splint maker's part.

Conformability or drape. Resistance to stretch and conformability or drape describe nearly the same characteristic; that is, if a material stretches easily, it will have better drape and conformability. This characteristic allows a material (generally the more plastic materials) to be laid on the body part, and with a minimum of handling, the material conforms. This conformability is caused by the pull of gravity on the warm material. Materials with a high degree of drape are not recommended for large splints or with uncooperative patients. They are ideal, however, for splinting postoperative cases where minimal pressure is desired and for dynamic splint bases where conformability secures the splint against migra-

tion (movement distally) when components are attached.

Memory. Memory is the ability of material to return to its original shape after it has been stretched and molded. The major advantage of a material's having excellent memory is that a splint can easily be repaired or remolded without the splint becoming thin and losing strength as well as aesthetic value. The disadvantage of a material with excellent memory is its tendency to return to its flat sheet state when an overstretched area is spot-heated for adjustment.

Rigidity versus flexibility. Rigidity and flexibility in cold splint material are terms describing the amount of resistance a material gives when force is applied to it. A highly rigid material is very resistive to applied force and may, with enough force, break. A highly flexible material bends easily when even small force is applied to it, and it is not apt to break under high stress. Materials are available that fall all along this continuum.

Generally, the thicker a thermoplastic and the more plastic its formula contains, the more rigid the material will be. The thermoplastics commonly used today come in thicknesses of $\frac{1}{16}$ inch (1.6 mm), $\frac{1}{12}$ inch (2.1 mm), $\frac{3}{32}$ inch (2.4 mm), $\frac{1}{8}$ inch (3.2 mm), and $\frac{3}{16}$ inch (4.8 mm). The thinner materials have less rigidity but generally more conformability when molded around small parts.

The thinner materials and the thermoplastics that contain rubber-like polymers in their formula tend to have greater flexibility in their molded state. Flexibility in a material allows for easier donning and doffing of circumferential splints and may be desirable for patients unable to tolerate the more unforgiving rigid materials.

Self-adherence. Self-adherence is the ability of the material to attach to itself when pressed together. Many materials are coated to resist accidental bonding and require solvents or surface scraping to remove the coating for a firmer bond. Uncoated materials, which require no solvents or scraping, have very strong bonding properties when two warm pieces are pressed together.

Self-sealing edges. Self-sealing edges are edges which round and seal themselves when heated material is cut. This characteristic produces smooth edges that require no additional finishing, which would add time to the fabrication process. Most plastic materials with little or no memory produce the smoothest, best sealed edges. Materials with memory, or those that have a high resistance to stretch, resist sealing and require additional finishing.

Choosing the Best Category of Material for the Splint

Although it is possible for an experienced splint fabricator to make many types of splints from the same material, it is better to choose the most appropriate category of material for the type of splint being made. The following listing is to be used as a guideline from which to start choosing materials for different applications. The availability of materials and the experience level of the therapist will further determine the most appropriate material.

Forearm and hand-based splints

Splints need close conformability around a part when they serve as a base for a dynamic splint, stabilize a part of the body, reduce contractures, remodel scar tissue, or immobilize to facilitate healing of an acute condition. Such splints should be made from a plastic, plastic and rubber-like, or soft elastic material. Where conformability is not crucial and the splint is being used for resting a flaccid or weak part of the body, it can be made from a rubber-like material. Such splints include positioning splints for burns and other acute trauma or postoperative splints, as well as functional position splints. If the splint is being used to position a spastic body part, it should also be made from a rubber-like material, which has the control necessary to withstand the forces of the spasticity during molding.

Large upper and lower extremity splints

Long splints fabricated for the elbow, shoulder, knee, or ankle should generally be made of rubber-like material, which has the control necessary for dealing with large pieces of material. Generally, such splints do not need to be highly conforming as they are molded over broad expanses of soft tissue. Care must be taken to relieve for bony prominences or provide padding to distribute pressure.

Circumferential splints

A splint designed to wrap all the way around the part should be fabricated from materials that have a high degree of memory and that tolerate stretching without the formation of thin spots. Elastics and certain rubberlike materials with memory work best. The materials should be highly perforated, thin, or able to be stretched in order to become evenly thin. After being stretched, these materials will cinch in around the body part but still allow sufficient flexibility for easy donning and doffing. These materials work very well for fracture bracing and for circumferential splints that are used for contracture reduction and for stabilizing or immobilizing joints. Another choice for making less restrictive circumferential splints is the use of semiflexible materials, which facilitate easy donning and doffing and allow for limited motion within the available arc of motion.

Serial splints

Serial splints that require frequent remolding to accommodate increases in joint range of motion should be made from a material that has considerable memory. Generally, elastics work best for these splints, because they have the most memory of any splint material category. Though they lack the memory of the elastics, several of the available rubber-like materials resist stretch to such a high degree that they do not thin with repeated remolding and are also recommended for serial splints.

Semiflexible splints

Materials used in the fabrication of semiflexible splints include neoprene, cotton duck, woven elastics, and thermoplastic-impregnated materials. Many of the commercially prefabricated splints are made from these materials because they present the broadest range of size adjustability and are less likely to require custom fabrication. It is highly recommended that even a prefabricated splint be custom fit by a therapist to ensure proper fit and adherence to an appropriate wearing schedule. A good rule to remember when fitting prefabricated, semiflexible supports is, "One-size-fits-all fits no one well."

WHAT TYPE OF TRACTION IS NEEDED FOR THE SPLINT?

Along the decision tree, once you have determined the purpose, design and material, you must then decide the type of force or traction to apply and how to apply it in order to meet your splinting goal. All splints provide traction through some kind of mechanism. The traction mechanism may be an outrigger, a spring, an elastic loop, a strap, a circumferential plastic splint, or a single-surface splint that uses a three-point design. The traction mechanism may be static or dynamic. If the mechanism moves, the splint is called a dynamic splint, and if the mechanism does not move, the splint is called a static splint. Thus, an outrigger and a spring are dynamic because they move, whereas an elastic strap (loop design) is static because it does not move, even when it is made of a resilient material that is frequently found in dynamic splints. The following section describes the various options for applying traction and discusses the appropriate uses of each option.

Dynamic traction

The purpose of dynamic splints is to mobilize a joint through the use of a moving elastic force attached to an outrigger, or through the use of a spring coil. Each mechanism of force has advantages and disadvantages that make it suited for some uses and ill-suited to others. The construction techniques differ substantially when using spring coils versus outriggers with elastic components. Thus, the indications for each style of splint vary.

Spring coils are best suited to assist weak muscles or substitute for paralyzed muscles (Fig. 19-27). Patients with weak or paralyzed muscles will likely require the splint for a long time and will wear it while working or performing their ADL. The low profile, lightweight construction of a coil splint is recommended because it is less likely to interfere with hand function. Spring coils retain their force and alignment over time and so are ideal for long-term conditions, because they rarely require adjustment.

Splints with outriggers are the optimal choice for

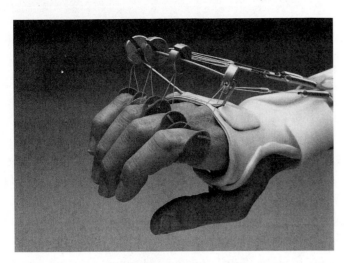

FIG. 19-37 Easily adjustable Phoenix outrigger with slotted pulleys allows for frequent changes in alignment.

splinting postoperative cases (Fig. 19-37). These splints allow for frequent adjustments to maintain correct positioning and to accommodate changes in bandage thickness and edema as the healing and rehabilitation progresses. The postoperative patient will likely only use the splint for a short time, generally four to six weeks. Such a patient will not be returning to normal functional activities with the affected hand during that time. Thus, the fact that an outrigger splint is bulky and more likely to limit function is relatively unimportant.

Finally, splints with outriggers are sometimes used for contracture reduction. For this purpose, they are generally most effective when used during the early stages of healing, when the contracture feels soft and is easy to reduce.[4] Frequently patients at this stage still have pain and inflammation. They cannot tolerate a rigid, static splint, but they will tolerate a light force provided by an outrigger.

Static traction

The overall purpose of static splints is to apply traction to immobilize or restrict motion, depending on the splint. When static splints immobilize, they are protecting, resting, or positioning. When they restrict, they are blocking motion, aligning joints, or limiting motion. When static splints are used to mobilize, they are used in either a serial static or static progressive fashion to reduce contractures and remodel scar.

Serial static traction

A serial static splint is fabricated by repeated adjustments that position a joint at its end range of motion each time, to achieve slow, progressive increases in range of motion. For example, a cylindrical cast (Fig. 19-22) made for gaining PIP extension, must be remade whenever the range of motion gains have ended with the current splint. Serial static splints are generally used to reduce flexion contractures.

Static progressive traction

A static progressive splint, often used to reduce extension contractures, requires a mechanism built into it for adjusting the amount of traction that is appropriate. Choosing the appropriate mechanism, be it a turnbuckle, Velcro strap, buckle, or rubber band, is dependent on availability, therapist experience, and the patient's ability to manage the mechanism. A good rule to follow is to choose the simplest component that will achieve the desired goal.

Serial static splints and static progressive splints each have certain advantages and disadvantages. Serial static splints are useful for difficult patients who have high muscle tone or who are cognitively impaired and would have problems with the adjustment mechanisms. Also, the therapist has the control necessary for patients who are noncompliant or who would be overly zealous and apply too much force.

The disadvantages are that (1) it requires more therapist time because it must be remolded many times and (2) if the patient does not remove it for several days, some range of motion may be lost in the direction opposite to that in which the splint is applying force.

The advantages of a static progressive splint are that (1) the therapist only has to make one splint and (2) reliable patients with normal muscle tone may make more rapid progress because they can tailor the adjustment to their own pace and tolerance. The disadvantage to a static progressive splint is that it cannot be used on the patient who has abnormal tone or who is unreliable.

USE OF SPLINTS TO REMODEL SCAR AND REDUCE CONTRACTURES

The presence of scar tissue is one of the major contributors to deformity. Anytime there is an insult to tissue, as occurs after an open injury or after surgery, scar tissue is produced by the body to heal the wound. The scar may be subcutaneous, superficial, or both. When it is subcutaneous, it often results in loss of motion because it acts like glue, keeping tissue planes from gliding. Scar also contracts, and when that contracture occurs over a joint, loss of joint motion results. To increase function, scar tissue must be remodeled; that is, it must be softened and lengthened. If the contracture is caused by shortened soft tissue that is not scar, that soft tissue must also be lengthened. The process is the same for scar or soft tissue.

There are two approaches to splinting for remodeling scar and reducing contractures. The first approach is to apply a good deal of force for a short period of time. The second approach is to apply a light force for a long period of time. Extensive literature supports the use of the second approach as the only safe, effective method.[3,4,5]

Two key concepts aid in understanding the different tissue responses to these two approaches. First, all materials, including human tissue, respond to applied stress. If considerable stress is applied over a long time and then relaxed, however, the tissue will no longer return to its original shape, but will adapt to the new shape. This phenomenon is called a plastic response in non-living tissue. In living tissue it is called creep.[2]

The second key concept is that of the elastic limit of tissue. Think of pulling on a rubber band. As the band is pulled, tension increases until the elastic limit is reached. If it is pulled beyond its elastic limit, the rubber band will break. In clinical terms, the end of the elastic limit is the point of tissue elongation that occurs just before the patient begins to feel pain, as opposed to discomfort. Stretching tissue beyond its elastic limit does not lead to permanent lengthening but instead to unwanted tearing and probable further tissue contracture.[2]

As Brand says, "if . . . living skin is held in only a slightly lengthened position, within its elastic limit, for a period of hours and days, the living cells will sense the strain and the collagen fibers will be actively and progressively absorbed and laid down again with modified bonding patterns with no creep and no inflammation."[2] Brand labels this response as tissue growth.[2]

It is not known exactly how long the gentle force must be applied for growth to occur. Brand states that the stimulus needs to be uninterrupted for hours at a time, nearly 24 hours a day.[3] Therapists may have to splint, or cast difficult contractures for up to five days in one position, to achieve results. Most contractures require far less time per day in a splint. Definitive studies have not yet given solid guidelines.

The effectiveness of splinting for remodeling scar and reducing contractures can be increased greatly by applying a deep heat modality, such as paraffin, before applying the splint. When tissue is unheated it is less elastic, meaning it has a great deal of tension and is difficult to elongate. With the application of heat, tissue becomes temporarily more elastic, meaning that the tension in the tissue is reduced and the tissue is much easier to elongate.

There are many approaches to splinting for remodeling scar and reducing contractures. They have all been discussed in previous sections. Three-point splints can be used for flexion contractures, loop splints for IP joint extension contractures, and outriggers for MCP extension contractures. Dynamic outriggers can be used for reducing early, soft contractures, particularly when the patient cannot tolerate a static splint. Finally static progressive splints or static splints can be used in a serial fashion.

USE OF SPLINTS FOR PAIN REDUCTION AND POSITIONING

Pain Reduction

Of the many uses of splints, perhaps the most common is to limit or reduce pain by providing rest and support. The most common splint prescriptions are written for splints to reduce the pain caused by the inflammatory processes of tendinitis and tenosynovitis or following sprain or strain injuries. The therapist has several decisions to make when determining how best to provide

support or protection to reduce pain and the likelihood of further injury.

Several questions help determine which splint will best serve the patient's need. First, the acute versus chronic nature of the pain must be considered. If the injury is due to an acute sprain, the choice may be for a more thoroughly immobilizing splint until pain and edema have subsided. If the pain is chronic in nature and due to the performance of a particular activity, a semiflexible splint may serve best. A semiflexible splint may sufficiently reduce pain by limiting range of motion, yet still allow function without increasing stress on unaffected joints or tissue.

A second question concerns the need for full-time splinting versus intermittent wear. In the presence of an acute injury with orthopedic involvement or tissue damage, the splint may not only need to immobilize, it may also serve to protect the part from further damage. Here, patient tolerance and compliance will in part determine material and design choice. The therapist may also need to consider the integrity of tissue and the need to accommodate bandages and bandage changes. If the splint is indicated only for intermittent wear, the design choice may be more dependent on the patient's ability to readily don and doff the splint. The choice of materials may be dictated by the functional needs of the patient. For intermittent splints used for vocational activities, lightweight, well-aerated materials may be indicated. For intermittent splints used for positioning, such as a resting splint designed to maintain functional position between exercise sessions, stronger materials may be indicated and perforations may not be necessary.

A third question of great import in deciding upon a splint design is, "What structures need to be immobilized or supported and which should be left free?" When providing protective or pain-reducing splints, care must be taken to splint only the involved structures and not impede motion elsewhere. If the purpose of the splint is to rest the tendons at the wrist to reduce inflammation, the splint must not limit CMC or MCP joint motion if these structures are not symptomatic. If used during the performance of ADL, splints that fully immobilize a joint may transfer stress to joints proximal or distal to the immobilized joint. For this reason, semiflexible splints that limit only end ranges of motion may be indicated during activity, while an immobilizing splint may be indicated for total rest at night.

Positioning

One of the splints most frequently fabricated by occupational therapists is the resting pan, which is used to maintain the hand in a functional position (Fig. 19-21). The purpose of this positioning splint is to maintain the soft tissues of the hand in midrange to maintain optimal mobility and prevent shortening of the soft tissue structures around the joints. Occasionally, positioning splints will be prescribed to position joints at end range to prevent contractures in the presence of severe tissue damage. Resting splints fitted on persons with burns are the prime example of this splint, because the MCP joints are positioned in full available flexion. The important decision here is to determine the optimal position for the most functional outcome.

Positioning splints may be fabricated for temporary use following surgery and may require frequent adjustment to accommodate for changes in edema and bandages. The choice of materials for these splints should be a material with memory that allows for remolding while keeping its thickness and strength. Resting splints fabricated for patients following a CVA will likely require only minimal adjustment, so more conforming plastic materials with little or no memory can be used. Further choices

of a dorsal-versus a volar-based splint and single-surface versus circumferential splint will depend on surgical and wound sites, need for ease of donning and doffing, and therapist and physician preference and experience.

SUMMARY

Section one of this chapter has introduced the basic concepts of splint design and problem solving that must precede the fabrication of a splint. The occupational therapist must bring to the splinting process a knowledge of anatomy, skills in assessing function, and the ability to determine the optimal intervention for each patient, whether it includes a splint or not.

CASE STUDIES

A great deal of information has been presented, including a decision tree to assist with the process of determining the optimal splint for a given purpose. To put this decision tree into practice, two cases are presented below with questions to lead you along branches of the tree.

Case study 1:
Mr. Smith is a 50-year-old male factory worker who had a surgical repair to the left index finger flexor digitorum profundus (FDP) tendon 3 months ago. The surgeon did not refer the patient for therapy until now. The repair was in zone II. The evaluation shows a 50° flexion contracture at the PIP joint. There is no active DIP flexion and only 20° of active PIP flexion when the finger touches the palm, although full passive flexion is available. These measurements indicate that the postoperative scarring is preventing FDP tendon gliding while also contracting the PIP joint into flexion.

Mr. Smith has returned to full-time work and must use both hands. He cannot wear a splint at work. Mr. Smith expresses a strong desire to regain the normal appearance of his hand and full function. He seems to have a very "macho" personality and feels that without pain, he will have no gain. His skin appears normal, as does his cognition.

As the therapist, you determine that a splint is needed as part of your program to remodel scar tissue, increase tendon gliding, and reduce contracture.
1. Is Mr. Smith a good candidate for splinting? Why?
2. Are there any foreseeable problems with applying a splint? If so, what are the problems and how would you handle them?
3. When must Mr. Smith wear the splint? What implications does that have for your splint?

Using the decision tree as a framework, continue to answer the following questions:
4. Will the purpose of the splint be to restrict, immobilize, or mobilize?
5. Which of the following design options will you choose?
   a. Will you use a three-point or a loop design? Why?

b. If you chose a three-point splint, will you make it single-surface or circumferential? Why?
c. If you chose a three-point splint, will you make it rigid or flexible? Why?
6. Which category of splint material will you use? Why?
7. Will you use dynamic traction?
   a. If so, will you use an outrigger or spring? Why?
   b. If not, Why?
   c. Will you use static traction? Why or why not?
   d. Will you use serial static traction? Why or why not?
   e. Will you use static progressive traction? Why or why not?
8. How will you determine the amount of force to use?
9. How long will you have the patient wear the splint during each 24-hour period?
10. What adjunct modality might you use before applying the splint?

Case study 2:
A patient is referred to you with a diagnosis of wrist pain and a prescription for a splint. Your evaluation of the patient reveals full range of motion of the wrist and all digits. Some pain is noted at both end ranges of flexion and extension. With the patient's wrist held at end range of flexion for one minute (Phalen's test for median nerve compression), some tingling is noted in the thumb and index finger, which subsides when flexion is released. The patient works in a warehouse alternately stocking shelves with small cans and applying can labels on an assembly line. The patient does report general aching and pain over the dorsum of the hand when working on the assembly line. The patient's job is dependent on completing a certain number of labels and cans within a given time and this requirement cannot be modified.

With this information, answer the questions given in each step of the decision tree to arrive at an answer for which if any splint to fit or fabricate.

CASE STUDY

The prescription from the physician includes a request for a splint, which, as the therapist, you feel is appropriate and necessary. Answer the first three questions and then proceed through the decision tree.

1. Is this patient a good candidate for splinting? What questions would you ask to determine this?
2. Are there any reasons why this patient should not be issued a splint? If yes, what might these reasons be and how might you deal with them?
3. What wearing schedule would you recommend and why?

Using the decision tree as a framework continue to answer the following questions:

4. Will the purpose of your splint be to restrict, immobilize, or mobilize?
5. In looking at design options, what will you choose and why? Three-point or loop design? Single-surface or circumferential? If you choose a three-point design, will it be rigid or flexible?
6. What category of splint material will you use and why?
7. Will the splint contain any components of dynamic, static, or static progressive traction? If yes, what type of traction and why?
8. How much force do you want the splint to apply and how will you determine if the amount of force is appropriate?
9. How long will your patient wear the splint per day and for how many days, weeks, or months will it be worn?
10. What other therapy interventions might you suggest and why?

Section 2 The balanced forearm orthosis and suspension sling

Carole Adler, Lorraine Williams Pedretti

The balanced forearm orthosis (BFO) and the suspension sling are both devices that support the upper extremity in a plane parallel to the floor. They are devices that facilitate useful upper extremity motion in the presence of substantial muscle weakness.

BALANCED FOREARM ORTHOSIS

The balanced forearm orthosis may also be called a mobile arm support or a ball-bearing feeder.[5] It is usually mounted on the wheelchair, but it can be mounted on a table or working surface. It consists of a trough that supports the user's forearm and a pivot and linkage system under the trough. This system can be preset and adjusted so that the user can produce elbow and shoulder motion with slight motions of the trunk or shoulder girdle[1] (Fig. 19-38).

Various BFO adjustments are possible, and these are individualized to suit the needs of the particular patient. The BFO provides assistance for shoulder and elbow movement by using gravity to aid lost muscle power. It provides a large, usable range of arm motion that would otherwise not be available to the patient. It helps support, assist, and strengthen weakened musculature and enables patients to perform simple activities of daily living (ADL) and leisure activities that they could not otherwise perform.[5]

CANDIDATES FOR USE OF THE BFO

Generally those patients with disabilities that result in muscle weakness (such as poliomyelitis, cervical spinal cord injuries, Guillain-Barré syndrome, muscular dystrophy, and amyotrophic lateral sclerosis) are candidates for BFO. If there is moderate to severe muscle weakness in the upper extremities (muscle grades trace [1] to fair [3] at the elbow and grades trace [1] to fair [3] at the shoulder) and limited endurance for sustained movement, the BFO could increase function.[6]

The patient must have a source of muscle power to initiate movement of the BFO. This source may be at the

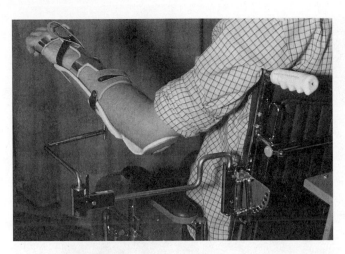

FIG. 19-38 Balanced forearm orthosis mounted on wheelchair with patient's arm positioned in forearm trough.

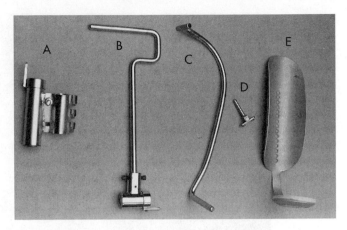

FIG. 19-39 Parts of BFO. **A,** Bracket assembly with stop. **B,** Proximal swivel arm and proximal ball bearing housing with stop. **C,** Distal swivel arm. **D,** Rocker arm assembly. **E,** Forearm trough.

trunk or shoulder. There should be adequate, pain-free range of motion (ROM) as follows: (1) shoulder flexion to 90°, abduction to 90°, external rotation to 30°, and internal rotation to 80°; (2) elbow flexion from 0° to 140°; (3) full forearm pronation from midposition and supination to midposition; and (4) hip flexion from 0° to 95°, required for the upright sitting position.[6]

The patient must have sufficient coordination to cope with and control movement of the freely swinging arms of the BFO. Involuntary movement, such as spasticity, substantially interferes with voluntary control of the upper extremity. In fact, because of its free movement, the BFO can actually increase involuntary movement.[6] There must be adequate trunk and neck stability provided by the patient's own muscle power or by outside support. A consistently stable sitting posture and good body alignment are key factors in the successful use of the BFO. The BFO works best when the user is sitting in an upright position with the trunk in midline. Successful use decreases as the user reclines.[6] Sitting tolerance and balance and gadget tolerance[5] must be adequate to engage in the training program and later make use of the BFO worthwhile.[2]

There must be sufficient motivation to use the BFO and adequate frustration tolerance to persevere at the training program until use is mastered.[2] It is important that the patient know the purpose in using the BFO. The patient and therapist should be aware that the active motion elicited will strengthen muscles and that the device may not necessarily be for permanent use.[6] Motivation to take care of personal needs, eat independently, enjoy avocational activities or operate a power wheelchair, which would otherwise be impossible, can be a determining factor in acceptance and mastery of the BFO. Because the BFO increases the overall width of a wheelchair, it is not functional for passing through standard-width doors. Successful experience with the BFO can be a motivating factor.[5,6]

PARTS OF THE BFO AND THEIR FUNCTIONS[5,6]

The most commonly used parts of a standard BFO are shown in Fig. 19-39. There are several types of BFO. Additional attachments and assisting devices are available to suit individual needs.[5,6] The semireclining, adjustable bracket assembly, *A,* holds the BFO to the wheelchair. It supports the proximal arm and controls the height of the BFO. It can be adjusted to assist horizontal movement at the shoulder and elbow. It may be adapted for use in the reclining position, but the upright position is most desirable.[2,6]

The standard proximal swivel arm, *B,* permits horizontal abduction and horizontal adduction at the shoulder and contains the distal ball bearings. Both the bracket assembly and the proximal ball-bearing housing have stops that can be set at any position on the circumference of the housing unit to limit horizontal motion. The proximal ball-bearing housing on the proximal swivel arm can also be tilted so that gravity assists elbow flexion or extension.[6] An additional option, the elevating proximal arm (Fig. 19-40), allows the patient with anterior or middle deltoids with a strength grade of F or 3 active assistance with shoulder abduction and flexion. A rubber band assist facilitates this action.

The distal swivel arm, *C,* which can be used with either the standard proximal or the elevating proximal arm, permits forearm motion in the horizontal plane. It supports the rocker arm assembly and forearm trough. Attached to the forearm trough is the rocker arm assembly, *D.* It is positioned in the distal swivel arm and permits vertical (hand-to-mouth) motions. It swivels to produce added horizontal motion. The forearm trough, *E,* supports the forearm. It offers stable elbow support but may limit elbow extension. The elbow dial can be bent to produce adjustments for comfort and vertical motion.[6] The assembled balanced forearm orthosis is shown in Fig. 19-41.

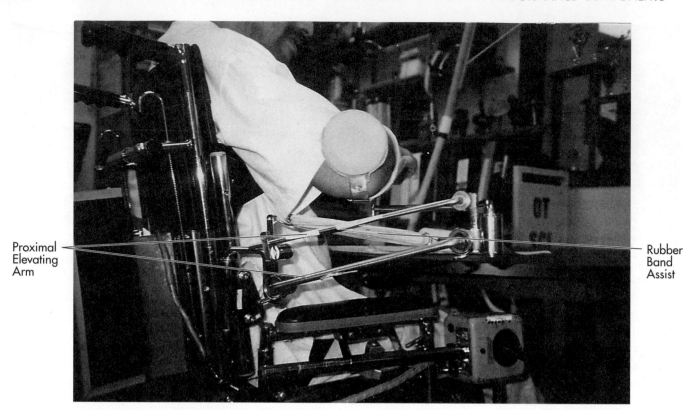

Proximal Elevating Arm

Rubber Band Assist

FIG. 19-40   Elevating proximal arm of BFO.

HOW THE BFO WORKS

The patient must have adequate voluntary muscle power to activate the BFO. Some source of power at the neck, trunk, shoulder girdle, shoulder, and elbow may serve alone or in combination to operate the device. Some controlling muscle in both elbow and shoulder is necessary if the user is to have control of motions in the horizontal plane across the midline of the body.[6]

The BFO allows horizontal and vertical motions. The device assists horizontal motions across the table top. Vertical movement allows table top–to–face activity. To assist horizontal motion the bracket assembly and the proximal ball-bearing housing on the proximal swivel arm can be adjusted to produce an inclined plane in the

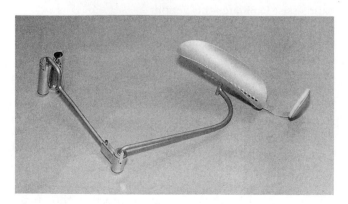

FIG. 19-41   Assembled BFO.

direction of horizontal abduction or horizontal adduction, as the need may be. Gravity then assists motion to the low point in the plane, and muscular effort must be exerted to return the arm to the high point of the plane.[6]

Adjustments for vertical motions are somewhat more complex. The rocker arm assembly is fastened to the underside of the forearm trough and acts as the fulcrum of this lever. There are several holes in the length of the forearm trough so that the fulcrum can be moved toward or away from the elbow (effort end). Any force applied by the user proximal to the fulcrum lifts the weight of the hand and anything in the hand toward the face. Shoulder elevation and depression are used to effect the vertical motions of the forearm trough. The distance of the fulcrum from the elbow determines whether the mechanical advantage is on the load side (hand) or effort side (elbow) of the lever.[6]

ADJUSTMENT AND CHECKOUT OF THE BFO[3,6]

To adjust the BFO the therapist must first (1) find the best position for the patient in the wheelchair; (2) choose the correct bracket assembly for the arm being fitted, because the right and left are not interchangeable; and (3) set the height of the bracket to position the whole BFO at the proper height. The forearm trough is then fitted to the patient. It is balanced for maximal range and force in vertical motion. The bracket is adjusted for maximal range and force in horizontal motion at the glenohumeral

BOX 19-1

1. Are the patient's hips set back in the chair?
2. Is the spine in good vertical alignment?
3. Is there good lateral trunk stability?
4. Are the chair seat and back adequate for comfort and stability?
5. Is the patient able to sit upright?
6. If the patient wears hand splints, are they on?
7. Does the patient have adequate passive ROM?
8. Is the bracket tight on the wheelchair and positioned perpendicular to the floor?
9. Is the bracket tight at the proper height so that the shoulders are not forced into elevation?
10. Is the proximal arm all the way down in the bracket?
11. Does the elbow dial clear the lap surface when the trough is in the UP position?
12. When the trough is in the UP position, is the patient's hand as close to the mouth as possible?
13. Can the patient obtain maximal active reach?
14. Is the trough the correct length? Does the distal end of the trough stop at the wrist joint?
15. Are the trough edges rolled so that they do not contact the forearm?
16. Is the elbow secure and comfortable in the elbow support?
17. Is the trough balanced correctly?
18. In vertical motion is the dial free of the distal arm?
19. Can the patient control motion of the proximal arm from either extreme?
20. Can the patient control motion of the distal arm from either extreme?
21. Can the patient control vertical motion of the trough from either extreme?
22. Have stops been applied to limit range, if necessary?
23. Can the patient lift a sufficient amount of weight to perform appropriate functional tasks?

joint. The therapist must then tilt the distal bearing, if necessary, to produce the maximal range and force in horizontal motion at the elbow joint. The therapist should then reevaluate range and force of combined horizontal motions of the glenohumeral and elbow joints and reevaluate the vertical motion of the trough. Some patients may require special attachments, such as straps, to stabilize the forearm in the trough.[6] The questions in Box 19-1 can serve as a guide for the therapist to determine the correctness of fit and adjustments of the BFO.[3]

TRAINING IN USE OF THE BFO

The therapist should be sure that supports are fitting well and correctly adjusted before attempting to instruct the patient in their use. If two BFOs are used, the patient should practice with one at a time until each is mastered. Bilateral use of BFOs requires considerable practice.

Early use includes training in vertical motions (external and internal rotation of the shoulder). External rotation is accomplished by depressing the shoulder to elevate the hand, shifting the body weight to the side of the BFO, rolling the shoulder back, tilting or turning the head toward the side of the device, or leaning backward. Internal rotation is accomplished by gravity, elevating the shoulder on the same side as the balance forearm orthosis, shifting the body weight to the opposite side from the device, rolling the shoulder forward, tilting and turning the head to the opposite side from the BFO, or leaning forward.

Work is started on horizontal adduction and abduction with the trough balanced at midposition. Then the patient can proceed to practice these motions with the trough at various heights between table top and head.

Practice progresses to include elbow flexion and extension with the trough at various heights. Activities that are designed to offer practice in the use of BFOs are arm-driven power wheelchair propulsion, typing or computer work, turning book pages, using the phone, grooming, hygiene at sink, and playing games such as checkers, cards, and puzzles.

The BFO offers the patient who demonstrates upper extremity weakness the necessary assistance to make maximal use of minimal muscle power. Once assembled, fitted, and adjusted it enables the patient to perform a variety of self-care and leisure activities that promote self-esteem and independence. The reader is referred to the references for more comprehensive discussion of BFOs and their use.[2,5,6]

SUSPENSION SLING

The suspension sling supports the upper extremity in a plane parallel to the floor. The suspension sling is used to facilitate horizontal movement during activity or exercise in which the force of gravity on the movement of the upper extremity needs to be minimized (Fig. 19-42).[4]

PARTS OF THE SUSPENSION SLING

A bracket *(A)* holds the suspension rod to the back of the wheelchair. The bracket can be adjusted to keep the top of the suspension rod parallel to the floor. It also allows for adjustments in height. The suspension sling is hung from the suspension rod *(D)* with a spring or a strap *(C)*. The length of the suspension device determines the height of the sling in relation to the user's body. The suspension device also swivels to eliminate friction or

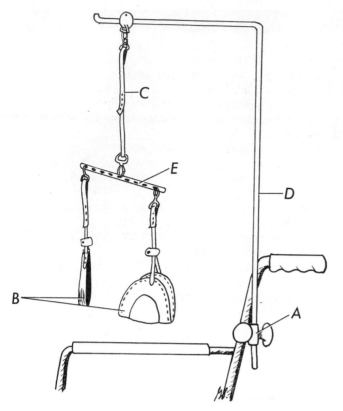

FIG. 19-42   Suspension sling. **A,** Bracket. **B,** Arm cuff. **C,** Suspension strap. **D,** Suspension rod. **E,** Horizontal supporting device for cuffs. (Modified with permission from Occupational Therapy Department, Rancho Los Amigos Hospital, Downey, Calif.)

twisting and to allow maximal mobility. If a spring suspension is used, it adds to the amount of motion that the user can produce in the sling but may decrease coordination.

The cuffs *(B)* of the suspension sling are fastened to a horizontal bar *(E)* that has holes along its entire length. These holes allow the cuffs of the sling to be placed for optimal balance to assist vertical or horizontal motions of the arm. A forearm trough, as used on the BFO, is sometimes substituted for the arm cuffs shown in Fig. 19-42, and the assembly is then referred to as a suspension feeder.[4]

USE OF THE SUSPENSION SLING

In many instances the suspension sling can be used with patients who have the same diagnoses as previously cited for the BFO, although somewhat greater muscle power and control is required for effective use. Use of the suspension sling may be initiated with enabling exercise to establish patterns of horizontal abduction and adduction, hand-to-body movements, and hand-to-face movements. Use may then progress to activities such as eating, hygiene at sink, table top communication skills, and leisure activities.

REVIEW QUESTIONS

SECTION 2
1. Which patients are good candidates for use of the BFO (in terms of disability or muscle grades)?
2. Which patients are poor candidates for use of the BFO? Why?
3. List the five criteria a patient must meet to use the BFO successfully.
4. What activities can be performed with the BFO that could not be performed without it?
5. List the three major steps in training the patient to use BFO.
6. List two ways external rotation motion can be accomplished.
7. List two ways internal rotation motion can be accomplished.
8. What are some activities that are good for practicing use of the BFO?
9. What is the primary purpose of the suspension sling?
10. List three purposeful activities that may be performed by patients with significant upper extremity dysfunction while using a suspension sling. Can you think of some that were not named in the text?
11. When is a elevating proximal arm the appropriate choice?

REFERENCES

SECTION 1: HAND SPLINTING
1. American Society of Hand Therapists: *Splint classification system,* Chicago, 1992, The Society.
2. Brand P: *Clinical mechanics of the hand,* ed 1, St Louis, 1985, CV Mosby.
3. Brand P: The forces of dynamic splinting: ten questions before applying a dynamic splint to the hand. In Hunter J, Schneider L, Mackin E, Callahan A: *Rehabilitation of the hand: surgery and therapy,* ed 3, St Louis, 1990, CV Mosby.
4. Colditz J: Dynamic splinting of the stiff hand. In Hunter J, Schneider L, Mackin E, Callahan A: *Rehabilitation of the hand: surgery and therapy,* ed 3, St Louis, 1990, CV Mosby.
5. Fess E: Principles and methods of splinting for mobilization of joints. In Hunter J, Schneider L, Mackin E, Callahan A: *Rehabilitation of the hand: surgery and therapy,* ed 3, St Louis, 1990, CV Mosby.
6. Fess E, Philips C: *Hand splinting: principles and methods,* St. Louis, 1987, CV Mosby.
7. Flatt AE: *Care of the arthritic hand,* St Louis, 1983, CV Mosby.

8. Hollister A, Giurintano D: How joints move. In Brand P, Hollister A: *Clinical mechanics of the hand,* ed 2, St Louis, 1993, CV Mosby.
9. McCollough N, Sarrafian S: Biomechanical analysis system. In *Atlas of orthotics, biomechanical principles and application,* St Louis, 1975, CV Mosby.
10. Strickland JW: Anatomy and kinesiology of the hand. In Fess E, Philips C: *Hand splinting: principles and methods,* St. Louis, 1987, CV Mosby.

SUGGESTED READINGS

Caillet R: *Hand pain and impairment,* ed 3, Philadelphia, 1982, FA Davis.
Hoppenfeld S: *Physical examination of the spine and extremities,* New York, 1976, Appleton-Century-Crofts.

Napier JR: The prehensile movements of the human hand, *J Bone Joint Surg* 38B(4), 1956.

REFERENCES

SECTION 2: BALANCED FOREARM ORTHOSIS AND SUSPENSION SLING

1. Bender LF: Upper extremity orthotics. In Kottke FJ, Lehmann JF: *Krusen's handbook of physical medicine and rehabilitation,* ed 4, Philadelphia, 1990, WB Saunders.
2. Dicus RG: Mobile arm supports. I. Downey, Calif, 1970, SRS Service Dept of Rancho Los Amigos Hospital (film).
3. Rancho Los Amigos Hospital: Check-out sheet for feeders. In Marshall E: *Occupational therapy management of physical dysfunction,* Loma Linda, Calif. 1981, Loma Linda University. (Distributed by Sammons, Inc, PO Box 386, Western Springs, IL 60558-0386.)
4. Rancho Los Amigos Hospital: Suspension feeders and slings: parts and their functions. In Marshall E: *Occupational therapy management of physical dysfunction,* Loma Linda, Calif, 1981, Loma Linda University. (Distributed by Sammons, Inc, Box 386, Western Springs, IL 60558-0386.)
5. Thenn JE: *Mobile arm support: installation and use,* San José, Calif, 1975, Self-published.
6. Wilson DJ, McKenzie MW, Barber LM: *Spinal cord injury: a treatment guide for occupational therapists,* rev ed, Thorofare, NJ, 1984, Slack.

CHAPTER 20

Neurophysiology for the Sensorimotor Approaches to Treatment

Guy L. McCormack, Fred Feuchter

The sensorimotor treatment approaches are used with patients who have central nervous system (CNS) dysfunction. The normal CNS functions to produce controlled, well-modulated movement through a balance between inhibition and facilitation of motor activities. In the damaged CNS, the inhibition and facilitation of motor responses are out of balance and do not work together to produce smooth, well-modulated movement.

In the sensorimotor approaches to treatment, it is assumed that specific, controlled sensory input can influence motor responses. Abnormal motor responses can be inhibited, and more normal motor responses can be learned by the CNS.

Many of the sensorimotor approaches to treatment use proprioceptive stimuli, such as stretching and resistance, to influence thresholds for inhibition and facilitation of movement.[94] Cutaneous stimulation, which has been found to increase stretch receptor sensitivity, may be combined with proprioceptive stimulation to facilitate voluntary contraction of specific muscles. Exteroceptive stimuli are used, for example, brushing to recruit touch receptors and icing or vibration to facilitate or inhibit muscle responses. Reflex mechanisms may be used in some approaches. Some of these are the tonic neck and lumbar reflexes, righting and protective reactions, and associated reactions.[89]

The purpose of this chapter is to provide an operational understanding of neurophysiology for the sensorimotor approaches to treatment discussed in Chapters 21 through 25. To treat persons who have neurologic dysfunctions effectively, occupational therapists should understand nervous system mechanisms (1) to help patients become able to perform functional activities and (2) to understand why certain motor disturbances exist.

REVIEW OF THE NERVOUS SYSTEM

The human nervous system has been described as the most complex structure in the universe.[75] Its functions in daily life are the manifestation of myriad biological interactions and processes. To understand the anatomical and physiological bases of its activities, neurobiologists have subdivided the nervous system into several parts, necessary because of its overwhelming complexity. The division into parts is artificial, however, because the anatomy and functions of the parts overlap considerably, and the parts are interdependent.

Those parts that are protected by bony structures, such as the cranium and vertebral canal, are called the *central nervous system* (CNS). The major functions of the CNS are receipt of information from bodily structures, central processing of the information, and sending commands to the periphery in the form of a response. Those parts that are found outside of the bony structures are referred to as the *peripheral nervous system* (PNS), whose major function is conduction of information from bodily structures to the CNS (afferent) and from the CNS to the body (efferent).

A second classification of structures is based on voluntary and involuntary activities. Those structures that regulate the viscera, largely involuntary and unconscious, constitute the *autonomic nervous system* (ANS), while those structures that regulate the skeletal muscles and skin, largely voluntary and conscious, make up the *somatic nervous system* (SNS). Both the ANS and SNS have central and peripheral elements. Careful analysis shows that our daily activities call into play all of these components, whose functions are linked to one another, as well as to other bodily regulators such as the endocrine and immune systems.

DIVISIONS OF THE NERVOUS SYSTEM
Central Nervous System
Spinal cord

The CNS consists of the spinal cord, brain stem, cerebellum, subcortical nuclei, and the cerebral cortex.[35,55] The spinal cord is phylogenetically older and less complex than other structures in the CNS. The spinal cord is less than an inch (2.54 cm) in diameter with enlargements in the lower cervical and in the lower lumbar regions to accommodate the outflow to the extremities. The spinal cord begins at the foramen magnum and extends caudally to vertebrae level L1 or L2.[73,95]

The spinal cord is functionally subdivided into segments. The spinal segments do not align opposite the corresponding vertebrae because the cord is about 9⅘ inches (25 cm) shorter, because of differential growth in fetal and neonatal life. There are 31 pairs of spinal nerves: 8 cervical, 12 thoracic, 5 lumbar, 5 sacral, and 1 coccygeal. Each spinal nerve has dorsal and ventral roots that form the sensory and motor components. All the sensory afferent fibers (somatic and visceral) enter the spinal cord by way of the dorsal roots. All motor fibers (efferent) exit the spinal cord via the ventral roots.

In a transverse section the spinal cord appears to have a butterfly-shaped area of gray substance surrounded by white matter. The white matter is composed of longitudinal ascending and descending fiber tracts connecting the brain to various spinal cord segments. The cell bodies of the efferent fibers are located in the ventral gray matter. The gray matter can be further subdivided into 10 laminae, each extending the length of the cord. The more dorsal laminae are concerned with sensory functions, whereas more ventrally located laminae are motor-related. Much of the gray matter consists of interneurons, which integrate sensory and motor functions with information descending from higher centers. The white matter of the spinal cord is divided into three pairs of funiculi (anterior, lateral, and dorsal).[72,86]

Some generalizations may be made about the descending and ascending tracts of the spinal cord. The anatomic positions occupied by the various fiber systems become important in consideration of the constellation of deficits resulting from partial injuries to the spinal cord. Functions may be lost or retained as determined by the site of the lesion. The anterolateral quadrant of the spinal cord contains the phylogenetically newer descending systems. These descending tracts are concerned with motor activity and are referred to as *pyramidal* or *extrapyramidal*.

The pyramidal tract is so-named because of the pyramid-shaped bulges formed where the descending fibers cross on the ventral surface of the medulla oblongata. The pyramidal tract comprises two pathways, the lateral and anterior corticospinal tracts, which are associated with finer movements of the distal limb musculature. These neurons tend to be excitatory to flexors and inhibitory to extensors.[93]

The extrapyramidal descending tracts include the rubrospinal and reticulospinal pathways, and tracts commonly associated with postural mechanisms, for example, the vestibulospinal and tectospinal tracts. These are phylogenetically older tracts and are located in anteromedial portions of the cord. Efferent impulses are transmitted along these tracts to be excitatory to extensor motor neurons and inhibitory to flexor motor neurons. There is also ample evidence to conclude that the descending pathways have important functions not related to motor activity. Some descending fibers are concerned with the transmission of sensory information at the spinal cord level, that is, to inhibit, amplify, or otherwise modulate activity of sensory nerves.

A similar relationship exists in the ascending sensory tracts. The anterolateral tracts (spinothalamic) are phylogenetically older and mediate pain, temperature, and crude touch along small-diameter fibers; they are considered to constitute a primitive protective system. Included in the vicinity are pathways that orient us to our environment: spinocerebellar (proprioceptive information from the limbs), spinoreticular (visceral information), spinotectal (head position information), and the spinoolivary tracts. Conversely, the dorsal columns of the spinal cord (medial lemniscal system) are present in the dorsal portion of white matter as two bundles, the fasciculus cuneatus (upper limb) and fasciculus gracilis (lower limb). They represent a newer sensory system conveying discriminative sensory information from the skin and deep structures to the cerebral cortex. This system is rapidly conducting because the fibers are large and well myelinated and undergo few synapses en route to the cortex.[5,93] The Lissauer fasciculus and the medial longitudinal fasciculus (MLF) are considered to be mixed tract systems. The Lissauer fasciculus is thought to convey fibers several segments up or down the cord, to integrate activity among many cord segments. The MLF contains many minor pathways that ascend or descend to various levels.

Brain stem

The brain stem is regarded as the center of sensory integration.[5] That is, all perceptual processes basic to learning are dependent on sensory integration at the brain stem level. The brain stem consists of the medulla oblongata, pons, midbrain, and thalamus.[82] All of the ascending and descending fiber pathways between spinal cord and cerebral cortex pass through the brain stem, providing ample opportunity for integration of information. In addition, the brain stem is the source of all but one of the cranial nerves. Parts of the brain stem are crucial to maintenance of consciousness, sleep, and alertness, and it participates in the regulation of the autonomic nervous system, along with the hypothalamus.

The lowest portion of the brain stem, the *medulla,* contains nuclei for five cranial nerves, the reticular formation, the vestibular system, and the respiratory and cardiac functions. All the major ascending and descending tracts pass through the medulla.[41] The *pons* is a large mass that lies above the medulla. The *pons* plays an important role as a relay station between the cerebral cortex and the cerebellum. The pons contains four cranial nerve nuclei, pontine nuclei, and major fiber tracts.[10,39]

The *midbrain* is a relatively short section of the brain stem but contains several important structures. Some of these structures are the corpora quadrigemina (superior and inferior colliculi), red nucleus, substantia nigra, crura cerebri, and cranial nerves III and IV.[39,72]

The brain stem is the source of the extrapyramidal motor pathways. Two tracts arising from the midbrain are the rubrospinal and tectospinal tracts. The reticulospinal pathway arises from both the pons and medulla, and the vestibulospinal pathway originates in the medulla.

Diencephalon

The diencephalon consists of four structures, each containing the term *thalamus*. The thalamus is a complex structure that makes up the rostral portion of the brain stem. With the exception of the olfactory system, all sensory information passes through the thalamus en route to the cerebral cortex.[83,93] The thalamus is regarded as a sensory relay station. In the past it was believed that the thalamus participated in the realization of crude sensation. However, it is now thought that the thalamus participates in refining or consolidating sensory information before it reaches the cortex.[83] Similarly, the anterior portions of the thalamus are involved in refining or consolidating motor information from the cerebellum and basal ganglia before sending it to the cerebral cortex. The thalamus may also play a role in emotion and behavior through its connections with the limbic system. Cerebral vascular accidents may cause destruction to parts of the thalamus resulting in thalamic syndrome. This condition can cause exaggerated pain or unpleasant sensations to nonnoxious stimuli.[20]

The *hypothalamus* lies inferior to the thalamus and forms the ventral floor of the third ventricle. Although the hypothalamus is only about the size of a fingernail, it exerts a direct or indirect influence on every function of the body.[74] Through widespread connections the hypothalamus coordinates the activities of the autonomic nervous system, the endocrine system, and the limbic system.[1,10,35,72,86] In short, the hypothalamus regulates emotions, sexual drive, hormones, eating, drinking, body temperature, sleeping and waking states, heart rate, and chemical balances.[82,83] The *subthalamus* and *epithalamus* are minor regions of the diencephalon. The subthalamus is associated with motor activity, and the epithalamus is concerned with diurnal and circadian rhythms and gonadal maturation.

Cerebellum

Cerebellum means "little brain," and it is appropriately named, comprising about 10% of the total weight of the brain. The cerebellum is located in the posterior cranial fossa and is attached to the pons, medulla, and midbrain by the cerebellar peduncles, which contain the fibers entering and exiting the cerebellum. Anatomically, the cerebellum consists of two *cerebellar hemispheres* joined by a narrow median strip called the *vermis*. The medial portions of the hemispheres adjacent to the vermis are known as the *paravermis*.

The hemispheres are divided into three lobes: anterior, posterior, and flocculonodular. It is more useful, however, to consider the functional divisions of the cerebellum. Based on a combination of criteria, including phylogenetic development and experimental studies of fiber tracts, the cerebellum can be divided into three functional zones, which correspond roughly, but not exactly, to the anatomical lobes. The *vestibulocerebellum* (archicerebellum) is phylogenetically the oldest region and corresponds to the flocculonodular lobe. It is related functionally to the vestibular system and controls balance and coordinates eye movements with movements of the head. The *spinocerebellum* (paleocerebellum), which comprises most of the anterior lobe, vermis, and paravermis, receives a variety of information from the spinal cord, mainly from the spinocerebellar tracts. It controls posture, muscle tone, and synergy during stereotyped movements such as walking. The *pontocerebellum* (neocerebellum) occupies the majority of tissue in the cerebellum, located in the large lateral regions of the hemispheres. It receives information from the cerebral cortex via the pontine nuclei. It coordinates the planning of movements and controls the muscle tone required for accurate nonstereotyped (i.e., learned) movements.[1,22,46]

Recent studies suggest other functional roles for the cerebellum. The cerebellum helps to regulate some aspects of the ANS, such as respiration, cardiovascular functions, and pupillary size. Another area influenced by the cerebellum is motor learning. It appears that cerebellar circuitry can be altered functionally by experience, and cerebellar lesions can interrupt certain kinds of motor learning.

Limbic system

The limbic system is a collection of interconnected structures in the cerebrum and diencephalon that contribute to emotional responses, affective behavior, and survival of the organism.[29] This system governs feeding, fighting, and reproductive behaviors. According to Moore, the limbic system integrates the newest cognitive structures in the cortex with the older reticular formation, sensorimotor systems, and primitive visceral structures.[70] Moore discussed the importance of the limbic system in rehabilitation techniques.[67]

The principle structures of the limbic system are the cingulate gyrus, septal area, insula, and temporal lobe structures, such as the parahippocampal gyrus, amygdala, and hippocampal formation.[1,39] The hypothalamus is also part of the limbic system. Although the individual areas of the limbic system are functionally diverse, serving emotional and motivational behavior on the one hand and learning and memory on the other, the high degree of interconnection suggests that these areas have an underlying unity. Although the limbic system is not directly connected to the motor systems, its emotional and behavioral components affect autonomic and somatic responses.

The system receives diverse multimodal sensory information and has a great deal of connectivity to the cerebral cortex and deeper brain structures, such as the hypothalamus. Anterior portions of the limbic system subserve affective behavior and visceromotor functions, and the posterior portions participate in temporary storage of information, including the encoding of spatial relations. Thus, emotional states can substantially influence learning and memory, and elements of learning and memory (habituation, orientation) can importantly alter emotional status and arousal. Two of the disorders involving portions of the limbic system are epilepsy and Alzheimer disease.

Basal ganglia

The basal ganglia are found deep within the cerebrum, the major structures of which are the caudate nucleus, putamen, and globus pallidus. The basal ganglia are also functionally related to the amygdaloid nucleus, claustrum, subthalamic nucleus, and substantia nigra.[1,23] The basal ganglia receive much input from the cerebral cortex and transmit it into many circuits and feedback loops. The output from the basal ganglia is focused mainly on the ventral anterior and lateral regions of the thalamus, similar to the cerebellum. Like the cerebellum, the basal ganglia play a role in the refinement of complex movement, automatic movement patterns, associated movements, and regulation of postural tone in antigravity muscles.[20,35] Unlike the cerebellum, because of their multiple connections with cortical structures, the basal ganglia are not associated with simple stereotyped movements, but rather movements within the context of complex behaviors that have cognitive, motivational, and sensory elements.

Cerebral cortex

The cortex makes up the outermost region of the cerebrum. It has been attributed to intellectual functions, memory storage, language, consciousness, perception, and complex motor activities.[23] The cortex is composed of six layers of densely packed neuron cell bodies. The cortex has been anatomically divided into four lobes and 52 distinct areas, based on types of cell groupings.[73] Some functions can be localized with precision to specific regions of the cerebral cortex, such as vision or speech, while others, like long-term memory, seem to be more diffusely represented within the cortex. Clinically, some of the most important areas include the primary motor strip (area 4), supplementary motor area (area 6), prefrontal cortex (areas 9 through 12), areas of Broca (areas 44 and 45), area of Wernicke (area 22), sensory strip (areas 1, 2, and 3), and supramarginal gyrus (area 40). Lesions to these areas result in profound sensory or motor dysfunction.[11,22]

In the past, the cerebral cortex has been mapped out by defining boundaries, structures, and functional units.[22,76] New techniques in visualizing brain structure and function, such as positron emission tomography (PET) scanning, have revealed considerable overlap of structural and functional capacities of the cerebral cortex and have shown that many regions participate cooperatively in human activities.[9,27,44,78,79] Cortical organization may be more plastic, or changeable, than previously believed, and neuroscientists have concluded that cortical representation on the brain is constantly being modified by interaction with the environment.

Peripheral Nervous System

By definition, the peripheral nervous system consists of those structures outside of the brain and spinal cord, such as spinal nerves and the cranial nerves. Several elements exist in both the CNS and PNS. For instance, alpha motor neurons are found in the ventral gray matter of the spinal cord, and their processes extend to the periphery. Sensory neurons, innervating peripheral structures, have processes that extend through the spinal cord all the way to the brain stem. There are 31 pairs of spinal nerves, related ganglia, and 12 pairs of cranial nerves.[39,72] The peripheral nerves contain motor (efferent), sensory (afferent), and autonomic components.

Sensory components

The sensory receptors (end organs) in the skin possess a certain amount of specificity in responding to different types of stimuli. Afferent impulses are transmitted along sensory fibers to the CNS. These nerve fibers vary greatly in their diameter and degree of myelination, which together determine conduction velocity.[73] Generally speaking, the greater the diameter of the fiber and the thicker the myelin sheath, the faster the rate of conduction.[23]

There are two classification schemes for nerve fibers. The first uses an alphabetical system consisting of three groups: A, B, and C. The A and B fibers are thicker in diameter and myelinated, whereas C fibers are thin and unmyelinated.[39] The A fibers are further divided into subgroups called alpha, beta, gamma, and delta. The A fibers contain two motor components: alpha fibers, which supply skeletal (extrafusal) muscle, and gamma fibers, which innervate muscle spindle (intrafusal) muscle. Beta and delta fibers convey information about fine touch and

TABLE 20-1 Nerve Fiber Classification

LETTER	ROMAN NUMERAL	FUNCTIONAL COMPONENT	FIBER DIAMETER (μm)*	CONDUCTION VELOCITY (m/sec)
A alpha (Aα)	Group I Ia	Primary muscle spindle ending (stretch)	12-22	70-120
A beta (Aβ)	Ib	Golgi tendon organ (contraction) and Ruffini endings	10-15	60-80
	Group II	Secondary sensory ending from muscle spindle (maintained stretch) Encapsulated endings	6-13	30-80
		Cutaneous afferents from skin and joints (joint position-pressure), Meissner corpuscles		
A gamma (Aγ)		Motor to muscle spindle (static-dynamic)	3-8	15-40
B		Motor; branch of alpha motor neuron	1-3	5-15
		Preganglionic autonomic efferents, some cranial nerves		
A delta	Group III	Bare nerve endings, cutaneous mechanoreceptors; cold and nociceptors	3-8	10-30
C fibers	Group IV	Unmyelinated, nonspecific sensory reception; cold, warm, and nociceptors, autonomous fibers	1-1.5	0.5-2.5

Adapted from Barr M, Kiernan S: The human nervous system, ed. 2, New York, 1993, Harper & Row.
* Micron millimeters.

sharp pain, respectively. B fibers are autonomic in function, and the C fibers convey diffuse, poorly localized pain.

The second classification pertains only to sensory fibers and uses Roman numerals to designate fiber size and fiber origin. This class includes group Ia for the primary ending of the muscle spindle; group Ib for the Golgi tendon organs; group II for secondary sensory endings from muscle spindles; group III for touch, pressure, pain, and temperature receptors; and group IV for nonspecific unmyelinated pain and temperature fibers. Table 20-1 summarizes the two classifications, giving their conduction velocities and differentiating the major modalities. Table 20-2 compares proprioception with pain and temperature.

Once stimuli have been transduced into sensory impulses, they are transmitted to the spinal cord by the fibers named previously. In the cord, the fibers may do

any or all of the following: cross to the opposite side, ascend the spinal cord, connect directly with a motor neuron, or connect with interneurons, some of which may have an inhibitory influence. The transfer of coded information from one neuron to another constitutes a synaptic transmission, which is largely a chemical process.

One of the ways the CNS generates motor activity in response to external stimuli is through reflex arcs[46] (Fig. 20-1). A reflex arc is a basic neuronal circuit consisting of at least five elements:

1. a receptor receiving the stimulus
2. an afferent fiber transmitting stimulus information to the CNS
3. a reflex center in the CNS where the stimulus can be influenced and distributed in several ways. The reflex center determines the complexity of the response to the stimulus.

TABLE 20-2 Comparison of Proprioception with Pain and Temperature

PROPRIOCEPTION		PAIN AND TEMPERATURE	
A ALPHA (I)	A ALPHA (III)	A DELTA (III)	C (IV)
Muscle stretch			
Muscle contraction	Muscle stretch		
	Position sense		
	Vibration		
	Velocity detection		
	Pressure	Cold	Cold
		Light touch	Touch
		Pain	Pain
			Warmth

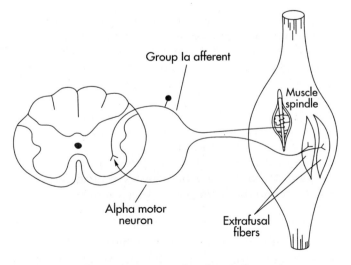

FIG. 20-1 Monosynaptic stretch reflex (reflex arc).

4. an efferent fiber to an effector organ
5. an effector organ, usually a muscle

Many of the somatic and autonomic functions mediated by the spinal cord are reflexogenic in nature. The combination and integration of many spinal cord reflexes forms the basis for development of more complex subroutines leading to familiar and automatic movements, such as walking.[20] If any of these components is destroyed, the reflex arc is abolished. Reflex arcs enable the nervous system to react to stimuli that may be potentially harmful without exerting conscious effort. Thus, touching the cornea of the eye results in a blink, touching a hot object results in a withdrawal reflex, and foreign objects in the windpipe produce coughing. The reflex arc is also used to examine the integrity of the nervous system or to elicit crude components of movement.[40]

Motor components

Alpha motor neurons are the largest of the anterior horn cells. They can be stimulated through the reflex arc by the Ia primary afferents and group II secondary afferents of the muscle spindles.[86] Alpha motor neurons are also influenced by higher centers and by fibers from the corticospinal, raphe spinal, reticulospinal, and lateral vestibulospinal tracts.[93] Whenever a motor act is elicited, either voluntary or reflexive, the impulse must travel to the muscle by way of an alpha motor neuron. Because the alpha motor neuron is the last remaining connection between the spinal cord and extrafusal muscle, it is called the "final common pathway."[22] If the cell body or axon of the alpha motor neuron is destroyed, the muscle is denervated, and the muscle becomes hypotonic. It will exhibit flaccid paralysis and atrophy, because of the loss of trophic effects exerted by the alpha motor neuron, constituting a lower motor neuron dysfunction. Efforts to activate that muscle through sensory stimulation are nonproductive unless some regeneration of the reflex arc has occurred.

Autonomic Nervous System

The autonomic nervous system regulates glands, viscera, smooth muscles, cardiac muscle, and reflexive mechanisms in the skin.[1,10,22] It functions predominantly at the subconscious level but is connected with conscious emotional states and influenced by events in the environment.[46,70,74] The control centers for the autonomic nervous system are located in the hypothalamus and the brain stem. Functionally, the autonomic nervous system consists of two divisions, the *sympathetic* and the *parasympathetic* systems. The two systems generally serve the same visceral organs but cause essentially opposite effects, counterbalancing each other's activities.

Sympathetic nervous system

The sympathetic nervous system mobilizes the body during extreme situations (such as fear, exercise, or rage), expending energy, redirecting blood flow to areas of intense activity, and shutting down functions in other areas. Motor innervation by the ANS requires a two-neuron chain in the periphery, as opposed to one neuron in the somatic motor system. These are referred to as preganglionic and postganglionic neurons. The cell bodies of preganglionic sympathetic neurons reside in the lateral horn of gray matter in the spinal cord segments T_1-L_2. They exit the spinal cord (thoracolumbar outflow) and enter the paravertebral ganglion chain (sympathetic chain) that runs adjacent to either side of the spinal column.[23,35]

The sympathetic chain extends from the top to the bottom of the spinal column, so that preganglionic fibers extend up or down the chain for considerable distances. At some point in the chain, the preganglionic fibers synapse with postganglionic neurons located in the paravertebral ganglia. The postganglionic cells send axons to innervate smooth muscles of all the organs. Each spinal nerve receives fibers from the sympathetic trunk ganglia, which are distributed to the blood vessels, erector pili muscles of hair, and secretory organs of the skin throughout the distribution of the nerve.[83] The viscera of the pelvic and abdominal cavities are innervated by sympathetic branches not associated with spinal nerves. In the abdomen and pelvis they are given the name of *splanchnic* nerves.[10] The splanchnic nerves carry preganglionic fibers to postganglionic neurons located in the prevertebral ganglia of the abdomen (celiac, superior mesenteric, and inferior mesenteric ganglia). Fibers from these ganglia follow the blood vessels and thus reach all of the abdominal and pelvis viscera (Fig. 20-2).

Norepinephrine is the primary neurotransmitter of postganglionic sympathetic nerves. Norepinephrine and substances with similar effects are termed *adrenergic*.[39] The principle receptors for the adrenergic system are classified as alpha and beta with subclassifications of each. These receptors are molecular sites on cell membranes in the viscera, where adrenergic neurotransmitters bind to produce their effects in tissues. The type and amount of receptors present determines the response of the target organ.

The sympathetic autonomic nervous system is stimulated when a person experiences strong emotions, such as fear and rage, and when he or she is exposed to cold or pain. The sympathetic system coordinates a generalized physiologic response, stimulating the adrenal glands to liberate norepinephrine and epinephrine into the bloodstream, which reinforces the effects of sympathetic neurons. As a result, the blood vessels in the skin and digestive systems constrict, and the blood vessels in the cardiac and skeletal muscles dilate. The bronchioles of the lungs and pupils of the eyes also dilate. Heart rate and force of contraction increase. The sweat, lacrimal, and salivary glands increase secretions.

These reactions are part of the organism's biologic response to situations that are perceived as potentially dangerous. When faced with tangible situations that are a

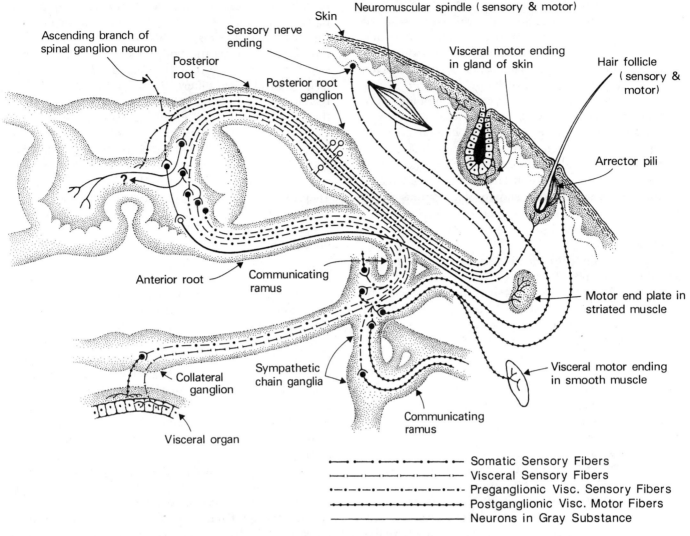

FIG. 20-2 Composite drawing showing traverse section of spinal cord, spinal nerve roots, posterior root ganglia, sympathetic ganglia, and various end organs. (Redrawn and expanded from Schaffer G, editor: *Morris' human anatomy*, New York, 1953, Blakiston.)

real threat to survival, the fight or flight response is appropriate. However, modern society produces many intangible stressors that generate prolonged sympathetic nervous system responses that cannot be acted upon through overt aggression. Many circumstances that cause no immediate harm can activate the autonomic nervous system, which does not differentiate between psychological and physical stressors. As a result, the biologic responses to psychological and physical circumstances may be the same.

Parasympathetic nervous system

In contrast, the major function of the parasympathetic nervous system is a "housekeeping" function, to monitor conditions and promote activity of the viscera, conserving energy.[41] In contrast to the sympathetic system, the parasympathetic system is limited in distribution to glands and viscera of the head, thorax, abdomen, and

pelvis. Peripheral tissues, blood vessels, and the skin have no significant parasympathetic innervation (except the head).

The preganglionic cell bodies arise from the craniosacral regions of the central nervous system. The cranial portion consists of cranial nerves III, VII, IX, and X. Cranial nerve X (vagus nerve) supplies the organs of the thorax and abdomen. The sacral portion arises from spinal segments *S2, S3,* and *S4.* The sacral division communicates with pelvic splanchnic nerves and supplies muscular walls of the colon, rectum, and urinary and reproductive organs. The parasympathetic motor system also is a two-neuron chain. The ganglia containing postganglionic cells are found in or near the walls of the organs innervated, however. The postganglionic terminals of the parasympathetic system liberate acetylcholine and are classified as cholinergic.[39]

The parasympathetic system can act simultaneously

with the sympathetic system during the fight or flight situation. During exaggerated fear the sacral segment may produce involuntary emptying of the bladder and rectum. In contrast to the sympathetic response, the parasympathetic system acts to dilate blood vessels in the skin and digestive tract, constrict bronchial tubes, contract the pupils of the eyes, and increase motility of the gastrointestinal tract. During sexual arousal the parasympathetic system controls penile and clitoral erection, while the sympathetic division mediates ejaculation.[35]

It has been found that the autonomic nervous system can be manipulated through facilitative and inhibitory techniques. Research has shown that various relaxation techniques, visualization, and biofeedback can reduce the activity level of the sympathetic nervous system.*

Anatomic and physiologic factors contributing to states of stress and relaxation have been described on a continuum.[37] The fight or flight state combines increased sympathetic activity, arousal of the cortex, and increased muscle tone. This state was termed the ergotropic response meaning moving in the direction of work. The other end of the continuum is a state that combines increased parasympathetic activity, cortical relaxation, and decreased muscle tone. This state has been termed the trophotropic end of the continuum. Benson, Beary, and Carol have renamed the trophotropic response as the relaxation response.[16]

In the process of using facilitative or inhibitory activities the therapist should determine where the patient's capabilities fall along this ergotropic-trophotropic continuum. If the goal is to reduce spasticity, the treatment activities should help move the patient toward the trophotropic (parasympathetic) end. However, if the goal is to promote learning or increase muscle, the activities should be stimulating and compatible with the ergotropic (sympathetic) response.

Research has revealed that the nervous system and the endocrine system respond simultaneously to stressful situations and are cooperative in their control of the body's systems.[26,52,74,77,92] In fact, their activities are so intricately interwoven that collectively they are now termed the neuroendocrine system. Endocrine secretions may alter activity in the CNS, and neural activity influences the endocrine organs, in turn. Additionally, some neurons secrete hormones directly into the blood. Thus, the view that the nervous and endocrine systems are separate and distinct entities is somewhat misleading.[26,37,48,60] The center that coordinates activity in the autonomic nervous system and the endocrine system is the hypothalamus.

The endocrine system plays an important role in the fight or flight response and other activities regulated by the ANS. For example, the adrenal glands release adrenalin (epinephrine) and noradrenalin (norepinephrine),

resulting in increased metabolic rate, cardiac output, and rapid respiration. The pancreas secretes insulin and glucagon to control levels of blood sugars for energy. The pineal gland acts as the body's clock, regulating menstrual cycles and the onset of maturation. The thymus gland is involved in differentiation and development of lymphocytes (functional cell of the immune system). The thyroid and parathyroid glands regulate the amount of calcium that is deposited in the bones and control its concentration in the blood. Much of the activity of the endocrine glands is controlled by the pituitary gland, which, in turn, is controlled by the hypothalamus. Therefore, the interactions of the endocrine and autonomic nervous systems, as well as the immune system, cooperatively affect the internal functions of the entire body.[1,10,35,65,74]

THE NEURON

The neuron is unique among all cells in the body because of its ability to transmit coded information from cell to cell and activate smooth and skeletal muscle. Each neuron varies in form and structure, depending on its role in the transport of information. Each neuron has a cell body containing a nucleus, dendrites that receive stimuli, an axon that conducts impulses away from the cell body, and axon terminals.[10] To convey information the neuron must have an excitable cell membrane and a system to synthesize and release neurotransmitter substances.[29,46]

The neuron has an excitable membrane that is activated by showers of neurotransmitters released by other neurons. Ionic differences between the interior of the cell and the fluid surrounding it determine the resting potential of the cell membrane. (An ion is a molecule that carries either a negative or positive electrical charge.) When a neuron membrane is excited by an outside stimulus, changes in potential occur along the cell membrane. If the stimulus is strong enough, the cell reaches its threshold and discharges an action potential (nerve impulse). The impulse then travels along the axon with a constant rate of speed until it reaches the terminal ending (synapse). A graded potential is a small change in resting potential and membrane voltage. It is not sufficient to discharge impulses along the axon but is carried by dendrites and cell bodies.[82]

Under some circumstances, several weak stimuli (subthreshold) may impinge on the neuron (spatial summation) to cause an action potential to develop. This phenomenon is called summation.[29] This concept is very important in therapy because it means that if the normal inputs to a neuron are destroyed, it may be possible to stimulate the cell to action potential by increasing the input to the neuron via alternative routes. If, for example, a traumatic lesion has destroyed neuronal circuits that normally stimulate a group of motor neurons to discharge, alternative pathways may be developed by consistent sensory stimulation. Neurons have the ability to adapt and change the direction of impulses through axon

---

* References 3, 14, 18, 21, 29, 59, 77, 80, 96.

collaterals.[81] Synaptic transmissions get stronger and more efficient with use.[71]

Neurotransmission

Neurotransmission represents the chemical aspect of interneuronal communication. It occurs between the presynaptic and postsynaptic membranes of two nerve cells. Normally there is a space or cleft between two communicating neurons called a synapse. A synapse can occur between an axon of the sending neuron and the dendrite, axon, or cell body of a receiving neuron. The transmission of information is propagated by a release of a chemical substance (neurotransmitter) that is capable of either increasing or decreasing the resting potential of the postsynaptic neuronal membrane.[72] If the neurotransmitter traverses the synapse and causes an action potential in the subsequent neuron, it is facilitative. If the neurotransmitter causes a hypopolarization of the postsynaptic cell membrane, however, it is inhibitory.[86]

There are hundreds, perhaps thousands, of different neurotransmitters in the human nervous system. Knowledge of neurotransmitters has increased dramatically in the last ten years and is a major focus of neuroscientific research. Neurotransmitters can be simple amino acids, short chains of amino acids called neuropeptides, proteins, or other more complex molecules. Neurons can release more than one type of neurotransmitter, and they have complex constellations of receptors for the various transmitters released from neighboring cells.

In addition to stimulating changes in the electrical potential of the membranes of target neurons, research has also shown that some substances released from neurons have long-lasting effects. They may change protein synthesis patterns in cells and determine whether or not certain genes are expressed. Various systems and assemblies within the nervous system exhibit different kinds of neurotransmitters, and certain types of nervous system dysfunctions have been related to altered levels of neurotransmitters. These findings present a new and exciting area of research, and many of the psychotropic drugs are suspected of altering the balances of certain neurotransmitters.

Synaptic junctions between neurons vary considerably throughout the nervous system. The average motor neuron may have about 6000 axon collateral synapses. Thus each neuron is capable of receiving several thousand messages from different sources. Generally speaking, sensory neurons conduct impulses in only one direction, away from the area in which the stimulus originated.[10]

According to Hinton[50] the latest findings suggest that neurons work cooperatively in networks requiring hundreds of millions of synapses between nerve cells at any given time. The complexity of these networks of neurons depends on the sophistication of the messages being transmitted. Neuronal networks feed information forward into higher level assemblies of neurons in various centers in the central nervous system. This arrangement allows neuronal pathways versatility to feed into a variety of feedback loops, allowing new information to go forward while sending back newly integrated information to locations where the original signals were produced.[50] Moore[69,70] suggests that this system allows neurons to anticipate, modify, and dampen synapses at each juncture.

The intensity of the stimulus may determine the action potential, yet the distance the impulse travels is dependent on the neuronal assembly receiving the communication.[39] Impulses can travel along several different circuits. Some neurons have many collateral branches that synapse with many neurons and form a divergent circuit to several regions of the nervous system. On the other hand, a single neuron may receive synaptic messages from several other neurons. This process is called *convergence*.[82] In this case the neuron must process both the excitatory and inhibitory impulses converging on it and decide to fire or inhibit the transmission. When the excitatory synapses predominate, action potentials are discharged and facilitation has occurred.

Another facilitative circuit is called positive feedback or reverberating excitation. Hypothetically, this action occurs in a circuit in which neurons further down the chain feed back excitation to the preceding neurons. Reverberating excitation occurs through axon collaterals and forms a continuous feedback loop, causing the neuron to discharge for a long time.[83] Reverberating circuits have been associated with short-term memory or arousal states generated within the reticular system.[46] It has been postulated that cutaneous stimulation (icing or brushing) may also initiate reverberating excitation.[53]

Neurons may also transmit through inhibitory circuits, which automatically suppress too much excitation. Typical inhibitory circuits include reciprocal inhibition through interneurons (Renshaw cells) or through groups of inhibitory neurons occupying parallel positions to excitatory neurons (surrounded inhibition).[82] Within the CNS there are regions in which inhibitory circuits play a greater role in suppressing excitatory impulses.[23] These neuronal circuits help to smooth out or prevent unwanted actions during movement. When the CNS is damaged, there is an imbalance between the excitatory and inhibitory circuits.[81] Consequently, patients may exhibit degrees of paralysis, alterations of reflex patterns, and changes in muscle tone.[40] When the inhibitory circuits are damaged, their dampening effects on excitatory neurons are "released." This phenomenon is called disinhibition. Clinically, it may be seen as spasticity, rigidity, tremors, or athetosis.

In summary, the concept of a single neuron conveying a message to a second single neuron is an extreme oversimplification of neuronal activity.* Although neurons are assembled into interactive circuits of thousands of cells, each with multiple connections, the activity of any one

---

* References 15, 27, 36, 69, 88, 90.

cell depends upon its complement of receptors for specific neurotransmitters. A cell's response to the showers of neurotransmitters it receives from its neighbors depends upon the type and amount of receptors that cell has for specific neurotransmitters.

Guyton[46] has described another phenomenon called rebound, which is related to fatigue of spinal level reflexes. Rebound occurs immediately after a reflex response has been evoked. Following the reflex response there is a period of fatigue, and the same reflex becomes more difficult to elicit. Strangely enough, reflexes of the antagonist muscles can be elicited more briskly. This response is a manifestation of reciprocal innervation and is a contributing factor to rhythmical movements. The term rebound has also been used to describe generalized reciprocal responses to prolonged use of thermal stimuli. For instance, if a patient stays in a heated therapeutic swimming pool too long, his biologic thermoregulatory system (posterior hypothalamus) may work as a thermostat and increase the activity in the parasympathetic nervous system, causing a state of relaxation. An hour later the autonomic nervous system can generate a sympathetic response, and the patient may become agitated and excitable and have an increase in muscle tone. This mechanism is not well understood and may be due to imbalances in types of neurotransmitters reactive to changes in body temperatures. Serotonin and norepinephrine levels have been associated with temperature, agitation, and changes in moods.[26,60,65]

The therapist must weigh the value of certain sensorimotor techniques with respect to long-term or short-term gains. Some inhibitory techniques, if used too long, can trigger a reciprocal sympathetic response. It should also be noted that high-intensity cutaneous stimulation can cause a similar rebound phenomenon.

MYELINATION

Myelin is a spirally deposited, fatlike substance that wraps around the axons of rapidly conducting nerve fibers.[10] It is produced by Schwann and oligodendroglial cells. The myelin sheath is important to the function of the nervous system because it increases the velocity of the impulses up to 100 times.[8,69] Myelination begins relatively late in development, not until the end of the third fetal month. Many of the tracts in the nervous system myelinate at different times. The vestibulospinal tract, tectospinal tract, and reflex arc begin myelination by the end of the fifth month.[29] The corticospinal tracts, which are responsible for voluntary skilled movements, continue myelination into the second year. Some areas of the reticular formation and the cerebellum continue to myelinate into early adulthood. The association fibers of the cortex may continue to myelinate throughout life.

Most myelinated nerve fibers exist predominantly in the cranial and spinal nerves. Therefore unmyelinated fibers are more abundant in the autonomic nervous system.[95] Evidence suggests that sensory stimulation during the developmental years may improve the myelination process.[91]

DENDRITIC GROWTH

Dendrites are the small branches (spines) projecting from the cell body of a neuron. Dendrites form synaptic connections with other neurons and function as receivers. Greenough[45] has conducted definitive studies with animal models to demonstrate the importance of environmental stimuli on the developing brain. The studies have shown that sensory stimulation promotes dendritic growth.[27] It is postulated that the proliferation of dendrites contributes to intelligence and adaptive behavior in humans.[71]

Current studies on the neurobiology of learning and memory continue to suggest that environmental stimuli contribute to the development of dendritic growth in specific regions of the brain.[6,7,9] Studies on the limbic system imply that the dendrites in both the hippocampus and the amygdala are associated with memory and learning.[90] This proposal suggests that subcortical dendritic growth in the hippocampus contributes to procedural or emotional memory that has been linked to the amygdala.

Dendritic growth also occurs before birth. Laboratory studies of animals found that when pregnant rats were exposed to an enriched environment, their offspring showed 10% to 16% greater dendritic growth in the cerebral cortex.[27]

NEUROPLASTICITY

Recent neuroscientific studies have demonstrated that the CNS has some capacity to adapt or recover from traumatic injury.[6,81] The ability of neurons to adapt depends on (1) activation of latent neurons that may have been previously suppressed, (2) ability of neurons adjacent to the lesion to sprout collateral axons that form new synapses, and (3) changes in neurotransmitter sensitivity. For example, denervated muscles can develop increased sensitivity to neurotransmitters through anatomic, physiologic, or biochemical changes. This phenomenon may be part of an adaptive process to compensate for loss of innervation.[6,7,91]

Research has shown that hormones influence neuroplasticity.[60,88] In animal studies the male sex hormones manufactured in the testes (androgens) have been shown to influence neuronal development. These hormones have also been found to influence the organization of spinal motor neurons. Thus, the ability of the nervous system to adapt to traumatic injury may depend on many chemical and physical changes in neuronal architecture. To compensate for a lesion the damaged nervous system must be "forced" into recovery. Studies have shown that when the damaged system is forced into action, it recovers to a greater extent. For instance, animals with lesions and hemiparetic extremities have shown better recovery when the uninvolved limbs are restrained and the affected limbs are forced into use.[6,7]

NEUROPHYSIOLOGICAL BASES FOR THE SENSORIMOTOR APPROACHES TO TREATMENT

MOTOR AND SENSORY ORGANIZATION OF THE CENTRAL NERVOUS SYSTEM

We have only a rudimentary knowledge of how the human brain produces voluntary, controlled movement, and how sensory information is utilized effectively in determining our responses to various stimuli. Sensory information is critical in the initiation, and correct performance, of both voluntary and involuntary motor responses. The determinants of activity in motor neurons can be very broadly divided into three overlapping groups:

1. *built-in patterns* of neural connections (i.e., reflex circuitry)
2. *descending pathways* that modulate the activity of motor neurons either directly or indirectly, and which may modulate activity in sensory pathways
3. *higher centers* that influence the activity of descending pathways, and which themselves are modulated by activity in ascending sensory pathways.

Motor Organization
Spinal cord

The circuitry of the spinal cord regulates the more primitive, stereotypical movements. These movements can be generated from muscles (myotatic, or stretch, reflex) or from sensory receptors in the skin (pain). Spinal reflexes are "phasic" in that they occur rapidly and extinguish very fast. These reflexes are believed to be primitive responses to potentially harmful stimuli. Therefore a painful stimulus or quick stretch produces a spinal level response. The spinal level reflexes include (1) flexor withdrawal, (2) crossed extension, (3) extensor thrust, (4) positive supporting reaction, (5) negative supporting reaction, and (6) cutaneous fusimotor reflexes. These reflexes are fairly predictable when elicited in infants or persons with CNS lesions. They demonstrate the principles of reciprocal innervation and autogenic inhibition. They are evoked by primary and secondary endings in muscle spindles, Golgi tendon organs, and nonspecific cutaneous receptors.

Lower brain stem

Motor activity in the lower brain stem includes the nuclei in the medulla and the facilitative portion of the reticular formation. These centers have long-lasting effects on posture and therefore are called tonic reflexes. For example, the nuclei for the vestibular system are constantly discharging into motor neuron pools of the spinal cord to sustain head and body alignment. The static labyrinthine reflex arises from the vestibule (utricle and saccule), which responds during changes in head position and linear acceleration. The kinetic labyrinth includes the three semicircular canals and responds to head movement and rotatory motions.

Reflexes involving the vestibular apparatus and semicircular canals regulate muscle tone (especially extensors) and balance reactions. In tonic neck reflexes, facilitative influences are exerted on limbs and postural muscles in response to stretch imposed on the neck muscles. The tonic lumbar reflex arises from joint and muscle proprioceptors in the lumbar segments. This reflex has symmetric and asymmetric components. The symmetric response occurs when the trunk is ventroflexed, causing flexion of all four extremities, and dorsiflexed, causing extension of all four extremities. The asymmetric response is stimulated by rotation or lateral flexion of the trunk. Trunk rotation to one side results in flexion of the ipsilateral upper extremity and extension of the lower extremity. Simultaneously the contralateral upper extremity extends and the lower extremity flexes. The opposite effects may contribute to the normal reciprocal movements of the limbs during gait pattern. Lateral flexion of the trunk results in ipsilateral upper extremity flexion and lower extremity extension. The contralateral response produces extension of the upper extremity and flexion of the lower. Lower brain stem reflexes include (1) tonic labyrinthine reflexes (static or kinetic), (2) tonic neck reflexes (asymmetric or symmetric), and (3) tonic lumbar reflexes. These reflexes arise from the proprioceptors in the neck muscles and trunk and the receptor organs in the vestibular apparatus.

Upper brain stem

The upper brain stem includes the midbrain and the diencephalon (hypothalamus and thalamus). This level participates in "tonically" induced reflexes for more refined postural adjustments. Because these reflexes assist with the maintenance of the upright position, they are called the righting or displacement reactions.[22] The upper brain stem includes labyrinthine righting, neck righting, body-and-head righting, and body-on-body righting reactions.

Central (higher) control centers

The integrated circuits between the cerebral cortex, basal ganglia, and cerebellum supply an added dimension to posture and movement. Much research has been done to single out the functions of these structures. Although investigators are not in full agreement, the higher control centers seem to work as feedback circuits to initiate and refine higher level motor functions. In general, skilled voluntary movement arises from the cerebral cortex. Descending impulses send collaterals to both the basal ganglia and the cerebellum. The basal ganglia are involved with the regulation of the more rhythmic automatic movement patterns.[23] The cerebellum tends to monitor the rate, range, force, and direction of movement. Therefore once the voluntary movement has been initiated by the cortex, the subcortical structures refine and feed back information during the motor act.[20,23]

The roles of the various regions of the human nervous system in motor activity do not subscribe solely to a linear or segmental organization.[36] In one sense, the components are organized hierarchically, as though premotor areas devise the plan for movement (based on incoming sensory data) and pass the information on to the motor cortex, which in turn issues motor commands down descending pathways. In another sense the components are organized in parallel, much as in the case of sensory pathways. Messages are conveyed to motor circuitry in the spinal cord not only from the motor cortex but also from premotor areas themselves. The cerebellum and basal ganglia are involved in various aspects of planning and monitoring movements but have no outputs of their own to the spinal cord. They act primarily by affecting motor and premotor areas of the cortex.

This extremely simplified overview of the central motor apparatus downplays the important role of sensory regulation of motor activity. The segmental approach has merit for helping to determine the origins of pathological signs and symptoms, either in motor-related structures (an example is Parkinson disease affecting the basal ganglia) or in sensory mechanisms (an example is ataxia from disease of the dorsal columns). Recent information suggests that the nervous system functions more holistically through resonance rather than segmental connection. Individual differences also need to be considered. No two nervous systems are entirely alike; each brain has its own uniqueness and functional signature.

Sensory Organization

Many of the techniques of the sensorimotor approaches to treatment are aimed at stimulating specific receptors and tract systems. There are four major tract systems through which sensory input travels from the periphery to the brain.[13,71]

Spinothalamic

The spinothalamic pathway has two major components. The *anterior spinothalamic* pathway conducts impulses related to the sensations of light, poorly localized (protopathic) touch. It is characterized by large, diffuse receptive fields, with poor localization and less precise qualities of tactile sensations. The *lateral spinothalamic* pathway is a phylogenetically newer tract in mammals and provides very precise sensation of pain and temperature. The distinction between anterior and lateral spinothalamic paths is now thought to have little anatomical significance; nor is their differentiation clearly defined functionally. The spinothalamic pathways as a whole can be considered to be involved in very sharp, precisely localized temperature sensations and "fast" pain (neospinothalamic path), poorly localized, aching "slow" pain (paleospinothalamic path), crude touch (protopathic touch), and visceral pain (spinoreticular path).

The first order neuron of this system enters the lateral portion of the dorsal horn of the spinal cord and synapses with interneurons. A second order neuron crosses to the opposite side of the cord and ascends in the spinothalamic tract to the thalamus. From the thalamus a third order neuron carries information to specific areas of the cerebral cortex. An important feature of this system is that it gives off numerous collaterals to the reticular activating system and other components of the reticular formation.[5,83,93] The third order neuron continues its ascent from the reticular formation to nonspecific nuclei of the thalamus. From there, other neurons terminate diffusely within many areas of the cerebral cortex. This second system involving the reticular formation may be the mechanism for dull pain coming from the viscera, poorly localized pain, and our emotional responses to pain because of cortical connections within the limbic system. In summary, the spinothalamic system serves a protective function that is both precise in localization and excitatory to the cortex because of its many collaterals in the reticular formation.

Lemniscal (dorsal columns)

The second system is phylogenetically advanced and is called epicritic because it has a high degree of specificity and carries discriminative sensory information. Anatomically, these sensory tracts occupy the dorsal funiculus of the spinal cord and are called the *lemniscal system,* or *dorsal columns.*[20] The lemniscal system contains fibers from the A alpha (group I) and A beta (group II) classifications. Because this system contains well-myelinated, thick fibers with few collaterals, it is a fast conducting system. The lemniscal system carries impulses from the discriminative receptors (Meissner corpuscles, pacinian corpuscles, and Ruffini end organs). Therefore this system mediates stereognosis, 2-point discrimination, pressure, vibration, and other senses of fine recognition, as well as conscious proprioception.

The lemniscal system is well defined. The first order neurons enter the medial portion of the dorsal root and ascend in the dorsal columns of the cord on the same side they enter. These fibers give off few collaterals to the reticular formation and synapse on the gracile and cuneate nuclei of the medulla. From the medulla, the second order neurons cross the midline and ascend to the ventral posterolateral nucleus of the thalamus. The third order neuron from the thalamus terminates in areas 3, 1, and 2 of the somatosensory cortex.[5,83,93]

Proprioceptive

The unconscious proprioceptive tracts make up the third sensory pathway. Proprioception refers to the conscious or unconscious awareness of body position and movement of bodily segments. The proprioceptive pathways are of particular interest to the occupational therapist because they regulate movements toward purposeful activities. Conscious proprioception is regulated by the lemniscal (dorsal column) system. This pathway begins in joint receptors and ends in the parietal lobe of the cerebral cortex where conscious awareness takes place. Conscious proprioception enables the cortex to refine voluntary movements for skillful activities.[22,35]

Unconscious proprioception is mediated by the spinocerebellar tracts. This pathway begins in the afferents of the muscle spindle and Golgi tendon organ and terminates in the cerebellum. Unconscious proprioception is concerned with muscle tension, muscle length, and speed of movement. The spinocerebellar tracts do not ascend to the cortex.[93] The cerebellum serves as a feedback mechanism for the motor cortex, however, so it can modify or correct voluntary movements as they are being initiated.[22]

Trigeminal

The trigeminal nerve (CN V) can be considered the fourth major sensory tract. The trigeminal nerve is unique in many ways, because it combines the functions of the lemniscal system, the spinothalamic system, and spinocerebellar systems into one nerve that serves the head, neck, and face. It is responsible for direct transmission of tactile, proprioceptive, pain, and temperature sensation in the skin of the facial region. (The posterior of the head and neck is supplied by C2, C3, and C4 of the cervical spinal roots).[13,83,95] Therefore the trigeminal nerve transmits information directly to brain stem sensory nuclei that are connected to the reticular formation, cerebellum, and thalamus, as are the other sensory pathways. Because the nerve supplies a large territory, its afferent fibers are separated into ophthalmic, maxillary, and mandibular divisions.

The trigeminal nerve is one of the earliest sensory roots to myelinate and respond to touch stimulation. Stimulation to the perioral area evokes a protective avoiding reaction at 7½ fetal weeks. The discriminative receptors begin their development and differentiation at about the fourth fetal month.[20] Because of the nerve's early ontogenetic development, some therapists using sensorimotor treatment approaches begin cutaneous stimulation to the trigeminal nerve. The motor branch of the trigeminal nerve supplies the muscles of mastication, the tensor tympani muscle of the ear, and the tensor veli palatini muscle of the soft palate.[23,55]

Dermatomes

With the exception of the facial region (covered by three branches of the trigeminal nerve), the skin of the body receives its sensory innervation in a segmental fashion by nerve roots of the spinal cord. The area of skin supplied by a single dorsal root and its ganglion constitutes a dermatome.[68] The dermatomes are arranged on the surface of the body in a sequence corresponding to the related spinal cord segments. Cutaneously, the highest dermatomal level represents the posterior of the head, whereas the lowest is in the anal region.[13] Fig. 20-3 shows the segmental arrangement of dermatomes from the neck down to the anal region. There is much overlap in the

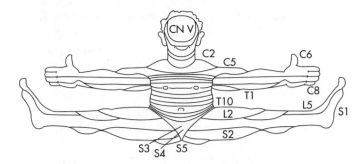

FIG. 20-3   Dermatomes (segmental levels).

segmental borders of the dermatomes, particularly in the trunk.

It is important for the occupational therapist to have a fundamental understanding of dermatomal segments. The spinal nerve that innervates each sensory dermatome also has a motor component for the respective segment. With respect to sensory functions, all areas of the skin are not alike. For example, the facial area and the volar surface of the hands contain a greater number of discriminative tactile receptors than the trunk. Dermatomes are important in evaluating the integrity of peripheral nerves and the spinal cord segments. In many cases cutaneous stimulation is applied dermatomally in an effort to activate selected myotomes or muscle groups.[44]

Receptors

The body contains many types of sensory receptors (end organs) that provide information about changes in the immediate environment. These end organs can be viewed therapeutically as portals through which stimuli can be systematically programmed into the nervous system. Although this information on sensory receptors is incomplete, it is important for the occupational therapist to have a basic understanding of the characteristics that these receptors possess. For the purposes of sensorimotor therapy, sensory receptors are classified into three categories in this discussion: (1) interoceptors, (2) exteroceptors, and (3) proprioceptors.

Interoceptors

Interoceptors monitor events within the body and are located within the walls of the respiratory, cardiovascular, gastrointestinal, and genitourinary systems.[95] Interoceptors can detect a variety of stimuli, such as distention of a cavity wall, or monitor pH levels in the bloodstream. Many interoceptors are activated during therapeutic activities.

The carotid sinus is a baroreceptor located in the walls of the carotid artery.[35,43] It is stimulated by blood pressure changes and linked to the parasympathetic nervous system. In therapy it is brought into action during inversion techniques.[29] Whenever the head approaches a position below the level of the shoulders, the increase in blood pressure distends the carotid sinus and fires impulses along the glossopharyngeal nerve (CN IX) to cardiovascular inhibitory centers of the vagus nerve, which in turn slows heart rate and reduces blood pressure.

This arrangement is a negative feedback system that must be used with caution. Clinicians have used the carotid sinus to reduce hypertension and to produce a state of generalized inhibition. The process of lowering the head below the level of the shoulders may also affect the chemistry of the brain.[57,97] There may indeed be many neurophysiologic advantages to the inverted position. It alleviates the gravitational forces on the vertebral column; it increases blood flow to the brain and facial muscles; and it promotes postural drainage of the venous, lymphatic, and respiratory systems.[46,71,86]

The mucous membranes of the oral cavity provide another area in which interoceptors are used for therapeutic intervention. The gums around the teeth are rich in sensory innervation from the trigeminal nerve.[43,95] The mucous membranes contain receptors that are stimulated by several modalities, such as temperature, touch, stretch, and taste. Stimulation to this area discharges impulses to the brain stem via the sensory components of the trigeminal nerve (CN V), facial nerve (CN VII), glossopharyngeal nerve (CN IX), and vagus nerve (CN X).[13] Occupational therapists use oral stimulation primarily for functional activities of daily living that are related to feeding.

Therapists have used cutaneous stimulation and vibration to affect the interoceptors in the wall of the bladder or detrusor muscle to facilitate or inhibit the micturition reflex. Stimulation has been applied dermatomally or to the skin directly over the bladder.[29] Montagu[66] describes the importance of sensory stimulation to the skin around the genitourinary organs in mammals. Shortly after birth, the mother cleans the neonate by licking. The stimulus is important to the development of normal bowel and bladder evacuation. A similar phenomenon has been observed in human children. Cutaneous stimulation over dermatome S2 on children with delayed sphincter control seems to alleviate bed-wetting and "accidents." These techniques should not be used without proper understanding of neurophysiology or supervision by a physician.

The use of temperature input is another way interoceptors are used in sensorimotor techniques. Neutral warmth and icing techniques not only influence cutaneous receptors but act on thermoregulatory centers in the spinal cord, brain stem, and hypothalamus.[12,83,95] Temperature input has been used primarily to reduce hypertonicity in skeletal muscles or for symptomatic pain. However, children exhibiting "tactile defensiveness" may benefit from a regimen that combines neutral warmth and skin exposure to cooler temperatures. The process needs further research but a systematic regimen of temperature changes should affect the receptors in

the hypothalamus, causing an increased threshold level to cutaneous stimuli.[29,82,83]

Exteroceptors

Exteroceptors are found immediately under the skin in the external mucous membranes or in special sense organs.[73,95] These receptors respond to stimuli that arise outside the body. Exteroceptors vary tremendously in their structure, function, and reaction to mechanical stimuli. Following is a brief summary of the primary cutaneous exteroceptors.

Free nerve endings. The subcutaneous tissues are richly innervated by free nerve endings. These are unencapsulated receptors with projecting, unmyelinated branches for sensory detection. Free nerve endings are widely distributed in the skin and viscera. They are thought to be nonspecific receptors for pain, crude touch, and temperature.[1] The free nerve endings associated with pain outnumber other receptors along the midline axis of the body.[71] Free nerve endings transmit impulses by way of unmyelinated C nerve fibers to the spinothalamic tracts (slow pain), others via myelinated faster conducting fibers (fast pain).[13] In general the free nerve endings involved with touch are rapidly adapting. Those that are associated with chronic pain syndromes are slowly adapting.[12,34,71] For therapeutic purposes free nerve endings are activated with thermal or brushing techniques and elicit primitive protective responses. Stimulation to free nerve endings can also cause states of arousal.[53] Also, some evidence supports the theory that forms of cutaneous stimulation such as ice packs and rubbing over the surface of the skin can alleviate acute pain.[34,63,64] It is also believed that free nerve endings, along with other receptors, can synapse with gamma motor neurons and bias the muscle spindle.

Hair end organs. Hair end organs are actually a type of free nerve ending that wraps around the base of a hair follicle.[73] These receptor organs are activated by the bending or displacement of hair. They are rapidly adapting and transmit impulses predominantly along A delta-size (group III) fibers.[71] In therapy, hair receptors are stimulated during light touch or stroking of the skin. Although they are rapidly adapting, hair end organs discharge into neuron pools that reach the reticular system and probably bias the muscle spindle through the fusimotor system. Part of the more primitive nervous system, hair end organs were used by our ancestors as sensory receptors to alert them to stimuli in close proximity to the skin.[39] In addition, they are neurologically related to the autonomic nervous system. Because primitive man had much more hair on the surface of his body, it acted as an insulator to the cold. When they were chilled, the arrector pili muscles attached to the hair follicles caused the hairs to fluff up and provide a thicker surface to contain body heat. Today the reminiscences of the hair follicles are seen as goose bumps when the body is exposed to cold.[74]

Meissner corpuscles. Meissner corpuscles are elongated, encapsulated end organs found just beneath the epidermis in hairless (glabrous) skin. Meissner corpuscles are the most superficial of all the cutaneous receptors. They are particularly abundant in the skin of the fingertips, tip of the tongue, lips, and pads of the feet.[93] Histologic studies show that these receptors maintain a close relationship with the skin. They are abundant on the fingertips of the hand and are arranged on the ridges of skin that make up the fingerprints.[91,93,95] The corpuscles are primarily rapidly adapting receptors that transmit along the thicker A beta (group II) fibers. Meissner corpuscles are largely responsible for fine tactile discrimination. They are very important in digital exploration and sensory substitution skills, such as reading braille. These receptors transmit discriminatory messages to the somatosensory cortex by way of the dorsal columns of the spinal cord.[73,93] Meissner corpuscles are rapidly adapting receptors with a small receptive field. They have also been found to be responsive to low frequency vibration.[25]

Pacinian corpuscles. Pacinian corpuscles are the largest encapsulated receptors (about the size of grains of rice) and are almost as widely distributed as free nerve endings. They are located in the deep layers of the skin —in viscera, mesenteries, ligaments, near blood vessels —and are embedded in the periosteum of long bones.[33,71] Histologic studies have shown that pacinian corpuscles are plentiful on the lateral margins of the digits but scarce in the central aspect of the palm of the hand and on the dorsum of the hand. Pacinian corpuscles are probably the most rapidly adapting receptors in the body.[73] They respond to deep pressure but are amazingly sensitive to slight indentations in the skin.[91] Pacinian corpuscles also discharge with a steady train of impulses when exposed to high frequency vibration. Therefore with vibratory stimuli the pacinian corpuscle is a slowly adapting receptor. Although the pacinian corpuscle fires when vibrated, it has not been demonstrated to play a role in the tonic vibration reflex.[45,93]

The pacinian discharges along fast-conducting A beta (group II) fibers to the dorsal columns of the spinal cord. Stimulation to a single corpuscle in the skin can excite an area of the postcentral gyrus of the cortex. It may also contribute to the inhibition of muscles when pressure is applied over tendinous insertions.[29] Furthermore, the pacinian corpuscle may play a role in the desensitization of hypersensitive skin in children who exhibit tactile defensiveness.[5] Research has shown that the pacinian corpuscle can suppress pain perception at the cutaneous level.[62,71]

Because the pacinian corpuscles transmit sensory impulses along thick fibers and synapse in the spinal cord at the substantia gelatinosa, they may indeed cause a condition of overload at this junction. According to the gate control theory, pain impulses travel along thin fibers and also synapse in the substantia gelatinosa. Also, increased sensory input carried along thick fibers can block the transmission of pain impulses that are carried along thin fibers.[63,64]

The hands, the soles of the feet, and the mesentery of the abdomen contain an abundance of pacinian corpuscles. Thus the sole of the foot and hand might be an excellent target area when using vibratory stimuli for sensory stimulation. The stimulation should be done with low frequency vibration and light pressure so that the positive supporting reaction is not elicited.

It has been observed in sensory integrative therapy that deep pressure and vibratory stimuli have a calming effect on children with attention deficit disorders.[5] It also appears that the pacinian corpuscles play a major role in this calming effect because they transmit impulses into the dorsal columns, which send fewer impulses into the excitatory cells of the reticular activating system. The dorsal columns also terminate in the cerebral cortex where synapses are made with association fibers and inhibitory networks.[71,86]

Merkel tactile disks. Merkel tactile disks are nonencapsulated receptors found in the deepest layer of the epidermis in hairless skin. These receptors are located most abundantly on the volar surface of the fingers, lips, and external genitalia. Merkel tactile disks are slowly adapting touch-pressure receptors. They transmit along A beta (group II) myelinated fibers.[73,93] These receptors are very sensitive to slow movements across the skin's surface. They have been related to the sense of tickle and pleasurable touch sensations.[91]

Proprioceptors

Proprioceptors monitor the awareness of position in space, posture, movement, and equilibrium reactions. These receptors are found in muscles, tendons, and joints. The process of proprioception can be conscious or subconscious. Conscious proprioceptors are discussed under kinesioceptors (joint receptors). Subconscious proprioception pertains to information received from muscle spindles, Golgi tendon organs, and the vestibular apparatus. Subconscious proprioception derived from Golgi tendon organs and muscle spindles transmits to the cerebellum. The vestibular apparatus may have connections to the cerebral cortex.[93]

Golgi tendon organs. Golgi tendon organs (GTO) are spindle-shaped receptors found in the musculotendinous region of the proximal and distal insertions.[10] In the past the GTO was believed to be a high-threshold protective receptor designed to inform the nervous system when muscle tension was reaching damaging proportions. More recent evidence has shown that the GTO has a greater sensitivity to muscle contraction.[62,69] Therefore it more specifically monitors the tendon tension and perhaps the force produced by muscle contraction rather than by muscle tension produced by stretch. In addition, the GTO appears to complement the action of the muscle spindle. For example, during isometric contraction of the biceps brachii, tendon tension is developed, and the GTO discharges (action potential). In contrast, the muscle spindle remains relatively silent because muscle length has not changed. If the same muscle (biceps brachii) is completely relaxed and passively stretched (elbow extended), the muscle spindle fires, and the GTO remains relatively silent because little tension is put on the tendon. Therefore the GTO and muscle spindle work collaboratively to inform the nervous system about the muscle length and tension.[73]

The GTO transmits along A beta (Ib) afferent fibers. It is a slowly adapting receptor that discharges at a rate nearly proportional to the tension of muscle contraction.[62] With respect to spinal reflexes the GTO is associated with autogenic inhibition,[46] which means that it can cause inhibition of the primary muscle that is contracting against resistance. This response occurs because the Ib fiber synapses with inhibitory interneurons in the spinal cord, which causes inhibition of the anterior horn cells that innervate the contracting muscle. Clinically, this phenomenon is seen as a sudden lengthening reaction.[22,40] It is commonly seen in patients with spasticity and is called the clasp-knife phenomenon.[23]

Golgi tendon organs are used to inhibit spasticity in adductors and superficial flexor muscles. This effect is obtained by teaching the patient to produce very small range contractions of the spastic muscle and its antagonist. Gravity should be eliminated, and small contractions should be done in several repetitions. A stimulus such as therapeutic vibration can be applied over the muscle bellies of the antagonistic abductor and extensor groups to promote isotonic contractions.[28] Other joint receptors may also contribute to this phenomenon.[68]

Muscle spindles. Muscle spindles are complex, encapsulated receptors that lie deep within skeletal muscle. Their principal function is to monitor changes in length of a muscle and the rate at which the length changes.[73]

Anatomically, the muscle spindle is a slender, encapsulated structure that houses four to six bundles of specialized muscle fibers called intrafusal muscle fibers (Fig. 20-4). There are two types of intrafusal fibers: nuclear chain and nuclear bag fibers.[4] Nuclear bag fibers have an enlarged, noncontractile central region containing many nuclei and tapered, contractile (plate) endings. The nuclear chain fibers are smaller and contain a single row of nuclei in the equatorial region. The muscle spindle receives motor innervation from gamma motor neurons.[65] The intrafusal fibers do not contribute to extrafusal muscle strength or joint movement but regulate the tension in the muscle spindle.[61] Hence, as the extrafusal fibers

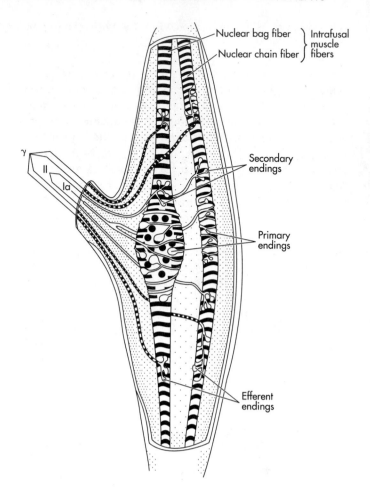

FIG. 20-4　Muscle spindle (sensory and motor attachments). (From Nolte J: *The human brain: an introduction to its functional anatomy,* St Louis, 1981, CV Mosby.)

contract, the intrafusal fibers contract concurrently to maintain some tension in the equatorial region and restore its sensitivity to stretch. In summary, the gamma motor neurons regulate the tension of the intrafusal fibers so that their sensitivity remains constant as the extrafusal fibers change their length.[4,62,85] (Fig. 20-5).

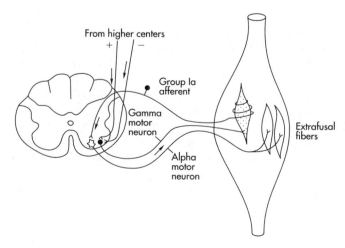

FIG. 20-5　Gamma loop (added gamma neuron to reflex arc).

The muscle spindle also contains two types of sensory endings. The first type is called the Ia primary fiber (annulospiral ending), which bifurcates within the spindle and wraps around the equatorial regions of both the nuclear bag and the nuclear chain. Because of this spiral arrangement, the Ia primary afferent is stretched like a spring when the equatorial region of the intrafusal muscle elongates. The Ia primary ending has a low threshold and is selectively sensitive to the onset of muscle stretch. The Ia primary afferent may be subdivided into phasic and tonic functions.[53] Therefore whenever the muscle is put through a quick stretch within normal range, it fires the Ia phasic component. The Ia tonic component is believed to originate around the nuclear chain fiber. Therefore the Ia tonic component is less sensitive to quick stretch but fires when the stretch is maintained in the submaximal range.[4,62,85]

A second afferent fiber wraps around the nuclear bag and nuclear chain adjacent to the equatorial region (predominantly on the nuclear chain fibers). This fiber was originally called the flower-spray ending because of its appearance. It is now called the secondary ending or group II fiber. The function of the secondary endings is not fully understood.[46] Classically, secondary endings are less sensitive to the onset of stretch but fire during maintained stretch, especially when the muscle is elongated to its maximal range[39,73] (Table 20-3). In classical theory, however, maintained stretch fires the secondary endings and produces facilitation of the flexor and inhibition of the extensor regardless of which muscle receives the stretch.[53]

The problem with this principle is determining which muscles are the physiologic flexors and which are the anatomic flexors. For example, by definition a physiologic extensor serves to elongate an extremity. Subsequently, if a person assumes the quadruped position with the palms of the hands flat on the floor and flexes the wrist, the forelimbs are elongated; physiologically, this elongation represents extension. Physiologic extensors can be regarded as "antigravity" muscles. In quadrupeds, anatomic extensors of the four limbs are also physiologic extensors (elongating the limb). In primates and humans, because of our arboreal evolution before ground dwelling, anatomic extensors of the lower limb are also physiologic extensors, but the upper limb is reversed. The anatomic flexors are equivalent to physiologic extensors, because they act against gravity (in tree-climbing). The relationship between extension of the lower limb and flexion of the upper limb probably contributes to position of the limbs assumed after a debilitating stroke.

The primary spinal level reflex associated with the muscle spindle is reciprocal innervation. This reflex is a basic stretch reflex in which one muscle group is facilitated and the opposing muscles are inhibited.[82] For example, when the biceps is stretched, it is facilitated, and the antagonist muscle (the triceps) is inhibited. This relationship is called reciprocal inhibition.[46,93]

Therapists have used the reflex functions of the muscle spindle in a number of ways. Because the Ia primary ending has a low threshold, it can be fired by quick stretch, vibration, tapping over the muscle belly, or any action that causes elongation of the extrafusal fibers.[37] The results are usually the same. The muscle receiving the stimulus is facilitated and the antagonist inhibited. The properties of the muscle spindle have been described in isolation. Yet in reality whenever a muscle is stretched or contracted, a multitude of skin and joint receptors are firing concurrently.

In addition, the person's emotional state affects the resting threshold of the muscle spindle. Emotional tension increases spasticity in persons with neurologic impairments. Other factors affecting the resting threshold of the muscle spindle are pain syndromes, gravitational forces or position in space, cold environments, distention in the bowel or bladder, excessive auditory stimuli, and medications such as muscle relaxants.[22,28,30,85] Therefore, many factors can affect the muscle spindle. The therapist should eliminate as many variables as possible before applying inhibitory and facilitative techniques.

Kinesioceptors

Kinesioceptors are joint receptors that represent the conscious division of proprioception because they transmit to the cerebral cortex. Anatomically, joint receptors are located in joint capsules, ligaments, and tendons. These include Ruffini end organs, Golgi-Mazzoni corpuscles, Vater-Pacini corpuscles, Golgi-type endings, and free nerve endings.

Ruffini end organs. Ruffini end organs are both joint receptors and cutaneous receptors. Many Ruffini receptors are found in the walls of the joint capsules.[93] These receptors respond vigorously at the beginning of joint movement, but their discharge rate declines in midrange and increases at the extremes of joint range. The current understanding of these receptors is that they fire when the skin is stretched and contribute little to proprioception because they monitor end points of joint range of motion and do not respond to midrange positions.[95]

TABLE 20-3	Muscle Spindle	
AFFERENT FIBERS		
Type Ia	Static (tonic)	Spiral endings
	Dynamic (phasic)	Nuclear bag fibers
Type II	Secondary endings	Polar endings
EFFERENT FIBERS		**TRAIL ENDINGS**
Static gamma		Chain fibers mainly
Dynamic gamma		Plate endings
		Bag fibers
B fibers alpha and gamma coactivation		
Alpha motorneuron		Extrafusal fibers

Golgi-Mazzoni corpuscles. Golgi-Mazzoni corpuscles are similar in appearance to pacinian corpuscles. They are small, encapsulated receptors found in joint capsules and tendon surfaces.[93,95] It is interesting to note that the Golgi-Mazzoni receptors are abundant in the connective tissues of the hands. These are rapidly adapting receptors that detect rapid joint movements.[73] They also discharge under deep pressure or vibratory stimuli.[62]

Vater-Pacini corpuscles. Vater-Pacini corpuscles are found in joint capsules and ligaments. They discharge at a greater rate as the joint reaches its maximal range of motion.[62] These receptors may serve a protective function to inform the cortex when the joint has reached its end position of range.

Golgi-Type endings. Golgi-type endings are a variation of the Golgi tendon organ found mostly in the joint ligaments. These receptors seem to monitor the rate of joint movement. They are slowly adapting and discharge most rapidly when joint movement is initiated.[13,93]

Free nerve endings support the joint receptors by providing a crude awareness of joint movement. Free nerve endings also mediate touch, pain, and temperature sensations in the joint region.[95]

The major function of joint receptors is to inform the nervous system about joint position, velocity of movement, and perhaps the direction of movement. At this time there is no evidence that joint receptors contribute to the force of muscle contraction.[73] Joint receptors supply the conscious awareness of joint position and joint movement.

As a group, joint receptors provide another means of sensory input. The therapist should incorporate activities that stress active range of motion and voluntary effort. Active movement generates much more neurologic activity. It requires a collaborative effort of receptors in the skin muscles and joints and sends a multitude of sensory stimuli to assemblies of neurons at the cortical level.

The proprioceptors provide conscious and unconscious awareness of proprioception through the lemniscal system and spinocerebellar pathways. While the lemniscal system is concerned solely with conscious proprioception, the spinocerebellar pathway, concerned mainly with unconscious proprioception, may also provide information to conscious pathways.

Cutaneous Reflex

An important concept in sensory stimulation is the existence of the cutaneous fusimotor reflex. This reflex was first demonstrated on polio patients by Kenny and later substantiated by Hagbarth.[47,57] In essence, studies have found that stimulation to certain areas of the skin can influence the specific muscles of the body. The cutaneous reflex is not a simple monosynaptic reflex arc. Instead, it is a polysynaptic system that entails cutaneous afferents, gamma motor neurons, and Ia afferents of the muscle spindle. Any stimulation to a dermatome discharges cutaneous receptors that synapse with gamma motor neurons at the same spinal segment in the ventral horn of the spinal cord. The gamma motor neurons cause intrafusal fibers to contract, causing the Ia afferents to discharge, which in turn sends impulses back into the spinal cord where they synapse with alpha motor neurons. If the stimulus is strong enough to cause the alpha motor neuron to discharge, a reflexive contraction or increase in tone occurs in the muscle innervated at that segmental level.

The activity of the cutaneous receptors and the gamma system is proportional to the intensity of the stimuli.[47,57] It should be emphasized, however, that the cutaneous stimulus should be applied to the dermatome that corresponds to the muscles to be activated. This technique seems to work best on the dermatomes that overlie the muscles to be activated. In patients with spinal cord injury or with CNS lesions, the response may be exaggerated because the supraspinal centers are detached or the excitatory neurons are disinhibited.

Special Sense Mechanisms

The special senses may be used in sensorimotor techniques, but specific procedures are limited. The following discussion outlines some of the salient features of the special sense organs and how they might be used in therapy.

Olfactory

The physiologic components of the olfactory system are not well understood. There are many theories about how smell is transduced into neuronal messages, but the scientific facts are somewhat limited. Basically, olfaction is a chemical process.[53] The receptors for smell are located in specialized epithelium in the roof of the nasal cavity. The olfactory epithelium contains three types of cells and small glands that secrete mucous substances for dissolving odorous materials. The receptor cells contain fine hairlike cilia, which are the most exposed nerve endings in the entire body. The olfactory epithelium is estimated to contain 100 million receptor cells, yet it occupies an area only the size of a dime.[35,46] The afferent fibers from these cells converge with the second order neurons in a ratio of 1000:1.[1]

The receptor cells for olfaction respond to a variety of stimuli. Some sources indicate that humans can distinguish between 2000 to 4000 different odors.[71] Each of these odors may generate different impulses from the olfactory receptors and pass directly to many regions of the brain. The principal regions are the temporal lobe of the cortex (area 28), structures in the limbic system, and subcortical nuclei and autonomic nuclei of the hypothalamus.[35,71] Furthermore, olfaction is the only sensory modality that bypasses the thalamus en route to the cortex.[43] So if the thalamus is damaged, olfactory stimulation can still reach certain portions of the CNS.

When using olfactory stimuli, the therapist should keep in mind that the receptors for smell adapt rather quickly. As many as 50% cease firing after the first few seconds of stimulation.[53] Therefore the strength of the odor has to be increased by about 30% to reactivate the adapted receptors. To allow for adaptation the therapist can use three vials of the same scent, each one containing a concentration 30% greater than the first. The therapist should start with a diluted scent first, then a solution of 60%, and last a solution of full strength. This process increases the times that the therapist can use a given scent for olfactory stimulation. Consequently, some noxious chemicals, such as ammonia and vinegar, cause irritation of the mucous linings in the nasal cavity, thereby causing more activity in the trigeminal nerve rather than the olfactory nerve. These odors are more useful for stimulating avoidance reactions or facial expressions. It should also be noted that olfactory stimuli go directly into the amygdala of the limbic system.[13,46,82,95] Responses to olfactory stimuli may also elicit emotional responses or primal behaviors associated with survival.

Gustatory

Gustation or taste is also a chemical process. However, the act of eating is a multisensory experience that uses somatosensory receptors as well. The taste receptors are located in the tongue, soft palate, and upper regions of the throat.[71] The tongue contains three different types of taste buds that occupy specific locations. Basically there are four primary taste sensations: sweet, sour, salty, and bitter. Many flavors are combinations of the four taste sensations,[84] but action potentials show the base of the tongue responds best to bitter, the outer edges to sour and salty, and the tip to sweet.[55]

The taste receptors transmit along the fibers of four cranial nerves: the glossopharyngeal (IX), trigeminal (V), facial (VII), and vagus (X). These cranial nerves transmit to nuclei in the brain stem, reticular formation, spinal and cranial reflex centers, thalamus, and regions of the parietal lobe of the cortex.[71,72]

Before beginning gustatory stimulation the therapist should evaluate swallowing and the gag reflexes to see if the glossopharyngeal (IX) and vagus (X) nerves are intact. Gustatory discrimination is similar to olfaction because it adapts readily and requires about a 30% change in concentration to distinguish differences.[45,82] Also, before a substance can be tasted, it must be somewhat water soluble. Therefore the therapist can use one of each primary flavor mixed in distilled water so the concentrations can be graded from weak to strong. Again the first solution should contain a 1:3 ratio, that is, one part flavor and three parts distilled water.

Three vials can be mixed for each taste stimulus. The second vial can contain a solution 30% stronger than the first, and the last can be full strength. These solutions can be applied to the tongue with an eye dropper so they contact specific portions of the tongue. For example, the sweet flavor can be made with low calorie sweeteners and distilled water. In this case the drops would be applied to the tip of the tongue. The sour taste can be made with vinegar and distilled water and applied to the middle sides of the tongue. Salt flavor can be made with table salt or sodium fluoride and applied to the anterior edges of the tongue.[12,71] Because bitter tastes are detected in lower concentrations and can trigger avoidance reactions, they should be used last. In addition, sour and bitter tastes may also elicit taste reflexes that stimulate the parotid and submaxillary glands to secrete saliva. This approach is a natural way of promoting swallowing, but it may dilute the taste stimuli.

Auditory

The auditory system enables the perception of events that are taking place at a distance. This sophisticated sense transduces sound waves into mechanical energy and ultimately neuronal impulses. The receptor cells for audition are housed in the cochlea in a structure called the organ of Corti.[13,71] This structure contains hair cells similar in appearance to the cells in the vestibular system. The impulses from the receptor cells pass along nerve fibers of the spiral ganglion through the nerve root of cranial nerve VIII to special nuclei in the superior portion of the medulla. Second order neurons project to the contralateral side of the brain stem or ascend ipsilaterally to the olivary and accessory nuclei. Still other collaterals synapse on neurons in the reticular system or ascend by way of the lateral lemniscus to the inferior colliculus. Third order neurons ascend to the medial geniculate body and then to the auditory cortex (Brodmann area 41).[10]

The auditory system has its own set of reflexes that are related to protective behavior. It connects to the reticular formation and evokes responses in the autonomic nervous system. In the midbrain the inferior colliculi feed into the tectospinal tract. This system is activated by sudden sounds, such as a car backfiring. Such a sound transmits auditory input to centers believed to trigger reflexive movements of the head, neck, and upper extremities.

The auditory system may be used with moderation in therapy, which does not imply that the therapist should use sudden sound stimuli to evoke reflex responses. Auditory stimuli feed into motor neuron pools that influence postural reflexes; the auditory stimuli going to the reticular formation may produce excitatory or inhibitory states, depending on the nature of the sound. For example, a novel sound stimulus tends to be excitatory. A constant sound stimulus, such as the waves of the ocean or city traffic, is suppressed by the reticular system. Soft melodic music is said to be restful, whereas "hard rock" music has an excitatory effect.

Some therapists use the sound of their voice as an inhibitory or excitatory stimulus. If the activity is designed to promote movement, the therapist can use simple, somewhat sharp, one-word commands, such as "reach," "pull," "stop," or "look." On the other hand, if the activity is designed to be inhibitory, the therapist should speak to the patient in a soft monotone. This approach is particularly helpful for elderly patients who have difficulty hearing sounds of high-pitched frequencies. Background music can be very beneficial with certain patient populations.[3,24,38]

Visual

The visual system is one of the most relied-on senses for orientation in space. Vision is a remarkable biochemical process that transduces light stimuli into neuronal impulses. Basically light is an electromagnetic energy that passes through the lens of the eye to be cast on the retina. The retina is actually an extension of the brain. It is composed of specialized receptor cells (rods and cones) and photopigments that absorb the light stimulus, causing an action potential, and impulses are conducted along visual pathways.[1,10]

The visual pathway projects posteriorly to form the fiber tracts of cranial nerve II where it becomes the optic nerve. The visual pathway can be very confusing because the retina of each eye contains fibers from the nasal portion that cross at the optic chiasm. The fibers arising from the temporal portions of each retina do not cross at the optic chiasm but continue uninterrupted to the lateral geniculate bodies of the thalamus. From this juncture the fibers proceed posteriorly until they terminate on the occipital lobes of the cortex. The visual cortex is composed of Brodmann area 17, which is the visual receptive area. Areas 18 and 19 are believed to be involved with visual reflexes and visual perception. Area 8 in the frontal lobe is associated with voluntary eye movements.[28]

The visual system mediates a number of protective and postural reflexes. For example, connections to the superior colliculus mediate reflexes for quick localization of potentially harmful stimuli. Connections to cranial nerves III, IV, VI, and the vestibular apparatus provide a stabilizing influence on the eyes during head rotation. Other visual reflexes may include the light reflex, visual fixation, convergence, accommodation, pupillary constriction, blinking, and ciliospinal reflex.[1,13] Much evidence suggests that the visual motor system is linked to chains of motor neurons that modulate posture and movement.[71] In essence the extraocular muscles direct the eyes toward a stimulus in the periphery. If the eyes are turned laterally to converge on the object in the visual field, the head rotates in an effort to center the eyes. Rotation of the neck sets off a volley of postural responses (tonic neck and righting reactions) that attempt to realign the trunk with the neck. Therefore the eyes lead, the head follows, and the trunk and limbs adjust accordingly.

Vestibular apparatus

The vestibular apparatus is classified as a proprioceptive organ.[23] It consists of three semicircular canals attached to a vestibule, which is further subdivided into the saccule and utricle (Fig. 20-6). The semicircular canal system is the kinetic labyrinth. This system is sensitive to head movement and rotatory acceleration or deceleration (spinning) (Fig. 20-7).[71,73] The vestibule (utricle and saccule) is regarded as the static labyrinth. This system is sensitive to head position and linear acceleration or deceleration.[83] The vestibular system acts as a complex relay center that influences many systems of the body. Thus vestibular stimulation has a profound influence on the development of the nervous system (Fig. 20-8).[5] As a proprioceptive organ, however, the vestibular system serves (1) to stabilize the position of the head in space, (2) to stabilize the position of the eyes in space during head movements, (3) to regulate posture and movement through tonic and phasic reflexes, and (4) to exert a powerful influence over the antigravity muscles of neck, trunk, and limbs.[71]

The receptor organs in the semicircular canals are the crista ampullaris. In the vestibule, the receptor organ is called the macula or otolith. The vestibular apparatus sends impulses to four nuclei in the upper medulla and disperses to centers throughout the nervous system. The descending tracts consist of the lateral and medial vestibulospinal tracts. Ascending fibers travel in the medial longitudinal fasciculus to extraocular muscles and other centers. Still other fibers connect with cranial nerves, the autonomic nervous system, and the cerebellum.[20,46,57]

The neurologic connections between the vestibular system and the cerebellum have many therapeutic impli-

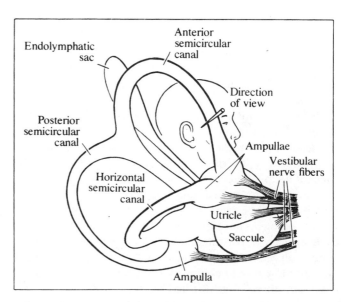

FIG. 20-6 Vestibular apparatus. (From Hardy M: *Structure of the vestibular apparatus,* New York, 1934, Anatomical Record.)

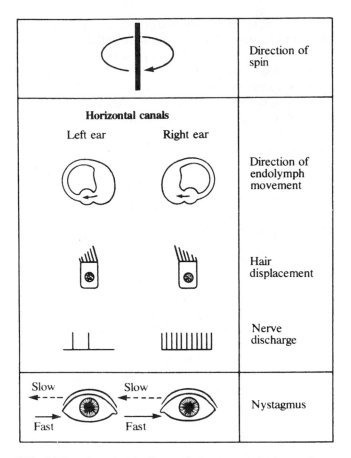

	Direction of spin
Horizontal canals Left ear Right ear	Direction of endolymph movement
	Hair displacement
	Nerve discharge
Slow Slow Fast Fast	Nystagmus

FIG. 20-7 Physiologic effects of spinning in clockwise direction. Endolymph remains inert on acceleration causing the hair cells in cristae ampularis to deflect to left. The endolymph in right ear is moving in direction of vestibule, and endolymph in left ear toward the semicircular canal. Nerve discharge is increased on right and decreased below resting level on left. After 20 seconds of continuous spinning, nerve discharge resumes resting level of activity because endolymph assumes same rate of movement in relationship to semicircular canals. When spinning stops, hair cells are deflected in opposite direction. Acceleration and deceleration cause greatest rate of nerve discharge. (Reprinted with permission from Selkurt E: *Basic physiology for the health sciences,* ed 2, Boston, 1982, Little, Brown.)

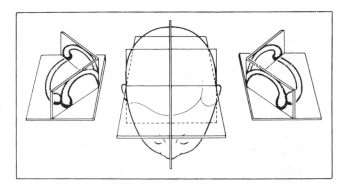

FIG. 20-8 Relationships of horizontal, anterior, and posterior semicircular canals. They detect motions in three dimensions of space and initiate vestibuloocular reflexes. (Reprinted with permission from Brown JL: Vestibular function. In Brobeck J, editor: *Best and Taylor's physiological basis of medical practices,* ed 10, Baltimore, 1979, Williams & Wilkins.)

cations. Slow rocking and inversion can reduce hypertonicity in some patients. More accelerated rocking, spinning, and movement in various directions can be useful for stimulating vestibuloproprioceptors for normal postural activity and balance mechanisms.[28,29,71]

THEORIES OF MOTOR CONTROL

Motor control theory is a developing body of knowledge that attempts to understand how humans learn through movement.[42,49] There is evidence to support the belief that the human motor control system is the result of millions of years of evolution. Fischbach[32] stated, "The machinery of the brain is constructed and maintained jointly by genes and experiences." The genes appear to provide the blueprints for motor control, and adaptations to the environment assure preservation in the day-to-day negotiations with the world. As a result of this dual influence, the human nervous system is thought to be the most complex structure in the universe. In total, the human nervous system consists of approximately a trillion cells, and about 100 billion of them are neurons.[75] The neurons in the central nervous system constitute a vast network of interconnections that are more or less genetically programmed biochemical microcircuits that give rise to memory, intelligence, creativity, emotion, and the various levels of consciousness of the human being.

Until recently, there has been an implicit assumption that the nervous system consists of linear pathways, which transmit along discrete tract systems that terminate on cell bodies in the cerebral cortex. Because the nervous system was thought to be an obligatory system, a motor response of some type was bound to ensue after a stimulus was applied.[19] This model, called the peripheral processing model, has been the basis of many of the sensorimotor approaches to treatment. Techniques that use peripheral sensory stimulation have value when used purely to elicit inhibitory and facilatative responses in skeletal muscles through reflex pathways. Basically, these peripheral processing approaches view the nervous system as a closed-loop system in which a stimulus applied to a peripheral receptor or end organ can cause action potential, which will evoke muscle responses that pave the way to motor learning. Simplistically, peripheral processing can be viewed as a "bottom-up" approach involving many neurogenic processes in a stimulus-response manner.

Most therapists who use various types of sensory stimuli to activate cutaneous receptors and proprioceptors realize, however, that the nervous system has many modulating and adapting mechanisms in place to alter and modify sensory input. This modulating system is called the central processing mechanism. Thus, the quality of the patient's prior thoughts, his or her trust in the therapist's clinical skills, the state of emotions and levels of stress, all affect the motor response.[87] This conscious override of peripheral stimuli, called central processing, appears to operate in a "top-down" fashion. Currently, there are three major models of motor control which address these contrasting views of the nature of motor behavior. They are 1) the reflex model, 2) the hierarchical model, and 3) the systems model.[51]

THE REFLEX MODEL

The reflex model suggests that controlled movement is preceded by stereotypic reflexive responses. The proponents of the reflex model proposed that movement is basically the summation of reflexes. In addition, sensory input regulates motor output and sensation is necessary for movement to take place. Thus the reflex model is placed in the category of the peripheral processing approach to understanding the nervous system.[17]

Therapists are questioning whether reflexes are truly the building blocks of movement or just one small component of a multimodality synthesis. The assumption that motor control develops in a cephalocaudal direction has been questioned. Recent evidence challenges the concept that motor skills are acquired in a predictable developmental sequence. In addition, if sensory stimulation is required for movement, why does movement occur spontaneously? Contrary to earlier beliefs about human development, motor control seems to follow a distal to proximal progression. For instance, the motor neuron — muscle connection develops first, followed by supraspinal pathways to spinal cord centers, and finally the peripheral sensory pathways establish connections to central control mechanisms.

THE HIERARCHICAL MODEL

The hierarchical model is based on the premise that there are central control mechanisms that separate reflex from voluntary control patterns.[56] According to this model, the control of movement is organized hierarchically with the spinal cord providing reflexive motor patterns, the brain stem providing tonic reflex control and integration, and the cerebral cortex superseding all lower structures with voluntary control mechanisms[31] (Table 20-4).

In this model it is assumed that normal movements are governed by centralized motor programs that determine muscle activation patterns derived from within the nervous system. Therefore, hyperreflexive movement disorders, such as spasticity, result from damage to higher level control releasing lower level or primitive reflexes from inhibition. In this view, voluntary movements are initiated internally and at will. As with the reflex model, the hierarchical model holds that stereotypic movements are governed by sensory input.

The hierarchical model sees the nervous system acting in an obligatory manner, with the motor system compelled to react. This obligatory response may also imply that the intensity and type of stimuli are directly related to the resulting motor response. The hierarchical model

allows for many levels of control, yet the emphasis remains on the spinal level being more reflexive and the higher cortical level being less automatic and more voluntary and superior in function. Using the hierarchical model, sensorimotor treatment approaches have been aimed at progressing from automatic control mechanisms to higher level voluntary control.

The critics of the hierarchical model argue that reflexes are not the building blocks of movement.[54] For example, the spinal cord level can dominate over higher centers of motor control in protective or spontaneous situations when a pain stimulus causes a withdrawal reflex. In this instance, the lower level motor response prevails to preserve the individual from immediate harm.[56,58]

THE SYSTEMS MODEL

The systems model proposes that motor control is determined by interactive systems, behavioral tasks, and adaptive and anticipatory mechanisms. This model is more holistic in that it recognizes the significance of internal and external stimuli coming to bear on motor output. The systems model also implies that nerve pathways are distributed in a parallel processing fashion. This means that instead of a formal chain of command that follows a linear serial pathway, motor control is accomplished by the integration along many different tract systems and feedback loops. An example is the act of reaching for and taking a bite out of an apple. The eyes have to see the apple, and the muscles must be regulated to reach for it; once in the hand, the tactile receptors and proprioceptors control the degree of grip on the apple and move it to the mouth where the smell, taste, and texture are all part of the experience being processed simultaneously along parallel pathways. This simple act is an example of multimodality synthesis.[2]

According to the systems model of motor control, movements are neither peripherally nor centrally controlled, but occur as a result of an integration and interaction among many systems. The systems model recognizes that motor control is influenced not only by intrinsic nervous system mechanisms, but also by mechanisms in the musculoskeletal system and other soft tissue structures. In this model, movement is the result of the interaction of many sensory modalities, each providing a different element of control. The systems model does not support the concept of higher or lower levels of motor control, but embraces a more concentric configuration that sees many systems overlapping to provide motor control. This model takes into account environmental influences, sensorimotor factors, musculoskeletal tissues, comparing, commanding and regulatory functions, and behavioral and emotional goals as well.[84]

Motor Control Theory and the Sensorimotor Approaches

The sensorimotor approaches to treatment had their foundations in the hierarchical and reflex models of

TABLE 20-4   Hierarchical Organization of Postural Reflexes

LEVEL	REFLEX	STIMULUS	RECEPTOR	MOTOR RESPONSE	PATHOLOGIC SIGN
Cerebral cortex (basal ganglia and cerebellum)	Optical righting	Visual cues	Eyes	Righting of head	Decorticate rigidity Spasticity Babinski sign Hoffmann sign Clasp-knife reflex
	Placing reaction Hopping reaction	Surface contact	Various proprioceptors*	Weight-bearing on palmar sole when placed on hard surface	
Upper brain stem (midbrain and diencephalon)	Labyrinthine righting	Tilt of body	Vestibular apparatus	Face vertical and mouth horizontal	
	Neck righting	Stetch of neck muscles	Muscle spindles	Rights body in respect to neck	Romberg sign Tremor
	Body on head righting	Pressure on side of body	Exteroceptors	Rights head in respect to gravity	Decerebrate rigidity
	Body on body reaction	Rotation of head or thorax	Exteroceptors	Rights head or thorax	
	Tonic lumbar reflex	Lateral flexion or rotation of trunk	Joint and muscle proprioceptors	Reciprocal movements of limbs, trunk, and pelvis for gait pattern	Ataxia Asynergies, weakness
Lower brain stem (medulla and reticular formation)	Tonic labyrinthine reflex (kinetic and static)	Head inversion (gravity)	Vestibular apparatus	Increased extensor tone	Vestibular shoot
	Tonic neck reflex	Rotation, flexion or extension of neck	Joint receptors Neck proprioceptors	Alterations in extensor or flexor tone of limbs	Asynergistic movements; tonic changes in muscle tone
Spinal cord (reflex arc)	Flexor withdrawal	Nociceptors	Exteroceptors	Withdrawal of stimulated extremity	
	Crossed extension	Nociceptors	Exteroceptors	Flexion of stimulated limb and extension-abduction of contralateral limb	
	Extensor thrust	Nociceptors	Exteroceptors	Extension-abduction of contrateral limb	
	Positive supporting reaction	Contact with sole or palm	Proprioceptors and distal flexors	Leg extended to support body	Marie-Foix reflex
	Negative supporting reaction	Stretch	Proprioceptors in extensors	Release of positive supporting reaction	Flexion reflex and clonus
	Cutaneous-fusimotor reflex	Cutaneous stimuli	Exteroceptors and spindle afferents	Prolonged increase in muscle tone at segmental level	Hyperreflexia Hypertonia Romberg sign Degrees of paralysis

*Pacinian corpuscles, Ruffini end organs, Golgi-Mazzoni muscle spindles, and several exteroceptors.

motor control. In these models it was assumed that (1) motor control and motor skill development were dependent upon reflexes that are organized in a hierarchical fashion and (2) motor output was dependent upon sensory input. The evolution of the systems model of motor control has brought these assumptions into question. Rather than think of these systems as mutually exclusive, they can be viewed as a continuum in which the earlier models rely heavily on sensory input and feedback to control motor behavior, whereas the systems model relies not only on sensory feedback to control motor be-

havior, but also relies heavily on feedback from nonsensory sources.

Therapists have observed that motor output is dependent, not only on sensory input and feedback, but also on the interaction of many other intrinsic and extrinsic factors. The systems model of motor control is in concert with a holistic view of human performance, motor learning principles, and evolving knowledge of neurophysiological mechanisms. The systems model of motor control does not negate the sensorimotor approaches. The theorists who developed the sensorimotor approaches considered the patient's interests, motivation, physiological and emotional states, and environment when applying the methodologies of their approaches. The sensorimotor approaches can be used in the context of the systems model, with sensory input as just one of many critical elements necessary for the achievement of motor control and motor learning.

SUMMARY

This chapter reviewed the divisions of the nervous system and explored the neurophysiological bases for the sensorimotor approaches to treatment, described in succeeding chapters. The motor and sensory organization of the nervous system, nervous system tracts, and various sensory receptors were discussed. Possible ways that sensorimotor techniques can be used to affect motor output through these nervous system mechanisms were explored.

The chapter concluded with a brief review of three models of motor control—the reflex model, the hierarchical model, and the systems model—and discussed some implications of the sensorimotor approaches in relation to these models.

Much is not known about how the nervous system develops, functions, or recovers from injury. Scientific research will yield more information in the future. Clinical research is needed to understand the efficacy of the sensorimotor approaches in relation to regaining motor control and motor learning after central nervous system dysfunction.

REVIEW QUESTIONS

1. What important role does the thalamus play in the mediation of sensory impulses?
2. What is the function of the limbic system? How is it important in rehabilitation techniques?
3. Why is the brain stem so important to sensorimotor integration?
4. What are the classifications of nerve fibers?
5. What is the primary function of the gamma loop (fusimotor neuron)?
6. Differentiate between the functions of the sympathetic and the parasympathetic branches of the autonomic nervous system.
7. Describe the two properties that a neuron must possess to convey information.
8. Explain the terms *reverberating, excitation,* and *disinhibited.*
9. List three factors associated with neuroplasticity.
10. Discuss how interoceptors are used in sensorimotor techniques.
11. Describe some of the therapeutic features associated with the pacinian corpuscle.
12. Contrast the basic functions of the Golgi tendon organ and the muscle spindle.
13. Describe the functions of the Ia afferent and secondary endings of the muscle spindle.
14. Describe the anatomic components of the static and kinetic labyrinthine systems.
15. List four functions of the vestibular system.

16. What are the functions of joint receptors?
17. Differentiate between the spinothalamic and the lemniscal tract systems.
18. Why is the trigeminal nerve considered to be an individual sensory tract system?
19. Describe how dermatomes relate to spinal cord segments and the topographic arrangement on the skin.
20. Describe the cutaneous reflex and its significance in sensorimotor therapy.
21. List the reflexes associated with each level of the nervous system.
22. Describe how the olfactory system can be used in sensorimotor therapy.
23. Discuss how gustation can be used in sensorimotor therapy.
24. How can auditory stimuli be used in sensorimotor therapy?
25. List the possible benefits of background music.
26. Describe the hierarchical model of motor control. On which premises is it based?
27. Describe the systems model of motor control.
28. How does the systems model differ from the reflex and hierarchical models?
29. Are the sensorimotor approaches to treatment useful in a systems model of motor control?
30. How can sensorimotor approach methodologies still be applicable in a systems model?

REFERENCES

1. Afifi A, Bergman R: *Basic neuroscience,* Baltimore, 1980, Urban and Schwarzenberg.
2. Almli CR, Finger S: Toward a definition of recovery of function. In LeVere TE, Almli RB, Stein DB, editors: *Brain injury and recovery: theoretical and controversial issues,* New York, 1988, Plenum.
3. Andrasik F: Relaxation and biofeedback for chronic headaches. In Holzman A, Turk K, editors: *Pain management: a handbook of psychological approaches,* New York, 1986, Pergamon Press.
4. Appelberg B, Beson P, LaPorte Y: Effects of dynamic and static fusimotor gamma fibers on the responses of primary and secondary endings, *J Physiol* 177:29, 1965.
5. Ayres J: *The development of sensory integrative theory and practice,* Dubuque, 1974, Kendall/Hunt.
6. Bach-y-Rita P: Central nervous system lesions: sprouting and unmasking in rehabilitation *Arch Phys Med Rehabil* 62:413, 1981.
7. Bach-y-Rita P, editor: *Recovery of function: theoretical considerations for brain injury rehabilitation,* Baltimore, 1980, University Park Press.
8. Balian R, Riggs H: *Myelination of the brain in the newborn,* Philadelphia, 1969, JB Lippincott.

9. Barnes J: Brain architecture: beyond genes, *Research News* 233(1):154-156, 1986.

10. Barr M, Kiernan S: *The human nervous system,* ed 2, New York, 1993, Harper & Row.

11. Basbaum A, Clanton C, Fields H: Opiate and stimulus produced analgesia: functional anatomy of a medullospinal pathway, *Proc Natl Acad Sci USA* 73:4685, 1976.

12. Basbaum A, Fields H: Endogenous pain control mechanisms: review and hypothesis, *Ann Neurol* 4:451, 1978.

13. Basmajian J: *Primary anatomy,* ed 7, Baltimore, 1976, Williams & Wilkins.

14. Battista J: The holistic paradigm and general systems theory, *Gen Systems J* 22:65, 1977.

15. Becker BO, Selden G: The body electric: electromagnetism and the foundation of life, New York, 1985, William Morrow.

16. Benson H: *The relaxation response,* New York, 1976, Avon Books.

17. Bobath K: The motor deficit in patients with cerebral palsy. In *Clinics in developmental medicine,* no. 23, London, 1966.

18. Boguslawski M: Therapeutic touch: a facilitator of pain relief, *Topics Clin Nurs* 2(1):27, 1980.

19. Brooks VB: *The neural basis of motor control,* New York, 1986, Oxford Press.

20. Brown D: *Neurosciences for allied health therapies,* St Louis, 1980, CV Mosby.

21. Bry A: *Visualization: directing the movies of the mind,* New York, 1979, Barnes & Noble Books.

22. Chusid J: *Correlative neuroanatomy and functional neurology,* ed 19, Los Altos, Calif, 1985, Lange Medical.

23. Clark R: *Clinical neuroanatomy and neurophysiology,* ed 5, Philadelphia, 1975, FA Davis.

24. Cock J: The therapeutic use of music: a literature review, *Nurs Forum* 20(3):252, 1981.

25. Cohen D, Palti B, Cuffen N, Schmid SJ: Magnetic fields produced by steady currents in the body, *Proceedings for the National Academy of Sciences* 77:1447-51, 1980.

26. Davis J: *Endorphins,* New York, 1983, Dial/Doubleday Books.

27. Diamond M: *Brain research and its implication for education,* California Infomedix Audiocassette, Physiology-Anatomy Department, University of California/Berkeley, 1987.

28. Downie P: *Cash's textbook of neurology for physiotherapists,* ed 4, Philadelphia, 1986, JB Lippincott.

29. Farber S: *Neurorehabilitation: a multisensory approach,* Philadelphia, 1982, WB Saunders.

30. Feigenson JS: Stroke rehabilitation: effectiveness, benefits and cost: some practical considerations, *Stroke* 10:1, 1979 (editorial).

31. Finger S, Stein DG, editors: *Supersensitivity as a recovery model: brain damage and recovery research and clinical perspectives,* New York, 1982, Academic Press.

32. Fischbach GD: Mind and brain, *Scientific American* 267(3):48-59, 1992.

33. Fitzgerald MJT: *Neuroanatomy: basis and clinical,* ed 2, London, 1992, Bailliere Tindall.

34. Fox E, Melzack R: Comparison of transcutaneous electrical stimulation and acupuncture in the treatment of chronic pain, *Adv Pain Research Ther* 2:797, 1976.

35. Gardner E: *Fundamentals of neurology,* ed 6, Philadelphia, 1975, WB Saunders.

36. Garfinkel A: Nonlinear dynamics of movement patterns, *Am J Physiol,* 245:438, 1984.

37. Gellhorn E: *Principles of autonomic-somatic integration,* Minneapolis, 1967, University of Minnesota Press.

38. Gernandy B, Harlow A: Spinal motor responses to acoustic stimulation, *Exp Neurol* 10:52, 1964.

39. Gilman S, Winans S: *Manter and Gatz's essentials of clinical neuroanatomy and neurophysiology,* ed 6, Philadelphia, 1982, FA Davis.

40. Gilroy J, Meyer JS: *Medical neurology,* ed 3, New York, 1979, Macmillan.

41. Goldberg S: *Clinical neuroanatomy made ridiculously simple,* Miami, 1979, Medical Master.

42. Gordon J: Assumptions underlying physical therapy intervention: theoretical and historical perspectives. In Carr JH, Shephard RB, Gordon J and associates, editors: *Movement science: foundations for physical therapy rehabilitation,* Rockville, Md, 1987, Aspen.

43. Goss CM: *Gray's anatomy,* ed 28, Philadelphia, 1970, Lea & Febiger.

44. Greenberg JH, Reivich M: Metabolic mapping of functional activity in human subjects with the fluorodeoxyglucose technique, *Science,* 212:678, 1981.

45. Greenough W: Experimental modification of the developing brain, *Am Sci* 63:30, 1975.

46. Guyton A: Structure and function of the nervous system, Philadelphia, 1972, WB Saunders.

47. Hagbarth KE: Excitatory and inhibitory skin areas for flexor and extensor motoneurons, *Acta Physiol Scand* 26:1, 1952.

48. Hammer S: The mind as healer, *Science Digest* 47-49, 1984.

49. Higgins S: Motor skill acquisition, *Phys Ther* 71(2):123-139, 1991.

50. Hinton GE: How neuronal networks learn from experience, *Scientific American,* 267:3, 144, 1992.

51. Horak FB, Anderson M: Preparatory postural activity associated with movement, *Phys Ther* 60:580, 1980.

52. Hughes J: Isolation of an endogenous compound from the brain with pharmacological properties similar to morphine, *Brain Res* 88:295, 1975.

53. Huss J: Sensorimotor treatment approaches. In Hopkins HL, Smith HD, editors: *Willard and Spackman's occupational therapy,* ed 6, Philadelphia, 1983, JB Lippincott.

54. Hutton RS, Atwater SW: Acute and chronic adaptations of muscle proprioceptors in response to increased use. *Sports Medicine* 14(6):106-121, 1992.

55. Jacob S, Francone C: *Structure and function in man,* Philadelphia, 1974, WB Saunders.

56. Kohl R, Sheal CH: PEW (1966) revisited: acquisition of hierarchical control as a function of observational practice, *J Motor Behav,* 24(3):247-260, 1992

57. Kottke FJ: The neurophysiology of motor function. In Kottke FJ, Lehmann JF: *Krusen's handbook of physical medicine and rehabilitation,* ed 4, Philadelphia, 1990, WB Saunders.

58. Lisberger SG, Segnowski TJ: Motor learning in a recurrent network model based on the vestibulo-ocular reflex, *Nature* 360(6100):159-161, 1992.

59. Locke S, Colligan D: Mind cures, *OMNI* 7(7):44, 1985.

60. Lundberg JM, Hokfelt T: Coexistence of peptides and classical neurotransmitters, *Trends Neurosci* 6(8):325, 1983.

61. Matthews PBC: *Mammalian muscle receptors and their central actions,* London, 1973, Edward Arnold.

62. McCloskey DI: Kinesthetic sensibility, *Physiol Rev* 58:763, 1978.

63. Melzack R: Trigger points and acupuncture points for pain: correlation and implications, *Pain* 3:3, 1977.

64. Melzack R: Myofascial trigger points: relationship to acupuncture and mechanisms of pain, *Arch Phys Med Rehabil* 82:47, 1981.

65. Merzennich M: The organization of neurotransmitters and receptors, *Science* 225:820, 1984.

66. Montagu A: *Touching: the human significance of the skin,* ed 2, San Francisco, 1978, Harper & Row.

67. Moore J: A new look at the nervous system in relation to rehabilitation techniques, *Am J Occup Ther* 22:6, 1965.

68. Moore J: The Golgi tendon organ and the muscle spindle, *Am J Occup Ther* 28:7, 1974.

69. Moore J: Recovery potentials following CNS lesions: a brief historical perspective in relationship to modern research data on neuroplasticity. *Am J Occup Ther* 40(7):459, 1986.

70. Moore JC: *Neuroanatomical considerations relating to recovery of function: theoretical considerations for brain injury rehabilitation,* Baltimore, 1980, University Park Press.

71. Mountcastle VB: *Medical physiology,* ed 14, St Louis, 1980, CV Mosby.

72. Noback C: *The human nervous system, basic principles of neurophysiology,* ed 2, New York, 1975, McGraw-Hill.

73. Nolte J: *The human brain: an introduction to its functional anatomy,* St Louis, 1981, CV Mosby.

74. Ornstein R: *The amazing brain,* Boston, 1984, Houghton-Mifflin.

75. Ornstein R, Swencionis C: *The healing brain: a scientific reader,* New York, 1990: Guilford Press.

76. Penfield W, Jasper H: *Epilepsy and the functional anatomy of the human brain,* Boston, 1954, Little, Brown.

77. Pert C: Brain and biochemistry, Washington, 3-N256 NIMH Audiocassette, Soundworks Box 75890, Washington (*Brain/Mind Bulletin*), 1986.

78. Phelps ME, Keihl DE, Maggiotta JC: Metabolic mapping of the brain's response to visual stimulation: studies in humans, *Science* 211(27):1445, 1981.

79. Phelps M, Kuhl D: Sex and handedness differences in cerebral blood flow during rest and cognitive activity, *Science* 217:13, 1982.

80. Prudden B: *Pain erasure,* New York, 1977, Ballantine Books.

81. Rosner BS: Recovery of function and localization of function in historical perspective. In Stein DG, Rosen JJ, Butlers N, editors: *Plasticity and recovery of function in the central nervous system,* New York, 1974, Academic Press.

82. Schmidt RA: *Sensory physiology,* New York, 1977, Springer-Verlag.

83. Schmidt RA: *Fundamentals of neurophysiology,* New York, 1978, Springer-Verlag.

84. Schmidt, RA: Motor learning principles for physical therapy. In MJ Lister, editor: Contemporary management of motor control problems. *Proceedings of the II Step Conference,* Alexandria, 1991, Foundation for Physical Therapy.

85. Scholz J, Campbell S: Muscle spindles and the regulation of movement, *Phys Ther* 60:1416, 1980.

86. Selkurt EE: *Basic physiology for the health sciences,* ed 2, Boston, 1982, Little, Brown.

87. Shea JB, Morgan RL: Contextual interference effects on the acquisition, retention and transfer of a motor skill, *J Experim Psychol* 5:179-187, 1979.

88. Snyder S: Neurosciences: an integrated discipline, *Science* 225:4668, 1984.

89. Stockmeyer SA: An interpretation of the approach of Rood to the treatment of neuromuscular dysfunction, *Am J Phys Med* 46:900, 1967.

90. Thompson R: The neurobiology of learning and memory, *Science* 233:941, 1986.

91. Vallbo A, Hagbarth H, Torebjard H: Somatosensory, proprioception sympathetic activity in human peripheral nerves, *Physiol Rev* 59:919, 1979.

92. Wechsler R: A new prescription: mind over malady, *Discover* 2(8):50, 1987.

93. Werner JK: *Neuroscience: a clinical perspective,* Philadelphia, 1980, WB Saunders.

94. Willard HL, Spackman CS, editors: *Occupational therapy,* ed 4, Philadelphia, 1971, JB Lippincott.

95. Williams P, Warwick R: Functional neuroanatomy of man. In Williams PL, Warwick R, editors: *Gray's anatomy (neurology section),* British ed 35. Philadelphia, 1975, WB Saunders.

96. Wolf SL: EMG biofeedback applications in physical rehabilitation: an overview, *Physiotherapy* 31:65, 1979.

97. Zajonic R: The face of emotion, *Science* 128(4):1443, 1985.

The Rood Approach to Treatment of Neuromuscular Dysfunction

Guy L. McCormack

The work of Margaret Rood evolved from developmental and neurophysiological literature of the 1930s.[96] Because of this literature, it was believed that: (1) motor output is dependent upon sensory input, (2) motor responses follow a normal development sequence, and (3) the psychic, somatic, and autonomic functions are interrelated. The first two assumptions have been disputed in recent years by newer models of motor control theory; the third assumption is still valid. Therefore, this chapter contains information that is undergoing scrutiny and may be refuted by current motor control theory. The information is important from an historical perspective in tracing the evolution of the sensorimotor approaches to treatment, however. Many of the techniques described in this chapter continue to be effective and can be appropriately used in the context of sensorimotor treatment and the development of motor control. Most therapists use a wide variety of treatment approaches and techniques, adapting to changing trends and theories and using therapeutic methods that have proved to be effective.

Margaret S. Rood was formally educated in both occupational and physical therapy. Her theory originated in the 1940s and underwent many revisions before she died. She did not write extensively; she seemed to prefer clinical teaching to disseminate her ideas. Most of the literature that describes the Rood approach is based on interpretations by accomplished physical and occupational therapists, such as Ayres,[5,6] Farber,[33,34] Heininger,[48] Randolph,[48] Huss,[54] and Stockmeyer.[96] They became experts in the neurosciences and were greatly influenced by Rood's work. Margaret Rood integrated neurophysiologic and developmental literature with clinical observations. At times her level of understanding was beyond the comprehension of the average clinician. Despite some controversy about the efficacy of Rood's techniques, current research in the neurosciences continues to support the importance of sensory stimulation.

The purpose of this chapter is to summarize the major tenets of Rood's theory and to suggest new considerations for the use of sensory stimulation in occupational therapy. Rood's basic assumption rested upon the belief that appropriate sensory stimulation can elicit specific motor responses. Rood combined controlled sensory stimulation with a sequence of positions and activities of normal ontogenetic motor development to achieve purposeful muscular responses.[54] Thus, according to Rood, muscle action could be "activated, facilitated and inhibited through the sensory system."[85,86]

ROOD'S THEORY

The goals and basic tenets of Rood's theory are summarized in the following discussion.

NORMALIZE MUSCLE TONE

Patients with neurologic dysfunction may have muscle tone ranging from hypotonic to hypertonic. Normalized muscle tone is a prerequisite to movement. Normal muscle tone flows smoothly and is constantly changing during a motor act. For example, to turn on the ignition of a car, one has to have fairly good eye-hand coordination, postural control of the trunk muscles, coinnervation of the proximal arm muscles, forearm pronation and supination, and moderately fine prehension and dexterity in the hands. Subsequently, the demands placed on the various muscle groups are different. Rood recognized this fact when she stated, "muscles have different duties," with some muscles predominantly used for heavy work and others for light work. The light work muscles (mobilizers) are primarily the flexors and adductors used for skilled movement patterns. The heavy work

TABLE 21-1 Characteristics of Heavy Work and Light Work Muscles

CHARACTERISTICS	HEAVY WORK (STABILIZERS)	LIGHT WORK (MOBILIZERS)
Function	Tonic position cocontraction (holding patterns and maintenance of posture)	Phasic movement (repetitive or rhythmic patterns of distal musculature and skilled movement)
Anatomy	Deep, close to bone and medial axis of body; fan-shaped with broad attachments	More superficial and lateral to midline axis; fusiform shaped, tendinous distal attachment
Fibers	Red fibers (aerobic); run obliquely, rich blood supply, low metabolic cost	White fibers (anaerobic), more energy; run parallel with long axis of muscle, high metabolic cost
Joints	Cross one major joint (uniarthrodial)	Cross two or more joints (multiarthrodial)
Specific muscles	Deep tonic extensors of neck and trunk, scapular adductors (rhomboid major and minor), downward rotators	Two joint extensors (longhead of the triceps brachii, gastrocnemius, flexors, and adductors)
Innervation	More reflexive (tonic) under extrapyramidal, vestibulospinal, reticulospinal, and medial motor system	More voluntary or willed under lateral corticospinal and rubrospinal tracts
Facilitation	Quick stretch, heavy joint compression and traction, pressure to skin surfaces bearing weight, static position of head in space; saccule and utricle of vestibular system	Quick stretch, nociceptive stimuli, light joint compression and traction, vibration, movement of head in space, (semicircular canals of vestibular system)
Exercise	Isometric resistance	Isometric or isotonic resistance
Testing	Inversion, joint compression of more than body weight	Quick stretch and light moving touch
Muscle innervation	Greater number of group II and fewer Golgi tendon organs	Greater number of Ia afferents

Modified from Farber S: *Sensorimotor evaluation and treatment procedures for allied health personnel.* Indianapolis, 1974, Indiana University & Purdue University at Indianapolis Medical Center; Rood M: Occupational therapy in the treatment of the cerebral palsied, *Phys Ther Rev* 32:220, 1952; Stockmeyer S: An interpretation of the approach of Rood to the treatment of neuromuscular dysfunction, NUSTEP proceedings, *Am J Phys Med* 46:900, 1967; Goff B: The Rood approach. In *Cash's textbook of neurology for physiotherapists,* ed 4, Philadelphia, 1986, JB Lippincott.

muscles (stabilizers) are principally the extensors and abductors used for postural support[41] (Table 21-1).

Rood[85] also believed that a voluntary motor act is based on inherent reflexes and on modification of those reflexes at higher centers. Therefore she began therapy by eliciting motor responses on a reflex level and incorporating developmental patterns to augment the motor response. The heavy work muscles are activated before the light work muscles except for the feeding and speech muscles.[84]

TREATMENT BEGINS AT THE DEVELOPMENTAL LEVEL OF FUNCTIONING

The patient is evaluated developmentally and treated in a sequential manner. The patient does not proceed to the next level of sensorimotor development until some measure of voluntary (supraspinal) control is achieved. This principle follows the cephalocaudal rule. Treatment begins from the head and proceeds downward segment by segment from the proximal to the distal to the sacral area. The flexors are stimulated first, the extensors second, the adductors third, and the abductors last.[96]

MOVEMENT IS DIRECTED TOWARD FUNCTIONAL GOALS

Rood realized that the patient's motivation plays an important role in rehabilitation. The patient must first accept the activity as a meaningful event. Second, the patient must develop a subcortical program in his or her central nervous system (CNS) to perform a motor act in a coordinated manner.

Neurologically, the pyramidal system (corticospinal) is used to control reflex activity and to perform isolated voluntary acts.[42,58] However, the coordination of the ago-

nist muscle, antagonist muscle, and synergies is a function of the extrapyramidal system. Complex motor patterns rely on subcortical centers for modification and correction so that the cortex can concentrate on the purpose of the act.[22] In addition, when the patient performs a willed movement with an intended goal, more neurons throughout the nervous system must discharge to initiate the task.[88]

REPETITION IS NECESSARY FOR THE RE-EDUCATION OF MUSCULAR RESPONSES

The importance of repetition to achieve coordination has been emphasized by Kottke.[58,59] Thousands of repetitions are required to formulate engrams. Engrams are interneuronal circuits involving specific neurons and muscles to perform a pattern of motor activity. Repetition, however, can be monotonous. Therefore activities that incorporate similar motor patterns add purpose and value to the exercise. Today, the relative merits of different patterns of repetition are being reexamined by experts in current learning theory.

PRINCIPLES OF TREATMENT

In a journal article in 1956 Rood[85] suggested four principles in the treatment of neuromuscular dysfunction. Following is an interpretation of those principles.

TONIC NECK AND LABYRINTHINE REFLEXES CAN ASSIST OR RETARD THE EFFECTS OF SENSORY STIMULATION

The tonic neck receptors lie in the muscles and skin of the neck region and respond to changes in the relationship of the head to the neck. The tonic neck reflexes

(TNR) are divided into symmetric and asymmetric.[49,52] According to Rood, the TNRs have a modifying influence on extensor tone, especially the "postural part." Fukuda[35] studied postural reflexes in humans and offered the following summary.

Dorsiflexion of the neck extends the upper extremities and flexes the lower extremities. Ventral flexion of the neck flexes the upper extremities and extends the lower extremities. Torsion or rotation of the neck toward one shoulder produces an increase in the extensor tone of the upper and lower extremities on the face side of that shoulder.

The labyrinthine receptors lie in the ampullae of the semicircular canals and in the vestibule.[22] These receptors are affected by the "position of the head in relation to gravity." Rood's description of labyrinthine influences on posture is not entirely clear.[84-86]

The following is a composite summary from several authors and is illustrated in Fig. 21-1 for clarification. In the normal upright bipedal stance (180°) (Fig. 21-1, A)

TNR and tonic labyrinthine reflexes (TLR) cause slight flexion of the elbow joint and extension of the lower limbs.[82] As the face moves clockwise to the quadruped position, the head is slightly tilted, decreasing the influences of the TNR and TLR[37,59] (Fig. 21-1, B).

In this position the vertebral column is almost horizontal, eliminating gravitational pressure on the intervertebral joints, and the face is looking downward, which reduces the activity of the TLR. In addition, weight-bearing is evenly distributed between the upper and lower extremities. If the subject assumes the quadruped position (Fig. 21-1, C) (−90°) in the horizontal plane and flexes or extends the neck, the TNRs prevail and the TLRs diminish.[77,82,98] If the subject assumes a position in which the head is lower than the shoulders (Fig. 21-1, D), extensor tone increases in selected muscles (extensor carpi ulnaris, extensor carpi radialis, and soleus).[95] A position of total inversion (Fig. 21-1, E) elicits righting reactions,[82,95,98] whereas a supine position with the head below the horizontal plane (Fig. 21-1, F and G) consti-

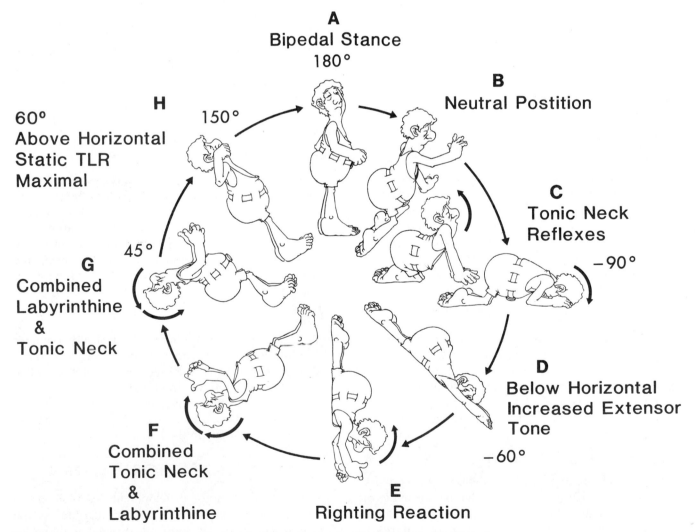

A
Bipedal Stance
180°

B
Neutral Postition

H
60° Above Horizontal Static TLR Maximal

150°

C
Tonic Neck Reflexes
−90°

45°

G
Combined Labyrinthine & Tonic Neck

D
Below Horizontal Increased Extensor Tone
−60°

F
Combined Tonic Neck & Labyrinthine

E
Righting Reaction

FIG. 21-1 Composite summary: tonic labyrinthine reflexes. **A,** Bipedal stance. **B,** Neutral position. **C,** Tonic neck reflexes (TNR). **D,** Below horizontal increased extensor tone. **E,** Righting reaction. **F,** Combined TNR and TLR. **G,** Combined TLR and TNR. **H,** Sixty degrees above horizontal static TLR maximum.

tutes a combined TNR and TLR.[55] A patient in the supine-semireclining position (Fig. 21-1, *H*) at 60° above horizontal is in a position that maximizes the static TLR.[59] This position causes abduction, flexion, and external rotation of the arms and increased extensor tone in the trunk and lower extremities. Hellebrant[49,50] and associates reported that this supine head-up position (45° to 60° above horizontal) suppresses the TNR.

Rood suggested that if the subject is lying on the side with the ear toward the earth's surface, "the arm and leg of the down side will exhibit extensor tone while the up side will be predominated by flexor tone."[85] The side-lying position is also used for the neurologically impaired patient to reduce the influences of the TLR and TNR.[41]

STIMULATION OF SPECIFIC RECEPTORS CAN PRODUCE THREE MAJOR REACTIONS

The three major reactions that can be produced by stimulation of specific receptors are homeostatic responses via the autonomic nervous system, reflexive-protective responses via spinal and brain stem circuits and adaptive responses that require greater integration of all regions of the nervous system.[3,43,100]

In 1970 Rood presented four rules of sensory input to clarify the procedure.[96] The first rule is, "A fast brief stimulus produces a large synchronous motor output. This type of stimulus is used to confirm that the reflex arc is intact." The second rule is, "A fast repetitive sensory input produces a maintained response." A stimulus, such as fast brushing with a battery-operated brush, activates nonspecific receptors that transmit impulses along the C fibers and probably the gamma fibers.[99] According to Rood, this stimulus feeds into the fusimotor system that can drive the alpha motor neuron of the muscle. The third rule is, "A maintained sensory input produces a maintained response." The force of gravity is an example of a maintained sensory input. Gravity is an everpresent force that has a constant effect on the sensory system. Whether standing, sitting, or lying, the exteroceptors of the skin are in contact with a surface, thus discharging impulses into the nervous system to reinforce the presence of gravity.[97] The fourth rule is, "Slow, rhythmical, repetitive sensory input deactivates body and mind." Any constant low-frequency stimuli, such as slow rocking in an easy chair, soft music, or even firm pressure to the upper lip, abdomen, soles of the feet or palms of the hands, activates the parasympathetic system, causing a generalized calming effect.

MUSCLES HAVE DIFFERENT DUTIES

Some muscles predominate as stabilizers (heavy work muscles), whereas other muscles undertake the duties of mobilization (light work muscles). According to Rood, both groups have distinct functions and characteristics. Table 21-1 summarizes the characteristics of the heavy work and light work muscles.

HEAVY WORK MUSCLES SHOULD BE INTEGRATED BEFORE LIGHT WORK MUSCLES

The principle of integrating heavy work muscles before light work muscles primarily refers to the use of the upper extremities. For example, fine fingertip manipulation is not functional if the proximal muscles are not strong enough to lift or stabilize the position of the arms.

SEQUENCE OF MOTOR DEVELOPMENT

Rood proposed four sequential phases of motor control.[6,85,86]

RECIPROCAL INHIBITION (INNERVATION)

Reciprocal inhibition is an early mobility pattern that subserves a protective function. It is a phasic (quick) type of movement that requires contraction of the agonist muscle as the antagonist muscle relaxes. This basic movement pattern is primarily a reflex governed by spinal and supraspinal centers.

CO-CONTRACTION (CO-INNERVATION)

Co-contraction or co-innervation provides stability and is considered to be a tonic (static) pattern. This pattern provides the ability to hold a position or an object for a longer duration. Co-contraction is defined as simultaneous contraction of the agonist muscle and antagonist muscle with the antagonist supreme.[34,48]

HEAVY WORK

Heavy work is described by Stockmeyer as "mobility superimposed on stability."[96] In this pattern the proximal muscles contract and move, and the distal segment is fixed. A good example is creeping. In the quadruped position the distal segments, wrist, and ankles are in a fixed position. The proximal joints, such as the neck and thorax, are stable whereas the shoulder and hip girdles are free to move.

SKILL

Skill is the highest level of motor control and combines the effort of mobility and stability.[37,85] To execute a skilled pattern, the proximal segment is stabilized while the distal segment moves freely. The art of oil painting demonstrates this pattern as the artist stands back from the canvas, holds his or her arm at full length, and manipulates the brush freely in the hand.

ONTOGENETIC MOTOR PATTERNS

The sequence of motor development described previously occurs as the patient is put through the skeletal function sequence that Rood called ontogenetic motor patterns.[41] The eight ontogenetic motor patterns are briefly described and related to their neurologic benefits

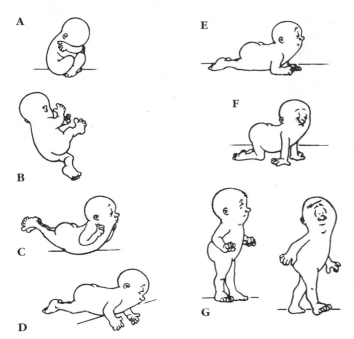

FIG. 21-2 Ontogenic motor patterns. **A,** Supine withdrawal. **B,** Rollover toward side-lying. **C,** Pivot prone. **D,** Neck contraction. **E,** Prone on elbows. **F,** Quadruped pattern. **G,** Static standing. **H,** Walking.

in the paragraphs that follow, they are illustrated in Fig. 21-2.

SUPINE WITHDRAWAL (SUPINE FLEXION)

Supine withdrawal is a total flexion response toward the vertebral level of T10. This position is protective because the flexion of the neck and the crossing of the arms and legs protects the anterior surface of the body. This position is a mobility posture requiring reciprocal innervation, yet it also requires heavy work of the proximal muscles and trunk.[85] Therapeutically, supine withdrawal aids in the integration of the TLR. Rood recommended this pattern for patients who do not have reciprocal flexion pattern and for patients dominated by extensor tone (Fig. 21-2, *A*).

ROLLOVER (TOWARD SIDE LYING)

When rolling over, the arm and leg flex on the same side of the body. This movement is a mobility pattern for the extremities and activates the lateral trunk musculature.[96] This pattern is encouraged for patients who are dominated by tonic reflex patterns in the supine position. The rolling action also stimulates the semicircular canals, which in turn activate the neck and extraocular muscles (Fig. 21-2, *B*).

PIVOT PRONE (PRONE EXTENSION)

The pivot-prone position demands a full range of extension of the neck, shoulders, trunk, and lower extremities. This pattern has been called both a mobility pattern and a stability pattern. The position is difficult to assume and

hold. Therefore it plays an important role in preparation for stability of the extensor muscles in the upright position. The pivot-prone position has been associated with the labyrinthine righting reaction of the head. The ability to maintain the position indicates integration of the symmetric TNRs and the TLRs (Fig. 21-2, *C*).

NECK CO-CONTRACTION (CO-INNERVATION)

Neck co-contraction is the first real stability pattern. In keeping with the cervicocaudal rule and cervicorostral rule, co-contraction of the neck precedes co-contraction of the trunk and extremities. As the head bobs up and down, the extensors and rotators are stretched. This action is said to activate both flexors and deep tonic extensors of the neck.[85] It is important to make sure the neck flexors are well established, however, before the prone position is assumed. To raise the head against gravity, the patient needs to have good co-contraction of the flexors and extensors of the neck.[33] Neurologically, this pattern elicits the tonic labyrinthine righting reaction when the face is perpendicular to the floor. As the head flexes, it stretches the proprioceptors in the neck and upper trapezius, causing them to contract against the forces of gravity.[77,82,83] This position also promotes neck stability and extraocular control (Fig. 21-2, *D*).

ON ELBOWS (PRONE ON ELBOWS)

Following co-contraction of the neck and prone extension, weight bearing on the elbows is the next pattern to achieve. Bearing weight on the elbows stretches the upper trunk musculature to influence stability of the scapular and glenohumeral regions. This position gives the patient better visibility of the environment and an opportunity to shift weight from side to side. It is also inhibitory to the symmetric TNR[3] (Fig. 21-2, *E*).

ALL FOURS (QUADRUPED POSITION)

The quadruped position follows stability of the neck and shoulders. The lower trunk and lower extremities are brought into a co-contraction pattern. Initially the position is static and the abdomen may sag at the T10 level, causing stretching of the trunk and limb girdles. This stretching develops co-contraction of the trunk flexors and extensors. Eventually weight shifting forward, backward, side to side, and diagonally provides a mobility superimposed on the stability phase. The weight shifting may be preparatory to equilibrium responses (Fig. 21-2, *F*).

STATIC STANDING

Assuming the upright bipedal position, static standing is thought to be a skill of the upper trunk because it frees the upper extremities for prehension and manipulation.[96] At first, weight is equally distributed on both legs and then weight shifting begins. This position brings in higher level integration, such as righting reactions and equilibrium reactions (Fig. 21-2, *G*).

WALKING

The gait pattern unites skill, mobility, and stability. According to Murray,[75] normal locomotion entails the ability to support the body weight, maintain balance, and execute the stepping motion. Walking includes a stance phase, push off, swing, heel strike, and stride length.[96] Walking is a sophisticated process requiring coordinated movement patterns of various parts of the body (Fig. 21-2, *H*).

SPECIFIC FACILITATION TECHNIQUES USED IN TREATMENT
CUTANEOUS FACILITATION

Cutaneous facilitation can be used to stimulate the exteroceptors of the skin.[3,81,100] *Exteroceptors* are those end organs located immediately under the skin in subcutaneous tissues or in external mucous membranes.[102] (See Chapter 20 for a discussion of specific exteroceptors.) Exteroceptors respond to stimuli arising from the external environment. In general, the exteroceptive system subserves protective withdrawal responses and produces states of alertness and rapid movements of the limbs.[6,16,31,37] The principal sensory modalities transmitted by the exteroceptive system are pain, temperature, and touch. These modalities are transmitted to the spinal cord along A delta (group III) and C fibers (group IV), which are thin, have little or no myelination, and are slow conductors. Nondiscriminative exteroceptive impulses travel to higher centers of the CNS by way of the spinothalamic and spinoreticular tracts. The more discriminative exteroceptive stimuli, vibration, stereognosis, and fine touch (conscious proprioception), ascend along the lemniscal (dorsal) columns.[2,31,34] Exteroceptive stimuli, such as icing and brushing, should be used judiciously because they have a profound effect on the reticular activating system and the autonomic nervous system.[48] Specific techniques of cutaneous facilitation are described later.

Light Moving Touch

Touch is important for normal growth and development.[72] Light touch stimuli send input to limbic structures and have been shown to increase corticosteroid levels in the bloodstream.[66,92] Corticosteroids aid in increasing resistance against disease, tissue repair, and fluid and electrolyte balance.[3,21] Rood used a light moving touch or stroking of the skin to activate the superficial mobilizing muscles. These muscles are classified as the light work group that perform skilled tasks.[83,84,96] Neurologically, the light stroke stimulus activates low threshold hair end organs and free nerve endings. The stimuli send impulses along A delta sensory fibers, which synapse with the fusimotor system. As a result, light moving touch causes reciprocal innervation, which is clinically seen as a phasic withdrawal response.[77] Light moving touch is applied with the fingertip, camel hair brush, or cotton swab.

Originally, the frequency of the touch stimulus was done "two times per second and at least ten times, and then repeated three to five times."[85] The formula now suggested is to apply three to five strokes and allow 30 seconds to elapse between strokes.[34,48] The 30-second rest period is important because it prevents a presynaptic inhibitory response called primary afferent *depolarization,* which is a synaptic mechanism that prevents overstimulation.[34,88] Light moving touch is applied to the facial region after firm pressure is maintained on the upper lip.[33] This causes a generalized inhibitory response before the light moving stimulus is applied to the perioral region. The first area stimulated is the area from the nose to the chin (perioral midline). The stimulus may have to be applied several times before a response is elicited. In infants the response may cause a flexion pattern of the upper and perhaps the lower extremities.[34]

A similar type of stimulus is to apply light stroking from the corner of the lip to the cheek (perioral lateral). This stimulus activates superficial musculature of the neck, and the head tilts laterally toward the side of the stimulus. In adults a unilateral flexion pattern can be facilitated by applying a light moving touch to the navel region or dermatome T10.[34,96] The stimulus is applied several times in a midline to lateral direction. Light moving touch can also be applied to the dorsal web spaces of the fingers and toes to elicit a withdrawal pattern of the extremities. More rapid results may be obtained if light moving touch is applied to the tips of the fingers or soles of the feet because it facilitates a 'tickle withdrawal response' of greater magnitude.[84,100]

Fast Brushing

In 1964 Rood introduced a battery-operated brush to stimulate the C fibers, which send many collaterals to the reticular activating system.[88,92] The stimulation to this system was reported to have its maximal effect 30 minutes after stimulation.[84] Therefore fast brushing was used before all other forms of stimulation because of its prolonged latency effect. Spicer and Matyas[94] compared brushing and icing as therapeutic modalities. They found brushing to be a better stimulus than icing, but the greatest effect occurs during the time the stimulation is applied. Neurologically, fast brushing is a nonspecific, high-intensity stimulus that increases the fusimotor activity of selected muscles.[59,77] The key to fast brushing is to apply it over the dermatomes of the same segment that supplies the muscle (myotome) to be facilitated.[41,96] Fig. 21-3 shows the anterior and posterior distribution of the dermatomes. Table 21-2 shows the spinal segment, the location of the dermatome, the muscles facilitated at the spinal level, and the primary function. The stimulus is applied for 3 to 5 seconds and repeated after 30 seconds have elapsed.[86] Fast brushing can be applied adjacent to

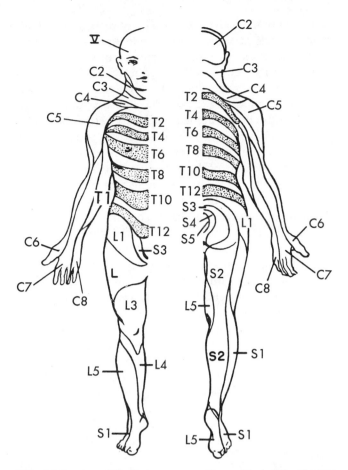

FIG. 21-3 A and **B,** Dermatomes. (From Clark RG: *Manter and Gatz's essentials of clinical neuroanatomy and neurophysiology.* ed 5, Philadelphia, 1975, FA Davis.)

the vertebral column over the posterior primary rami to facilitate the deep tonic muscles of the back[96] (Fig. 21-4). Figure 21-5 shows brushing in the web spaces of the dorsum of the hand, a technique purported to increase proximal support. Heininger and Randolph[48] have suggested that the inverted position is more effective for this purpose. The anterior primary rami can also be brushed to tonically facilitate the superficial muscles. Again the stimulus is applied to the dermatomal segment (T2 to T12) that corresponds to specific muscle groups.[85] Brushing appears to work best on isolated muscle groups where the dermatome lies over the muscle to be facilitated.[54]

Fast brushing is contraindicated for certain areas of the skin. The outer ring of the trigeminal nerve where C2 dermatome begins has a tremendous overlap of free nerve endings.[34,36] This area also has an extensive input to the reticular system. These fibers also transmit to the parasympathetic branch of the autonomic nervous system, causing a generalized inhibitory response.[34,100] Facial brushing should be avoided on patients with high cervical spinal cord or brain stem injuries because of autonomic dysreflexia and the possibility of inducing a deep state of unconsciousness.[11]

The pinna of the ear also has an abundant nerve supply. It receives sensory fibers from the trigeminal, facial, and vagus cranial nerves as well as the auricular and occipital nerves that surface from C2 and C3 spinal segments.[23,26,27] Dermatomal skin areas L1 and L2 connect with sympathetic fibers in the spinal cord and innervate the detrussor urinae. Fast brushing to this area can cause

TABLE 21-2	Dermatomes		
SPINAL SEGMENT	DERMATOME LOCATION	MUSCLES FACILITATED	FUNCTION
CN V	Anterior facial region	Mastication	Ingestion
C3	Neck region	Sternocleidomastoid, upper trapezius	Head control
C4	Upper shoulder region	Trapezius (diaphragm)	Head control
C5	Lateral aspect of shoulder	Deltoid, biceps, rhomboid major and minor	Elbow flexion
C6	Thumb and radial forearm	Extensor carpi radialis, biceps	Shoulder abduction, wrist extension
C7	Middle finger	Triceps, extensors of wrist and fingers	Wrist flexion, finger extension
C8	Little finger, ulnar forearm	Flexor of wrist and fingers	C8 finger flexion
T1	Axilla and proximal medial arm	Hand intrinsics	Abduction and adduction of fingers
T2-12	Thorax	Intercostals	Respiration
L1-2	Inside of thigh	Cremasteric reflex, accessory muscles	Elevation of scrotum
T4,T6	Nipple line	Intercostals	Respiration
T7-11	Midchest region Lower rib	Abdominal wall, abdominal muscles	T5-7 superficial abdominal reflex
T10	Umbilicus	Psoas, iliacus	Leg flexion
L2	Proximal anterior thigh	Iliopsoas, adductors of thigh	Reflex voiding
L3-4	Anterior knee	Quadriceps, tibialis anterior, detrusor urinae	Hip flexion, extensors of knee, abductors of thigh
L5	Great toe	Lateral hamstrings	Flexion at knee, toe extension
L5-S1	Foot region	Gastrocnemius, soleus, extensor digitorum longus	Flexor withdrawal, urinary retention
S2	Narrow band of posterior thigh	Small muscles of foot (flexor digitorum, flexor hallucis)	Bladder retention

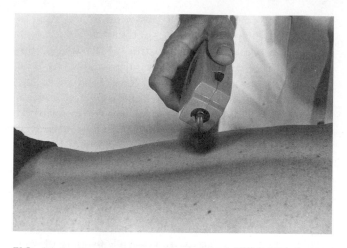

FIG. 21-4   Fast brushing to deep proximal muscles.

voiding. Stimulation to dermatomes S2 to S4 can improve bladder retention in incontinent patients. This technique appears to work as an overflow mechanism similar to the referred pain phenomenon. The smooth muscle of the bladder responds to a stretch reflex controlled by the proprioceptors in its wall.[39] Fast brushing over dermatome S2 to S4 sends impulses to the proprioceptors of the sphincter muscle, thereby causing involuntary constriction of the sphincter muscles.[96]

Fast brushing also should be used with caution on infants and children with flaccid paralysis. These children have underdeveloped nervous systems, and autonomic nervous system responses are not yet well developed.[41]

Icing

Ice is an extreme in thermal facilitation and has been used for facilitation of muscle activity and autonomic nervous system responses.[84] Unfortunately, icing is a powerful stimulus and the results are not predictable. Rood described three uses for icing.[84,85]

First, A icing or quick icing is used for patients who

exhibit hypotonia and are in a state of relaxation. A icing probably activates the more myelinated A delta fibers, causing a reflex withdrawal response in the superficial muscles.[96] The ice is applied to the skin in three quick swipes and the water blotted with a terry cloth towel after each swipe (Fig. 21-6). To elicit a withdrawal response of the limbs, the ice is applied to the dorsal web spaces or the palms and soles of the hands and feet[86] (Fig. 21-7). Ice also alerts the mental processes if applied to the palmar surfaces of the fingertips.[41] Second, C icing is a high-intensity nociceptive stimulus that affects the nonspecific C fibers.[86] This type of icing is used to facilitate maintained postural responses. The ice cube is pressed to the skin of a dermatome serving the same spinal segment as the target muscles to be stimulated, and the excess water is blotted away. The response may take as long as 30 minutes because it must travel through spinal circuits and the reticular activating system.[86] Third, autonomic icing is a stimulus affecting the sympathetic nervous system and probably influences glandular output of the thyroid and adrenal glands.[85] For example, Fig. 21-8 shows C icing to activate the diaphragm for stimulating respiration. This area needs more research.

Rood described the use of ice to promote the reciprocal pattern between the diaphragm and the abdominal muscles.[51] Ice is administered to the upper right quad-

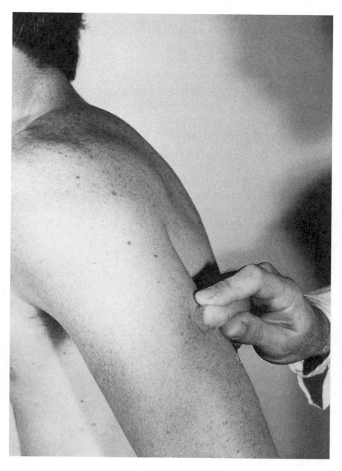

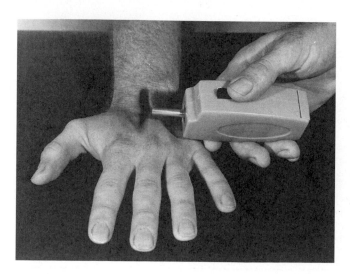

FIG. 21-5   Fast brushing to web spaces of fingers.

FIG. 21-6   A icing.

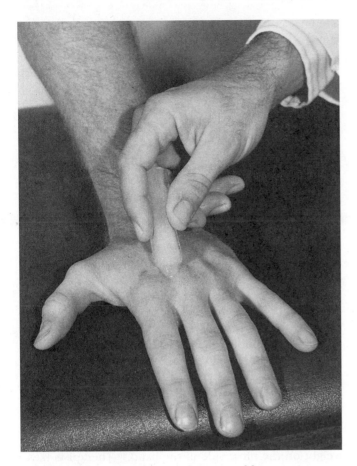

FIG. 21-7 A icing to dorsal web spaces of fingers.

rant of the abdomen (T7 through T9) along the angle of the lower rib. The stimulus is applied briefly two or three times from midline to the lateral direction. As the ice melts, the water should be blotted instead of stroked.[85] This technique has been reported to increase breathing patterns, voice production, and general vitality.[84]

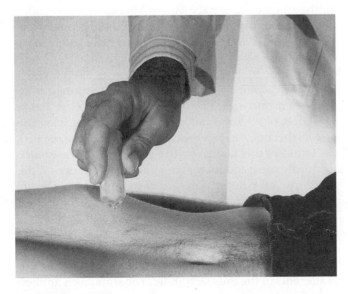

FIG. 21-8 C icing.

Ice chips have been used inside the mouth to stimulate the mucosa, to facilitate closure of the mouth, and to aid swallowing.[54] Ice can be used safely on the inner walls of the cheeks and the posterior of the tongue because fewer nerve endings are in this area.[24] In some patients ice applied to the lips can cause opening of the mouth.[34] Application of ice for 2 or 3 seconds to the upper sternal notch may induce swallowing in patients with dysphagia.[34]

Icing should be used more selectively than fast brushing. Aside from the mucosa of the mouth, ice should never be applied above the neck to the trigeminal nerve distribution or to the pinna of the ear. Furthermore, ice should not be applied along the midline axis of the body. The midline axis contains a greater concentration of free nerve endings and a greater capacity to feed into the sympathetic outflow of the autonomic nervous system.[24] In patients with spinal cord injury at the level of C4, C5, icing along midline may cause autonomic dysreflexia, which can bring on seizures, palpitations of the heart, and vasoconstriction.

Icing also should be avoided in patients with a history of cardiovascular problems. If ice is applied to the region of the left shoulder, angina or heart arrhythmia may occur. If applied behind the ear, ice can facilitate a sudden lowering of blood pressure.[41]

In general, the exteroceptive stimulation can be unpredictable. It is a divergent system that recruits other neurons and can cause discharge long after the stimulus is applied.[44] In the 1970s Rood began to abandon the use of exteroceptive stimuli and endorsed the use of proprioceptive input.[48]

PROPRIOCEPTIVE FACILITORY TECHNIQUES

Proprioceptive stimulation refers to the facilitation of muscle spindles, Golgi tendon organs, joint receptors, and the vestibular apparatus.[65,69,102] In general, proprioceptive stimulation gives the therapist more control over the motor response. Proprioceptors adapt more slowly than exteroceptors and can produce sustained postural patterns.[16] There is little or no recruitment in the proprioceptive system. Therefore the motor response lasts as long as the stimulus is applied.[32,88]

Heavy Joint Compression

Heavy joint compression is defined as joint compression greater than body weight applied through the longitudinal axis of the bone.[6] The amount of force is more than that of the normal body weight above the supporting joint[34,48] (Fig. 21-9). Heavy joint compression is used to facilitate cocontraction at the joint undergoing compression. This approach can be combined with developmental patterns, such as prone on elbows, quadruped (Fig. 21-10), sitting, and standing positions. The joint compression may be done manually by the therapist or with weighted wrist cuffs or sandbags. Clinically, joint compression is most effective when applied through the lon-

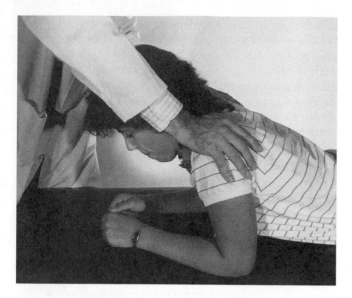

FIG. 21-9 Heavy joint compression.

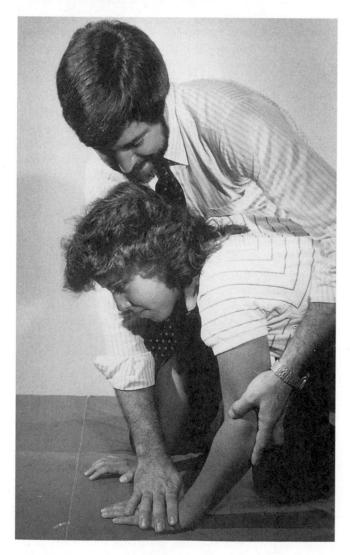

FIG. 21-10 Joint compression to elbow with stretch to wrist extensors in quadraped position.

gitudinal axis of long bones such as the humerus (glenohumeral joint) and the femur (acetabulum).

Stretch

Stretch is a physiologic stimulus used to activate the proprioceptors in selected muscles of the body.[85] Quick stretch employs the principles of reciprocal innervation. The muscle undergoing stretch is facilitated through the Ia afferent of the muscle spindle and by alpha motor neurons. Quick stretch is applied by holding the proximal bony prominences of the limb to be stretched while moving the distal joint in one direction. For example, the elbow joint is secured while the forearm is pushed into flexion to stretch the triceps. The response is immediate and short-lived. Quick stretch is used on light work muscle groups, such as physiologic flexors and adductors.[41,96]

Intrinsic Stretch

Intrinsic stretch pertains to Rood's use of the intrinsic muscles to promote stability of the scapulohumeral region.[96] For example, in the on-elbows position, shoulder stability can be enhanced if the patient engages in an activity requiring a resistive grasp. Resistance is a form of stretching because it increases fusimotor activity of the muscle spindle. Another variation of this principle can be used in the quadruped position if the patient bears more weight on the ulnar side of the hand.[96] Therapists have used cones, float trowels, and horizontal bars angled downward toward the ulnar side of the forearm to distribute more weight on that side of the patient's wrist toward the pisiform bone.[34,41,96]

Secondary Ending Stretch

Rood combined resistance and maintained stretch to facilitate developmental muscle patterns. For instance, to promote the supine withdrawal pattern, the patient is placed supine on a mat with the knees flexed and feet flat on the supporting surface. A small book is placed under the head and a folded towel under the lumbosacral region. The book and towel put the deep extensor muscles on full stretch. In principle, anytime a muscle is put on full stretch, it fires the secondary endings, which is always facilitory to the flexors and inhibitory to the extensors regardless of which muscle is being stretched.[48,54,96] Rood called this procedure "driving the flexors through the extensors." To reinforce the reciprocal action of this maneuver the patient offers resistance to the flexors, adductors, and internal rotators of the shoulders by compressing a device, such as a bicycle pump. This technique is very good for integrating the tonic labyrinthine reflex in the supine position.[6]

Stretch Pressure

Stretch pressure affects both the exteroceptors and the Ia afferents of the muscle spindle. The stimulus is applied by placing the pads of the thumbs and index and middle fingers on the skin over a superficial muscle. Firm downward pressure and stretching motion is achieved as the thumb moves away from the fingers.[33,34] The degree of pressure and stretch should be sufficient to cause deformation of the skin and stretch the underlying muscle fibers. The stimulus should not exceed 3 seconds. This technique can be applied dermatomally or directly over the muscle belly. Because this stimulus is offensive to some patients, a lubricant can be used to reduce the friction on the skin.

Resistance

Rood used heavy resistance to stimulate both primary and secondary endings of the muscle spindle. Resistance is used in an isotonic fashion in developmental patterns to influence the stabilizer muscles. According to Stockmeyer,[96] resistance to contraction of muscles in the shortened range facilitates muscle spindle afferents in the deeper, tonic postural muscles. Fast brushing is used over the stabilizers before resistance is applied to maximize the response. Farber[34] uses quick stretch before resistance to increase the responsiveness of the muscle spindle. In addition, when a muscle contracts against resistance, it assumes a shortened length that causes the muscle spindles to contract so they readjust to the shorter length. This process is called biasing the muscle spindle so it is more sensitive to stretch. Intermittent resistance graded to the desired motion is better than manual stretching for alleviating tight muscles.[65,68,85]

Tapping

The tapping technique is done by tapping over the belly of a muscle with the fingertips. The therapist percusses 3 to 5 times over the muscle to be facilitated. This may be done before or during the time a patient is voluntarily contracting the muscle. This stimulus acts on the afferents of the muscle spindle and increases the tone of the underlying skeletal muscle.

Vestibular Stimulation

Vestibular stimulation is a powerful proprioceptive input.[27] The static labyrinthine system can be used to promote extensor patterns of the neck, trunk, and extremities.[105] The kinetic labyrinth can be used to elicit phasic subcortical responses, such as protective extension.[35] Jones and Watt[55] studied muscular responses to unexpected falls in human subjects. Their findings demonstrate that the vestibular system activates the antigravity muscles and their antagonists before the stretch reflex of the muscle spindles.

The vestibular system is a divergent system that affects tone, balance, directionality, protective responses, cranial nerve function, bilateral integration, auditory-language development, and eye pursuits.[22,48,105] The vestibular system is stimulated during linear acceleration and deceleration in horizontal and vertical planes and angular acceleration and deceleration, such as spinning, rolling, and swinging. Vestibular stimulation can be either facilitative or inhibitory, depending on the rate of stimulation. Fast rocking tends to stimulate, whereas slow rhythmic rocking tends to relax.[5,6]

Inversion

Rood encouraged the use of the inverted position to alter muscle tone in selected muscles. In the inverted position the static vestibular system produces increased tonicity of the muscles of the neck, midline trunk extensors, and selected extensors in the limbs.[48] Tokizane[98] used human subjects to study the effects of head position on selected skeletal muscles. His findings indicate that extensor tone is maximized in certain muscles in the head-down position, whereas extensor tone is minimized in those muscles in the upright position. For best results, the head must be in normal alignment with the neck. If the neck is flexed or extended, the TNR interferes with the response.[82,98]

Inversion should be used with extreme care for patients with cardiovascular diseases. As the head approaches a point below the level of the shoulders, baroreceptors in the carotid sinus are stimulated by blood pressure changes. This positioning produces a physiologic response through the parasympathetic nervous system and reduces blood pressure, decreases muscle tone, and promotes generalized relaxation. Inversion techniques can be combined with vibration or neck compression to change tone in selected muscles.[34,48]

Therapeutic Vibration

Vibration may be defined as a series of rapid touch stimuli. Therapeutic vibration has been used for tactile stimulation, to desensitize hypersensitive skin, and to produce tonal changes in muscles.[34,48,54] Vibratory stimuli applied over a muscle belly activate the Ia afferent of muscle spindle, thereby causing contraction of that muscle, inhibition of its antagonist muscle, and suppression of the stretch reflex (Fig. 21-11). This response is called the tonic vibration reflex and is best elicited with a high-frequency vibrator that delivers 100 to 300 cycles per second. A low-frequency vibrator that delivers 50 to 60 cycles per second can be used to fire subcutaneous encapsulated receptors called pacinian corpuscles.[102] These receptors send impulses along the dorsal columns to higher centers of the nervous system in which the vibratory sense is consciously perceived.[1] Pacinian corpuscles do not elicit the tonic vibration reflex but may play a role in the suppression of pain perception at the cutaneous level.[8-12,65,68]

Because vibration is a proprioceptive therapeutic modality, it has a short latency period and lasts only as long as the stimulus is applied.[8-12] To elicit the tonic vibration reflex, the vibrator should be applied over the muscle

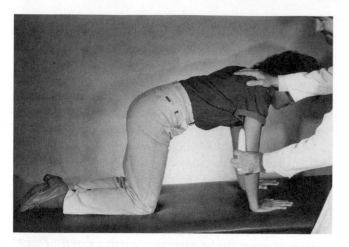

FIG. 21-11   Vibration combined with joint compression.

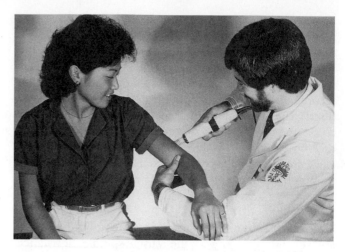

FIG. 21-12   Vibration with pressure to muscle insertion.

belly, parallel with the muscle fibers. If the vibrator is placed over the tendon, it may conduct along the bone and stimulate adjoining muscles. The muscle should be on stretch or contracting when the vibration is applied[45] (Fig. 21-12). The vibrator should be applied with light pressure because deep pressure is inhibitory and may interfere with the results. The duration of vibration should not exceed 1 to 2 minutes per application because heat friction will result.[11] The position of the patient may also be a factor. The prone position may be best while vibrating flexor muscle groups, and the supine position may enhance extensor muscle groups.[8-12]

Temperature may also be a factor when using vibration. For example, ice compresses applied to painful joints may slow nerve conduction and have a dampening effect on the tonic vibration reflex. If the patient is in a cool environment, however, the lower temperature may increase the activity of the sympathetic nervous system, increase muscle tone, and maximize the tonic vibration reflex. When using vibration for cutaneous stimulation, it is best to have the patient in a warm environment because the skin receptors are at a lower threshold for firing.[33,37]

The results of vibration are also influenced by the patient's response to the stimulus or his or her emotional state.[13] If the patient is depressed or angry, the tonic vibration reflex may be less effective than when the patient is calm. Certain medications such as muscle relaxants and barbiturates can block synaptic transmission at the myoneural junction or in the fusimotor system. These medications also decrease the tonic vibration reflex.[8-12] Vibration should not be used with children less than 3 years of age. Vibration is a powerful stimulus and the CNS is not well myelinated in children.[106] In addition, vibration should not be applied near joints in children, because it may interfere with bone cells in the growth (epiphyseal) plate.[45] In persons over 65 years of age, the skin is thinner and the blood vessels, bones, and organs are more susceptible to vibratory stimuli. With extrapyramidal or cerebellar lesions, vibration may increase tremors, promote irregular muscle tone, or impair the action of synergies.[8-12]

The electrical vibrator can be a useful tool when properly applied. More research needs to be done on vibration, and therapists should be properly trained before using vibration on patients with neurologic dysfunction.

Osteopressure

Pressure on bony prominences has been used with some success to facilitate or inhibit voluntary muscles.[85] It is not clear whether the stimulus is affecting the nerve network in the periosteum of the bone or the subcutaneous pressure receptors (pacinian corpuscle) of the skin. According to Rood, osteopressure produces a slower reaction and needs to be preceded by a light moving touch stimulus. For example, if light moving touch is applied to dermatome C7 of the arm and pressure applied over the lateral epicondyle of the elbow, the arm extends.[85] Pressure on the medial aspect of the malleolus facilitates the lateral dorsiflexors, whereas pressure on the lateral malleolus facilitates the medial dorsiflexors and inhibits the calf muscles.[86] The light moving touch is probably applied to dermatomes L3 and L4. This technique needs further research verification before it can be used as an effective treatment modality.

Pressure on or near bony prominences also may affect acupressure points. Traditional Chinese medicine recognizes two points located below the medial and lateral malleolus bones of the ankle joint, which are anatomically the same locations described by Rood. According to Chinese medicine, these points contribute to the promotion of deep sleep and correct insomnia.[53,67] Therefore, the mechanism that explains why osteopressure works remains obscure.

SPECIFIC INHIBITION TECHNIQUES USED IN TREATMENT

NEUTRAL WARMTH

The neutral warmth technique most likely affects the temperature receptors of the hypothalamus and stimulates the parasympathetic nervous system.[88] Neutral warmth can be used for patients with hypertonia, particularly spasticity and rigidity. It may also be helpful for children with attention deficit disorders.[34]

The procedure entails having the patient assume a recumbent position while the entire body is wrapped in a cotton blanket or comforter for approximately 5 to 10 minutes. Neutral warmth provides a moderate amount of heat that is homeostatically compatible with the receptors of the hypothalamus. The patient usually feels relaxed and muscle tone is decreased.[33,54]

GENTLE SHAKING OR ROCKING

Gentle shaking or rocking is a generalized inhibitory technique that uses light joint compression and traction of the cervical vertebrae and slow rhythmic circumduction of the head. The patient lies in the supine position, and the therapist places the palm of the right hand under the occiput of the head. The left hand is positioned on top of the patient's head. The neck is held in slight flexion and the head is slowly moved in a circumferential pattern (Fig. 21-13). The head is moved slowly and rhythmically as light joint compression is applied down through the cervical vertebrae with the left hand.[34] As the slow circumduction continues, the therapist uses the right hand to apply gentle traction by placing the fingertips under the ridge of the occipital bone and applying a slight pulling action after each light compression of the cervical vertebrae. The emphasis should be on a slow continuous motion to elicit a relaxation response.

This motion affects the proprioceptors of the neck and the vestibular apparatus because the joint receptors

between the cervical vertebrae and the muscle spindles in the neck muscles are facilitated.[22,100] The slow circumduction of the neck causes the hair cells in the semicircular canals and in the vestibule to alter their rate of discharge. A similar technique can be applied to the shoulder and pelvic girdles to promote segmental relaxation of the upper extremities.

For the upper extremity, the patient lies in a supine position, and the therapist slides the left hand between the patient's left arm and chest (axilla) so that the hand is facing upward and supporting just beneath the scapula. The therapist places the right hand on the patient's left shoulder. With the left hand supporting below the scapula and the right hand firmly placed on top of the left shoulder, the therapist gently rotates the upper region of the shoulder backward (posteriorly). The shoulder may be rotated backward about 4 times, depending on the patient's shoulder mobility and the presence of pain in the shoulder. The immediate response is that the left shoulder will appear to be lower and fully resting on the supporting surface below. This technique should be used on the patient's right shoulder to promote symmetry and also works well for patients with a spastic scapula. It slowly relaxes and mobilizes the scapula so it can glide along with the upper extremity. These procedures are continued until relaxation can be palpated in the muscles or observed in the patient's posture.

To apply gentle shaking and rocking to the pelvic girdle, the patient continues to lie in the supine position. The therapist stands over or straddles the patient so his or her hands can be placed around the lateral aspects of the pelvic girdle. The thumbs are placed on the pelvic crest and the fingertips under the gluteal muscles. Thus, the therapist can lift and gently rotate the pelvis from side to side.

The lower extremities can be relaxed in the following manner. The patient remains in the supine position, and the therapist moves to the bottom of the feet. The therapist places the palms of the hands under the patient's heels and slowly lifts the legs about 12 inches off the mat. At the same time, the therapist leans backward to put slight traction on the legs. As the therapist lowers the legs to the mat, they can be jiggled laterally in a scissoring fashion.

In addition, when the legs are slowly lowered to the mat, the therapist's hands remain under the heels (Achilles tendon) and carefully jiggle the patient's entire body toward the head and feet. This slow jiggling motion is very relaxing and allows the patient's body to become evenly distributed on the surface below.

SLOW STROKING

Slow stroking has been described as an inhibitory technique. The patient lies in the prone position while the therapist provides rhythmic, moving, deep pressure over the dorsal distribution of the primary posterior rami of the spine. The therapist applies fingertip pressure on

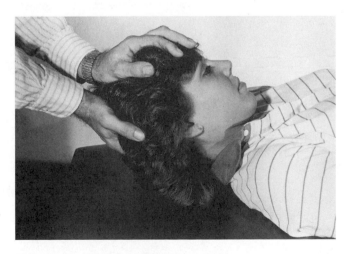

FIG. 21-13   Gentle shaking and rocking.

both sides of the spinous process to affect the nerve endings and the sympathetic outflow of the autonomic nervous system. The stroking action is done slowly and continuously from the occiput to the coccyx. The hands are alternated so that as one hand reaches the bottom of the spine, the other is starting downward from the top.[34,48,54]

Several variations of slow stroking have been used by therapists. To achieve the best results, a lubricant such as hand cream can be used to prevent friction on the skin. Some therapists use the ends of the flexed proximal interphalangeal (PIP) joints of the index and long finger to provide firm and continuous downward pressure to both sides of the spinous process. Other therapists apply the ulnar side of the hands in a cascading motion with alternating pressure from the neck region to the lumbar area.

These inhibition techniques have been found to be clinically beneficial when accompanied by soft music. Music also has been used as a closure technique following sensory integrative therapy to calm children after vestibular and proprioceptive facilitation. This procedure should not exceed 3 minutes, because it may cause a rebound phenomenon, resulting in excitation of the sympathetic branch of the autonomic nervous system.[96]

SLOW ROLLING

The patient is placed in a side-lying position. (The hemiplegic patient should first lie with the uninvolved side down.) The therapist kneels behind the patient and places one hand on the rib cage or shoulder and the other hand on the lateral aspect of the patient's pelvis (Fig. 21-14, *A*). The patient is rolled slowly from a side-lying position to a prone position and back again in a rhythmic fashion[33,34] (Fig. 21-14, *B*). In addition to rolling the entire body from lying on the side toward a prone position, the therapist can incorporate some slow rotational movements between the hip and the trunk. This technique should be used on both sides of the body. With some patients it is necessary to place a pillow between the knees or under the head to prevent friction and malalignment of the body.

LIGHT JOINT COMPRESSION (APPROXIMATION)

Joint compression of body weight or less than body weight can be used to inhibit spastic muscles around a joint.[86] This technique may be used with hemiplegic patients to alleviate pain and to offset temporarily the muscle imbalance around the shoulder joint.[34] The patient can be sitting or lying in the supine position. The therapist places one hand over the patient's shoulder and the other hand under the flexed elbow joint. The arm is abducted 35 to 45° and a compression force of body weight or less is applied through the longitudinal axis of the humerus.[6] This procedure compresses both the glenohumeral joint and the articulation between the humerus and ulna. Moreover, if applied properly this technique compresses two joints, but has the most dramatic effect on the shoulder.

Once the muscles begin to relax, the therapist can slowly and gently circumduct the humerus in small circles to reduce pain and stiffness in the shoulder joint.[34] Joint compression of the shoulder and elbow joints also can be achieved when the patient is in the on-elbows position.[96] Light joint compression is also beneficial when applied through the longitudinal axis of the wrist and elbow joints.[34] The therapist places one hand behind the elbow and places the patient's forearm in midposition; the wrist joint is extended, and compression is applied through the heel of the patient's hand. Joint compression has its greatest effect during the time that the stimulus is applied.[100]

TENDINOUS PRESSURE

Manual pressure applied to the tendinous insertion of a muscle or across long tendons produces an inhibitory effect.[6,48] This pressure has a dramatic effect on spastic or

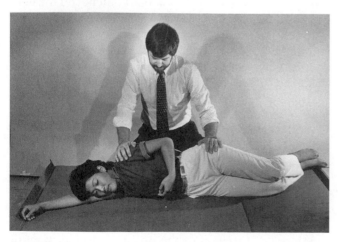

A

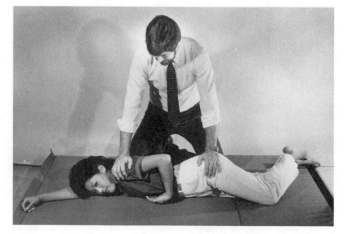

B

FIG. 21-14   **A** and **B,** Slow rolling.

tight muscle groups in which the tendons are accessible to the forces of pressure. Pressure provided by hard surfaces is preferable to that provided by soft surfaces.[26] Therefore many therapists use a hard cone in the hand with the tapered end toward the thumb side to inhibit the flexors.[33] A hard surface over the anterior aspect of the forearm is inhibitory to the extrinsic flexors of the hand.[86] This principle has been used in a number of orthotic devices to manage muscle imbalance and contractures provided by spasticity. It is postulated that the pacinian corpuscle is responsible for the inhibition of the muscle.[99] The Golgi tendon organ, however, may also play a role in this response, because it is located in the musculotendinous insertions and monitors tendon tension.[73]

MAINTAINED STRETCH

Rood recommended positioning hypertonic extremities in the elongated position for various periods to cause lengthening of the muscle spindles.[68,86] The rationale for this is to reset or bias the afferents of the muscle spindle to a longer position so that they are less sensitive to stretching. Rood did not advocate passive stretch for tight muscles. Instead, she recommended maintained stretch in the lengthened position for the stronger agonist muscle to increase the threshold of the muscle spindles. The antagonist muscle is then facilitated by cutaneous stimulation to offset the muscle imbalance.[85] Rood also used autogenic inhibition through the Golgi tendon organ to reciprocally facilitate the antagonist muscle.[84,86]

Goff[41] suggests that spasticity is reduced if the patient is taught to practice very small range contractions of isolated muscles and their antagonists. If these contractions are done repeatedly with no resistance and with gravity eliminated, spasticity can be reduced, especially in extensor and abductor muscles.

ROCKING IN DEVELOPMENTAL PATTERNS

In keeping with the developmental sequence and the concept of mobility superimposed on stability, Rood encouraged movement as the patient gained mastery of the static position.[96] Developmentally, the patient first must assume and be able to achieve a static position and then integrate coordinated movements while maintaining the posture, which Rood referred to as the development of "skill." For example, in the quadruped position, the patient shifts weight to a three-point stance so that one hand is free to reach forward to grasp and explore. Movement may begin by shifting the weight forward and backward. The shifting may progress to side-to-side and diagonal patterns as the patient becomes comfortable with the rhythmic movements.[34]

Hemiplegic patients are assisted in the quadruped position by achieving stability of the involved elbow (Fig. 21-10) when the therapist applies pressure and stretch to the triceps brachii and anconeus. As the therapist applies compression that is greater than body weight to facilitate cocontraction, the pressure exerted on the extended wrist and heel of the hand inhibits the wrist flexors. Light moving touch over the dorsum of the hand is done to promote finger extension.[86] Rocking in the quadruped

---

TABLE 21-3 Effects of Proprioceptive Facilitation

STIMULUS	LIGHT WORK (MOBILIZERS) (FLEXORS AND ADDUCTORS)	HEAVY WORK (STABILIZERS) (EXTENSORS AND ABDUCTORS)
Quick stretch	Excitation of Ia afferents in muscles stretched and inhibition in antagonist (reciprocal innervation)	Not applicable
Full stretch in maximum range	Not applicable	Inhibition of group II or secondary ending of muscles on stretch and synergic muscles; excitation in antagonistic flexors of adductors
Joint compression (approximation)	Reduction of spasticity in flexor and adductor group	Promotes cocontraction especially facilitative to one joint extensors
Tendinous pressure over insertion of superficial muscles	Inhibition of tone in long flexors of elbow, fingers, and thumb	Not applicable
Vibration (musculotendinous insertion with the muscle on stretch or working)	Facilitation of underlying muscle via Ia afferents (tonic vibration reflex)	Facilitation via Ia afferents (prior positioning and cutaneous brushing enhances its effect)
Firm pressure over palmar surface of metacarpals	Reduces tonicity in long flexors of fingers and thumb	Allows extensors to facilitate a more normal release pattern
Outside muscle resistance	Facilitation to muscle being resisted	Sustained contraction if applied proximally; cocontraction if applied distally
Active muscle setting; small range contractions with gravity eliminated (no resistance)	Inhibition via Golgi tendon organs (Ib); reduction of spasticity in flexor and adductor muscles	Facilitation; isotonic contraction of antagonistic extensor and abductor muscles
Input from semicircular canals, e.g., movement of head in space	Facilitation; protective responses in limb muscles	Increased tone in postural muscles
Input from utricle and saccule, ie, static position of the head in space	Slight changes in tone depending on position of head	Facilitation predominantly to specific extensor muscles

position should first be done with the neck in a straight normal relationship to the body so that the proprioceptors of the neck do not influence the tonicity of the limbs.[32] As the patient moves in an anteroposterior plane, the shoulder and pelvic girdles are mobilized. Later in treatment the therapist may want to incorporate flexion, extension, and rotation of the neck as a reflex inhibition measure.[77] Table 21-3 (see p. 391) summarizes the effects of proprioceptive facilitation.

SPECIAL SENSES FOR FACILITATION OR INHIBITION

Rood suggested the use of olfactory and gustatory stimuli to facilitate cranial nerves and to influence the autonomic nervous system.[84,86] In principle, pleasant odors such as vanilla and banana oil may have a calming effect or evoke strong moods. Unpleasant odors such as sulfur and fresh horseradish can produce primitive protective responses such as sneezing and choking.[34] Rood used noxious substances such as ammonia and vinegar to affect the trigeminal nerve, which activates the muscles of mastication.[96]

Warm liquids may be calming to the oral musculature, whereas sweet foods or sour tastes can stimulate the salivary glands.[44] As with other stimuli, the intensity of warm liquids and sweet and sour tastes can be gauged to facilitate or inhibit the CNS. Rood[84-86] did not provide specific guidelines for the stimulation of special senses.

The importance of using many sensory modalities in the rehabilitation of neurologic dysfunction is emphasized by several therapists.[5,33,48] In theory, the CNS retains its capacity to produce adaptive changes to stimuli throughout life.[24,106] Bach-y-Rita[7] has suggested that a process called "sensory substitution" can compensate for the loss of a particular sensory modality. Sensory substitution is the process in which a blind person uses the tactile sense instead of vision in reading braille. Another example is the stroke patient who sees four objects on a table and with the eyes closed can identify the objects correctly by using the sense of touch alone. Farber[34] refers to this phenomenon as "cross-modal" stimulation. Regardless of what it is called, the ability to learn and relearn depends on the integration of sensory input. Rood's basic hypothesis, that sensory stimulation can elicit specific motor responses, continues to gain credence in the realm of physical medicine and rehabilitation.

APPLICATION OF THE ROOD APPROACH IN OCCUPATIONAL THERAPY

The occupational therapist uses the previously described techniques primarily to prepare the patient for purposeful activities. Patients who have undergone severe neurologic damage usually do not have voluntary control over their muscles. The motor responses exhibited by the patient may begin with primitive reflexive motions. There-

fore the therapist may consider beginning with the ontogenetic developmental patterns. During this phase of rehabilitation, the therapist must carefully select the pattern to be trained and must control extraneous conditions. Next, the desired motor patterns should be done passively by the therapist and reinforced by sensory stimulation. The motor patterns should be repeated until the patient can actively perform the pattern in a slow, accurate manner. The speed of the movement should not be increased until precision is accomplished. The therapist should avoid fatiguing the patient and should not allow incorrect patterns to develop. Thousands of correct repetitions may be necessary before the speed and force of contraction are increased.[58,59]

As the patient gains mastery of a motor pattern, the therapist should introduce purposeful activities into the repertoire. Hence, a basic tenet of the Rood approach is that activity should be purposeful. The introduction of purposeful activities adds meaning and relevance to the endeavor. Routine exercises and neurophysiologic techniques alone can become redundant, and the patient may reach a plateau too early in therapeutic progression.

ONTOGENETIC MOTOR PATTERNS WITH ACTIVITIES
Supine Withdrawal

The therapist may use an activity that promotes elbow flexion or shoulder adduction. The patient may squeeze an accordion or a large balloon to add resistance and to reinforce the pattern. An easel or macramé frame may be set up in such a way that the patient can lie supine, reach forward toward the midline, and paint an oil painting or tie cords for plant hangers. Certain leather craft projects and numerous minor crafts could be manipulated in this pattern. The incentive for the patient is an end product that can adorn his or her room or be given to a relative or friend.

Rollover

The rollover pattern can be promoted by placing an object on either side of the patient so he or she has to fixate visually on the object and to roll to reach for it. It is best to minimize extraneous demands and external stimuli in the room so the patient can concentrate on the task at hand. The therapist may begin the rollover pattern by having the patient lie on an equilibrium board tilted slightly to one side to remove some of the gravitational demands. Objects such as a cassette tape recorder or remote control for a television or video game can provide an incentive to roll, reach, and manipulate an object.

Pivot Prone

The pivot-prone position is a stability pattern that places demands on the proximal extensor muscles. Scooter board activities are ideal for this pattern because the patient must lift the extremities against gravity. The scooter board may be equipped with a rope-and-pulley system so the board can accelerate and decelerate forward and backward. This linear movement (forward and backward) stimulates the vestibular apparatus and enhances the tonicity of the extensor muscles. The prone-extension pattern (pivot prone) also can be reinforced with activities that provide light resistance. The patient can lie prone on a soft bolster (suspended or on a mat) and manipulate strings attached to bells or talking toys. The object of this activity is to entice the patient into looking up so that his or her neck extends and the arms pull backward away from the midline axis.

Neck Co-contraction

Neck co-contraction can be reinforced by positioning the patient in the prone position on a firm surface such as a table. The head and neck should extend off the end of the table so the weight is distributed on the patient's chest region. In this position, the patient can suck through a straw to pick up objects and transfer them from one container to another. The object of the sucking action is to reinforce neck co-contraction. For an advanced activity, table tennis balls marked with numbers could be placed in a pan of water. The object is to pick up these balls by sucking through the straw. The score board can be positioned on the wall in front of the patient so he or she has to extend the neck and look up to see the score.

On Elbows

A patient on his or her elbows is in a position that is conducive to many activities. The patient may be positioned on a mat in front of a video game monitor. The control handle is placed near the midline so that the patient can use either hand to manipulate the controls. This activity provides concentration and fine eye-hand manipulation as the patient bears weight on the elbows. A number of minor crafts, games, and puzzles can be integrated into this pattern.

All Fours (Quadruped)

The quadruped position does not allow freedom of the hands for manipulation unless the patient can shift weight to a three-point stance. Thus if the patient can support his or her body weight on the knees and one hand, he or she can use one hand to draw or manipulate objects. In an effort to produce mobility in the quadruped position, the patient can support half of the body weight on a scooter board. For example, the hands and anterior part of the body can rest on the scooter board while the lower extremities provide forward propulsion. This activity does not provide coordination and reciprocal movements between the upper and lower extremities but does afford mobility and exploration of the environment. In addition, when the knees are resting on the scooter board and the upper limbs are used for propulsion, the patient is receiving some of the benefits of inversion.

Static Standing

Standing provides the best position for activities of daily living (ADL) and purposeful activities. In this position, the arms are free to explore and manipulate while the task of weight-bearing is placed on the legs. The patient can begin with light resistive activities on a high bench and proceed to resistive crafts, such as woodworking, leather crafts, and ceramics. As the patient develops stability in standing and in activities that require weight shift and equilibrium, the responses can be integrated into the repertory of motor skills.

Walking

Walking is the skilled level of mobility. The upright bipedal position requires an integration of many components of the CNS. The physical therapist usually undertakes the responsibility of gait training, whereas the occupational therapist provides purposeful activities to encourage walking for ADL, such as grocery shopping, visiting neighbors, and to facilitate the cardiovascular system. The occupational and physical therapists should work together closely on walking skills so the patient can receive a well-coordinated treatment plan.

NEW CONCEPTS FOR SENSORY STIMULATION

If Margaret Rood's work is accepted from an historical perspective, some useful principles for sensorimotor stimulation can be extracted from it. When these techniques are used today, most therapists provide sensory stimulation first to the proprioceptors by using joint compression, vibration, vestibular input, and manual pressure to the muscle bellies. Cutaneous or exteroceptive input is used more sparingly. Ice, if used as a stimulus, is used only on the extremities.

Margaret S. Rood was a pioneer in the field of sensory stimulation. She laid down the foundation for the use of sensory stimulation as it is known today and she integrated neurophysiology with clinical techniques. Current research, however, warrants a new look at sensory stimulation and its implications as a therapeutic modality. The following are new concepts to consider.

First, sensory stimulation or touch has been found to be more complicated than simply facilitating receptors beneath the skin. A stimulus applied to the skin sets off a cascade of biochemical and neuroendocrinologic events more pervasive and complex than previously imagined.[25,28,66,80] Up to this time, sensory stimulation in occupational therapy has focused on neuromuscular and possibly psychosocial responses.[6,34,48] Today, growing evidence exists that touch or sensory stimulation has an integrating effect on many organ systems and homeostatic mechanisms throughout the body.[87,89,101] In the health care delivery context, five types of touch (sensory stimulation) have been identified.[87,101]

Social touch is skin-to-skin contact for the development of human relationships. Much has been written about the importance of touch in infancy and throughout life for human growth and development.[15,72,81] It is commonly agreed that social touch promotes social bonds, attachment, and emotional well-being.

Passive touch pertains to a sensory stimulus that is applied to the patient's skin to facilitate specific receptors and tract systems. For example, when fast brushing is applied dermatomally, a reflex arc is set off, which facilitates muscles of a myotome that serve the same spinal segment.[41]

Active touch provides the patient with the opportunity for manual exploration in which the receptors in the skin, joints, and muscles must function collaboratively to obtain information about the activity or the environment. Occupational therapy provides active touch experiences by engaging the patient in purposeful activities.[5,78]

Comforting touch is often used by care givers for the purpose of assisting the patient to cope with dysfunction and its related stressors.[28] A touch on the shoulder for encouragement and holding the patient's hand are immeasurable therapeutic tools. Studies have shown that patients have a greater need for this type of touch during illness.[17-19]

Procedural touch is the result of science and technology in Western medicine. Health professionals are trained to use touch to evaluate, monitor, diagnose, and treat illnesses. According to Morse,[74] the intent of this type of touch is to perform a procedure or activity that is important to the patient's physical health. Procedural touch may be perceived by the patient as routine, directive, and controlling. Studies have shown that taking the pulse and measuring blood pressure in intensive care units has profound negative influences on the patient's heart rate and other physiologic responses.[19,66,71,101]

This brief overview of the types of sensory stimulation shows that touch is much more complicated than mastering the application of a technique. For instance, the patient's perception of touch can influence the response to the stimulus. Experimental evidence indicates that the precondition of the nervous system (that is, the patient's emotional state before touch) affects the neurologic tract systems and biochemical responses.[25,40,57,89] If the patient perceives the stimulus as being potentially harmful, the sympathetic branch of the autonomic nervous system is more likely to prevail and release catecholamines and various biogenic amines causing fight-or-flight responses.[40,71,93,101] Therefore, it is important for the therapist to set up the emotional climate that is conducive to the desired response before the stimulus is applied. For example, if the patient is overly anxious about a noxious stimulus such as ice, the therapist should explain what will take place and should incorporate relaxation techniques such as deep breathing to induce relaxation responses.[25,47]

Scientific information is emerging about the skin that will have enormous influences on patient care in the future. Traditional concepts about the skin have suggested that it is the largest organ of the body, the first line of defense against infectious organisms, and a vehicle of communication.[38,57] New concepts of the human skin

suggest even more profound characteristics. For example, the skin can be considered the organ of health. A study conducted at Ohio State University involved feeding rabbits a high-cholesterol diet.[76] After being fed the unhealthy diet for a period of time the rabbits were sacrificed and their coronary arteries examined for arteriosclerotic plaque. One subset of rabbits had 60% less fat build-up in their arteries than that of the others. The only variable in this subset was that the attendant made a practice of taking this group out of their cages and petting them. The researchers replicated the study 3 times, and each time the subgroup that was touched had significantly less arteriorsclerosis.[30,76]

Similar results are reported on human subjects. Medalie and Goldboust[70] conducted a study involving 10,000 males with arteriosclerotic heart disease. The researchers found that the patients who had loving, supportive, and caring spouses reported an incidence of angina that was only half that of the group as a whole. Another study conducted at the University of Miami Medical School examined the effects of touch on premature infants.[14] The experimental group received gentle stroking and passive range of motion. The control group received the normal treatment and care. As result, the experimental group showed a 47% greater weight gain per day with the same caloric intake. The infants who received gentle stroking required an average of 6 days less hospitalization at a savings of $3000 per child.

The literature also suggests that the skin influences internal homeostasis. It is well documented that the skin is the primary transducer of information to the nervous system. Rood's focus on neuromuscular dysfunction through sensory stimulation is still of major interest to occupational therapists. Research continues to suggest that certain types of sensory stimulation may be linked to facilitation of regional areas of the nervous system. Stimuli of long duration, high frequency, and strong intensity excite a greater number of neurons in the spinal thalamic system and limbic system. Sensory stimuli to areas of rich innervation, such as the face and hands, transmit to specific cell bodies in the cortex and association fibers.[19,90] Also, evidence exists that the skin is connected to internal organs through complex reflex arcs.[20,29,67,80] In fact, many diseases of internal organs manifest on the surface of the skin like a mirror reflecting disturbances within. Liver deficiency results in a characteristic waxy yellow skin, and heart disease causes cyanosis.[67]

This reflex arc phenomenon is best illustrated by referred pain. Dysfunction in an internal organ manifests as pain on the surface of the skin at a location some distance from the organ. For instance, pain arising from the stomach is transmitted to the skin of the upper abdomen and the adjacent part of the back. An explanation for this phenomenon is that the stomach and the skin areas are supplied by the same nerve segment (T7 and T8). An old remedy for stomach discomfort was a hot water bottle placed over the skin area where the pain was referred.[9] The reduction of pain indicates the presence of cutaneous-visceral reflexes transmitted by way of the nervous system.[38,67,88]

Rood's approaches were based on passive touch and sensory stimulation applied to specific dermatomal areas of the skin. The long-term effects on internal organs have not yet been fully determined, but some research is showing positive effects of sensory stimulation because of the release of catecholamines, which are organic compounds known to stimulate the nervous and cardiovascular systems, metabolic rates, temperature, and smooth muscle.[63,71,89,104]

Researchers drawing on data from psychology, neurobiology, and immunology are developing a new discipline called psychoneuroimmunology.[64,102] They are demonstrating that stimulation to the skin not only sends messages to the central nervous system but to the endocrine and immune systems as well. Studies conducted by Pertovaara[79] have shown that *neuropeptides* (small chains of amino acids including endorphins) play a prominent role throughout the body. To date, neuropeptides have been associated with pain, anxiety, pleasure, appetite, learning, and a variety of moods. Movement and sensory stimulation have been found to trigger mechanisms in the brain to release neuropeptides into the bloodstream.[93] In the bloodstream, neuropeptides direct the movement of the key components of the immune systems, the *monocytes* (macrophages). These specialized white blood cells are crucial to wound healing and elimination of foreign bodies, and they communicate with B cells and T cells to combat disease.[46,64,103]

Neuropeptides are also the neurotransmitters of emotions and are greatly influenced by the patient's attitude. A positive attitude toward wellness increases the patient's chances for recovery from a catastrophic illness.[46,64] Blood tests show that patients who cope poorly with illnesses have less active immune cells than those with a more positive attitude,[46,64] which explains why mental imagery has been beneficial to terminal cancer patients. The occupational therapist can use imagery and metaphors with sensory stimulation to potentiate these effects. Carl Simonton's book, *Getting Well Again* (Bantam, 1982), and Norman Cousins' work, *Anatomy of an Illness* (Bantam, 1992), offer many strategies for clinical practice. According to Pertovaara, neuropeptides are strategically located throughout the body. For example, breathing techniques used in relaxation may release neuropeptides in the brain stem nuclei, which probably explains why deep breathing alters pain thresholds and levels of consciousness.[93] Breathing techniques were not suggested in Rood's original work. Yet clinical experience with children and adults has shown that inhibitory techniques such as slow stroking or gentle shaking and rocking are more effective when the patient uses deep breathing and visualization.[4,34,91]

The clinical signs of inhibition were not well outlined in Rood's work. Today, when using holistic and inhibitory techniques, the therapist can gauge the effectiveness of the techniques by observing the following:

1. If the eyes are open, the size of the pupils may constrict, indicating a parasympathetic response. In some patients, the eyes remain partly open and the pupils appear fixed or glazed when they are inhibited. The most important eye signs are the rapid eye movements (REM). This eye flutter is indicative of an altered state of consciousness. REMs are a natural occurrence during sleep and dreaming.[61,91]

2. The patient's respirations change because breathing is influenced by both the autonomic and the voluntary nervous systems. For some patients the respirations slow down and deepen. This response may be preceded by large inspirations and expirations as if to blow off tension.[61,91,101]

3. A third manifestation to note is change in voice quality. Sometimes the therapist needs to elicit a verbal response by asking, "How are you doing?" The patient's voice takes on a quality and vitality different from before the inhibition or relaxation techniques began.[61,91]

4. A fourth clinical sign often noticed is the presence of gurgling or rumbling sounds (called borborygmus) created by the gastrointestinal tract. This sign is a good one because an increase in stomach motility indicates a parasympathetic response.

5. Changes in skin tone caused by dilation of the peripheral vascular system may be observed.

6. Muscle jerks unrelated to neurologic movement disorders also are observed. These muscle jerks may appear as minor twitches, as seen in a person about to fall asleep.

It is important for the therapist to monitor these responses. Allowing the patient to get too inhibited decreases purposeful neuromuscular responses.

The skin senses both pleasure or pain and a whole gamut of sensations in between. According to Smith,[91] memories and emotions can be triggered during various forms of cutaneous stimulation. The physiologic mechanism for this phenomenon is unknown at present, but possibly neuropeptides are involved.[46,57,64,93] Neuropeptides have an influence on learning, moods, and emotions. Therefore, as the therapist is using sensory stimulation techniques, the patient may suddenly remember a past event or experience changes in emotions. The therapist should not brush aside these psychological responses. Although the therapist is working on a physical response, the importance of the emotional response should not be underemphasized. The patient should feel free to discuss psychosocial matters with a nonjudgmental therapist. Because the occupational therapist is trained to work with the whole person and because research indicates that the body is not biochemically separated from the mind, a holistic approach to treatment is feasible. Furthermore, the discussion of emotions or stressors related to the physical disability may help the patient develop coping mechanisms and a better attitude about the disability.[17,46,57,74]

Another new concept is that the skin is incredibly dynamic. With the exception of the cornea and mucous membranes, the skin is one of the fastest growing tissues in the body.[29] A completely new skin is developed every 4 to 6 weeks. Radiographic studies have shown that 98% of the body's atoms are renewed each year, and the atoms of the skin are the first to be exchanged.[30] Some researchers are referring to the human body as a complex energy field.*

An approach to working with the skin's bioelectric energy was developed by Doris Krieger in the field of nursing.[47,56,60-62] Since 1977, several studies have confirmed the efficacy of her technique, called *therapeutic touch.* According to this theory, each person is composed of a complex energy field and forms of life energy. These fields of energy not only run through the skin, body, and bones but also are in constant interaction and exchange with surrounding energy fields in the environment. Therapeutic touch is performed by directing the life energy through the hands of the therapist to the patient, who may then internalize it or use it to restore balance and promote self-regulation of healing.[56]

At first, this concept was very controversial and regarded as little more than mysticism and nonscience. Several well-controlled studies have revealed, however, that subjects receiving therapeutic touch (TT) recorded increased hemoglobin levels, which bring more oxygen

---

* References 20, 53, 56, 62, 80, 91.

to tissues, increased relaxation responses verified by electroencephalograph readings, reduction of orthopedically related pain, and a balance of positively and negatively charged ions.[47,56,60-62] The practice of therapeutic touch goes beyond the scope of this chapter but it can be used effectively before touch and sensory stimulation. To date, one of the most important findings of this research is that touch is biochemically and psychologically more beneficial when the therapist performs it with unconditional kindness or with the intent to help or heal.[61,91]

Studies show that when the person performing therapeutic touch is mentally preoccupied, the physiologic benefits are significantly diminished.[56] In my opinion, the occupational therapy concept called *therapeutic use of self* is synonymous with the intent of therapeutic touch. It also appears that we are connected in ways that are not fully understood. Therefore, when applying any procedure in occupational therapy, the therapist should have clear intentions to help the person and keep in mind that the activity or modality is only a medium through which to communicate.

This brief review of the literature has revealed many new possibilities for sensory stimulation as a modality for treatment. The Rood approach to the use of sensory stimulation has opened the door to many possibilities. New avenues can be explored to expand the basic tenets of Rood's work. Occupational therapists should continue to use sensory stimulation with confidence while keeping a cautious eye on new research literature for scientific verification of sensorimotor techniques.

REVIEW QUESTIONS

1. List the four goals of the Rood approach.
2. Differentiate between the motor responses elicited by the TNR and TLR.
3. What are the three major reactions produced by sensory stimulation?
4. Describe the four rules for sensory stimulation.
5. List the four sequences of motor development.
6. Describe the eight ontogenetic motor patterns.
7. Differentiate between exteroceptive and proprioceptive stimulation.
8. Which nerve fibers carry pain, temperature, and light touch?
9. Which nerve fibers carry conscious and subconscious proprioceptive messages?
10. Contrast the functions of the stabilizer and mobilizer muscles.
11. How often is the light touch

stimulus applied and what happens if it is applied too often?
12. How long should fast brushing be applied to the skin?
13. Why should fast brushing be applied according to dermatomal segments?
14. List the skin areas in which fast brushing is contraindicated.
15. Describe the uses of C icing, A icing, and autonomic icing and the principal motor responses elicited by each.
16. Discuss the advantages of proprioceptive stimulation over cutaneous stimulation.
17. How is heavy joint compression differentiated from light joint compression?
18. Describe how inversion is used as a therapeutic modality.
19. Explain how therapeutic vibration can be used to activate muscles and cutaneous receptors.
20. Discuss three methods of reducing muscle tone.
21. List five types of touch and describe the benefits or adverse effects of each.
22. Discuss the potential benefits of therapeutic touch.
23. Under what conditions is therapeutic touch most beneficial to the patient?

REFERENCES

1. Abbruzzese G and associates: Excitation from skin receptors contributing to the tonic vibration reflex in man, *Brain Res* 150:194, 1978.
2. Afifi A, Bergman R: *Basic neuroscience,* Munich, 1980, Verlag Urban und Schwarzenberg.
3. Alpern M, Lawrence N, Wolsk D: *Sensory processes,* Belmont, Calif, 1976, Brooks/Cole.

4. Androsik F: Relaxation and biofeedback for chronic headaches. In Halzman A, Turk D, editors: *Pain management: a handbook of psychological treatment approaches,* New York, 1986, Pergamon Press.

5. Ayres J: *Sensory integration and learning disorders,* Los Angeles, 1972, Western Psychological Services.

6. Ayres J: *The development of sensory integrative theory and practice,* Dubuque, Iowa, 1974, Kendall/Hunt.

7. Bach-y-Rita P: *Sensory substitution in rehabilitation of the neurological patient,* Oxford, England, 1983, Basil Blackwell.

8. Barr ML: *The human nervous system,* ed 2, New York, 1974, Harper & Row.

9. Beeson P, McDermott W: *The textbook of medicine,* Philadelphia, 1979, WB Saunders.

10. Bishop B: Vibratory stimulation. I. *Phys Ther* 54:1273, 1974.

11. Bishop B: Vibratory stimulation. II. *Phys Ther* 55:29, 1975.

12. Bishop B: Vibratory stimulation. III. *Phys Ther* 55:139, 1975.

13. Bishop B: Spasticity: its physiology and management. I, II, and III. *Phys Ther* 57:4, 1977.

14. Bower B: Different strokes, *Science News* 128:301, 1985.

15. Bowlby J: The nature of the child's tie to his mother, *Int J Psychoanal* 39:350, 1958.

16. Buchwald J: Exteroceptive reflexes and movement, *Am J Phys Med* 46:121, 1967.

17. Burnside IM: Caring for the aged: touching is talking, *Am J Nurs* 73:2060, 1973.

18. Burton A, Heller L: The touching of the body, *Psychoanal Rev* 51:122, 1964.

19. Buschsbaum M, Pfefferbaum A: Individual differences in stimulus intensity response, *Psychophysiology* 8:600, 1971.

20. Capra F: The Tao of physics, Boulder, Colo, 1975, Shambhala Publications.

21. Chusid JG: *Correlative neuroanatomy and functional neurology,* ed 18, Los Altos, Calif, 1982, Lange Medical Publications.

22. Clark B: The vestibular system. In Mussen PH, Rosenzweig MR, editors: *Annual review of psychology,* New York, 1970, Harper & Row.

23. Clark R: *Manter and Gatz's essentials of clinical neuroanatomy and neurophysiology,* ed 5, Philadelphia, 1975, FA Davis.

24. Colavila F: *Sensory changes in the elderly,* Springfield, Ill, 1978, Charles C Thomas.

25. Day F: The patient's perception of touch. In Anderson D, Bergersen M, Duffey M and associates, editors: *Current concepts in clinical nursing,* St Louis, 1973, CV Mosby.

26. Dayhoof N: Re-thinking stroke: soft or hard devices to position hands? *Am J Nurs* 7:1142, 1975.

27. DeQuiros JB: Diagnosis of vestibular disorders in the learning disabled, *J Learning Disabilities* 9:50, 1974.

28. Dominion J: The psychological significance of touch, *Nurs Times* 67:896, 1971.

29. Dossey L: The biodance in space, time, and medicine, Boulder, Colo, 1982, Shambhala Publications.

30. Dossey L: The skin: what is it? *Topics Clin Nurs* 5:1, 1983.

31. Eldred E: The dual sensory role of muscle spindles, *Phys Ther* 45:290, 1965.

32. Eldred E: Peripheral receptors: their excitation and relation to reflex patterns, *Am J Phys Med* 46:69, 1967.

33. Farber S: *Sensorimotor evaluation and treatment procedures for allied health personnel,* Indianapolis, 1974, Indiana University & Purdue University Medical Center.

34. Farber S: *Neurorehabilitation: a multisensory approach,* Philadelphia, 1982, WB Saunders.

35. Fukuda T: Studies on human dynamic postures from the viewpoint of postural reflexes, *Acta Otolaryngol* 161(suppl):8, 1961.

36. Fulton JF: *Physiology of the nervous system,* vol 179, ed 3, New York, 1949, Oxford University Press.

37. Gardner E: *Fundamentals of neurology,* ed 6, Philadelphia, 1975, WB Saunders.

38. Geldard F: *The human senses,* New York, 1972, John Wiley & Sons.

39. Gilman S, Winans S: *Essentials of clinical neuroanatomy and neurophysiology,* ed 6, Philadelphia, 1982, FA Davis.

40. Glick G, Brauwald E: Relative roles of the sympathetic and parasympathetic system in the reflex control of heart rate, *Circ Res* 16:363, 1965.

41. Goff B: The Rood approach. In *Cash's textbook of neurology for physiotherapists,* ed 4, Philadelphia, 1986, JB Lippincott.

42. Goldberg S: *Clinical neuroanatomy made ridiculously simple,* Miami, 1979, Medical Master.

43. Greenberg JH, Reivich A, Alavi A, Hand P: Metabolic mapping of functional activity in human subjects with the fluorodeoxyglucose technique, *Science* 212:678, 1981.

44. Guyton A: *Structure and function of the nervous system,* Philadelphia, 1972, WB Saunders.

45. Hagbarth KE, Edlund G: The muscle vibrator: a useful tool in neurological therapeutic work, *Scand J Rehabil Med* 1:26, 1969.

46. Hammer S: The mind as healer, *Science Digest* 47, April 1984.

47. Heidt P: Effect of therapeutic touch on anxiety level in hospitalized patients, *Nurs Res* 30(1):32, 1981.

48. Heininger M, Randolph S: *Neurophysiological concepts in human behavior,* St Louis, 1981, CV Mosby.

49. Hellebrandt F, Schade M, Carns M: Methods of evoking the tonic neck reflexes in normal human subjects, *Am J Phys Med* 41:89, 1962.

50. Hellebrandt F and associates: Tonic neck reflexes in exercise of stress in man, *Am J Phys Med* 35:144, 1956.

51. Henderson A, Coryell J: *The body senses and perceptual deficit: Proceedings of the Occupational Therapy Symposium,* Boston, 1973.

52. Hirt S: The tonic neck reflex mechanism in the normal human adult, *Am J Phys Med* 46:362, 1967.

53. Holbrook B: *The stone monkey: an alternative Chinese scientific reality*, New York, 1981, William Morrow.

54. Huss AJ: Sensorimotor approaches. In Hopkins H, Smith H, editors: *Willard and Spackman's occupational therapy*, ed 5, Philadelphia, 1978, JB Lippincott.

55. Jones GM, Watt D: Muscular control of landing from unexpected falls in man, *J Physiol (London)* 219:729, 1971.

56. Keller E, Bzdek V: Effects of therapeutic touch on tension headache pain, *Nurs Res* 35(2):101, 1986.

57. Kenshalo D: *Sensory functions of the skin of humans*, New York, 1977, Plenum Press.

58. Kottke F: From reflex to skill: the training of coordination, *Arch Phys Med Rehabil* 61:551, 1980.

59. Kottke F, Stillwell K, Lehmann J: *Krusen's handbook of physical medicine and rehabilitation*, ed 3, Philadelphia, 1982, WB Saunders.

60. Krieger D: Healing by the laying on of hands as a facilitator of bioenergetic change: the response of in vivo hemoglobin, *Psychenergetic Systems* 1:121, 1976.

61. Krieger D: *The therapeutic touch: how to help your hands to help or heal*, Englewood Cliffs, NJ, 1979, Prentice-Hall Books.

62. Krieger D, Peper E, Ancoli S: Therapeutic touch: searching for evidence of physiological change, *Am J Nurs* 79:660, 1979.

63. Lagercrantz H, Slotkin T: The stress of being born, *Scientific American*: 254(4):100, 1986.

64. Locke S, Colligan D: Mind cures, *OMNI* 7:(7)44, 1986.

65. Loeb GE, Hoffer JA: *Muscle spindle function: in muscle receptors in movement control*, London, 1981, Macmillan Publishing.

66. Lynch JJ, Thomas SA, Mills ME and associates: The effects of human contact on cardiac arrhythmia in coronary care patients, *J Neurol Ment Dis* 158:88, 1974.

67. Mann F: *Acupuncture: the ancient Chinese art of healing*, New York, 1972, Vintage Books-Random House.

68. Matthews PBC: Muscle spindles and their motor control, *Physiol Rev* 44:219, 1964.

69. McCloskey DI: Kinesthetic sensibility, *Physiol Rev* 58:763, 1978.

70. Medalie JH, Goldbourt U: Angina pectoris among 10,000 men with psychosocial and other risk factors as evidenced by a multivariate analysis of a five year incidence study, *Am J Med* 60(6):920, 1978.

71. Mills ME, Thomas SA, Lynch JJ, Katcher AH: Effect of pulse palpation on cardiac arrhythmia in coronary care patients, *Nurs Res* 25:378, 1976.

72. Montague A: *Touching: the significance of the sin*, ed 2, San Francisco, 1978, Harper & Row.

73. Moore J: The Golgi tendon organ and the muscle spindle, *Am J Occup Ther* 28:415, 1974.

74. Morse JM: An ethnoscientific analysis of comfort: a preliminary investigation, *Nursing Papers* 15:6, 1983.

75. Murray MP: Gait as a total pattern of movement, *Am J Phys Med* 46:290, 1967.

76. Nerem RM, Levesque MJ, Cornhill JF: Social environment as a factor in diet-induced atherosclerosis, *Science* 208(4451):1475, 1980.

77. Payton R, Hirt E, Newtown G, editors: *Scientific basis for neurophysiologic approaches to therapeutic exercise: an anthology*, ed 2, Philadelphia, 1978, FA Davis.

78. Pedretti LW: *Occupational therapy: practice skills for dysfunction*, St Louis, 1981, CV Mosby.

79. Pertovaara M: Modification of human pain threshold by specific tactile receptors, *Acta Physiol Scand* 107:339, 1979.

80. Randolph G: Therapeutic and physical touch: physiological response to stressful stimuli, *Nurs Res* 33(1):33, 1984.

81. Rausch P: A tactile and kinesthetic stimulation program for premature infants. In Brown C, editor: *The many facets of touch*, Special issue, Skillman, NJ, 1984, Johnson & Johnson.

82. Roberts T: *Neurophysiology of postural mechanisms*, New York, 1976, Plenum.

83. Rood M: Occupational therapy in the treatment of the cerebral palsied, *Phys Ther Rev* 32:220, 1952.

84. Rood M: Neurophysiological reactions as a basis for physical therapy, *Phys Ther Rev* 34:444, 1954.

85. Rood M: Neurophysiological mechanisms utilized in the treatment of neuromuscular dysfunction, *Am J Occup Ther* 10:4, 1956.

86. Rood M: The use of sensory receptors to activate, facilitate and inhibit motor response, automatic and somatic, in developmental sequence. In Sattely C, editor: *Approaches to the treatment of patients with neuromuscular dysfunction*, Dubuque, Iowa, 1962, Wm C Brown Book.

87. Rose S: Preterm responses of passive, active and social touch. In Brown C, editor: *The many facets of touch*, Special issue, Skillman, NJ, 1984, Johnson & Johnson.

88. Schmidt R: *Fundamentals of sensory physiology*, New York, 1978, Springer-Verlag.

89. Schwartz P, Malliani A: Electrical alteration of the T wave: clinical and experimental evidence of its relationship with the sympathetic nervous system and with the long Q-T syndrome, *Am Heart J* 89:45, 1976.

90. Sinclair D: *Cutaneous sensation*, New York, 1967, Oxford University Press.

91. Smith F: *Inner bridges: a guide to energy movement and body structure*, Atlanta, Georgia, 1986, Humanic, New Age.

92. Smythies JR: *Brain mechanisms and behavior*, ed 2, New York, 1970, Academic Press.

93. Snyder S: Neurosciences: an integrative discipline, *Science* 225(4468):1255, 1984.

94. Spicer SD, Matyas TA: Facilitation of the tonic vibration reflex (TVR) by cutaneous stimulation, *Am J Phys Med* 59:223, 1980.

95. Stejskal L: Postural reflexes in man, *Am J Phys Med* 58:1, 1979.

96. Stockmeyer S: An interpretation of the approach of Rood to the treatment of neuromuscular dysfunction, NUSTEP proceedings, *Am J Phys Med* 46:900, 1967.

97. Taubes G: An electrifying possibility, *Discover* 7(4):22, 1986.

98. Tokizane T and associates: Electromyographic studies on tonic neck, lumbar and labyrinthine reflexes in normal persons, *Jpn J Physiol* 2:30, 1951.

99. Trombly CA, Scott AD: *Occupational therapy for physical dysfunction,* Baltimore, 1977, Williams & Wilkins.

100. Vallbo A and associates: Somatosensory proprioceptive and sympathetic activity in human peripheral nerves, *Physiol Rev* 4:59, 1979.

101. Weiss S: Psychophysiological effects of caregiver touch on incidence of cardiac dysrhythmia, *Heart and Lung,* 15(5):495, 1986.

102. Werner J: *Neuroscience: a clinical perspective,* Philadelphia, 1980, WB Saunders.

103. Weschsler R: A new prescription: mind over malady, *Discover* 2(8): 50, 1987.

104. Williams P, Warwick R: *Functional neuroanatomy of man,* Philadelphia, 1975, WB Saunders.

105. Wilson VJ, Paterson BW: The role of the vestibular system in posture and movement. In Mountcastle V, editor: *Medical physiology,* ed 14, St Louis, 1979, CV Mosby.

106. Yakovlev P, Lecours A: *Regional development of the brain in early life,* vol 3, Oxford, 1967, Minkowski Blackwell Scientific Publications.

Movement Therapy: The Brunnstrom Approach to Treatment of Hemiplegia

Lorraine Williams Pedretti

PROFILE

Signe Brunnstrom was a physical therapist from Sweden. Her practice, teaching, and theory development in the United States extended from the World War II years through the 1970s. Her clinical observation and research at major treatment and educational institutions were done primarily in the Northeast and led to the development of the treatment approach that she called *movement therapy*. It was the first systematic approach to the treatment of motor dysfunction after cerebral vascular accident (CVA). Brunnstrom published three major works in the United States. She coauthored a book with Donald Kerr, *Training the Lower Extremity Amputee*, and later published the well-known *Clinical Kinesiology*. Her third book was *Movement Therapy in Hemiplegia*, published in 1970, in which she described movement therapy, also known as the *Brunnstrom approach* to the treatment of hemiplegia. Signe Brunnstrom died in February, 1988.[10]

Movement Therapy in Hemiplegia has been a primary reference for this chapter.[3] The theoretical foundations, treatment goals, and methods are intended as an overview and introduction to some of the procedures that the new practitioner may find helpful. To learn the details of the treatment approach and additional procedures, the reader is referred to the original source for further study.

THEORETICAL FOUNDATIONS

Brunnstrom evolved her treatment approach on the basis of an extensive review of the literature in neurophysiology, central nervous system (CNS) mechanisms, effects of CNS damage, sensory systems and related topics, plus clinical observation and application of training procedures.[3]

The work of several major theorists, such as Gellhorn, Denny-Brown, Hagbarth, Jackson, Magnus, and Sherrington, served as the foundation for the treatment approach. A few of the important concepts are summarized briefly here. Sherrington, whose work dates to the late 1800s, stated that afferent-efferent (sensory-motor) mechanisms in phylogenesis are retained in man. He stated that these mechanisms served as the basis for the evolutionary process that resulted in man's movements being more voluntary than automatic, as seen in lower animals. Sherrington postulated that sensory denervation abolished all voluntary movement and that sensation was necessary for effective movement.[3]

In the early 1900s Magnus stated that peripheral influences continuously affect the CNS and may work together to facilitate a movement or exert opposite influences that compete with each other. Magnus demonstrated in experimental animals that the same stimulus may evoke opposite motor responses, depending on the position of the responding part.[3] The studies of Magnus support the hypothesis that sensory stimuli and positioning can be used to influence motor function.

In the late 1800s Hughlings Jackson described the successive levels of CNS integration. He postulated that the spinal cord and cranial nerve nuclei are located at the lowest motor centers and that muscles in all parts of the body are represented at this level, but few movement combinations are possible. Movements are simple and more automatic than voluntary at this level. He described the middle motor centers in the Rolandic region of the brain. All the muscles represented at the lowest motor centers also are represented here. More complex movements are possible, however, but movement is still more automatic than voluntary at the middle motor centers. Jackson stated that the frontal lobes contain the highest motor centers, along with corresponding sensory centers. The body parts represented at the middle and lowest motor centers are represented here in a still more complex manner than before. This level subserves complex voluntary movement.[11]

Jackson hypothesized that the damaged CNS has undergone an "evolution in reverse." The same reflexes present in earlier phylogenesis and ontogenesis are present once again after CNS damage. Therefore, these reflexes were considered normal for the regressed CNS. Jackson also stated that reflexes are precursors of purposeful movement and that they support purposeful movement.[3] Brunnstrom's treatment approach is based on Jackson's hypotheses. These hypotheses are being modified by newer concepts in neurophysiology.[6,7] The behavioral responses that Brunnstrom observed continue to be valid however, and many aspects of the treatment approach are very useful.

The successive levels of CNS integration and the reflexes and reactions thought to be integrated at each level were summarized as follows:

- Spinal level (apedal): flexor withdrawal, extensor thrust, crossed extension
- Brain stem level (apedal): tonic neck reflexes (TNRs), tonic labyrinthine reflex (TLR), associated reactions, positive and negative supporting reactions
- Midbrain level (quadrupedal): neck righting, body righting, labyrinthine righting, optical righting, amphibian reaction, Moro reflex
- Cortical level (bipedal): equilibrium reactions[5]

Twitchell described a sequence of motor recovery after CVA. He hypothesized that recovery after CVA constitutes a reversal of the regression of CNS function. He stated that primitive responses are the bases for the evolution of more elaborate motor responses. Twitchell also noted that all proprioceptive responses are influenced by neck- and body-righting reactions, reflexes, and tactile stimulation. He replicated Sherrington's study and concluded that (1) sensation is critical to movement, (2) without sensation a limb is essentially useless, (3) preservation of cutaneous sensation in the hand is indispensable for motor function of the upper limb, and (4) movements of the upper limb, particularly grasp function, are directed by contactual stimuli. The recovery process after CVA described by Twitchell is summarized sequentially by the following characteristics:

1. Flaccidity
2. Stretch reflexes
3. Complex proprioceptive reactions such as the proximal traction response
4. Limb synergies with ability to use these movement patterns
5. Decline in spasticity
6. Improvement of willed movement and ability to be influenced by tactile stimuli[12]

Brunnstrom subscribed to the concept that the damaged CNS has undergone an evolution in reverse and regressed to phylogenetically older patterns of movement. These include the *limb synergies,* gross patterns of limb flexion and extension that are primitive spinal cord patterns, and primitive reflexes.[2,3] These primitive movement patterns were thought to be modified in man through the influence of higher centers of nervous system control during development. After CVA, they returned to their primitive, stereotyped character. When the influence of higher centers is disturbed or destroyed, reflexes present in early life (such as TNRs, tonic lumbar reflex, and TLR) reappear, and normal deep tendon reflexes (DTR) become exaggerated. The TNRs, TLR, and tonic lumbar reflex are considered 'normal' when, as in hemiplegia, the central nervous system (CNS) has regressed to an earlier developmental stage.[3]

The Brunnstrom approach to the treatment of hemiplegia is based on the use of motor patterns available to the patient at any point in the recovery process. It enhances progress through the stages of recovery toward more normal and complex movement patterns. Brunnstrom saw synergies, reflexes, and other abnormal movement patterns as a normal part of the process that the patient must go through before normal voluntary movement can occur.

Synergistic movements are used by normal persons all of the time, but they are controlled, occur in a wide variety of patterns, and can be modified or stopped at will. Brunnstrom maintained that the synergies appear to constitute a necessary intermediate stage for further recovery. Gross movement synergies of flexion and extension always precede the restoration of advanced motor functioning following hemiplegia.[3] Therefore during the early stages of recovery (stages 1 to 3), Brunnstrom maintained that the patient should be aided to gain control of the limb synergies and that selected afferent stimuli (TNRs, TLR, cutaneous and stretch stimuli, and positioning and associated reactions) can be advantageous in helping the patient to initiate and gain control of movement. Once the synergies can be performed voluntarily with some ease, they are modified, and simple to complex movement combinations can be performed (stages 4 and 5), which deviate from the stereotypical synergy patterns of flexion and extension.[3]

The advisability of using reflexes, synergies, and associated reactions to effect motion was challenged by Bobath.[1] It is argued that no pathologic responses should be used in training for fear that by repeated use the efferent pathways will become too readily available for use at the expense of normal pathways.[2,3] Brunnstrom, however, concluded that the opposite was true. She maintained that during the early stages of recovery, the development of the synergies should be facilitated. The use of selected exteroceptive and proprioceptive stimuli is justified for this purpose.[2,3] Both Bobath and Brunnstrom based their hypotheses on neurophysiology. Brunnstrom proposed that the approaches may not be as opposed as they appear. She stated that at an early recovery stage, only re-flex movement is available and is considered normal, whereas at later stages, reflex activity is inhibited and more normal movement is possible. Brunnstrom proposed that both approaches can be useful if applied to a specific patient at a specific time.[3]

THE LIMB SYNERGIES

A *limb synergy* of flexion or extension, seen in hemiplegia, is a group of muscles acting as a bound unit in a primitive and stereotypical manner.[3] The muscles are neurophysiologically linked and cannot act alone or perform all of their functions. If one muscle in the synergy is activated, each muscle in the synergy responds partially or completely. The patient thus cannot perform isolated movements when bound by these synergies.

The flexor synergy of the upper limb consists of scapular adduction and elevation, shoulder abduction and external rotation, elbow flexion, forearm supination, wrist flexion, and finger flexion. Hypertonicity (spasticity) is usually greatest in the elbow flexion component, and least in shoulder abduction and external rotation (Fig. 22-1). The extensor synergy consists of scapula abduction and depression, shoulder adduction and internal rotation, elbow extension, forearm pronation, and wrist and finger flexion or extension. Shoulder adduction and internal rotation are usually the most hypertonic components of the extensor synergy, with much less tone in the elbow extension component (Fig. 22-2).

In the lower limb the flexor synergy consists of hip flexion and abduction and external rotation, knee flexion, ankle dorsiflexion and inversion, and toe extension. Hip flexion is usually the component with the highest tone, and hip abduction and external rotation are the components with the least tone. The extensor synergy is composed of hip adduction, extension, and internal rotation; knee extension; ankle plantar flexion and inversion; and toe flexion. Hip adduction, knee extension, and ankle plantar flexion are usually the most hypertonic

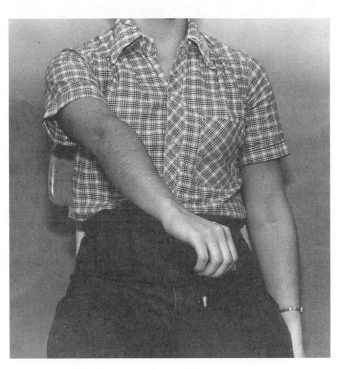

FIG. 22-2 Extensor synergy of upper limb in hemiplegia.

components, whereas hip extension and internal rotation are usually less so.

CHARACTERISTICS OF SYNERGISTIC MOVEMENT

The flexor synergy dominates in the arm, and the extensor synergy dominates in the leg. Performance of synergistic movement, either reflexively or voluntarily, may be influenced by the postural mechanism. When the patient performs the synergy, the components with the greatest degree of hypertonicity are often most apparent, rather than the entire classic patterns described previously. By the same token, the resting posture of the limb, particularly the arm, is usually characterized by a position that represents the most hypertonic components of both flexor and extensor synergies, that is, shoulder adduction, elbow flexion, forearm pronation, and wrist and finger flexion. With facilitation or voluntary effort, however, the more classic synergy pattern can usually be evoked.[3]

MOTOR RECOVERY PROCESS

Following CVA resulting in hemiplegia, Brunnstrom observed that the patient progresses through a series of recovery steps or stages in a fairly stereotypical fashion (Table 22-1). The progress through these stages may be rapid or slow.

The recovery follows an ontogenetic process, usually proximal to distal so that shoulder movement can be expected before hand movement. Flexion patterns occur before extension patterns in the upper limb. Reflex motion occurs before controlled, volitional movement, and

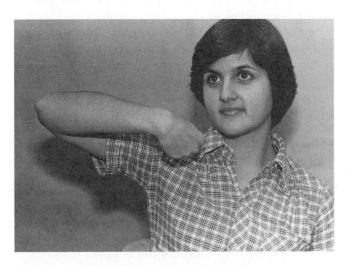

FIG. 22-1 Flexor synergy of upper limb in hemiplegia.

TABLE 22-1   Motor Recovery Following Cerebrovascular Accident

STAGE	CHARACTERISTICS		
	Leg	Arm	Hand*
1	Flaccidity	Flaccidity; inability to perform any movements	No hand function
2	Spasticity develops; minimal voluntary movements	Beginning development of spasticity; limb synergies or some of their components begin to appear as associated reactions	Gross grasp beginning; minimal finger flexion possible
3	Spasticity peaks; flexion and extension synergy present; hip-knee-ankle flexion in sitting and standing	Spasticity increasing; synergy patterns or some of their components can be performed voluntarily	Gross grasp, hook grasp possible; no release
4	Knee flexion past 90° in sitting, with foot sliding backward on floor; dorsiflexion with heel on floor and knee flexed to 90°	Spasticity declining; movement combinations deviating from synergies are now possible	Gross grasp present; lateral prehension developing; small amount of finger extension and some thumb movement possible
5	Knee flexion with hip extended in standing; ankle dorsiflexion with hip and knee extended	Synergies no longer dominant; more movement combinations deviating from synergies performed with greater ease	Palmar prehension, spherical and cylindrical grasp and release possible
6	Hip abduction in sitting or standing; reciprocal internal and external rotation of hip combined with inversion and eversion of ankle in sitting	Spasticity absent except when performing rapid movements; isolated joint movements performed with ease	All types of prehension, individual finger motion, and full range of voluntary extension possible

From Brunnstrom S: *Movement therapy in hemiplegia.* New York, 1970, Harper & Row.
* NOTE: Recovery of hand function is variable and may not parallel the six recovery stages of the arm.

gross movement patterns can be performed before isolated, selective movement.[3]

Recovery may cease at any stage and is influenced by factors such as sensation, perception, cognition, motivation, affective states, and concomitant medical problems. Few patients make a very good recovery of arm function, and the greatest loss is usually in the wrist and hand.

It should be noted that no two patients are exactly alike. There is much individual variation in the characteristic motor disturbances and the recovery process among patients. The motor behavior and recovery process described represent common characteristics that may be observed in most persons after CVA occurs.[3]

DEFINITIONS OF TERMS

Some definitions of terms are necessary before the discussion of treatment principles that follows. *Associated reactions* are movements seen on the affected side in response to voluntary forceful movements in other parts of the body.[3] Resistance to flexion movements of the normal upper extremity usually evokes a flexion synergy or some of its components in the affected upper extremity. By the same token, resistance to extension on the sound side evokes extension on the affected side. In the lower extremities the responses are reversed. Resisted flexion of the normal limb evokes extension of the affected limb and vice versa.[9]

Homolateral limb synkinesis is a mutual dependency between the synergies of the affected upper and lower limbs. The same or similar motion occurs in the limb on the same side of the body. For example, efforts at flexion

of the affected upper extremity evoke flexion of the lower extremity.[3,9] The mirroring of movements attempted or performed on the affected side by the unaffected side, perhaps in an effort to facilitate the movement, is called *imitation synkinesis.*[3]

Several specialized reactions can be noted in the hemiplegic hand. These are the proximal traction response, grasp reflex, instinctive grasp reaction, instinctive avoiding reaction, and the Souques finger phenomenon. The *proximal traction response* is elicited by a stretch to the flexor muscles of one joint of the upper limb, which evokes contraction of all flexors of that limb, including the fingers. This response may therefore be used to elicit the flexion synergy. To elicit the *grasp reflex,* deep pressure is applied to the palm and moved distally over the hand and fingers, mostly on the radial side. The responses are complex but in general adduction and flexion of the digits are present. The *instinctive grasp reaction* is differentiated by Brunnstrom from the grasp reflex. It is a closure of the hand in response to contact of a stationary object with the palm of the hand. The person is unable to release the object-stimulus once the fist has been closed.

A hyperextension reaction of the fingers and thumb in response to forward-upward elevation of the arm is the *instinctive avoiding reaction.* Brunnstrom reported that, with the arm in this position, stroking distally over the palm and attempting to reach out and grasp an object resulted in an exaggeration of the reaction. The automatic extension of the fingers when the shoulder is flexed is known as the *Souques' finger phenomenon* and can be observed in some but not all patients with hemiplegia. Brunnstrom found that although this phenomenon may not be exhibited, the elevated position of the affected arm is favorable for the facilitation of finger extension.[3]

MOTOR EVALUATION OF THE PATIENT WITH HEMIPLEGIA

Brunnstrom in *Movement Therapy in Hemiplegia* described an evaluation procedure that assesses muscle tone, stage of recovery, movement patterns, motor speed, and prehension patterns of the upper extremity.[3] The evaluation is based on the recovery stages after the onset of hemiplegia. The test requires the patient to perform motor acts that are graduated in complexity and require increasingly finer neuromuscular control.

Progress through the recovery stages is gradual, and signs of two stages may be apparent at any given time in the patient's recovery. Because it is not possible to establish an absolute demarcation between one recovery stage and the next, the patient may be classified as stages 2 and 3 or 3 and 4, for example. This rating indicates progression from one stage to the next. The Hemiplegia Classification and Progress Record is presented in Fig. 22-3. The reader should refer to this form while reading the directions for test administration, which have been summarized from *Movement Therapy in Hemiplegia*.[3]

GROSS SENSORY TESTING

Sensory evaluation precedes motor evaluation and includes assessment of passive motion sense and touch localization in the hand. Tests of passive motion sense of the shoulder, elbow, forearm, wrist, and fingers are carried out by procedures similar to those described in Chapter 13. Results are recorded on the first and second pages of the form (shown in Fig. 22-3, *A* and *B*).

Fingertip recognition is evaluated by asking the patient to localize touch stimuli to specific fingers. The patient is seated with forearms pronated and resting on a pillow in the lap. The test is given with the vision occluded after a rehearsal in full view. The palmar surface of the fingertips is lightly touched with a pencil eraser in a random sequence. The patient must indicate which finger is being touched. Results are recorded on the second page of the form (Fig. 22-3, *B*).

MOTOR TESTS, UPPER EXTREMITY

The patient is classified as being in recovery stage 1 when no voluntary movement of the affected arm can be initiated.[3] The examiner should move the limb passively through the synergy patterns and assess the degree of resistance to passive movement. The patient should be asked to attempt movement during these maneuvers. During recovery stage 1 the limb is predominantly flaccid and feels heavy, there is little or no resistance to passive movement, and the patient is unable to initiate or effect any movement voluntarily.

During recovery stage 2 tone begins to increase, and the limb synergies or some of their components may be evoked on voluntary effort or as associated reactions. The flexor synergy usually appears first.[3] The therapist may again move the limb passively, alternating between flexor and extensor synergy patterns. The therapist should ask the patient to help in the movements. Thus it is possible to assess the degree of hypertonicity and to assess whether the subject's voluntary efforts are evoking any movement responses.

During recovery stage 3, hypertonicity is increased and may be marked. The limb synergies or some of their components are performed voluntarily, though with much effort and cognitive control. The patient may remain at this stage for a long time, and severely involved patients may never progress beyond it. The pectoralis major, pronators, and wrist and finger flexors may be very spastic, causing limited performance of their antagonists.

The patient is seated, and the complete flexor synergy is demonstrated by the therapist. The patient is asked to perform the movement pattern with the unaffected side to demonstrate that the directions are understood. The patient is then asked to perform the movement pattern with the affected side after a command such as "touch your ear" or "touch your mouth," which gives purpose and direction to the effort. A similar procedure is used to evaluate performance of the extensor synergy. The patient is asked to reach forward and downward to touch the therapist's hand, which is held between the patient's knees. The responses may be influenced by the predominant hypertonicity seen in components of each of the synergies. For instance, the very spastic pectoralis major and elbow flexors may predominate during the patient's efforts and result in the patient reaching across the thorax to touch the opposite shoulder. The status of the synergies is recorded on the evaluation form in terms of the active joint range achieved for each motion in the pattern. The joint ranges are estimated and recorded as 0, ¼, ½, ¾, or full range.

When the patient has reached recovery stage 4, there is a decrease in spasticity, and the patient is capable of performing gross movement combinations that deviate from the limb synergies. Brunnstrom chose three movements to represent stage 4. These are (1) placing the hand behind the body to touch the sacral region, (2) raising the arm forward to 90° of shoulder flexion with elbow extended, and (3) pronating and supinating the forearm with the elbow flexed to 90° and stabilized close to the side of the body. The patient performs all of the movements while seated, and as in all test items, no facilitation is allowed. During the test for pronation-supination, bilateral performance is allowed so that the therapist can compare the two sides.

Further decrease of hypertonicity and ability to perform more complex combinations of movement characterize recovery stage 5. The patient is relatively free of

HEMIPLEGIA CLASSIFICATION AND PROGRESS RECORD

Upper limb-test sitting

Name_____ Age _____ Date of onset_____ Side affected _____

Date _____

____ Passive motion sense: Shoulder _____ Elbow _____

____ Pronation-supination _____ Wrist flexion-extension _____

____ 1.   NO MOVEMENT INITIATED OR ELICITED _____

____ 2.   SYNERGIES OR COMPONENTS FIRST APPEARING.   Spasticity developing_____
____   Flexor synergy_____
____   Extensor synergy_____

____ 3.   SYNERGIES OR COMPONENTS INITIATED VOLUNTARILY. Spasticity marked_____

FLEXOR SYNERGY		ACTIVE JOINT RANGE		REMARKS
____ Shoulder girdle	Elevation			
	Retraction			
____ Shoulder joint	Hyperextension Abduction			
____	External rotation			
____ Elbow	Flexion			
____ Forearm	Pronation			
EXTENSOR SYNERGY				
____ Shoulder	Pectoralis major			
____ Elbow	Extension			
____ Forearm	Pronation			
4. MOVEMENTS DEVIATING	Hand to sacral region			
____ FROM BASIC SYNERGIES.	Raise arm forward-horizontally			
____ Spasticity decreasing	Pronate-supinate elbow at 90 degrees			
5. RELATIVE IN-DEPENDENCE	Raise arm sideways -horizontally			
____ OF BASIC SYNERGIES.	Raise arm over head			
____ Spasticity waning	Pronate-supinate elbow extended			
6. MOVEMENT COORDINATION NEAR NORMAL. Spasticity minimal				

A

FIG. 22-3   *A, B, C,* Hemiplegia classification and progress record. (From Brunnstrom S: *Movement therapy in hemiplegia,* New York, 1970, Harper & Row.)

the influence of the limb synergies and performs the stage 4 movements with greater ease. Three movements chosen to represent stage 5 are (1) raising the arm to 90° of shoulder abduction with the elbow extended and forearm pronated, (2) raising the arm forward, as in stage 4, but above 90° of shoulder flexion, and (3) pronating and supinating the forearm with the elbow extended. The third movement is performed with the arm in the forward or side horizontal position and is not isolated from shoulder internal and external rotation.

Persons who progess to recovery stage 6 are able to perform isolated joint motions and demonstrate coordination that is comparable or nearly comparable to that of the unaffected side. On close observation the trained observer may detect some awkwardness of movement, and there may be some incoordination when rapid movement is attempted. The patient may be evaluated while performing a variety of daily living tasks, provided that recovery of hand function has kept pace with recovery of arm function.

HEMIPLEGIA CLASSIFICATION AND PROGRESS RECORD

Upper limb-test sitting cont'd

Name_____

Date_____

SPEED TESTS FOR Classes 4, 5, 6   Strokes per 5 seconds

Hand from lap to chin	Normal		
	Affected		
Hand from lap to opposite knee	Normal		
	Affected		

___ Passive motion sense, digits_____

___ Fingertip recognition_____

___ Wrist stabilization for grasp   1. Elbow extended_____

              2. Elbow flexed_____

___ Wrist flexion and extension   1. Elbow extended_____

___ Fist closed   2. Elbow flexed_____

___ Wrist circumduction_____

DIGITS

___ Mass grasp_____ Dynamometer test   Normal_____lb.
                                                    Affected_____lb.

___ Mass extension _____

___ Hook grasp (handbag, 2 lb.)_____

___ Lateral prehension (card)_____

___ Palmar prehension (pencil)_____

___ Cylindrical grasp (small jar)_____

___ Spherical grasp (ball)_____ Catch_____ Throw_____

___ Indiv. thumb movements, hands in lap ulnar side down   1. Vertical movements_____
                              2. Horizontal movements_____

___ Individual finger movements_____

___ Button and
___ unbutton shirt   Using both hands_____
                 Using affected hand only_____

___ Other skilled activities_____

B

FIG. 22-3 *cont'd.* For legend see opposite page.

The tests of motor speed on the second page of the evaluation form (Fig. 22-3, *B*) may be used to assess hypertonicity during any recovery stage, provided that the patient has enough range of active motion to perform the necessary movement. The tests are especially useful in stages 4, 5, and 6. The normal side is tested first for comparison; then the affected side is tested. The two movements that are tested are (1) hand to chin and (2) hand to opposite knee. The patient is seated in a sturdy chair without armrests. The trunk should be stabilized against the back of the chair, and the head should be erect. The hand is closed, but not tightly, and rests in the lap. For the hand-to-chin test the forearm is at 0° neutral between pronation and supination. The therapist asks the patient to bring the hand from lap to chin as rapidly as possible, first with the unaffected side and then with the affected side, and records the number of full back-and-forth movements accomplished in 5 seconds. If speed is slow because of marked spasticity, half movements may be counted. The same procedure is followed for the hand-to-opposite knee test, except that the forearm is positioned in full pronation on the lap. The hand is moved from the lap to the opposite knee, using full range of elbow extension. These two tests measure the hypertonicity of elbow flexors and extensors.

Wrist stabilization, which is automatic during normal grasp, is often lacking after a stroke. Therefore it is important to evaluate wrist stabilization during fist closure.

HEMIPLEGIA CLASSIFICATION AND PROGRESS RECORD

Trunk and lower limb

Name_____ Evaluation date_____

SUPINE

Passive motion sense   Hip_____ Knee_____

Ankle_____ Big toe_____

Flexor synergy_____

Extensor synergy_____

Hip: Abduction_____ Adduction_____

SITTING ON CHAIR	STANDING
Trunk balance (no back support)	With_____ without_____ support Balance, normal limb sec.
Sole sensation Correct (no. of answers) Incorrect	Double scale (a) _____ (b) _____ reading†
Hip-knee-ankle flexion	Hip-knee-ankle flexion
Knee flexion-extension small range	Knee flexion-extension small range
Knee flexion beyond 90°	Knee flexion hip extended
Ankle, isolated dorsiflexion	Ankle, isolated dorsiflexion
Reciprocal hamstring action*	Hip abduction knee extended

AMBULATION   Evaluation date_____

Brace?_____ Cane?_____ In parallel bars_____

Supported_____ Escorted_____ Alone_____

Arm in sling_____ Arm swings loosely_____ Elbow held flexed_____

Arm swings near normal_____

GAIT ANALYSIS   Evaluation date_____

STANCE PHASE   SWING PHASE

Ankle_____   _____

Knee_____   _____

Hip_____   _____

Walking cadence: Steps per min.   Speed: Feet per min.

*Inward and outward rotation at knee with inversion-eversion at ankle.
†Recorded as normal/affected; (a) preferred stance, (b) weight shift on affected limb.

C

FIG. 22-3 *cont'd.* For legend see p. 406.

This test is done with the elbow both flexed and extended. During the recovery stages when the synergies are dominant, the wrist tends to flex when the elbow flexes. The patient is asked to make a fist while the elbow is extended across the front of the body. The patient is then asked to make a fist while the elbow is flexed at the side of the body. Whether the wrist remains stabilized in the neutral position or extends slightly is observed. This test is followed by a request for wrist flexion and extension with the fist closed. The patient holds an object such as a wide (1¾ inches, or 4.5 cm) dowel, and extends and flexes the wrist. This is done in the elbow-extended and elbow-flexed positions as on the previous test.

Circumduction of the wrist indicates significant recovery to the advanced stages. When evaluating the ability to perform this movement, the therapist should stabilize the forearm in pronation. The upper arm should be stabilized against the trunk.

Mass grasp is tested with a dynamometer, which measures pounds of pressure of grasp strength. The normal side is tested first; then the affected side is tested, and the results are recorded for comparison. Mass extension is evaluated by asking the patient to release and actively extend the fingers to the degree possible. Whether active extension was accomplished and the approximate amount of range achieved should be noted on the form. Active release to full range of extension is very difficult for many persons with CVA.

All types of prehension are evaluated in order of their difficulty. Everyday tasks that require the particular prehension pattern should be used. Hook grasp may be assessed by asking the patient to hold a handled bag. Holding a card demands lateral prehension. Palmar prehension is required for grasping a pencil. Cylindrical grasp may be assessed by asking the patient to hold a small, narrow jar. Grasping a ball requires spherical grasp. The patient's ability to catch and throw the ball may be observed. These activities are difficult for persons with hemiplegia, because they require rapid grasp and release, coordination of the entire limb, and time-space judgment. In all the prehension tests the normal side should be observed first for purposes of comparison.

Individual thumb movements are evaluated with the patient's hand resting in the lap, ulnar side down. The normal side is observed first; then the affected side is observed. The patient is asked to move the thumb up and down (flexion-extension) and side to side (adduction-abduction).

Individual finger movements are evaluated by asking the patient to tap the index and middle fingers on the tabletop or on a pillow held in the lap. Isolated control of metacarpophalangeal (MP) flexion and extension is assessed and noted on the evaluation form.

Fine, coordinated use of the affected hand and arm and of both hands together usually is indicative of advanced recovery. Subjects who have succeeded well at the prehension tests may be asked to button and unbutton a shirt, first using both hands, then using the affected hand only. Other skilled activities, such as writing, threading a needle, removing a small bottle cap, and picking up and placing ¼-inch (0.6 cm) mosaic tiles, may be used further to test skilled hand use.

MOTOR TESTS, TRUNK AND LOWER EXTREMITY

To evaluate trunk and lower extremity function the patient is tested first in the supine position, then in the sitting position, and then in the standing position. If the patient is ambulatory, a gait analysis is made (Fig. 22-3, *C*). Tests in the supine position include tests of passive motion sense, flexor and extensor synergies, and hip abduction and adduction. In the sitting position trunk balance, sole sensation, and specific movements of the lower limb are tested. These tests include hip-knee-ankle flexion, knee flexion and extension in small range, knee flexion beyond 90°, isolated ankle dorsiflexion, and reciprocal hamstring action (inward and outward rotation

at the knee with inversion-eversion at the ankle). In the standing position balance and selected movements are evaluated. These tests are hip-knee-ankle flexion, knee flexion-extension in small range, knee flexion with the hip extended, isolated ankle dorsiflexion, and hip abduction with the knee extended. The lower extremity evaluation concludes with a gait analysis, including timed walking cadence.[3] The physical and occupational therapists should perform the motor evaluation cooperatively and use an integrated approach in treatment, which incorporates upper limb, trunk, and lower limb function, according to prescribed treatment goals.

GENERAL PRINCIPLES OF FACILITATING MOTOR FUNCTION

The goal of Brunnstrom's movement therapy is to facilitate the patient's progress through the recovery stages that occur after onset of hemiplegia (Table 22-1). Use of the available afferent-efferent mechanisms of control is the means for attainment of this goal. Some of these mechanisms are summarized here.

Postural and attitudinal reflexes are used as means to increase or decrease tone in specific muscles.[9] For instance, changes in head and body position can influence muscle tone by evoking the tonic reflexes, such as the TNRs, tonic lumbar reflex, TLR, and equilibrium and protective reactions. Associated reactions may be used to initiate or elicit synergies in the early stages of recovery by giving resistance to the contralateral muscle group on the normal side. Efforts at flexion synergy of the affected leg may be used to elicit a flexor synergy of the arm through homolateral limb synkinesis.

Stimulating the skin over a muscle by rubbing with the fingertips produces contraction of that muscle and facilitation of the synergy to which the muscle belongs. An example is briskly stimulating the triceps muscle during other efforts at performance of the extensor synergy, which enhances elbow extension and amplifies the synergy pattern. Muscle contraction is facilitated when muscles are placed in their lengthened position, and the quick stretch of a muscle facilitates its contraction and inhibits its antagonist. Resistance facilitates the contraction of muscles resisted. Synergistic movement may be augmented by the voluntary effort of the patient. Visual stimulation through the use of mirrors, videotape of self, and movement of parts can facilitate motion in some patients as can auditory stimuli in the forms of loud and repetitive commands to perform the desired movement.

The strongest component of a synergy pattern inhibits its antagonist through reciprocal innervation. It follows that if relaxation of the stronger or spastic muscle can be effected, it may be possible to evoke some activity in the weaker antagonist, which may appear to be functionless because of its inability to overcome the very hypertonic agonist.[2,9]

GENERAL TREATMENT GOALS AND METHODS

Before the initiation of any intervention strategies, the occupational and physical therapists must make a thorough evaluation of the motor, sensory, perceptual, and cognitive functions of the patient. The motor evaluation yields information about stage of recovery, muscle tone, passive motion sense, hand function, sitting and standing balance, leg function, and ambulation. The treatment goals and methods summarized are directed primarily to the rehabilitation of the upper extremity. The point at which the therapist initiates treatment depends on the stage of recovery and muscle tone of the individual patient.

BED POSITIONING

Proper bed positioning begins immediately after the onset of the stroke when the patient is in the flaccid stage.[3] During this period the limbs can be placed in the most favorable positions without interference from hypertonic muscles. Correct bed positioning is often the responsibility of the nurse; therefore it is essential that the physical therapist or occupational therapist provide information about the influence of the limb synergies on bed postures.

If left unsupervised, the lower limb tends to assume a position of hip external rotation and abduction and knee flexion. This posture is partly a result of mechanical influences on the flaccid limb; that is, the weight of the part tends to pull the hip into external rotation. Neurologically, this position mimics the flexor synergy of the lower extremity. The advent of muscular tension in the flexor and abductor muscle groups of the hip and the flexor group of the knee contributes to the posture of the lower extremity as described previously.

If the extensor synergy is developed in the lower extremity, a different position may be present. Hypertonicity of the extensor muscles usually exceeds that of the flexor muscles in the lower limb. In this case the posture of the lower extremity is characterized by extension and adduction at the hip, knee extension, and ankle plantar flexion. If adductor spasticity is severe, the patient may habitually place the unaffected leg under the affected leg, which allows the affected limb to adduct even more and results in a crossed-limb posture.

If the extensor synergy dominates in the lower limb, the recommended bed position in the supine position is slight flexion of the hip and knee maintained by a small pillow under the knee. Lateral support of the leg at the knee with pillows or a rolled blanket or bolster should be provided to prevent abduction and external rotation. The bed clothes should be supported to prevent them from resting on the foot. This helps to prevent excessive ankle plantar flexion. The position of slight flexion at the hip and knee is beneficial because it has an inhibitory effect on the extensor muscles of the knee and ankle, counteracting the development of severe hypertonicity in these muscles, which hinders ambulation.

If the flexor synergy dominates in the lower limb, the knee must be maintained in extension. Hip external rotation can be prevented with supports as described previously. The choice of bed position is determined on an individual basis. The position selected should be opposite the pattern of the greatest amount of muscle tone to effect the inhibition of excessive hypertonicity.

The affected upper extremity is supported on a pillow in a position comfortable for the patient. Abduction of the humerus in relation to the scapula should be avoided, because in this position the stabilizing action of the lower portion of the glenoid fossa on the humeral head is reduced and the superior portion of the joint capsule is slackened. This position can predispose the humeral head to downward subluxation. In handling the patient, traction on the affected upper extremity is to be avoided. The patient is instructed to use the unaffected hand to support the affected arm when moving about in bed.

BED MOBILITY

Turning toward the affected side is easier than turning toward the unaffected side, because it requires little activity of the affected limb(s). The affected arm is placed close to the body, and the patient rolls over the affected arm when turning. Turning toward the unaffected side requires muscular effort of the affected limbs. The unaffected arm can be used to elevate the affected arm to a vertical position over the face, with the shoulder in 80 or 90° of flexion and the elbow fully extended. The affected lower extremity is positioned in partial flexion at the knee and hip and can be stabilized in this position momentarily by the therapist. The patient turns by swinging the arms and the affected knee across the body toward the unaffected side. The movements of the limbs assist in the turn of the upper body and pelvis. When control improves, the patient can carry out the maneuver independently in one smooth, continuous movement to turn from the supine position to the side-lying position on the unaffected side.

TRUNK MOVEMENT AND BALANCE

One of the early goals in treatment is for the patient to achieve good trunk or sitting balance. Most persons with hemiplegia demonstrate "listing" to the affected side, which may result in a fall when the appropriate equilibrium responses do not occur. To evoke balance responses the therapist deliberately disturbs the patient's erect sitting posture in forward-backward and side-to-side direction while the patient sits on a chair, edge of a bed, or mat table. The patient is prepared for the procedure with an explanation and is pushed, at first gently, then more vigorously. The patient may support the affected arm by cradling it to protect the shoulder. This prevents the patient from grasping the supporting surface during the procedure. Later the therapist initiates and assists the patient with bending the trunk directly forward and obliquely forward. The patient sits and supports the affected arm as previously described. The therapist's hands are held under the patient's elbows. The therapist may use the knees to stabilize the patient's knees if balance is poor. In this position the therapist guides the patient while inclining the trunk forward and obliquely and attains some passive glenohumeral and scapular motion at the same time.

Trunk rotation is encouraged in a similar manner, with the therapist sitting in front of the patient or standing behind and supporting the patient's arms as before. Trunk rotation is first performed through a limited range and is gently guided by the therapist. The range is gradually increased. Some neck mobilization may be attained almost automatically during these maneuvers. As the trunk rotates, the patient cradles the affected arm and swings the arms rhythmically from side to side to achieve shoulder abduction and adduction alternately as the trunk rotates. The shoulder components of the flexor and extensor synergies might be evoked during these procedures through the TNR and tonic lumbar reflexes.[3]

SHOULDER RANGE OF MOTION

A second important early goal in treatment is to maintain or achieve pain-free range of motion (ROM) at the glenohumeral joint. There appears to be a relationship between the shoulder pain, so common in patients with hemiplegia, and the stretching of spastic muscles around the shoulder joint. Traditional forced passive exercise procedures may actually produce this stretching and contribute to the development of pain. Such exercise is harmful and contraindicated. Once the patient has experienced the pain, the anticipation of it increases the muscular tension that in turn decreases the joint mobility and increases the pain experienced on passive motion. Therefore the shoulder joint should be mobilized through guided trunk motion without forceful stretching of hypertonic musculature about the shoulder and shoulder girdle.

The patient sits erect, cradling the affected arm. The therapist supports the arms under the elbows while the patient leans forward. The more the patient leans, the greater the range of shoulder flexion that can be obtained. The therapist guides the arms gently and passively into shoulder flexion while the patient's attention is focused on the trunk motion. In a similar fashion the therapist can guide the arms into abduction and adduction while the patient rotates the trunk from side to side. The asymmetric tonic neck reflex (ATNR) and tonic lumbar reflex facilitate relaxation of muscles during this maneuver. When the patient is confident that the shoulder can be moved painlessly, active-

assisted movements of the arm in relation to the trunk can begin.

First, the patient moves both shoulders into elevation and depression and scapula adduction and abduction. These movements are then combined with glenohumeral movements. The arm is supported by the therapist from behind, with the shoulder between forward flexion and abduction, the elbow flexed less than 90°, and the wrist supported in slight extension. The therapist may ask the patient to elevate the shoulders while tapping the upper trapezius with the fingertips. At the same time the therapist is assisting the patient to elevate the arm as well. Active shoulder elevation tends to elicit other components of the flexor synergy that in turn tends to inhibit the very hypertonic adduction component of the extensor synergy (pectoralis major), allowing the therapist to elevate the arm into abduction by small degrees each time the patient repeats the active shoulder girdle elevation. The procedure is repeated, and the therapist gives the appropriate verbal commands "pull up, let go."

The abduction movement is at an oblique angle between forward flexion and full abduction. Sideward abduction with the arm in the same plane as the trunk is likely to be painful and should be avoided. Alternate pronation and supination of the forearm by the therapist should accompany the elevation and lowering of the arm throughout the procedure. The forearm should be supinated when the shoulder is elevated and pronated when the arm is lowered. Head rotation to the normal side inhibits activity in the pectoralis major muscle through the ATNR. When abduction movement above the horizontal has been accomplished without pain, the patient can be directed to reach overhead and straighten out the elbow if there has been sufficient recovery to do so. The patient is directed to rotate the head to the affected side to facilitate the elbow extension while observing the movement of the arm.

These techniques result in increased ROM at the shoulder and also help the development of the flexor synergy. A small ROM in the path of the extensor synergy should be performed between the patient's efforts at flexion so that both synergies are developed. As training progresses, greater emphasis is placed on the development of the extensor synergy.

SHOULDER SUBLUXATION

Glenohumeral subluxation appears to be a result of dysfunction of the following rotator cuff muscles: supraspinatus, infraspinatus, teres minor, and subscapularis. Activation of these muscles in treatment is necessary if subluxation is to be minimized or prevented. Function of the supraspinatus muscle is particularly important for the prevention of subluxation. Slings have been used in an effort to hold the humeral head in the glenoid fossa, but they do not in any way activate the muscles needed to protect the integrity of the shoulder joint.[3] The use of slings has been found to be of little value and may actually be harmful.[4] A more complete discussion of shoulder problems and slings appears in Chapter 24.

METHODS OF TREATMENT
UPPER LIMB TRAINING

The training procedures for improving arm function are geared to the patient's recovery stage. During stages 1 and 2 when the arm is essentially flaccid or some components of the synergy patterns are beginning to appear, the aim is to elicit muscle tone and the synergy patterns on a reflex basis. This improvement is accomplished through a variety of facilitation procedures. Associated reactions and tonic reflexes may be employed to influence tone and evoke reflexive movement. The proximal traction response may be used to activate the flexor synergy. Tapping over the upper and middle trapezius, rhomboids, and biceps may elicit components of the flexor synergy. Tapping over the triceps and stretching of the serratus anterior may activate components of the extensor synergy. Passive movement alternately through each of the synergy patterns is not only an excellent means for maintaining ROM of several joints but provides the patient with proprioceptive and visual feedback for the desired patterns of early movement. Quick stretch and surface stroking of the skin over them are also used to activate muscles.

These methods are not employed in any set order or routine but are selected to suit the particular responses of each individual patient. Because the flexor synergy usually appears first, it may be useful to begin trying to elicit the flexor patterns. This attempt should be followed immediately with facilitation of the extensor synergy components, which tend to be weaker and more difficult to perform in later stages of recovery.[3,8]

When the patient has recovered to stages 2 and 3, the synergies or their components are present and may be performed voluntarily. Hypertonicity is developing and reaches its peak in stage 3. During this period the aim is for the patient to achieve voluntary control of the synergy patterns. This goal is reached by repetitious alternating performance of the synergy patterns, first with the assistance and facilitation of the therapist. Facilitation is provided through resistance to voluntary motion, verbal commands, tapping, and cutaneous stimulation. This step is followed by voluntary repetition of the synergy patterns without the facilitation and, finally, concentration on the components of the synergies from proximal to distal with, then without, facilitation.

Bilateral rowing movements with the therapist holding the patient's hands are a useful activity for reciprocal motion of the synergies that should be started during this time. Weight-bearing on the affected arm may be employed to reinforce elbow extension. The patient uses the normal hand to guide the affected hand, fist clenched, to a low stool positioned in front of him or her.

A sandbag or cushion is placed on the stool and a concavity is made in it to accommodate the fist. The patient's body weight is shifted to the affected arm and the weight bearing facilitates elbow extensors.[3,8]

The treatment aim during stages 4 and 5 is to break away from the synergies by mixing components from antagonistic synergies to perform new and increasingly complex patterns of movement. One means for accomplishing this goal is to use skateboard or powder board exercises in arcs of movement to get elbow flexion, combined with shoulder horizontal adduction and forearm pronation, and alternating with shoulder horizontal abduction and elbow extension with forearm supination (Fig. 22-4). Later the patient may be able to perform the more complex figure-of-eight pattern on the skateboard or powder board. In the final recovery stages 5 and 6, increasingly complex movement combinations and isolated motions are possible. The aims in treatment are to achieve ease in performance of movement combinations and isolated motion and to increase speed of movement.

It should be noted that the hemiplegic upper extremity seldom makes a full recovery. If voluntary and spontaneous movement is possible, the patient should be trained to use the limb as an assist to the sound arm to the extent possible in bilateral activities.

HAND TRAINING

Methods for retraining hand function are treated separately, because recovery of hand function does not always coincide with arm recovery. Hand retraining commensurate with the recovery status of the patient should be carried out continuously.

The first goal of hand retraining is to achieve mass grasp. The proximal traction response and grasp reflex may be used to elicit early grasp movement on a reflex level. During the proximal traction response maneuver the therapist should maintain the patient's wrist in extension and give the command "squeeze."

Because the normal association between wrist exten-

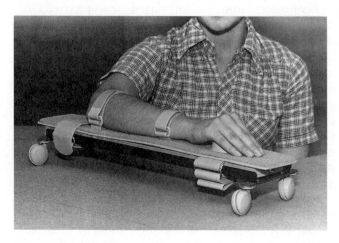

FIG. 22-4 Skateboard exercises for synergy or combined movement patterns.

sion and grasp is disturbed, the second goal is to achieve wrist fixation for grasp. Wrist extension often accompanies the extensor synergy. Wrist extension can be evoked if the therapist applies resistance to the proximal palm or fist while supporting the arm in the position described earlier for elevation of the arm into abduction. Percussion of the wrist extensors with the elbow in extension and arm elevated and supported by the therapist can activate wrist extension. The proximal portion of the extensors are tapped, and the therapist directs the patient to squeeze simultaneously. The commands to "squeeze" and "stop squeezing" are given at appropriate points in the facilitation procedures.

During the wrist extension and fist closure the therapist carries the elbow forward into extension. During the wrist and finger relaxation the therapist carries the elbow back into flexion. While the patient is maintaining fist closure, the therapist may withdraw the wrist support and give the command "hold." The therapist may continue tapping the wrist extensors while the patient attempts to hold the posture. The goal is to synchronize the muscles for fist closure with wrist extension.

This procedure should be alternated with a command to "stop squeezing," and the wrist should be allowed to drop and fingers to open while the elbow is moved into flexion. These steps are alternated and the wrist extension–fist closure is performed gradually with increasing amounts of elbow flexion so that the patient can learn to grasp with wrist stabilization when the arm is in a variety of positions.

A third objective in hand retraining is to achieve active release of grasp. This movement is difficult, because there is usually a considerable degree of hypertonicity in the flexor muscles of the hand. A release of tension in the finger flexors, then, is primary to the achievement of any active finger extension. Active grasp should be alternated with manipulations to release tension in the flexors. The therapist sits facing the patient and pulls the thumb out of the palm by gripping the thenar eminence. The forearm is supinated. The wrist is allowed to remain in slight flexion. The therapist maintains the grasp around the thumb and alternately pronates and supinates the forearm with emphasis on supination. Pressure on the thumb is decreased during pronation and increased during supination. Cutaneous stimulation is given to the dorsum of the hand and wrist when the forearm is supinated. This manipulation is likely to develop some tension in the finger extensors, and the fingers extend. The patient may actually participate in opening the hand when the forearm is supinated. Strong efforts on the part of the patient may evoke flexion instead, however, and should be avoided.

If this manipulation is inadequate, stretch of the finger extensors may be used. With the therapist and patient positioned and the hand manipulated as just described, the therapist uses the free hand for distally directed, rapid stroking movements over the proximal phalanges of the affected hand. This action causes momentary flexion of the MP joints, which then bounce back into partial extension. The stroking movement is performed so that the proximal, then distal interphalangeal (IP) joints are included. The movement is performed rapidly and continuously, causing rapid flexion and then bounce back of MP and IP joints. The fingers become extended, and the finger flexors are relaxed because they are reciprocally inhibited by the stretch reflex response in the extensors. If the flexors are stretched or stroking is performed over the palmar surface of the fingers, the spasticity returns to the finger flexors, and they act to close the hand.[3] For this reason the fingers should not be pulled into extension.

Active finger extension may be further facilitated by the use of a finger extension exercise glove with rubber bands, which the patient uses while the hand is manipulated into supination with the thumb pulled out of the palm as described earlier (Fig. 22-5). Elevation above the horizontal position evokes the extensor reflexes of the fingers. After flexor spasticity has been decreased by the maneuvers just described, the therapist stands on the affected side and maintains the thumb in abduction and extension and the forearm in pronation. The fingers are kept in extension by pressure over the IP joints and stabilization of the fingertips. The grip on the thumb is released, and the arm is raised above the horizontal position.

The therapist strokes distally over the IP joints with the heel of the hand. The fingers extend or hyperextend, and the therapist gradually discontinues contact with the patient's hand. If the patient is ready, slight voluntary mental effort can be superimposed on the reflex extension, which may bring about additional extension of the fingers. If the forearm is supinated while the arm is elevated, thumb extension is enhanced. The hand should be positioned overhead for this maneuver. To facilitate extension of the fourth and fifth fingers, the forearm should be pronated as the arm is elevated and friction should be applied over the ulnar side of the dorsum of the forearm.

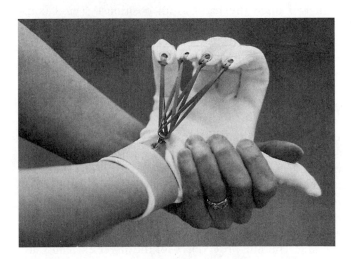

FIG. 22-5   Finger extension exercise glove.

When reflex extension of the fingers is well established, alternate fist opening and closing can begin. The arm is lowered passively, and the elbow is flexed. The forearm and wrist are supported, and the patient is asked to squeeze, then stop squeezing. As soon as the fingers relax, the manipulations to facilitate finger extension are carried out. These two steps are alternated, and the patient's voluntary efforts are superimposed on the reflex activity so that the movements begin to assume a semivoluntary character. Semivoluntary finger extension is influenced by the position of the limb and appears to be linked to gross movements other than the synergy patterns. Voluntary movements of the thumb appear when semivoluntary mass extension becomes possible.

Once the flexor muscles have been relaxed, the hand can be placed in the patient's lap, ulnar side down, and the patient can attempt to move the thumb away from the first finger, a preliminary for lateral prehension. The therapist may stimulate the tendons of the abductor pollicis and the extensor pollicis brevis by tapping or friction at the point where they pass over the wrist to enhance the patient's effort. The patient can learn to twiddle the thumbs to attain further control of thumb motion. The patient folds hands, wrists slightly flexed, and moves the thumbs around each other. Initially the normal thumb may push the other around, but the involved thumb may begin to participate actively. The willed effort, visual input, and sensory feedback from affected and unaffected sides contribute to the development of this movement.

During treatment sessions the patient must be comfortable and relaxed. The patient's willed efforts must be slight because too much effort may evoke a flexor response rather than the desired extensor response. Excessive muscle tension in the limb and entire body must be avoided or finger extension will not occur.

Many patients with hemiplegia never achieve good voluntary extension or coordinated, fine hand motions. If semivoluntary extension can be well established, however, voluntary extension usually follows so that the patient can open the hand in all positions.[3] The accomplishment of palmar prehension and fine hand movements requires the achievement of voluntary opening of the hand, opposition of the thumb to the fingers, and ability to release objects in contact with the palm of the hand.

LOWER LIMB TRAINING

Lower limb training is directed toward restoring safe standing and the development of a gait pattern that is as nearly normal as possible. The goal is to modify the gross movement synergies and facilitate movement combinations that are more nearly like those used during normal ambulation. Lower limb training includes trunk balance and activation of specific muscle groups followed by gait training. Training procedures for the lower extremity are primarily the domain of the physical therapist. When training the patient in functional activities, however, the occupational therapist can use procedures that are in concert with the work of the physical therapist. For example, transfer training, dressing, toileting, and ambulating about in the occupational therapy clinic involve the lower limb. Therefore it is important for the occupational therapist to know which training procedures are in progress, which movement patterns are to be encouraged or inhibited, and which methods facilitate the desired gait pattern when assisting or accompanying the patient during functional tasks.

OCCUPATIONAL THERAPY APPLICATIONS

Controlled movements achieved in upper limb training have more significance if the patient can use them for functional activities. Even with limited control, the affected limb can be used in many ways to assist with function. Encouraging the use of the affected arm in everyday activities decreases the possibility of the patient functioning strictly as a one-handed person.

During stages 3 and 4 when the patient has voluntary control of the synergies and may begin to use movement combinations that deviate from the synergies, the occupational therapist should help the patient to use the newly learned movement for functional and purposeful activities. Some of the activities that can be adapted to use the synergy patterns or gross combined movement patterns are skateboard or powder board exercises (see Fig. 22-4), sanding, leather lacing, braid weaving, finger painting, sponging off tabletops, and using a push broom or carpet sweeper. Activities that demand too much conscious effort tend to increase fatigue and hypertonicity and should be avoided.

Brunnstrom[3] described several possible uses for the flexor and extensor synergies in stage 3. The extensor synergy may be used to stabilize an object on a table while the unaffected arm is performing a task. Examples are stabilizing stationery while writing letters or stabilizing fabric for sewing. The extensor synergy may also be used to stabilize a jar against the body while unscrewing the lid or to hold a handbag or newspaper under the arm. When pushing the affected arm through the sleeve of a garment, the garment can be positioned so that the arm follows the path of the extensor synergy. The forearm must be pronated first, however, to facilitate elbow extension.

The flexor synergy or its components may be used to carry a coat or handbag over the forearm and to hold a toothbrush while the unaffected hand squeezes the toothpaste, for example. Bilateral pushing and pulling activities that alternate the paths of both synergies may be helpful for some patients, for example, sweeping, vacuuming, and dusting. Such activities may be performed with the unaffected hand stabilizing the affected one. The affected hand may be more a hindrance than a help until greater control is gained. Strongly motivated patients will try to use available movements under the guidance and encouragement of the occupational therapist.

To promote transition from stage 3 to stage 4, movement combinations are facilitated and practiced in upper limb training. These movements are hand to chin, hand to ear on the same side and opposite side, hand to opposite elbow, hand to opposite shoulder, hand to forehead, hand to top of head, hand to back of head, and stroking movements from top to back of head and from dorsum of the forearm to the shoulder and toward the neck on the normal side. As soon as possible, these movement patterns should be translated to functional activities. Success at functional tasks increases motivation and establishes a purpose for the training. Also contact with body parts where sensation is intact is instrumental in guiding the hand to its goal. Examples of application of these movements to function are hand-to-mouth motions used in eating finger foods, combing hair, washing the face, washing the unaffected arm, and reaching the opposite axilla for washing or application of deodorant.[3] The therapist's role is to analyze activities for movement patterns that are possible for the patient to perform, and to select activities with the patient that have meaning and are interesting.

At this time the occupational therapist should stress the use of any voluntary movement of the affected limb in performance of activities of daily living. Using the arm for dressing and hygiene skills translates the movements to purposeful use. The patient's sensory status, and not only on the motor recovery achieved, will influence the degree to which purposeful, spontaneous use of the arm is possible. If the patient surpasses stage 4, the number of activities that can be performed increases, and more movement combinations are possible. The involvement of the affected limbs in activities of daily living should be encouraged. The activities mentioned earlier can be performed now in their usual manner and can be graded to demand finer and more complex movement patterns. Gardening, furniture refinishing, leather tooling, rolling out dough, sweeping, dusting, and washing dishes are a few of the activities that may enlist the use of the affected arm purposefully if hand recovery is adequate.

SUMMARY

Signe Brunnstrom was a physical therapist who developed a treatment approach for CVA called *movement therapy*. The approach is based in neurophysiological principles of successive levels of CNS integration. Brunnstrom described stages of motor recovery following CVA and developed treatment methods designed to enhance the progress of the patient from one stage to the next toward higher and higher levels of motor skill. Her approach uses techniques of facilitation such as synergies, reflexes, associated reactions, resistance, tapping, and stretch.

The use of reflexes or synergisitic movement in treatment is controversial and the concept of the hierarchical organization of the nervous system has been modified in neurophysiology in recent years. However, Brunnstrom's observations of motor recovery and motor behavior are valid and the techniques are useful in treatment. Some similarities can be seen between Brunnstrom's methods and those of other sensorimotor theorists. The evaluation of motor recovery and elements of treatment methodology continue to be used in the treatment of CVA.

REVIEW QUESTIONS

1. List the stages of recovery of arm function after CVA, as described by Brunnstrom.
2. List the motions in the flexor and extensor synergies of the arm, and draw stick figures to illustrate the positions.
3. What is the most hypertonic component of the flexor synergy of the arm?
4. What is the least hypertonic component of the extensor synergy of the arm?
5. What is the basis of the Brunnstrom approach to the treatment of hemiplegia?
6. For what purposes does Brunnstrom recommend the use of reflexes and associated reactions in the early recovery stages after onset of hemiplegia?
7. Define or describe the following terms: limb synergy, associated reactions, imitation synkinesis, proximal traction response, grasp reflex, and the Souques' finger phenomenon.
8. Describe or demonstrate the procedure that Brunnstrom recommended to maintain or achieve pain-free ROM at the glenohumeral joint.
9. What is the aim of treatment for functional recovery of the arm during stages 1 and 2? Stages 2 and 3? Stages 3 and 4?
10. List two treatment methods that could be used to achieve each of the aims in question 9.
11. Describe three activities other than those listed in the text that may be used in occupational therapy to enhance voluntary control of the flexor and extensor synergies.
12. What is the effect of the proximal traction response on muscle function?
13. Describe or demonstrate the procedure that Brunnstrom recommends to establish wrist fixation in association with grasp.
14. Describe the procedure that may be used to relax spastic finger flexion and facilitate finger extension.

15. Which muscle group is thought to play a substantial role in maintaining glenohumeral joint stability?
16. Describe proper bed positioning for the patient with a dominant extensor synergy of the leg. What is the rationale for this position?

REFERENCES

1. Bobath B: *Adult hemiplegia: evaluation and treatment,* London, 1978, Wm Heinemann Medical Books.
2. Brunnstrom S: Motor behavior in adult hemiplegic patients, *Am J Occup Ther* 15:6, 1961.
3. Brunnstrom S: *Movement therapy in hemiplegia,* New York, 1970, Harper & Row.
4. Cailliet R: *The shoulder in hemiplegia,* Philadelphia, 1980, FA Davis.
5. Fiorentino MR: *Reflex testing methods for evaluating CNS development,* Springfield, Ill, 1973, Charles C Thomas.
6. Ghez C: The control of movement. In Kandel ER, Schwartz JH, Jessel TM: *Principles of neural science,* New York, 1991, Elsevier.
7. Giuliani CA: Theories of motor control: new concepts for physical therapy. In *Contemporary management of motor control problems: proceedings of the II Step Conference,* Alexandria, Va, 1991, Foundation for Physical Therapy.
8. Perry C: Principles and techniques of the Brunnstrom approach to the treatment of hemiplegia, *Am J Phys Med* 46:789, 1967.
9. Sawner K: *Brunnstrom approach to treatment of adult patients with hemiplegia: rationale for facilitation procedures,* Buffalo, State University of New York. Unpublished manuscript, 1969.
10. Schleichkorn J: *Signe Brunnstrom, physical therapy pioneer, master clinician and humanitarian,* Thorofare, NJ, 1990, Slack.
11. Taylor J, editor: Selected writings of Hughlings Jackson. New York, 1958, Basic Books (abstract). Cited in Brunnstrom S: *Movement therapy in hemiplegia,* New York, 1970, Harper & Row.
12. Twitchell TE: The restoration of motor function following hemiplegia in man, *Brain* 74:443-480, 1951 (abstract). Cited in Brunnstrom S: *Movement therapy in hemiplegia,* New York, 1970, Harper & Row.

The Proprioceptive Neuromuscular Facilitation Approach

Sara A. Pope-Davis

The purpose of this chapter is to introduce the reader to proprioceptive neuromuscular facilitation (PNF) and its application to evaluation and treatment in occupational therapy (OT). The basic principles, diagonal patterns, and a few of the more commonly used facilitation techniques are presented here. A case study is used to apply the concepts discussed. To use PNF effectively, it is necessary to understand normal development, learn the motor skills to use the techniques, and apply the concepts and techniques to OT activities. This chapter should form the basis for further reading and training under the supervision of a therapist experienced in PNF.

Proprioceptive neuromuscular facilitation is based on normal movement and motor development. In normal motor activity the brain registers total movement and not individual muscle action.[12] Encompassed in the PNF approach are mass movement patterns that are spiral and diagonal in nature and that resemble movement seen in functional activities. In this multisensory approach, facilitation techniques are superimposed on movement patterns and postures through the therapist's manual contacts, verbal commands, and visual cues. PNF is effective in the treatment of numerous conditions, including Parkinson disease, spinal cord injury, arthritis, stroke, head injury, and hand injuries.

HISTORY

Proprioceptive neuromuscular facilitation originated with Dr. Herman Kabat, physician and neurophysiologist, in the 1940s. He applied neurophysiologic principles, based on the work of Sherrington, to the treatment of paralysis secondary to poliomyelitis and multiple sclerosis. In 1948 Kabat and Henry Kaiser founded the Kabat-Keiser Institute in Vallejo, California. Here he worked with physical therapist Margaret Knott to develop the PNF method of treatment. By 1951 the diagonal patterns and several techniques were established. Essentially no new techniques have been developed since 1951, although new methods have been applied. PNF is now used to treat numerous neurologic and orthopedic conditions.

In 1952 Dorothy Voss, a physical therapist, joined the staff at Kaiser-Kabat Institute. She and Knott undertook the teaching and supervision of staff therapists. In 1954 Knott and Voss presented the first two-week course in Vallejo. Two years later, the first edition of *Proprioceptive Neuromuscular Facilitation* by Margaret Knott and Dorothy Voss was published by Harper & Row.

During this same period several reports in the *American Journal of Occupational Therapy* described PNF and its application to OT treatment.* It was not until 1974 that the first PNF course for occupational therapists, taught by Dorothy Voss, was offered at Northwestern University. Since then Beverly Myers, an occupational therapist, and others have offered courses for occupational therapists throughout the United States. In 1984 PNF was first taught concurrently to both physical and occupational therapists at the Rehabilitation Institute in Chicago.[15,22] Today combined courses are offered throughout the United States.

PRINCIPLES OF TREATMENT

Voss presented 11 principles of treatment at the Northwestern University Special Therapeutic Exercise Project

I want to thank Beverly Myers and Diane Harsch for their assistance in reviewing and editing this chapter. I also want to thank Barbara Gale for using her technical skills to take photographs for the illustrations and Diane Harsch for her patience in posing for them.

*References 3, 5, 6, 13, 19, 23.

in 1966. These principles were developed from concepts in the fields of neurophysiology, motor learning, and motor behavior.[20]

1. *All human beings have potentials that have not been fully developed.* This philosophy is the underlying basis of PNF. Therefore, in evaluation and treatment planning, the patient's abilities and potentials are emphasized. For example, the patient who has weakness on one side of his body can use the intact side to assist the weaker part. Likewise, the hemiplegic patient who has a flaccid arm can use the intact head, neck, and trunk musculature to begin reinforcement of the weak arm in weight-bearing activities.

2. *Normal motor development proceeds in a cervicocaudal and proximodistal direction.* In evaluation and treatment the cervicocaudal and proximodistal direction is followed. When severe disability is present, attention is given to the head and neck region, with its visual, auditory, and vestibular receptors, and to the upper trunk and extremities. If the superior region is intact, an effective source of reinforcement for the inferior region is available.[22] The proximodistal direction is followed by developing adequate function in the head, neck, and trunk before developing function in the extremities. This approach is of particular importance in treatment that often facilitates fine motor coordination in the upper extremities. Unless there is adequate control in the head, neck, and trunk region, fine motor skills cannot be developed effectively.

3. *Early motor behavior is dominated by reflex activity. Mature motor behavior is supported or reinforced by postural reflexes.* As the human being matures, primitive reflexes are integrated and available for reinforcement to allow for progressive development such as rolling, crawling, and sitting. Reflexes also have been noted to have an effect on tone changes in the extremities. Hellebrandt and associates[10] studied the effect of the tonic neck reflex (TNR) and the asymmetric tonic neck reflex (ATNR) on changes in tone and movement in the extremities of normal adults. They found that head and neck movement significantly affected arm and leg movement. In applying this finding to treatment, weak elbow extensors can be reinforced with the ATNR by having the patient look toward the side of weakness. Likewise, the patient can be assisted in assuming postures with the influence of reflex support. For example, the body-on-body righting reflex supports assuming side-sitting from the side-lying position.

4. *Early motor behavior is characterized by spontaneous movement, which oscillates between extremes of flexion and extension. These movements are rhythmic and reversing in character.*

In treatment it is important to attend to both directions of movement. When working with the patient on getting up from a chair, attention also must be given to sitting back down. Often with an injury the eccentric contraction (sitting down) is readily lost and becomes very difficult for the patient to regain. If not properly treated, the patient may be left with inadequate motor control to sit down smoothly and thus may "drop" into a chair. Similarly, in activities of daily living (ADL) training, the patient must learn how to get undressed as well as dressed.

5. *Developing motor behavior is expressed in an orderly sequence of total patterns of movement and posture.* In the normal infant the sequence of total patterns is demonstrated through the progression of locomotion. The infant learns to roll, to crawl, to creep, and finally to stand and walk. Throughout these stages of locomotion the infant also learns to use the extremities in different patterns and within different postures. Initially the hands are used for reaching and grasping within the most supported postures such as supine and prone. As postural control develops, the infant begins to use the hands in side-lying, sitting, and standing. To maximize motor performance, the patient should be given opportunities to work in a variety of developmental postures.

The use of extremities in total patterns requires interaction with component patterns of the head, neck, and trunk. For example, in swinging a tennis racquet in a forehand stroke, the arm and the head, neck, and trunk move in the direction of the swing. Without the interaction of the distal and proximal components, movement becomes less powerful and less coordinated.

6. *The growth of motor behavior has cyclic trends as evidenced by shifts between flexor and extensor dominance.* The shifts between antagonists help to develop muscle balance and control. One of the main goals of the PNF treatment approach is to establish a balance between antagonists. Developmentally the infant establishes this balance before creeping, that is, when rocking forward (extensor dominant) and backward (flexor dominant) on hands and knees. Postural control and balance must be achieved before movement can begin in this position. In treatment it is important to establish a balance between antagonistic muscles by first observing where imbalance exists and then facilitating the weaker component. For example, if the stroke patient demonstrates a flexor synergy (flexor dominant), extension should be facilitated.

7. *Normal motor development has an orderly sequence but lacks a step-by-step quality. Overlapping occurs. The child does not perfect perform-*

ance of one activity before beginning another more advanced activity. In trying to ascertain in which total pattern to position the patient, normal motor development should be heeded. If one technique or developmental posture is not effective in obtaining the desired result, it may be necessary to try the activity in another developmental posture. For example, if an ataxic patient is unable to write while sitting, it may be necessary to practice writing in a more supported posture, such as prone on elbows. Just as the infant reverts to a more secure posture when attempting a complex fine motor task, so must the patient. On the other hand, if the patient has not perfected a motor activity such as walking on level surfaces, he or she may benefit from attempting a higher level activity such as walking up or down stairs, which in turn can improve ambulation on level surfaces. Moving up and down the developmental sequence is a natural occurence and allows multiple and varied opportunities for practicing motor activities. The cognitive demands of the task in relation to the developmental posture also must be considered. When the patient's position is varied, either by changing the base of support or shifting weight on different extremities, the quality of visual and cognitive processing is influenced.[1]

8. *Locomotion depends upon reciprocal contraction of flexors and extensors, and the maintenance of posture requires continual adjustment for nuances of imbalance. Antagonistic pairs of movements, reflexes, muscles, and joint motion interact as necessary to the movement or posture.* This principle restates one of the main objectives of PNF—to achieve a balance between antagonists. An example of imbalance is the head-injured patient who is unable to maintain adequate sitting balance for a table top cognitive activity because of a dominance of trunk extensor tone. Another example is the hemiplegic patient with tight finger flexors secondary to flexor dominant tone in the hand. In treatment, emphasis is placed on correcting the imbalances. In the presence of spasticity first the spasticity is inhibited and then the antagonistic muscles, reflexes, and postures are facilitated.

9. *Improvement in motor ability is dependent upon motor learning.* Multisensory input from the therapist facilitates the patient's motor learning and is an integral part of the PNF approach. For example, the therapist may work with a patient on a shoulder flexion activity such as reaching into the cabinet for a cup. The therapist may say, "Reach for the cup," to add verbal input. This approach also encourages the patient to look in the direction of the movement to allow vision to enhance the motor response. Thus tactile, auditory, and visual input are used. Motor learning has occurred when these external cues are no longer needed for adequate performance.

10. *Frequency of stimulation and repetitive activity are used to promote and for retention of motor learning, and for the development of strength and endurance.* Just as the therapist who is learning PNF needs the opportunity to practice the techniques, the patient needs the opportunity to practice new motor skills. In the process of development, the infant constantly repeats a motor skill in many settings and developmental postures until it is mastered, as becomes apparent to anyone who watches a child learning to walk. Numerous attempts fail, but efforts are repeated until the skill is mastered. After the activity is learned, it becomes part of the child. He or she is able to use it automatically and deliberately as the occasion demands.[22] The same is true for the person learning to play the piano or to play tennis. Without the opportunity to practice, motor learning cannot successfully occur.

11. *Goal-directed activities coupled with techniques of facilitation are used to hasten learning of total patterns of walking and self-care activities.* When applying facilitation techniques to self-care the objective is improved functional ability, but improvement is obtained by more than instruction and practice alone. Correction of deficiencies is accomplished by directly applying manual contacts and techniques to facilitate a desired response.[11] In treatment this approach may mean applying stretch to finger extensors to facilitate release of an object or providing joint approximation through the shoulders and pelvis of an ataxic patient to provide stability while standing to wash dishes.

MOTOR LEARNING

As discussed previously, motor learning requires a multisensory approach. Auditory, visual, and tactile systems are all used to achieve the desired response. The correct combination of sensory input with each patient should be ascertained, implemented, and altered as the patient progresses. The developmental level of the patient and the ability to cooperate also should be taken into consideration.[22] The approach used with an aphasic patient differs from the approach used with a hand-injured patient. Similarly the approach with a child varies greatly from that with an adult.

AUDITORY

Verbal commands should be brief and clear. Timing of the command is important so that it does not come too early or too late in relation to the motor act. Tone of voice may influence the quality of the patient's response. Buchwald[4] states that tones of moderate intensity evoke gamma motor neuron activity and that louder tones can alter alpha motor neuron activity. Strong sharp commands simulate a stress situation and are used when maximal stimulation of motor response is desired. A soft tone of voice is used to offer reassurance and to encourage a smooth movement, as in the presence of pain. When a patient is giving the best effort, a moderate tone can be used.[22]

Another effect of auditory feedback on motor performance was studied by Loomis and Boersma.[14] They used a "verbal mediation" strategy to teach patients with right CVA wheelchair safety before transferring out of the chair. They taught patients to say aloud the steps required to leave the wheelchair safely and independently. They found that only patients who used verbal mediation learned the wheelchair drill sufficiently to perform safe and independent transfers. Their retention of the sequence also was better, suggesting that verbal mediation is beneficial in reaching independence with better sequencing and fewer errors.

VISUAL

Visual stimuli assist in initiation and coordination of movement. Visual input should be monitored to ensure that the patient is tracking in the direction of movement. For example, the therapist's position is important because the patient often uses the therapist's movement or position as a visual cue. If the desired direction of movement is forward, the therapist should be positioned diagonally in front of the patient. In addition to the therapist's position, placement of the OT activity also should be considered. If the treatment goal is to increase head, neck, and trunk rotation to the left, the activity is placed in front and to the left of the patient. Because OT is activity-oriented, an abundance of visual stimuli is offered to the patient.

TACTILE

Developmentally, the tactile system matures before the auditory and visual systems.[7] Furthermore, the tactile system is more efficient because it has both temporal and spatial discrimination abilities as opposed to the visual system, which can make only spatial discriminations, and the auditory system, which can make only temporal discriminations.[8] Affolter[2] states that during development, processing of tactile-kinesthetic information can be considered fundamental for building cognitive and emotional experience. Looking at and listening to the world does not result in change. The world cannot be touched without some change, however. A Chinese proverb often cited at PNF courses reinforces this viewpoint: I listen and I forget, I see and I remember, I do and I understand.

It is important for the patient to feel movement patterns that are coordinated and balanced. With the PNF approach, tactile input is supplied through the therapist's manual contacts to guide and reinforce the desired response. This approach may mean gently touching the patient to guide movement, using stretch to initiate movement, and providing resistance to strengthen movement. The type and extent of manual contacts depend on the patient's clinical status, which is determined through evaluation and reevaluation. For example, use of stretch or resistance in the presence of musculoskeletal instability may be contraindicated. Likewise, stretch or resistance should be avoided if they cause increased pain or tone imbalance.

To increase speed and accuracy in motor performance, the patient needs the opportunity to practice. Through repetition, habit patterns that occur automatically without voluntary effort are established. The PNF approach uses the concepts of part-task and whole-task practice. In other words, to learn the whole task, emphasis is placed on the parts of the task that the patient is unable to perform independently. The term *stepwise procedures* is descriptive of the emphasis on a part of the task during performance of the whole.[22] Performance of each part of the task is improved by practice, combined with appropriate sensory cues and techniques of facilitation. For example, the patient learning to transfer from a wheelchair to a tub bench may have difficulty lifting the leg over the tub rim. This part of the task should be practiced, with repetition and facilitation techniques to the hip flexors, during performance of the transfer. When the transfer becomes smooth and coordinated, it is no longer necessary to practice each part individually.

In summation, several components are necessary for motor learning to occur. In the PNF treatment approach, these components include multisensory input from the therapist's verbal commands, visual cues, and manual contacts. Touch is the most efficient form of stimulation and provides the opportunity for the patient to feel normal movement. The patient must practice motor activities in varying situations with immediate and constant feedback given.

EVALUATION

Evaluation of the patient requires astute observational skills and knowledge of normal movement. An initial evaluation is completed to determine the patient's abilities, deficiencies, and potential. After the treatment plan is established, ongoing assessment of the patient is necessary to ascertain the effectiveness of treatment and to make modifications as the patient changes.

The PNF evaluation follows a sequence from proximal to distal. First vital and related functions are considered, such as breathing, swallowing, voice production, facial and oral musculature, and visual/ocular control. Any impairment or weakness in these functions is noted.

The head and neck region is observed next. Deficiencies in this area directly affect the upper trunk and extremities. Head and neck positions are observed in varying postures and total patterns during functional activities. It is important to note (1) dominance of tone (flexor or extensor), (2) alignment (midline or shift to one side), and (3) stability/mobility (more or less needed).[15]

After observation of the head and neck region, the evaluation proceeds to the following parts of the body: upper trunk, upper extremities, lower trunk, and lower extremities. Each segment is evaluated individually in specific movement patterns, as well as in developmental activities in which interaction of body segments occurs. For example, shoulder flexion can be observed in an individual upper extremity movement pattern as well as during a total developmental pattern such as rolling.

During assessment of developmental activities and postures, the following issues should be addressed:

1. Is there a need for more stability or mobility?
2. Is there a balance between flexors and extensors, or is one more dominant?
3. Is the patient able to move in all directions?
4. What are the major limitations (weakness, incoordination, spasticity, contractures)?
5. Is the patient able to assume a posture and to maintain it? If not, which total pattern or postures are inadequate?
6. Are the inadequacies more proximal or distal?
7. Which sensory input does the patient respond to most effectively (auditory, visual, tactile)?
8. Which techniques of facilitation does the patient respond to best?

Finally, the patient is observed during self-care and other ADL to determine whether performance of individual and total patterns is adequate within the context of a functional activity. The patient's performance may vary from one setting to another. After the patient leaves the structured setting of the OT or PT (physical therapy) clinic for the less structured home or community environment, deterioration of motor performance is not unusual. Thus the treatment plan must accommodate for practice of motor performance in a variety of settings in locations appropriate to the specific activity.

TREATMENT IMPLEMENTATION

After evaluation, a treatment plan is developed, which includes goals that the patient hopes to accomplish. The techniques and procedures that have the most favorable influence on movement and posture are used. Similarly, appropriate total patterns and patterns of facilitation are selected to enhance performance.

DIAGONAL PATTERNS

The diagonal patterns used in the PNF approach are mass movement patterns observed in most functional activities. Part of the challenge in OT evaluation and treatment is recognizing the diagonal patterns in activities of daily living. Knowledge of the diagonals is necessary to identify areas of deficiency. Two diagonal motions are present for each major part of the body: head and neck, upper and lower trunk, and extremities. Each diagonal pattern has a flexion and extension component together with rotation and movement away from or toward the midline.

The head, neck, and trunk patterns are referred to as (a) flexion with rotation to the right or left and (b) extension with rotation to the right or left. These proximal patterns combine with the extremity diagonals. The upper and lower extremity diagonals are described according to the three movement components at the shoulder and hip: (1) flexion/extension, (2) abduction/adduction, and (3) external/internal rotation. Voss[20] introduced shorter descriptions for the extremity patterns in 1967 and referred to them as diagonal 1 (D_1) flexion/extension and diagonal 2 (D_2) flexion/extension. The reference points for flexion and extension are the shoulder and hip joints of the upper and lower extremities, respectively.

The movements associated with each diagonal and examples of these patterns seen in self-care and other ADL follow. Note that in functional activities, not all components of the pattern or full range of motion are necessarily seen. Furthermore, the diagonals interact during functional movement, changing from one pattern or combination to another, when they cross the transverse and sagittal planes of the body.[17]

Unilateral Patterns

1. UE (upper extremity) D_1 flexion (antagonist of D_1 extension). Scapula elevation, abduction, and rotation; shoulder flexion, adduction, and external rotation; elbow in flexion or extension; forearm supination; wrist flexion to the radial side; finger flexion and adduction; thumb adduction (Fig. 23-1, *A*). Examples in functional activity: hand-to-mouth motion in feeding, tennis forehand, combing hair on left side of head with right hand (Fig. 23-2, *A*), rolling from supine to prone.

2. UE D_1 extension (antagonist of D_1 flexion). Scapula depression, adduction, and rotation; shoulder extension, abduction, and internal rotation; elbow in flexion or extension; forearm pronation; wrist extension to the ulnar side; finger extension and abduction; thumb in palmar abduction (Fig. 23-1, *B*). Examples in functional activity; pushing a car door open from the inside (Fig. 23-2, *B*), tennis backhand stroke, rolling from prone to supine.

3. UE D_2 flexion (antagonist of D_2 extension). Scapula elevation, adduction, and rotation; shoulder flexion, abduction, and external rotation; elbow in flexion or extension; forearm supination; wrist extension to the radial side; finger extension and abduction; thumb extension (Fig. 23-3, *A*). Examples in functional activity: combing hair on right side of head with right hand (Fig. 23-4, *A*), lifting racquet in tennis serve, back stroke in swimming.

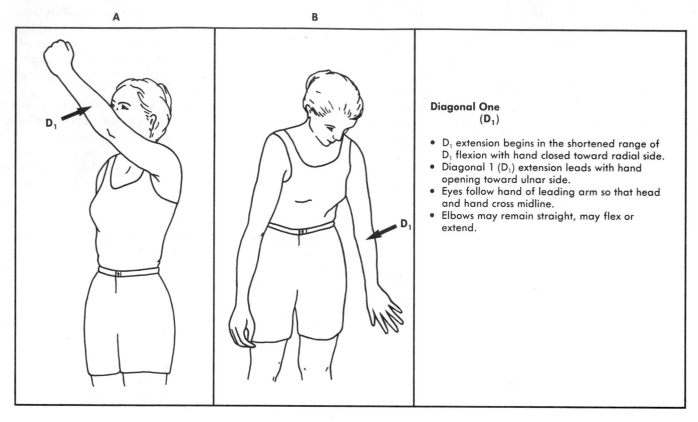

**Diagonal One
(D₁)**

- D₁ extension begins in the shortened range of D₁ flexion with hand closed toward radial side.
- Diagonal 1 (D₁) extension leads with hand opening toward ulnar side.
- Eyes follow hand of leading arm so that head and hand cross midline.
- Elbows may remain straight, may flex or extend.

FIG. 23-1   A, UE D₁ flexion pattern. **B,** UE D₁ extension pattern. (From Myers BJ: Unit I: PNF diagonal patterns and their application to functional activities, videotape study guide, Rehabilitation Institute of Chicago, 1982.)

4. UE D₂ extension (antagonist of D₂ flexion). Scapula depression, abduction, and rotation; shoulder extension, adduction, and internal rotation; elbow in flexion or extension; forearm pronation; wrist flexion to the ulnar side; finger flexion and adduction; thumb opposition (Fig. 23-3, *B*). Examples in functional activity: pitching a baseball, hitting ball in tennis serve, buttoning pants on left side with right hand (Fig. 23-4, *B*).

The rotational component in lower extremity D₁ flexion and extension parallel the upper extremity patterns.

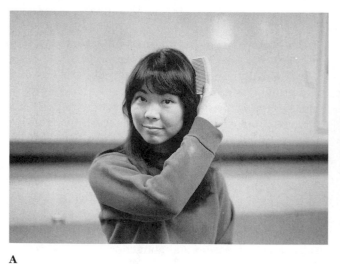

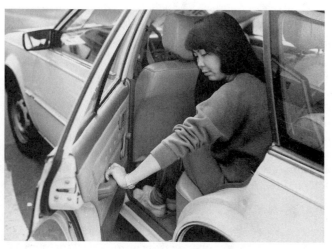

FIG. 23-2   A, UE D₁ flexion pattern is used in combing hair, opposite side. **B,** UE D₁ extension pattern is used in pushing a car door open.

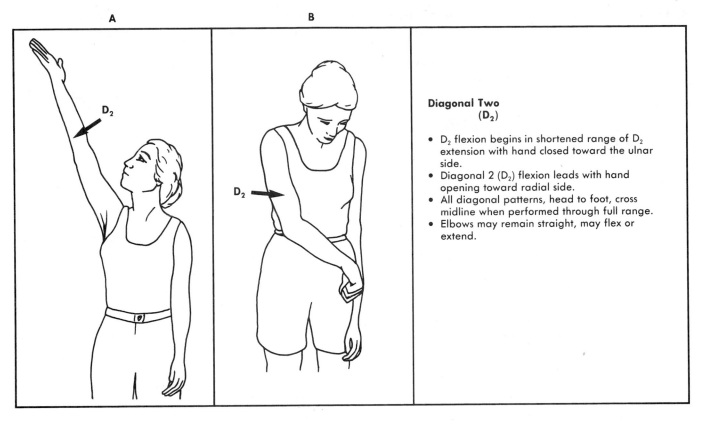

**Diagonal Two
(D₂)**

- D₂ flexion begins in shortened range of D₂ extension with hand closed toward the ulnar side.
- Diagonal 2 (D₂) flexion leads with hand opening toward radial side.
- All diagonal patterns, head to foot, cross midline when performed through full range.
- Elbows may remain straight, may flex or extend.

FIG. 23-3   A, UE D₂ flexion pattern. **B,** UE D₂ extension pattern. (From Myers BJ: Unit I: PNF diagonal patterns and their application to functional activities, videotape study guide, Rehabilitation Institute of Chicago, 1982.)

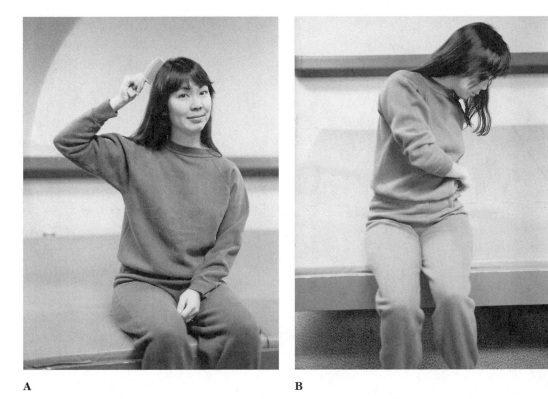

A   **B**

FIG. 23-4   A, UE D₂ flexion pattern is used in combing hair, same side. **B,** UE D₂ extension pattern is used in buttoning trousers, opposite side.

5. LE (lower extremity) D₁ flexion (antagonist of D₁ extension). Hip flexion, adduction, and external rotation; knee in flexion or extension; ankle and foot dorsiflexion with inversion and toe extension. Examples in functional activity: kicking a soccer ball, rolling from supine to prone, putting on a shoe with leg crossed (Fig. 23-5, *A*).

6. LE D₁ extension (antagonist of D₁ flexion). Hip extension, abduction, and internal rotation; knee in flexion or extension; ankle and foot plantar flexion with eversion and toe flexion. Examples in functional activity: putting leg into pants (Fig. 23-5, *B*), rolling from prone to supine.

The rotational component of lower extremity D₂ flexion and extension is opposite to the upper extremity patterns.

7. LE D₂ flexion (antagonist of D₂ extension). Hip flexion, abduction, and internal rotation; knee in flexion or extension; ankle and foot dorsiflexion with eversion and toe extension. Examples in functional activity: karate kick (Fig. 23-6, *A*), drawing the heels up during the breaststroke in swimming.

8. LE D₂ extension (antagonist of D₂ flexion). Hip extension, adduction and external rotation: knee in flexion or extension; ankle and foot plantar flexion with in-

version and toe flexion. Examples of functional activity: push-off in gait, the kick during the breaststroke in swimming, long sitting with legs crossed (Fig. 23-6, *B*).

Bilateral Patterns

Movements in the extremities may be reinforced by combining diagonals in bilateral patterns as follows:

1. Symmetric patterns. Paired extremities perform like movements at the same time (Fig. 23-7, *A*). Examples: bilateral symmetric D₁ extension, such as pushing off a chair to stand (Fig. 23-8, *A*); bilateral symmetric D₂ extension, such as starting to take off a pullover sweater (Fig. 23-8, *B*); bilateral symmetric D₂ flexion, such as reaching to lift a large item off a high shelf (Fig. 23-8, *C*). Bilateral symmetric upper extremity patterns facilitate trunk flexion and extension.

2. Asymmetric patterns. Paired extremities perform movements toward one side of the body at the same time which facilitates trunk rotation. (Fig. 23-7, *B*). The asymmetric patterns can be performed with the arms in contact such as in the chopping and lifting patterns in which greater trunk rotation is seen (Figs. 23-9 and 23-10, *A, B*). Furthermore, with the arms in contact, self-touching occurs, which is frequently observed in the presence of pain or in reinforcement of a motion when greater control or power is needed.[22] This phenomenon is observed

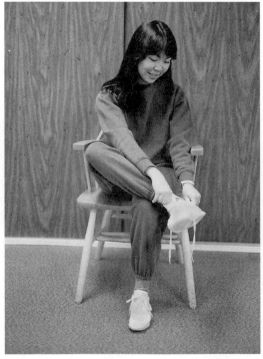

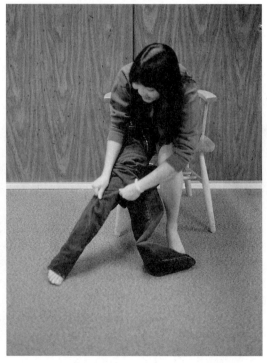

A   **B**

FIG. 23-5 A, LE D₁ flexion pattern is demonstrated in crossed leg when putting on shoe. **B,** LE D₁ extension pattern is used when pulling on trousers.

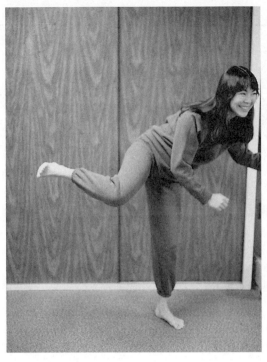 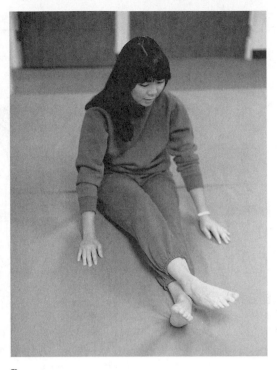

A B

FIG. 23-6 **A,** LE D_2 flexion pattern is shown in karate kick. **B,** LE D_2 extension pattern is used in long sitting with legs crossed.

in the baseball player at bat and in the tennis player who uses a two-handed backhand to increase control and power. Examples: bilateral asymmetric flexion to the left, with the left arm in D_2 flexion and the right arm in D_1 flexion, such as putting on a left earring (Fig. 23-11); bilateral asymmetric extension to the left, with the right arm in D_2 extension and the left arm in D_1 extension, such as zipping a left side zipper.

3. Reciprocal patterns. Paired extremities perform movements in opposite directions at the same time (Fig. 23-7, *C*). Reciprocal patterns have a stabilizing effect on the head, neck, and trunk, because movement of the extremities is in the opposite direction while head and neck remain in midline. In reciprocal patterns, the paired extremities move in opposite directions simultaneously, either in the same diagonal or in combined diagonals. During activities requiring high-level balance, the reciprocal patterns come into play with one extremity in D_1 extension and the other extremity in D_2 flexion. Examples: pitching in baseball, walking, sidestroke in swimming, and walking a balance beam with one extremity in a diagonal flexion pattern and the other in a diagonal extension pattern (Fig. 23-12).

Combined Movements of Upper and Lower Extremities

Interaction of the upper and lower extremities results in (1) ipsilateral patterns with extremities of the same side

moving in the same direction at the same time, (2) contralateral patterns with extremities of the opposite sides moving in the same direction at the same time, and (3) diagonal reciprocal patterns with contralateral extremities moving in the same direction at the same time while opposite contralateral extremities move in the opposite direction (Fig. 23-7, *D–F*).

The combined movements of the upper and lower extremities are observed in activities such as crawling and walking. Awareness of these patterns is important in the evaluation of the patient's motor skills. The ipsilateral patterns are more primitive developmentally and indicate lack of bilateral integration. Less rotation also is observed in ipsilateral patterns. Therefore, the goal in treatment is to progress from ipsilateral to contralateral to diagonal reciprocal patterns.

There are several advantages to using the diagonal patterns in treatment. First, crossing of midline occurs. This movement is of particular importance in the remediation of perceptual motor deficits such as unilateral neglect in which integration of both sides of the body and awareness of the neglected side are treatment goals. Second, each muscle has an optimal pattern in which it functions. For example, the patient who has weak thumb opposition benefits from active movement in D_2 extension. Similarly, D_1 extension is the optimal pattern for ulnar wrist extension. Third, the diagonal patterns use groups of muscles, which is typical of movement seen in functional activities. For example, in eating, the hand-to-

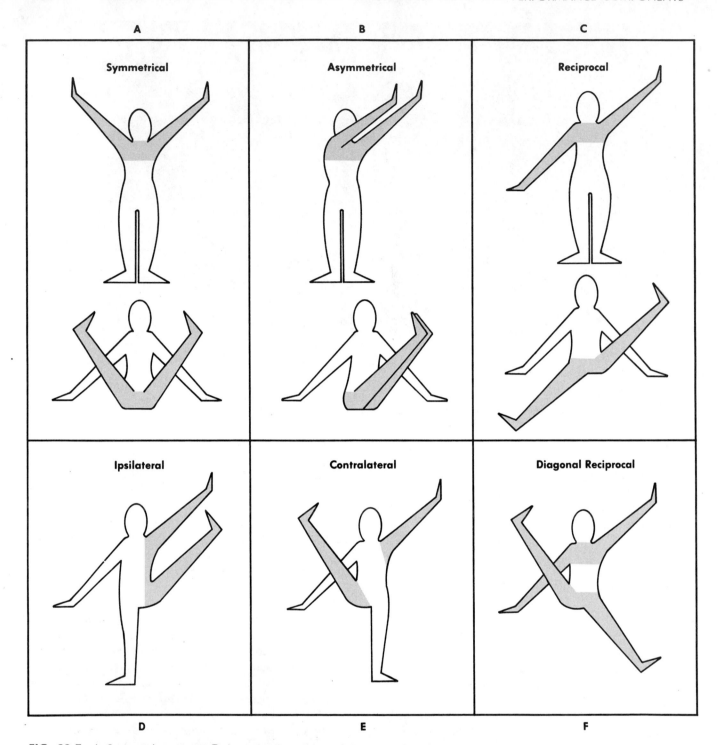

FIG. 23-7   **A,** Symmetric patterns. **B,** Asymmetric patterns. **C,** Reciprocal patterns. **D,** Ipsilateral pattern. **E,** Contralateral pattern. **F,** Diagonal reciprocal pattern. (From Myers BJ: Unit I: PNF diagonal patterns and their application to functional activities, videotape study guide, Rehabilitation Institute of Chicago, 1982.)

mouth action is accomplished in one mass movement pattern (D_1 flexion) that uses several muscles simultaneously. Therefore, movement in the diagonals is more efficient than movement performed at each joint separately. Finally, rotation is always a component in the diagonals (trunk rotation to the left or right and forearm pronation/supination). With an injury or the aging process, rotation frequently is impaired and can be facilitated with movement in the diagonals. In treatment, attention should be given to placement of activities so that movement occurs in the diagonal. For example, if the patient is working on a wood-sanding project, trunk rotation with extension can be facilitated by placing the project on an inclined plane in a diagonal.

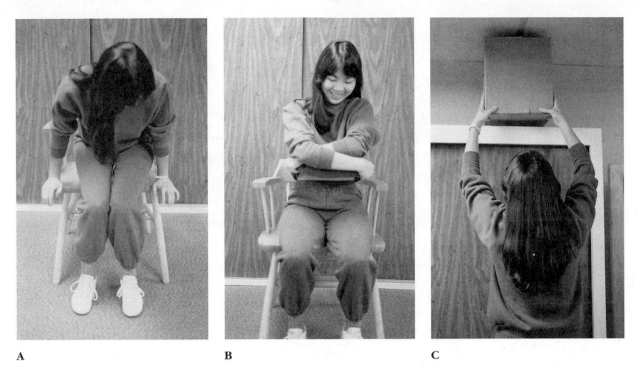

A   B   C

FIG. 23-8   **A,** UE bilateral symmetric D_1 extension pattern is shown in pushing off from chair.
B, UE bilateral symmetric D_2 extension pattern is used when starting to take off pullover shirt.
C, UE bilateral symmetric D_2 flexion pattern is used when reaching to lift box off high shelf.

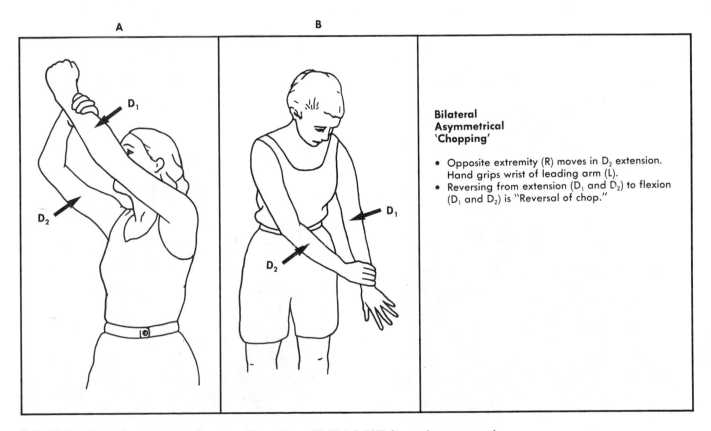

**Bilateral
Asymmetrical
'Chopping'**

- Opposite extremity (R) moves in D_2 extension. Hand grips wrist of leading arm (L).
- Reversing from extension (D_1 and D_2) to flexion (D_1 and D_2) is "Reversal of chop."

FIG. 23-9   Bilateral asymmetric chopping. (From Myers BJ: Unit I: PNF diagonal patterns and their application to functional activities, videotape study guide, Rehabilitation Institute of Chicago, 1982.)

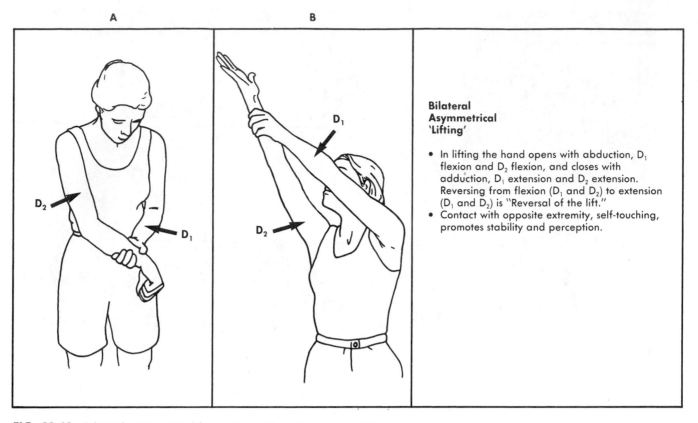

Bilateral Asymmetrical 'Lifting'

- In lifting the hand opens with abduction, D_1 flexion and D_2 flexion, and closes with adduction, D_1 extension and D_2 extension. Reversing from flexion (D_1 and D_2) to extension (D_1 and D_2) is "Reversal of the lift."
- Contact with opposite extremity, self-touching, promotes stability and perception.

FIG. 23-10 Bilateral asymmetric lifting. (From Myers BJ: Unit I: PNF diagonal patterns and their application to functional activities, videotape study guide, Rehabilitation Institute of Chicago, 1982.)

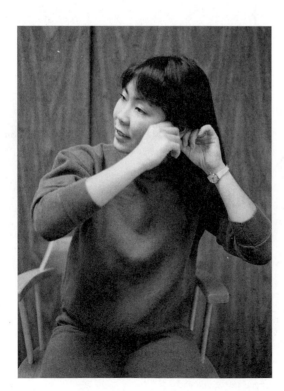

FIG. 23-11 Putting on earring requires use of UE bilateral asymmetric flexion pattern.

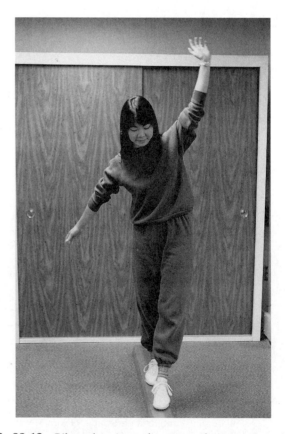

FIG. 23-12 Bilateral reciprocal pattern of upper extremities is used to walk balance beam.

TOTAL PATTERNS

In PNF, developmental postures also are called *total patterns* of movement and posture.[16] Total patterns require interaction between proximal (head, neck, and trunk) and distal (extremity) components. The assumption as well as the maintenance of postures is important. When posture cannot be sustained, emphasis should be placed on the *assumption* of posture.[21] In other words, before the patient can be expected to sustain a sitting posture, he or she must have ability in lower developmental total patterns of movement, such as rolling and moving from side-lying to side-sitting.

Active assumption of postures can be included in OT activities. For example, a reaching and placing activity could be set up so that the patient must reach for the object in supine posture and place the object in side-lying posture. The use of total patterns also can reinforce individual extremity movements. For example, in an activity such as wiping a table top, wrist extension is reinforced while the patient leans forward over the supporting arm.

Several facts support the use of total patterns in the PNF treatment approach.[16] First, total patterns of movement and posture are experienced as part of the normal developmental process in all human beings. Therefore, recapitulation of these postures is meaningful to the patient and acquired with less difficulty. Second, movement in and out of total patterns and the ability to sustain postures enhance components of normal development, such as reflex integration and support, balance between antagonists, and development of motor control in a cephalocaudal, proximodistal direction. Third, use of total patterns improves the ability to assume and maintain postures, which is important in all functional activities.

The sequence and procedures for assisting patients to the developmental postures were developed by Voss. In 1981 Myers developed a videotape showing use of the sequence and procedures in OT.[16] Refer to this video for further information on application of the total patterns and postures to OT.

PROCEDURES

Proprioceptive neuromuscular facilitation techniques are superimposed on movement and posture. Among these techniques are basic procedures considered essential to the PNF approach. Two procedures, verbal commands and visual cues, have been discussed previously. Other procedures are described in the following sections.

Manual contacts refer to the placement of the therapist's hands on the patient and are most effective when applied directly to the skin. Pressure from the therapist's touch is used as a facilitating mechanism and serves as a sensory cue to help the patient understand the direction of the anticipated movement.[22] The amount of pressure applied depends on the specific technique being used and the desired response. Location of manual contacts is chosen according to the groups of muscles, tendons, and joints responsible for the desired movement patterns. If the patient is having difficulty reaching to comb the back of the hair because of scapular weakness, the desired movement pattern is D_2 flexion. Manual contacts should be on the posterior surface of the scapula to reinforce the muscles that elevate, adduct, and rotate the scapula.

Stretch is used to initiate voluntary movement and enhance speed of response and strength in weak muscles. This procedures is based on Sherrington's neurophysiologic principle of reciprocal innervation.[18] When a muscle is stretched, the Ia and II fibers in the muscle spindle send excitatory messages to the alpha motor neurons, which innervate the stretched muscle. Inhibitory messages are sent to the antagonistic muscle simultaneously.[7]

When stretch is used in the PNF approach, the part to be facilitated is placed in the extreme lengthened range of the desired pattern (or where tension is felt on all muscle components of a given pattern). This range is the completely shortened range of the antagonistic pattern. Special attention is given to the rotatory component of the pattern because it is responsible for elongation of the fibers of the muscles in a given pattern. After the correct position for the stretch stimulus has been achieved, stretch is superimposed on the pattern. The patient should attempt the movement at the exact time that the stretch reflex is elicited. The use of verbal commands also should coincide with the application of stretch to reinforce the movement. Discrimination should be exercised when using stretch to prevent increasing pain or muscle imbalances.

Traction facilitates the joint receptors by creating a separation of the joint surfaces. It is thought that traction promotes movement and is used for pulling motion.[22] In activities such as carrying a heavy suitcase or pulling open a jammed door, traction can be felt on joint surfaces. Although traction may be contraindicated in patients with acute symptoms, such as after surgery or a fracture, it can sometimes provide relief of pain and promote greater range of motion in painful joints.

Approximation facilitates joint receptors by creating a compression of joint surfaces. It promotes stability and postural control and is used for pushing motion.[22] Approximation is usually superimposed on a weight-bearing posture. For example, to enhance postural control in prone on elbows, approximation may be given through the shoulders in a downward direction.

Maximal resistance is a procedure that applies Sherrington's principle of irradiation, namely, that stronger muscles and patterns reinforce weaker components.[18] This procedure is frequently misunderstood and applied incorrectly. It is defined as the greatest amount of resistance that can be applied to an active contraction allowing full range of motion to occur or to an isometric contraction without defeating or breaking the patient's hold.[22] It is *not* the greatest amount of resistance that the therapist can apply. The objective is to obtain maximal effort on the part of the patient, because strength is increased by movement against resistance that requires maximal effort.[9]

If the resistance applied by the therapist results in uncoordinated or jerky movement or if it breaks the patient's hold, too much resistance has been given. Movement against maximal resistance should be slow and smooth. To use this technique effectively, the therapist must sense the appropriate amount of resistance. For patients with neurologic impairment or pain, the resistance may be very light, and is probably maximal for the patient's needs. The therapist's manual contacts may offer light resistance that actually assists by providing the patient with a way to track the desired movement. In the presence of spasticity, resistance may increase existing muscle imbalance and needs to be monitored. For example, if an increase in finger flexor spasticity is noted with resisted rocking in the hands-knees position, resistance should be decreased or eliminated, or an alternate position used.

TECHNIQUES

Specific techniques are used in conjunction with these basic procedures. A few have been selected for discussion. These techniques are divided into three categories: those directed to the agonist, those that are a reversal of the antagonists, and those that promote relaxation.[22]

Techniques Directed to the Agonist

Repeated contractions is a technique based on the assumption that repetition of an activity is necessary for motor learning and helps develop strength, range of motion, and endurance. The patient's voluntary movement is facilitated with stretch and resistance using isometric and isotonic contractions. Repeated contractions could be used to increase trunk flexion with rotation in the patient who has difficulty reaching to put on a pair of shoes from the sitting position. The patient bends forward as far as possible. At the point when active motion weakens, he or she is asked to "hold" with an isometric contraction. This action is followed by isotonic contractions, facilitated by stretch, as the patient is asked to "reach toward your feet." This sequence is repeated until fatigue is evident or the patient is able to reach the feet. The pattern can be reinforced further by asking the patient to hold with another isometric contraction at the end of the sequence.

Rhythmic initiation is used to improve the ability to initiate movement, a problem that may be seen with Parkinson disease or apraxia. This technique involves voluntary relaxation, passive movement, and repeated isotonic contractions of the agonistic pattern. The verbal command is, "Relax and let me move you." As relaxation is felt, the command is, "Now you do it with me." After several repetitions of active movement, resistance can be given to reinforce the movement. Rhythmic initiation

allows the patient to feel the pattern prior to active movement. Thus the proprioceptive and kinesthetic senses are enhanced.

Reversal of Antagonists Techniques

Reversal of antagonists techniques employ a characteristic of normal development, namely, that movement is reversing and changes direction. These techniques are based on Sherrington's principle of successive induction in which the stronger antagonist facilitates the weaker agonist.[18] The agonist is facilitated through resistance to the antagonist. The contraction of the antagonist can be isotonic, isometric, or a combination. In patients in whom resistance of antagonists increases symptoms such as pain and spasticity, these techniques may be contraindicated. For example, the facilitation of finger extension (agonist) would not be effectively achieved through resistance applied to spastic finger flexors (antagonist). In this situation, finger extension may be better facilitated through the use of repeated contractions, in which the emphasis is only on the extensor surface.

Slow reversal is an isotonic contraction (against resistance) of the antagonist followed by an isotonic contraction (against resistance) of the agonist. *Slow reversal-hold* is the same sequence, with an isometric contraction at the end of the range. For the patient who has difficulty reaching his mouth for oral hygiene because of weakness in the D_1 flexion pattern, the slow reversal procedure is as follows: an isotonic contraction against resistance in D_1 extension with verbal command "push down and out" followed by an isotonic contraction of D_1 flexion against resistance with verbal command "pull up and across." An increase or build-up of power in the agonist should be felt with each successive isotonic contraction.

Rhythmic stabilization is used to increase stability by eliciting simultaneous isometric contractions of antagonistic muscle groups. Cocontraction results if the patient is not allowed to relax. Because this technique requires repeated isometric contractions, increased circulation or the tendency to hold one's breath or both occurs. Therefore, rhythmic stabilization may be contraindicated for patients with cardiac involvement, and no more than three or four repetitions should be done at a time.

Manual contacts are applied on both agonist and antagonist muscles with resistance given simultaneously. The patient is asked to hold the contraction against graded resistance. Without allowing the patient to relax, manual contacts are switched to opposite surfaces. Rhythmic stabilization is useful with patients lacking postural control because of ataxia or proximal weakness. Used intermittently during an activity requiring postural stability, such as meal preparation in standing posture, this technique enhances muscle balance, endurance, and control of movement.

Relaxation Techniques

Relaxation techniques are an effective means of increasing range of motion, particularly in the presence of pain or spasticity, which may be increased by passive stretch.

Contract-relax involves an isotonic contraction of the antagonistic pattern against maximal resistance and only the rotational component of the diagonal movement is allowed to occur. This action is followed by relaxation, then passive movement into the agonistic pattern. This procedure is repeated at each point in the range of motion in which limitation is felt to occur.[22] Contact-relax is used when no active range in the agonistic pattern is present.

Hold-relax is performed in the same sequence as contract-relax but involves an isometric contraction of the antagonist, followed by relaxation, then active movement into the agonistic pattern. Because this technique involves an isometric contraction against resistance, it is particularly beneficial in the presence of pain or acute orthopedic conditions. For the reflex sympathetic dystrophy (RSD) patient who has pain with shoulder flexion, abduction, and external rotation, the therapist asks the patient to hold against resistance in the D_2 extension pattern, followed by active movement into the D_2 flexion pattern. This technique is beneficial for the RSD patient during self-care activities such as shampooing hair and zipping a shirt in back.

Slow reversal-hold-relax begins with an isotonic contraction, followed by an isometric contraction, then by relaxation of the antagonistic pattern, and then by active movement of the agonistic pattern. When the patient has the ability actively to move the agonist, the technique is preferred. For example, to increase active elbow extension in the presence of tight elbow flexors, the therapist asks the patient to perform D_1 flexion with elbow flexion as resistance is applied to the elbow flexors. When the range of motion is complete, the patient is asked to hold with an isometric contraction followed immediately by relaxation. When relaxation is felt, the patient moves actively into D_1 extension with elbow extension. This technique helps to increase elbow extension for such activities as reaching to lock the wheelchair brakes or picking up an object off the floor.

Rhythmic rotation is effective in decreasing spasticity and increasing range of motion. The therapist passively moves the body part in the desired pattern. When tightness or restriction of movement is felt, the therapist rotates the body part slowly and rhythmically in both directions. After relaxation is felt, the therapist continues to move the body part into the newly available range. This technique is effective in preparing the paraplegic patient with lower extremity spasticity or clonus to put on a pair of pants and also in preparing for splint fabrication on a spastic extremity.

SUMMARY

Emphasis in the PNF approach is on the patient's abilities and potential so that strengths assist weaker components. Strengths and deficiencies are evaluated and addressed in treatment within total patterns of movement and posture. A battery of techniques is superimosed on these total patterns to enhance motor response and facilitate motor learning.

Proprioceptive neuromuscular facilitation uses multisensory input. Coordination and timing of sensory input are important in eliciting the desired response from the patient. The patient's performance should be monitored and sensory input adjusted accordingly.

To use PNF effectively, an understanding of the developmental sequence and the components of normal movement is necessary. Second, it is necessary to learn the diagonal patterns and how they are used in ADL. Third, the therapist must know when and how to use the techniques of facilitation and relaxation, which requires observation and practice under the supervision of an experienced PNF therapist. Finally, the therapist applies patterns and techniques of facilitation to OT evaluation and treatment.

CASE STUDY

A 50-year-old woman was referred to OT with a right cerebral vascular accident (CVA) resulting in left hemiplegia. Before the CVA, she had a history of hypertension but otherwise good health. Referral to OT was made 10 days after onset for evaluation and treatment in ADL, visual perceptual skills, and left upper extremity function.

Evaluation

Initial evaluation revealed intact vital and related functions, such as oral/facial musculature and swallowing. Voice production was good. Patient had a tendency to hold her breath during activities, and subsequent decreased endurance was noted. Visual tracking was impaired with inability to scan past midline and apparent left side neglect.

Head and neck were observed to be frequently rotated to the right and slightly flexed because of weak extensors. Trunk was noted to be asymmetric in sitting posture with most of the weight supported on the right side. Posture was flexed because of weak extensors. Static sitting balance was fair and dynamic sitting balance was poor, with patient listing forward and left.

Right arm was normal in sensation and strength, although motor planning was impaired. Left arm was essentially flaccid with impaired sensation of light touch, pain, and proprioception. Patient complained of mild glenohumeral pain during passive movement at end ranges of shoulder abduction and flexion. Scapular instability was noted. No active movement could be elicited in left arm.

Perceptual evaluation showed apraxia (especially during activities requiring crossing of midline), and left side neglect. Patient was alert and oriented with good attention span and memory. Carryover in tasks was adequate.

Patient needed moderate assistance in ADL and moderate to maximum assistance with transfers. Impaired balance and apraxia were most limiting factors in performance of ADL.

Treatment implementation

Following cervicocaudal direction of development, alignment of head and neck was appropriate starting point for treatment. Left side awareness, sitting posture, and trunk balance were directly influenced by position of head and neck. Before the start of self-care activities patient performed head and neck patterns of flexion and extension with rotation. To reinforce rotation to left, therapist was positioned to left of patient. Clothing and hygiene articles also were placed to left of patient.

Lack of trunk control was another problem. During bending activities patient reported fear of falling and was unsure of her ability to return to upright position. Consequently, she had difficulty leaning forward to transfer from wheelchair. Slow reversal-hold technique was used to reinforce trunk patterns during ADL. For example, as patient prepared to don her left pant leg, therapist was positioned in front and to left of patient. Manual contacts were on anterior aspect of either scapula. Therapist moved with patient and applied resistance as she leaned forward to don her pants. At end of the range, patient was instructed to hold with isometric contraction. After pants were donned, manual contacts switched to posterior surface of either scapula. Resistance was applied as patient returned to upright position. Verbal command was, "look up and over your right shoulder." When patient was upright she was again instructed to hold with isometric contraction. In addition to reinforcing trunk control, this technique alleviated patient's fear of leaning forward, because therapist was in continual contact with patient.

An indirect benefit of the flexion and extension patterns of the head, neck, and trunk was reinforcement of respiration. Patient was encouraged to inhale during extension and exhale during flexion. This approach eliminated the patient's tendency to hold her breath.

Treatment consisted of total patterns and techniques to facilitate proximal stability in left upper extremity and provide proprioceptive input. Weight-bearing activities were selected because no active movement was available in the left arm. Patient performed perceptual tasks in diagonal patterns with right upper extremity, such as a mosaic tile design, paper and pencil activities and board games. These activities were performed to include side-lying posture on left elbow, prone posture on elbows, side-sitting posture with weight on left arm, and all fours. To reinforce stability at the shoulder girdle, approximation and rhythmic stabilization were used with manual contacts at both shoulders and then shoulder and pelvis. Performance of perceptual tasks in diagonals improved patient's motor planning, left-side awareness, and trunk rotation.

Patient was instructed in bilateral asymmetric chopping and lifting patterns to support scapula and left upper extremity in rolling and other activities. These also enhanced left-side awareness and trunk rotation. To facilitate scapular movement during chop and lift patterns, therapist applied stretch to initiate movement followed by slow reversal technique. In preparation for lift pattern, manual contacts were placed on posterior surface of scapula. Stretch was applied in lengthened range. As patient initiated lifting pattern, resistance was given and maintained throughout range. This procedure was repeated for antagonistic or reverse of lift pattern with manual contacts switching to anterior surface of scapula.

About 3 to 4 weeks after injury, patient was able to initiate left upper extremity movement in synergy with predominance of flexor tone. Weight-bearing activities and rhythmic rotation were helpful in normalizing tone, and both techniques were used with ADL such as dressing and bathing. Wrist and finger extensions were facilitated in the D_1 extension and D_2 flexion patterns using repeated contractions.

Results

Reevaluation after 5 weeks of OT revealed increased endurance and ability to coordinate breathing with activity, and consistency in crossing midline during visual scanning activities. Patient was able to turn head and neck to the left without cues from therapist. Fear of falling forward with bending had diminished, and patient automatically turned her head to look up and over her shoulder to reinforce assumption of upright position. As trunk strength continued to improve, reinforcement with head and neck rotation was no longer necessary. Visual tracking alone, in direction of movement, was sufficient to reinforce assumption of upright position. Eventually patient was able to obtain an upright position without apparent visual or head and neck reinforcement. Sitting balance improved with bilateral weight bearing through both hips. Shoulder pain decreased and scapular stability improved during weight-bearing activities. Patient initiated left upper extremity movement out of flexor synergy pattern. Right upper extremity motor planning was within functional limits for ADL. Transfers and self-care required only minimal assistance, and cues were no longer needed for left upper extremity awareness.

REVIEW QUESTIONS

1. Give examples of how the TNR and the ATNR reinforce motor performance.
2. Is rolling from prone to supine a flexor- or extensor-dominant activity?
3. In the presence of pain, what tone of voice should be used when giving verbal commands?
4. Discuss the significance of auditory, visual, and tactile input in motor learning.
5. Which upper extremity diagonal pattern is used for the hand-to-mouth phase of eating? For zipping front-opening pants?
6. Discuss the advantages of using the chop and life patterns.
7. Which trunk pattern is used when donning a left sock?
8. List three advantages of using the diagonal patterns.
9. What is the developmental sequence of total patterns?
10. If a patient needs more stability, which of the following total patterns should be chosen: side-lying or prone posture on elbows?
11. Which PNF technique facilitates postural control and cocontraction?
12. Discuss the neurophysiologic principles of Sherrington upon which the PNF techniques of facilitation are based.
13. What is an effective technique to prepare the patient with upper extremity flexor spasticity to don a shirt?
14. Define maximal resistance.
15. Name two PNF techniques that facilitate initiation of movement.

REFERENCES

1. Abreu BF, Toglia JP: Cognitive rehabilitation: a model for occupational therapy, *Am J Occup Ther* 41(7):439, 1987.
2. Affolter F: Perceptual processes as prerequisites for complex human behavior, *Int Rehabil Med* 3(1):3, 1981.
3. Ayres JA: Proprioceptive neuromuscular facilitation elicited through the upper extremities. I. Background 9(1):1. II. Application 9(2):57. III. Specific application to occupational therapy, *Am J Occup Ther* 9(3):121, 1955.
4. Buchwald JS: Exteroceptive reflexes and movement, *Am J Phys Med* 46(1):121, 1967.
5. Carroll J: The utilization of reinforcement techniques in the program for the hemiplegic, *Am J Occup Ther* 4(5):211, 1950.
6. Cooke DM: The effects of resistance on multiple sclerosis patients with intention tremor, *Am J Occup Ther* 12(2):89, 1958.
7. Farber SD: *Neurorehabilitation: a multisensory approach,* Philadelphia, 1982, WB Saunders.
8. Hagbarth KE: Excitatory and inhibitory skin areas for flexor and extensor mononeurons, *Acta Physiol Scand* 26(suppl 94):1, 1952.
9. Hellebrandt FA: Physiology. In Delorme TL, Watkins AL: *Progressive resistance exercise,* New York, 1951, Appleton, Century, & Crofts.
10. Hellebrandt FA, Schade M, Carns ML: Methods of evoking the tonic neck reflexes in normal human subjects, *Am J Phys Med* 4(90):139, 1962.
11. Humphrey TL, Huddleston OL: Applying facilitation techniques to self care training, *Phys Ther Rev* 38(9):605, 1958.
12. Jackson JH: Selected writings, vol 1, London, 1931, Hodder & Staughton (edited by J Taylor).
13. Kabat H, Rosenberg D: Concepts and techniques of occupational therapy neuromuscular disorders, *Am J Occup Ther* 4(1):6, 1950.
14. Loomis JE, Boersma FJ: Training right brain damaged patients in a wheelchair task: case studies using verbal mediation, *Physiother Can* 34(4):204, 1982.
15. Myers BJ: *Proprioceptive neuromuscular facilitation: concepts and application in occupational therapy as taught by Voss. Notes from course at Rehabilitation Institute of Chicago, September 8–12, 1980.*
16. Myers BJ: *Assisting to postures and application in occupational therapy activities,* Chicago, Rehabilitation Institute of Chicago, 1981 (videotape).
17. Myers BJ: *PNF: patterns and application in occupational therapy,* Chicago, Rehabilitation Institute of Chicago, 1981 (videotape).
18. Sherrington C: *The integrative action of the nervous system,* New Haven, 1961, Yale University Press.
19. Voss DE: Application of patterns and techniques in occupational therapy, *Am J Occup Ther* 8(4):191, 1959.
20. Voss DE: Proprioceptive neuromuscular facilitation, *Am J Phys Med* 46(1):838, 1967.
21. Voss DE: Proprioceptive neuromuscular facilitation: the PNF method. In Pearson PH, Williams CE, editors: *Physical therapy services in the developmental disabilities,* Springfield, Ill, 1972, Charles C Thomas.
22. Voss DE, Ionta MK, Myers BJ: *Proprioceptive neuromuscular facilitation,* ed 3, Philadelphia, 1985, Harper & Row.
23. Whitaker EW: A suggested treatment in occupational therapy for patients with multiple sclerosis, *Am J Occup Ther* 4(6):247, 1950.

Neurodevelopmental Treatment of Adult Hemiplegia: The Bobath Approach

Jan Zaret Davis

The ultimate goal of occupational therapy for the patient with hemiplegia is to regain as much independence as possible, under safe conditions, regardless of the therapy setting or length of treatment. A foundation of treatment should be established that will allow the patient to make positive changes beyond the time limitations of therapy. It is often the case that changes occur for many months or even years following a cerebrovascular accident (CVA). Working within the confines of the current health care system, most therapists will not have the opportunity to follow a patient throughout the recovery process. The limitations of a therapist's time with the patient should not dictate the theme of the treatment program.

Occupational therapists want to establish a program that facilitates optimal learning and promotes recovery. Neurodevelopmental treatment (NDT) provides a sound foundation for such a program. First developed in the 1940s by Berta Bobath, a physical therapist, and her husband, Dr. Karel Bobath,[2] NDT is based on normal development and movement. The term *neurodevelopmental treatment* was first coined by the Bobaths from their work with children with cerebral palsy. Also known as the Bobath approach, NDT has been used successfully in the treatment of adult hemiplegia.

During recovery a patient typically overuses the uninvolved side, compensating for the loss of sensory and motor function on the hemiplegic side. Resulting problems in posture, alignment, balance, strength, tone, and coordination often lead to less effective patterns of movement and may eventually cause orthopedic problems, pain, or decreased safety. If patients are trained only in the use of adaptive equipment, compensatory movement is reinforced and potential for obtaining the highest level of function is hindered.

In NDT the therapist develops a program to help the patient avoid these abnormal patterns of movement. The program provides a foundation that promotes the highest level of functional recovery based on relearning normal movement, rather than on compensation. NDT techniques are intended for more than just the movements of an arm or leg; the person is treated by encouraging the use of both sides of the body. One of the central principles of NDT is that alignment and symmetry of the trunk and pelvis are necessary for good alignment and symmetry of the extremities. Adaptive equipment is used when absolutely necessary for safety, but not as a first resort and not as a replacement for treatment.

With good handling and treatment skills, the occupational therapist can facilitate positive changes for the patient with hemiplegia at any stage of recovery. It is important to know what to avoid in treatment as well as what to promote and facilitate. Therapists must become efficient in problem solving and prioritizing patient needs to design an effective treatment program that will best serve the needs of the patient throughout recovery.

TYPICAL PROBLEMS OF HEMIPLEGIA
MOTOR PROBLEMS

The major motor problem in hemiplegia is the lack of postural control affecting voluntary movement. Flaccidity is most common at the onset of a CVA. During this time the patient is often passive, displaying low endurance and low tolerance to activity. This condition may last a few days or as long as several months. Although the patient displays no movement in the affected extremities at this time, a proper treatment program can have a strong impact on the eventual functional outcome.[2]

Following the flaccid stage, patients enter a stage of

mixed tone, displaying a combination of flaccidity and spasticity. For example, the upper extremity may have an increase in tone proximally (scapular retraction, depression and/or downward rotation, internal rotation of the humerus) but a decrease in tone distally (at the wrist, hand, and/or fingers). It is during the mixed tone phase that trauma to the shoulder is common. If treatment does not address the problems of high tone at this stage, the patient progresses to the next stage.

Spasticity is the most commonly identified problem and the most difficult motor problem to treat following a CVA. If not treated correctly, spasticity can progress until independent living is nearly impossible. Spasticity interferes with the patient's selective motor function. It produces abnormal sensory feedback and contributes to weakness of the antagonist muscles. It can cause contractures, pain, and an all-consuming fear in many patients. Fear, pain, and spasticity are often so intertwined that they cause a vicious cycle. The spasticity causes an increase in pain, which causes an increase in fear, which in turn increases the amount of spasticity.[5]

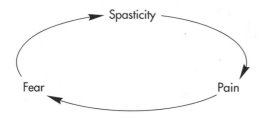

If measures are taken to reduce pain and fear, the therapist has a much better chance for success with the methods used to reduce spasticity. Other factors that can influence the amount of spasticity are emotional stress, physical effort (on the hemiplegic side or the nonaffected side), temperature, and the rate at which an activity is done.

The typical posture in the adult patient with hemiplegia (Fig. 24-1) can be described as follows:
- Head: lateral flexion toward the involved side with rotation away from the involved side
- Upper extremity: a combination of the strongest components of the flexion and extension synergies
  1. Scapula — depression, retraction
  2. Shoulder — adduction, internal rotation
  3. Elbow — flexion
  4. Forearm — pronation
  5. Wrist — flexion, ulnar deviation
  6. Fingers — flexion
- Trunk: lateral flexion toward the involved side (trunk shortening)
- Lower extremity: typical posture in adult with hemiplegia is the extension synergy
  1. Pelvis — posterior elevation, retraction
  2. Hip — internal rotation, adduction, extension
  3. Knee — extension
  4. Ankle — plantar flexion, supination, inversion
  5. Toes — flexion

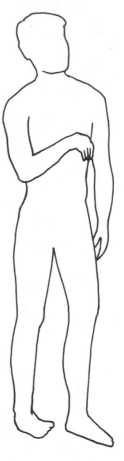

FIG. 24-1   Typical posture of adult with hemiplegia in standing position. (Courtesy of Graphic Arts Department, Harmarville Rehabilitation Center, Pittsburgh, Pa.)

ADDITIONAL PROBLEMS

In addition to motor problems, patients often have many problems that can be debilitating either alone or in combination. The following are some of the most common problems.

Weight-bearing. Most patients avoid bearing weight on the affected side of the body. Instead of the weight being equally distributed over both hips (in sitting) or over both feet (in standing), it is usually shifted to the nonhemiplegic side. Many factors make weight-bearing difficult over the weak side. Loss of sensation, loss of strength, and fear of falling contribute to this problem.

Fear. Fear may be the most debilitating factor for many patients. Fear magnifies other problems that cause the patient to be dependent rather than independent. Fear can be caused by loss of sensation, poor balance reactions, lack of protective extension (fear of falling), and perceptual or cognitive problems. Fear is a major factor influencing spasticity.[5]

Sensory loss. Sensory loss may include loss of stereognosis, kinesthetic awareness, light touch, and pressure. A patient's extremity can remain useless because of sensory loss even though there is good motor control.[2,5]

Neglect. Unilateral neglect can be a combination of one or more of the following: sensory loss, perceptual or cognitive dysfunction, or visual field deficit (homonymous hemianopsia). The patient may have good motor recovery but is unable to use it functionally because of the neglect.[1,5]

Many other problems are related to CVA, such as aphasia, apraxia, and a variety of perceptual motor problems. These conditions are discussed in Chapter 41.

EVALUATING THE PATIENT

When evaluating the patient, emphasis is placed on the quality of movement, that is, the way the patient moves. The therapist observes coordination, changes of tone, and postural reactions rather than looking at specific muscles and joints.[2] It is imperative for the therapist to have knowledge of normal posture and movement to identify patterns that may be abnormal. Each patient presents a different picture based upon age, premorbid physical condition, and normal degenerative changes.

THE IMPORTANCE OF OBSERVATION

Good observation skills are the foundation for a good evaluation. Therapists must learn to be very specific in their observations and in their analysis of these observations. Although certain characteristics are common to most patients with hemiplegia, each patient demonstrates a unique set of problems. Therapists with the most advanced skills see problems that others may miss.

BASIC OBSERVATION PROCESS

In evaluations, patients must be observed from the front, back, and side. Most information about patient *symmetry* is gained by observing both the hemiplegic and nonhemiplegic sides, from head to toe. Observations should be both static and dynamic, that is, (1) with the patient sitting, standing, or supine in a *static* position; and (2) while the patient tries to move for *dynamic* changes in the trunk, head/neck, and both upper extremities.

To evaluate *asymmetry* in posture, pelvic, and shoulder girdle, the patient should be in an upright position. If the patient is unable to maintain the sitting posture, evaluation may be in a supine position, but observations will be limited. It helps to have the patient's shirt off to detect asymmetries in the trunk, shoulder girdle, and upper extremities. For privacy, the therapist may want to do this evaluation in the patient's room. It is also helpful to keep a tank top in the OT department for female patients. Outpatients often wear a bathing suit, halter top, or tank top under their shirts.

A good way to structure observation is to imagine reference lines, as shown in Fig. 24-2, which will help to identify deviations. The first line of reference is vertical at

Observation Guide

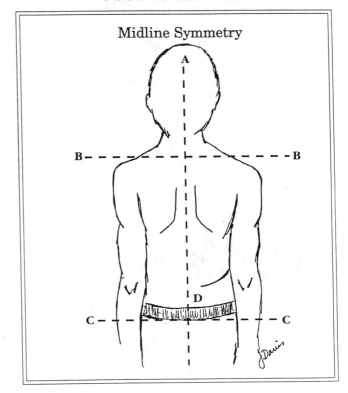

Look for:
• unilateral creases, folds
• equal weight-bearing

Check:
• distances
• head position
• height of shoulders
• symmetry of trunk

FIG. 24-2 Observation guide. (Reprinted with permission, International Clinical Educators, Inc., 1993.)

midline, Fig. 24-2, *A.* Look for asymmetries by comparing the right and left sides of the patient. Is the head centered in midline? Are the medial borders of both scapulae equidistant from the spine? Is the trunk shifted to one side? Next visualize a level, horizontal line at the top of the shoulders, Fig. 24-2, *B.* Is one shoulder higher than the other? Is one shoulder abnormally high *or* the other abnormally low? The third reference is a level horizontal line at the height of the hips, Fig. 24-2, *C.* Is one hip higher or lower? Is the patient bearing weight equally over both hips? The therapist also should look for unilateral creases or folds on the trunk, Fig. 24-2, *D,* which might indicate additional problem areas.

It is important to remember that observations of asymmetry do not necessarily indicate what the problem is; it indicates only that there is a problem. To understand the cause of the problem, the therapist continues the evaluation.

Never assume the obvious. Now the detective work begins as the pieces of the puzzle come together. In problem solving, information from observations is combined with information about the medical history and premorbid conditions, and most important, handling by the therapist.

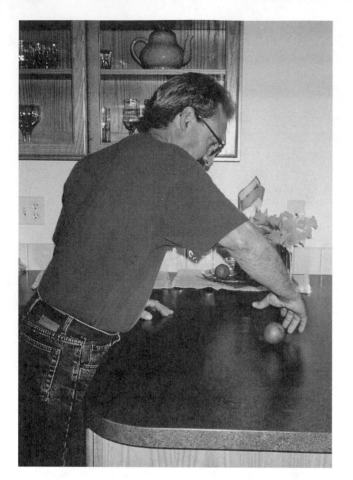

FIG. 24-3 Patient reaching forward using abnormal movement patterns.

and everyone has associated movements at one time or another. They are most commonly identified in children; for example, when cutting with scissors, the child's tongue protrudes. The patient may use compensatory movements or movements influenced by abnormal synergy patterns. These abnormal patterns of movement, called *associated reactions,* can be caused by (1) excessive effort on the sound side that "overflow" to the weak side or by (2) excessive effort on the weak side, which causes a synergy pattern. Associated reactions are abnormal and should be discouraged or inhibited.[6]

By comparing the patient's movement pattern to the normal pattern, the therapist can identify problem areas interfering with normal movement. For example, when the patient with a hemiplegic arm reaches for an object, the shoulder elevates and retracts, the elbow maintains a flexed position, and the forearm is in partial pronation with wrist and finger flexion; the trunk flexes forward to position the hand nearer the object (Fig. 24-3). In comparison, a normal pattern of movement might display trunk stability with scapular protraction, selective elbow extension with pronation, wrist extension, and finger flexion (Fig. 24-4). The therapist must thoroughly understand the components of normal movement to compare it to abnormal movement for effective evaluation. Table

To identify the underlying cause when asymmetries are noted, the affected limb is taken through passive range of motion. It is important for the therapist to move the upper extremity within normal patterns of movement and in normal alignment to avoid orthopedic problems (microtearing of structures or impingement). Any pain or discomfort upon movement should be noted; never move the limb past the point of pain or discomfort. If able, the patient should be asked to describe the pain (stabbing, aching, dull, pulling) and show its specific location. This information will help in determining the cause of the pain.

As the patient is passively moved, the therapist feels deviations from normal. If resistance is felt, patient probably has abnormally high tone. It is important to take the limb slowly through range to prevent a quick stretch followed by clonus, which increases the problem of high tone. If no resistance is felt but the arm feels heavy, patient probably has abnormally low tone.

For dynamical evaluation, the therapist observes any movement initiated by the patient on the weak side. As the patient attempts to move the weak side, sometimes the strong side attempts to make the same movements. This effect is called *associated movement.* It is normal,

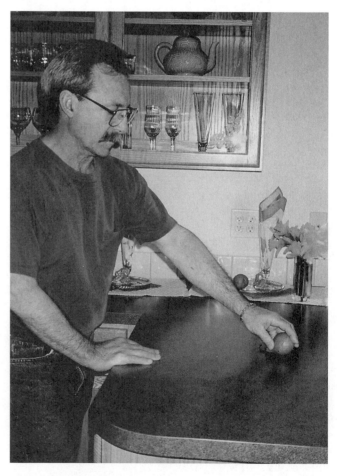

FIG. 24-4 Patient using normal movement patterns while reaching forward with the uninvolved side.

TABLE 24-1	Observations and Possible Causes	

STRUCTURED OBSERVATION (STATIC)

AREA OBSERVED	OBSERVATION	POSSIBLE CAUSES OF PROBLEM*
Head	Lateral flexion to affected side	Shortened upper trapezius; poor head righting; midline orientation deficit
Shoulder	Hemiplegic shoulder lower	Weak trunk with lateral flexion to the hemi side; low tone in shoulder girdle with arm hanging to the side; increased tone in depression and downward rotation of the scapula
	Nonaffected shoulder higher	Bracing/holding with strong side caused by poor sitting balance, weak trunk control, or fear
Scapular position	Downward rotation of scapula	Increased tone of muscles acting on scapular downward rotation (rhomboids, levator scapulae, serratus anterior); decreased tone of stabilizing muscles of the scapula allowing it to fall into downward rotation
	Winging of the scapula	Weakness of serratus ant.; increased tone of the subscapularis pulling the scapula and causing it to wing
Trunk	Unilateral crease on affected side	Lateral flexion of trunk caused by weak abdominals or increased tone in scapular retraction and depression with pelvic retraction and elevation causing shortening on the hemi side

*These are some examples. A problem may have one or more causes.

24-1 lists a few common problems observed during static evaluation, along with their possible causes.

INTEGRATING EVALUATION AND TREATMENT

The information collected while observing the patient both statically and dynamically is followed by identifying specific problem areas. Next the therapist determines what to do in treatment. According to Bobath, "Every evaluation is a treatment and every treatment is an evaluation".[2]

The primary goal of NDT is to relearn normal movements. The methods used are intended to treat the person as a whole, encouraging the use of both sides of the body. The patient uses less adaptive equipment (for example, slings, braces, and canes) and is more able to move about freely with more normal muscle tone.[2] This approach creates a better atmosphere for the psychosocial adjustment to family and everyday living. The more normal a person appears to others, with less deformity from spasticity, the better he or she is accepted.

FLUCTUATIONS IN TONE ARE NORMAL

Under stressful conditions anyone's muscle tone might be higher (e.g., when presenting a paper in front of the class for the first time); tone may be lower after a big lunch or when the instructor turns down the lights. Patients, on the other hand, demonstrate abnormally high tone and abnormally low tone. It is the therapist's job to determine where the patient displays abnormally high or low tone and then implement a treatment program designed to normalize tone. Decreasing abnormally high tone is called *inhibition;* increasing abnormally low tone is called *facilitation.* NDT uses patterns of movement that are opposite to spastic patterns and are guided by

the therapist from key points of control. Abnormal patterns (synergies) must be suppressed or inhibited before normal, selective isolated movement can take place. It is impossible to superimpose normal movement on abnormal tone.[2]

Normalization of muscle tone may be accomplished by using one or more of the following techniques:[2,5,7]

1. weight-bearing over the affected side
2. trunk rotation
3. scapular protraction
4. anterior pelvic tilt/position pelvis forward
5. facilitation of slow, controlled movements
6. proper positioning

These six techniques, discussed in the paragraphs that follow, provide the foundation for treatment of the adult patient with hemiplegia using the Bobath (NDT) approach. The techniques are most effective and provide the best potential in rehabilitation when they are started in the acute phase, but can be useful in any phase of the treatment program.

SPECIFICS OF NDT TREATMENT

Weight-Bearing over the Affected Side

Weight bearing over the hemiplegic side is the most effective way of normalizing tone. With patients displaying low tone it is facilitative, and with patients displaying high tone it can be inhibitory. Weight-bearing not only helps to normalize tone, it also provides sensory input to the hemiplegic side through proprioception. Additionally this approach improves the patient's awareness of that side and helps to decrease neglect. As the awareness of the weak side improves, the patient often is less fearful, thus establishing a better foundation for the recovery process.

The positive effects of weight-bearing can be observed in nearly every stage of recovery. Correct weight-bearing can be as simple as positioning the patient in side-lying on the hemiplegic side in bed, or as difficult as the facilitation of stance phase in gait training. When weight-bearing is introduced early, the benefits can be seen throughout the rehabilitation program. The patient should be taught to bear weight equally through both hips in sitting and through both feet in standing.

Weight-bearing through the upper extremity in sitting or standing can help to normalize tone throughout the upper extremity (UE). It is most effective with patients displaying a flexion synergy of the upper extremity. The patient can be brought into a weight bearing position before or during treatment in functional daily living tasks.

Before weight-bearing through the UE, the UE and shoulder girdle must be prepared. The therapist must make sure the scapula is gliding in forward protraction, elevation, and upward rotation. Following mobilization of the scapula, the patient's hand should be placed on the mat or bench several inches away from the hip. (If the hand is placed next to the hip, extreme hyperextension of the wrist can occur). The humerus is in external rotation with the elbow in extension. As the patient shifts weight over the hemiplegic side, the therapist should be careful not to allow internal rotation of the upper arm and not to allow the elbow to collapse. Do not allow weight-bearing if the patient complains of pain or if the hand is edematous. The patient should not be allowed to hang on the arm in weight-bearing, but instead, should move the body over the arm to normalize tone without putting undue stress on the joint (Fig. 24-5).

When facilitating weight-bearing during functional activities, it is normal to allow the elbow to bend slightly. The best rule of thumb is to check the position normally assumed for activity, and then see if the patient's position is similar.

Trunk Rotation

Trunk rotation, or dissociation of upper and lower trunk, is another very effective way of normalizing tone and facilitating normal movement throughout the upper and lower extremities. Patients with hemiplegia often move in a blocklike pattern, with little separation of shoulder girdle and pelvic girdle. To facilitate normal movement, the therapist should set up activities to stimulate or facilitate trunk rotation, which activates trunk musculature and aids in trunk stability. Without stabilization of the trunk, the patient will be unable to use the upper extremities effectively.

When facilitating trunk rotation in sitting or standing, take the opportunity to vary the height of the task. This approach helps to incorporate not only the rotational components of movement, but mobilizes the shoulder girdle and pelvic girdle as well and improves weight shift to the hemiplegic side. Additional benefits from activities facilitating trunk rotation include the following: increased sensory input to the hemiplegic side, improved

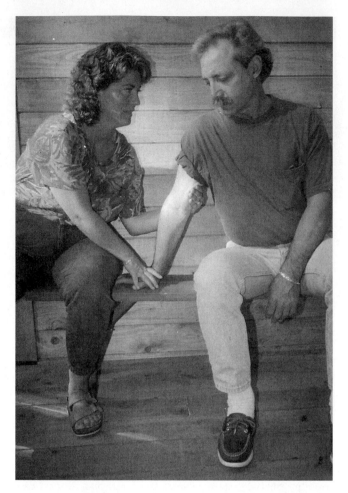

FIG. 24-5   Proper position for weight-bearing over hemiplegic side.

awareness of the hemiplegic side and trained compensation for visual field deficit (Figs. 24-6, 24-7, 24-8). It is easiest and most effective to facilitate trunk rotation during functional daily activities.

Scapular Protraction

Scapular protraction benefits patients displaying a flexion synergy of the upper extremity. High tone involving finger flexion, wrist flexion, and/or elbow flexion with either supination or pronation of the forearm can be difficult to inhibit. It is important for the therapist to remember the basic principle of treatment and work proximal to distal. Before trying to pry open clenched fingers, first bring the scapula into forward protraction. *Do not pull on the arm;* instead, gently cradle the arm while placing the other hand along the medial border of the scapula and bring the scapula forward. Once the scapula is forward, maintain the position for a few seconds before returning the arm to the starting position. Remember never to force the arm into scapular retraction.

Position Pelvis Forward

The neutral position of the pelvis is the preferred sitting position for patients with hemiplegia. The posterior pel-

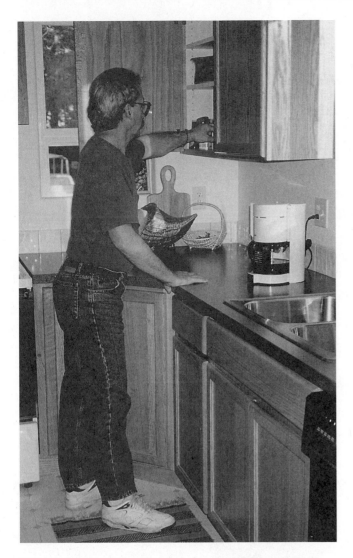

FIG. 24-6 Trunk rotation, side to side, to a high surface.

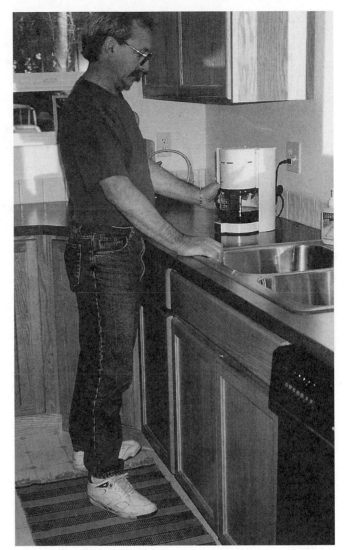

FIG. 24-7 Trunk rotation, side to side, to counter height.

vic tilt is a position in which patients are often seen; they look as though they are sliding out of the wheelchair. Sitting in this position encourages abnormal posture resulting in increased hip extension (often associated with extension synergy of the lower extremity) and rounding of the upper thoracic region (kyphosis) with resultant head and neck extension. This posture has an adverse affect on swallowing (see Chapter 11), impedes normal/proper alignment of the scapula and humerus, and encourages flexion synergy of the upper extremity. Proper alignment of pelvis, shoulder, and head position in sitting can be attained by bringing the pelvis forward into a more neutral position.

In addition to facilitating the pelvis into a more forward position, the therapist can bring the patient forward to help inhibit extensor tone at the hip. The patient should be sitting with both feet flat on the floor. The therapist is on the weak side and helps guide the patient's hands toward the shoes. The benefits are that this position: (1) inhibits extension synergy of the lower extremity, (2) promotes weight-bearing equally through both lower extremities, (3) permits gravity assistance in bringing both scapulae into forward protraction, (4) facilitates thoracic and neck extension for patients who fall forward in a sitting position, (5) helps to decrease the fear factor for patients fearful of coming forward.

Facilitation of Slow, Controlled Movements

Slow, controlled movements benefit patients with high tone. When patients move too quickly, slow them down. Whether they are doing home exercise programs, changing position (e.g., moving from side-lying to sitting or coming from sit to stand), or trying to use the affected upper extremity functionally, quick movements increase tone and tend to set off an associated reaction resulting in a flexion synergy of the UE. To be most effective in tone normalization, the patient must be taught to use slower and more controlled movements. Another basic treatment principle is that the therapist must act as the patient's biofeedback. The therapist must give feedback ap-

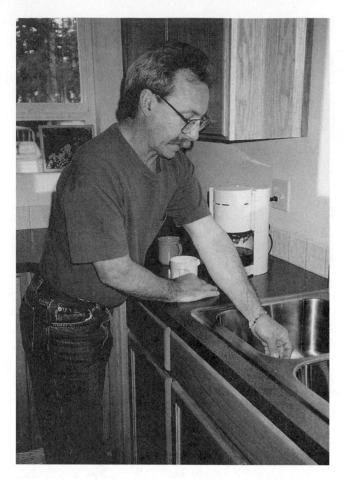

FIG. 24-8 Trunk rotation, side to side, to a lower surface.

propriate to the patient's response. The patient is told that he or she has done something well if it is so; otherwise, the patient will not learn to distinguish proper movements from compensatory movements.

Proper Positioning

Proper position of the patient in side-lying, supine, sitting, or standing facilitates more normal movement throughout the recovery process. Abnormal postures manifested in flexion or extension synergies of the upper or lower extremities promote compensatory movement and should be avoided. Proper positioning in bed is extremely important during the acute stage, but is effective at any stage of recovery. In sitting, avoid excessive posterior pelvic tilt, lower extremity external rotation, asymmetry of the trunk and head, and scapular retraction. The patient should have the feet flat on the floor, hips near 90° of flexion, knees and ankles less than 90° of flexion, and trunk extended (discourage thoracic flexion). The head should be in midline and arm fully supported when working at the table. In standing the head should be in midline, trunk symmetric, and weight equally distributed on both lower extremities.[2]

INCORPORATING THE UPPER EXTREMITY INTO ACTIVITY

There are three ways to incorporate the involved upper extremity into functional activities: (1) weight-bearing through the involved upper extremity (Fig. 24-9), (2) bilateral activities, and (3) guiding. Weight-bearing was discussed previously. Bilateral activities with hands clasped together (Fig. 24-10) are used to increase awareness of the hemiplegic side, increase sensory input to the hemiplegic side, bring the affected arm into the visual field, begin purposeful movement of the hemiplegic arm, discourage flexion synergy by protraction of the scapula and extension of the elbow and wrist, develop abduction of fingers and thumb that discourages spasticity of the hand, and teach the patient reflex inhibiting patterns which can be performed without any help. Guiding of the patient's hand (Fig. 24-11) through normal patterns of movement during functional activities can be done by placing the therapist's hand over the patient's hand with firm but not forceful movements.[6]

Each therapeutic activity can be done sitting or standing, depending on the patient's level of function. At

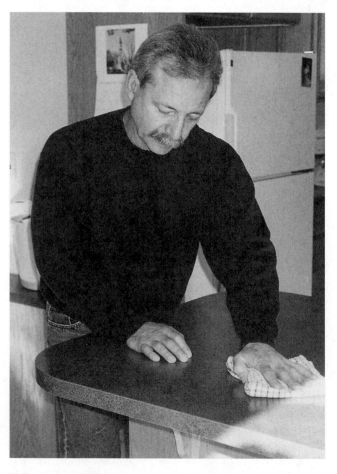

FIG. 24-9 Proper position for weight-bearing over hemiplegic side during functional activity.

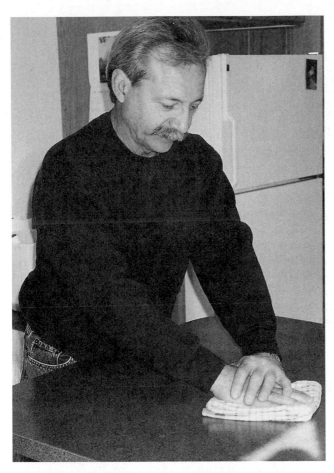

FIG. 24-10   Bilateral use of UE during functional activity.

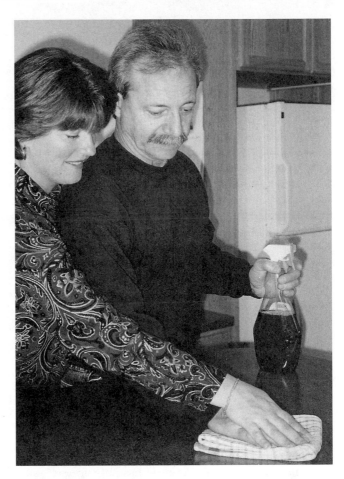

FIG. 24-11   Guiding UE during functional activity.

every possible opportunity the patient should be treated in a straight chair (or standing) rather than the wheelchair to obtain maximal benefit. During NDT the therapist must give specific feedback to the patient whether he or she is moving correctly (normally) or incorrectly (abnormally, with compensatory movements). If the patient is unable to move selectively when the therapist asks, the therapist should take the patient through the normal pattern of movement either during isolated movement or during functional activities/tasks so that the patient can experience the movement.

NDT IN EVERYDAY LIVING

It can be difficult to bridge the gap between facilitation of selective upper extremity control and incorporating these movements and NDT principles into daily living skills. The patient's inability to function independently is extremely complex involving much more than just movement/motor control. Problems of perception, cognition, sensation, motor planning, and language can complicate the rehabilitation process, making it especially difficult for the therapist to treat something as specific and refined as motor control.

SELECTING A THERAPEUTIC ACTIVITY

To incorporate the desired movement into functional activity, think of a functional activity that will require or elicit the same movement. There are a great number of variations on normal movement. If a patient attempts the task with a movement sequence different from your own, your job is to determine if it is abnormal or just a variation on normal. This task sounds very simple, but it is critical to bridging the gap between movement and function.

The best learning experiences come from real-life situations that are practical, functional, and familiar.[1] Contrived (simulated) activities are exercises or tasks that have little or no direct relation to real-life situations; they weaken the carry-over from movement to functional performance. Stacking cones, using parquetry cubes, or tossing beanbags are contrived activities that are often difficult for perceptually disturbed patients to translate to functionally significant tasks. It is much easier for patients to attend to, and be motivated by, activities that are purposeful and relate to real-life situations. When a patient relates to an activity, more normal movement patterns are displayed as well as increased attention and endurance.

A primary goal of therapy is independence. A great deal of treatment is often spent in practicing skills that don't relate to actual daily tasks or routines. Teaching problem solving, however, allows the patient to transfer and adapt those skills to any situation. In rehabilitation programs, therapists must make sure they are teaching problem solving rather than splinter skills with very little, if any, carry-over. Part of problem solving is in anticipating problems before they occur. Therapists are often guilty of planning an activity that is contrived or fixes a problem before the patient has an opportunity to solve it. This approach does not encourage learning and does not promote carry-over into functional daily life tasks.

When selecting a functional activity, ask the following questions:

- Is the activity meaningful to the patient?
- Does the patient see the purpose of the activity?
- Does the activity require problem solving?

The answer is "yes" to all questions for the most effective activities.

INITIATING TREATMENT

Introduce the patient to the activity. If possible have the patient take part in the preparation (for example, help get the supplies from the cupboard) because additional cues from the environment often help the patient understand what is expected (especially for patients with aphasia). Get the patient in a good starting position. Be exact: feet flat on the floor, good base of support, good pelvic alignment with trunk, shoulder, neck, and head position. As the patient moves through the functional activity, facilitate/inhibit/guide as needed to elicit normal movement patterns. Don't just modify the patient's movements; modify the activity to elicit better movements, or modify the position of the patient to elicit more appropriate movements. Monitor the speed of movement; a good pace is usually slightly slower than normal. Patients need time to process incoming information as well as motor responses. Increase the difficulty of the activities as the patient improves to stimulate both problem solving and motor skills.

A number of factors influence the patient's quality of movement within a functional context:

1. how the patient is positioned, and on what surface(s)
2. the patient's base of support
3. the patient's response when the base of support changes, check for any associated reactions
4. where the activity is set up in relation to the patient (to facilitate the desired movement and weight shift)
5. where weight shifts are initiated
6. physical properties of the objects to be manipulated

As the patient moves within the context of function, the therapist gains additional information and insight into the patient's problem areas. Observe where the difficulties are, and be specific.

During each treatment, the therapist should constantly be asking the following questions:

1. Was the patient able to do the task?
2. How did the patient do the task?
3. Which components appeared to be normal?
4. Which components were in abnormal movement patterns?

Break down the activity. What is lacking? Movement? Stability? Weight Shift? Sensation? Motor Planning? Redefine priorities in treatment as new problem areas are identified.

NDT IN ACUTE CARE, REHABILITATION, OR LONG-TERM CARE

NDT is more than muscle reeducation for a specific limb; it is a 24-hour management of the patient with hemiplegia. NDT principles should be incorporated into the daily management of the patient, whether in the hospital, in long-term care (skilled nursing facility), or at home. The following tips help the patient to (1) become more aware of the hemiplegic side, (2) better integrate both sides of the body, and (3) increase sensory stimulation to the hemiplegic side. By following these tips, family members as well as all members of the health care team can help to prevent or minimize some problems that are characteristic of hemiplegia.

Room arrangement. The hemiplegic side of the patient should face the source of stimulation. The patient's hemiplegic side should face the door and be positioned so that the telephone, the nightstand, and the television encourage the patient to turn toward that side, thus increasing integration of both sides of the body (Fig. 24-12). The one exception is the call light for the nurse.[4,6]

Approach. Always approach the patient from the hemiplegic side to encourage eye contact. Sometimes the patient has difficulty turning the head and may need assistance. The therapist should simply assist the patient by

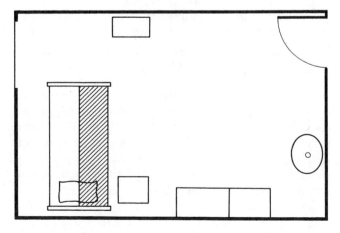

FIG. 24-12 Room arranged so that patient must turn to affected side. Shaded area represents affected side of body.

gently but firmly turning the head until he or she is able to establish eye contact. Family members can be encouraged to give tactile input to the patient by holding his or her hand or stroking his or her arm.

Naming. During nursing tasks such as washing, name each body part to increase awareness of it.

Encouraging independence. The patient should begin to assist in simple ADL. If the patient is unable to complete a task independently, the therapist or caregiver can guide the patient's hands to feel movement pattern necessary to complete an activity. This approach encourages the patient to learn to carry out the task sooner.[1]

In each medical setting the roles of occupational therapy and physical therapy may differ slightly. Yet the methods described are imperative for proper patient treatment, and all persons in professional services should be aware of them and be able to apply them appropriately. The Bobaths strongly emphasized that this approach is not a series of exercises and the upper and lower extremities must not be treated independently.[2] The occupational therapist must be constantly aware of the tonus, motor patterns, positions, and reflex mechanisms of both the upper and lower extremities.

BED POSITIONING

The patient should be properly positioned (Figs. 24-13, 24-14, 24-15). The benefits from patients being positioned in this manner are as follows: (1) weight-bearing normalizes tone and inhibits spasticity; (2) weight-bearing increases awareness of the hemiplegic side, increasing sensory input; (3) weight-bearing on the weak side helps the patient to be less fearful; and (4) lengthening of the hemiplegic side inhibits spasticity.

The three basic positions are listed in order of their therapeutic value: lying on the hemiplegic side, lying on the nonhemiplegic side, and lying supine. Patients should be repositioned as often as nursing procedures require (usually every 2 hours) for the prevention of decubiti.

Lying on the hemiplegic side. This position is preferred for the hemiplegic patient.[2,7] (Fig. 24-13). The patient's back should be parallel with the edge of the bed. The head is placed on the pillow symmetrically but not in extreme flexion. The shoulder is fully protracted with at least 90° of shoulder flexion (less than 90° encourages a flexion synergy). The forearm is supinated and the elbow is flexed. The hand is placed under the pillow. An alternative position is with the elbow extended and the wrist either supported on the bed or slightly off the bed, which

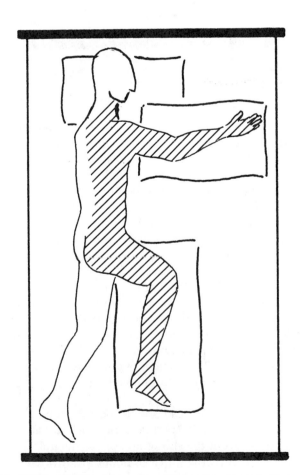

FIG. 24-13   Bed position when lying on affected side.   **FIG. 24-14**   Bed position when lying on unaffected side.

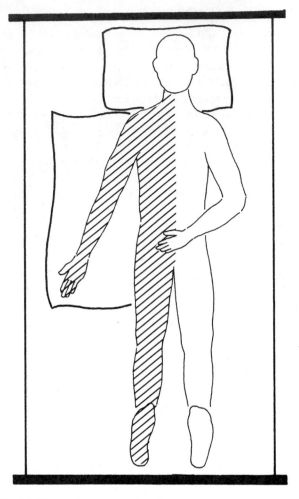

FIG. 24-15 Bed position when lying supine.

encourages wrist extension. These positions are familiar to most patients and encourage external rotation at the shoulder. The nonaffected leg is placed on a pillow. The affected leg is slightly flexed at the knee with hip extension. A pillow can be placed behind the patient to prevent rolling onto the back.

Lying on the nonhemiplegic side. In this position (Fig. 24-14), the back should be parallel with the edge of the bed.[2,5] The head is placed symmetrically on the pillow. The shoulder is in full protraction with the shoulder in at least 90° of flexion. The arm and hand are fully supported on a pillow. The wrist should not be allowed to drop off the pillow into flexion. The affected lower extremity is in hip flexion and knee flexion and fully supported on a pillow. The foot and ankle must be supported to keep the foot from inverting.

Lying supine. The head should be symmetric on the pillow (Fig. 24-15).[2,5] The body and trunk are also symmetric to prevent the shortening of the hemiplegic side of the trunk. A pillow is placed under the affected shoulder, supporting the shoulder so it is no more than level

with the nonhemiplegic shoulder. If higher, an anterior subluxation may occur at the glenohumeral joint. The affected arm is fully supported, with the elbow extended and forearm in supination and entirely supported on a pillow in elevation. A small pillow can be placed under the hip to reduce retraction of the pelvis. *Do not place a pillow under the knees or a footboard at the end of the bed,* because the former encourages knee flexion contractures and the latter encourages an extension synergy of the lower extremity.

DRESSING ACTIVITIES

Dressing and grooming activities are a part of every occupational therapy program. It is purposeful, functional, familiar to the patient, and necessary to improve the patient's level of independence. Relearning how to dress oneself can be one of the most frustrating activities requested of the patient. Dressing requires not only trunk stability in sitting, it also requires the ability to do motor planning, sequencing, and problem solving. It is one of the most difficult tasks required by the occupational therapist, yet it is nearly always the first one introduced.[1] With that in mind, while working on dressing training, the therapist should grade the activity to sitting balance, endurance, frustration level, and cognitive-perceptual status. The following method is an example of how the principles of NDT can be used in ADL training. The facilitation of each task should be modified to fit each patient's abilities and problem areas.

As the patient learns to bear weight over both hips in sitting and to shift weight to either side (or forward), as necessary, he or she moves more normally and with less compensation. The patient learns to inhibit his or her own spasticity. The procedure breaks up typical hemiplegic patterns of lower extremity extension synergy and upper extremity flexion synergy. Using the NDT approach, dressing is learned faster than by traditional, one-handed methods, especially for patients with perceptual problems. The patient learns to carry over techniques of inhibition into daily living skills.

Tips. The patient should not attempt to get dressed in bed. Instead the patient should be seated on a chair, preferably a straight chair next to the bed. The therapist should *always* assist from the affected side. Always begin dressing with the hemiplegic side. The same sequence in dressing is maintained to increase learning.

PROCEDURES

Donning Shirt (Figs 24-16, 24-17)
1. Position shirt across patient's knees with armhole visible and sleeve between knees (Fig. 24-16).
2. Bend forward at hips (inhibiting extension synergy of the lower extremity), placing affected hand in sleeve (Fig. 24-17).
3. Arm drops into sleeve; shoulder protraction and gravity inhibit upper extremity flexion synergy.

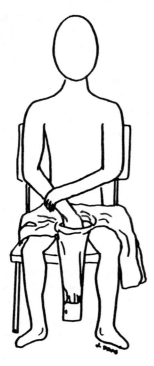

FIG. 24-16   Dressing training. Shirt positioned across patient's knees, armhole visible, and sleeve dropped between knees.

4. Bring collar to neck.
5. Sit upright, dress nonhemiplegic side.
6. Button shirt from bottom to top.

Donning Underclothes and Pants (Fig. 24-18)

1. Clasp hands and cross affected leg over nonhemiplegic leg. (Therapist helps when needed.)
2. Release hands. Hemiplegic arm can dangle and should not be trapped in lap. When able, the patient can use the affected hand as needed.
3. Pull pant leg over hemiplegic foot.

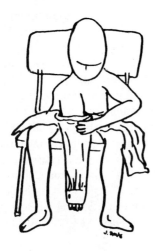

FIG. 24-17   Patient bends forward at hips (inhibiting extension synergy of lower extremity) and places affected hand into sleeve.

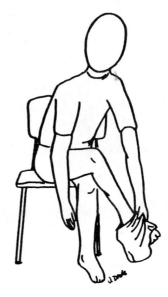

FIG. 24-18   Proper position while putting on pants and underclothes.

4. Clasp hands to uncross leg.
5. Place nonhemiplegic foot in pant leg (no need to cross legs). This step is difficult, because the patient must bear weight on hemiplegic side.
6. Pull pants to knees.
7. While holding onto waistband, patient stands with therapist's help.
8. Zip and snap pants.
9. Therapist helps patient return to sitting position.

Donning Shoes and Socks (Fig. 24-19)

1. Clasp hands and cross legs (as before).
2. Put sock and shoe on hemiplegic foot.
3. Cross nonhemiplegic leg, put on sock and shoe.

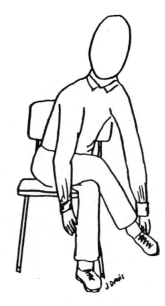

FIG. 24-19   Proper position while putting on shoes and socks.

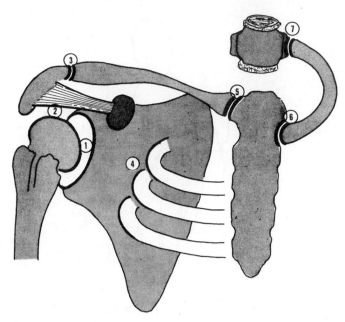

FIG. 24-20 Composite drawing of shoulder girdle. (From Cailliet R: *The shoulder in hemiplegia,* Philadelphia, 1980. FA Davis.

THE SHOULDER IN HEMIPLEGIA

Problems of the hemiplegic shoulder are often frustrating and confusing to the occupational therapist. Pain can hinder the entire rehabilitation program. The responsibility of the therapist is to learn how to evaluate these problems and prepare a treatment program that is effective in dealing with them. It is important to understand the basic anatomy and functional mechanism of the shoulder girdle. Those interested in expanding their knowledge in this area are directed to readings from the references, particularly *The Shoulder in Hemiplegia,* by Rene Cailliet.[3] The shoulder girdle is made up of seven joints (Fig. 24-20): (1) glenohumeral, (2) suprahumeral, (3) acromioclavicular, (4) scapulocostal, (5) sternoclavicular, (6) costosternal, and (7) costovertebral.

To have full pain-free range of motion (ROM), all seven joints need to work synchronously. The glenohumeral joint allows for considerable mobility but lacks stability. It is dependent on the proper alignment of the scapula and humerus for mechanical support, as well as muscular support from the supraspinatus.

It is important to understand the relationship of the scapula to the humerus and its significance in pain-free shoulder flexion and abduction. When the arm is raised in forward flexion or abduction, the scapula must glide and rotate upward. The humerus and the scapula work in unison; more specifically, they work in a 2:1 ratio pattern. In other words, if the shoulder moves 90° of abduction, the humerus moves 60° and the scapula moves 30°. Another possibility is 180° of shoulder flexion in which the humerus moves 120° and the scapula moves 60° (again, a 2:1 ratio).[3]

If for any reason the arm is raised in shoulder flexion or abduction without the scapula gliding along, joint trauma and pain can occur. The therapist must be aware of this effect and take it into consideration during ROM, ADL, transfers, and all other activities.

In the hemiplegic shoulder, the scapula can fall into downward rotation because of a heavy, flaccid upper extremity or because the muscles that move the scapula in downward rotation (rhomboids, latissimus dorsi, and levator scapulae) are spastic. This condition makes it difficult for the scapula to glide upward, which is necessary for pain-free movement. The scapula must first be mobilized and the spasticity reduced to regain the ROM and allow for selective movement. The arm must never be raised over 90° before the scapula has been mobilized and the therapist can feel its gliding movements. Even in a seemingly flaccid arm, the scapula can be influenced by spasticity of the rhomboids, trapezius, and latissimus dorsi. The techniques previously described assist the therapist.

Because the hemiplegic shoulder can often be pulled back into retraction, the emphasis of treatment is placed on forward gliding of the scapula. By protracting the scapula, the patient is able to reduce the hypertonicity of the upper extremity, allowing for more isolated movement and selective control. When the spasticity is too strong for the patient to obtain protraction of the shoulder, the therapist must assist. The therapist should use reflex inhibiting patterns to control and reduce spasticity. As Bobath stated, "The main reflex inhibiting pattern counteracting spasticity in the trunk and arm is the extension of neck and spine and external rotation of the arm at the shoulder with elbow extended. Further reduction of flexor spasticity can be obtained by adding extension of the wrist with supination and abduction of the thumb."[2]

SUBLUXATION

Many professionals are particularly concerned about the subluxed shoulder. Numerous efforts are made to protect the shoulder and prevent subluxation, but subluxation cannot be prevented. If the muscles around the shoulder girdle (which are attached to the humerus and scapula) are weak enough, the shoulder will be subluxed. Slings do not help subluxation. They keep the arm in a poor position and may contribute to pain and swelling. Subluxation itself does not cause pain. The pain is caused by improper handling of a subluxed arm. Forcing the head of the humerus back into place can cause trauma and pain. Doing standard ROM procedures on an arm without a gliding scapula can also cause pain. Treatment of the subluxed arm should include proper sitting, weight-bearing, mobilization of the scapula, and proper positioning in bed (Figs. 24-13, 24-14, 24-15).

SLINGS

The application of a sling to the hemiplegic arm is a source of considerable controversy. It has been demonstrated over the past several years that "the commonly used hemiplegic sling has no appreciable effect on ultimate ROM, subluxation, pain, or peripheral nerve traction injury."[9] It has also been stated that "there is no need to support a pain free shoulder in order to prevent or correct subluxation since the sling does not prevent, improve, cure or reduce such a deformity."[8] The use of a sling on the hemiplegic arm can actually contribute to subluxation and lead to a painful, disabling condition called shoulder-hand syndrome. It is important to realize that when a patient wears a sling, the arm is supported in a position that is compatible with the typical hemiplegic posture and discourages the patient from using the arm either bilaterally or unilaterally. Even the sling previously described by the Bobaths is no longer being used.[2] This sling was found to hinder the circulation of the arm and push the head of the humerus into lateral subluxation as well.

If the patient has a painful shoulder or swollen hand, a thorough evaluation should be done to determine the cause. Then appropriate treatment can be started.

PREPARING THE PATIENT FOR HOME

The benefits of the treatment program are lost if the patient is not adequately prepared for returning home. This preparation should include (1) prescribing a home exercise program, (2) family education, and (3) communication with the follow-up therapist when applicable. The hospital or clinic is a very secure setting, and it is very important that both the patient and family feel comfortable and confident on the return home. The home exercise program is important to maintain mobility and movement. The therapist should select exercises that can be done easily and correctly without assistance. If stress or excessive effort is used to complete the exercises, the patient is likely to form bad habits, and spasticity will increase.

After the selection of exercises the therapist must train the patient in each of them. To encourage consistency, the patient should follow the same sequence of exercises each day. This program should begin long before discharge from occupational therapy so that it is a well-established part of the daily routine.

Each exercise should be written down in the proper sequence, including how often the exercises should be done (for example, twice a day), the number of repetitions (for example, 10 times each), with diagrams if necessary. Some family members have found videotape to be especially helpful in following through with a home program. During a treatment session the therapist can videotape the home program (exercises, bed positioning, or other tasks important to continue at home); the family then has a copy to use at home.

Next, the family should be trained so that they are also well acquainted with each exercise. Thus they can guide the home program properly. For best results in family teaching, the occupational therapist should (1) demonstrate and explain the importance of tasks; (2) emphasize each major point (for example, position of arm and placement of hands); (3) have the family work with the patient under the therapist's guidance; and (4) repeat instructions as often as needed until the family and patient are confident enough to do the exercises at home alone.

Family education should include a home exercise program and ADL training in areas of dressing, eating, grooming, hygiene, bathing, transfers, and cooking. This program should also include instruction in proper position (lying, sitting, and standing) and proper use of equipment. Before discharge from the treatment center the therapist should give the family his or her name and telephone number at work, set up a date for a reevaluation if necessary, and contact the therapist treating the patient following discharge from the treatment facility to ensure proper carry-over.

SUMMARY

Neurodevelopmental treatment, developed by Karel and Berta Bobath, is used successfully in the treatment of adult hemiplegia. Treatment emphasis is on relearning normal movement while avoiding abnormal movement patterns. Quality of movement, control, and coordination are emphasized by using treatment methods to normalize abnormal muscle tone and to avoid abnormal patterns of movement.

REVIEW QUESTIONS

1. What is the primary goal of the NDT approach?
2. List three advantages of the NDT approach stated in the text.
3. Describe and assume the typical posture of the adult patient with hemiplegia.
4. What is the key element of an NDT evaluation?
5. List four factors that can cause or increase spasticity.
6. Describe the observation process using the NDT approach in evaluating a patient.
7. Why is skilled observation critical to treatment effectiveness?
8. Describe the elements of the vicious cycle that may contribute to the maintenance of spasticity.
9. What are some of the possible causes of asymmetrical shoulder height observed in the patient with hemiplegia?
10. List and describe at least three treatment methods designed to normalize tone and promote normal movement.
11. What are the purposes of trunk rotation? Bilateral activities?

12. Describe recommended positioning and mobilization procedures to prevent shoulder pain and severe spasticity around the shoulder and shoulder girdle.
13. How can the affected upper extremity be incorporated into activity? What effects will this approach have?
14. Why is it important to use functional activities from real life in the treatment program?
15. List at least four factors that will influence the quality of the patient's movement when performing functional activities.
16. How should the therapist evaluate the effectiveness of the treatment session?
17. Describe and assume the recommended positions for the patient with hemiplegia in supine, prone, and side-lying on the affected and unaffected sides. What is the rationale for these postures?
18. When using the NDT approach, what is the recommended method for donning a shirt? Try this method for putting on your own shirt, then teach it to another person.
19. Why is scapula protraction stressed in positioning and movement of the hemiplegic arm?
20. What are some possible causes of shoulder subluxation in hemiplegia?
21. What is the recommended treatment for should subluxation in the NDT approach?
22. Why is the common hemiplegic sling contraindicated?
23. What is the role of the occupational therapist in preparing the patient to go home?

REFERENCES

1. Affolter F: *Perceptual processes as requisites for complex human behavior,* Bern, Switzerland, 1980, Hans Huber.
2. Bobath B: *Adult hemiplegia: evaluation and treatment,* London, 1978, William Heinemann Medical Books.
3. Cailliet R: *The shoulder in hemiplegia,* Philadelphia, 1980, FA Davis.
4. Cash J: *Neurology for physiotherapists,* London, 1977, Faber & Faber.
5. Davies P: *Treatment techniques for adult hemiplegia: study course,* Valens Switzerland, 1979, Klinik Valens.
6. Davies P: *Steps to follow,* Berlin, 1985, Springer-Verlag.
7. Eggers O: *Occupational therapy in the treatment of adult hemiplegia,* Rockville, Md, 1984, Aspen Systems.
8. Friedland F: Physical therapy. In Licht & S, editor: *Stroke and its rehabilitation,* Baltimore, 1975, Williams & Williams.
9. Hurd MM, Farrell KH, Waylonis FW: Shoulder sling for hemiplegia: friend or foe? *Arch Phys Med Rehab* 55:519, 1974.

The Affolter Approach to Treatment: A Perceptual-Cognitive Perspective of Function

Karin Berglund Bonfils

This chapter introduces an innovative perceptual-cognitive approach developed in Switzerland by Felicie Affolter. Affolter holds degrees in child psychology; education of normal, deaf, and language-disordered children; audiology; and language pathology and speech sciences. She studied with Jean Piaget and uses his interaction model of development as a foundation for her theory. Affolter is the founder of the Center for Perceptually Disturbed Children and Adults in St. Gallen, Switzerland. During the last 28 years, she and Walter Bischofberger have conducted research specifically involving development based on tactile-kinesthetic interaction.

This introduction to the Affolter theory and treatment approach is designed to give the student food for thought about the process of cognitive-perceptual development and the relationship that exists between tactile-kinesthetic (T-K) input and problem-solving skills in daily life. This practical technique emphasizes evaluation and treatment in realistic situations using functional and age-appropriate activities. It has been successfully used in the treatment of coma recovery, cerebral vascular accident (CVA), traumatic brain injury, and other neurological deficits including Alzheimer's disease and aging issues, pervasive developmental disorder and autism, and learning disabilities. The Affolter concept challenges the clinician to take a hands-on functional approach in the treatment of tactile-kinesthetic perceptual deficits in addition to using the standard evaluations and assessments for visual and auditory perceptual processing.

Affolter has developed the treatment technique of nonverbal guiding to facilitate perceptual-cognitive interaction. Therapy is geared toward emphasizing appropriate input through a problem-solving process rather than focusing on output and successful completion of a product. In using this treatment technique, specific guidelines should be carefully followed and continually practiced. This chapter should form the basis for further reading and training under the direct supervision of an experienced therapist who has been trained in the Affolter approach. It is beneficial for the student to refer to Piaget's developmental framework, to continue investigation and research of the tactile-kinesthetic sense, and begin to develop a critical analytical eye in the observation of both normal and deviant behaviors.

UNDERSTANDING PERCEPTION AND COGNITION IN FUNCTIONAL TERMS

It is very important to explore and understand the definition and clinical interpretation of the term *perception* and its relationship with *cognition*. Webster's defines perception as "a mental image; awareness of the elements of the environment through physical sensation; an impression of an object obtained by the use of senses; physical sensation interpreted in the light of experience."[10] According to Affolter, "Whenever we speak about perception, in its broadest sense, we refer to the input of stimuli over the different sensory modalities which allows us to relate to the exterior world or our surroundings."[2] We use our sense of touch, vision, hearing, taste and smell to learn about our environment and ourselves. A person needs to interact with the environment to know where he or she is in relation to the world, situation, or activity.

Interaction requires adequate exploration of the situa-

Dr. Felicie Affolter is gratefully acknowledged for reviewing this chapter.

tion. Through research, Affolter has concluded that "the tactile-kinesthetic sensory system provides the information which is essential for interaction and through the process of interaction the development of more complex performances. Visual and auditory information are secondary for interaction. Research has shown that patients who fail in complex human behavior also fail in processing tactile-kinesthetic information from their environment."[3] Webster's defines *cognition* as "knowledge; the process of knowing in the broadest sense, including perception, memory and judgment; the result of such a process; perception."[10] Cognitive specialists have broken down the concept of cognition to include arousal, attention, orientation, initiation, sequencing, problem solving, memory, distractibility, impulsivity, and inhibition. Components of safety judgment, reasoning, organization, planning, and processing time are carefully assessed. A person must be able to perceive the self in relation to the world, however, if there is to be progress in these components.

Very little is known about T-K information processing. Historically, most perception research has centered on visual processing; therefore many people assume that perception is mainly influenced by vision. Research in tactile-kinesthetic information has been minimal; until recently, the significance of changes in resistance (contrast) through the use of touch has been greatly underestimated. "The tactile-kinesthetic system appears to offer unique information about environmental qualities that is missing in the information provided by the other sensory systems."[3] It receives information through perceived amounts of changes in resistance during activities involving interaction, which leads to cause-and-effect relationships. "The T-K system is unique among the sensory systems in the sense of being the only one that relates directly to reality. One's looking at the world does not alter it. Listening does not change the world either. However one can scarcely touch the world without changing it."[3] The tactile system provides feedback to the patient. Cause and effect between actions and objects within the environment leads to perceptual inferences. "Perceptual inferences are the ability to predict or anticipate changes before an action occurs. . . . Individuals are continually using their storage of experiences to compare and contrast gathered sensory data from actual situations. In other words, people cannot perceive or have a perception of something without having some experience upon which to base it."[7] Affolter and Stricker[3] maintain that "interaction between the environment and the individual requires contact. Contact means to be 'in touch with.' To be in touch or in contact with can be realized only through the tactile-kinesthetic sensory system."

CURRENT RESEARCH IN CHILD DEVELOPMENT

Affolter and Bischofberger have conducted research on normal infants and children, profoundly deaf children, blind children, and those who are both deaf and blind (both longitudinal and cross-sectional studies). Affolter concluded that normal and profoundly deaf children progress along the same developmental hierarchy at a similar rate.[1] Blind and deaf and blind children also follow the same pattern, except at a slower rate. All children who deviated from the normal developmental pattern had in common a lack of adequate tactile-kinesthetic input (information based on touch and movement).[1] Children with severe hearing impairment develop as normal children do, and performances that do not require auditory information processing show the same sequence of stages.[1] Investigations suggested that children with language disabilities, and learning-disturbed children with or without hearing loss, exhibit perceptual disturbances that are tactile-kinesthetic or intermodal rather than visual.[1,3] Research findings support the hypothesis that neither hearing nor vision is necessary for adequate interaction with the environment, but tactile-kinesthetic information is absolutely essential.

Until 3 months of age, an infant's behavior is mostly sensory-specific, meaning he or she uses one sense at a time to process information. The child usually either sees, hears, smells, or touches. It isn't until approximately 3 months of age that a baby shows integration of the senses occuring frequently. This integration is referred to as intermodal organization. The infant can then look and touch, or touch and look, hear and look, smell and look, etc. Integrating the senses allows the child to explore cause-and-effect relationships and interact in problem-solving situations. Babies learn about themselves in relation to their world by searching, moving, and exploring in the environment. What happens to the babies who are somewhat or totally unable to search, move, or explore with their bodies in the environment? These are some of the questions Affolter set out to answer in her research.

Affolter noticed a distinct similarity in behavior of children lacking adequate tactile-kinesthetic information and children and adults who suffered from traumatic brain injury, stroke, learning disability, and other neurological anomalies including aging. Many of these individuals have difficulty with movement and adaptation of muscle tone because of paralysis, spasticity, decreased balance, and incoordination; they are often unable to explore their environment effectively or efficiently. Their inability to explore is often coupled with peculiar hand usage or abnormal body movement. Furthermore, patients who have these types of diagnoses often resort to sensory-specific behavior similar to the 3-month-old infant. A person who has had a stroke and frequently closes the eyes during functional activities may be misinterpreted as being tired, depressed, or unmotivated when he or she is actually blocking out at least one of the senses (vision) to enhance the most primitive sense, the tactile-kinesthetic sense. It is often necessary to block out one stimulus to attend to the other. "If perception is disturbed, information is not processed properly and learning, if it takes place at all, is slow, unreliable, deviant and mainly frustrating. Analysis of activities with brain damaged adults and children show strong evidence that they often fail in searching for tactile kinesthetic information in goal oriented tasks, leading to frustration with consequent behavioral as well as safety issues."[6]

THE IMPORTANCE OF PROBLEM SOLVING IN PERCEPTUAL PROCESSING

One cannot solve problems of daily living without the ability to perceive. Problem solving always deals with a goal. In solving a problem an individual must be able to do the following:

1. evaluate (based on the information present)
2. build a hypothesis
3. act
4. use feedback[6]

Problem solving includes several levels of planning, from simple to complex. The first level is that of planning step-by-step. To solve a problem, a person must recognize that a problem or situation exists. It is important to determine if the patient is working on a step-by-step level, because many are not. A patient must be able to plan step-by-step or carry out an activity in an actual situation with all necessary information and/or objects within the perceptual field.[7] The most important detail to remember in assisting the patient to solve problems is that the therapist or person guiding needs to offer the patient possibilities, not solutions.

It is the therapist's role to facilitate exploration of a situation. In coma stimulation, assessment of a patient's ability to perceive or recognize has always been somewhat difficult and often frustrating to assess or facilitate. In traditional sensory stimulation, how do we know that a patient recognizes a specific smell, a visual stimulus, or the ringing of a bell? Health professionals have relied on facial grimace in response to a noxious stimulus, turning of the head, or visual tracking, which is often inconsistent or unreliable. When a patient is guided nonverbally through a familar task (hair brushing, for example), many signs of recognition may be observed. The patient may react initially with an increase in tone in response to unexpected input or an unfamiliar situation (Fig. 25-1, *A*). As the infomation is processed and assimilated, often the patient's muscle tone becomes more normal, and frequently the patient begins to take over purposeful move-

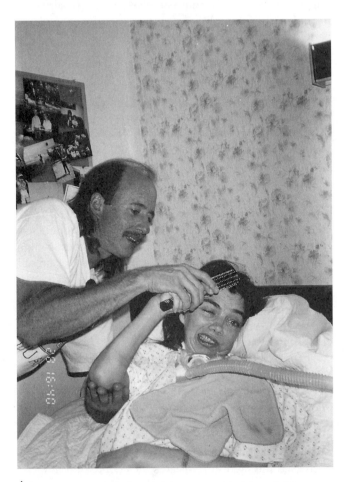

A

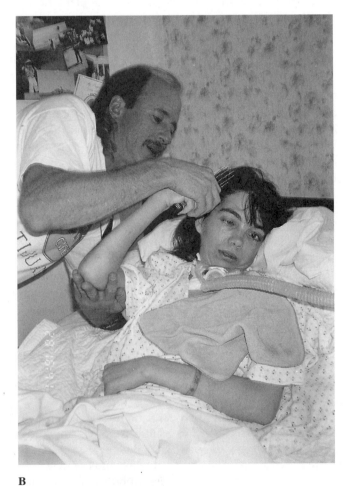

B

FIG. 25-1   A, Patient in coma is guided through task of hairbrushing. Patient may initially exhibit increase in tone (observed in facial musculature) in response to unfamiliar or unexpected input. **B,** As information is processed and assimilated, patient's tone normalizes and she begins taking over purposeful movement.

ment as a sign of recognition (Fig. 25-1, *B*). The goal is not for the patient to brush hair independently, but to provide information about the situation.

An additional example of a patient working on or near a recognition level is that of an adult male patient who has aphasia and is set up for a grooming and hygiene activity in the bathroom. The instruction to the patient is that he is to begin brushing his teeth. All of the objects are within his visual field. The patient acknowledges the request, but never initiates the task. Perhaps he has a questionable look on his face, or he may even refuse to do the task. The therapist begins to guide him through the appropriate steps nonverbally, and as the patient picks up the toothbrush and toothpaste, he exclaims, "oh," as if to express that now he recognizes what to do. He begins to take over the movement the therapist has initiated. Every time the therapist observes a breakdown in motor movement or hesitation in the appropriate sequence for the task, he or she immediately assists him by guiding as needed. Perhaps he is ready to bring the toothbrush to his mouth, but brings it toward his hair as if it were a comb. In this situation, it is possible he has not recognized the tool (apraxia). The therapist can intervene without words by redirecting his hand to his mouth. She doesn't have to bring the mistake to his attention verbally, which is often humiliating. The task is completed and the problem solved together. The patient's brain received the correct information, interrupting the old engram and replacing it with a new one. Talking may be initiated after the task, and the tools, objects, and sequence of the steps used in the activity should be integrated into conversation. This approach is an excellent way to check recognition, to assess memory, and also to incorporate the speech therapist as part of an interdisciplinary team.

A higher level of planning means that patients can plan for an event without visual, verbal, or other cues. Most therapists operate on such a production level when they are familiar with the situation or activity and can organize, plan, prepare, and follow the appropriate sequences using normal movement patterns to meet the goal. If there is a breakdown in any of these processes, therapists too move back to a step-by-step level and must seek assistance to reach the goal. Perhaps the therapist looks up the instructions and reverts back to the step-by-step procedures. Working on a high production level requires the ability to evaluate, hypothesize, act, and respond accordingly. It is consequently a very demanding level of performance.

Therapists frequently expect patients to work on such a high production level when they are often not ready. For example, it is common to ask a patient to plan a meal, write down all the steps in the activity, and compile a list of utensils needed. If a patient is exhibiting any difficulty in recognition of familiar activities, including anticipating and sequencing steps, he or she is still working at a step-by-step level. Perhaps instead this patient should prepare the food item first with guided assistance as appropriate, and then compile a list of utensils used and a list of steps taken. For those patients who appear to be operating on a high level in familiar situations, it is important to assess their function in unfamiliar situations, because this is where breakdown often occurs. The ultimate goal in therapy is for the patient to reach the high planning level of complex production. "Planning is based on past experience situations and sequences of action which are internalized, stored and retrieved. For the therapist, this means that the patient must get essential experiences along the way in order to build up production level experiences."[7]

SIGNS AND SYMPTOMS OF DIFFICULTY WITH PERCEPTUAL-COGNITIVE PROCESSING

One of the problems facing psychologists attempting to understand perception is that the process of perception cannot be witnessed. Only the behavior is observed.[6] In a hospital or home setting it is devastating to observe the breakdown of perceptual-cognitive processes during a patient's activities of daily living. An obvious example is the patient who wishes to get up out of bed, but stares at the therapist for a clue on how to begin, or the patient who turns on the electric razor and puts it in his mouth, takes a comb and attempts to brush his teeth, or puts his arm through the leg of his trousers. These behaviors are classified as types of apraxia and are described in Chapter 14. A patient exhibiting any kind of apraxia is struggling with a perceptual deficit, which must be addressed with a functional approach. Many times patients exhibit other behaviors that may not be so obvious to the untrained eye and are often misinterpreted. A patient may refuse to participate, confabulate, become easily frustrated and even agitated, shut the eyes, or look away. These behaviors are often interpreted as lack of motivation, unwillingness to participate, aggressiveness and agitation, sometimes the patient is thought to be asleep, depressed, or over medicated.

The ability to perceive is based on interaction with the environment and the ability to integrate information received by the senses.[2] It is important to determine which senses a patient uses in searching for information about the environment or situation. Often a patient doesn't search for information, for example, in the presence of paralysis, spasticity, or incoordination. A patient with hemiplegia may experience a significant change in the way he or she moves and explores the environment. The decreased interaction translates into decreased information sent to and processed by the brain. A deviance in searching for information may also be observed in the quality of touch. A patient with perceptual deficits develops a unique way of touching and searching, which may result in asymmetrical body movements, peculiar hand and finger movements, or lower extremity gait deviances.

There are two typical personality behaviors displayed by individuals with perceptual processing problems. They can be described as hectic and quiet patterns. A person with perceptual processing problems will exhibit many of the following behavior characteristics.

THE HECTIC INDIVIDUAL

The hectic individual often searches for maximum amounts of resistance in the shortest time possible.[2] The searching is frequently exhibited in the fingertips where touching is quick and hard. The following behaviors may be observed:

- quick, brief actions often combined with constant movement
- evokes labels such as aggressive, hyperactive, and tactile defensive by therapists and care givers
- difficulties attending to tasks
- release by throwing instead of putting or placing an object down
- unintentional breakage of objects, frequent hurting of others
- movement through free space without use of support as a reference
- use of one hand instead of two in bimanual activities, two fingers instead of five in gross manipulative skills[2]
- incessant talking, often with poor pragmatic speech (impractical, out of context)
- difficulty licking and sipping, preference for biting and sucking instead

THE QUIET INDIVIDUAL

The quiet individual often does not initiate or search in exploration of the environment. The quality of touch is less than adequate and ineffective. Behaviors that may be observed include the following:

- poor initiation
- limited participation, preference for observing
- compensation, takes more time than usual
- self-limitations that protect him or her from sensory overload
- frequent frustration, which leads to lack of self-confidence
- preference for minimal changes occurring in the environment; prefers what is familiar[2]
- whines and complains

The following behaviors may be observed both in hectic and quiet individuals:

- poor orientation to time and space
- difficulty assessing and detecting danger
- causative actions not correspondent to situations[2]

THE EVALUATION PROCESS

Currently, the evaluation of patient behavior is based on observation and interpretation. Good observation skills are critical in evaluating patient behavior. Health care professionals are quick to interpret behavior, but it is important to remember that every person observing certain behavior in a certain situation may have a different interpretation of the behavior itself, and each interpretation may be valid. A simple way to keep observations separate from interpretations is to document them separately. Always attach a situation to the observed behavior. In treatment often it is the environment or situation (input) that can be adapted to minimize or change the behavior.

In evaluating an individual's perceptual processing skills, the most important component is that the patient needs to be participating in a functional problem-solving activity. Self-feeding is one of the first functional activities necessary to evaluate. Is the patient able to eat independently? The process involves attending to the activity (the plate) within the environment (the table and room), as well as shifting attention between the plate, the utensil, and the different foods on the plate. It involves (1) the sequence of deciding what to pick up with the utensil and when the movement will be initiated, (2) the process of holding the utensil and using it to transport the food to the mouth, (3) the process of anticipating when the food will meet the mouth and coordinating the sequence of movements necessary in managing the food in the mouth, and (4) the process of swallowing. There is variation each time in the choice of movement, deciding to switch the fork from the right to the left hand, for example, or choosing a different food on the plate.

The therapist should observe the patient before offering assistance. Does the patient show any signs of recognizing the task or problem to be solved? Can the patient initiate the appropriate steps necessary in the sequence of events to meet the goal? Can motor skills be combined with perceptual-cognitive skills to reach the goal? (Many times a patient cannot think and do at the same time.) If the patient needs assistance, how much assistance? What is the quality of touch, manipulation, grasp, and release? How does the patient use the body and adapt muscle tone during the activity? How does performance affect facial tone, oral motor function, and communication skills? Evaluation needs to continue every time the patient is seen, because changes always occur. Every treatment should begin with evaluation, using observation and interpretation.

If the patient needs assistance, the therapist should use guiding techniques. Often a patient immediately responds to the input by adjusting body tone and exhibiting attention and sustained focus on the task, usually followed by increased eye-hand coordination, hand-mouth coordination, and oral-motor coordination. A patient who is unable to eat independently may begin to take over the purposeful movement and start to self-feed during the guiding process. Families are often available when meals or snacks are served, and it is a perfect time to invite nonverbal interaction between individuals and begin family education (Fig. 25-2).

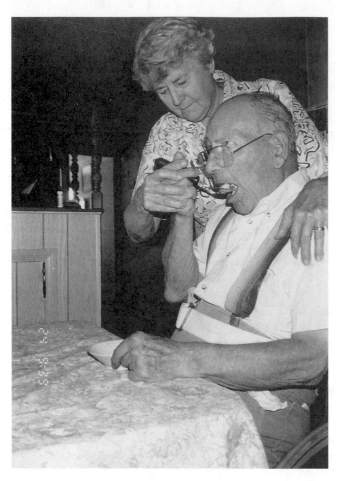

FIG. 25-2   Facilitation of self-feeding through guiding. Patient stabilizes bowl with left hand while wife assists by guiding right hand, inhibiting flexor synergy pattern. As patient processes tactile input, eyes gaze away. Mouth opens in anticipation of food on utensil.

TREATMENT: MEANINGFUL ACTIVITY

Learning requires the creation of appropriate situations and the interaction between the patient and the environment. Activities must be meaningful to the patient as well as age-appropriate. It is easier for patients to be motivated by functional activities that are purposeful and that relate to real-life situations.[7] As Noble said, "Simple situations involving self care, meal preparation and household or work related tasks are valuable tools that will afford the individual the opportunity to reconnect with the previously learned and automatic motor, perceptual, cognitive, social and emotional skills. These tasks contain all the vital components of treatment activities for which we search our cabinets and imaginations on a daily basis."[8]

The environment is a critical factor as well. Grooming and hygiene are much more meaningful when performed in the bathroom, dressing in a bedroom, meal preparation in the kitchen. When the activity is meaningful, the patient is motivated to complete the task (Fig. 25-3). It is

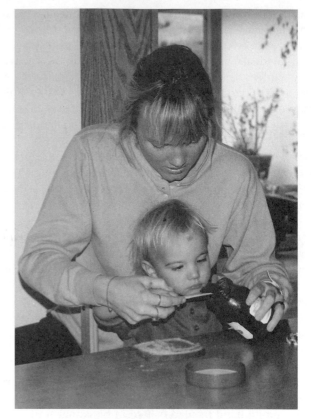

A

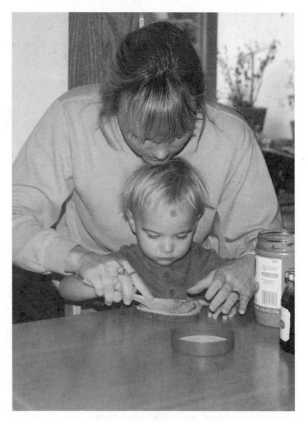

B

FIG. 25-3   **A,** T-K input during an event facilitates attention, focus, and eye-hand coordination. **B,** Meaningful activity motivates child to complete task.

inappropriate to use pegs, cones, beanbags, or simulated situations during the process of guiding. Stacking cones may be an acceptable nonpurposeful activity for increasing range of motion, but not for facilitation of perceptual processing. Wiping a counter top that is not dirty is also nonpurposeful. In both of these situations, there is no problem to be solved. As Parkinson said, "Choosing the right activity and then continuing to treat effectively within the activity requires a considerable amount of skill."[9]

As health care providers, occupational therapists constantly face limited treatment time. All too often a patient is scheduled for therapy, but conflicts arise. Perhaps there is an appointment scheduled for medical testing, or the patient is very tired and needs to go back to bed. The pleasure about guiding as a perceptual facilitation technique is that these moments no longer need to be considered wasted time. If the patient is too tired to participate in treatment the therapist can assist the patient into bed, guiding him or her to lock the wheelchair brakes (Fig. 25-4). Rather than telling the patient to lock the brake in preparation to transfer, he or she is guided

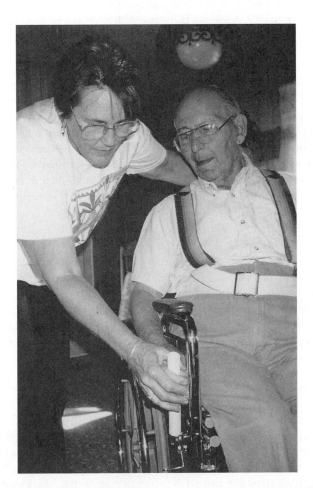

FIG. 25-4 Locking wheelchair brakes incorporates guiding into daily routine. Patient has hemiparesis, hemianopsia, and apraxia. Maximal tactile input through guiding facilitates purposeful and controlled movement, right regard, and eye-hand coordination.

through the process nonverbally. The goal is still meaningful and perceptual-cognitive facilitation took place in the most appropriate circumstance.

Often valuable treatment time is lost when the therapist attempts to set up an activity, clean up, or demonstrate while the patient waits. The alternative is to involve the patient in the process. Guide the patient to gather the equipment or take the tools out of the tool box. Open the drawers and put things away together. This approach integrates the components of problems faced in real life including organization and preparation. Things don't always go as planned, and we often must make detours to meet the original goals. Did the patient spill the juice? Use guiding to get the sponge or mop, and go through the entire process that anyone needs to go through to get the job done, nonverbally.

Therapists take great care in setting up situations to be successful experiences, but it is often the little mistakes that lead to the most learning. "Therapists often see a problem arise before the patient and they will "fix it" before the problem happens . . . before the patient has the opportunity to solve the problem in the situation. This deprives patients of an opportunity to learn and add to the repertoire of experience."[7] If the patient is about to spill, the best decision may be to allow the patient to spill rather than avoid it. Use the opportunity to take care of the problem and clean up together. The therapist needs to be aware that change is not always measured by his or her concept of success. "Error must be allowed within limitation. A patient must learn to adapt to different situations, modify his behavior and movement, and change his strategy."[9] Change is a process that comes about with challenges.

THE USE OF GUIDING IN PERCEPTUAL-COGNITIVE FACILITATION

Affolter developed the treatment technique of guiding as a way for therapists to assist their patients in perceiving the environment, by physically guiding patients' hands and bodies in functional activities. Because the clinician's hands are directly guiding the patient, therapists receive concrete information about the patient and his or her ability to attend to tasks, anticipate sequencing, solve problems, adjust muscle tone, and much more. The goal in guiding is input rather than output. Guiding can be facilitated in many different ways. There is maximal assist (heavy) guiding, and moderate and minimal assist (light) guiding. These terms have been adopted in the Affolter approach as a way to document patient performance using the present documentation system in most clinical settings.

The amount of tactile-kinesthetic information given depends upon the body tone of the patient in any given moment. Body tone changes in direct relationship to input and can fluctuate throughout an activity. It also varies in different positions and situations. Therefore, the amount of guiding continually fluctuates. Guiding should produce regular, harmonious movements of exploration —not too slow, not too fast. The goal of treatment is to search with the patient for tactile-kinesthetic information while exploring and solving problems of daily living.

The traditional approach in assisting a patient in a functional activity has been for the therapist to give the patient verbal instructions. In using the Affolter approach it is imperative that the search for information be nonverbal, communicating only through the T-K sense. Refraining from speaking is very nontypical in traditional therapeutic approaches, but it is one of the most important aspects in using the technique correctly. By refraining from speaking during guiding, the patient is given the best opportunity to process information without extra stimuli. Language is made up of symbols. When the patient is able to process incoming stimuli and assimilate the information to past experience, the language-impaired patient will often produce spontaneous, appropriate, and articulate speech.

Although instructions are not necessary in preparation to guide, at times it may be appropriate to say, "I am going to guide you by moving your hands (or body) with my hands. I am not going to tell you with words what I want you to do. Listen to my hands." Sometimes it is not possible or appropriate to communicate this thought to the patient, for example, if the patient is having difficulty with language reception or if there is a cultural language barrier. Often this approach is just a matter of seizing the opportunity to assist the patient at just the right time to take care of the task together without the necessity of verbal input. The result is a nonverbal understanding between the patient and therapist based on personal respect. The following is an actual example:

Mr. M. is a 68-year-old who underwent heart transplant surgery and sustained a left cerebral vascular accident during the procedure. This CVA resulted in severe motor deficits and postural insecurity as well as severe receptive and expressive aphasia. He was understandably frustrated with the communication deficits but was also very afraid to move, often resisting transfers and training in dressing and self-care. The staff used short, simple phrases and gestures in attempting to teach transfer techniques. Mr. M. tried very hard to watch the therapists and guess at what they wanted him to do. Reliability was less than 25%, and the therapists felt that the patient would often nod his head yes or no in attempts to please the staff, not really comprehending the task or instructions. He remained at a maximal assist level for several weeks and did not seem to be following through with any of the techniques. Physicians questioned his potential for progress. Then a therapist familiar with the Affolter approach guided Mr. M nonverbally through a transfer from the wheelchair to a mat and proceeded to guide him through removing his shoes in preparation for a mat program. This activity demanded a considerable amount of trunk control. Mr. M attended to the task with focus and intent and was able to anticipate the movements and follow the nonverbal cues with surprising accuracy of approximately 75%. His transfer improved immediately to a moderate, almost minimal, assist and there was much less of a hesitation to lean forward during the transfer. Once on the mat, the therapist guided Mr. M.'s hands along the surface of his legs to reach his shoelaces, and he followed right along, never having heard a verbal instruction. His tone adapted accordingly and it was obvious by observation as well as the tactile cues the therapist received that the patient did not feel uncomfortable about leaning so far forward. He assisted in the crossing of his legs (which requires weight shifting) and eventually removed both shoes and socks. At the end of the task Mr. M. looked at the therapist, smiled and made an OK sign with his fingers indicating that he enjoyed the activity, he understood and followed the nonverbal cues, and he knew without external feedback that he had been successful.

Guiding needs to be performed in contact with a reference of support. This means moving a patient's body along a surface, as opposed to moving through the air. In guiding Mr. M. to untie his shoelaces, the therapist used the patient's own body as a reference of support and guided his hands along the surface of his legs. In a grooming and hygiene activity, when reaching toward the faucet to turn the water on a patient should be guided along the edge of the sink, in contact with the surface. This movement allows the patient the opportunity to explore the environment and perceive how far the sink is from the body, how far the faucet is from the sink, etc. When tone normalizes, a patient can then be guided through the air, as this is more typical of normal movement.

Guiding must also use familiar and functional problem-solving activities. Stacking cones, using parquetry cubes, or tossing bean bags are difficult activities for perceptually disturbed patients to translate into functional significance.[7] Using daily events that are familiar to the patient offers some regularity and predictability within the situation. At the same time variations of environment, positions, sequencing, and material being used can be easily integrated into the regularity of the daily routine.

When guiding a patient, it is important to realize that perception has no dominance. It does not occur specifically in the left hemisphere or right hemisphere; it involves the whole brain. Therefore, guiding should involve the whole body, not just one side of the body. Guiding needs to be bilateral, moving each extremity, one at a time, as opposed to both extremities at once. One hand is the stabilizer while the other hand moves. If there is paralysis, would the therapist guide a nonfunctional extremity or a patient who does not seem aroused or alert? The answer is YES! The goal in guiding is not to facilitate movement, but purely to provide the patient with familiar sensory input. A right hand–dominant patient with left hemiplegia may be guided to cut an orange using not only the right upper extremity but also the left upper extremity, not with the expectation that the knife will be held independently or that the patient will learn how to cut with his left hand. The patient may never do these things, but may take over some of the purposeful movement if the brain recognized this information from past experience. Once the orange is cut, there is a change in the shape of the orange and it is wet, perhaps sticky. It has an incredible smell. The orange slice can even be guided to touch the lips of the patient to allow a hand/object-to-mouth experience as well as the taste. This action facilitates intermodal integration of some of the other senses. Without ever saying a word, the patient has been given the opportunity to develop a picture and perceive the task of cutting an orange. "In perception, connections are always being made between present stimuli and stored stimuli of the past. Assimilation means the process of integrating incoming stimuli to past experience."[7] When a patient can use stored information in a similar situation, learning has taken place.

EVALUATING EFFECTIVENESS OF TREATMENT

In evaluating effectiveness of treatment, therapy has to initiate learning in the patient. The patient must be challenged enough so that learning occurs, yet assisted enough to minimize frustration and failure. It is the therapist's responsibility to help patients reach their optimum level of performance when guiding them. This level is described by Affolter as the performance ceiling[7] and occurs when the patient is working at or near peak performance and is attending to the task and motivated to continue. The therapist can estimate the patient's actual performance level by observing attentiveness and muscle tone while carrying out tasks during therapy. Patients are working at their performance ceiling when some of the following characteristics are observed:[4,5,7]

- silence while the patient is guided
- an intent facial expression
- appropriate eye contact for the task
- normalization of muscle tone (i.e., a patient with very low tone may increase tone or a patient who is hypertonic may become more normal in muscle tone)

The patient's behavior provides feedback to the therapist regarding how appropriate the activity is for optimal learning.[5,7] The patient may (1) become panicked, fearful, or agitated; (2) complain of unrelated aches and pains; (3) talk about irrelevant topics; or (4) simply stop attending to the task.[5] It does not help to point out when the patient has been successful or unsuccessful. The patient must interpret the tactile-kinesthetic information independently to judge the effectiveness of the performance. "When working at his individual peak performance level the patient recognizes his successful performance and is motivated to continue to work the task."[4]

Attention and input are maximal when a perceiver has to perform at the limit or at a ceiling level of his performance. Watch a child walking down the street. The child will not be content to walk nicely on the sidewalk. The child will always look for some difficulty to overcome; a wall to climb, a fence to jump over, or a curb to skip along. Usually, children are quite skilled at finding something that is not too easy and yet not too

difficult. This captures the essence of what is meant by performance ceiling . . . performance ceiling is that level of performance whereby one can estimate the amount of difficulty in a situation, and attempt to solve it. But there must still be some risk; an unknown factor to measure one's own skill against, a problem to overcome and master.[3]

THE ROOT OF DEVELOPMENT

Research findings have revealed that patients with brain injury or other neurological deficits have difficulty in processing tactile-kinesthetic information.[3] These findings are supported by clinical observations of touching deviances.[2] Difficulties or deviances in touching have consequences in daily life because most of our daily life interaction requires touching. Affolter explains this effect using the analogy of a plant. "Failure to interact or difficulty with touching will make the root of the plant sick so that it is not able to grow adequately. The sickness in the root explains the failure in more complex developmental skills, language acquisition, reading and writing problems, attention span, etc. The plant may continue to grow, but in treating the plant, it is not enough to nurture the leaves or branches. We have to work on the root. This means we have to involve the patients in daily life events and provide better tactile-kinesthetic information when interacting by planning the environment, and by guiding if possible, the patient during the event. Working in this way should improve tactile-kinesthetic experience in daily life interaction, thus improve the growth of the root and enhance more adequate development of complex developmental skills."[2]

Although Affolter's model differs from neurodevelopmental treatment (NDT) criteria, many of the basic NDT principles can be applied in clinical situations when planning the environment for interactive guiding experiences. As stated in Chapter 24, throughout the treatment session the therapist must continually observe not only what the patient is doing, but also how he or she is doing it. The primary goal of NDT is to normalize muscle tone and relearn normal movements during activities of daily living. This goal is accomplished by proper positioning, weight-bearing, inhibition or facilitation of the trunk and upper and lower extremities with integration of balance, rhythm, and velocity during dynamic movement. Proper positioning and guidance through components of normal movements during grooming, dressing, and transfers help to trigger automatic responses and previously learned skills improving stability, efficiency, and quality in functional movement. "For carry-over to occur, the patient must take over management of himself within each session. A change and recognition must occur at some level of his central nervous system that requires the patient's own muscle activity. . . . A patient feels the movement and can immediately begin to help and be active in the movement. Then he takes the movement over and makes it his own."[9]

The primary goal of the Affolter approach is to provide adequate input in searching for information and exploring the environment. When guiding is incorporated into the therapeutic treatment program, careful attention must be paid to preparing the patient for the activity by proper positioning. Positioning is one key to stability, support, and effective function during an activity. As guiding occurs and the patient receives adequate T-K input, it can be expected that an improvement of perceptual organization will be followed by an improvement of complex human performances.[3] When the patient is guided in a meaningful activity, often he or she gazes away as the information is being processed (Fig. 25-2), but as the information starts to become familiar, facilitation of eye-hand coordination takes place (Figs. 25-3, *A* and *B* and 25-4). Hand-mouth coordination and changes in facial tonus also occur as objects are explored and brought to the mouth. Grasp, release, reaching, transporting, displacing, filling, and emptying through exploration of the environment facilitates spatial awareness, adaptation of muscle tone, and balance reactions.

EDUCATION: A VITAL COMPONENT FOR OPTIMAL FUNCTION

Perceptual-cognitive facilitation should happen regularly, throughout every waking hour of the patient's day, which requires collaboration with the treatment team as well as the family. Cotreatment should include both the OT and PT or any other discipline including speech, recreation therapy, nursing, and psychology, as well as teachers and support staff. If recovery is going to occur, it appears most likely to happen when there is a real need to do problem solving and to move.

Educating families, care givers, educators, and the community about perceptual processing is a vital role that the occupational therapist can play. Families are in desperate need of information that helps them understand the confusing behavior they witness. Teaching them about perception in terms of problem solving helps them to process the situations they observe every day. Families often struggle with lack of functional information about how they can help in the healing process. Taking a family member through the same nonverbal guided experience as the patient provides the feel of the tactile-kinesthetic experience. The family member can feel the correct amount of input and experience the process of problem solving first hand.[5] When the activity is meaningful, the family member has a greater possibility of being able to follow through with the information learned.

SUMMARY

Occupational therapists must learn to observe carefully and interpret individual behavior and recognize the importance of interactive problem solving in perceptual processing. Affolter's research suggests the necessity for continuation and extension of the present studies to gain more knowledge about the tactile-kinesthetic system. This applied knowledge will assist occupational therapists and other health care professionals in the identification of children with developmental deviances at an early age, analysis of behavior with learning disabled and brain-injured persons, and development of effective, efficient and individual therapeutic interventions with a focus on function and carry-over. This technique is used with all ages, many different diagnoses, and may be incorporated into many different lifestyles respecting every language and culture. The Affolter approach offers unlimited opportunities to faciltate optimal perceptual input emphasizing tactile exploration through realistic learning situations.

REVIEW QUESTIONS

1. Define perception.
2. What kind of information is needed for adequate interaction and thus stimulates the growth of the root for development and complex human performances?
3. What is the primary reason for perceptual processing deficits?
4. List 4 prerequisites for problem solving.
5. What is the goal of using guiding when a patient is interacting in daily life events?
6. List 2 typical personality behaviors and corresponding symptoms displayed by individuals with perceptual processing problems.
7. What is the difference between observation and interpretation?
8. List at least 3 rules to follow in guiding.
9. Describe performance ceiling level when a patient is guided.
10. How often should guiding occur?

REFERENCES

1. Affolter F: The development of perceptual processes and problem solving activities in normal, hearing impaired and language-disturbed children. In Martin DS, editor: *Cognition, education, and deafness: directions for research and instruction*, Washington, DC, 1987, Gallaudet College Press.
2. Affolter FD: Perception, Interaction and Language, Interaction of Daily Living as the Root of Development. Berlin, Germany, 1991. Springer-Verlag.
3. Affolter F, Stricker E, editors: Perceptual processes as prerequisites for complex human behavior: a theoretical model and its application to therapy. Bern, Switzerland, 1980, Hans Huber.

4. Davies P: Steps to follow, Berlin, West Germany, 1985, Springer-Verlag.
5. Davies P: Starting again, Berlin, Germany, 1994, Springer-Verlag.
6. Davies P, Sonderegger H: An advanced course: treatment of traumatic brain injury and other severe brain lesions, Presented at Meadowbrook Neurologic Care Center, San José, Calif, 1993.
7. Davis JZ: The Affolter method: A model for treating perceptual disturbances in the hemiplegic and brain injured patient, *OT Practice* 3(4):30-38, 1992.
8. Noble CR: An analysis of the process and learning involved in activities of daily living, *O T Forum* 2(10): 3-4, 1987.
9. Parkinson T: Carry-over with NDT in limited time frames, *NDTA Network* 3:1-3, 1994.
10. *Webster's New World Dictionary, Third College Edition,* New York, 1988, Simon & Shuster.

SUGGESTED READINGS

Arabit LL: The Affolter concept: guiding patients through rehab, *OT Week* 8(14):24-26, 1994.
Arnadottir G: *The brain and behavior: assessing cortical dysfunction through activities of daily living (ADL),* St Louis, Mo. 1990, CV Mosby.
Bobath B: *Adult hemiplegia: evaluation and treatment,* London, England, 1978, William Heinemann.
Davies P: *Right in the middle: selective trunk activity in the treatment of adult hemiplagia,* Berlin, Germany, 1990, Springer-Verlag.
Montagu A: *Touching, the human significance of the skin,* New York, 1986, Harper & Row.
Rudolph M: Affolter method guides therapy, *Advance for OTs,* 7(2), 1991.

CHAPTER 26

Activities of Daily Living

Diane Foti, Lorraine Williams Pedretti, Susan Lillie

Section 1   Self-care/home management

Diane Foti, Lorraine Williams Pedretti

ctivities of daily living (ADL) and instrumental activities of daily living (I-ADL) are tasks of self-maintenance, mobility, communication, home management and community living that enable an individual to achieve personal independence.[10,14] Evaluation and training in the performance of these important life tasks have long been important aspects of occupational therapy programs in virtually every type of healthcare service. Loss of ability to care for personal needs and to manage the environment can result in loss of self-esteem, a deep sense of dependence, and even feelings of infantilism. Family roles are also disrupted, requiring partners to assume the function of caregiver, when a person loses the ability to perform ADL or I-ADL independently.[19]

The role of occupational therapy is to assess ADL and I-ADL performance skills, determine problems that interfere with independence, determine treatment objectives, and provide training or equipment to increase independence. The occupational therapist may also be involved in removing or reducing physical, cognitive, social, and emotional barriers that are interfering with performance. The need to learn new methods or use assistive devices to perform daily tasks may be temporary or permanent, depending on the particular dysfunction and the prognosis for recovery.

DEFINITION OF ADL AND I-ADL

Daily activities can be separated into two areas: activities of daily living and instrumental activities of daily living. ADL require basic skills whereas I-ADL require more advanced problem-solving skills, social skills, and more complex environmental interactions. ADL tasks include mobility, self-care, communication, management of environmental hardware and devices, and sexual expression.

I-ADL include home management and community living skills, health management, and safety preparedness (Table 26-1).

EVALUATION OF PERFORMANCE AREAS

ADL is one of the major performance areas in the occupational performance model discussed in Chapter 1. A comprehensive evaluation of performance skills should include assessment of the client's abilities and limitations in (1) work and productive activities, (2) play/leisure, and (3) activities of daily living or self-maintenance. A primary purpose of occupational therapy is to facilitate skill in performance of these essential tasks of living. It is important to help the individual with a disability to balance activity in each of these three performance areas according to his or her personality, skills, limitations, needs, cultural values, and lifestyle.

The therapist's evaluation of the client's performance profile could begin with the charting of a daily or weekly schedule (see Chapter 4), an activities configuration, an interest checklist, or an occupational role history.[6,9,21,23,28] The activities configuration protocol can be used to gather data about the client's values, education, work history, and vocational interests and plans. The interest checklist can be used to determine degree of interest in five categories of activities: (1) manual skills, (2) physical sports, (3) social recreation, (4) activities of daily living (ADL), and (5) cultural and educational activities.[21] The occupational role history is used to indicate

TABLE 26-1 Activities in ADL and I-ADL	
ACTIVITIES OF DAILY LIVING (ADL)	**INSTRUMENTAL ACTIVITIES OF DAILY LIVING (I-ADL)**
MOBILITY	**HOME MANAGEMENT**
Bed mobility	Shopping
Wheelchair mobility	Meal planning
Transfers	Meal preparation
Ambulation	Cleaning
	Laundry
	Child care
	Recycling
SELF-CARE	**COMMUNITY LIVING SKILLS**
Dressing	
Self-feeding	Money/financial management
Toileting	Use of public transportation
Bathing	Driving
Grooming	Shopping
	Access to recreation activities
COMMUNICATION	**HEALTH MANAGEMENT**
Writing	Handling medication
Typing/computer use	Knowing health risks
Telephoning	Making medical appointments
Using special communication devices	
ENVIRONMENTAL HARDWARE	**SAFETY MANAGEMENT**
Keys	Fire safety awareness
Faucets	Ability to call 911
Light switches	Response to smoke detector
Windows/doors	Identification of dangerous situations
	ENVIRONMENTAL HARDWARE
	Vacuum cleaner
	Can opener
	Stove/oven
	Refrigerator
	Microwave oven

the balance between work and leisure roles.[9] Although the interest checklist and the occupational role history were developed for a psychiatric population, they can be adapted for application to clients with a physical dysfunction.

Occupational therapists focusing on remedying specific performance components may fail to integrate these components with the development of occupational role performance. A performance component goal of increasing fine motor control, for example, may include independence with sewing, handling clothing fasteners, or improving computer keyboard skills. Improvement in these skills improves occupational role performance. The outcome of improving a performance component should be linked to a functional task.

An interview and performance evaluation can yield a well-rounded picture of the client's occupational performance. Deficits and imbalances in occupational performance will be apparent. The performance evaluation is fundamental to the development of a comprehensive treatment plan, which deals with performance components that underlie those skills. The performance evaluations to be addressed in this chapter are for ADL, I-ADL, and driving. Resources to improve access or ability to participate in play and leisure activities are also presented.

Work evaluation is assessment of specific work skills using a real or simulated work situation.[15] Work habits and attitudes are also observed and evaluated. Work evaluation may be carried out by the occupational therapist. (Work evaluation and work hardening programs are discussed in Chapter 30.)

FACTORS TO CONSIDER IN ADL AND I-ADL EVALUATION AND TRAINING

Before commencing ADL/I-ADL performance evaluation and training, the occupational therapist must assess performance components and consider several factors about the client and the individual's environment. Physical resources, such as strength, range of motion (ROM), coordination, sensation, and balance, should be evaluated to determine potential skills and deficits in ADL performance and possible need for special equipment. Perceptual and cognitive functions should be evaluated to determine potential for learning ADL skills. General mobility in bed or wheelchair or ambulation should be assessed.

In addition to these relatively concrete and objective evaluations, the occupational therapist should be familiar with the client's culture and its values and mores in relation to self-care, the sick role, family assistance, and independence. The values of the client and the client's peer group and culture should be important considerations in selecting objectives and initial activities in the ADL program. The balance of activities in the client's day, which demand time and energy, may influence how many ADL can be performed independently.

The environment to which the client will return is an important consideration. Will the client live alone or with his or her family or a roommate? Will the client go to a skilled nursing facility or to a board and care home permanently or temporarily? Will the client return to work and community activities? The type and amount of assistance available in the home environment must be considered if the appropriate caregiver is to receive orientation and training in the appropriate supervision and assistance required.

The finances available for assistant care, special equipment, and home modifications are important considerations. For example, a wheelchair-bound client who is wealthy may be willing and able to make major modifications in the home, such as installing an elevator, lowering kitchen counters, widening doorways, and replacing deep pile carpeting to accommodate a wheelchair lifestyle. A client with fewer financial resources may need the assistance of an occupational therapist in making less costly modifications, such as removing scatter rugs and door sills, installing a plywood ramp at the entrance, and attaching a handheld shower head to the bathtub faucet.

The ultimate goal of any ADL and I-ADL training program is for the client to achieve the maximal level of independence. It is important to note that this level is different for each client. For the client with mild muscle weakness in one arm caused by a peripheral neuropathy, complete independence in ADL may be the maximal, whereas for the individual with a high-level quadriplegia, self-feeding, oral hygiene, and communication activities with devices and assistance may be the maximal level of independence that can be expected. Therefore the potential for independence depends on each client's unique personal needs, values, capabilities, limitations, and environmental resources.

Independence is a strong value in the American culture. It should not be pursued solely on that basis, however, or because it is a value of the rehabilitation personnel or family or friends of the client. Achieving independence must be important to the client and within the realm of possibility.

ADL AND I-ADL EVALUATION
GENERAL PROCEDURE

When data have been gathered about the client's physical, psychosocial, and environmental resources, the feasibility of ADL evaluation or training should be determined by the occupational therapist in concert with the client, supervising physician, and other members of the rehabilitation team. In some instances ADL should be delayed because of limitations of the client or in favor of more immediate treatment objectives that require the client's energy and participation.

Evaluation of ADL and I-ADL performance is often initiated with an interview, using a checklist as a guide for questioning the client about individual capabilities and limitations. Several types of ADL/I-ADL checklists and evaluations are available, but they all cover similar categories and performance tasks.[5]

The interview may serve as a screening device to determine the need for further assessment by observation of performance. This need is determined by the therapist based on knowledge of the client, the dysfunction, and previous evaluations. A partial or complete performance evaluation is invaluable in assessing ADL performance. The expression, "One look is worth a thousand words" applies well here. The interview alone, as a measure of performance, can lead to inaccurate assumptions because the client may recall his or her performance before the onset of the dysfunction, may have some confusion or memory loss, and may overestimate or underestimate

individual abilities because there has been little opportunity to perform routine ADL since the onset of the physical dysfunction.

Ideally the occupational therapist should conduct the performance evaluation when and where the activities to be evaluated usually take place. For example, a dressing evaluation could be arranged early in the morning in the treatment facility when the client is dressed by nursing personnel or in the client's home. Self-feeding evaluation should occur at regular meal hours. If this timing is not possible, the evaluation may be conducted during regular treatment sessions in the occupational therapy clinic under simulated conditions. Requiring the client to perform routine self-maintenance tasks at irregular times in an artificial environment can contribute to a lack of carry-over, especially for those clients who have difficulty generalizing learning.

The therapist should select relatively simple and safe tasks from the ADL/I-ADL checklist and should progress to more difficult and complex items. The evaluation should not be completed at one time, because this approach would cause fatigue and create an artificial situation. Those tasks that would be unsafe or very obviously cannot be performed should be omitted and the appropriate notation made on the evaluation form.

During the performance evaluation the therapist should observe the methods that the client is using or attempting to use to accomplish the task and try to determine causes of performance problems. Common causes include weakness, spasticity, involuntary motion, perceptual deficits, and low endurance. If problems and their causes can be identified, the therapist has a good foundation for establishing training objectives, priorities, methods, and need for assistive devices.

Other very important aspects of this evaluation that should not be overlooked are the client's need for respect and privacy and the ongoing interaction between the client and the therapist. The client's feelings about having his or her body viewed and touched should be respected. Privacy should be maintained for toileting, grooming, and dressing tasks. The therapist with whom the client is most familiar and comfortable may be the appropriate person to conduct the ADL evaluation and training. As the therapist interacts with the client during performance of daily living tasks, it may be possible to elicit the client's attitudes and feelings about the particular tasks, priorities in training, dependence and independence, and cultural, family, and personal values and customs regarding performance of daily living activities.

RECORDING RESULTS OF ADL EVALUATION

During the interview and performance evaluation the therapist makes appropriate notations on the checklists. These may include separate checklists for self-care, home management, mobility, and home environment evaluations. When describing levels of independence occupational therapists often use terms like moderate independence, maximal assistance, and minimal skill. These quantitative terms have little meaning to the reader unless they are defined or supporting statements are included in progress summaries to give specific meaning for each. It also should be specified whether the level of independence refers to a single activity, a category of activities such as dressing, or all ADL. In designating levels of independence an agreed-on performance scale should be used to mark the ADL checklist. The following general categories and their definitions are suggested:

1. Independent: can perform the activity or activities without cuing, supervision, or assistance, with or without assistive devices, at normal or near normal speeds
2. Supervised: can perform the activity alone but needs someone available for safety
3. Minimal assistance: supervision, cuing, or less than 20% physical assistance
4. Moderate assistance: supervision, cuing, and 20% to 50% physical assistance
5. Maximal assistance: supervision, cuing, and 50% to 80% physical assistance
6. Dependent: can perform only one or two steps of the activity or very few activities independently, may fatigue easily and perform very slowly, may require elaborate equipment and devices to perform basic skills such as feeding, needs more than 80% physical assistance

These definitions are broad and general. They can be modified to suit the program plan and approach of the particular treatment facility.

The information is then summarized succinctly for inclusion in the client's permanent records so that interested professional coworkers can refer to it. A sample case study, with ADL and home management checklists, and summaries of an initial evaluation and progress report are included in Figs. 26-1 and 26-2. The reader should keep in mind that the evaluation and progress summaries relate to the ADL portion of the treatment program only.

INSTRUMENTAL ACTIVITIES OF DAILY LIVING
HOME MANAGEMENT EVALUATION

Home management tasks are evaluated similarly to self-care tasks. The client should first be interviewed to elicit a description of the home and former and present home management responsibilities. Those tasks that the client needs to perform when returning home, as well as those that he or she would like to perform, should be ascertained during the interview. If the client has a communication disorder or a cognitive deficit, aid from friends or family members may be enlisted to get the information needed. The client may also be questioned about his or her ability to perform each task on the activities list. The evaluation is much more meaningful and accurate, how-

---

Sample case study

J.V. is a 48-year-old married woman who suffered a cerebral thrombosis resulting in a CVA 6 months ago. She lives in a modest home with her husband and teenage daughter and was a full-time homemaker before the onset of her stroke. She was a cheerful and active woman who enjoyed cooking, baking, gardening, and visiting her neighbors and friends. The stroke resulted in the disturbance of cerebellar and brain stem functions. J.V. has a severe motor apraxia for speech, cannot close her mouth, drools, and walks with a broad-based ataxic gait. Since the onset of her disability J.V. has been very depressed, weeps frequently, is dependent for much of her self-care, and sits idly for long periods of time. She was referred to occupational therapy for evaluation and training in ADL, adjustment to disability, and development of drooling and swallowing control to facilitate feeding.

SAMPLE ADL PROGRESS REPORT

J.V. has attended occupational therapy 3 times weekly for 3 weeks since the initial evaluation. Further evaluation of self-care skills revealed that J.V. is capable of some hygiene skills, except a tub bath, nail care, hair care, and makeup application. However, at home she remains al-

most entirely dependent on Mr. V. for self-care, while crying and complaining of feeling weak.

Home management evaluation revealed considerable difficulty with most tasks except table setting, dusting, dishwashing, and sweeping, which she can perform if given cues and supervision. Performance of more complex tasks is limited by psychomotor retardation, incoordination, distractibility, inability to sequence a process, and apraxia for fine hand activities. It was necessary to supervise J.V. closely and give step-by-step instructions while she performed household tasks. A few simple homemaking tasks were performed for several training sessions, but performance did not improve.

J.V. appears to be very depressed and lacks intrinsic motivation. It was suggested to her family that they offer less assistance for self-care, and involve her with them in household tasks that she can perform, under their supervision, if possible.

The occupational therapy program will continue with greater emphasis on achieving control of mouth musculature, a primary goal of J.V. ADL training will be delayed until J.V. is moving toward the achievement of this primary goal.

FIG. 26-1 ADL evaluation. (Adapted from *Activities of daily living evaluation form 461-1,* Hartford, Conn, 1963, The Hartford Easter Seal Rehabilitation Center.)

OCCUPATIONAL THERAPY DEPARTMENT

ACTIVITIES OF DAILY LIVING EVALUATION

Name __J. V.__ Age __48__ Diagnosis __CVA__ Dom. __Right__

Disability __Bilateral incoordination, ataxia, apraxia of mouth musculature__

Mode of ambulation __Independent__

Grading key:
I = Independent
MiA = Minimal assistance
MoA = Moderate assistance
MaA = Maximal assistance
D = Dependent
NA = Not applicable
O = Not evaluated

TRANSFERS AND AMBULATION

	Date	Independent	Assisted	Dependent
Tub or shower	8/1			D
Toilet	8/1		MiA	
Wheelchair	NA			
Bed and chair		I		
Ambulation			MiA	
Wheelchair management	NA			
Car			MiA	

BALANCE FOR FUNCTION

	Adequate	Inadequate
Sitting	I	
Standing	I	
Walking		MiA

ADL SKILLS

EATING	Date	8/1	8/25			REMARKS
		Grade				
Butter bread		I				
Cut meat		I				
Eat with spoon		I				
Eat with fork		I				
Drink with straw		D				Mouth apraxia
Drink with glass		D				prevents performance
Drink with cup		D				of these activities
Pour from pitcher		D				

UNDRESS	Date	8/1	8/25			REMARKS
Pants or shorts		I				Is physically
Girdle or garter belt		MoA				capable of
Brassiere		MiA				performing the
Slip or undershirt		I				activities as
Dress		I				indicated but
Skirt		I				Mr. V. reports
Blouse or shirt		I				that J.V. is
Slacks or trousers		I				dependent on him
Bandana or necktie		NA				for much assistance,
Stockings		MoA				pleading fatigue,
Nightclothes		I				whining, and
Hair net		NA				crying for help
Housecoat/bathrobe		I				
Jacket		I				
Belt and/or suspenders		I				
Hat		I				
Coat		I				
Sweater		I				
Mittens or gloves		I				
Glasses		NA				
Brace		NA				
Shoes		MoA				
Socks		MoA				
Overshoes		MoA				

DRESS	Date	8/1	8/25			REMARKS
Pants or shorts		MiA				
Girdle or garter belt		MoA				
Brassiere		MoA				
Slip or undershirt		I				
Dress		I				
Skirt		I				
Blouse or shirt		I				
Slacks or trousers		I				
Bandana or necktie		NA				
Stockings		MoA				
Nightclothes		I				
Hair net		NA				
Housecoat/bathrobe		I				
Jacket		I				
Belt and/or suspenders		I				
Hat		I				
Coat		I				
Sweater		I				
Mittens or gloves		NA				
Glasses		NA				
Brace		NA				
Shoes		MoA				
Socks		MoA				
Overshoes		MoA				

FASTENINGS	Date	8/1	8/25			REMARKS
		Grade				
Button		I				
Snap		MoA				
Zipper		MiA				
Hook and eye		MaA				
Garters		D				
Lace		D				
Untie shoes		D				
Velcro		MiA				

HYGIENE	Date	8/1	8/25			REMARKS
Blow nose		O	I			
Wash face, hands		O	I			
Wash extremities, back		O	MaA			
Brush teeth or dentures		O	I			
Brush or comb hair		O	I			
Set hair		O	D			
Shave or put on makeup		O	MiA			
Clean fingernails		O	I, D			
Trim fingernails, toenails		O	D			
Apply deodorant		O	I			
Shampoo hair		O	D			
Use toilet paper		O	I			
Use tampon or sanitary napkin		O	NA			

COMMUNICATION	Date	8/1	8/25			REMARKS
Verbal		D				
Read		I				
Hold book		I				
Turn page		I				
Write		I				Writes name and
Use telephone		D				few words
Type		D				

HAND ACTIVITIES	Date	8/1	8/25			REMARKS
Handle money		O				
Handle mail		O				
Use of scissors		O				
Open cans, bottles, jars		O				
Tie package		O				
Sew (baste)		O				
Sew button, hook and eye		O				
Polish shoes		O				
Sharpen pencil		O				
Seal and open letter		O				
Open box		O				

COMBINED PERFORMANCE ACTIVITIES	Date	8/1	8/25			REMARKS
Open-close refrigerator		O	I			
Open-close door		O	I			
Remove and replace objects		O	I			
Carry objects during locomotion		O				
Pick up object from floor		O	D			
Remove, replace light bulb		O	D			
Plug in cord		O	O			

OPERATE	Date	8/1	8/25			REMARKS
		Grade				
Light switches		O	I			
Doorbell		O	I			
Door locks and handles		O	O			
Faucets		O	I			
Raise-lower window shades		O	O			
Raise-lower venetian blinds		O	O			
Raise-lower window		O	O			
Open-close drawer		O	I			
Hang up garment		O	I			

SUMMARY OF EVALUATION RESULTS

Date __8/1__

Intact	Impaired		REMARKS
		SENSORY STATUS	
X		Touch	
X		Pain	
X		Temperature	
	X	Position sense	More marked on left
	X	Olfaction	
	X	Stereognosis	More marked on left
	X	Visual fields (hemianopsia)	
		PERCEPTUAL/CONCEPTUAL TESTS	
X		Follow directions	Verbal
X		Visual spatial (form)	
	X	Visual spatial (block design)	Minimal impairment
X		Make change	
	X	Geometric figures (copy)	Some difficulty with triangle & diamond square, circle, triangle, diamond
	X	Praxis	Mild apraxia evident on fine hand activities
		FUNCTIONAL RANGE OF MOTION	
X		Comb hair—two hands	
X		Feed self	
X		Button collar button	
X		Tie apron behind back	
X		Button back buttons	
X		Button cuffs	
X		Zip side zipper	
	X	Tie shoes	Poor balance limits
	X	Stoop	Reach and bending for these activities
	X	Reach shelf	

FIG. 26-1 *cont'd.* For legend see opposite page.

OCCUPATIONAL THERAPY DEPARTMENT

ACTIVITIES OF HOME MANAGEMENT

Name _J.V._ Date _8/25_

Address _Anytown, U.S.A._

Age _48_ Weight _135_ Height _5'5"_ Role in family _Wife, mother_

Diagnosis _CVA_ Disability _Bilateral ataxia, apraxia of mouth musculature_

Mode of ambulation _Independent, no aids, mild ataxic gait_

Limitations or contraindications for activity_____

DESCRIPTION OF HOME
1. Private house _✓_
   No. of rooms _6_ - kitchen, dining room, living room, 3 bedrooms
   No. of floors _2_
   Stairs _14_ - bedrooms on second floor
   Elevators _O_

2. Apartment house _____
   No. of rooms _____
   No. of floors _____
   Stairs _____
   Elevators _____

3. Diagram of home layout (attach to completed form)

Will patient be required to perform the following activities? If not, who will perform?
Meal preparation _No_ _Daughter_
Baking _No_ _Daughter (J.V. used to bake a lot)_
Serving _Yes_
Wash dishes _Yes_
Marketing _No_ _Husband_
Child care _No_
   (under 4 years)
Washing _Yes_
Hanging clothes _NA_ _Has dryer_
Ironing _No_ _Daughter_
Cleaning _Yes_ _Light cleaning_
Sewing _No_ _Does not sew_
Hobbies or _Yes_ _Baking and gardening would be desirable activities_
   special interest

Does patient really like housework? _No_
Sitting position: Chair _X_ Stool _X_ Wheelchair _NA_
Standing position: Braces _NA_ Crutches _NA_ Canes _NA_
Handedness: Dominant hand _Right_ Two hands _X_ One hand only_____ Assistive_____

Continued.

Grading key: I = Independent
 MiA = Minimal assistance
 MoA = Moderate assistance
 MaA = Maximal assistance
 D = Dependent
 O = Not evaluated

CLEANING ACTIVITIES	Date	8/25				REMARKS
		Grade				
Pick up object from floor		D				
Wipe up spills		D				
Make bed (daily)		D				
Use dust mop		I				
Shake dust mop		D				
Dust low surfaces		I				
Dust high surfaces		D				
Mop kitchen floor		D				
Sweep with broom		I				
Use dust pan and broom		MiA				
Use vacuum cleaner		O				
Use vacuum cleaner attachments		D				
Carry light cleaning tools		I				
Use carpet sweeper		I				
Clean bathtub		D				
Change sheets on bed		D				
Carry pail of water		D				

MEAL PREPARATION	Date	8/25				REMARKS
Turn off water		I				
Turn off gas or electric range		I				
Light gas with match		D				
Pour hot water from pan to cup		D				
Open packaged goods		I				
Carry pan from sink to range		D				
Use can opener		D				
Handle milk bottle		I				
Dispose of garbage		D				
Remove things from refrigerator		D				
Bend to low cupboards		D				
Reach to high cupboards		O				
Peel vegetables		D				
Cut up vegetables		D				
Handle sharp tools safely		D				
Break eggs		D				
Stir against resistance		D				
Measure flour		D				
Use eggbeater		D				
Use electric mixer		D				
Remove batter to pan		I				
Open oven door		D				
Carry pan to oven and put in		O				
Remove hot pan from oven to table		D				
Roll cookie dough or piecrust						

Continued.

MEAL SERVICE	Date	8/25			REMARKS
Set table for four		I			
Carry four glasses of water to table		D			
Carry hot casserole to table		D			
Clear table		I			
Scrape and stack dishes		I			
Wash dishes (light soil)		I			
Wipe silver		I			
Wash pots and pans		MiA			
Wipe up range and work areas		MoA			
Wring out dishcloth		I			

LAUNDRY	Date	8/25			REMARKS
Wash lingerie (by hand)		D			
Wring out, squeeze dry		D			
Hang on rack to dry		I			
Sprinkle clothes		I			
Iron blouse or slip		D			
Fold blouse or slip					
Use washing machine					

SEWING	Date	8/25			REMARKS
Thread needle and make knot					
Sew on buttons					
Mend rip					
Darn socks					
Use sewing machine					
Crochet					
Knit					
Embroider					
Cut with shears					

HEAVY HOUSEHOLD ACTIVITIES. WHO WILL DO THESE?					
	Date	8/25			REMARKS
Wash household laundry					
Hang clothes					
Clean range					
Clean refrigerator					
Wax floors					
Marketing					
Turn mattresses					
Wash windows					
Put up curtains					

WORK HEIGHTS

SITTING/STANDING
Best height for Wheelchair_____ Chair _X_ Stool _X_
   Ironing _17½" seated_
   Mixing _26" on high stool at counter_
   Dish washing _26" on high stool at counter_
   General work
Maximal depth of counter area (normal reach) _25"_
Maximal useful height above work surface _33" if standing_
Maximal useful height without counter surface _68" if standing_
Maximal reach below counter area _20" if standing_
Best height for chair _17½"-can be used at adjustable ironing board_
Best height for stool with back support _24"-can be used at sink or food preparation counter_

SUGGESTIONS FOR HOME MODIFICATION
Remove scatter rugs in bedroom
Install guard rail on both sides of toilet
Install grab bars on wall next to bathtub
Place nonskid strips on bottom of bathtub

FIG. 26-2 Activities of home management. (Adapted from *Activities of home management form,* Occupational Therapy Department, University Hospital, Ohio State University, Columbus.)

ever, if the interview is followed by a performance evaluation in the ADL kitchen or apartment of the treatment facility or in the client's home if possible.

It is assumed that at this point the therapist has already evaluated motor, sensory, perceptual, and cognitive skills. Consequently the therapist should select tasks and exercise safety precautions consistent with the client's capabilities and limitations. The initial tasks should be simple one- or two-step procedures that are not hazardous, such as wiping a dish, sponging off a table, and turning the water on and off. As the evaluation progresses, tasks graded in complexity and involving safety precautions should be performed, such as making a sandwich and a cup of coffee and vacuuming the carpet.

Home management skills apply to women, men, and sometimes adolescents and children. Individuals may live independently or share home management responsibilities with their partners. In some homes it is necessary for a role reversal to occur after the onset of a physical disability, and the partner who usually stays at home may seek employment outside the home, while the disabled individual remains at home.

If a client will be home alone, there are several basic ADL and I-ADL skills needed for safety and independence. Minimal ADL skills include independence with toileting, transfers or alternative plan to allow for rest periods, and use of the telephone or special call system in case of emergency. Minimal I-ADL skills required to stay at home alone include the ability to (1) prepare or retrieve a simple meal, (2) employ safety precautions and exhibit good judgment, (3) take medication, and (4) get emergency aid if needed. The occupational therapist can evaluate potential for remaining at home alone through the activities of home management evaluation. Safety management as listed in Table 26-1 is also evaluated as a part of the home management evaluation.

A child with a permanent disability also needs to be considered for evaluation and training for I-ADL skills as he or she develops and matures with a growing need for independence.

HOME EVALUATION

When discharge from the treatment facility is anticipated, a home evaluation should be carried out to facilitate the client's maximal independence in the living environment. Ideally it should be performed by the physical and occupational therapists together on a visit to the client's home with the client and family members or housemates present. Budget and time factors may not allow two professional workers to go to the client's home, however. Therefore either the physical or occupational therapist should be able to perform the evaluation, or the evaluation may be referred to the home health agency that will provide home care services to the client.

The client and a family member should be interviewed to determine the client's and family's expectations and the roles the client will assume in the home and community. The cultural or family values regarding a disabled member may influence role expectations and whether or not independence will be encouraged. Willingness and financial ability to make modifications in the home can also be determined.[27]

Sufficient time should be scheduled for the home visit so that the client can demonstrate the required transfer and mobility skills. The therapist may also wish to ask the client to demonstrate selected self-care and home management tasks in the home environment. During the evaluation the client should use the ambulation aids and any assistive devices that he or she is accustomed to using. The therapist should bring a tape measure to measure width of doorways, height of stairs, height of bed, and other dimensions.

The therapist can begin by explaining the purposes and procedure of the home evaluation to the client and others present, if not done before the visit. The therapist can proceed to take the required measurements while surveying the general arrangement of rooms, furniture, and appliances. It may be helpful to sketch the size and arrangement of rooms for later reference and attach these to the home evaluation checklist (Fig. 26-3). For more information on a variety of checklists see Letts and associates.[18] Next the client demonstrates mobility and transfer skills, essential self-care and home management tasks. The client's ability to use the entrance to the home and to transfer to and from an automobile, if it is to be used, should be included in the home evaluation.

During the performance evaluation the therapist should observe safety factors, ease of mobility and performance, and limitations imposed by the environment. If the client requires assistance for transfers and other activities, the caregiver should be instructed in the methods that are appropriate. The client may also be instructed in methods to improve maneuverability and simplify performance of tasks in a small space.

At the end of the evaluation the therapist can make a list of problems, modifications recommended, and additional safety equipment and/or assistive devices. The most common changes are installation of a ramp or railings at the entrance to the home; removal of scatter rugs, extra furniture, and bric-a-brac; removal of doorsills; addition of safety grab bars around the toilet and bathtub; rearrangement of furniture to accommodate a wheelchair; rearrangement of kitchen storage; and lowering of the clothes rod in the closet.[27]

Access into the bathroom and maneuvering with a wheelchair or walker are common problems. Frequently a bedside commode is recommended until a bathroom can be made accessible or modified to allow for independence with toileting (Fig. 26-4). Shower seats can be used in the tub, if a client can transfer over the edge of the tub or also may be used in a shower. A transfer tub bench (Fig. 26-5) is recommended for individuals who cannot

HOME EVALUATION CHECKLIST

Name_____ Date_____
Address_____
Diagnosis_____

Mobility Status
- ☐ ambulatory, no device ☐ walker
- ☐ cane ☐ wheelchair

Exterior

Home located on
- ☐ level surface
- ☐ hill

Type of House
- ☐ owns house ☐ mobile home
- ☐ apartment ☐ board and care

Number of floors
- ☐ one story ☐ split level
- ☐ two story

Driveway surface
- ☐ inclined ☐ smooth
- ☐ level ☐ rough

Is the DRIVEWAY negotiable? ☐ yes ☐ no
Is the GARAGE accessible? ☐ yes ☐ no

Entrance

Accessible entrances
- ☐ front ☐ side
- ☐ back

Steps
- number _____
- height of each _____
- width _____
- depth _____

Are there HANDRAILS? ☐ yes ☐ no

If yes, where are they located? ☐ left ☐ right

HANDRAIL height from step surface? _____

If no, how much room is available for HANDRAILS? _____

Are landings negotiable? ☐ yes ☐ no

Briefly describe any problems with LANDINGS:_____
_____

Ramps ☐ yes ☐ no
- ☐ front ☐ back
- height _____
- width _____
- length _____

Are there HANDRAILS? ☐ yes ☐ no
If yes, where are they located? ☐ left ☐ right height_____
If no ramp, how much room is available for one? _____

Porch
- width _____
- length _____
- Level at threshold? ☐ yes ☐ no

Door
- width _____
- threshold height _____ Negotiable? ☐ yes ☐ no
- ☐ swing in
- ☐ swing out
- ☐ sliding

Interior

Living Room

Is furniture arranged for easy maneuverability? ☐ yes ☐ no

Is frequently used furniture accessible ☐ yes ☐ no

Type of floor covering: _____

Comments _____

Hallways

Can wheelchair or walking aide be maneuvered in hallway? ☐ yes ☐ no
- hall width _____
- door width _____
- Sharp turns ☐ yes ☐ no

Steps? ☐ yes ☐ no
- number

Are there HANDRAILS? ☐ yes ☐ no
If yes, where are they located? ☐ left ☐ right height_____

Bedroom
- ☐ single
- ☐ shared

Is there room for a W/C? ☐ yes ☐ no

Door:
- width _____
- threshold height _____ Negotiable? ☐ yes ☐ no
- ☐ swing in
- ☐ swing out

Bed:
- ☐ twin
- ☐ double
- ☐ queen
- ☐ king
- ☐ hospital bed

Overall height _____ Accessible? ☐ yes ☐ no

Would hospital bed fit into room if needed? ☐ yes ☐ no

Clothing:

Are drawers accessible? ☐ yes ☐ no
☐ on right ☐ on left

Is closet accessible? ☐ yes ☐ no
☐ on right ☐ on left

Comments: _____

Bathroom

Door:
- width _____
- threshold height _____ Negotiable? ☐ yes ☐ no

Tub:
- height, floor-rim _____
- height, tub bottom rim _____
- tub width inside _____
- glass doors? ☐ yes ☐ no
- width of tub doors _____
- overhead shower? ☐ yes ☐ no
- Is tub accessible? ☐ yes ☐ no

Stall Shower: ☐ yes ☐ no
- door width _____
- height of bottom rim _____
- accessible? ☐ yes ☐ no

Sink:
- height _____
- faucet type _____
- ☐ open
- ☐ closed
- accessible? ☐ yes ☐ no

Toilet:
- height from floor _____
- location of toilet paper _____
- distance from toilet to side wall L _____
  R _____

Grabbars: ☐ yes ☐ no
- Location _____

Comments: _____

Kitchen

Door:
- width _____
- threshold height _____ Negotiable? ☐ yes ☐ no

Stove:
- height _____
- Location of controls ☐ front ☐ back
- Is stove accessible for use? ☐ yes ☐ no

Oven:
- Height from floor to door hinge & door handle _____
- Location of oven _____

Sink:
- Will w/c fit underneath? ☐ yes ☐ no
- Type of faucets _____

Cupboards:
- accessible from w/c? ☐ yes ☐ no

Refrigerator:
- hinges on ☐ left ☐ right
- accessible from w/c? ☐ yes ☐ no

Switches / Outlets:
- accessible? ☐ yes ☐ no

Kitchen Table:
- height from floor _____
- accessible? ☐ yes ☐ no

Comments: _____

Laundry

Door: width _____
- threshold height _____ Negotiable? ☐ yes ☐ no

Steps: ☐ yes ☐ no
- number _____
- height _____
- width _____

Are there HANDRAILS? ☐ yes ☐ no
If yes, where are they located? ☐ left ☐ right height_____

FIG. 26-3 Home visit checklist. (Adapted from *Occupational/physical therapy home evaluation form,* Ralph K. Davies Medical Center, San Francisco, and *Occupational therapy home evaluation form,* Alta Bates Hospital, Albany, Calif., 1993.)

Washer:
- ☐ Topload
- ☐ Front load
- accessible?   ☐ yes   ☐ no

Dryer:
- ☐ Topload
- ☐ Front load
- accessible?   ☐ yes   ☐ no

Safety

Throw rugs
☐ yes   ☐ no
Location _____

Phone
accessible?   ☐ yes   ☐ no
Location _____

Emergency phone numbers
☐ yes   ☐ no
Location _____

Mailbox
accessible?   ☐ yes   ☐ no
Location _____

Thermostat
accessible?   ☐ yes   ☐ no
Location _____

Electric Outlets / switches
accessible?   ☐ yes   ☐ no

Imperfect floor?
☐ yes   ☐ no
Location _____

Sharp Edged furniture?
☐ yes   ☐ no
Location _____

Insulated hot water pipes: ☐ yes   ☐ no
Location _____

Cluttered areas?
☐ yes   ☐ no
Location _____

Fire extinguisher?
☐ yes   ☐ no
Location _____

Equipment present: _____
_____
_____

Problem list: _____
_____
_____
_____

Recommendations for modifications: _____
_____
_____
_____
_____

Equipment Recommendations: _____
_____
_____

FIG. 26-3   *cont'd.* For legend see opposite page.

safely or independently step over the edge of the tub. Installation of a handheld shower increases access to the water and also eliminates risky turns and standing while bathing.

When the home evaluation is completed, the therapist should write a report summarizing the information on the form and describing the client's performance in the home. The report should conclude with a summary of the environmental barriers and the client's functional limitations encountered. Recommendations should include equipment or alterations with specifics in terms of size, building specifications, costs, and sources. Recommendations may also include further functional goals to improve independence in the individual's home environment.

These recommendations are carefully reviewed with the client and family. This review is done with tact and diplomacy in a way that gives them options and freedom to refuse or consider alternative possibilities. Family finances may limit carrying out needed changes. The social worker may be involved in working out funding for needed equipment and alterations, and the client should be made aware of this service when cost is discussed.[27]

The therapist should include recommendations regarding the feasibility of the client's discharge to the home environment or remaining in or managing the home alone, if applicable. If there is a question regarding the client's ability to return home safely and independently, the home evaluation summary should include the functional skills the client needs to return home.

If a home visit is not possible, much of the information can be gained by interviewing the client and family member(s) following a trial home visit. The family member or caregiver may be instructed to complete the home visit checklist and provide photographs or sketches of the rooms and their arrangements. Problems encountered by the client during the home visit should be discussed and the necessary recommendations for their solution made, as described earlier.[27]

COMMUNITY LIVING SKILLS
Money and Financial Management

If the client is to resume management of money and financial matters independently, a cognitive and perceptual evaluation that accurately assesses these skills should be implemented. Because some persons with physical disabilities also have concurrent involvement of cognition and perception, the level of impairment should be determined. Caregivers may require training if the role of financial manager is new and must be assumed. The client may be capable of handling only small amounts of money or may need retraining with activities that require money management, such as shopping, balancing a checkbook, or making a budget. If a physical limitation is involved, adaptive writing devices can be introduced to allow the client to handle the paperwork aspects of money management.

Community Mobility

Some clients are fortunate enough to be able to drive and to adapt their own vehicle or purchase an adapted van

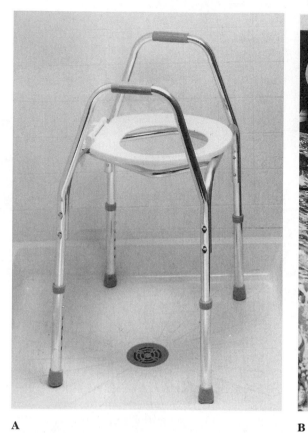

A

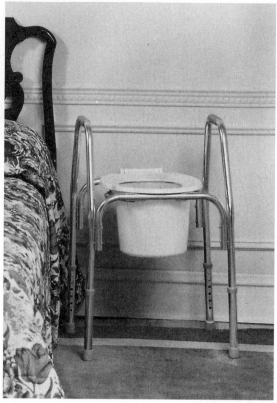

B

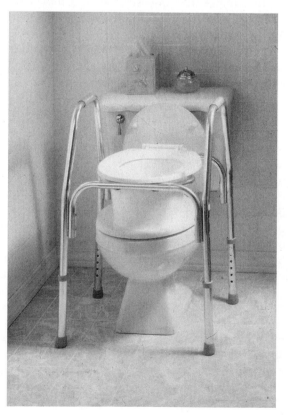

C

FIG. 26-4   All-purpose commode is provided by Sammons, Inc., a BISSELL Inc. Company. **A,** In shower. **B,** At bedside. **C,** Over toilet.

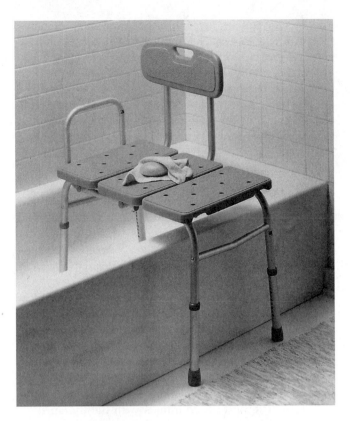

FIG. 26-5   Transfer tub bench is provided by Sammons, Inc., a BISSELL Inc. Company.

(Section 2 of this chapter). The client who does not meet these criteria must learn to use public transportation or to get around the community on foot or in a wheelchair. In this case, the occupational therapist must assess the client's physical, perceptual, cognitive, and social capabilities to be independent and safe with community mobility.

Physical capabilities to be considered are (1) whether the client has the endurance to be mobile in the community without fatigue, and (2) whether the client is sufficiently independent with the walker, cane, crutch, or wheelchair skills and transfers needed to go beyond the home environment. These skills include managing uneven pavement, curbs, and inclines and crossing the street. Other skills to be evaluated before considering community mobility are how to (1) handle money, (2) carry objects in a wheelchair or with a walker, and (3) manage toileting in a public restroom.

Cognitive skills require the client to be geographically oriented; if taking a bus, to know how to read a schedule and map or know how to get directions; and to have good problem-solving skills if a problem should occur in the community. If the disability is new, the client may be developing new social skills, which will initially be stretched to the limit once out in the community — for example, learning how to be assertive to get an accessible table at a restaurant, getting assistance with unreachable items in the grocery store, and getting comfortable with a new body image within the able-bodied community.

The client's community environment also needs to be assessed. For example, is the neighborhood safe enough for an individual who might be vulnerable because of physical limitations? What is the terrain like? Are there curb cut-outs? Are the sidewalks smooth and even? How far away are the closest store and bus stop?

Accessibility of community transportation should also be considered. Some communities have door-to-door cab and van service, which have certain restrictions. Some of these restrictions include the need to arrange transportation one week in advance, the ability to get out the front door and to the curb independently, and the ability to transfer independently into the vehicle. If a public bus is to be used by the client, he must learn how to use the electric lifts and how to lock a wheelchair into place. Because all bus stops are not wheelchair-accessible, the neighboring bus stops need to be evaluated.

Community mobility requires preplanning by the occupational therapist and the client, accurate assessment of the client's abilities and knowledge of potential physical, cognitive, and social barriers that may be encountered. A valuable resource by Armstrong and Lauzen, *Community Integration Program,*[2] provides practical treatment protocols to establish a community living skills program. Attaining independence in community mobility is worth the investment because it allows the client to expand life tasks beyond those in the home and interact with the community.

HEALTH MANAGEMENT

Health management includes the client's ability to understand the medical condition and make decisions to maintain good health. Some very practical aspects of health management include the client's ability to handle medications, know when to call a physician, and how to make medical appointments. The evaluation of the client's ability to perform these activities may not be completed solely by the occupational therapist but will probably include other team members such as the nurse and the physician.

Performance components must be assessed in light of the skills required for each task. The occupational therapy assessment can be helpful in determining which aspects of the task need to be modified for the client to be independent. For example, the occupational therapist can work jointly with a nurse to ensure that a client with hemiplegia and diabetes can manage the insulin shots. The OT evaluation considers the client's cognitive and perceptual abilities to make judgments about drawing the insulin out of the bottle, measuring the insulin, and injecting the insulin. Physical concerns are how to stabilize the insulin bottle and handle the syringe with one hand. Other medication management may involve only how the client is able to open the medication and measure it if liquid.

The occupational therapist may also evaluate and train the client in other skills. Examples include using the phone, finding the appropriate phone numbers, and providing the needed information to make a medical appointment.

Health management is an issue for the client and entire health care team. The occupational therapist plays an important role because of the scope of the ADL and I-ADL evaluation, which may identify and help resolve problems related to health management.

ADL AND I-ADL TRAINING

If, after evaluation, it is determined that ADL/I-ADL training is to be initiated, it is important to establish appropriate short- and long-term objectives, based on the evaluation and on the client's priorities and potential for independence. The following sequence of training for self-care activities is suggested: feeding, grooming, continence, transfer skills, toileting, undressing, dressing, and bathing. This sequence is based on the normal development of self-care independence in children.[27] It provides a good guide but may have to be modified to accommodate the specific dysfunction and the capabilities, limitations, and personal priorities of the client.

The occupational therapist should estimate which ADL/I-ADL tasks are possible and which are impossible for the client to achieve. The therapist should explore with the client the use of alternate methods of performing the activities and the use of any assistive devices that may be helpful. He or she should determine for which tasks the client requires assistance and how much should be given. It may not be possible to estimate these factors until training is underway.

The ADL/I-ADL training program may be graded by beginning with a few simple tasks and gradually increasing the number and complexity of tasks. Training should progress from dependent to assisted to supervised to, independent, with or without assistive devices.[27] The rate at which grading can occur depends on the client's potential for recovery, endurance, skills, and motivation.

METHODS OF TEACHING ADL

The methods of teaching the client to perform daily living tasks must be tailored to suit each client's learning style and ability. The client who is alert and grasps instructions quickly may be able to perform an entire process after a brief demonstration and verbal instruction. Clients who have perceptual problems, poor memory, and difficulty following instructions of any kind require a more concrete, step-by-step approach, reducing the amount of assistance gradually as success is achieved. For these persons it is important to break down the activity into small steps and progress through them slowly, one at a time. Slow demonstration by the therapist of the task or step in the same plane and in the same manner in which the client is expected to perform is very helpful. Verbal instructions to accompany the demonstration

may or may not be helpful, depending on the client's receptive language skills and ability to process and integrate two modes of sensory information simultaneously.

Touching body parts to be moved, dressed, bathed, or positioned, passive movement of the part through the desired pattern to achieve a step or a task, and gentle manual guidance through the task are helpful tactile and kinesthetic modes of instruction (see Chapters 7 and 25). These techniques can augment or replace demonstration and verbal instruction, depending on the client's best avenues of learning. It is necessary to perform a step or complete task repetitiously to achieve skill, speed, and retention of learning. Tasks may be repeated several times during the same training session, if time and the client's physical and emotional tolerance allow, or they may be repeated on a daily basis until desired retention or level of skill is achieved.

The process of "backward chaining" can be used in teaching ADL skills. In this method the therapist assists the client until the last step of the process is reached. The client then performs this step independently, which affords a sense of success and completion. When the last step is mastered, the therapist assists until the last two steps are reached and the client then completes these two steps. The process continues with the therapist offering less and less assistance and the client performing successive steps of the task, from last to first, independently. This method is particularly useful in training clients with brain damage.[27]

Before beginning training in any ADL, the therapist must prepare by providing adequate space and arranging equipment, materials, and furniture for maximal convenience and safety. The therapist should be thoroughly familiar with the task to be performed and any special methods or assistive devices that will be used in its performance. The practitioner should be able to perform the task, as he or she expects the client to perform it, skillfully. After preparation the activity is presented to the client, usually in one or more modes of guidance, demonstration, and verbal instruction described earlier. The client then performs the activity either along with the therapist or immediately after being shown, with the amount of supervision and assistance required. Performance is modified and corrected as needed, and the process is repeated to ensure learning.

Because other staff or family members are frequently the individuals reinforcing the newly learned skills, family training is critical to reinforce learning and ensure the client carries over the skills from previous treatment sessions. In the final phase of instruction, when the client has mastered one or more tasks, he or she is asked to perform them independently. The therapist should check on performance in progress and later arrange to check on adequacy of performance and carry-over of learning with nursing personnel, the caregiver, or the supervising family members.[12]

RECORDING PROGRESS IN ADL PERFORMANCE

The ADL checklists used to record performance on the initial evaluation usually have one or more spaces for recording changes in abilities and results of reevaluation during the training process. The sample checklist given earlier in this chapter is so designed and filled out (Fig. 26-1). Progress is usually summarized for inclusion in the medical record. The progress record should summarize changes in the client's abilities and current level of independence and should also estimate the client's potential for further independence, attitude, motivation for ADL training, and future goals for the ADL program. The progress record should also relate the client's current level of independence or level of assistance needed to discharge plans. For example, if a client continues to need moderate assistance with self-care he or she may need to hire an attendant, or the occupational therapist may justify a need for ongoing treatment when the client has potential for further independence.

SPECIFIC ADL TECHNIQUES

In many instances specific techniques to solve specific ADL problems are not possible. Rather the occupational therapist may have to explore a variety of methods or assistive devices to reach a solution. It is sometimes necessary for the therapist to design a special device, method, splint, or piece of equipment to make a particular activity possible for the client to perform. Many of the assistive devices available today through rehabilitation equipment companies were first conceived and made by occupational therapists and clients. Many of the special methods used to perform specific activities also evolved through trial-and-error approaches of therapists and their clients. Clients often have good suggestions for therapists, because they live with the limitation and are confronted regularly with the need to adapt the performance of daily tasks.

The purpose of the following summary of techniques is to give the reader some general ideas about how to solve ADL problems for specific classifications of dysfunctions. The reader is referred to the references at the end of this chapter for more specific instruction in ADL methods.

LIMITED ROM AND/OR STRENGTH

The major problem for persons with limited joint ROM is to compensate for the lack of reach and joint excursion through such means as environmental adaptation and assistive devices. Individuals who lack muscle strength may require some of the same devices or techniques to compensate and to conserve energy. Some adaptations and devices are outlined here.[20,22,24,27]

Dressing Activities

The following are general suggestions for facilitating dressing:

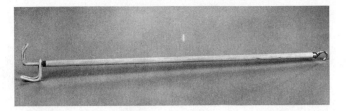

FIG. 26-6   Dressing stick or reacher is provided by Sammons, Inc., a BISSELL Inc. Company.

1. Use front-opening garments, one size larger than needed and made of fabrics that have some stretch.
2. Use dressing sticks with a garter on one end and a neoprene-covered coat hook on the other (Fig. 26-6) for pushing and pulling garments off and on feet and legs and to push a shirt or blouse over the head. Use a pair of dowels with a cup hook on end of each to pull socks on if a loop tape is sewn to the tops of the socks.
3. Use larger buttons or zippers with a loop on the pull tab.
4. Replace buttons, snaps, hooks, and eyes with Velcro or zippers (for those clients who cannot manage traditional fastenings).
5. Eliminate the need to bend to tie shoelaces or to use finger joints in this fine activity by using elastic shoelaces or other adapted shoe fasteners.
6. Facilitate donning stockings without bending to the feet by using stocking aids made of garters attached to long webbing straps or by buying those that are commercially available (Fig. 26-7).
7. Use one of several types of commercially available buttonhooks (Fig. 26-8) if finger ROM is limited.
8. Use reachers (Fig. 26-9) for picking up socks and shoes, arranging clothes, removing clothes from hangers, picking up objects on the floor, and donning pants.

Eating Activities

The following are assistive devices that can facilitate feeding:

1. Built-up handles on eating utensils can accommodate limited grasp or prehension (Fig. 26-10).

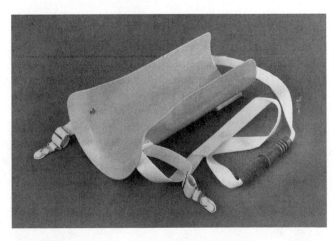

FIG. 26-7   Sock aid is provided by Sammons, Inc., a BISSELL Inc. Company.

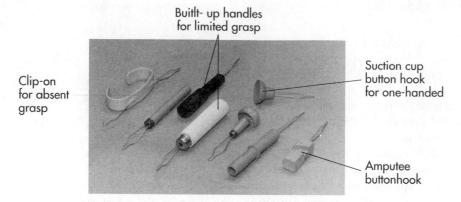

FIG. 26-8   Buttonhooks to accommodate limited or special types of grasp or amputation.

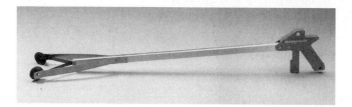

FIG. 26-9   Extended handled reacher.

2. Elongated or specially curved handles on spoons and forks may be needed to reach the mouth. A swivel spoon or spoon-fork combination can compensate for limited supination (Fig. 26-11).
3. Long plastic straws and straw clips on glasses or cups can be used if neck, elbow, or shoulder ROM limits hand-to-mouth motion or if grasp is inadequate to hold the cup or glass.
4. Universal cuffs or utensil holders can be used if grasp is very limited and built-up handles do not work (Fig. 26-12).
5. Plate guards or scoop dishes may be useful to prevent food from slipping off the plate.

Hygiene and Grooming

Environmental adaptations that can facilitate bathing and grooming are:

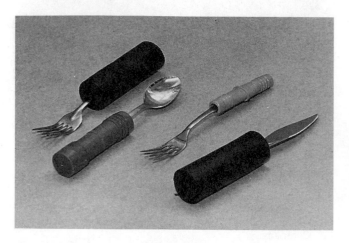

FIG. 26-10   Eating utensils with built-up handles.

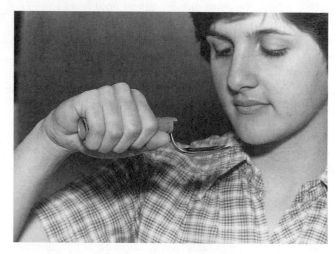

FIG. 26-11   Swivel spoon compensates for limited supination or incoordination.

1. A handheld shower head on flexible hose for bathing and shampooing hair can eliminate the need to stand in the shower and offers the user control of the direction of the spray. The handle can be built up or adapted for limited grasp.
2. A long-handled bath brush or sponge with a soap holder (Fig. 26-13) or long cloth scrubber can allow the user to reach legs, feet, and back. A wash mitt (Fig. 26-14) and soap on a rope can aid limited grasp.
3. A position-adjustable hair dryer described by Feldmeier and Poole[8] may be helpful for those who prefer a hair style more elaborate than one that can be air-dried. This device is useful for clients with limited ROM, upper extremity

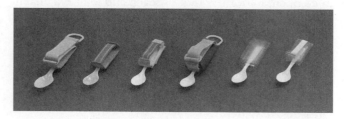

FIG. 26-12   Utensil holders/universal cuffs are provided by Sammons, Inc., a BISSELL Inc. Company.

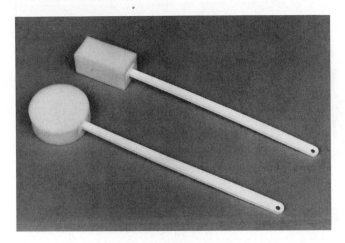

FIG. 26-13   Long-handled bath sponges are provided by Sammons, Inc., a BISSELL Inc. Company.

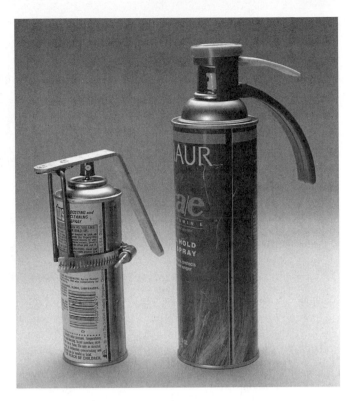

FIG. 26-15   Spray can adapters are provided by Sammons, Inc., a BISSELL Inc. Company.

weakness, incoordination, or use of only one upper extremity. The dryer is adapted from a desk lamp with spring-balanced arms and a tension control knob at each joint. The lamp is removed and the hair dryer is fastened to the spring-balanced arms. The device is mounted on a table or counter top and can be adjusted for various heights and direction of air flow. It frees the client's hands to manage brushes or combs used to style the hair. The reader is referred to the original source for specifications for constructing this device.[8]

4. Long handles on comb, brush, toothbrush, lipstick, mascara brush, and safety or electric razor may be useful for limited hand-to-head or hand-to-face movements. Extensions may be constructed from inexpensive wooden dowels or pieces of PVC pipe found in local hardware stores.

5. Spray deodorant, hair spray, and spray powder or perfume can extend the reach by the distance the material sprays.

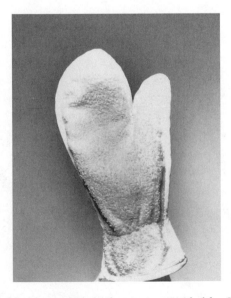

FIG. 26-14   Terry cloth bath mitt is provided by Sammons, Inc., a BISSELL Inc. Company.

Special adaptations may be required by some persons to operate the spray mechanism (Fig. 26-15).

6. Electric toothbrushes and a Water-Pik may be easier to manage than a standard toothbrush.

7. A short reacher can extend reach for using toilet paper. Several types of toilet aids are available in catalogues that sell assistive devices.

8. Dressing sticks can be used to pull garments up after using the toilet. An alternative is the use of a long piece of elastic or webbing with garters on each end that can be hung around the neck and fastened to pants or panties, preventing them from slipping to the floor during use of the toilet.

9. Safety rails (Fig. 26-16) can be used for bathtub transfers, and safety mats or strips can be placed in the bathtub bottom to prevent slipping.

10. A transfer tub bench (shown previously in Fig. 26-5), shower stool, or regular chair set in the bathtub or shower stall can eliminate the need to sit on the bathtub bottom or stand to shower, thus increasing safety.

11. Grab bars can be installed to prevent falls and ease transfers.

Communication and Environmental Hardware Adaptations

The following are examples of environmental adaptations that can facilitate communication and hardware management:

1. Extended or built-up handles on faucets can accommodate limited grasp.

2. Telephones should be placed within easy reach. A clip-type receiver holder (Fig. 26-17), extended receiver holder, speaker phone, or voice-activated phone (Fig. 26-18) may be

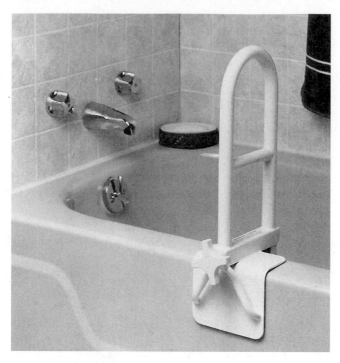

FIG. 26-16   Bathtub safety rail is provided by Sammons, Inc., a BISSELL Inc. Company.

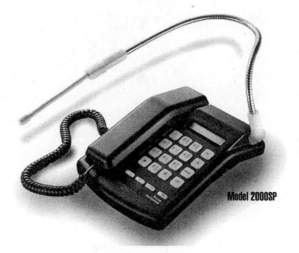

FIG. 26-18   Voice activated speaker phone. (Reproduced with permission of Temasek Telephone Inc., 260 E. Grand Ave. #19, So. San Francisco, CA 94080.)

necessary. A dialing stick or push-button phone are other adaptations.

3. Built-up pens and pencils to accommodate limited grasp and prehension can be used. A Wanchik writer and several other commercially available or custom fabricated writing aids are possible (Fig. 26-19).
4. Electric typewriters or personal computers and book holders can facilitate communication for those with limited or painful joints.
5. Lever-type doorknob extensions (Fig. 26-20), car door openers, and adapted key holders can compensate for hand limitations.

Mobility and Transfer Skills

The individual who has limited ROM without significant muscle weakness may benefit from the following assistive devices:

1. A glider chair that is operated by the feet can facilitate transportation if hip, hand, and arm motion is limited.

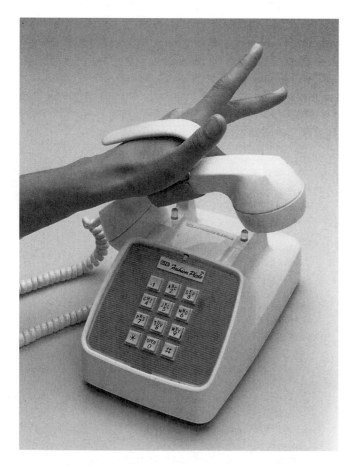

FIG. 26-17   Telephone clip holder is provided by Sammons, Inc., a BISSELL Inc. Company.

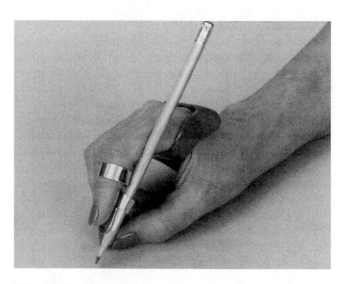

FIG. 26-19   Wanchik writing aid is provided by Sammons, Inc., a BISSELL Inc. Company.

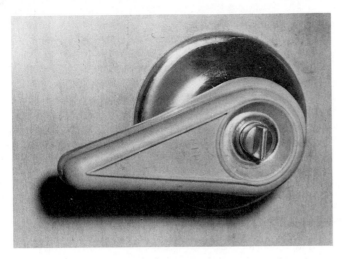

FIG. 26-20 Rubber doorknob extension is provided by Sammons, Inc., a BISSELL Inc. Company.

2. Platform crutches can prevent stress on hand or finger joints and accommodate limited grasp.
3. Enlarged grips on crutches, canes, and walkers can accommodate limited grasp.
4. A raised toilet seat can be used if hip and knee motion is limited.
5. A walker with padded grips and forearm troughs can be used if marked hand, forearm, or elbow joint limitations are present.
6. A walker or crutch bag or basket can facilitate the carrying of objects.

Home Management Activities

Home management activities can be facilitated by a wide variety of environmental adaptations, assistive devices, energy conservation methods, and work simplification techniques.[16,24] The principles of joint protection are essential for those with rheumatoid arthritis. These principles are discussed in Chapter 34. The following are suggestions to facilitate home management for persons with limited ROM:

1. Store frequently used items on the first shelves of cabinets just above and below counters or on counters where possible.
2. Use a high stool to work comfortably at counter height or attach a drop-leaf table to the wall for planning and meal preparation area if a wheelchair is used.
3. Use a utility cart of comfortable height to transport several items at once.
4. Use reachers to get lightweight items (for example, cereal box) from high shelves.
5. Stabilize mixing bowls and dishes with nonslip mats.
6. Use lightweight utensils, such as plastic or aluminum bowls and aluminum pots.
7. Use electric can openers and electric mixers.
8. Use electric scissors or adapted loop scissors to open packages (Fig. 26-21).
9. Eliminate bending by using extended and flexible plastic handles on dust mops, brooms and dustpans.
10. Use adapted knives for cutting (Fig. 26-22).
11. Use pull-out shelves to organize cupboards and eliminate bending.

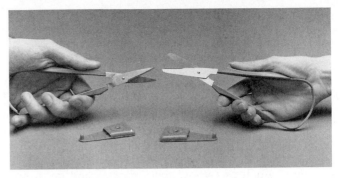

FIG. 26-21 Loop scissors are provided by Sammons, Inc., a BISSELL Inc. Company.

12. Eliminate bending by using wall ovens, countertop broilers, and microwave ovens.
13. Eliminate leaning and bending by using a top-loading automatic washer and elevated dryer. Wheelchair users can benefit from front-loading appliances.
14. Use an adjustable ironing board to make it possible to sit while ironing.
15. Elevate the playpen and diaper table and use a bathinette or a plastic tub on the kitchen counter for bathing to reduce the amount of bending and reaching for the ambulatory mother during child care. The crib mattress can be in a raised position until the child is 3 or 4 months of age.
16. Use larger and looser fitting garments with Velcro fastenings on children.
17. Use a reacher to pick up clothing and children's toys.

PROBLEMS OF INCOORDINATION[1,20,27]

Incoordination in the form of tremors or ataxia or athetoid or choreiform movements can result from a variety of central nervous system (CNS) disorders, such as Parkinson disease, multiple sclerosis, cerebral palsy, and head injuries. The major problems encountered in ADL performance are safety and adequate stability of gait, body parts, and objects to complete the tasks.

The degree of incoordinated movement may be influenced by fatigue, emotional factors, and fears. The

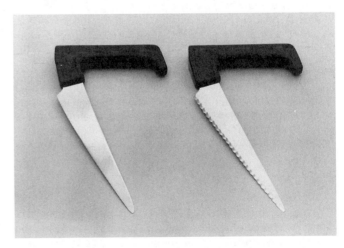

FIG. 26-22 Right-angle knife is provided by Sammons, Inc., a BISSELL Inc. Company.

client must be taught appropriate energy conservation and work simplification techniques along with appropriate work pacing and safety methods to avoid the fatigue and apprehension that could increase incoordination and affect performance.

When muscle weakness is not a major deficit for the individual with incoordination, the use of weighted devices can help with stabilization of objects. A Velcro-fastened weight can be attached to the client's arm to decrease ataxia, or the device being used can be weighted, such as eating utensils, pens, and cups. Another technique that can be used throughout all ADL tasks is stabilizing the involved upper extremity. This technique is accomplished by propping the elbow on a counter or table top, pivoting from the elbow and only moving the forearm, wrist and hand in the activity. Stabilizing the arm reduces some of the incoordination and may allow the individual to accomplish gross and fine motor movements without assistive devices.

Dressing Activities

Potential dressing difficulties can be reduced by using the following adaptations:

1. Front-opening garments that fit loosely can facilitate donning and removing garments.
2. Large buttons, Velcro, or zippers with loops on the tab can facilitate opening and closing fasteners. A buttonhook with a large, weighted handle may be helpful.
3. Elastic shoelaces, Velcro closures, other adapted shoe closures, and slip-on shoes eliminate the need for bow tying.
4. Trousers with elastic tops for women or Velcro closures for men are easier to manage than those with hooks, buttons, and zippers.
5. Brassieres with front openings or Velcro replacements for the usual hook and eye may facilitate donning and removing this garment. A slipover elastic-type brassiere or bra-slip combination also may eliminate the need to manage brassiere fastenings. Regular brassieres may be fastened in front at waist level, then slipped around to the back and the arms put into the straps, which are then worked up over the shoulders.
6. Clip-on ties can be used by men.
7. Dressing should be performed while sitting on or in bed or in a wheelchair or chair with arms to avoid balance problems.

Eating Activities

For clients with problems of incoordination, eating can be a challenge. Lack of control during eating is not only frustrating but can cause embarrassment and social rejection. Therefore it is important to make eating safe, pleasurable, and as neat as possible. The following are some suggestions for achieving this goal:

1. Use plate stabilizers, such as nonskid mats, suction bases, or even damp dishtowels.
2. Use a plate guard or scoop dish to prevent pushing food off the plate. The plate guard can be carried away from home and clipped to any ordinary dinner plate (Fig. 26-23).
3. Prevent spills during the plate-to-mouth excursion by using weighted or swivel utensils to offer stability. Weighted cuffs

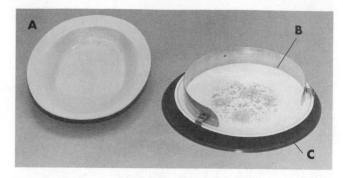

FIG. 26-23   **A,** Scoop dish. **B,** Plate with plate guard. **C,** Nonskid mat.

may be placed on the forearm to decrease involuntary movement (Fig. 26-24).
4. Use long plastic straws with a straw clip on a glass or cup with a weighted bottom to eliminate the need to carry the glass or cup to the mouth, thus avoiding spills. Plastic cups with covers and spouts may be used for the same purpose.
5. Use a resistance or friction-type arm brace similar to a mobile arm support, which was shown by Holser and associates[11] to help control patterns of involuntary movement during feeding activities of adults with cerebral palsy and athetosis. Such a brace may help many clients with severe incoordination to achieve some degree of independence in feeding.

Hygiene and Grooming

Stabilization and handling of toilet articles may be achieved by the following suggestions:

1. Articles such as razor, lipstick, and toothbrush can be attached to a cord if frequent dropping is a problem. An electric toothbrush may be more easily managed than a regular one.
2. Weighted wrist cuffs may be helpful during the finer hygiene activities, such as applying make-up, shaving, and hair care.

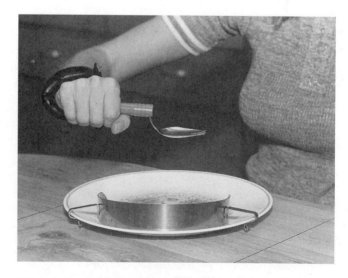

FIG. 26-24   Weighted wrist cuff and swivel utensil can sometimes compensate for incoordination or involuntary motion and limited supination.

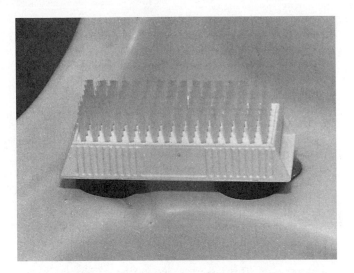

FIG. 26-25 Suction brush attached to bathroom sink for dentures or fingernails. Can also be used in kitchen to wash vegetables and fruit.

3. The position-adjustable hair dryer described earlier for clients with limited ROM can be useful for clients with incoordination as well.[8]
4. An electric razor rather than a blade razor offers stability and safety. A strap around the razor and hand can prevent dropping.
5. A suction brush attached to the sink or counter can be used for nail or denture care (Fig. 26-25).
6. Soap should be on a rope and can be worn around the neck or hung over a bathtub or shower fixture during bath or shower to keep it within easy reach. A leg from a pair of pantyhose with a bar of soap in the toe may be tied over a faucet to keep soap within reach and will stretch for use.
7. An emery board or small piece of wood with fine sandpaper glued to it can be fastened to the table top for filing nails. A nail clipper can also be stabilized in the same manner.
8. Large roll-on deodorants are preferable to sprays or creams.
9. Sanitary pads that stick to undergarments may be easier to manage than tampons.
10. A bath mitt with a pocket to hold the soap can be used for washing and eliminates the need for frequent soaping and rinsing and wringing a washcloth.
11. Nonskid mats should be used inside and outside the bathtub during bathing. Their suction bases should be fastened securely to the floor and bathtub before use. Safety grab bars should be installed on the wall next to the bathtub or fastened to the edge of the bathtub. A bathtub seat or shower chair provides more safety than standing while showering or transferring to a bathtub bottom. Many uncoordinated clients require supervisory assistance during this hazardous activity. Sponge bathing while seated at a bathroom sink may substitute for bathing or showering several times a week.

Communication and Environmental Hardware Adaptations

The following adaptations can facilitate communication for clients who have incoordination:

1. Doorknobs may be managed more easily if adapted with lever-type handles or covered with rubber or friction tape (Fig. 26-20).
2. A holder for a telephone receiver, large button phones, or speaker phones may be helpful.
3. Writing may be managed by using a weighted, enlarged pencil or pen. An electric typewriter or computer with a keyboard guard is a very helpful aid to communication. A computer mouse may frequently be substituted for the keyboard.
4. Keys may be managed by placing them on an adapted key holder that is rigid and offers more leverage for turning the key. Inserting the key in the keyhole may be very difficult, however, unless the incoordination is relatively mild.
5. Extended lever-type faucets are easier to manage than knobs that turn and push-pull spigots. To prevent burns during bathing and kitchen activities, cold water should be turned on first and hot water added gradually.
6. Lamps that require a wall switch only, light touch to turn on, or a signal-type device can eliminate turning a small switch.

Mobility and Transfers

Clients with problems of incoordination may use a variety of ambulation aids, depending on the type and severity of incoordination. In degenerative diseases it is sometimes necessary to help the client recognize the need for and to accept ambulation aids. This problem may mean graduation from a cane to crutches to a walker and finally to a wheelchair for some persons. Clients with incoordination can improve stability and mobility by the following suggestions:

1. Instead of lifting objects, slide them on floors or counters.
2. Use suitable ambulation aids.
3. Use a utility cart, preferably a custom-made cart that is heavy and has some friction on the wheels.
4. Remove doorsills, throw rugs, and thick carpeting.
5. Install banisters on indoor and outdoor staircases.
6. Substitute ramps for stairs wherever possible.

Home Management Activities[16,20,27]

It is important for the occupational therapist to make a careful assessment of homemaking activities performance to determine (1) which activities can be done safely, (2) which activities can be done safely if modified or adapted, and (3) which activities cannot be done adequately or safely and should be assigned to someone else. The major problems are stabilization of foods and equipment to prevent spilling and accidents and the safe handling of appliances, pots, pans, and household tools to prevent cuts, burns, bruises, electric shock, and falls. The following are suggestions for the facilitation of home management tasks:

1. Use a wheelchair and wheelchair lapboard, even if ambulation is possible with devices. The wheelchair saves energy and increases stability if balance and gait are unsteady.
2. If possible, use convenience and prepared foods to eliminate as many processes as possible, for example peeling, chopping, slicing, and mixing.
3. Use easy-open containers or store foods in plastic containers once opened. A jar opener is also useful.
4. Use heavy utensils, mixing bowls, and pots and pans to increase stability.
5. Use nonskid mats on work surfaces.

6. Use electrical appliances such as crock pots, electric fry pans, toaster-ovens, and microwave or convection ovens because they are safer than using the range.

7. Use a blender and countertop mixer, because they are safer than handheld mixers and easier than mixing with a spoon or whisk.

8. If possible, adjust work heights of counters, sink, and range to minimize leaning, bending, reaching, and lifting, whether the client is standing or using a wheelchair.

9. Use long oven mitts, which are safer than potholders.

10. Use pots, pans, casserole dishes, and appliances with bilateral handles, because they may be easier to manage than those with one handle.

11. Use a cutting board with stainless steel nails (Fig. 26-26) to stabilize meats and vegetables while cutting. When not in use the nails should be covered with a large cork. The bottom of the board should have suction cups or should be covered with stair tread, or the board should be placed on a nonskid mat to prevent slippage when in use.

12. Use heavy dinnerware, which may be easier to handle, because it offers stability and control to the distal part of the upper extremity. On the other hand, unbreakable dinnerware may be more practical if dropping and breakage are problems.

13. Cover the sink, utility cart, and countertops with protective rubber mats or mesh matting to stabilize items.

14. Use a serrated knife for cutting and chopping, because it is easier to control.

15. Use a steamer basket or deep-fry basket for preparing boiled foods to eliminate the need to carry and drain pots with hot liquids in them.

16. Use tongs to turn foods during cooking and to serve foods, because they may offer more control and stability than a fork, spatula, or serving spoon.

17. Use blunt-ended loop scissors to open packages.

18. Vacuum with a heavy upright cleaner, which may be easier for the ambulatory client. The wheelchair user may be able to manage a lightweight tank-type vacuum cleaner or electric broom.

19. Use dust mitts for dusting.

20. Eliminate fragile knickknacks, unstable lamps, and dainty doilies.

21. Eliminate ironing by using no-iron fabrics or a timed dryer or by assigning this task to other members of the household.

22. Use front-loading washers, a laundry cart on wheels, and premeasured detergents, bleaches, and fabric softeners.

23. Sit while working with an infant and use foam-rubber bath aids, an infant bath seat, and a wide, padded dressing table with safety straps with Velcro fastening to offer enough stability for bathing, dressing, and diapering an infant. (Child care may not be possible unless the incoordination is mild.)

24. Use disposable diapers with tape fasteners, because they are easier to manage than cloth diapers and pins.

25. Do not feed the infant with a spoon or fork unless the incoordination is very mild or does not affect the upper extremities. This task may need to be performed by another household member.

26. Provide clothing for the child that is large, loose, with Velcro fastenings, and made of nonslippery stretch fabrics.

HEMIPLEGIA OR USE OF ONLY ONE UPPER EXTREMITY[1,16,20,27]

Suggestions for performing daily living skills apply to persons with hemiplegia, unilateral upper extremity amputations, and temporary disorders, such as fractures, burns, and peripheral neuropathic conditions which can result in the dysfunction of one upper extremity.

The client with hemiplegia requires specialized methods of teaching and many have greater difficulty in learning and performing one-handed skills than those with orthopedic or lower motor neuron dysfunction. Because the trunk and leg are involved, as well as the arm, ambulation and balance difficulties may exist. Also, sensory, perceptual, cognitive, and speech disorders may be present in a mild to severe degree. These disorders affect the ability to learn and retain learning and performance. Finally, the presence of motor and ideational apraxia sometimes seen in this group of clients can have a profound effect on the potential for learning new motor skills and remembering old ones. Therefore, the client with normal perception and cognition and the use of one upper extremity may learn the techniques quickly and easily. The client with hemiplegia needs to be evaluated for sensory, perceptual, and cognitive deficits to determine potential for ADL performance and to establish appropriate teaching methods (previously described) to facilitate learning.

The major problems for the one-handed worker are reduction of work speed and dexterity, stabilization to substitute for the role normally assumed by the nondominant arm. The major problems for the individual with hemiplegia are balance and precautions relative to sensory, perceptual, and cognitive losses.

Dressing Activities

If balance is a problem, dressing should be done while seated in a locked wheelchair or sturdy armchair. Clothing should be

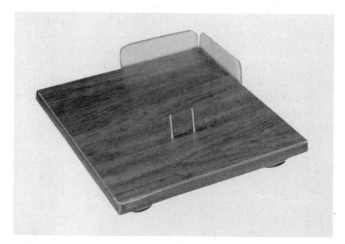

FIG. 26-26 Cutting board with stainless steel nails, suction cup feet, and corner for stabilizing bread is useful for patients with incoordination or use of one hand. (Provided by Sammons, Inc., a BISSELL Inc. Company.)

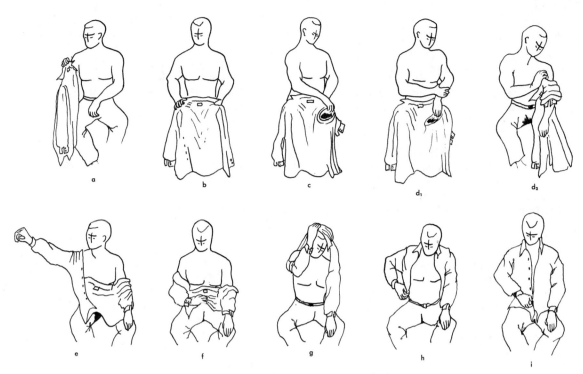

FIG. 26-27   Steps in donning a shirt: method I. (Reproduced with permission of Christine Shaw, Metro Health Center for Rehabilitation, Metro Health Medical Center, Cleveland, Ohio.)

within easy reach. Reaching tongs may be helpful for securing articles and assisting in some dressing activities. Assistive devices should be minimal for dressing and other ADL.

One-handed dressing techniques: * Dressing techniques for the client with hemiplegia that employ neurodevelopmental (Bobath) treatment principles are discussed in Chapter 24. The following one-handed dressing techniques can facilitate dressing for persons with use of one upper extremity. A general rule is to begin with the affected arm or leg first when donning clothing. When removing clothing start with the unaffected extremity.

Front-opening shirts may be managed by any one of three methods. The first method can be used for jackets, robes, and front-opening dresses.

Method I

Donning Shirt (Fig. 26-27)

1. Grasp shirt collar with normal hand and shake out twists (*a*).
2. Position shirt on lap with inside up and collar toward chest (*b*).
3. Position sleeve opening on affected side so it is as large as possible and close to affected hand, which is resting on lap (*c*).

---

* Summarized from *Activities of daily living for clients with incoordination, limited range of motion, paraplegia, quadriplegia, and hemiplegia,* Cleveland, 1989, Metro Health Center for Rehabilitation, Metro Health Medical Center, Unpublished.

4. Using normal hand, place affected hand in sleeve opening and work sleeve over elbow by pulling on garment (*d₁, d₂*).
5. Put normal arm into its sleeve and raise up to slide or shake sleeve into position past elbow (*e*).
6. With normal hand, gather shirt up middle of back from hem to collar and raise shirt over head (*f*).
7. Lean forward, duck head, and pass shirt over it (*g*).
8. With normal hand, adjust shirt by leaning forward and working it down past both shoulders. Reach in back and pull shirttail down (*h*).
9. Line shirt fronts up for buttoning and begin with bottom button (*i*). Button sleeve cuff of affected arm. Sleeve cuff of unaffected arm may be prebuttoned if cuff opening is large. Button may be sewn on with elastic thread or sewn onto a small tab of elastic and fastened inside shirt cuff. A small button attached to crocheted loop of elastic thread is another opton. Slip button on loop through buttonhole in garment so that elastic loop is inside. Stretch elastic loop to fit around original cuff button. This simple device can be transferred to each garment and positioned before shirt is put on. Loop stretches to accommodate width of hand as it is pushed through end of sleeve.[26]

Removing Shirt

1. Unbutton shirt.
2. Lean forward.
3. With normal hand, grasp collar or gather material up in back from collar to hem.
4. Lean forward, duck head, and pull shirt over head.
5. Remove sleeve from normal arm and then from affected arm.

Method II

Donning Shirt

Method II may be used by clients who get shirt twisted or have trouble sliding the sleeve down onto normal arm.

1. Position shirt as described in Method I, steps 1 to 3.
2. With normal hand place involved hand into shirt sleeve opening and work sleeve onto hand, but do not pull up over elbow.
3. Put normal arm into sleeve and bring arm out to 180° of abduction. Tension of fabric from normal arm to wrist of affected arm will bring sleeve into position.
4. Lower arm and work sleeve on affected arm up over elbow.
5. Continue as in steps 6 through 9 of method I.

Removing Shirt

1. Unbutton shirt.
2. With normal hand, push shirt off shoulders, first on affected side, then on normal side.
3. Pull on cuff of normal side with normal hand.
4. Work sleeve off by alternately shrugging shoulder and pulling down on cuff.
5. Lean forward, bring shirt around back, and pull sleeve off affected arm.

Method III

Donning Shirt (Fig. 26-28)

1. Position shirt and work onto arm as described in method I, steps 1 to 4.
2. Pull sleeve on affected arm up to shoulder *(a)*.
3. With normal hand, grasp tip of collar that is on normal side, lean forward, and bring arm over and behind head to carry shirt around to normal side *(b)*.
4. Put normal arm into sleeve opening, directing it up and out *(c)*.
5. Adjust and button as described in method I, steps 8 and 9.

Removing Shirt

The shirt may be removed using the procedure described previously for method II.

Variation for donning pullover shirt

1. Position shirt on lap, bottom toward chest and label facing down.
2. With normal hand, roll up bottom edge of shirt back up to sleeve on affected side.

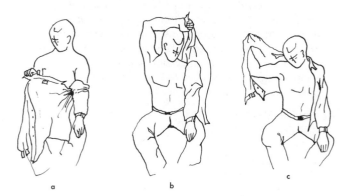

FIG. 26-28   Steps in donning a shirt: method III. (Reproduced with permission of Christine Shaw, Metro Health Center for Rehabilitation, Metro Health Medical Center, Cleveland, Ohio.)

3. Position sleeve opening so it is as large as possible and use normal hand to place affected hand into sleeve opening. Pull shirt up onto arm past elbow.
4. Insert normal arm into sleeve.
5. Adjust shirt on affected side up and onto shoulder.
6. Gather shirt back with normal hand, lean forward, duck head, and pass shirt over head.
7. Adjust shirt.

Variation for removing pullover shirt

1. Gather shirt up with normal hand, starting at top back.
2. Lean forward, duck head, and pull gathered back fabric over head.
3. Remove from normal arm and then affected arm.

Trousers may be managed by one of the following methods, which may be adapted for shorts and women's panties as well. It is recommended that trousers have a well-constructed button fly front opening, which may be easier to manage than a zipper. Velcro may be used to replace buttons and zippers. Trousers should be worn in a size slightly larger than worn previously and should have a wide opening at the ankles. They should be put on after the socks have been put on but before the shoes are put on. If the client is dressing in a wheelchair, feet should be placed flat on the floor, not on the footrests of the wheelchair.

Method I

Donning Trousers (Fig. 26-29)

1. Sit in sturdy armchair or in locked wheelchair *(a)*.
2. Position normal leg in front of midline of body with knee flexed to 90°. Using normal hand reach forward and grasp ankle of affected leg or sock around ankle *(b₁)*. Lift affected leg over normal leg to crossed position *(b₂)*.
3. Slip trousers onto affected leg up to position where foot is completely inside of trouser leg *(c)*. Do not pull up above knee or difficulty will be encountered in inserting normal leg.
4. Uncross affected leg by grasping ankle or portion of sock around ankle *(d)*.
5. Insert normal leg and work trousers up onto hips as far as possible *(e₁, e₂)*.
6. To prevent trousers from dropping when pulling pants over hips, place affected hand in pocket or place one finger of affected hand into belt loop. If able to do so safely, stand and pull trousers over hips *(f₁, f₂)*.
7. If standing balance is good, remain standing to pull up zipper or button *(f₃)*. Sit down to button front *(g)*.

Removing Trousers

1. Unfasten trousers and work down on hips as far as possible while seated.
2. Stand, letting trousers drop past hips or work them down past hips.
3. Remove trousers from normal leg.
4. Sit and cross affected leg over normal leg, remove trousers, and uncross leg.

Method II

Donning Trousers

Method II is used for clients who are in wheelchairs with brakes locked and footrests swung away or who are in sturdy straight

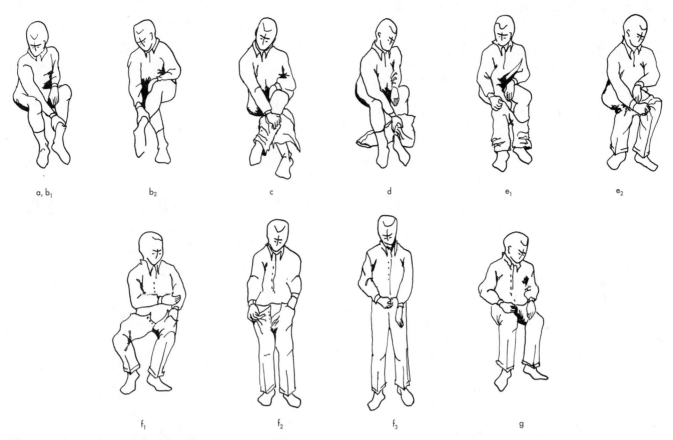

FIG. 26-29   Steps in donning trousers: method I. (Reproduced with permission of Christine Shaw, Metro Health Center for Rehabilitation, Metro Health Medical Center, Cleveland, Ohio.)

armchairs positioned with back against wall and for clients who cannot stand independently.

1. Position trousers on legs as in method I, steps 1 through 5.
2. Elevate hips by leaning back against chair and pushing down against the floor with normal leg. As hips are raised, work trousers over hips with normal hand.
3. Lower hips back into chair and fasten trousers.

Removing Trousers

1. Unfasten trousers and work down on hips as far as possible while sitting.
2. Lean back against chair, push down against floor with normal leg to elevate hips, and with normal arm work trousers down past hips.
3. Proceed as in method I, steps 3 and 4.

Method III

Donning Trousers

Method III is for clients who are in a recumbent position. It is more difficult to perform than those methods done sitting. If possible, bed should be raised to semireclining position for partial sitting.

1. Using normal hand, place affected leg in bent position and cross over normal leg, which may be partially bent to prevent affected leg from slipping.
2. Position trousers and work onto affected leg first, up to the knee. Then uncross leg.

3. Insert normal leg, and work trousers up onto hips as far as possible.
4. With normal leg bent, press down with foot and shoulder to elevate hips from bed and with normal arm pull trousers over hips or work trousers up over hips by rolling from side to side.
5. Fasten trousers.

Removing Trousers

1. Hike hips as in putting trousers on in method III, step 4.
2. Work trousers down past hips, remove unaffected leg, and then remove affected leg.

Clothing items, such as brassieres, neckties, socks, stockings, and braces, may be difficult to manage with one hand. The following methods are recommended:

BRASSIERE

Donning

1. Tuck one end of brassiere into pants, girdle, or skirt waistband, and wrap other end around waist (wrapping toward affected side may be easiest). Hook brassiere in front at waist level and slip fastener around to back (at waistline level).
2. Place affected arm through shoulder strap, and then place normal arm through other strap.
3. Work straps up over shoulders. Pull strap on affected side up over shoulder with normal arm. Put normal arm through its

strap and work up over shoulder by directing arm up and out and pulling with hand.

4. Use normal hand to adjust breasts in brassiere cups. NOTE: It is helpful if brassiere has elastic straps and is made of stretch fabric. If there is some function in affected hand, a fabric loop may be sewn to back of brassiere near fastener. Affected thumb may be slipped through loop to stabilize brassiere while normal hand fastens it. All elastic brassieres, prefastened or without fasteners, may be put on adapting method I for shirts described previously. Front opening bras may also be adapted with a loop for the affected hand with some gross arm function.

Removing

1. Slip straps down off shoulders, normal side first.
2. Work straps down over arms and off hands.
3. Slip brassiere around to front with normal arm.
4. Unfasten and remove.

NECKTIE

Donning

Clip-on neckties are attractive and convenient. If conventional tie is used, the following method is recommended:

1. Place collar of shirt in up position and bring necktie around neck and adjust so that smaller end is at desired length when tie is completed.
2. Fasten small end to shirt front with tie clasp or spring clip clothespin.
3. Loop long end around short end (one complete loop) and bring up between V at neck. Then bring tip down through loop at front and adjust tie, using ring and little fingers to hold tie end and thumb and forefingers to slide knot up tightly.

Removing

Pull knot at front of neck until small end slips up enough for tie to be slipped over head. Tie may be hung up in this state and replaced by slipping it over head around upturned collar, and knot tightened as described in step 3 of donning necktie.

SOCKS OR STOCKINGS

Donning

1. Sit in straight armchair or in wheelchair with brakes locked, feet on the floor and footrest swung away.
2. With normal leg directly in front of midline of body, cross affected leg over it.
3. Open top of stocking by inserting thumb and first two fingers near cuff and spreading fingers apart.
4. Work stocking onto foot before pulling over heel. Care should be taken to eliminate wrinkles.
5. Work stocking up over leg. Shift weight from side to side to adjust stocking around thigh.
6. Thigh-high stockings with an elastic band at the top are often an acceptable substitute for panty hose, especially for the nonambulatory individual.
7. Panty hose may be donned and doffed as a pair of slacks, except the legs would be gathered up one at a time before placing feet into the leg holes.

Removing

1. Work socks or stockings down as far as possible with normal arm.

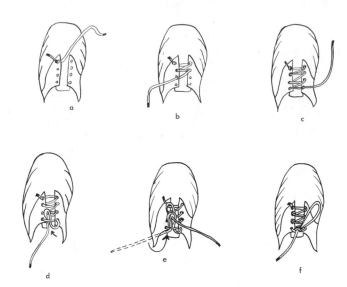

FIG. 26-30 One-hand shoe-tying method. (Reproduced with permission of Christine Shaw, Metro Health Center for Rehabilitation, Metro Health Medical Center, Cleveland, Ohio.)

2. Cross affected leg over normal one as described in step 2 of putting on socks or stockings.
3. Remove sock or stocking from affected leg. Dressing stick may be required by some clients to push sock or stocking off heel and off foot.
4. Lift normal leg to comfortable height or to seat level and remove sock or stocking from foot.

SHOES

If possible select slip-on shoes to eliminate lacing and tying. If an individual uses an ankle-foot orthosis (AFO) or short leg brace, shoes with fasteners are usually needed.

1. Use elastic laces and leave shoes tied.
2. Use adapted shoe fasteners such as "kno-bows."
3. Use one handed shoe-tying techniques (Fig. 26-30).
4. It is possible to learn to tie a standard bow with one hand but it requires excellent visual perceptual and motor planning skills along with much repetition.

ANKLE-FOOT ORTHOSIS (AFO)

An AFO is frequently used by the individual with hemiplegia who lacks adequate ankle dorsiflexion to walk safely and efficiently. It can be donned in this way:

Donning (Fig. 26-31)

1. Sit in straight armchair or wheelchair with brakes locked and feet on the floor (a). The fasteners are loosened and tongue of the shoe pulled back to allow the AFO to fit into the shoe (b).
2. AFO and shoe are placed on the floor between the legs but closer to the affected leg, facing up (c).
3. With the unaffected hand, lift the affected leg behind the knee and place toes into the shoe (d).
4. Reach down with unaffected hand and lift AFO by the upright. Simultaneously use the unaffected foot against the affected heel to keep the shoe and AFO together (e).

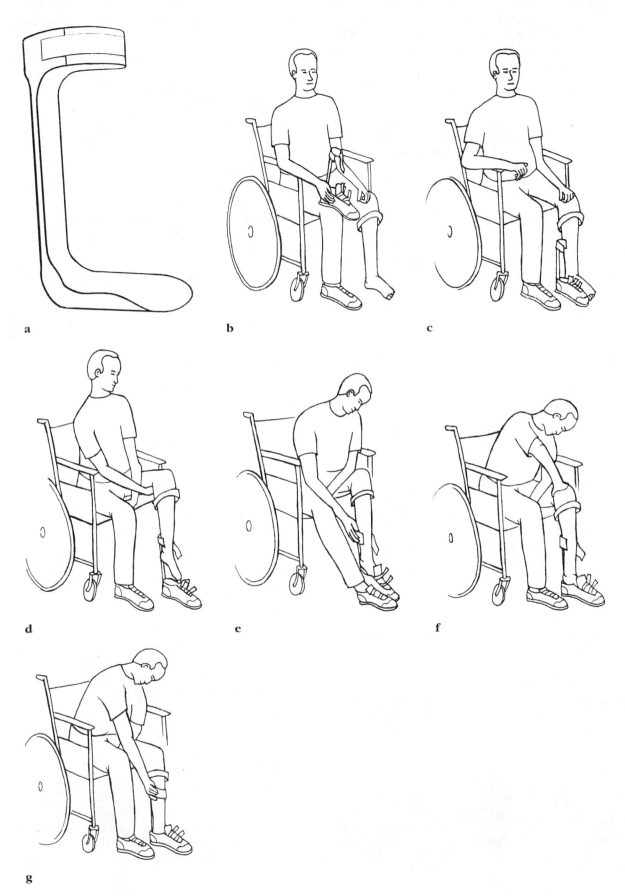

FIG. 26-31   Steps in donning ankle-foot orthosis.

5. The heel will not be pushed into the shoe at this point. With the unaffected hand apply pressure directly downward on the affected knee to force the heel into the shoe, if leg strength is not sufficient *(f)*.

6. Fasten Velcro calf strap and fasten shoes *(g)*. The affected leg may be placed on a footstool to assist with reaching shoe fasteners.

7. To fasten shoes, one-handed bow-tying may be used; elastic shoelaces, Velcro-fastened shoes, or other commercially available shoe fasteners may be required if the client is unable to tie shoes.

Removing

Variation I

1. While seated as for donning an AFO, cross affected leg over normal leg.
2. Unfasten straps and laces with normal hand.
3. Push down on AFO upright until shoe is off foot.

Variation II

1. Unfasten straps and laces.
2. Straighten affected leg by putting normal foot behind heel of shoe and pushing affected leg forward.
3. Push down on AFO upright with hand and at same time push foreword on heel of AFO shoe with normal foot.

Eating Activities

The main problem encountered by the one-handed individual is managing a knife and fork simultaneously for meat cutting. This problem can be solved by the use of a rocker knife for cutting meat and other foods (Fig. 26-32). It cuts with a rocking motion rather than a slicing back and forth action. Use of a rocking motion with a standard table knife or a sharp paring knife may be adequate to accomplish cutting tender meats and foods. If such a knife is used, the client is taught to hold the knife handle between the thumb and the third, fourth, and fifth fingers, and the index finger is extended along the top of the knife blade. The knife point is placed in the food in a vertical position, and then the blade is brought down to cut the food. The rocking motion, using wrist flexion and extension, is continued until the food is cut.

The occupational therapist should keep in mind that one-handed meat cutting involves learning a new motor pattern. This skill may be difficult for clients with hemiplegia and apraxia.

Hygiene and Grooming Activities

With some assistive devices and the use of alternate methods, hygiene and grooming activities can be accomplished by those with the use of one hand or one side of the body. The following are suggestions for achieving hygiene and grooming with one hand:

1. Use an electric razor rather than a safety razor.
2. Use a bathtub seat or chair in the shower stall, bathmat, wash mitt, long-handled bath sponge, safety rails on the bathtub or wall, soap on a rope or suction soap holder, and suction brush for fingernail care.
3. Sponge bathe while sitting at the lavatory, using the wash mitt, suction brush, and suction soap holder. The uninvolved forearm and hand may be washed by placing a soaped washcloth on the thigh and rubbing the hand and forearm on the cloth.
4. Use the position-adjustable hair dryer previously described. Such a device frees the unaffected upper extremity to hold a brush or comb to style the hair during blow-drying.[8]
5. Care for fingernails as described previously for clients with incoordination.
6. Use spray deodorants rather than creams or roll-ons, because sprays can be applied more easily to the uninvolved underarm.
7. Use a suction denture brush for care of dentures. The suction fingernail brush may also serve this purpose (shown in Fig. 26-23).

Communication and Environmental Hardware

The following are suggestions to facilitate writing, reading, and using the telephone:

1. The primary problem in writing is stabilization of the paper or tablet. This problem can be overcome by using a clipboard or paperweight or by taping the paper to the writing surface. In some instances the affected arm may be positioned on the table top to stabilize the paper passively.
2. If dominance must be shifted to the nondominant extremity, writing practice may be necessary to improve speed and coordination. One-handed writing and typing instruction manuals are available.
3. Book holders may be used to stabilize a book while reading or holding copy for typing and writing practice. A soft pillow will easily stabilize a book while the person is seated in an easy chair.
4. The telephone is managed by lifting the receiver to listen for the dial tone, setting it down, dialing or pressing the buttons, then lifting the receiver to the ear. To write while using the telephone, a stand or shoulder telephone receiver holder must be used. A speaker phone can also leave hands free to take messages.

Mobility and Transfers

Principles of transfer techniques for clients with hemiplegia are described in Chapter 27.

Home Management Activities

Many assistive devices are available to facilitate home management activities.[16] Various factors determine how many home management activities can realistically be performed, which methods can be used, and how many assistive devices can be managed. These factors include (1) whether the client is disabled by the loss of function of one arm and hand, as in amputation or a peripheral neuropathic condition, or (2) whether both arm and leg are affected along with possible visual, perceptual, and cognitive dysfunctions, as in hemiplegia. The reader is referred to the references listed at the end of this chapter for

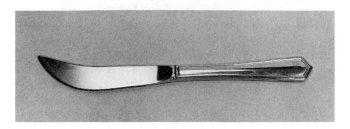

FIG. 26-32 One-handed rocker knife is provided by Sammons, Inc., a BISSELL Inc. Company.

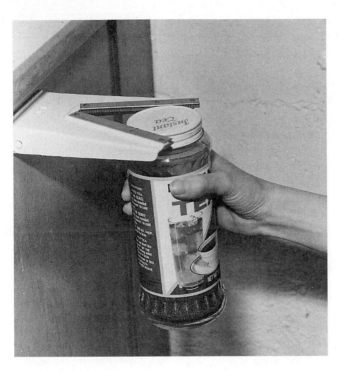

FIG. 26-33 Zim jar opener.

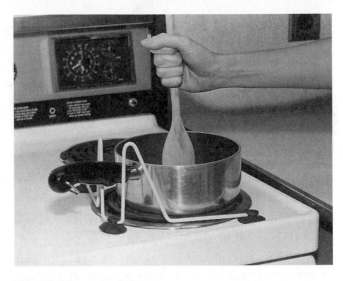

FIG. 26-34 Pan stabilizer.

details of home management with one hand. The following are some suggestions for home management for the client with use of one hand:[16]

1. Stabilization of items is a major problem for the one-handed homemaker. Stabilize foods for cutting and peeling by using a board with two stainless steel or aluminum nails in it. A raised corner on the board stabilizes bread for making sandwiches or spreading butter. Suction cups or a rubber mat under the board will keep it from slipping. Rubber stair tread may be glued to the bottom of the board (Fig. 26-26).

2. Use sponge cloths, nonskid mats or pads, wet dishcloths, or suction devices to keep pots, bowls, and dishes from turning or sliding during food preparation.

3. To open a jar, stabilize it between the knees or in a partially opened drawer while leaning against it. Break the air seal by sliding a pop bottle opener under the lid until the air is released, then use a Zim jar opener (Fig. 26-33).

4. Open boxes, sealed paper, and plastic bags by stabilizing between the knees or in a drawer as just described, and cut open with household shears. Special box and bag openers are also available from ADL equipment vendors.

5. Open an egg by holding it firmly in the palm of the hand, hitting it in the center against the edge of the bowl, and then using the thumb and index finger to push the top half of the shell up and the ring and little finger to push the lower half down. Separate whites from yolks by using an egg separator or a funnel.

6. Eliminate the need to stabilize the standard grater by using a grater with suction feet or use an electric countertop mincer instead.

7. Stabilize pots on counter or range for mixing or stirring by using a pan holder with suction feet (Fig. 26-34).

8. Eliminate the need to use handcranked or electric can

openers requiring two hands by using a one-handed electric can opener.

9. Use a utility cart to carry items from one place to another. A cart that is weighted or constructed of wood may be used as a minimal support during ambulation for some clients.

10. Transfer clothes to and from the washer or dryer by using a clothes carrier on wheels.

11. Use electrical appliances, such as a lightweight electrical hand mixer, blender, and food processor, which can be managed with one hand and save time and energy. Safety factors and judgment need to be evaluated carefully when electrical appliances are considered.

12. Floor care becomes a greater problem if ambulation and balance are affected as well as one arm. For those clients with involvement of one arm only, a standard dust mop, carpet sweeper, or upright vacuum cleaner should present no problem. A self-wringing mop may be used if the mop handle is stabilized under the arm and the wringing lever operated with the normal arm. Clients with balance and ambulation problems may manage some floor care from a sitting position. Dust mopping or using a carpet sweeper may be possible if gait and balance are fairly good without the aid of a cane.

These are just a few of the possibilities to solve home management problems for one-handed individuals. The occupational therapist must evaluate each client to determine how the dysfunction affects performance of homemaking activities. One-handed techniques take more time and may be difficult for some clients to master. Activities should be paced to accommodate the client's physical endurance and tolerance for one-handed performance and use of special devices. Work simplification and energy conservation techniques should be employed. New techniques and devices should be introduced on a graded basis as the client masters one technique and device and then another. Family members need to be oriented to the client's skills, special methods used, and work schedule. The therapist with the family and client may facilitate the planning of homemaking responsibilities to be shared by other family members and the supervision of the client, if that is needed. If special equipment and assistive devices are needed for ADL, it is advisable to acquire these through the health agency, if possible. The therapist can then train the client and demonstrate their use to a family member before these items are used at home. Following training the occupational therapist should provide the client with sources to replace items independently, such as a consumer catalogue of adaptive equipment.

ADL FOR WHEELCHAIR-BOUND INDIVIDUALS WITH GOOD-TO-NORMAL ARM FUNCTION (PARAPLEGIA)

Clients who are confined to a wheelchair need to find ways to perform ADL from a seated position, to transport objects, and to adapt in an environment designed for standing and walking. Given normal upper extremity function, the wheelchair ambulator can probably perform independently. The client should have a stable spine and mobility precautions should be clearly identified.

Dressing Activities*

It is recommended that wheelchair-bound clients put on clothing in this order: stockings, undergarments, braces (if worn), trousers or slacks, shoes, shirt, or dress.

TROUSERS

Donning

Trousers and slacks are easier to fasten if they button or zip in front. If braces are worn, zippers in side seams may be helpful. Wide-bottom slacks of stretch fabric are recommended. Procedure for putting on trousers, shorts, slacks, and underwear is as follows:

1. Use side rails or trapeze to help pull up to sitting position.
2. Sit on bed and reach forward to feet or sit on bed and pull knees into flexed position.
3. Holding top of trousers flip pants down to feet.
4. Work pant legs over feet and pull up to hips. Crossing ankles may help get pants on over heels.
5. In semireclining position roll from hip to hip and pull up garment.
6. Reaching tongs may be helpful to pull garment up or position garment on feet if there is impaired balance or range of motion in the lower extremities or trunk.

Removing

Remove pants or underwear by reversing procedure for putting on. Dressing sticks may be helpful to push pants off feet.

---

* Summarized from *Activities of daily living for clients with incoordination, limited range of motion, paraplegia, quadriplegia, and hemiplegia,* Cleveland, 1989, Metro Health Center for Rehabilitation, Metro Health Medical Center, Unpublished.

SOCKS OR STOCKINGS

Soft stretch socks or stockings are recommended. Panty hose that are slightly large may be useful. Elastic garters or stockings with elastic tops should be avoided because of potential skin breakdown. Dressing sticks or a stocking device may be helpful to some clients.

Donning

1. Put on socks or stockings while seated on bed.
2. Pull one leg into flexion with one hand and cross over the other leg.
3. Use other hand to slip sock or stocking over foot and pull it on.

Removing

Remove socks or stockings by flexing leg as described for donning, pushing sock or stocking down over heel. Dressing sticks may be needed to push sock or stocking off heel and toe and to retrieve it.

SLIPS AND SKIRTS

Slips and skirts slightly larger than usually worn are recommended. A-line, wraparound, and full skirts are easier to manage and look better on a person seated in a wheelchair than narrow skirts.

Donning

1. Sit on bed, slip garment over head, and let it drop to waist.
2. In semireclining position, roll from hip to hip and pull garment down over hips and thighs.

Removing

1. In sitting or semireclining position, unfasten garment.
2. Roll from hip to hip, pulling garment up to waist level.
3. Pull garment off over head.

SHIRTS

Fabrics should be wrinkle-resistant, smooth, and durable. Roomy sleeves and backs and full shirts are more suitable styles than closely fitted garments.

Donning

Shirts, pajama jackets, robes, and dresses opening completely down front may be put on while client is seated in wheelchair. If it is necessary to dress while in bed, the following procedure can be used:

1. Balance body by putting palms of hands on mattress on either side of body. If balance is poor, assistance may be needed or bed backrest may be elevated. (If backrest cannot be elevated, one or two pillows may be used to support back.) With backrest elevated, both hands are available.
2. If difficulty is encountered in customary methods of applying garment, open garment on lap with collar toward chest. Put arms into sleeves and pull up over elbows. Then hold on to shirttail or back of dress, pull garment over head, adjust, and button.

Removing

1. Sitting in wheelchair or bed, open fastener.
2. Remove garment in usual manner.

3. If usual manner is not feasible, grasp collar with one hand while balancing with other hand. Gather material up from collar to hem.
4. Lean forward, duck head, and pull shirt over head.
5. Remove sleeve from supporting arm and then from working arm.

SHOES

Donning

If an individual has sensory loss and is at risk for bruising during transfers shoes should be donned in bed. Shoes may be applied by one of the following variations:

Variation I

1. In sitting position on bed, pull one knee at a time into flexed position with hands.
2. While supporting leg in flexed position with one hand, use free hand to put on shoe.

Variation II

1. Sit on edge of bed or in wheelchair for back support.
2. Bend one knee up to flexed position, supporting leg with arm, and with free hand slip shoe on.

Variation III

1. Sit on edge of bed or in wheelchair for back support.
2. Cross one leg over other and slip shoe on.
3. Put foot on footrest and push down on knee to push foot into shoe.

Removing

1. Flex or cross leg as described for appropriate variation.
2. For variations I and II remove shoe with one hand while supporting flexed leg with other hand.
3. For variation III remove shoe from crossed leg with one hand while maintaining balance with other hand, if necessary.

Eating Activities

Eating activities should present no special problem for the wheelchair-bound person with good to normal arm function. Wheelchairs with desk arms and swing-away footrests are recommended so that it is possible to sit close to the table.

Hygiene and Grooming

Face and oral hygiene and arm and upper body care should present no problem. Reachers may be helpful to secure towels, washcloths, make-up, deodorant, and shaving supplies from storage areas, if necessary. Tub baths or showers require some special equipment. Transfer techniques for toilet and bathtub are discussed in Chapter 27. The following are suggestions for facilitating bathing activities:

1. Use a handheld shower head and keep a finger over the spray to determine sudden temperature changes in water.
2. Use long-handled bath brushes with soap insert for ease in reaching all parts of the body.
3. Use soap bars attached to a cord around the neck.
4. For sponge bath in wheelchair, cover the chair with a sheet of plastic.
5. Use shower chairs or bathtub seats.
6. Increase safety during transfers by installing grab bars on wall near bathtub or shower and on bathtub.

7. Fit bathtub or shower bottom with nonskid mat or adhesive material.
8. Remove doors on the bathtub and replace with a shower curtain to increase safety and ease of transfers.

Communication and Environmental Hardware

With the exception of reaching difficulties in some situations, use of the telephone should present no problem. Short-handled reachers may be used to grasp the receiver from the cradle. Touching key pad could be accomplished with a short, rubber-tipped, ¼-inch dowel stick. A cordless telephone would eliminate reaching except when the phone needed recharging. Use of writing implements, typewriter, tape recorder, and personal computer should be easily possible for these clients. Managing doors may present some difficulties. If the door opens toward the person, opening it can be managed by the following procedure:

1. If doorknob is on right, approach door from right, and turn doorknob with left hand.
2. Open door as far as possible and move wheelchair close enough so that it helps keep door open.
3. Holding door open with left hand, turn wheelchair with right hand and wheel through door.
4. Start closing door when halfway through.

If the door is very heavy and opens out or away from the person, the following procedure is recommended:

1. Back up to door so knob can be turned with right hand.
2. Open door and back through so that big wheels keep it open.
3. Also use left elbow to keep door open.
4. Wheel backward with right hand.[4]

Mobility and Transfers

Principles of transfer techniques are discussed in Chapter 27.

Home Management Activities[16]

When performing homemaking activities from a wheelchair, the major problems are work heights, adequate space for maneuverability, access to storage areas, and transfer of supplies, equipment, and materials from place to place. If funds are available for kitchen remodeling, lowering counters and range to a comfortable height for wheelchair use is recommended. Such extensive adaptation is often not feasible, however. Suggestions for home management are as follows:

1. Remove cabinet doors to eliminate the need to maneuver around them for opening and closing. Frequently used items should be stored toward the front of easy-to-reach cabinets above and below the counter surfaces.
2. If entrance and inside doors are not wide enough, use a device to reduce wheelchair width or make doors slightly wider by removing strips along the door jambs. Offset hinges can replace standard door hinges and increase the door jam width by 2 inches (Fig. 26-35).
3. Increase the user's height with a wheelchair cushion so that standard counters may be used.
4. Use detachable desk arms and swing-away detachable footrests to allow the wheelchair user to get as close as possible to counters and tables and also to stand at counters, if that is possible (Fig. 26-36).
5. Transport items safely and easily by using a wheelchair lapboard. The lapboard may also serve as a work surface for

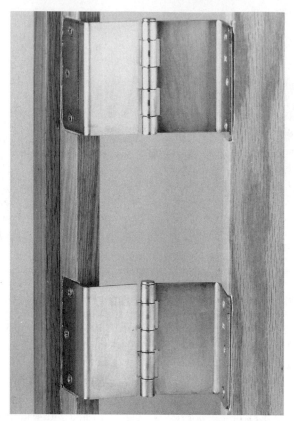

A

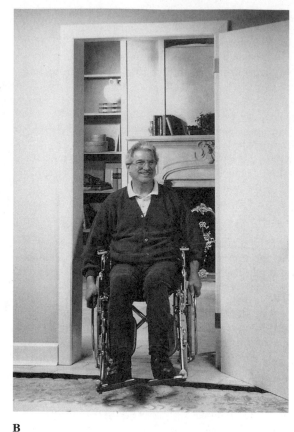

B

FIG. 26-35 **A,** Offset hinges. **B,** Offset hinges widen doorway for wheelchair user (Provided by Sammons, Inc., a BISSELL Inc. Company.

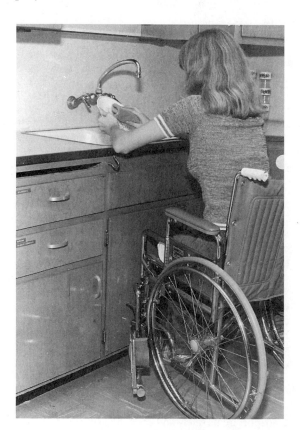

FIG. 26-36 Wheelchair footrests are swung away to allow close access to sink.

preparing food and drying dishes. It also protects the lap from injury from hot pans and prevents utensils from falling into the lap (Fig. 26-37).

6. Fasten a drop-leaf board to a bare wall or slide-out board under a counter to give the wheelchair homemaker one work surface that is a comfortable height in a kitchen that is otherwise standard.

7. Fit cabinets with custom- or ready-made lazy Susans or pull-out shelves to eliminate need to reach to rear space (Fig. 26-38).

8. Ranges ideally should be at a lower level than standard height. If this arrangement is not possible, place the controls at the front of the range, and hang a mirror angled at the proper degree over the range so that the homemaker can see contents of pots.

9. Substitute small electric cooking units and microwave ovens for the range if it is not safely manageable.

10. Use front-loading washers and dryers.

11. Vacuum carpets with a carpet sweeper or tank-type cleaner that rolls easily and is lightweight or self-propelled. A retractable cord may be helpful to prevent tangling of cord in wheels.

ADL FOR THE WHEELCHAIR-BOUND INDIVIDUAL WITH UPPER EXTREMITY WEAKNESS (QUADRIPLEGIA)

In general, persons with muscle function from spinal cord levels C7 and C8 can follow many of the methods just described for paraplegia, except for fine motor tasks

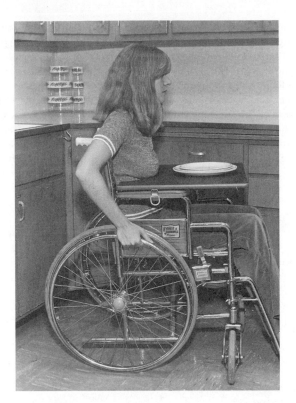

FIG. 26-37   Wheelchair lapboard is used to transport items.

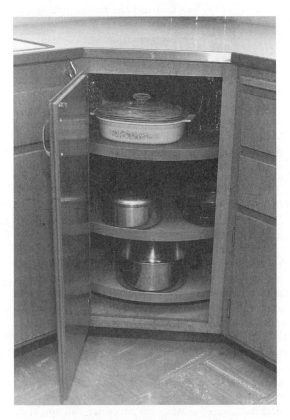

FIG. 26-38   Lazy Susan in kitchen storage cabinet.

such as buttoning or typing. Individuals with muscle function from C6 can be relatively independent with adaptations and assistive devices, whereas those with muscle function from C4 and C5 will require considerable special equipment and assistance. Clients with muscle function from C6 may benefit from the use of a wrist-driven flexor hinge splint. Externally powered splints and arm braces or mobile arm supports are recommended for C3, C4, and C5 levels of muscle function (refer to Chapters 19 and 40).[1]

Dressing Activities
Criteria

Training in dressing can be commenced when the spine is stable.[3,25] Minimal criteria for upper extremity dressing are (1) fair to good muscle strength in deltoids, upper and middle trapezii, shoulder rotators, rhomboids, biceps, supinators, and radial wrist extensors; (2) ROM of 0 to 90° in shoulder flexion and abduction, 0 to 80° in shoulder internal rotation, 0 to 30° in external rotation, and 15 to 140° in elbow flexion; (3) sitting balance in bed or wheelchair, which may be achieved with the assistance of bedrails, an electric hospital bed, or wheelchair safety belt; and (4) finger prehension achieved with adequate tenodesis grasp or wrist-driven flexor-hinge splint.

Additional criteria for dressing the lower extremities are (1) fair to good muscle strength in pectoralis major and minor, serratus anterior, and rhomboid major and minor; (2) ROM of 0 to 120° in knee flexion, 0 to 110° in hip flexion, and 0 to 80° in hip external rotation; (3) body control for transfer from bed to wheelchair with minimal assistance; (4) ability to roll from side to side, balance in side-lying, or turning from supine position to prone position and back; and (5) vital capacity of 50% or better.[25]

Contraindications. Dressing is contraindicated if any of the following factors are present: (1) unstable spine at site of injury, (2) pressure sores or tendency for skin breakdown during rolling, scooting, and transferring, (3) uncontrollable muscle spasms in legs, and (4) less than 50% vital capacity.[3,25]

Sequence of dressing. The recommended sequence for training to dress is to put on underwear and trousers while still in bed, then transfer to a wheelchair and put on shirts, socks, and shoes.[25] Some clients may wish to put the socks on before the trousers, because they may help the feet to slip through the trouser legs more easily.

Expected proficiency. Total dressing, which includes both upper and lower extremity dressing skills, can be achieved by clients with spinal cord lesions at C7 and below. Total dressing can be achieved by clients with lesions at C6, but lower extremity dressing may be difficult or impractical in terms of time and energy for these clients. Upper extremity dressing can be achieved by clients with lesions at C5 to C6 with some exceptions. It is difficult or impossible for these clients to put on a brassiere, tuck a shirt or blouse into a waistband, or fasten buttons on shirt fronts and cuffs. Factors such as age, physical proportions, coordination, concomitant medical problems, and motivation will affect the degree of proficiency in dressing skills that can be achieved by any client.[3]

Types of clothing. Clothing should be loose and have front openings. Trousers need to be a size larger than usually worn to accommodate the urine collection device or leg braces if worn. Wraparound skirts and rubber pants are helpful for women. The fasteners that are easiest to manage are zippers and Velcro closures. Because the client with quadriplegia often uses the thumb as a hook to manage clothing, loops attached to zipper pulls, undershorts, and even the back of the shoes can be helpful. Belt loops on trousers are used for pulling and should be reinforced. Brassieres should have stretch straps and no boning in them. Front-opening brassiere styles can be adapted by fastening loops and adding Velcro closures; back-opening styles can have loops added at each side of the fastening.

Shoes can be one-half to one size larger than normally worn to accommodate edema and spasticity and to avoid pressure sores. Shoe fasteners can be adapted with Velcro, elastic shoelaces, large buckles, or flip-back tongue closure. Loose woolen or cotton socks without elastic cuffs should be used initially. As skill is gained, nylon socks, which tend to stick to the skin, may be possible. If neckties are used, the clip-on type or a regular tie that has been preknotted and can be slipped over the head may be manageable for some clients.[3,25]

The following techniques can facilitate dressing for persons with upper extremity weakness.

TROUSERS AND UNDERSHORTS

Donning

1. Sit on bed with bedrails up. Trousers are positioned at foot of bed with trouser legs over end of bed and front side up.[25]
2. Sit up and lift one knee at a time by hooking right hand under right knee to pull leg into flexion, then put trousers over right foot. Return right leg to extension or semiextended position while repeating procedure with left hand and left knee.[3] If unable to maintain leg in flexion by holding with one arm or through advantageous use of spasticity, dressing band may be used. This device is a piece of elasticized webbing that has been sewn into a figure-eight pattern, with one small loop and one large loop. The small loop is hooked around the foot and the large hoop is anchored over the knee. Band is measured for individual client so that its length is appropriate to maintain desired amount of knee flexion. Once the trousers are in place, knee loop is pushed off knee and dressing band is removed from foot with dressing stick.[7]
3. Work trousers up legs, using patting and sliding motions with palms of hands.
4. While still sitting with pants to midcalf height, insert dressing stick in front belt loop. Dressing stick is gripped by slip-

ping its loop over wrist. Pull on dressing stick while extending trunk, returning to supine position. Return to sitting position and repeat this procedure, pulling on dressing sticks and maneuvering trousers up to thigh level.[25] If balance is adequate, an alternative is for client to remain sitting and lean on left elbow and pull trousers over right buttock, then reverse process for other side. Another alternative is for client to remain in supine position and roll to one side; throw opposite arm behind back; hook thumb in waistband, belt loop, or pocket; and pull trousers up over hips. These maneuvers can be repeated as often as necessary to get trousers over buttocks.[3]

5. Using palms of hands in pushing and smoothing motions, straighten the trouser legs.
6. In supine position, fasten trouser placket by hooking thumb in loop on zipper pull, patting Velcro closed, or using hand splints and buttonhooks if there are buttons.[3,25]

Variation

Substitute the following for step 2:
Sit up and lift one knee at a time by hooking right hand under right knee to pull leg into flexion, then cross the foot over the opposite leg above the knee. This position frees the foot to place the trousers more easily and requires less trunk balance. Continue with all other steps.

Removing

1. Lying supine in bed with bedrails up, unfasten belt and placket fasteners.
2. Placing thumbs in belt loops, waistband, or pockets, work trousers past hips by stabilizing arms in shoulder extension and scooting body toward head of bed.
3. Use arms as described in step 2 and roll from side to side to get trousers past buttocks.
4. Coming to sitting position and alternately pulling legs into flexion, push trousers down legs.[25]
5. Trousers can be pushed off over feet with dressing stick or by hooking thumbs in waistband.

CARDIGANS OR PULLOVER GARMENTS

Cardigan and pullover garments include blouses, vests, sweaters, skirts, and front-opening dresses.[3,25] Upper extremity dressing is frequently performed in the wheelchair for greater trunk stability. Procedure for putting on these garments is as follows:

Donning

1. Garment is positioned across thighs with back facing up and neck toward knees.
2. Place both arms under back of garment and in armholes.
3. Push sleeves up onto arms past elbows.
4. Using a wrist extension grip, hook thumbs under garment back and gather material up from neck to hem.
5. To pass garment over head, adduct and externally rotate shoulders and flex elbows while flexing head forward.
6. When garment is over head, relax shoulders and wrists, and remove hands from back of garment. Most of material will be gathered up at neck, across shoulders, and under arms.
7. To work garment down over body, shrug shoulders, lean forward, and use elbow flexion and wrist extension. Use wheelchair arms for balance if necessary. Additional maneu-

vers to accomplish task are to hook wrists into sleeves and pull material free from underarms or lean forward, reach back, and slide hand against material to aid in pulling garment down.

8. Garment can be buttoned from bottom to top with aid of button hook and wrist-driven flexor hinge splint if hand function is inadequate.

Removing

1. Sit in wheelchair and wear wrist-driven flexor hinge splints. Unfasten buttons (if any) while wearing splints and using buttonhook. Remove splints for remaining steps.
2. For pullover garments, hook thumb in back of neckline, extend wrist, and pull garment over head while turning head toward side of raised arm. Maintain balance by resting against opposite wheelchair armrest or pushing on thigh with extended arm.
3. For cardigan garments, hook thumb in opposite armhole and push sleeve down arm. Elevation and depression of shoulders with trunk rotation can be used to get garment to slip down arms as far as possible.
4. Hold one cuff with opposite thumb while elbow is flexed to pull arm out of sleeve.

BRASSIERE (BACK-OPENING)

Donning

1. Place brassiere across lap with straps toward knees and inside facing up.
2. Using a right-to-left procedure, hold end of brassiere closest to right side with hand or reacher and pass brassiere around back from right to left. Lean against brassiere at back to hold it in place, while hooking thumb of left hand in a loop that has been attached near brassiere fastener. Hook right thumb in a similar loop on right side and fasten brassiere in front at waist level.
3. Hook right thumb in edge of brassiere. Using wrist extension, elbow flexion, shoulder adduction, and internal rotation, brassiere is rotated around body so that front of brassiere is in front of body.
4. While leaning on one forearm, hook opposite thumb in front end of strap and pull strap over shoulder, then repeat procedure on other side.[3,25]

Removing

1. Hook thumb under opposite brassiere strap, and push down over shoulder while elevating shoulder.
2. Pull arm out of strap, and repeat procedure for other arm.
3. Push brassiere down to waist level, and turn around as described previously to bring fasteners to front.
4. Unfasten brassiere.

Alternatives for a back-opening bra are (1) a front-opening bra with loops for using a wrist extension grip or (2) a fully elastic bra that has no fasteners and can be donned like a pullover sweater.

SOCKS

Donning

1. Sit in wheelchair or on bed if balance is adequate in cross-legged position with one ankle crossed over opposite knee.

2. Pull sock over foot with wrist extension grip and patting movements with palm of hand.[3,25]
3. If trunk balance is inadequate and cross-legged position cannot be maintained, prop foot on stool, chair, or open drawer while opposite arm is around upright of wheelchair for balance. Wheelchair safety belt or leaning against wheelchair armrest on one side are alternatives to maintain balance.
4. Use stocking aid or sock cone (Fig. 26-7) to assist in putting on socks while in this position. Powder sock cone (to reduce friction) and apply sock to it by using thumbs and palms of hands to smooth sock out on cone.
5. Place cord loops of sock cone around the wrist or thumb and throw cone beyond foot.
6. Maneuver cone over toes by pulling cords using elbow flexion. Insert foot as far as possible into cone.
7. To remove cone from sock after foot has been inserted, move heel forward off wheelchair footrest. Use wrist extension (of hand not operating sock cone) behind knee and continue pulling cords of cone until it is removed and sock is in place on foot. Use palms to smooth sock with patting and stroking motion.[25]
8. Two loops can also be sewn on either side of the top of the sock so that thumbs can be hooked into the loops and the socks pulled on.

Removing

1. While sitting in wheelchair or lying in bed, use dressing stick or long-handled shoehorn to push sock down over heel. Cross legs if possible.
2. Use dressing stick with cup hook on end to pull sock off toes.[4]

SHOES

Donning

1. Use same position for donning socks as for putting on shoes.
2. Use extended-handle dressing aid and insert it into tongue of shoe; then place shoe opening over toes. Remove dressing aid from shoe, and dangle shoe on toes.
3. Using palm of hand on sole of shoe, pull shoe toward heel of foot. One hand is used to stabilize leg while other pushes against sole of shoe to work shoe onto foot. Use thenar eminence and sides of hand for this pushing motion.
4. With feet flat on floor or on wheelchair footrest and knees flexed 90°, place a long-handled shoehorn in heel of shoe and press down on flexed knee.
5. Fasten shoes.[25]

Removing

1. Sitting in wheelchair with legs crossed as described previously, unfasten shoes.
2. Use shoehorn or dressing stick to push on heel counter of shoe, dislodging it from heel; then shoe will drop or can be pushed to floor with dressing stick.[25]

Eating Activities

Eating may be assisted by a variety of devices, depending on the level of muscle function.[1] Levels C5 and above require mobile arm supports or externally powered splints and braces. A wrist splint and universal cuff may be used together if a wrist-driven flexor hinge splint is not used. The univeral cuff holds the eating utensil, and

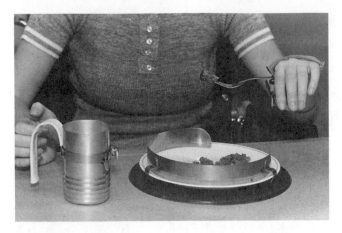

FIG. 26-39 Self-feeding with aid of universal cuff, plate guard, nonskid mat, and clip-type cup holder to compensate for absent grasp.

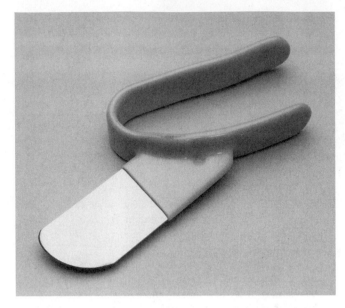

FIG. 26-41   Quad-quip knife.

the splint stabilizes the wrist. A nonskid mat and a plate with plate guard may provide adequate stability of the plate for pushing and picking up food (Fig. 26-39).

The spoon plate is an option for independent feeding for clients with high spinal cord injuries. It is a portable device that can be adjusted in height to the level of the client's mouth. The plate is made of a high-temperature thermoplastic and is formed over a mold that has a rim bowled to the approximate depth and length of a spoon. The client rotates the device with mouth and neck control. Food is removed from the rim of the plate with the mouth. Successful use of the device depends on adequate oral control, head and trunk control, and motivation. The reader is referred to the original source for information on making or obtaining this device.[29] Also available for client's who have no use of their upper extremeties is the electric self-feeder which requires only slight head motion and is activated by a chin switch (Fig. 26-40).

A regular or swivel spoon/fork combination can be used when there is minimal muscle function (C4 to C5). A long plastic straw with a straw clip to stabilize it in the cup or glass eliminates the need for picking up these drinking vessels. A bilateral or unilateral clip-type holder on a glass or cup makes it possible for many persons with hand and arm weakness to manage liquids without a straw.

Built-up utensils may be useful for those with some functional grasp or tenodesis grasp. Cutting food may be managed with a quad-quip knife if arm strength is adequate to manage the device (Fig. 26-41).

Hygiene and Grooming[1]

General suggestions to facilitate hygiene and grooming are as follows:

1. Use a shower or bathtub seat and transfer board for transfers.
2. Extend reach by using long-handled bath sponges with loop handle or built-up handle.
3. Eliminate need to grasp washcloth by using bath mitts.
4. Hold comb and toothbrush with a universal cuff.[1]
5. Use the position-adjustable hair dryer previously described.[8] Use a universal cuff to hold brush or comb for hair styling while using this mounted hair dryer.
6. Use a clip-type holder for electric razor.
7. Suppository inserters can be used by persons with quadriplegia who can manage bowel care independently.
8. Use skin inspection mirror with long stem and looped handle for independent skin inspection (Fig. 26-42). Devices and methods selected must be adapted to the degree of weakness for each client.
9. Adapted legbag clamps to empty catheter legbags are also available for individuals with limited hand function. Elastic legbag straps may also be replaced with Velcro straps.

Communication and Environmental Hardware

The following are suggestions for facilitating communication:

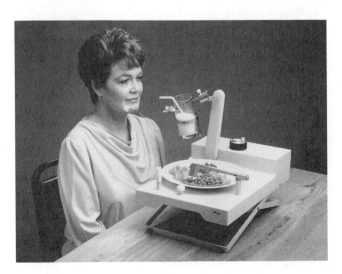

FIG. 26-40   Electric self-feeder is provided by Sammons, Inc., a BISSELL Inc. Company.

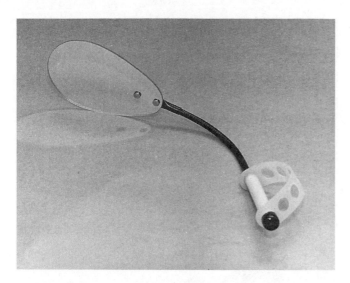

FIG. 26-42 Skin inspection mirror.

1. Turn pages with an electric page turner, mouth stick, or head wand if hand and arm function are inadequate (Fig. 26-43).
2. Insert pen, pencil, typing stick, or paintbrush in a universal cuff that has been positioned with the opening on the ulnar side of the palm for typing, writing, operating a tape recorder, and painting (Fig. 26-44).
3. Touch telephone key pad with the universal cuff and a pencil positioned with eraser down. The receiver may need to be stationed in a telephone arm and positioned for listening or adapted with telephone clip holder (Fig. 26-17). Special adaptations are available to substitute for the need to replace the receiver in the cradle. For clients with no arm function, a speaker phone can be used along with a mouthstick to push the button to initiate a call. The operator assists with dialing. A voice-activated phone is also available for individuals with little to no upper extremity function (Fig. 26-18).
4. Use personal computers, word processors, or electric typewriters. A computer mouse may be substituted for use of the keyboard.
5. Built-up pencils and pens or special pencil holders are needed for clients with hand weakness. The Wanchik writer is an effective adaptive writing device (Fig. 26-19).
6. Sophisticated electronic communications devices operated by mouth, pneumatic controls, and head control are available for clients with no upper extremity function.[27]
7. Kelly[13] described two mouthsticks and a cassette tape holder that allow C3, C4, or C5 quadriplegic clients to operate a tape recorder or radio independently. The first mouthstick, a rod about 19¹¹⁄₁₆ inches (50 cm) long with a friction

FIG. 26-43 Wand mouthstick is provided by Sammons, Inc., a BISSELL Inc. Company.

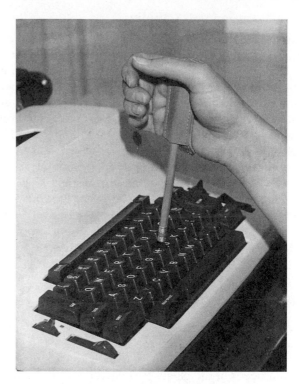

FIG. 26-44 Typing with aid of utensil holder and typing stick.

tip, is used to depress the operating buttons and adjust the volume and selector dials of the radio. The second mouthstick is a metal rod that separates into two prongs at its end. These prongs are 4 inches (about 10.2 cm) apart, and the mouthstick is used to place the cassettes from the cassette holder to the tape recorder and remove the cassettes from the recorder. The cassette tape stand has eight levels and is designed to hold eight tapes. It is a vertical stand made of metal and tilted backward to a 70° angle. The reader is referred to the original source for specifications on construction of these devices.[13]

8. Environmental controls allow for easy operation from a panel designed to run multiple devices such as televisions, radios, lights, telephones, intercoms, and hospital beds. (See Chapter 28.)

Mobility and Transfers

Principles of wheelchair transfer techniques for the individual with quadriplegia are discussed in Chapter 27. Mobility depends on degree of weakness. Electric wheelchairs operated by hand, chin, or pneumatic controls have greatly increased the mobility of persons with severe upper and lower extremity weakness. Vans fitted with wheelchair lifts and stabilizing devices have made it possible for such clients to be transported to pursue community, vocational, educational, and avocational activities with an assistant. In addition, adaptations for hand controls have made it possible for many clients with function of at least C6 level to drive independently.

Home Management Activities

Many individuals with upper extremity weakness who are bound to wheelchair ambulation are dependent or partially dependent for homemaking activities. Clients with muscle function of C6 or better may be independent for light homemaking with appropriate devices, adaptations, and safety awareness. Many of the suggestions for wheelchair maneuverability and environmental adaptation outlined for the paraplegic apply here as well. In addition, the client with upper extremity weakness needs to use lightweight equipment and special devices. The *Mealtime Manual for People With Disability and the Aging* compiled by Judith Lannefeld Klinger[16] contains many excellent specific suggestions that apply to the homemaker with weak upper extremities.

ACCESS TO RECREATION AND LEISURE ACTIVITIES

A well-rounded occupational therapy treatment program should focus not only on basic self-care tasks and home management but also on the recreation and leisure interests and needs of the client. Participation in recreational activities frequently holds intrinsic value for the client, helps boost self-esteem, and may be important in the social life of the client, family, and friends.[5]

The assessment needs to include previous activities,[5] new activities the client is willing to learn, and the client's potential for participating in the activities. To determine the client's interests, the therapist could use the interest checklist and activities configuration described previously in this chapter.

The occupational therapist's role varies according to the type of program, where services are offered, and whether a recreation therapist is available. The occupational therapist may function as a resource person referring the client to resouces in the community, may refer the client to a recreation therapist, or may actually teach the client some leisure tasks. Caregiver education is an important component because (1) the client may be dependent on the caregiver to purchase items that facilitate participation in a leisure activity or (2) the caregiver may need to learn new methods to help the client get involved in leisure activities.

Community resources vary but some areas offer activities and provide services to meet the needs of the physically limited individual. Some examples are sailing, skiing, white water rafting, camping, wheelchair basketball, and travel agencies that specialize in planning trips for the physically challenged person.

Adaptive equipment for leisure activities is also available. Some examples of equipment include adapted bicycle units to attach to wheelchairs, swimming aids, adapted bowling equipment, and fishing equipment to attach to a wheelchair or use with one hand (Fig. 26-45). For more sedentary activities there are card holders, automatic card shufflers, pneumatic video game controls,

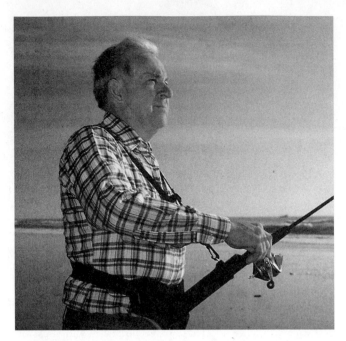

FIG. 26-45   Angler's rod holder. (Reproduced with permission, Don Krebs' Access to Recreation, Adaptive Recreation Equipment for the Physically Challenged, 2509 E. Thousand Oaks Blvd, Suite 430, Thousand Oaks, CA.)

camera holders to attach to a wheelchair, and needlework tools for one-handed use. To support return to gardening, which may be a household management task or for others a leisure task, there is adaptive equipment for those who have difficulty bending, reaching, and grasping tools.*

Although occupational therapy may initially focus on ADL and I-ADL tasks, the client will eventually want to begin considering involvement in recreation and leisure activities. If the occupational therapist is knowledgeable about regional resources and adaptive equipment for leisure activities, he or she may function as a resource person to help the client resume a balance of activities.

SUMMARY

ADL and I-ADL are tasks of self-maintenance, mobility, communication, home management, and community living that enable a person to function independently and assume important occupational roles.

ADL is one of the performance areas in the occupational performance model. Occupational therapists routinely evaluate performance in ADL to assess clients' levels of functional independence. Evaluation is carried out by interview and observation of performance. Results of the evaluation and ongoing progress are recorded

---

* Access to Recreation, Inc., 2509 E. Thousand Oaks Blvd., Suite 430, Thousand Oaks, CA (D. Krebs, President).[17]

on one of many available ADL checklists, the content of which is summarized for the permanent medical record.

Treatment is directed at training in independent living skills with activities such as eating, dressing, mobility, home management, communication, and community liv-ing skills. The occupational therapist can include in the treatment program special equipment and many methods for performing activities of daily living with specific functional problems.

Section 2   Driving with a physical dysfunction

Susan M. Lillie

DRIVING EVALUATION
IMPORTANCE OF DRIVING

Driving is an essential ADL in today's society, playing a pivotal role in personal independence, employment, and aging. A driver's license symbolizes a rite of passage to adulthood for the teenager, independence for leisure activities and employment opportunities for the adult, and wellness and competence for the older adult. The ability to drive is regarded as instrumental in obtaining and maintaining an independent lifestyle.

Driving requires continuous integration of visual, motor, cognitive, and perceptual skills at a high level of functioning. A complex task, driving carries more implications for harm than other ADL, which is one reason evaluation programs have proliferated in recent years.

Occupational therapists play a vital role in assessing driving potential by combining theoretical approaches with clinical testing and functional assessment. Analysis of activity and occupational role performance provide a framework within which to approach driver assessment. The education and training in physical measurement, visual-perceptual skills, cognitive skills, adaptive devices, and psychosocial functioning make occupational therapists uniquely suited to conduct driver evaluations.

PURPOSE OF DRIVING EVALUATION

The purpose of a driving evaluation is to assess a person's ability to drive. The ability to drive is often disrupted by a medical condition, disability, or factor of aging. Driver evaluations also help determine the most appropriate vehicle for an individual, and the adaptive equipment and training necessary to drive safely.

Driver evaluation programs vary greatly in the types of services offered. Some programs offer clinical assess-ment or simulator road tests. These programs are valuable in general problem identification, but research shows these results do not predict road performance. A comprehensive driver evaluation program includes clinical, stationary, and behind-the-wheel performance testing in a special evaluation vehicle.[8,14,15]

CANDIDATES FOR EVALUATION

Health care professionals, including physicians, therapists, and case managers, play an important role in identifying those individuals requiring a driver evaluation. The purpose of the referral is most frequently to promote independent driving. Driver assessments are costly[4] and are generally not covered by insurance or Medicaid plans. By thoroughly screening referrals for appropriateness, therapists conserve patient resources and provide cost-effective treatment. A referral to a qualified driver evaluation program should be made in the following situations:

- The patient, family, or health care professional expresses concerns about the driver's safety or competence.
- The patient has limitations that preclude use of the standard driving pattern of 2-handed steering and right foot on the gas and brake pedals.
- The patient has neuromuscular weakness or disease (e.g., MS, MD, or polio).
- The patient has a neurological condition (e.g., TBI, CVA, CP, peripheral neuropathy, Parkinson disease, tumor, or dementia).
- The patient has impaired or low vision.

OLDER DRIVERS

Older drivers are increasing in numbers with the graying of America, causing possibly unfounded concern amongst legislators and public policy makers. To date, research has not identified those skills or qualities that make an older driver incompetent.[7,9,10,11,17] Older adults have different driving habits and patterns, but most are within the continuum of safe driving performance.[10] It is suspected that within the older driver category, those with multiple medical conditions may be the at-risk group that requires a screening and/or evaluation process.

To an older person, loss of a license has considerable psychological impact.[5] Some older drivers report they would rather die than not drive again. Evaluation of older drivers with consideration of graded licenses to prolong driving within safe limitations will enable more older adults to maintain self-sufficiency and independence.[5]

Theoretical Constructs

Occupational role assessment and activity analysis are necessary steps in providing a thorough driver evaluation. Application of the principles of activity analysis reduces the task of driving to its component parts. Once identified, each of the component skills can be assessed separately, and then during the on-road test, the ability of the individual to coordinate these skills into the integrated task of driving is evaluated.

Occupational role theory is also helpful in driver assessment. Examination of the roles a person performed before the onset of physical dysfunction and the roles the person will resume can affect vehicle selection and driving equipment. Roles held by the driver (e.g., parent, student, homemaker, and employee) require activity analysis to provide additional information. A person who travels to multiple job sites, for example, may need to transfer several times each day, which directly affects fatigue level and joint viability. Use of airports or businesses that have parking structures or covered parking makes vehicle height a critical factor in accessibility. A parent may need to fasten the car seat of a toddler or supervise other children while managing predriving tasks. In each of these examples, vehicle selection and driving equipment may be affected by life roles.

A holistic viewpoint is also integral to the driver evaluation. A person's psychological state, coping strategies, acceptance of disability, tolerance of technology, and lifestyle can impact the evaluation process. Because of these and other complex issues involved in a driver evaluation, the State of California Department of Rehabilitation recommends that therapists conducting driving evaluations have a minimum of 2 years experience in physical disabilities, knowledge of adaptive equipment, driving systems, and equipment vendors.[15]

DRIVING EVALUATION COMPONENTS
CLINICAL ASSESSMENT

The clinical assessment is also referred to as a prescreening or predriving evaluation. A screening process used to identify strengths and problem areas related to driving,

the clinical assessment begins with a review of medical information, medication and side effects, episodes of seizure or loss of consciousness, mobility status, social history, vocational history, driving history, and purpose of the evaluation. Reviewing the information before the client's appointment is helpful and can lead to other pertinent questions that require answers before the evaluation.

It should be clear whether a patient's condition is stable or improving. Patients with progressive conditions may be able to drive, but additional medical data is usually required. The rate and history of decline is instrumental in building in safety margins and designing a driving system that can accommodate future changes in condition.

The clinical assessment can be performed solely by the occupational therapist[14,15] or by many members of the rehabilitation team.[4] In both models, the clinical evaluation includes the same basic components of vision, motor function, cognition, and visual perceptual skills.

Vision Screening

Visual testing should be conducted first to ascertain the driver candidate's visual acuity to eliminate impaired acuity as a factor. Standards for far acuity vary among the states, but 20/40 to 20/50 is generally the cutoff point before the motor vehicles department requires lenses from a vision specialist. Although acuity has not been related to accident rate, it is a universal standard applied by motor vehicle departments.

A comprehensive vision screening is important because vision is the primary sense used to gather information required for driving-related decision making. A comprehensive vision screening includes near and far acuities, phoria or alignment, saccades, oculomotor pursuits, range of motion, convergence, and field of vision.[3,6,14,16] Glare recovery is recommended by some and is helpful for the older adult evaluation. A vision screening is useful for identifying gross deficits, but is not to be considered diagnostic in nature.[3]

Physical Measurements

Muscle strength, active range of motion (ROM), grip, and reaction time are frequently cited as the basic abilities requiring measurement.[9,15,16,18] Head and trunk control, balance, and endurance are also important. Other areas that provide critical information when neurological disturbances are present include quality of selective movement, muscle tone, and coordination. Specialized measurements, such as steering wheel force readings with a torque wrench or push/pull motions with a Chatillon scale provide objective data in selecting more complex modifications for driving, such as the level of resistance required for steering or braking.

Cognitive and Visual-Perceptual Skills

Driving requires adequate, reliable perception of a rapidly changing environment, blending both cognitive and visual-perceptual skills. There is still no clear evidence that any one test identifies at-risk drivers or predicts driving competence.[7] Properly used and selected, however, cognitive and visual-perceptual testing assists the driver evaluator in identifying problem areas and more safely managing the behind-the-wheel segment.

Evaluation methods include observation, functional task performance, pencil and paper tasks, computerized assessment programs, and video tests.[18] Cognitive areas requiring assessment include selective and divided attention, decision making, safety judgment, planning ahead, and awareness of how the disability affects driving safety. Visual-perceptual components include visual organization, visual search and scanning, spatial relations, directionality, and visual processing speed.[8,9,15,18] These areas overlap and blur, making problem identification a challenge even to experienced therapists.

STATIONARY ASSESSMENT

The stationary component evaluates the predriving tasks and equipment setup in the static position. The vehicle for evaluation must be chosen first because of variations in the driver station, including steering resistance; gas/brake pedal angle, size, and resistance; seating; and overall layout. A stationary assessment worksheet or checklist is suggested to ensure all essential elements of the task of driving are included routinely.

Predriving Tasks

Predriving tasks include mobility to the vehicle, inserting and turning a key (or keyless entry operation), opening and closing the door, entering and exiting the vehicle, loading and unloading mobility devices (cane, walker, wheelchair), adjusting the driver seat, adjusting the mirrors, and fastening the seatbelt (and chest strap when needed). Adaptive devices to facilitate independence in predriving tasks include special key holders, loops for lower extremity management, a wheelchair strap to extend reach for wheelchair loading, and modifications for independent retrieval of the seatbelt. Mechanical devices enable some patients to manage mobility equipment independently and continue to use their car, truck, or minivan without expensive modifications. Because the effectiveness of adaptive devices varies with different products, a trial-and-error approach is appropriate in selecting the proper adaptive device or equipment for a patient.

Steps in Equipment Selection

The first step in the primary control assessment phase is to achieve optimal positioning of the driver, whether from the vehicle's driver seat or from a wheelchair. Positioning is important for optimal upper extremity function and safety. Poor trunk stability may require special positioning devices or the use of an upper torso or chest strap.[1,2] All securement devices (seatbelts, chest straps) should be in place before proceeding to primary control assessment, because these stability devices can inhibit reach or alter substitution patterns used by a patient.

Equipment setups proceed in a logical progression, starting with the primary controls. Primary controls are those devices that control the steering, accelerator, and braking of a vehicle. Steering is the first primary control assessed, followed by the gas and brake controls. All other controls, such as turn signals, horn, and headlights, are secondary controls. It is vital to safety that the driver be able to access the horn, windshield wiper, turn signals, and dimmer switch quickly and efficiently with the vehicle in motion.[13]

The State of California's Department of Rehabilitation Guidelines require that recommendations for adaptive equipment be made only when a driver can demonstrate the ability to use the "same general type of device" in a behind-the-wheel assessment.[16] This quality assurance and liability protection measure serves to protect the patient and driver evaluator as well as preventing costly (and potentially dangerous) equipment mistakes.

Steering Options

Whether the driver uses two-handed steering techniques (i.e., hand-over-hand, shuffling, or feeding the wheel) or one-handed steering with a steering device, smooth, controlled steering is the goal. When steering is done single-handedly, a steering device is recommended for safety to maintain control of the wheel at all times. Without such a device, driving with one hand requires "palming" of the steering wheel during turns, when the palm rests on the rim of the wheel, rather than locking through grip or pinch. One-handed steering by palming the wheel is not recommended. Additionally, a driver generally has to make a turn more slowly when palming the wheel, sometimes well below the speed of the flow of traffic, to manage the turn. Use of a steering device (spinner knob, v-grip, tripin, palmar cuff, or amputee ring) allows a driver to maintain smoother control of the steering wheel. A steering device provides constant control of the steering wheel and the ability to make turns quickly and efficiently.

Additional modifications include smaller diameter steering wheels and reduced levels of steering resistance, but both require meticulous evaluation for safety. Smaller diameter steering wheels are harder to turn and require low or zero effort modifications to enable a patient to turn the steering wheel efficiently. The Veteran's Administration or each state Department of Rehabilitation regulations can assist in the selection process for steering setup. Only after the steering setup is determined does the process move to the accelerator and brake controls.

Accelerator and Brake Controls

Modified accelerator and brake controls can be installed in most vehicles. Simple modifications, such as pedal extensions, can be installed on both the accelerator and brake pedals to compensate for limited reach. In the case

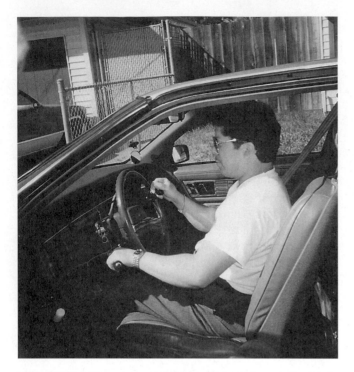

FIG. 26-46 Basic setup for paraplegic includes spinner knob steering device for right hand steering, push-right-angle-pull hand control to operate gas and brake, and extended brake handle to set parking brake.

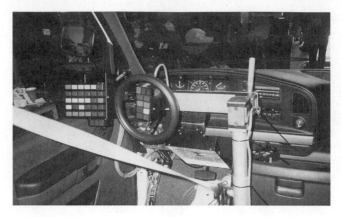

FIG. 26-47 Driving Systems Incorporated (dSi) and joystick systems combine gas, brake, and steering functions onto one lever. These sophisticated unilever systems enable many persons with severe disabilities (arthrogryposis, C5 quadriplegia, muscle diseases) to drive.

of a person with a significant right hemiplegia, however, the right foot is unable to operate the standard pedals. A left sided accelerator pedal can be used to compensate by placing the pedal to the left of the standard gas pedal; the left foot can then operate gas and brakes safely. When the lower extremities lack adequate motor control or are paralyzed, a device called a hand control allows operation of the accelerator and brake pedal with an upper extremity (Fig. 26-46).

Hand controls can use rotary, push/pull, push/pull down, or side-to-side motions to apply pressure to the accelerator and the brake. The occupational therapist must know an individual's medical condition, predict potential problems with motion specific to the hand control, and then select which hand control is most appropriate for evaluation. For example, if a person has severe arthritis in the hand or carpal tunnel syndrome, the rotary-style hand control could exacerbate the symptoms.

High tech gas/brake controls, operated by vacuum, pneumatics, or computer, allow more disabled persons to drive than ever before by requiring less ROM to activate the device (Fig. 26-47). This specialized area of driver evaluation requires advanced training in addition to keeping abreast of technological advances, and mobility seating system trends.

VEHICLE SELECTION
Car Consideration

A basic level of service for a driver evaluation program is the car evaluation. A car is generally appropriate if a per-

son can enter and exit the vehicle independently and load mobility equipment devices. Transfer methods include the stand pivot, bent pivot, sliding board, and upper extremity depression. A person using the sliding board or upper extremity depression method must be able to transfer up inclines because transferring from a car to a wheelchair is generally in an upward direction. When loading equipment manually is not feasible, independence can sometimes be obtained by using a mechanical device to perform the task. This process becomes complicated because all vehicles and mechanical aids are not compatible; one generalization is that compact and subcompact vehicles are usually too small to accommodate these mechanical wheelchair-loading aids.

The standard car recommendation is a 2-door vehicle with power steering, power brakes, and automatic transmission. Bench seats are easiest to transfer into, but are rapidly disappearing from automotive designs. Bucket or semibucket seats are more common and becoming the standard. Gearshift levers positioned in a central console between the driver and passenger seats can be problematic, interfering not only with transfers, but also requiring dexterity to depress the gear shift release button to shift gears. Those with hand impairments may do better with a gearshift lever mounted on the steering column.

Van Considerations

Two types of drivers utilize vans: those transferring to a driver seat and those driving from their wheelchairs. Drivers must choose between full size vans and minivans. Evaluations for those driving from their wheelchairs are more complex and require greater skill because of increased variables that affect driving performance and equipment selection.

Entry into a van requires a mechanical lift for most people using a wheelchair or scooter. Mechanical lifts can be mounted on the rear or side of a full-size van or the side of a minivan. Lifts fall into two basic categories:

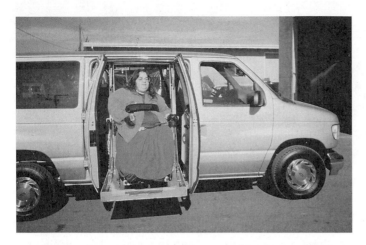

FIG. 26-48 Platform-sytle lift can be located at side or rear of van. Additional entry headroom, obtained through lowered floor, allows this client to see out windshield when driving from her power wheelchair.

rotary or swing-in style lifts and platform-style lifts (Fig. 26-48). Each lift has unique characteristics, strengths, and drawbacks.[12] Minivans also have fully automatic mechanical ramps for independent entry and exit (Fig. 26-49). The therapist must provide a safe and compatible match between lift choice, parking needs, and lifestyle. Restrictions by each state's Department of Vocational Rehabilitation can also influence vehicle and equipment selections for those patients funded by these agencies.

Behind-the-Wheel Assessment

Once the driver has been set up with primary controls in the evaluation vehicle, the ability to use these controls must be verified through actual driving, commonly called the behind-the-wheel or on-road portion of the evaluation. Sometimes several driving equipment setups are attempted during the behind-the-wheel session before the right combination for safe driving is determined.

Road Test Components

The industry standard is to accept the on-road driving test as the optimal measure of driving compe-

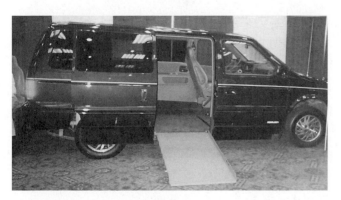

FIG. 26-49 Minivan conversions have access ramp in lieu of lift, along with 10-inch floor drop. Airbag system lowers van to decrease ramp angle for easier entry and exit.

tence.[3,7,10,11,15] Therefore, a decision made on a person's license, when based on an actual road test, is considered a sound decision. Efforts are being made to standardize the behind-the-wheel test and scoring system to improve validity and interrater reliability.

For safety and comprehensive testing, it is recommended that the moving vehicle portions of a driver evaluation include two staff members, the driver instructor/educator and the driving evaluator/observer. The driving instructor, in the front passenger seat, can be a state licensed instructor or a therapist with special training,[2,15] while the driving evaluator, usually an occupational therapist, sits in the back seat. The driving instructor tells the patient where to drive, instructs in use of adaptive driving equipment, maintains vehicle control by intervening when necessary, and keeps the vehicle occupants safe by adhering to laws and rules of the road. The evaluator observes the task of driving, takes written notes, and completes a scoring sheet. The driving instructor and evaluator work as a team and both must be able to stand behind recommended driving and equipment modification recommendations. A standardized or consistent score sheet to score drivers is recommended for objectivity and data comparison.

The Driving Route

Driving routes should incorporate a sampling of road conditions, traffic patterns, and unusual settings common to that region. The assessment route needs to progress through faster and more congested traffic and various traffic conditions to obtain information on the driver's skills in a wide variety of conditions. The driving route should be graded and allow the patient time to become familiar with the evaluation vehicle and adaptive equipment. This period of learning and accommodation will be longer for novice or apprehensive drivers. Driving performance scores should reflect physical management of the vehicle, ability to use the adaptive equipment,[1] interaction with other traffic, adherence to rules of the road, and safety judgment.[7,14,17]

Recommendations for Driving

After the drive test is completed, the driving team reviews the results with the patient. Asking the patient for feedback first provides valuable perspective on the patient's insight. All recommendations for driving should be made in writing to the patient and submitted to medical records. The comprehensive driving report

. . . shall contain a summary of the clinical assessment and a statement of the client's potential to be a safe and independent driver. The report should specify the type of vehicle which is necessary, the modifications required, other adaptive equipment required, vendor sources, and special instructions or problems. The report shall make recommendations on the type of follow-up required, what to look for, and who is best suited to provide the follow-up services. The report should also estimate the amount of driver's training needed, what specific areas of training should be emphasized, and where the training is available.*

The Unsafe Driver

One of the most difficult tasks facing a driver evaluator is notifying a driver candidate and the family that the person cannot drive safely. The decision to rate a driver as unsafe results in immediate dependency and transportation issues that have no easy solution. It is important to develop the skill of listening to the driver's response and frustration while remaining firm in the decision. Referring the driver to the motor vehicle department for a photo ID card and providing materials on alternative transportation, such as mass transit or paratransit systems, is another means of assisting the patient at the current level of functioning.

LEGAL ISSUES AND PUBLIC POLICY
STATE LAWS PERTAINING TO THERAPISTS

Therapists and physicians need to be aware of their state's laws concerning medical conditions and driving. Most states do not require the reporting of medical conditions, seizures, or loss of consciousness to the motor vehicles department.[9,11,17] Instead, most states rely on

---

* From *Statement of Assurances for Providers of Driver Evaluation Services,* State of California Department of Rehabilitation Mobility Evaluation Program, Downey, Calif, 1990, page 6.

voluntary reporting of medical conditions by the driver having the condition. While some states advocate reporting by family, physician, or law enforcement, not all states provide immunity for such reporting. Once identified to the motor vehicle department, the patient undergoes a license review that varies from state to state.

Laws affecting the legality of the therapist in the driver instructor role also vary by state. Some states allow the therapist to conduct training without being a licensed driver trainer. Other states allow therapists legally to perform the driver instructor role for evaluations only, while ongoing driver instructor training requires the state driver instructor license. Therapists must know their state's regulations and not exceed them. Because some states allow therapists to conduct driver training without driver instructor education, additional education and training should be sought to minimize liability and ensure that skills meet industry standards.

PUBLIC POLICY DEVELOPMENT

Department of Motor Vehicle Medical Advisory Boards have been reactivated across the country in response to public safety concerns and policy needs. As occupational therapists start to be recognized for their expertise and contributions in driver safety, more therapists are being appointed to medical advisory boards in the 50 states. Therapists add a valuable functionally-based perspective to driver evaluation that aids sound development of public policy and licensing decisions.

REVIEW QUESTIONS

SECTION 1: SELF-CARE/HOME MANAGEMENT

1. Define activities of daily living and instrumental activities of daily living. List three classifications of tasks that may be considered in each category.
2. What is the role of occupational therapy in restoring ADL and I-ADL independence?
3. List at least three activities that are considered self-care skills, three mobility skills, three communication skills, three home management skills and three community living skills.
4. List three factors that the occupational therapist must consider before commencing ADL performance evaluation and training. Describe how each could limit or effect ADL performance.

5. What is the ultimate goal of the ADL and I-ADL training program?
6. Discuss the concept of maximal independence, as defined in the text.
7. List the general steps in the procedure for ADL evaluation.
8. Describe how the occupational therapist can use the ADL checklist.
9. List the steps in the activities of home management evaluation.
10. What is the purpose of the home evaluation?
11. List the steps in the home evaluation.
12. Who should be involved in a comprehensive home evaluation?
13. What kinds of things are assessed in a home evaluation?
14. How does the therapist record and report results of the home evaluation and make the necessary recommendations?

15. Describe the role of the occupational therapist in the driving evaluation.
16. List eight criteria that can be used to select potential candidates for driving.
17. List six physical and performance skills that can help to determine driving potential.
18. How does the occupational therapist, with the client, select ADL and I-ADL training objectives after an evaluation?
19. Describe three approaches to teaching ADL skills to a client with perception or memory deficits.
20. List the important factors to include in an ADL progress report.
21. Describe the levels of independence, as defined in the text.
22. Describe how the occupational therapist may help facilitate the client's participation in leisure activities.
23. Give an example of health and safety management issue.

EXERCISES

SECTION 1

1. Demonstrate the use of at least three assistive devices mentioned in the text.
2. Teach another person to don a shirt, using one hand.
3. Teach another person how to don and remove trousers, as if he or she had hemiplegia.
4. Teach another person how to don and remove trousers, as if the legs were paralyzed.

REVIEW QUESTIONS

SECTION 2: DRIVING WITH A PHYSICAL DYSFUNCTION

1. What is the importance of driving to the adolescent, adult, and older adult?
2. What are some of the physical and psychological skills required for safe driving?
3. List the purposes of the driving evaluation.
4. What criteria are used to determine candidates for driving evaluation?
5. How do occupational roles affect the driving evaluation?
6. List and describe the components of the driving evaluation.
7. What are the elements of vision screening for driving?
8. Which physical capacities are evaluated in the predriving assessment?
9. List the cognitive and visual-perceptual components for evaluation.
10. What is evaluated in the pre-driving tasks portion of the driving assessment?
11. How is appropriate adapted equipment selected?
12. List 5 steering devices available.
13. Why is palming the wheel not advisable for steering?
14. List at least three ways to modify accelerator and brake controls.
15. If a car is selected as the vehicle of choice, what is the type usually recommended?
16. What are the components of the behind-the-wheel and on-road components of the assessment?
17. What legal issues must be considered by the occupational therapist performing a driving assessment?
18. What skills should the occupational therapist possess if he or she plans to become a driving evaluator?

REFERENCES

SECTION 1: ACTIVITIES OF DAILY LIVING

1. *Activities of daily living for patients with incoordination, limited range of motion, paraplegia, quadriplegia, and hemiplegia,* Cleveland, 1968, Rev. 1989, Metro Health Center for Rehabilitation, Metro Health Medical Center, Unpublished.
2. Armstrong M, Lauzen S: *Community Integration Program,* ed 2, Washington, 1994, Idyll Arbor.
3. Bromley I: *Tetraplegia and paraplegia: a guide for physiotherapists,* ed 2, London, 1981, Churchill Livingstone.
4. Buchwald E: *Physical rehabilitation for daily living,* New York, 1952, McGraw-Hill.
5. Christiansen C: Occupational performance assessement. In Christiansen C, Baum C, editors: *Occupational therapy overcoming human performance deficits,* Thorofare, NJ, 1991, Slack.
6. Cynkin S, Robinson AM: *Occupational therapy and activities health: toward health through activities,* Boston, 1990, Little, Brown.
7. Easton LW, Horan AL: Dressing band, *Am J Occup Ther* 33:656, 1979.
8. Feldmeier DM, Poole JL: The position-adjustable hair dryer, *Am J Occup Ther* 41:246, 1987.
9. Florey LL, Michelman SM: Occupational role history: a screening tool for psychiatric occupational therapy, *Am J Occup Ther* 36:301, 1982.
10. Guerette P, Moran W: ADL awareness, *Team Rehab Report* June, 1994.
11. Holser P, Jones M, Ilanit T: A study of the upper extremity control brace, *Am J Occup Ther* 16:170, 1962.
12. Hopkins HL, Smith HD, Tiffany EG: Therapeutic application of activity. In Hopkins HL, Smith HD, editors: *Willard and Spackman's occupational therapy,* ed 6, Philadelphia, 1983, JB Lippincott.
13. Kelly SN: Adaptations for independent use of cassette tape recorder/radio by high-level quadriplegic patients, *Am J Occup Ther* 37:766, 1983.
14. Kemp BJ, Mitchell JM: Functional assessment in geriatric mental health. In JE Birren and associates, editors: *Handbook of Mental Health and Aging,* 2nd ed, San Diego, 1992, Academic Press.
15. Kester DL: Prevocational and vocational assessment. In Hopkins HL, Smith HD, editors: *Willard and Spackman's occupational therapy,* ed 6, Philadelphia, 1983, JB Lippincott.
16. Klinger JL: *Mealtime manual for people with disabilities and the aging,* Camden, NJ, 1978, Campbell Soup.
17. Krebs D: Access to recreation: adaptive recreation equipment for the physically challenged, Thousand Oaks, Calif, 1995, Access to Recreation.
18. Letts L, Law M, Rigby P and associates: Person-environment assessments in occupational therapy, *Am J Occup Ther* 48:608-618, 1994.
19. Malick MH, Almasy BS: Assessment and evaluation: life work tasks. In Hopkins HL, Smith HD, editors: *Willard and Spackman's occupational therapy,* ed 6, Philadelphia, 1983, JB Lippincott.
20. Malick MH, Almasy BS: Activities of daily living and homemaking. In Hopkins HL, Smith HD, editors: *Willard and Spackman's occupational therapy,* ed 7, Philadelphia, 1988, JB Lippincott.

21. Matsusuyu J: The interest checklist, *Am J Occup Ther* 23:323, 1969.
22. Melvin JL: *Rheumatic disease: occupational therapy and rehabilitation,* ed 2, Philadelphia, 1982, FA Davis.
23. Moorhead L: The occupational history, *Am J Occup Ther* 23:329, 1969.
24. The Professional Manual Subcommittee of the Educational Committee, Allied Health Professional Section of the Arthritis Foundation: *Arthritis manual for allied health professionals,* New York, 1973, The Arthritis Foundation.
25. Runge M: Self-dressing techniques for clients with spinal cord injury, *Am J Occup Ther* 21:367, 1967.
26. Sokaler R: A buttoning aid, *Am J Occup Ther* 35:737, 1981.
27. Trombly CA: Activities of daily living. In Trombly CA, editor: *Occupational therapy for physical dysfunction,* ed 2, Baltimore, 1983, Williams & Wilkins.
28. Watanabe S: Activities configuration: regional institute on the evaluation process, *Final Rep. RSA-123-T-68,* New York, 1968, American Occupational Therapy Association.
29. Wykoff E, Mitani M: The spoon plate: a self-feeding device, *Am J Occup Ther* 36:333, 1982.

REFERENCES

SECTION 2: DRIVING WITH A PHYSICAL DYSFUNCTION

1. Babirad J: Considerations in seating and positioning severely disabled drivers, *Assist Technol* 1:31-37, 1989.
2. Blanc C, Hunt JT: Getting in gear, *Team Rehab Report* 33-39, August, 1994.
3. Bouska MJ, Gallaway M: Primary visual deficits in adults with brain damage: management in occupational therapy, *Occup Ther Pract* 3(1):1-11, 1991.
4. Breske S: The drive for independence, *Advance/Rehab* 3(8):10-19, 1994.
5. *Graduated driver licensing creating mobility choices: PF5078(793)· D15109,* Washington, DC, 1993, American Association of Retired Persons.
6. Hopewell CA: Head injury rehabilitation: adaptive driving after TBI. In Burke WH and associates, editors: The HDI professional series on traumatic brain injury, No. 5, Houston, 1988, HDI.
7. Janke MK: *Age-related disabilities that may impair drivers and their assessment,* Sacramento, Calif, 1994, State of California Department of Motor Vehicles.
8. Latson LF: Overview of disabled drivers' evaluation process, *Physical Disabilities Special Interest Section Newsletter,* 10(4), 1987, American Occupational Therapy Association.
9. Lillie SM: Evaluation for driving. In Yoshikawa TT, editor: *Ambulatory geriatric care,* St Louis, 1993, Mosby-Year Book.
10. Odenheimer GL: *Cognitive dysfunction and driving abilities,* Presentation to the annual meeting of the American Geriatrics Society, Atlanta, May 18, 1990.
11. Odenheimer GL and associates: Performance-based driving evaluation of the elderly driver: safety, reliability, and validity, *J Geront Med Sci* 49(4):M153-M159, 1994.
12. Perr A, Barnicle K: Van lifts: the ups and downs and ins and outs, *TeamRehab Report* 49-53, June, 1993.
13. Roush L, Koppa R: A survey of activation importance of individual secondary controls in modified vehicles, Human Factors Program, Safety Division, Texas Transportation Institute, Texas A & M University, January, 1992
14. Sabo S, Shipp M: *Disabilities and their implications for driving,* Ruston, La, 1989, Louisiana Tech University Center for Rehabilitation Sciences and Biomedical Engineering.
15. Statement of assurances for providers of driver evaluation services, State of California Department of Rehabilitation Mobility Evaluation Program, Downey, Calif, 1990.
16. Strano CM: Driver evaluation and training of the physically disabled driver: additional comments, *Physical Disabilities Special Interest Section Newsletter,* 10(4), 1987, American Occupational Therapy Association.
17. Summary of proceedings of the Conference on Driver Competency Assessment, CAL-DMV-RSS-91-132, Sacramento, 1993, State of California Department of Motor Vehicles, Program and Policy Administration, Research and Development Section.
18. Taira ED, editor: *Assessing the driving ability of the elderly,* Binghamton, NY, 1989, Hayworth Press.

Wheelchair Assessment and Transfers

Carole Adler, Michelle Tipton-Burton

WHEELCHAIRS

A wheelchair can be the primary means of ambulation for someone with a permanent or progressive disability such as cerebral palsy, brain injury, spinal cord injury, multiple sclerosis, or muscular dystrophy. It may be required as a temporary means of mobility for someone with a short-term illness or orthopedic problem. In addition to mobility, the wheelchair can substantially influence the total body positioning, skin integrity, overall function, and general well-being of the patient. Regardless of the patient's diagnosis, the occupational therapist must understand the complexity of wheelchair technology, available options and modifications, the evaluation and measuring process, the use and care, and the process by which this equipment is funded.

Wheelchairs have evolved considerably in recent years. There have been significant advances in powered and manual wheelchair technology by manufacturers and service providers. Products are constantly changing, and although many of the improvements result from user recommendations, the therapists who prescribe the equipment have had influence as well.

Occupational therapists and/or physical therapists, depending on their respective roles at the treatment facility, are usually responsible for evaluating, measuring, and selecting a wheelchair for the patient. They also teach wheelchair safety and mobility. Because of the increasingly sophisticated nature and variety of power and manual wheelchairs, it is advisable to include on the ordering team an experienced and knowledgeable rehabilitation technology supplier (RTS) and a durable medical equipment (DME) supplier. They are proficient in ordering custom items and can offer an objective and broad mechanical perspective on the availability and appropriateness of the options being considered. It is the RTS who will be the patient's resource for repairs and reordering when returning to the community.

Whether the patient requires a noncustom rental wheelchair for temporary use or a custom wheelchair for use over many years, an individualized prescription clearly outlining the specific features of the chair is needed to ensure optimal performance, mobility and enhancement of function. A wheelchair that has been prescribed by an inexperienced or nonclinical person is potentially hazardous to the patient. An ill-fitting wheelchair can, in fact, contribute to unnecessary fatigue, skin breakdown, and trunk or extremity deformity, and can inhibit function.[4] A wheelchair is an extension of the patient's body[6] and should act to facilitate good alignment, mobility, and function rather than inhibit these features.

WHEELCHAIR EVALUATION[1]

The therapist has considerable responsibility in recommending the wheelchair appropriate to meet not only immediate needs but long-term needs as well. When evaluating for a wheelchair, the therapist must know the patient and have a broad perspective of the patient's clinical, functional, and environmental needs. Careful evaluation of physical status must include the following: the specific diagnosis, prognosis, and current and future problems that may affect wheelchair use (such as age, spasticity, loss of ROM, muscle weakness, and endurance). Functional use of the wheelchair in a variety of environments must be considered. See Box 27-1 for questions to ask before making specific recommendations.

All data must be considered before making recommendations. The information must be weighed for advantages and disadvantages and how these are integrated with the entire system before preparing the final prescription.

The therapist must develop a good working relationship with the equipment supplier and the reimbursement sources to facilitate payment of the most appropriate mobility system for the patient. Verbal and written skills must be developed to communicate clearly throughout the entire assessment and treatment process.

BOX 27-1

QUESTIONS TO ASK BEFORE MAKING SPECIFIC RECOMMENDATIONS

What is the specific disability?

What is the prognosis?

Is ROM limited?

Is strength or endurance limited?

How will the patient propel the chair?

How old is the patient?

How long is the patient expected to use the wheelchair?

What was the patient's lifestyle and how has it changed?

Is the patient active or sedentary?

How will the dimensions of the chair affect the patient's ability to transfer to various surfaces?

What is the maneuverability of the wheelchair in the patient's home: entrance, door width, turning radius in bathroom and hallways, floor surfaces?

What is the ratio of indoor to outdoor activities?

Where will the wheelchair be primarily used: in the home, at school, work, the community?

Which mode of transportation will be used? Will the patient be driving from the wheelchair? How will it be loaded and unloaded from the car?

Which special needs exist in the work or school environment, for example, work heights, available assistance, accessibility of toilet facilities, parking facilities?

Does the patient participate in indoor or outdoor sports activities?

How will the wheelchair affect the patient psychologically?

Who will pay for the wheelchair?

Can accessories and special modifications be justified or are they luxury items?

What are the patient's resources for equipment maintenance?

An in-depth awareness of the patient's specific reimbursement requirements and documentation with thorough justification of medical necessity is imperative for authorization of payment. Therapists must substantiate clearly why particular features of a wheelchair are being recommended. They must be aware of standard versus "up charge" items, their cost, and how they will affect the end product.[1]

WHEELCHAIR ORDERING CONSIDERATIONS[1,4,7]

The following sequence of evaluation considerations should be carefully thought about when assessing a wheelchair and before determining a specific brand and specifications.

PROPELLING THE WHEELCHAIR

Propelling a wheelchair may be accomplished in a variety of ways, depending on the physical capacities of the user. If the patient is capable of self-propulsion using the arms on the rear wheels of the wheelchair, it is to be assumed that there is sufficient bilateral grasp, arm strength, and physical endurance to maneuver the chair independently over varied terrain throughout the day.[7] An assortment of push rims is available to facilitate self-propelling depending on the user's arm and grip strength. A patient with hemiplegia may propel a wheelchair using the unaffected arm and the ipsilateral leg to maneuver the wheelchair.

If independence in mobility is to be achieved, a power wheelchair should be considered for those with minimal or no use of the upper extremities, limited endurance, or inaccessible outdoor terrain.[7] Power chairs can be belt- or direct-drive, have a wide variety of features and programmability, can be driven by foot, arm, head, or neck or be pneumatically controlled. A person with the most severe disability can drive a power wheelchair given today's sophisticated technology.

If the chair is to be caregiver-propelled, then consideration must be given to ease of maneuverability and handling by the caregiver as well as the positioning and mobility needs of the patient.

Regardless of the method of propulsion, serious consideration must be given to the impact that the chair has on the patient's current and future mobility and positioning needs. In addition, lifestyle and environment, available resources such as ability to maintain the chair, transportation options, and available reimbursement sources are major determining factors.

RENTAL VERSUS PURCHASE

The therapist should know about how long the patient will require the chair and whether the chair should be rented or purchased, which will affect the type of chair being considered. This decision is based on several clinical and functional issues. A rental chair is appropriate for short-term or temporary use, such as when the patient's clinical picture, functional status, or body size are changing. Rental chairs may be necessary when the permanent wheelchair is being repaired. A rental wheelchair also may be useful when the patient cannot accept a wheelchair and needs to experience it initially as a temporary piece of equipment. Often it is not known what the eventual functional outcome will be. In that case a chair can be rented for several months until a reevaluation determines whether a permanent chair will be necessary.[1]

A permanent wheelchair is indicated for the full-time user and for the patient with a progressive need for a wheelchair over a long period of time. It may be indicated when custom features are required and also when body size is changing such as in the growing child.[1]

FRAME STYLE

Once method of propulsion and permanence of chair have been determined, there are several wheelchair frame styles to consider. The frame style must be selected before specific dimensions and brand names can be determined. The therapist needs to be aware of the various features, advantages and disadvantages, and how these features will affect the patient in every aspect of his of her life both from a short-term and long-term perspective.

WHEELCHAIR SELECTION[1]

The following considerations regarding patient needs should be carefully assessed before determining the specific type of chair:

Manual versus Electric (Fig. 27-1)
Manual (Fig. 27-1, *A*)

Does the user have sufficient strength and endurance to propel chair?

Does manual mobility enhance functional independence and cardiovascular conditioning of user?

Does the user require manual mobility as an exercise modality?

Does user demonstrate insufficient cognitive ability to propel an electric wheelchair safely?

Will caregiver be propelling the chair at any time?

Electric (Fig. 27-1, *B*)

Does the user demonstrate insufficient endurance and functional ability to propel manual wheelchair independently?

Does the user demonstrate progressive functional loss, making powered mobility an energy-conserving option?

Is powered mobility required to increase independence at school, work, and in the community?

Does the user demonstrate cognitive and perceptual ability to operate a power-driven system safely?

Does the user or caregiver demonstrate responsibility for care and maintenance of equipment?

Is a van available for transportation?

Manual Recline versus Power Recline (Fig. 27-2)
Manual recline (Fig. 27-2, *A*)

Is the patient unable to sit upright secondary to hip contractures, poor balance, fatigue?

Is a caregiver available to assist with weight shifts and position changes?

Is relative ease of maintenance a concern?

Is cost a consideration?

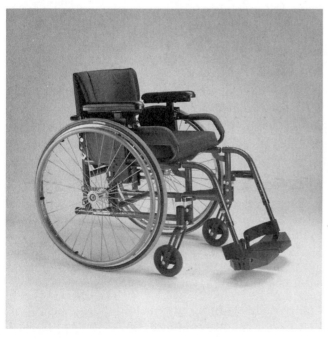

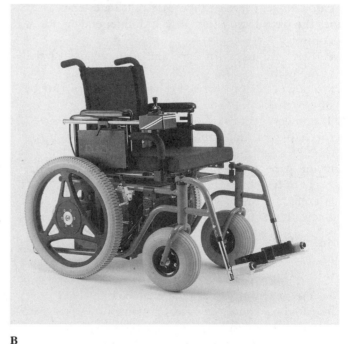

A   **B**

FIG. 27-1 Manual vs. electric wheelchair. **A,** Rigid frame chair with swing-away footrests. **B,** Power-driven wheelchair with hand control. (Photos courtesy of Quickie Designs.)

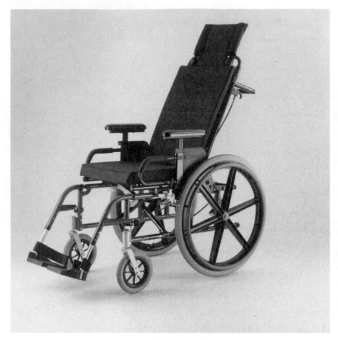
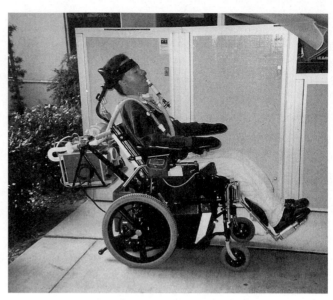

A   **B**

FIG. 27-2 Manual recline vs. power recline wheelchair. **A,** Reclining back on folding frame. (Photo courtesy of Quickie Designs.) **B,** Power recliner with chin control on electric wheelchair.

Power recline (power only) (Fig. 27-2, *B*)

Does the patient have the potential to operate independently?

Are independent weight shifts and position changes indicated for skin care and increased sitting tolerance?

Does the user demonstrate safe and independent use of controls?

Are there resources for care and maintenance of the equipment?

Will a power recline decrease or make more efficient use of caregiver time?

Will a power recline reduce the need for transfers to bed for catheterizations and rest periods throughout the day?

Will the patient require quick position changes in the event of hypotension and dysreflexia?

Has a reimbursement source been identified for this relatively "high tech" and therefore expensive feature?

Folding Versus Rigid Manual Wheelchairs (Fig. 27-3)
Folding (Fig. 27-3, *A*)

Does the patient prefer a traditional-looking chair?

Is the folding frame required for transport, storage, or home accessibility?

Which footrest style is necessary for transfers, desk clearance, and other daily living skills? Elevating footrests may be available only on folding frames.

Is patient or caregiver able to load and fit into necessary vehicles?

Most equipment suppliers have knowledge and a variety of brands available. Frame weight can range between 28 and 50 pounds depending on size and accessories. Frame adjustments and custom options depend on the model.

Rigid (Fig. 27-3, *B*)

Does the user or caregiver have the upper extremity function and balance to load and unload the nonfolding frame from a vehicle?

Will the user benefit from limited maintenance responsibilities because there are few moving parts?

Footrest options are limited and the frame is lighter weight (20 to 35 pounds). Features include adjustable seat angle, rear axle, caster mount, and back height. Efficient frame design maximizes performance. There are options in frame material composition, frame colors, and aesthetics. These chairs are usually custom ordered; availability and expertise are usually limited to custom rehabilitation technology suppliers.

Lightweight (Folding or Nonfolding) versus Standard Weight (Folding)
Lightweight (under 35 pounds, Fig. 27-3, *A*)

Does user have trunk balance and equilibrium necessary to handle lighter frame weight?

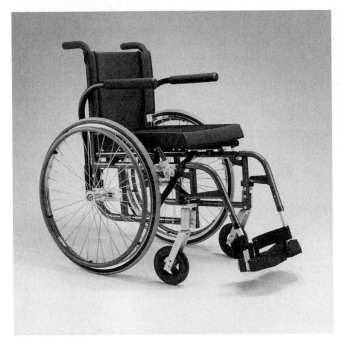

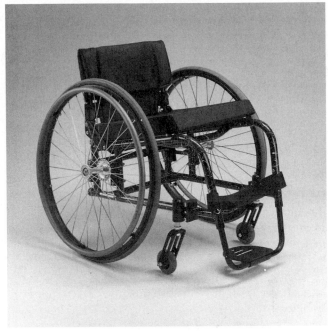

A

B

FIG. 27-3 Folding vs. rigid wheelchair. **A,** Lightweight folding frame with swing-away footrests. **B,** Rigid (nonfolding) aluminum frame with tapered front end and solid foot cradle. (Photo courtesy of Quickie Designs.)

Does lighter weight enhance mobility by reducing fatigue of the user?

Do lightweight parts such as armrests and footrests provide ease of management during daily living skills?

Are custom features necessary, for example, adjustable height back, seat angle, axle mount?

Standard weight (over 35 pounds, Fig. 27-4)

Does the user require the stability of a standard weight chair?

Does the user have the ability to propel a standard weight chair?

Can caregiver manage the increased weight when loading the wheelchair and fitting into a vehicle?

Will the increased weight of parts be unimportant during daily living skills?

Custom options are limited, and these wheelchairs are usually less expensive (except heavy-duty models).

Bottom of the Line versus Top of the Line

The price range, durability/warranty, and standard and custom features within a specific manufacturer's brand line must be considered.

Bottom of the line

Is the chair required only for part-time use?

Does the user have a limited life expectancy?

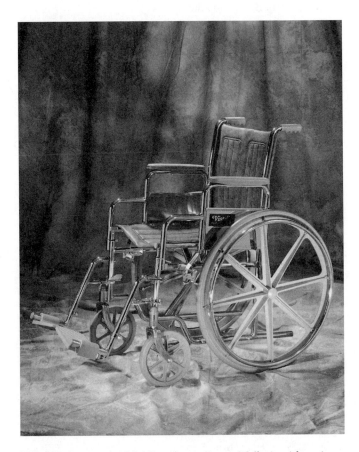

FIG. 27-4 Standard folding frame (over 35 lbs.) with swing-away footrests. (Photo courtesy of Everest and Jennings, Inc.)

Is the chair required as a second or transportion chair, used only 10% to 20% of the time?

Will the chair be primarily for indoor or sedentary use?

Will the chair be propelled only by the care giver?

Are custom features or specifications not necessary?

Is substantial durability unimportant?

For bottom of the line wheelchairs, limited warranty is available on the frame. They may be indicated because of reimbursement limitations. Limited sizes and options and adjustability are available. These cost considerably less than top of the line wheelchairs.

Top of the line

Will patient be a full-time user?

Is there a good prognosis for long-term use of the wheel-chair?

Will this be the primary wheelchair?

Is the user active both indoors and outdoors?

Will this frame style improve prognosis for independent mobility?

Is the user a growing adolescent or does he or she have a progressive disorder requiring later modification?

Are custom features, specifications, or positioning devices required?

For top of the line wheelchairs, there is a long-term warranty on the frame. Custom specifications, options, and adjustability are available.

WHEELCHAIR MEASUREMENT PROCEDURE (Fig. 27-5)[1,6]

Measurements should be determined with the patient seated on a mat table. The patient is measured in the style of chair and with the cushion that most closely resembles

those being ordered. If the patient will wear a brace or body jacket or require any additional devices in the chair, these should be in place during the measurement. Observation skills are very important during this process. *Do not go by measurements alone. "Eyeball" entire body position every step of the way.*

Seat Width (Fig. 27-5, *A*)

Objectives. (1) To distribute the patient's weight over the widest possible surface and (2) to Keep the overall width of the chair as narrow as possible.

Measure. Across the widest part of either the thighs or hips while patient is sitting in a chair comparable to that expected.

Wheelchair clearance W/C. Add ½ to 1 inch on each side of the hip or thigh measurement taken. Consider how increasing overall width of chair will affect accessibility.

Check. Flat palm of hand between the patient's hip/thigh and wheelchair skirt and armrest.

Consider

- User's potential weight gain or loss.
- Accessibility of varied environments.
- Overall width of wheelchair.

Seat Depth (Fig. 27-5, *B*)

Objective. To distribute the body weight along the sitting surface by bearing weight along the entire length of thigh to just behind the knee. This approach is necessary to assist in prevention of pressure sores on the buttocks and for optimal muscle tone normalization throughout the entire body.

Measure. From the rear of buttocks to inside of bent knee. W/C clearance: 1 to 2 inches less than the measurement for *B*.

Check. Clearance behind the knees to prevent contact of front edge of seat upholstery with the popliteal space.

Consider

- Braces or back inserts that may be pushing the patient forward.
- Postural changes throughout the day from fatigue or spasticity.
- Thigh length discrepancy; the depth of the seat may be different for each leg.
- If considering a power recliner, assume the patient will slide forward slightly throughout the day and make depth adjustments accordingly.
- Seat depth may need to be shortened to allow independent propulsion with the lower extremities.

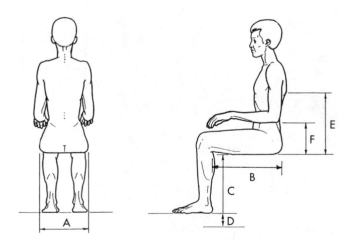

FIG. 27-5 What and where to measure. **A,** Seat width. **B,** Seat depth. **C,** Seat height from floor. **D,** Footrest clearance. **E,** Back height. **F,** Arm rest height. (Adapted from Wilson A and McFarland SR, *Wheelchairs: a prescription guide*, pg. 29, Charlottesville, Va, 1986, *Rehabilitation Press.*)

Seat Height from Floor and Foot Adjustment (Fig. 27-5, C, D)

Objectives. (1) To support patient's body while maintaining thighs parallel to the floor (Fig. 27-5, C) and (2) to elevate foot plates to provide ground clearance over varied surfaces and curb cuts (Fig. 27-5, D)

Measure. Top of the seat post to the floor. Popliteal fossa to the bottom of the heel.

W/C clearance. The patient's thighs are parallel to the floor so the body weight is distributed evenly along entire depth of seat. The lowest point of footplates must clear the floor by at least 2 inches.

Check. Slip fingers under patient's thighs at front edge of seat upholstery. Note: A custom seat height may be needed to obtain footrest clearance. An inch of increased seat height raises the footplate one inch.

Consider
- If the knees are too high, increased pressure at ischial tuberosities puts patient at risk for skin breakdown and pelvic deformity.
- Sitting too high off the ground can impair the patient's center of gravity, seat height for transfers, and visibility if driving a van from the wheelchair.

Back Height (Fig. 27-5, E)

Objective. To provide back support consistent with physical and functional needs. It should be low enough for maximal function and high enough for maximal support.

Measure. For full trunk support, measure from top of the seat post to top of the shoulders. For minimum trunk support, top of back upholstery should permit free arm movement and no skin or scapular irritation while providing good total body alignment.

Check. The patient is not being pushed forward because the back is too high or leaning backward over top of the upholstery because back is too low.

Consider
- Adjustable-height backs (usually 4-inch range).
- Adjustable upholstery.
- Lumbar support or other commercially available or custom back insert to prevent kyphosis, scoliosis, or other long-term trunk deformity.

Arm Height (Fig. 27-5, F)

Objectives. To (1) maintain posture and balance, (2) to provide support and alignment for upper extremities, and (3) to allow change in position by pushing down on armrests.

Measure. With patient in comfortable position, measure from seat post to bottom of bent elbow.

W/C clearance. The height of the top of arm rest should be 1 inch higher than height from seat post to patient's elbow.

Check. Posture should look correct. The shoulders should not slouch forward or be subluxed or forced into elevation when in normal sitting posture with flexed elbows slightly forward on armrests.

Consider
- Other uses of armrests such as to increase functional reach or to hold a cushion in place.
- Certain styles of armrests can increase overall width of chair.
- Are armrests necessary at all?
- The patient's ability to remove and replace armrest from chair independently.

Review all measurements against standards for a particular model of chair. Manufacturers have listings of standard dimensions available and the cost for custom modifications.

The goals in pediatric wheelchair ordering, as in all wheelchair ordering, should focus on obtaining a proper fit and facilitating optimal function. Very rarely does a standard wheelchair meet the fitting requirements of a child. The selection of size is variable: therefore custom seating systems specific to the pediatric population are available. A secondary goal is to consider a chair that will accommodate the child's growth.

For children under 5 years of age, a decision must be made whether to use a stroller base versus a standard wheelchair base. Considerations are the child's ability to propel the chair relative to the developmental level and the parent's preference for a stroller or a wheelchair.

There are many variables to consider when customizing a wheelchair frame. Consult with an experienced RTS or the wheelchair manufacturer before assuming a custom request will be successful.

ADDITIONAL SEATING AND POSITIONING CONSIDERATIONS[1]

A wheelchair evaluation is not complete until seat cushion, back support, and any other positioning devices and the integration of those parts are carefully thought out, regardless of the diagnosis. It is essential that the therapist appreciate the impact that optimal body alignment has on skin integrity, tone normalization, overall funtional ability, and general well-being. Following are the goals of a comprehensive seating and positioning assessment.

Prevention of deformity. By providing a symmetrical base of support, proper skeletal alignment is preserved, discouraging spinal curvature and other body deformities.

Tone normalization. By providing proper body alignment, and bilateral weight bearing and adaptive devices as needed, tone normalization can be maximized.

Pressure management. Pressure sores can be caused by improper alignment and an inappropriate sitting surface. The proper seat cushion can provide comfort, assist in trunk and pelvic alignment, and create a surface that minimizes pressure, heat, and shearing, the primary causes of skin breakdown.

Promotion of function. Pelvic and trunk stability is necessary to free the upper extremity for participation in all functional activities including wheelchair mobility and daily living skills.

Maximum sitting tolerance. Wheelchair sitting tolerance will increase as support, comfort, and symmetrical weight-bearing are provided.

Optimal respiratory function. Support in an erect, well aligned position can decrease compression of the diaphragm and thus contribute to an increase in vital capacity.

Provision for proper body alignment. Good body alignment is necessary for prevention of deformity, normalization of tone, and to promote movement. The patient should be able not only to propel the wheelchair, but also to move around within the wheelchair.

A wide variety of seating and positioning equipment is available for all levels of disability. Custom modifications are continually being designed to meet a variety of patient needs. In addition, technology in this area is ever-growing, and interest in wheelchair technology as a professional specialty is growing as well. Skill of clinicians in this field, however, ranges from negligible to extensive. Though an integral aspect of any wheelchair evaluation, the scope of seating and positioning equipment is much greater than can be addressed in this chapter. The reader is referred to the suggested reading list at the end of this chapter for additional resources.

ACCESSORIES[1,7]

Once the measurements and additional positioning devices have been determined, there is a wide variety of accessories available to meet a patient's individual needs. It is extremely important to understand the function of each accessory and how it interfaces with the rest of the chair and seating and positioning equipment.

Armrests come in fixed, flip-up, detachable, desk, standard, reclining, and tubular styles. The fixed armrest is a continuous part of the frame and is not detachable. It limits proximity to table, counter, and desk surfaces and prohibits side transfers. Flip-up, detachable desk and standard length arms are removable and allow for side-approach transfers. Reclining arms are attached to the back post and recline with the back of the chair. Tubular arms are found on lightweight frames.

Footrests may be standard, swinging detachable, solid cradle, and elevating. The standard footrests are fixed to the wheelchair frame and do not move. They prevent the person from getting close to counters and may make some types of transfers more difficult. The swinging detachable footrests can be moved to the side of the chair or removed entirely from the chair. They allow a closer approach to bed, bathtub, and counters, and when removed, reduce the overall wheelchair length and weight for easy loading into a car. They lock into place on the chair with a locking device.[7] A solid cradle footrest is found on rigid lightweight chairs and is not removable. Elevating legrests are available for those patients with conditions such as edema, an arthrodesed knee, and orthopedic problems.

The footplates may have heel loops and toe straps to aid in securing the foot on the footplate.[7] A calf strap can be used on a solid cradle or where additional support behind the calf is necessary. Additional accessories can include the following: seat belts, various brake styles, brake extensions, antitip devices, caster locks, arm supports, and head supports.

PREPARING THE PRESCRIPTION

Once specific measurements, modifications, and accessories have been determined, the wheelchair prescription must be completed. It should be concise and very specific so that everything requested can be accurately interpreted by the equipment supplier, who will be submitting a sales contract for payment authorization. Before and after pictures can be very helpful in illustrating medical necessity. It is important that the requirements for payment authorization from a particular reimbursement source are known so that medical necessity can be demonstrated. The therapist must be very aware of the cost of everything being requested and why it is necessary. Payment can be denied if the need for every item and modification requested is not clearly substantiated.

Before delivery of the wheelchair to the patient, the therapist should check the chair to the specific prescription and ensure that all specifications and accessories are correct. When ordering a custom chair, it is recommended that the patient be fitted by the ordering therapist to ensure that the chair fits and that it provides all the elements that were expected when the prescription was generated.

WHEELCHAIR SAFETY

Elements of safety for the wheelchair user and the caregiver are as follows:

1. Brakes should be locked during all transfers.
2. Foot plates should never be stood on and during most transfers are in the UP position.
3. In most transfers it is an advantage to have footrests swung away if possible.
4. If a caregiver is pushing the chair, he or she should be sure that the patient's elbows are not protruding from the armrests and the hands are not on the hand rims. If approaching from behind to assist in moving the wheelchair, the caregiver should inform the patient of this intent and check the position of the feet and arms before proceeding.
5. If the caregiver wishes to push the patient up a ramp, he or she should move in a normal, forward direction. If the ramp is negotiated independently, the patient should lean slightly forward while propelling the wheelchair up the incline.[8]
6. If the caregiver wishes to push the patient down a ramp, he or she should tilt the wheelchair backward by pushing the foot down on the tipping levers to its balance position, which is a tilt of approximately 30°. Then the caregiver should ease the wheelchair down the ramp in a forward direction, while maintaining the chair in its balance position. The caregiver should keep his or her knees slightly bent and the back straight.[8] The caregiver may also move down the ramp backward while the patient maintains some control of the large wheels to prevent rapid backward motion. This approach is useful if the grade is relatively steep. Ramps with only a slight grade can also be managed in a forward direction if the caregiver maintains grasp and pull on the hand grips, and the patient again maintains some control of the big wheels to prevent rapid forward motion. If the ramp is negotiated independently, the patient should move down the ramp facing forward while leaning backward slightly and maintaining control of speed by grasping the hand rims. Gloves may be helpful to reduce the effect of friction.[8]
7. A caregiver can manage ascending curbs by approaching them forward, tipping the wheelchair back, and pushing the foot down on the tipping levers, thus lifting the front casters onto the curb and pushing forward. The large wheels then are in contact with the curb and roll on with ease as the chair is lifted slightly onto the curb.
8. To descend the curb using a forward approach the wheelchair is tilted backward, and the large wheels are rolled off the curb in a controlled manner while the front casters are tilted up. When the large wheels are off the curb, the assistant can slowly reduce the tilt of the wheelchair until the casters are once again on the street surface. The curb may be descended using a backward approach. The assistant can move him or herself and the chair around as the curb is approached and pull the wheelchair to the edge of the curb. Standing below the curb, the assistant can guide the large wheels off the curb by slowly pulling the wheelchair backward until it begins to descend. After the large wheels are safely on the street surface, the assistant can tilt the chair back to clear the casters, move backward, lower the casters to the street surface, and then turn around.[8]

With good strength and coordination, many patients can be trained to manage curbs independently. To mount and descend a curb, the patient must have an good bilateral grip, arm strength, and balance. To mount the curb, the patient tilts the chair onto the rear wheels and pushes forward until the front wheels hang over the curb, then lowers them gently. The patient then leans forward and forcefully pushes forward on the hand rims to bring the rear wheels up on the pavement. To descend a curb, the patient should lean forward and push slowly backward until the rear and then the front wheels roll down the curb.[3]

The ability to lift the front casters off the ground and balance on the rear wheels ("pop a wheelie") is a beneficial skill and expands the patient's independence in the community for curb management and in rural settings for movement over grassy, sandy, or rough terrain. Patients who have good grip, arm strength, and balance usually can master this skill and perform safely. The technique involves being able to tilt the chair on the rear wheels, balance the chair on the rear wheels, and move and turn the chair on the rear wheels. The patient should not attempt to perform these maneuvers without instruction and training in the proper techniques, which are beyond the scope of this chapter. Refer to the references for specific instructions on teaching these skills.[3]

TRANSFER TECHNIQUES

Transferring is the process of a patient moving from one surface to another. In addition, transfering includes the sequence of events that must occur both before and after the move such as the pretransfer sequence of bed mobility and the posttransfer phase of wheelchair positioning. Assuming that a patient has some physical and/or cognitive limitations, it will be necessary for the therapist to assist in or supervise a transfer. Many therapists question which transfer type and technique to employ or feel perplexed when a particular one does not succeed with the patient. It is important to remember that each patient, therapist, and situation is different. The techniques outlined in this chapter are not all-inclusive, but are basic ones with generalized principles. Each transfer must be adapted for the particular patient and his or her needs. Directions for some transfer techniques that are most commonly employed in practice are outlined. These are the stand pivot, bent pivot, and two-person transfers.

PRELIMINARY CONCEPTS

It is important for the therapist to be aware of the following concepts when selecting and carrying out transfer techniques to ensure safety for both the patient and self.

1. The therapist should be aware of the patient's assets

and limitations, especially his or her physical, cognitive, perceptual, and behavioral abilities and deficits.

2. The therapist should know his or her own physical abilities and limitations and whether he or she can communicate clear, sequential instructions to the patient (and eventually the long-term caregiver of the patient).

3. The therapist should be aware of and use correct moving and lifting techniques.

GUIDELINES FOR USING PROPER MECHANICS[2]

The therapist should be aware of the principles of basic body mechanics.

1. Get close to the patient or move the patient closer to you.
2. Square off with the patient (face head on).
3. Bend knees: use your legs, not your back.
4. Keep a neutral spine (not bent or arched back).
5. Keep a wide base of support.
6. Keep your heels down.
7. Don't tackle more than you can handle; ask for help.
8. Don't combine movements. Avoid rotating at the same time as bending forward or backward.

The therapist should consider the following questions before performing a transfer:

1. What medical precautions affect patient's mobility or method of transfer?
2. Can the transfer be performed safely by one person or is assistance required?
3. Has enough time been allotted for safe execution of a transfer? Are you in a hurry?
4. Does the patient understand what is going to happen? If not, does he or she demonstrate fear or confusion? Is there preparation for this limitation?
5. Is the equipment that the patient is being transferred to or from in good working order and in a locked position?
6. What is height of bed (or surface) in relation to the wheelchair? Can the heights be adjusted?
7. Is all equipment placed in correct position?
8. Is all unnecessary bedding and equipment moved out of the way so you are working without obstructions?
9. Is the patient dressed properly in case you need to use a waistband to assist? If not, do you need a transfer belt or other assistance?
10. What are the other components of the transfer, such as leg management and bed mobility?

It is important for the therapist to be familiar with as many types of transfers as possible so that each situation can be resolved as it arises.

Many classifications of transfers exist, based on the amount of therapist participation. Classifications range from dependent, in which the patient is unable to participate and the therapist moves the patient, to independent, in which the patient moves independently while the therapist merely supervises, observes, or provides input for appropriate technique as related to the patient's disability.

Before attempting to move a patient, it is important to understand the biomechanics of movement and the effect the patient's center of positioning mass has on transfers.

PRINCIPLES OF BODY POSITIONING[5]

Pelvic tilt. Generally after the acute onset of a disability or prolonged time spent in bed, patients assume a posterior pelvic tilt (i.e., a slouched position with lumbar flexion). This posture in turn moves the center of mass back toward the buttocks. The therapist may need to verbally cue or assist the patient into a neutral or slightly anterior pelvic tilt position to move the center of mass forward over the center of the patient's body (Fig. 27-6).

Trunk alignment. It may be observed that the patient's trunk alignment is shifted either to the right or the left side. If the therapist assists in moving the patient while his or her weight is shifted to one side, the movement could throw both the patient and the therapist off balance. The patient may need verbal cues or physical assistance to come to and maintain a midline trunk position before and during the transfer.

Weight shifting. To initiate the transfer the patient's weight needs to be shifted forward, unweighting the buttocks. This movement allows the patient to stand, partially stand, or be pivoted by the therapist. This step must be performed regardless of the type of transfer.

Extremity positioning. The patient's feet must be placed firmly on the floor with ankles stabilized and with knees aligned at 90° flexion over the feet. This position allows the weight to be shifted easily onto and over the feet. Heels must be pointing toward the surface to which the patient is transferring. The patient should either be barefoot or have shoes on to prevent slipping out of position. Feet can easily pivot in this position and risk of twisting or injuring an ankle or knee is minimized.

Upper extremities. The patient's arms must be in a safe position or in a position where he or she can assist in the transfer. If one or both of the upper extremities is nonfunctional, the arms should be placed in a safe position that will not be in the way during the transfer (e.g., patient's lap). If the patient has partial or full movement, motor control, and/or strength, he or she can assist in the transfer either by reaching toward the surface to be reached or pushing off from the surface to be left. The therapist's decision is based on prior knowledge of the patient's motor function.

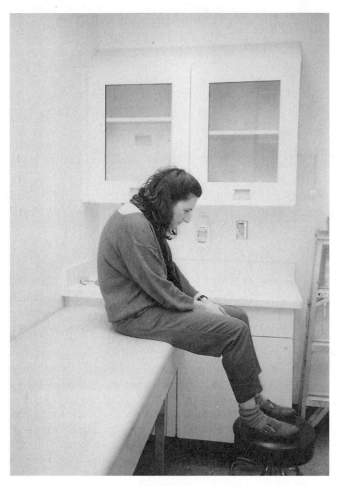

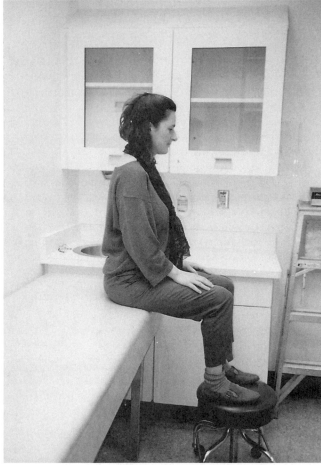

A   B

FIG. 27-6   A, Posterior pelvic tilt. **B,** Neutral pelvic position.

PREPARING THE EQUIPMENT AND THE PATIENT FOR THE TRANSFER

It is important to realize that the transfer process includes setting up the environment, positioning the wheelchair, and assisting the patient into a pretransfer position. The following is a general overview of these steps.

Positioning the Wheelchair
1. Place the wheelchair at approximately a 45° angle to the surface to which the patient is transferring.
2. Lock the brakes.
3. Place both the patient's feet firmly on the floor, hip width apart and with knees over the feet.
4. Remove the armrest closer to the bed.
5. Remove the wheelchair seatbelt.

Bed Mobility in Preparation for the Transfer

Rolling
1. Before rolling, the therapist may need to put his or her hand under the scapula on the weak side and gently mobilize it forward to prevent the patient from rolling onto the shoulder, causing potential pain and/or injury.

2. Assist the patient in clasping the strong hand around the wrist of the weak arm, and lift upper extremities towards ceiling.
3. Flex the knees.
4. The therapist may assist the patient to roll onto his or her side by moving the arms, then legs, and by holding one hand at the scapula area and the other at the hip, guiding the roll.

Sitting up at the edge of bed
1. Bring the patient's feet off edge of bed.
2. Assist the patient to lift the head and push up.
3. Shift the patient's body to upright sitting position.
4. Place the patient's hands on the bed at the sides of his or her body to help maintain balance.

Scooting to the edge of the bed
When working with an individual who has stroke or traumatic brain injury, walk patient's hips towards the edge of the bed. Shift the patient's weight to the unaffected side, position your hand behind the opposite buttock and guide forward. Shift weight to the affected side and repeat the procedure if necessary. Move forward until the patient's feet are flat on the floor.

In the case of an individual with spinal cord injury the therapist grasps the patient's legs from behind the knees and pulls the patient forward, placing feet firmly on floor and being sure that ankles are in a neutral position.

STAND PIVOT TRANSFERS

The stand pivot transfer requires the patient to be able to come to a standing position and pivot on one or both feet. It is most commonly used with those patients who have hemiplegia, hemiparesis, or general loss of strength or balance.

Wheelchair to Bed/Mat Transfer (Fig. 27-7)

1. Assist the patient to scoot to the edge of the surface and put the feet flat on the floor. Ankles are pointed towards surface to which the patient is transferring.
2. The therapist stands on the patient's affected side with hands either on the patient's scapulae or around the waist or hips. The therapist stabilizes the patient's foot and knee with his or her own foot and knee. The therapist assists by guiding the patient forward as the buttocks are lifted up and toward the transfer surface (Fig. 27-7, A).
3. The patient either reaches toward the surface to which he or she is transferring or pushes off the surface from which he or she transferring (Fig. 27-7, B).
4. The therapist guides the patient toward the transfer surface and gently assists him or her down to a sitting position (Fig. 27-7, C).

Variations: Stand/Ambulate Transfer

This transfer is generally used when a patient can take small steps towards the surface goal rather than pivoting around. The therapist intervention may range from physical assistance to accommodate for potential loss of balance to facilitation of near

normal movement, equal weight-bearing, and maintenance of appropriate posture for those with hemiplegia or hemiparesis. If a patient demonstrates impaired cognition and/or behavior deficit including impulsiveness and poor safety judgment, the therapist may need to provide verbal cues or physical guiding.

SLIDING BOARD TRANSFERS

Sliding Board transfers are best used with those who cannot bear weight on the lower extremities and who have weakness or poor endurance in their upper extremities. The transfer requires the use of upper extremity strength and is most often employed with persons who have lower extremity amputations or individuals with spinal cord injuries who have adequate upper extremity strength.

Method (Fig. 27-8)

1. Position and setup wheelchair as previously outlined.
2. Lift up the leg closer to the transfer surface. Place the board midthigh between the buttocks and knee, angled toward the opposite hip. The board must be firmly under the thigh and firmly on the surface to which the patient is transferring.
3. The therapist blocks the patient's knees with his or her knees.
4. The patient places one hand on the edge of the board, the other hand on the wheelchair seat.
5. The patient leans forward.
6. The patient transfers the upper body weight in the direction opposite to which he or she is going. The patient should use both arms to push along board. Upper extremity strength and the patient's balance are used to scoot along the sliding board.

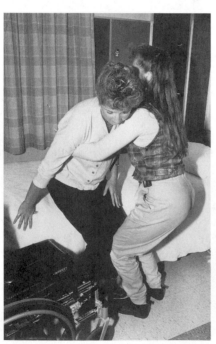
A

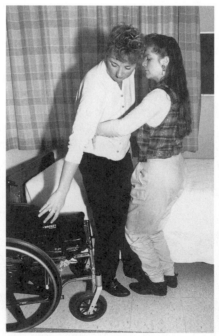
B

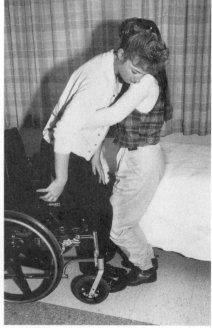
C

FIG. 27-7 Standing pivot transfer; wheelchair to bed, assisted. **A,** Therapist stands on patient's affected side, stabilizes patient's foot and knee. She assists by guiding patient forward and initiates lifting buttocks up. **B,** Patient reaches toward transfer surface. **C,** Therapist guides the patient towards transfer surface. (Photos: Luis Gonzalez, SCVMC.)

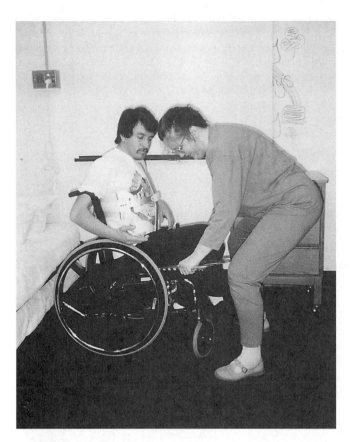

FIG. 27-8 Positioning sliding board. Lift leg closest to transfer surface. Place board midthigh between buttocks and knee angled toward opposite hip.

7. The therapist can assist by putting his or her hands on the patient's waist or scapulae and helping the person shift weight forward and/or slide across board as needed.

BENT PIVOT TRANSFER: BED TO WHEELCHAIR (Fig. 27-9)

The bent pivot transfer is used when the patient cannot initiate or maintain a standing position. A therapist often prefers to keep a patient in the bent knee position to maintain equal weight-bearing, provide optimal trunk and lower extremity support, and for a safer and easier therapist-assisted transfer.

Procedure

1. Assist patient to scoot to edge of bed until both feet are flat on the floor. The therapist grasps the patient around the waist or hips or even under the buttocks if a moderate or maximal amount of assistance is required.
2. Guide the patient's trunk into a midline position.
3. Shift the weight forward from the buttocks toward and over the patient's feet (Fig. 27-9, *A*).
4. Have the patient either reach toward the surface he or she is transferring to or push from surface transferring from (Fig. 27-9, *B*).
5. The therapist assists by guiding and pivoting patient around toward the transfer surface (Fig. 27-9, *C*).

Depending on the amount of assistance required, the pivoting portion can be done in 2 or 3 steps, while repositioning self and patient's lower extremities between steps. The therapist has a variety of choices of where to hold or grasp the patient during the bent pivot transfer, depending on the weight and

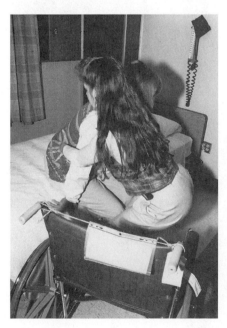
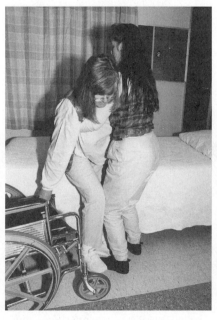
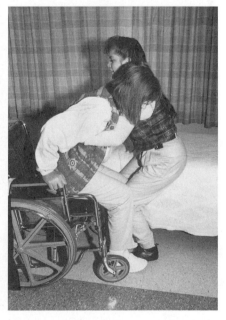

A   B   C

FIG. 27-9 Bent pivot transfer; bed to wheelchair. **A,** Therapist grasps patient around trunk and assists in shifting patient's weight forward over feet. **B,** Patient reaches towards wheelchair. **C,** Therapist assists patient down toward sitting position. (Photos: Luis Gonzalez, SCVMC.)

height of the patient in relation to the therapist and the patient's ability to assist in the transfer. Variations include using both hands and arms at the waist, or trunk, or one or both hands under the buttocks. The therapist never grasps under the patient's weak arm or grasps the weak arm, which may cause significant injury because of weak musculature and poor stability around the shoulder girdle. The choice is made with consideration to proper body mechanics. Trial and error of technique is advised to allow for optimal facilitation of patient independence, safety, and the therapist's proper body mechanics.

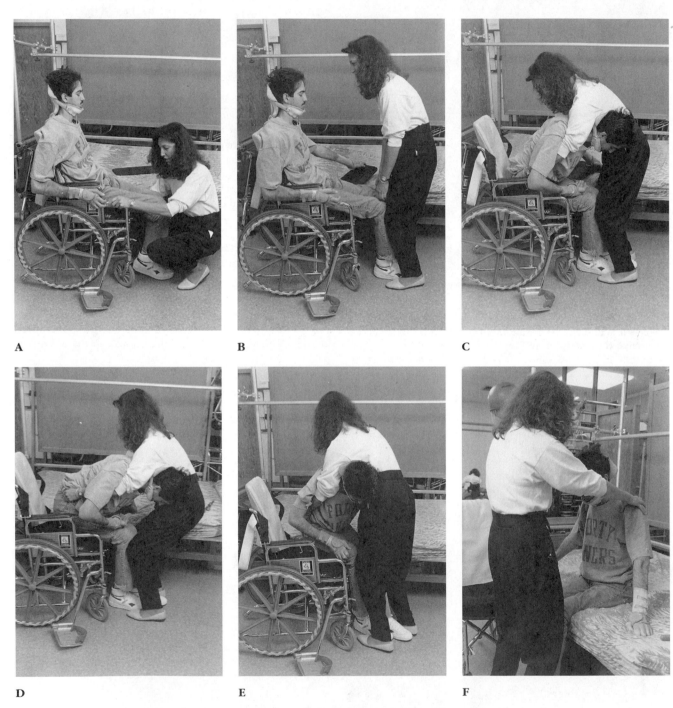

A   **B**   **C**

D   **E**   **F**

FIG. 27-10   Wheelchair to bed, sliding board transfer. **A,** Therapist positions wheelchair and patient and pulls patient forward in chair. **B,** Therapist stabilizes patient's knees and feet after placing sliding board. **C,** Therapist grasps patient's pants at lowest point of buttocks. **D,** Therapist rocks with patient and shifts his weight over his feet, making sure her back remains straight. **E,** Therapist pivots with patient and moves him onto sliding board. **F,** Patient is stabilized on bed.

DEPENDENT TRANSFERS[2]

The dependent transfer is designed for use with the patient who has minimal to no functional ability. If this transfer is performed incorrectly, it is potentially hazardous for both therapist and patient. This transfer should be practiced with able-bodied persons and used initially with the patient only when another person is available to assist.

The purpose of the dependent transfer is to move the patient from surface to surface. The requirements are that the patient be cooperative and willing to follow instructions. The therapist should be keenly aware of correct body mechanics as well as his or her own physical limitations. With heavy patients, it is always best to use the two-person transfer or at least have a second person available to spot the transfer.

Wheelchair-to-Bed Sliding Board Dependent Transfer (Fig. 27-10, A-F)

The procedure for transferring the patient from wheelchair to bed is as follows:

1. Set up wheelchair as described previously.
2. The therapist positions the patient's feet together on the floor directly under the knees and swings the outside footrest away. The therapist grasps the patient's legs from behind the knees and pulls the patient slightly forward in the wheelchair so that the buttocks will clear the big wheel when the transfer is made (Fig. 27-10, A).
3. A sliding board should be placed under the patient's inside thigh, midway between the buttocks and the knee, to form a bridge from the bed to the wheelchair. The sliding board is angled toward the patient's opposite hip.
4. The therapist then stabilizes the patient's feet by placing his or her own feet laterally around the patient's feet.
5. The therapist stabilizes the patient's knees by placing his or her knees firmly against the anterolateral aspect of the patient's knees (Fig. 27-10, B).
6. The therapist assists the patient to lean over the knees by pulling him or her forward from the shoulders. The patient's head and trunk should lean opposite the direction of the transfer. The patient's hands can rest on the lap.
7. The therapist reaches under the patient's outside arm and grasps the waistband of the trousers or under the buttock. On the other side, the therapist reaches over the patient's back and grasps the waistband or under the buttock (Fig. 27-10, C).
8. After the therapist's arms are correctly positioned, they are locked to stabilize the patient's trunk. The therapist keeps the knees slightly bent and braces them firmly against the patient's knees.
9. The therapist then gently rocks with the patient to gain some momentum and prepare to move after the count of three. Both therapist and patient count to three aloud. On three, with the therapist's knees held tightly against the patient's knees, the patient's weight is transferred over his or her feet. The therapist's back must be kept straight to maintain good body mechanics (Fig. 27-10, D).
10. The therapist pivots with the patient and moves him or her onto the sliding board (Fig. 27-10, E). The therapist repositions himself or herself and the patient's feet and repeats

the pivot until the patient is firmly seated on the bed surface, perpendicular to the edge of the mattress and as far back as possible. This step usually can be achieved in two or three stages (Fig. 27-10, F).
11. The therapist can secure the patient on the bed by easing him or her against the back of an elevated bed or on the mattress in a side-lying position, then by lifting the legs onto the bed.

This transfer can be adapted to move the patient to other surfaces. It should be attempted only when therapist and patient feel secure with the wheelchair to bed transfer.

Two-Person Dependent Transfers

Bent pivot: with or without a sliding board bed to wheelchair (Fig. 27-11)

A bent pivot transfer is used to allow increased therapist interaction and support. It allows the therapist greater control of the patient's trunk and buttocks during the transfer. This technique can also be employed during a two-person dependent transfer. It is often used with neurologically involved patients because trunk flexion and equal weight-bearing are often desirable with this diagnosis:

1. Set the wheelchair up as described previously.
2. One therapist assumes a position in front of the patient and the other in back.
3. The therapist in front assists in walking the patient's hips forward until the feet are flat or floor.
4. The same therapist then stabilizes the patient's knees and feet by placing his or her knees and feet lateral to each of the patient's.
5. The therapist in back positions self squarely behind the patient's buttocks, grasping either the patient's waistband or placing his or her hands under the buttocks. Proper body mechanics are maintained (Fig. 27-11, A).
6. The therapist in front moves the patient's trunk into a midline position, grasps the patient around the waist or hips and guides the patient to lean forward and shift weight forward over the feet and off the buttocks. The patient's head and trunk should lean in the direction opposite the transfer. The patient's hands can rest on the lap (Fig. 27-11, B).
7. As the therapist in front shifts the patient's weight forward, the one in back shifts the patient's buttocks in the direction of the transfer. This step can be done in 2 or 3 steps, making sure the patient's buttocks land on a safe, solid surface. The therapists reposition themselves and patient to maintain safe and proper body mechanics (Fig. 27-11, C).
8. The therapists make sure they coordinate the time of the transfer with the patient and one another by counting to three aloud and instructing the team to initiate the transfer on three.

Mechanical Lift Transfer

Some patients, because of body size, degree of disability, or the health and well-being of the caregiver, require the use of a mechanical lift. A variety of mechanical lifting devices can be used to transfer patients of any weight (Fig. 27-12, A and B). A properly trained caregiver, even one who is considerably smaller than the patient, can learn to use the mechanical lift safely and independently.[8] The patient's physical size, environment in which the lift will be used, and the uses to which the lift will be put must be considered to order the appropriate mechanical

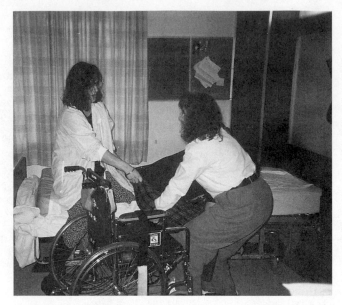

A

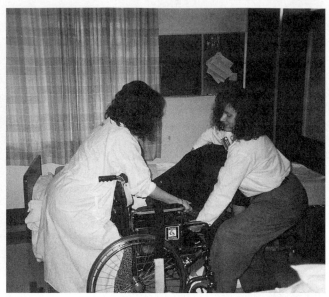

B

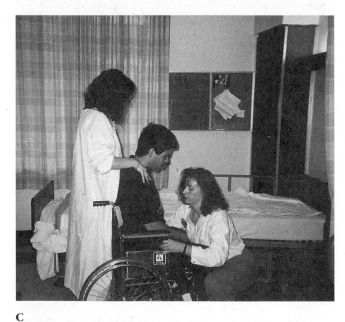

C

FIG. 27-11 Two-person dependent transfer, bed to wheelchair. **A,** One therapist positions self in front of patient blocking feet and knees. The therapist in back positions self behind patient's buttocks and assists by lifting. **B,** Person in front rocks patient forward and unweights buttocks as the back therapist shifts buttocks towards wheelchair. **C,** Both therapists position patient in upright, midline position in wheelchair. Seat belt is secured and positioning devices added.

lift. The patient and caregiver should demonstrate safe use of the lift to the therapist before prescribing it.

TRANSFERS TO HOUSEHOLD SURFACES

Sofa/chair (Fig. 27-13). Wheelchair to sofa and chair transfers are similar to wheelchair to bed transfers, however, the following should be assessed.

The therapist and patient need to be aware that the chair may be light and less stable than a bed or wheelchair. When transferring to the chair, the patient needs to be instructed to reach for the seat of the chair. Reaching for the arm rest or back of chair should be avoided because this action may cause the chair to tip over. When moving from a chair to the wheelchair, the patient should use a hand to push off from the seat of the chair as

he or she comes to standing. Standing from a chair is often more difficult if the chair is low or the seat cushions are soft. Dense cushions may be added to increase height and provide a firm surface to which to transfer.

Toilet. In general, wheelchair to toilet transfers are difficult because of the confined space in most bathrooms. Attempt to position the wheelchair next to or at an acute angle to the toilet. An analysis of the space around the toilet and wheelchair is made to ensure no obstacles are present. To increase independence of the patient during this transfer, adaptive devices can be added such as grab bars and/or raised toilet seats. The patient can use these devices to support self during transfers and maintain an even level surface to which to transfer.

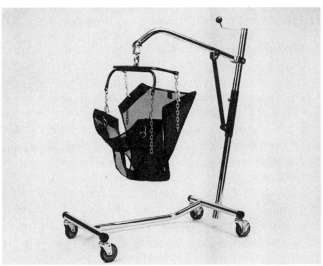

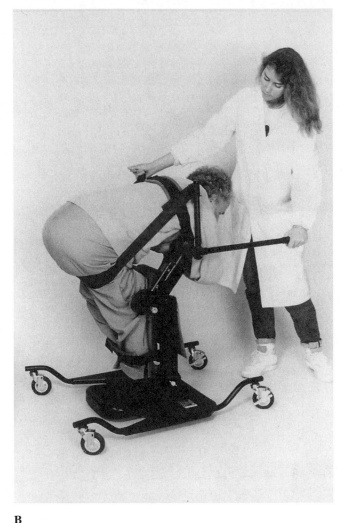

A   **B**

FIG. 27-12   A, Traditional boom-style mechanical lift. (Photo courtesy of Trans-Aid Lifts, Sunrise Medical.) **B,** Alternative patient lift. (Photo courtesy of EZ- Pivot, Rand-Scott.)

Bathtub. The occupational therapist should be most cautious when assessing or teaching bathtub transfers because the bathtub is considered one of the most hazardous areas of the home. Wheelchair to the bottom of the bathtub transfers are extremely difficult and used with patients who have good bilateral strength and motor control of the upper extremities (e.g, patients with paraplegia and lower extremity amputation). A commercially produced bath bench, bath chair or a well-secured straight-back chair is commonly used by therapists for seated bathing. Therefore, whether a standing pivot, bent pivot, or sliding board transfer is performed, the technique is similar to a wheelchair to chair transfer. The transfer may be complicated, however, by the confined space, the slick bathtub surfaces, and the bathtub wall between the wheelchair and the bathtub seat.

If a standing pivot transfer is employed, it is recommended that the locked wheelchair be placed at a 45° angle to the bathtub if possible. The patient should stand, pivot, sit on the bathtub chair, and then place the lower extremities into the bathtub.

If a bent pivot or sliding board transfer is used, the wheelchair is placed next to the bathtub with the armrest removed. The transfer tub bench may be used, which removes the need for a sliding board. This approach allows the wheelchair to be placed right next to the bench, allowing a safe and easy transfer of the buttocks to the seat. Then the lower extremities can be assisted into the bathtub.

In general, the patient may exit by first placing his or her feet securely outside the bathtub on a nonskid floor surface and then performing a standing or seated transfer back to the wheelchair.

CAR TRANSFERS

A car transfer is often the most challenging for therapists because it involves trial-and-error methods to develop a technique that is not only safe, but also easy for the patient and caregiver to carry out. The therapist often uses the patient's existing transfer technique. The patient's size, degree of disability, and vehicle style (2-door vs. 4-door) must be considered. These factors will affect

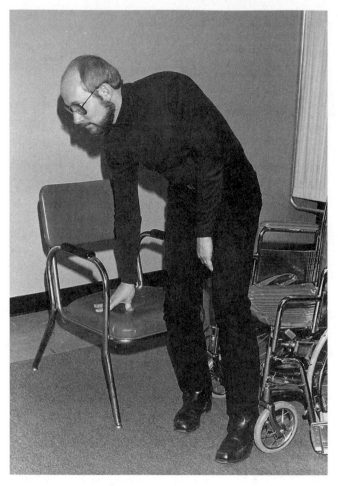

FIG. 27-13 Patient in midtransfer, reaches for seat of chair, pivots, and lowers body to sitting.

level of independence and may necessitate a change in the usual technique to allow for a safe, easy transfer.

In general, it is difficult to get a wheelchair close enough to the car seat, especially with four-door vehicles.

1. Car seats are often much lower than standard wheelchair seat height, which makes the uneven transfer much more difficult, especially from the car seat to the wheelchair.
2. Occasionally, patients may have orthopedic injuries that require use of a brace such as a halo body jacket or lower extremity cast or splint. The therapist often must alter technique to accommodate these devices.
3. The therapist may suggest use of the sliding board for this transfer to compensate for the large gap between transfer surfaces.
4. Because uphill transfers are difficult and level of assistance may increase for this transfer, the therapist may choose a two-person assist vs. one-person assist transfer to ensure a safe and smooth technique.

SUMMARY

A wheelchair that fits well and can be managed safely and easily by its user and caregiver is one of the most important factors in the patient's ability to perform activities of daily living with maximal independence.[6] Each wheelchair user must learn the capabilities and limitations of the wheelchair and safe methods of performing ADL. If there is a caregiver, he or she needs to be thoroughly familiar with safe and correct techniques of handling the wheelchair and the patient.

Transfer skills are among the most important activities that must be mastered by the wheelchair user. The ability to transfer increases the possibility of mobility and travel. Yet transfers can be hazardous. Safe methods must be learned and followed.[8] Several basic transfer techniques were outlined in this chapter. Additional methods and more detailed training and instructions are available, as cited previously.

It should be recognized that many wheelchair users with exceptional abilities have developed unique methods of wheelchair management. Although such innovative approaches may work well for the person who has devised and mastered them, they cannot be considered basic procedures that can be learned by everyone.[8]

REVIEW QUESTIONS

1. What is the objective in measuring seat width?
2. What is the danger of having a wheelchair seat that is too deep?
3. What is the minimal distance for safety from the floor to the bottom of the wheelchair step plate?
4. List three types of wheelchair frames and the general uses of each.
5. Describe three types of wheelchair propulsion systems and tell when each would be used.
6. What are the advantages of detachable desk arms and swing-away footrests?
7. Discuss the factors for consideration before wheelchair selection.
8. Name and discuss the rationale for at least three general wheelchair safety principles.
9. Describe or demonstrate how to descend a curb in a wheelchair with the help of an assistant.
10. Describe or demonstrate how to descend a ramp in a wheelchair with the help of an assistant.
11. List four safety principles for correct moving and lifting technique during wheelchair transfers.
12. Describe or demonstrate the basic standing pivot transfer from a bed to a wheelchair.
13. Describe or demonstrate the wheelchair to bed transfer, using a sliding board.
14. Describe the correct placement of a sliding board before a transfer.
15. In what circumstances would you use a sliding board transfer technique?

16. List the requirements for patient and therapist to perform the dependent transfer safely and correctly.
17. List two potential problems and solutions that can occur with the wheelchair to car transfer.
18. When is the mechanical lift transfer most appropriate?

REFERENCES

1. Adler C, *Wheelchairs and seat cushions: a comprehensive guide for evaluation and ordering,* San José, 1987, Santa Clara County, Santa Clara Valley Medical Center, Occupational Therapy Department.
2. Adler C, Musik D, Tipton-Burton M, *Body mechanics and transfers, multidisciplinary cross training manual,* San José, Calif, 1994, Santa Clara Valley Medical Center.
3. Bromley I: *Tetraplegia and paraplegia: a guide for physiotherapists,* ed 3, London, 1985, Churchill Livingstone.
4. Pezenik D, Itoh M, Lee M: Wheelchair prescription. In Ruskin AP: *Current therapy in physiatry,* Philadelphia, 1984, WB Saunders.
5. Physical Therapy Dept., *Lifting and moving techniques,* San José, Calif, 1985, Santa Clara Valley Medical Center.
6. *Wheelchair prescription: measuring the patient* (Booklet no. 1), Camarillo, Calif, 1979, Everest and Jennings.
7. *Wheelchair prescription: wheelchair selection,* (Booklet no. 2), Camarillo, Calif, 1979, Everest and Jennings.
8. *Wheelchair prescription: safety and handling* (Booklet no 3), Camarillo, Calif, 1983, Everest and Jennings.
9. Wilson AB, McFarland SR: *Wheelchairs, a prescription guide,* Charlottesville, Va, 1992, Rehabilitation Press.

SUGGESTED READINGS

1. Bergen A, Presperin J, Tallman T: *Positioning for function,* Valhalla, New York, 1990, Valhalla Rehabilitation Publications.
2. Davies PM: *Steps to follow: a guide to the treatment of adult hemiplegia,* New York, 1985, Springer-Verlag.
3. Ford JR, Duckworth B: *Physical management for the quadriplegic patient,* Philadelphia, 1974, FA Davis.
4. Gee ZL, Passarella PM: *Nursing care of the stroke patient: a therapeutic approach,* Pittsburgh, Pa, 1985, A.R.E.N. Publications.
5. Hill J P, editor: *Spinal cord injury: a guide to functional outcomes in occupational therapy,* Rockville, Md, 1986, Aspen.

Electronic Assistive Technologies in Occupational Therapy Practice

Albert M. Cook, Susan M. Hussey

This chapter is about electronic assistive devices and the role they play in the lives of people who have disabilities. As such, it is also a chapter about the role electronic assistive technologies play in the lives of practicing occupational therapists. Electronic assistive technologies have a relatively brief history, which parallels the development of electronics in general. As the complexity, power, and flexibility of electronic devices have increased, so have the capabilities of electronic assistive technologies. Today virtually all of these devices contain at least one microcomputer, and their capabilities are much greater than even five years ago. The key to successful application of electronic assistive devices for persons who have disabilities, however, lies in a thorough understanding of the user's needs, the context in which the technology will be used, and the skills the person brings to the task. The development of this base of understanding is very much in the domain of occupational therapy practice.

DEFINITION OF ASSISTIVE TECHNOLOGIES

One widely used definition of assistive technologies is that provided in PL (public law) 100-407, the Technical Assistance to the States Act in the United States. The definition of an assistive technology device is as follows:

Any item, piece of equipment or product system whether acquired commercially off the shelf, modified, or customized that is used to increase or improve functional capabilities of individuals with disabilities.

This definition has also been incorporated into other legislation in the United States and is used as a working definition in other countries as well. Note that the definition includes commercial, modified, and customized devices. Thus, products made for the general population can be included. This definition specifies functional capabilities of individuals with disabilities. The use of assistive technology devices to increase functional capabilities brings them within the context of occupational therapy practice.

FRAMEWORK FOR APPLYING ASSISTIVE TECHNOLOGIES

When a person with a disability is faced with an activity in a given context, he or she may require assistive technologies to facilitate the performance. The human activity assistive technology (HAAT) model is shown in Fig. 28-1.[12] The major benefit of this model is that it shows the relationship of the assistive technologies to the other three components. The HAAT model will form the framework for a discussion of electronic assistive technologies.

Each of the components shown in Fig. 28-1 plays a unique part in the total assistive technology system. The specification of a system begins with a need by the human to perform an activity such as cooking, writing, or playing tennis, which defines the goal of the assistive technology system. Each activity is carried out within a context, which includes social and cultural aspects as well as environments and physical conditions (e.g., temperature, noise level, lighting). The combination of the activity and the context determines which human skills are required to achieve the specified goals.

When human skills to complete a task are lacking, the occupational therapist looks at ways to make adaptations so that the desired goal is achieved. Electronic assistive technologies may be used as part of this adaptation. An electronic assistive technology device is matched to the capabilities of the human and then used to accomplish the desired activity.

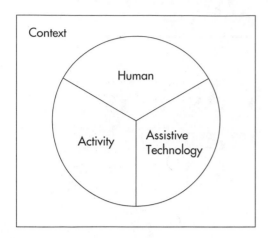

FIG. 28-1   Human Activity Assistive Technology (HAAT) Model. (From Cook Am, Hussey SM: *Assistive technologies: principles and practice,* St Louis, Mosby-Yearbook.)

The major components of the assistive technology system are shown in Fig. 28-2. The human/technology interface component facilitates interaction between the human and the assistive technology, and it forms the boundary between these two parts of the HAAT model. The human-technology interaction is two-way, that is, information may be directed from the human to the technology or vice versa. The technology facilitates functional performance through the activity output component. The processor receives information from the human via the human/technology interface. This information is translated into signals that control the activity

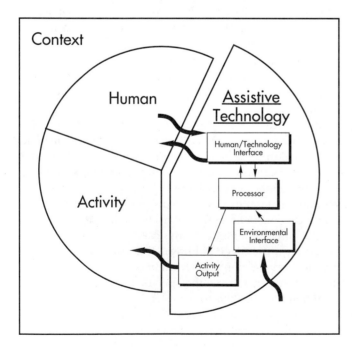

FIG. 28-2   Flow of information between assistive technologies and other components of HAAT model. (From Cook AM, Hussey SM: *Assistive technologies: principles and practice,* St Louis, 1995, Mosby-Yearbook.)

output. Assistive technologies such as sensory aids must also be capable of detecting external environmental data through an environmental interface. The external data are interpreted and formatted by the processor so they can be provided to the user through the human/technology interface.

Not all assistive technologies have all of the components shown in Fig. 28-2, but they all have at least three components (usually they have either the activity output or the environmental sensor). This HAAT model can also be applied to nonelectronic assistive technologies (e.g., manual wheelchairs and other aids to daily living).[12]

The interaction among the components of the HAAT model can be illustrated by the following example.[12] Tony needs to write reports. Thus writing is his activity. He is required to accomplish this task as part of his work, which specifies part of the context. Because of a spinal cord injury, Tony is unable to use his hands, but he is able to speak clearly. A voice recognition system (the assistive technology) is obtained for him. This system allows Tony to use his skills (speaking) to accomplish the activity (writing) by translating what Tony says into computer-recognizable characters. As Tony speaks, the assistive technology recognizes what is said and sends it to the computer as if it had been typed. Because there are other workers in the office, Tony uses a noise canceling microphone to avoid errors in voice recognition, and he works in a cubicle to avoid bothering other workers. These features further define the context of this system. Tony's assistive technology system consists of the activity (writing), the context (at work in a noisy office), the human skills (speaking), and the assistive technology (voice recognition).

For any other individual, one or more parts of this system may be different. For example, another person may be able to type, but only with an enlarged keyboard. Another person may need to write at home, rather than at work. Thus each assistive technology system is unique.

SERVICE DELIVERY IN ASSISTIVE TECHNOLOGY

There is a basic process by which assistive technology devices and services are delivered to the consumer.[12] Many professionals can be involved in assistive technology delivery including occupational and physical therapists, speech/language pathologists, special educators, and rehabilitation engineers. Collectively these individuals are referred to as assistive technology practitioners (ATPs). The first step in the service delivery process is referral and intake, in which an ATP is contacted because the consumer has identified a need for which assistive technology intervention might be helpful. The ATP then gathers basic information and determines whether there is a match between the type of services provided and the identified needs of the consumer. Funding for the services to be provided is then sought.

If the criteria for intake are met, then the evaluation phase begins. This stage is similar to that carried out in other areas of occupational therapy. There are some important differences in both the procedures and the results of the evaluation process, however, because of the involvement of assistive technologies. One of the most important steps in the evaluation process is needs identification. It is particularly important that the needs be related to the capabilities of potential assistive technologies. The evaluation continues with an assessment of the consumer's sensory, physical, and central processing skills as they relate to the use of assistive technologies. The major way in which assessment for assistive technologies differs from assessment to determine a therapeutic regime is in the purpose of the evaluation. The primary purpose of assistive technology intervention is not remediation or rehabilitation of an impairment, but rather the provision of hard and soft technologies that enable an individual with a disability to function in activities of daily living.

The needs identification and skills evaluation define the activity and human operator portions of the HAAT model. Once these are clearly known, assistive technologies can be matched with the needs of the consumer consistent with his or her skills. Generally a trial evaluation of these technologies takes place to ensure that the match is appropriate and likely to lead to effective functional outcomes. This matching process is another distinguishing feature of assistive technology service delivery, and it requires that the assistive technology team be aware of available devices and their characteristics. The evaluation results are summarized and recommendations for technologies are made based on consensus among those involved. A written report is generally prepared for the funding source, school or work site, residence staff or family, and other professionals working with the consumer.

An important part of the report is a description of the plan for acquiring the technologies, installing or setting them up, and training the consumer and care providers. This portion of the service delivery process is often referred to as the implementation phase. At this phase, the recommended equipment is ordered, modified, and fabricated as necessary, set up, and delivered to the consumer. Training activities are extremely important, and for complex electronic assistive technologies can take many hours of practice and tutoring. Training is not only necessary to understand basic operation of the device, but also to develop strategies for using the device effectively.

Once the device has been delivered and training has been completed, the effectiveness of the system as a whole is evaluated during the follow-up phase. During this period an assessment is made of whether the goals of facilitating or enabling a particular activity are being met through the assistive technology intervention. The final phase of the service delivery process, the follow-along phase, provides for the ATP to contact the consumer to see whether further assistive technology intervention is necessary as needs, goals, and skills change in the future. Changes in the consumer's skills, needs, or contexts of use may indicate a need for further assistive technology intervention. Changes in the technology may also create new opportunities for independence by the consumer. In either case, the consumer is brought back to the referral and intake phase, and the process (wholly or partially) is repeated.

CONTROL INTERFACES FOR ELECTRONIC ASSISTIVE TECHNOLOGIES

Three elements make up the human/technology interface: the control interface, the selection set, and the selection method.[12] The control interface forms the boundary between the user and an electronic or mechanical assistive technology device. This interface allows the individual to operate or control the device. For electronic assistive technology systems, control interfaces include joysticks for powered wheelchairs, keyboards for computers and communication devices, and single switches used to control household devices such as lights or radios.

The selection set is a presentation of the items from which the user makes choices. The elements in the selection set correspond to the elements of a specific activity output (Fig. 28-2). Selection sets may consist of written letters, words and sentences, symbols used to represent ideas, computer icons, or line drawings/pictures. They may be presented in visual (e.g., letters on keys), tactile (e.g., Braille), or auditory (e.g., voice synthesis) forms. The user makes selections using the control interface through direct selection and indirect selection.[12] For any particular application the three elements of the human/technology interface are chosen based on the best match to the consumer's skills (motor, sensory, linguistic, and cognitive).[12]

The fastest and easiest selection method to understand and use is direct selection. In this method every choice in the selection set is available at all times, and the user merely chooses the one he or she wants. Indirect selection methods were developed to provide access for individuals who lacked the motor skills to use direct selection. Indirect selection methods are scanning, directed scanning, and coded access. Each of the indirect selection methods involves one or more intermediate steps between the consumer's action and the actual selection. One of the most common methods is scanning. Although there are a variety of implementations of scanning, they all rely on the basic principle of presenting the selection set to the user sequentially and having the user indicate the desired selection, often by a single movement of some body part.

Because scanning is inherently slow, there have been

a number of approaches that increase the rate of selection. The most common is group item scanning. In this method, the selection set items are first scanned in groups, and the user chooses the group in which the choice selection appears. The device then scans that group item by item and the user makes a final choice of the desired item. In rotary scanning, the scanned elements are arranged in a circle; in linear scanning, they are arranged in a straight line. If they are placed in a rectangular matrix, the group item scan becomes a row/column scan because the groups are rows and the columns contain the individual elements. Vanderheiden and Lloyd[25] describe a variety of other scanning strategies. Single switch scanning requires good visual tracking skills and the ability to attend and sequence. On the other hand, this type of scanning requires very little motor control to make a selection.

In a combined approach, called directed scanning, the user first activates the control interface to select the direction (vertically or horizontally) in which the selection set is scanned by the device. The user then sends a signal to the processor (Fig. 28-2) to make the selection when the desired choice is reached. This signal is either generated by pausing at the choice, an acceptance time, or activating another control interface to indicate the choice. Joysticks or other arrays of switches (2 to 8 switches) are the control interfaces typically used with directed scanning. This indirect selection approach takes advantage of greater user motor skills (i.e., the ability to move a joystick in one of four directions or activate one of four switches) to increase selection rate.

Coded access requires the individual to use a unique sequence of movements to select a code corresponding to each item in the selection set. These movements constitute a set of intermediate steps that are required to make the selection using either a single switch or an array of switches as the control interface. There are several examples of coded access used in assistive technologies. One is Morse code, in which the selection set is the alphabet. An intermediate step (e.g., holding longer [dash] or shorter [dot] or hitting one switch for short and one for long) is necessary in order to make a selection. Because of its early use in telegraphy, a major goal in the development of Morse code was its efficiency, which was achieved by assigning the most frequently used letters to the shortest codes (e.g., *e* is one dot, *t* is one dash). This efficiency can be very useful in augmentative communication and computer access.

A second example of coded access used for computer input is Darci code,* which is based on an eight-way switch code. The eight-way switch is similar to a four-position switched joystick with the diagonal positions used as additional switch positions. With this code, letters are generated by moving the switch to specific loca-

tions (e.g., upper left, then to lower right, then to the center) to select a specific letter. It is this sequence of movements that tells the processor which letter has been selected. Because codes are usually memorized, this method does not require that a selection set be visually displayed and therefore has advantages for persons with visual limitations. Coded access also requires less physical skill than direct selection, and the timing of the input is under the control of the user rather than the device. Coded access requires more cognitive skill, however, especially memory and sequencing, than other methods.

Control enhancers are aids that extend the motor capabilities of the human to allow activation of a control interface. Examples of control enhancers are arm supports (see Chapter 19), mouthsticks, and head or hand pointers. For example, if a consumer lacks sufficient fine hand control to press the keys on a keyboard, a control enhancer such as a hand pointer may enable the consumer to use the keyboard for direct selection. In other cases, a control enhancer such as a mobile arm support may be used to reduce fatigue by making the task physically easier.

METHODS OF ACTIVATION FOR CONTROL INTERFACES

Control interfaces may be characterized by the way in which the consumer activates them.[12] Three types of action by the user can activate the control interface: movement, respiration, and phonation as detailed in Table 28-1. Movements can be sent and detected in several ways, also shown in Table 28-1. First, a force may be generated by the movement and detected by the control interface. Mechanical control interfaces (e.g., switches, keyboard keys, joysticks, mouse, and trackball) comprise the largest category of control interfaces. The switches vary in the anatomic site to be used (some are very specific, others more general), the amount of force required, the sensory feedback provided, and the mounting arrangement for easy access by the consumer.

Electromagnetic control interfaces also can be used to detect movement at a distance through either light or radio frequency (rf) energy. These interfaces include head-mounted light sources or detectors and transmitters used with environmental control systems for remote control. The third type of movement detection is electrical. These detectors are sensitive to electricity generated by the body. Switches of this type require no force; just a light touch sends an electrical impulse. A common example of this type of interface is buttons on some elevators.

The second type of body-generated signal is respiration or ventilation, which is detected by measuring either air flow or air pressure using what is called a sip-and-puff switch. Switch arrays are manufactured in one of two ways. Either a group of single switches is mounted on one plate or a special construction is designed to allow multiple outputs. An example of the former is two sip-

---

* WesTest Engineering Corp, Bountiful, Utah.

TABLE 28-1	Methods of Activation	
SIGNAL SENT	**SIGNAL DETECTED**	**EXAMPLES**
1. Movement (eye, head, tongue, arms, legs)	1a. Mechanical: application of force	1a. Joystick, keyboard, tread switch
	1b. Electromagnetic: receipt of electromagnetic energy such as light or radio waves	1b. Light pointer, light detector, remote radio transmitter
	1c. Electrical: detection of electrical signals from the surface of the body	1c. EMG,* EOG,† capacitive or contact switch
	1d. Proximity: movement close to the detector, but without contact	1d. Heat-sensitive switches
2. Respiration (inhalation/expiration)	2. Pneumatic: detection of respiratory air flow or pressure	2. Puff and sip
3. Phonation	3. Sounds or words: detection of articulated sounds or speech	3. Sound switch, whistle switch, speech recognition

Adapted from Cook AM, Hussey SM: *Assistive technologies: principles and practices,* St Louis, 1995, Mosby-Yearbook, p. 324.
* Electromyograph, which records electrical impulses from skeletal muscles.
† Electrooculograph, which records tracings of eye movement.

and-puff switches mounted sided by side for wheelchair control. An example of a special construction is the eight-way switch described for use with Darci code.

Control Interfaces for Direct Selection

The most common control interface for direct selection is the keyboard. There are many different types of keyboards, however, and each requires certain skills. Some consumers have limited range of movement but fine motor control is good. In this case a contracted keyboard is more useful than the standard keyboard. Other individuals have difficulty accessing small targets, but they have good range of movement. An expanded keyboard, in which the size of each key can be up to several inches, may allow direct selection in this case. Keys can be used individually or they can be redefined to form larger keys. Different keyboard layouts can also be used (e.g., for left hand or right hand only typing). It is also possible to make the keys in different sizes and different shapes on the same keyboard. Touch screens are available on both desktop and portable computers. Using this control interface, the user chooses from the selection set by touching the icon for the item on the screen. Other screens allow the user to point at the item. This method can be cognitvely easier for some consumers.

The other common control interface for direct selection in general-purpose computers is a mouse. Alternative pointing interfaces often used in assistive technologies to replace the traditional mouse include the trackball, head-controlled mouse, continuous joystick, and the arrow keys on the keypad (called mouse keys). In each case, a pointer on the screen is moved by changing the position of the pointing device. Once the pointer is moved to the desired item, the user can make a selection by either pausing for a preset time (called acceptance time selection) or pressing a switch (called manual selection).

The sensory feedback provided by the particular type of pointing device can vary widely, which affects the user's performance. Successful pointing device use also requires considerable coordination between the body site executing pointer movement and the eyes following the pointer on the screen and locating the targets. The pointer characteristics must be matched to the user's skills and needs.[12]

Voice recognition, in which the individual uses sounds, letters, or words as a selection method, is another alternative to keyboard input. In most systems the voice recognition is speaker-dependent, and the user either "trains" the system to recognize his or her voice by producing several samples of the same element or the system adapts to the consumer through use.[6] Speaker-independent systems recognize speech patterns of different individuals without training.[14] These systems are developed using samples of speech from hundreds of people and information provided by phonologists on the various pronunciations of words; the total recognition vocabulary is generally small.[6] Voice recognition is used in assistive technology applications for computer access, wheelchair control and environmental control systems.

Control Interfaces for Indirect Access

Indirect methods of selection use a single switch or an array of switches and require less motor skill on the part of the consumer. Most switches require mechanical activation. Usually single switches are activated by the hand, head, arm, leg, or foot. Switch arrays, including some joysticks, are generally activated by hand, foot, or head movement (e.g., chin). Pneumatic switches include sip-and-puff or pillow switches. Sip-and-puff switches are activated by blowing air into the switch or sucking air out of it. In some cases it is possible to vary the amount of air pressure to the switch to generate different commands. Pillow switches are activated by squeezing (e.g., with a hand bulb). Some electrical switches detect muscle electrical activity (EMGs) or eye movement (EOG) by attaching electrodes to the skin. Cook and Hussey[12] and Bergen and associates[7] describe a variety of interfaces used for indirect selection.

When scan is used, selection techniques include automatic (the user stops the cursor at the desired element), step (the user moves the cursor one element at a time), and inverse (the user holds a switch to move the cursor and releases it to stop the cursor). Each of these places different motor demands on the user, and it is important to match the selection technique to the user's skills.

COMPUTER ACCESS BY PERSONS WITH DISABILITIES

Computer use by persons who have disabilities has opened up new opportunities for education, employment, and recreation. Persons who have disabilities use both stand-alone computers, such as those used in general business and educational applications, and special-purpose computers built into assistive devices. In both cases the computer offers (1) flexibility (multiple options with the same hardware), (2) adaptability (as user's skills change over time), (3) customization to a specific user and need (e.g., settings of scanning rate in augmentative communication, acceleration rate on powered wheelchair), and (4) specific applications and/or upgrades based on software rather than hardware (e.g., augmentative communication application software and upgrades, specific user profile of speed and acceleration parameters in a powered wheelchair controller).[12] Despite these advantages, computer use is often difficult for individuals who have motor and/or sensory impairments. To use a computer successfully, an individual must have sensory and perceptual abilities for processing computer outputs, motor control for generating input to the computer, and cognitive skills (i.e., problem solving, decision making, memory, language) for understanding the computer functions. If a person with one or more disabilities has difficulty carrying out these functions, the computer can be adapted to facilitate its use.

The major functional components of a standard (non-adapted) computer system are shown in Fig. 28-3. The central processing unit (CPU) portion of the computer is capable of executing a set of instructions assembled in the form of a program, accepting input and sending output, and transferring information among the components. There are several ways in which computers store information, data, and instructions. Electronic circuits are used for temporary storage (i.e., only as long as the power is on) in random access memory (RAM) and for permanent storage in read only memory (ROM). Computers also have an additional type of storage which uses magnetic media in either floppy disk (removable) or hard disk form.

Compact disk-read only memory (CD-ROM) uses optical rather than magnetic means to store data. These disks, similar to the CDs used for audio recording, can store music and pictures in addition to very large amounts of data. The most common user input to general-purpose computers is via either a keyboard or mouse. As stated

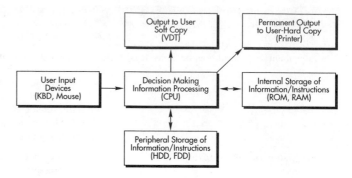

FIG. 28-3 Major functional components of standard (non-adapted) computer system. (From Cook AM, Hussey SM: *Assistive technologies: principles and practice,* St Louis, 1995, Mosby-Yearbook.)

previously, many alternatives are available. User output from the computer is typically provided by either a video display terminal (VDT), which shows soft copy, or a printer, which produces a printout called hard copy.

A human operator interacts with a computer via a communication channel called the computer user interface. Two types of user interfaces are typically used in computer applications. The command line interface (CLI) is based on the use of a marker (called a cursor) that shows where input information will appear on the VDT. As Hayes[17] points out, this interface is ideally suited to short commands and the use of text rather than graphics. The CLI can be slow for individuals who have difficulty with keyboard entry, but it is easier for individuals who have visual limitation because all text can be spoken with a voice synthesizer. The CLI is used in the MS-DOS operating system.*

The other common user interface is the graphical user interface (GUI), which is based on the use of a mouse pointer that controls movement around the screen, one or more graphical menu bars and one or more windows that provide a menu of choices.[17] Entries are made through movement of the pointer to a desired item by a mouse or other device and then pressing a button to choose the item. Because the GUI uses a menu approach for item selection, it reduces the number of keyboard entries required. For persons with limited motor skills, this approach reduces effort and increases accuracy. The use of icons generally helps with recall and ease of use because the operator doesn't need to remember as many commands, and icons make it possible for persons who can't read to use the interface. These features can be very helpful to persons who have difficulty with keyboard entry. However, the graphical nature of the GUI makes adaptation for persons with visual impairments much more difficult than for the CLI. This is primarily because the GUI environment is not easily converted to voice (e.g., synthesized speech) or tactile (e.g., Braille) output.

---

* Microsoft Corp., Redmond, Wash.

A virtual keyboard is an image of the keyboard on the video screen. The image is divided into "keys," each of which is labeled with an alphanumeric character, special character, or function. The user selects a character or function by positioning the cursor inside the desired "key" with a pointing device. Once the cursor is positioned, the user makes the selection either by activating another switch or holding the cursor on the choice until it is accepted by the device. There are many virtual keyboard programs, which can be used with either Apple IIgs computers, Macintoshes, or IBM-compatible PCs.[3,4]

ADAPTATIONS OF COMPUTER INPUTS

Computer input can be adapted in many ways depending on the needs of the consumer. Many of these adaptations are mandated by Section 508 of the Rehabilitation Act in the United States (PL 99-506, 1986). The most common problems experienced by persons with disabilities when using a standard keyboard are shown in Table 28-2 together with typical hardware and software solutions. For the IBM and compatible PCs these software adaptations are included in Access DOS* and Access Pack for Windows.† For the Apple Macintosh, the software adaptations are built into the operating system, and for commercial keyboard alternatives (often called emulators) an assisted keyboard method is used to accomplish the basic need shown in Table 28-2.

The most common alternatives to the standard keyboard are expanded or contracted keyboards and voice recognition. A common alternative to the standard mouse is the use of the keyboard arrow keys to move the on-screen pointer, listed in Table 28-2 as mouse keys. Other alternative pointing devices such as a trackball, joystick, or head pointer can also be used.

Concept keyboards can increase access for persons who have cognitive difficulties. These keyboards replace the letters and numbers of the keyboard with pictures, symbols, or words that represent the concepts required by the software program. For example, a program designed to teach monetary concepts might use a concept keyboard in which each key is a coin, rather than a number or letter. The user can push on the coin and have that amount entered into the program.

To use many of the alternative control interfaces (such as an expanded keyboard or a single switch) to access a computer, a general input device emulating interface or *GIDEI* is used. The GIDEI is a special-purpose processor that translates the signals from the control interface into those required for input to the computer. For example, if the computer application requires the use of [ESC] or [DEL] keys, the GIDEI must provide a way for the control interface to generate these key commands. Each commercially available GIDEI has a set of features that allows

TABLE 28-2 Basic Adaptations to Standard Keyboard and Mouse

PROBLEM	SOFTWARE APPROACH	HARDWARE APPROACH
Modifier key cannot be used at same time as another key	Sticky keys	Mechanical latch
User cannot release key before it starts to repeat	Repeat keys	Keyguard
User accidentally hits wrong keys	Slow keys Bounce keys	Keyguard, template, shield
User cannot easily point with hand or finger	NONE	Typing aid, mouth stick, head pointer
User cannot manipulate mouse	Mouse keys	Trackball, head sensor, joystick
User wants to use augmentative communication device as input	Serial keys	GIDEI

Sticky keys: user can press modifier key, then press second key without holding both down simultaneously

Repeat keys: user can adjust how long key must be held before it begins to repeat

Slow keys: key must be held for certain duration before character is entered into computer; that is, user can release an incorrect key before it is entered

Bounce keys: prevent double characters from being entered if the user bounces on key when pressing and releasing

Mouse keys: arrow keys substitute for mouse movements

Serial keys: allow any serial input to replace mouse and keyboard

Adapted from Cook AM, Hussey SM: *Assistive technologies: principles and practices,* St Louis, 1995, Mosby-Yearbook, p. 392.

the computer to be altered for a given application to match the needs of a specific consumer. This set of features is called a setup and consists of three basic elements: (1) an input method, (2) overlays, and (3) a set of options. As shown in Fig. 28-4, each setup is used with an application program.[12] The setup shown in Fig. 28-4, *A,* is intended to be used for text entry in a business environment with application software comprising a word processor, a spreadsheet program, and a database program. For a single switch user, the overlay on the screen is a scanning array with special characters, as shown in 28-4, *B.* The second setup, shown in Fig. 28-4, *C* and *D,* is for a young child who is using any of a wide range of software programs that require selection of an answer by matching a pointer with the correct numbers, letters, shapes, words, or pictures. Often one key (e.g., [RIGHT ARROW]) is used to move the cursor and another key (e.g., [RETURN]) selects the one the student believes is correct. Since the user is likely to be a prereader, the speech overlay helps to identify the possible choices. Speech is also used as a reinforcer when the choice is made. Cook and Hussey[12] describe several commercially available GIDEIs.

* IBM, Armonk, NY.
† Microsoft Corp., Redmond, Wash.

	METHOD	OVERLAY	OPTIONS	APPLICATION
A	Virtual Keyboard	User: Qwerty Layout Computer: Same Speech: No	Speed of Mouse • • •	Business, productivity software (word processing, spreadsheet, etc.)
B	Single Switch Scanning	User: ETA Array Computer: Same Speech: No	Rate • • •	
C	Expanded Keyboard	User: [→] [STOP] Computer: Arrow, Return Speech: "This one", "Next one"	Speech Slowdown •	Early education matching task with arrow and return
D	Single Switch Scanning	User: [- →] [OK] Computer: Arrow, Return Speech: "This one", "Next one"	Rate Speech Slowdown	

FIG. 28-4 Elements of general input device emulating interface (GIDEI). (From Cook AM, Hussey SM: *Assistive technologies: principles and practice,* St Louis, 1995, Mosby-Yearbook.)

ADAPTATIONS OF COMPUTER OUTPUTS

Standard visual display devices and printers are often not suitable for use by persons who have visual impairments. In the case of low vision, the standard size, contrast, and spacing of the displayed information is inadequate. For individuals who are blind, alternative computer outputs based on either audition (hearing) or tactile (feeling) modes are used. Persons who are deaf or hard of hearing may experience difficulties in recognizing auditory computer outputs such as beeps. Adaptations that facilitate some of these functions, and which are included in AcessDOS and AccessWindows,* are shown in Table 28-3. ToggleKeys uses a beep to replace light indicators on keys such as CAPS LOCK. SoundSentry replaces auditory tones with flashing lights or cursors. These adaptations are also required by Section 508 of the Rehabilitation Act.

Low Vision Adaptations

The major problem with visual computer displays for individuals with low vision is that the text characters and icons are not easily readable. The three factors that affect the readability of text characters are as follows: (1) size (vertical height), (2) spacing (horizontal distance between letters and width of letters), and (3) contrast (the relationship of background and foreground color). Brown[10] has identified the capabilities of an ideal low vision system for computer output. The most important are compatibility with all commercial software programs, adjustability for level of magnification, inclusion of both text and graphics, and compatibility with different types of video display terminals. Several commercial adaptations that allow persons with low vision to access

---

TABLE 28-3 Simple Adaptations for Sensory Impairment

NEED ADDRESSED	SOFTWARE APPROACH
User cannot see lights showing status of caps lock, num lock, etc.	ToggleKeys
User cannot hear beeps signaling change of operation or error during program operation	SoundSentry

From Cook AM, Hussey SM: *Assistive technologies: principles and practices,* St Louis, 1995, Mosby-Yearbook, p. 408.
Software modifications developed at the Trace Center University of Wisconsin, Madison. These are included as before market modifications to DOS, OS/2, or Windows in some personal computers and are available as after market versions in others.

the computer screen are described by Goodrich and McKinley.[15] Software programs that are built into the computer operating system, such as Closeview* for the Apple Macintosh, are the most cost-effective. Magnifiers and filters, which are attached in front of the VDT screen, also provide enlargement of text and graphics, but limited magnification (about 2X) and distortion are major problems. Software programs purchased separately from the computer vendor offer wider range of magnification and have more features than built-in software programs. Several commercial products are discussed by Cook and Hussey.[12] Adaptations that include both hardware and software generally provide the greatest compatibility, but at the highest cost.

Hard copy (printer) output may also need to be altered for persons with low vision. For enlarged print, the most common approach uses a large font on a printer. The formatting (e.g., to avoid breaking words at the end of a line) is accomplished by special large print software programs.

Alternatives to Visual Output for Individuals Who Are Blind

For individuals who are blind, computer outputs must be provided in either auditory or tactile form or both. Auditory output is typically provided through systems that use voice synthesis, generally referred to as screen readers. Brown[10] has also identified the capabilities of an ideal screen reader. The most important features are compatibility with all commercial software, capability of accessing both text and graphics, and hardware compatibility with a range of voice synthesizers. Several commercial screen reader systems are available.[12] Screen readers are ideally suited for applications that consist of a CLI and text only. The use of graphics, such as with the GUI, adds considerable complexity to the screen reader

---

* Microsoft Corp., Redmond, Wash.

* Berkeley Systems, Berkeley, Calif.

system. In this case it is necessary to speak the names of icons, to locate which screen window is open, and to provide a spatial representation of the entire screen using auditory information only. Boyd, Boyd, and Vanderheiden[9] describe the fundamental screen reader approaches used for access to the GUI.

Tactile presentation of information is the other major alternative to visual output for persons who are blind. Tactile information can be presented in one of two ways: (1) tactile facsimile and (2) Braille.[12] Tactile facsimile is the provision of a tactile image of the letter using vibrating pins incorporated into the Optacon II.* Braille output is based on a pattern of six or eight dot cells. Both paper and electromechanical (often called paperless) formats are available for Braille. To use the Optacon II or a Braille cell array with a computer, interface software is required. It is also possible to use a combination of Braille or tactile facsimile with speech synthesis to maximize the information provided to the user who is blind.[24]

AUGMENTATIVE AND ALTERNATIVE COMMUNICATION

The term augmentative and alternative communication (AAC) is used to describe any communication that requires something other than the person's own body, for example, a pen or pencil, a letter or picture communication board, typewriter, or electronic communication device. There are two basic communication needs that lead to the use of augmentative and alternative communication systems: conversation and graphics.[11]

Conversational needs are those that would typically be accomplished using speech if it were available. Conversational use typically focuses on interaction between two or more people. Light[19] describes four types of communicative interaction: (1) expression of needs and wants, (2) information transfer, (3) social closeness, and (4) social etiquette. Each has unique features that dictate the AAC characteristics to be included. Because speech allows communication at a rapid rate, between 150 and 175 words per minute,[20] an individual using an AAC system must be as rapid as possible. In all AAC systems, some form of letter or symbol selection is required, and in many cases persons who are unable to speak use a keyboard to type their messages, which are then spoken by an AAC device. Limited motor skills can result in considerably lower rates of communication than for speech (as low as a few words per minute). Cook and Hussey[12] describe other relationshps between AAC characteristics and effective conversational skills.

Graphic communication describes all the things that are normally done using a pencil and paper, typewriter, word processor, calculator, and other similar tools, and it includes writing, mathematics, and drawing and/or plotting. Each serves a different need and therefore AAC devices designed to meet each type of need have different characteristics.[12] For example, all AAC systems for writing must be capable of providing a hard copy printout, in either normal text (letters, numbers, and special characters) or special symbols. If spelling is difficult for the user, some devices allow the selection of whole words which are then output to a printer. Although it is possible to learn basic arithmetic without being able to write the numbers, it is much more difficult. AAC systems used for math allow the cursor to move from left to right as the user enters numbers to be added, but once there is a column of numbers, the cursor moves right to left for entering the sum. Special symbols (e.g., greek letters), and superscripts and subscripts are also required for more advanced mathematics. AAC device characteristics required for drawing include cursor movement in all four directions; choice of colors, line widths, and other features; and the ability to save a drawing for later editing.

Table 28-4 shows three major groupings of AAC device characteristics, which correspond to the assistive technology component of the HAAT model (Fig. 28-2): (1) human/technology interface, (2) processor, and (3) activity output. The human/technology interface includes a user control interface and an optional user display to provide feedback for self-correction. For AAC systems, the processor has several specific functions: (1) selection technique, (2) rate enhancement and vocabulary expansion, (3) vocabulary storage, and (4) output control. The activity output is conversational and/or graphic communication, and this activity can take place in many different settings.

The human/technology component was discussed

TABLE 28-4	**Characteristics of Augmentative Communication Systems**	
HUMAN/ TECHNOLOGY INTERFACE	**PROCESSOR**	**ACTIVITY OUTPUTS**
Control interface	1. Selection method: Selection technique Selection set	Partner: Visual Voice Print
User visual display		External device: Serial Parallel
	2. Rate enhancement and vocabulary expansion: Codes Prediction Levels	
	3. Vocabulary storage	
	4. Text editing	
	5. Output control	

From Cook AM, Hussey SM: *Assistive technologies: principles and practices,* St Louis, 1995, Mosby-Yearbook, p. 482.

___
* Telesensory, Mountain View, Calif.

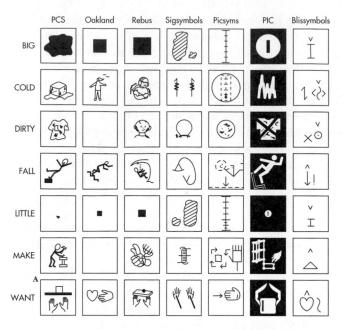

FIG. 28-5 Typical symbols in AAC systems. (From Blackstone S: *Augmentative communication,* Rockville, Md, 1986, American Speech Language Hearing Association. In Cook AM, Hussey SM: *Assistive technologies: principles and practice,* St Louis, 1995, Mosby-Yearbook.)

earlier in this chapter. One important feature for AAC devices is the use of special symbols in the selection set. Examples of symbols typically used in AAC systems are shown in Fig. 28-5. In addition, text characters and multiple-meaning icons* are frequently used. All of the selection methods discussed earlier are available in AAC devices.

To maximize the production of output, AAC devices use techniques called rate enhancement. This term is used here to refer to all approaches that result in the number of characters generated being greater than the number of selections the individual makes. Rate enhancement techniques can be grouped into two broad categories: (1) encoding techniques, and (2) prediction techniques. Several types of codes are currently used in AAC devices. Numeric codes can be related to words or complete phrases or sentences. When the user enters one or more numbers, the device outputs the complete stored vocabulary item, which can save many entries by the user.

Abbreviation expansion is a technique in which a shortened form of a word or phrase (the abbreviation) stands for the entire word or phrase (the expansion). When an abbreviation is entered, it is automatically expanded by the device into the desired word or phrase. For example, if the user typed the abbreviation ASAP, the device would expand it to "as soon as possible." Vanderheiden and Kelso[23] discuss the major features of abbrevi-

ation expansion systems and the strategies for developing stored vocabulary using this approach.

An alternative approach, called semantic encoding,[5] encodes words, sentences, and phrases on the basis of their meaning. In this approach, pictorial representations (icons) are used in place of numerical or letter codes. If the icons are carefully chosen, they can make recall much easier. For example, using a picture of an apple for food and a sun rising for morning, then selecting apple and sunrise as a code for "What's for breakfast?" is easier to remember than an arbitrary numeric or letter code for the same phrase.

It is also possible to realize substantial increases in rate by using word prediction or word completion techniques with any selection method.[22] Devices that use these techniques typically display a list of the most likely words based on the letters that have previously been entered. The user selects the desired word, if it is listed, by entering a number listed next to the word. If the desired word is not displayed, the user continues to enter letters, and the listed words change to correspond to the entered letters. In many devices, the word prediction or completion ranking of the presented list is changed, based on the user's frequency of use. This feature is referred to as an adaptive system.

Newell and associates[21] demonstrated that word completion and word prediction devices can also contribute to the development of writing skills. The long-term use of these devices resulted in improvements in spelling and the intelligibility of written work for children and adults who had poor literacy skills.

Some AAC devices include both abbreviation expansion and word prediction, allowing the user access to the strengths of each approach. Abbreviations are more direct, because the user can merely enter the code and immediately get the desired word, and AAC devices allow complete phrases and sentences. Predictions are easier to use because they do not require memorization of codes.

A very different approach is to model conversational acts and build typical sequences of such acts into the AAC system. One approach, called CHAT (for Conversation Helped by Automatic Talk), is based on the premise that each keystroke should produce a complete "speech act" (an utterance with a purpose).[1] CHAT breaks the conversation into five discrete sections: (1) greetings, (2) small talk, (3) main section, (4) wrap-up remarks, and (5) farewells. CHAT also allows the superimposition of mood on the other features: polite, informal, humorous, or angry. The user of CHAT is presented with the conversational sections in the order listed. Pressing one key generates a complete phrase for each section of the conversation. The user can also override the automatic choice with either a filler (e.g., "That's nice", "I don't think so") or with a typed message. Alm, Arnott, and Newell[2] present the details of the CHAT software program. The essential features of CHAT are available for the

---

* Minsymbols, Prentke Romich Co., Wooster, Ohio.

IBM PC or compatible computers and as Talk: About for the Macintosh computer.*

The term vocabulary expansion refers to methods by which the available vocabulary can be increased. One method of vocabulary expansion is by the use of levels. In this technique, multiple language items can be stored and retrieved from one location.[18] Storage or retrieval is accomplished by selecting the level and then selecting the location. If the device has more than a few levels, it can be difficult visually to display all of the items represented by that location. This problem can be addressed by using dynamic communication displays, which change the displayed selection set when a new level is selected. The displayed information is changed based on previous entries. For example, a general selection set might consist of categories such as work, home, food, clothing, greetings, or similar classifications. If one of these is chosen, either by touching the display surface directly or by scanning, a new selection set is displayed. For example, a variety of food-related items and activities (eat, drink, ice cream, pasta, etc.) might follow the choice of foods from the general selection set. Thus the user does not have to remember what is on each level.

Vocabulary storage refers to both the basic selection set (e.g., the letters of the alphabet) and specific words, phrases, or sentences used for specific applications. Many manufacturers include prestored vocabularies of various types. Today selection and storage of vocabulary for easy retrieval is an involved process. Beukelman and Mirenda[8] describe a variety of approaches.

To describe present augmentative communication devices, Cook and Hussey[12] derived five categories as follows: (1) simple scanners, (2) simple voice output, (3) direct selection, spelling, (4) direct selection with rate enhancement, and (5) multiple selection method with rate enhancement. Simple scanners are generally operated by a single switch (although some use multiple switch directed scanning), and a light indicates the output selection. Devices in this category generally do not have voice output as a standard feature. Simple voice output devices were all developed to provide a limited vocabulary, easy-to-use output generated by direct selection. Speech is typically stored using digital recording. Some devices in this category have rate enhancement (e.g., levels, simple codes, or key sequences), and vocabulary storage varies from a low of 8 or 16 utterances to over 100. Direct selection, spelling-only devices are distinguished by their small size, built-in printer, and minimal (if any) rate enhancement and vocabulary expansion.

The last two categories include today's most sophisticated electronic devices. These devices include all of the rate enhancement and vocabulary expansion techniques that have been discussed. Some are software programs written for laptop or notebook general-purpose computers; others have specially designed computer hardware and software programs. The last two categories are distinguished by the flexibility in control interfaces and selection methods. The multiple selection method devices in the last category allow many different types of control interfaces and selection methods. Selection methods available on some or all of these devices include the following: scanning, directed scanning, Morse code (one- and two-switch), and direct selection via light pointers (typically attached to the user's head). Cook and Hussey[12] describe commercial examples in each of these categories.

ENVIRONMENTAL CONTROL UNITS

One activity output is manipulation. This term refers to those activities that are normally accomplished using the upper extremities, particularly the fingers and hands (e.g., reading a book, feeding oneself). Assistive technologies that aid manipulation may be simple mechanical aids (e.g., reachers, enlarged handle eating utensils), special-purpose electromechanical devices (e.g., page turners or feeders), or general-purpose devices (e.g., environmental control units and robotics). In this chapter only electronic devices for manipulation are discussed. The others are described elsewhere in this book and in Cook and Hussey.[12]

Many objects that need to be manipulated are electrical appliances (e.g., television, room lights, fans, blenders and food processors), which are powered from standard house wiring (110 volts AC, in North America). The assistive devices used to control them are called environmental control units (ECUs). A typical ECU for turning appliances on and off is shown in Fig. 28-6. The user control interface may be a keypad as shown or a single switch with an indirect selection method. The appliances are plugged into modules controlled by the ECU. The most common type of ON/OFF module is the X-10.* ECUs can be remotely controlled using one of three methods. The most common is infrared (IR) transmission like that used in most TV remote units. A second method, also sometimes used for TV control, is ultrasound transmission. The third method, often used in garage door openers, is radio frequency (RF) transmission. IR and ultrasound require that the user control interface shown in Fig. 28-6 be aimed directly at the distribution and control unit along a path often called line of sight. RF transmission does not have this requirement.

The system of Fig. 28-6 may be modified to include remote control over TV or VCR functions such as volume control, channel selection, play, fast forward, and reverse. In this case the level (for volume) or number (for channel) is under the control of the user. Often these functions are incorporated into ECUs by modifying stan-

---

* Don Johnston Developmental Equipment, Inc., Wauconda, Ill.

* X-10 Powerhouse System, Northvale, NJ.

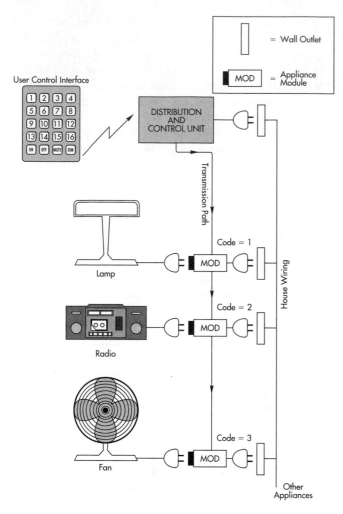

FIG. 28-6 Environmental control unit that uses individual appliance control modules plugged into house wiring and remote control from user control interface to ECU. (From Cook AM, Hussey SM: *Assistive technologies: principles and practice,* St Louis, 1995, Mosby-Yearbook.)

Persons with physical disabilities of the upper extremities often have difficulty in carrying out the tasks associated with telephone use, including the following: lifting the handset, dialing, holding the handset while talking, and replacing the handset in its cradle. There are several options for accomplishing these tasks. Nonelectronic methods such as mouthsticks or head pointers can be used to press a button to open a line on a speaker phone, dial, and hang up. ECUs perform these telephone tasks electronically. For persons who require single-switch access to the system, the control interface is connected to a control unit that also interfaces with a display and with standard telephone electronics. A typical approach is for the device to display numbers sequentially; the user presses a switch when the number to be dialed appears. By repeating this process, any phone number can be entered and then sent through the standard telephone electronics for automatic dialing. Because many persons with disabilities respond slowly, all practical systems use stored numbers and automatic dialing. Another unique feature is the inclusion of a HELP or EMERGENCY phone number which can be dialed quickly. Most systems have a capacity of 50 to 100 stored numbers. Some telephones are IR controlled and they can be included with ECUs that learn device codes.

The assessment of consumers for the specification of ECUs is described by Dickey and Shealy.[13] The steps involved are those described previously, but they are specifically related to ECU use. Gross[16] presents a detailed case study of the process of selecting and implementing an ECU for a person with a high level spinal cord injury.

SUMMARY

A basic framework for viewing assistive technologies, the HAAT model, has been described and the most commonly used electronic assistive technologies were introduced. The area of assistive technology is becoming increasingly integrated into occupational therapy practice. This trend is expected to continue with many of the advancements in the application of assistive technologies coming from this field.

dard TV or VCR remote controls by merely adding a single switch to the remote control or by more elaborate adaptations, which allow indirect selection. Universal remote controls that can "learn" the signal for a particular TV or VCR which allow several appliances to be controlled from the same ECU. Cook and Hussey[12] describe several commercial approaches to this type of ECU.

REVIEW QUESTIONS

1. What is the definition of *assistive technologies* according to PL 100-407?
2. What is the purpose of assistive technologies in the rehabilitation of persons with disabilities? How is occupational therapy concerned with the assessment and delivery of assistive technologies?
3. What are the components of the HAAT model?
4. Describe and give an example of the interaction between the components of the HAAT model.
5. Which professional disciplines might be involved in assistive technology delivery to the patient or client?
6. List the steps in the process of service delivery and describe the components of each step.
7. What is meant by control interface?
8. Give some examples of control interfaces.
9. What is meant by the selection set? Give examples of different types of selection sets.

10. Compare the selection methods described. What are the advantages and disadvantages of each in relation to the user's capabilities?
11. How are control interfaces activated? Give examples of each method.
12. Discuss the types of disabilities for which each type of control interface is most likely to be used.
13. What is a virtual keyboard? How does it work?
14. Name two alternatives to the standard computer keyboard.
15. What is a GIDEI? Why is it necessary?
16. List and describe at least two types of computer outputs.
17. Define *augmentative and alternative communication.*
18. How is vocabulary expansion accomplished?
19. What is an environmental control unit?
20. What kinds of household devices can be operated by an environmental control unit (ECU)?
21. How are ECUs controlled?

REFERENCES

1. Alm N, Newell AF, Arnott JL: A communication aid which models conversational patterns, *Proc. 10th Ann. Conf. Rehab. Engr.,* 127-129, 1987.
2. Alm N, Arnott JL, Newell AF: Prediction of conversational momentum in an augmentative communication system, *Communications of the ACM* 35(5):46-57, 1992.
3. Anson D: Presentation to RESNA workshop on instructional materials development, RESNA 13th Annual Conference, Washington, DC, 1990.
4. Anson D: Virtual keyboard techniques, *Occup Ther Forum* 6(3):1-7, 1991.
5. Baker B: Minspeak, *Byte,* 7:186-202, 1982.
6. Baker JM: How to achieve recognition: a tutorial/status report on automatic speech recognition. *Speech Technology,* Fall, 1981, pgs. 30-31, 36-43.
7. Bergen AF, Presperin J, Tallman T: Positioning for function: wheelchairs and other assistive technologies, Valhalla, NY, 1990, Valhalla Rehabilitation Publications.
8. Beukelman DR, Mirenda P: *Augmentative and alternative communication, management of severe communication disorders in children and adults,* Baltimore, 1992, Paul H. Brooks.
9. Boyd LH, Boyd WL, Vanderheiden GC: The graphical user interface: crisis, danger, and opportunity, *Jour Visual Impair Blindness* 84(10):496-502, 1990.
10. Brown C: Computer access in higher education for students with disabilities, ed 2, Monterey, Calif, 1989, US Department of Education.
11. Cook AM: Communication devices. In Webster JG, editor: *Encyclopedia of medical devices and instrumentation,* New York, 1988, John Wiley and Sons.
12. Cook AM, Hussey SM: *Assistive technologies: principles and practice,* St Louis, 1995, Mosby-Yearbook.
13. Dickey R, Shealey SH: Using technology to control the environment, *Am J Occup Ther* 41(11):717-721, 1987.
14. Gallant JA: Speech-recognition products, *EDN* January 19, 1989, pgs. 112-122.
15. Goodrich GL, McKinley JL: A guide to large print computer access, *J Vision Rehabilitation* 1(2):29-40, 1987.
16. Gross K: Controlling the environment, *Team Rehab Report* 3(6):14-16, 1992.
17. Hayes F: From TTY to VDT, *Byte* 15(4):205-211, 1990.
18. Kraat A, Stiver-Kogut M: Features of portable communication devices, Wilmington, Del, 1991, Applied Science and Engineering Laboratories, University of Delaware.
19. Light J: Interaction involving individuals using augmentative and alternative communication systems: State of the art and future directions, *Augmentative and Alternative Communication* 4(2):66-82, 1988.
20. Miller GA: *Language and speech,* San Francisco, 1981, Freeman.
21. Newell AF, Arnot JL, Booth L and associates: Effect of the "PAL" word prediction system on the quality and quantity of text generation, *Augmentative and Alternative Communication* 8(4):304-311, 1992.
22. Swiffin AL, Arnott JL, Pickering AA, Newell AF: Adaptive and predictive techniques in a communication prosthesis, *Augmentative and Alternative Communication* 3(4):181-191, 1987.
23. Vanderheiden GC, Kelso DP: Comparative analysis of fixed-vocabulary communication acceleration techniques, *Augmentative and Alternative Communication* 3:196-206, 1987.
24. Vanderheiden GC, Kunz DC: Systems 3: an interface to graphic computers for blind users, RESNA 13th Annual Conference 259-260, Washington, DC, 1990.
25. Vanderheiden GC, Lloyd LL: Communication systems and their components. In Blackstone S, Bruskin D: *Augmentative communication: an introduction,* Rockville, Md, 1986, American Speech-Language and Hearing Association.

Americans with Disabilities Act: Accommodating Persons with Disabilities

Patricia Smith

It is estimated that 43 million Americans have physical or mental disabilities. During the 25 years from 1965 to 1990 there was a 400% increase in the number of severely disabled people between the ages of 17 and 44.[4] Many of these people were employed before their disability; they seldom returned to their former place of employment or to a new employment setting, however. Although the majority of people with disabilities want to work, two-thirds of all disabled Americans between the ages of 16 and 64 are not working.[7]

People with disabilities, as a group, have frequently been subjected to discrimination and have faced barriers to employment and to use of transportation, public services, and telecommunications. The costs to society have been staggering in terms of economic and social costs and have undermined national efforts to educate, rehabilitate, and employ persons with disabilities. When these barriers are removed society benefits from the skills, talents, and purchasing power of these citizens, and the individuals are able to lead more productive and fulfilling lives.

HISTORY OF LEGISLATION

The Americans with Disabilities Act (ADA) gives civil rights protection to persons with disabilities similar to the protections provided to all persons on the basis of race, sex, national origin, age, and religion.[2] The ADA was modeled after the Civil Rights act of 1964, which prohibited discrimination against handicapped persons who were beneficiaries of programs or activities receiving federal funds or employees of federal contractors and federal employees. The ADA does not preempt any federal, state, or local law that provides greater or equal protection for the rights of persons with disabilities. The ADA guarantees equal opportunity for persons with disabilities in public accommodations, employment, transportation, state and local government services, and telecommunications. It was passed by Congress and signed into law on July 26, 1990, by President George Bush.[2]

In 1991 the Civil Rights Act was signed into law.[5] It amends the Civil Rights Act of 1964 and strengthens and improves federal civil rights laws. It prohibits discrimination on the basis of race, color, gender, age, and national origin. It provides for damages in cases of intentional discrimination. Whereas the ADA provides for monetary and injunctive relief, back pay, future pay, lost benefits and attorneys fees for persons proving discrimination, the Civil Rights Act of 1991 permits substantial awards of compensatory and punitive damages to victims of intentional discrimination. In addition to actual dollar losses, compensatory damages might include awards for emotional pain and suffering and for loss of enjoyment of life. Employers who are shown to have acted with malice and indifference to these federally protected rights may also be subject to fines of up to $300,000.00 if the employer has more than 500 employees. Smaller employers are also subject to large fines if they do not make a good-faith effort to comply with the law.

THE AMERICANS WITH DISABILITIES ACT[2]

The ADA is comprised of five sections, called titles. Each Title has an effective date and lists specific entities covered, regulatory and enforcement agencies, remedies, and exceptions. Title I concerns employment, Title II concerns public services, Title III covers public accommodations, Title IV relates to telecommunications, and Title V deals with a wide range of other topics concerning implementation of the law. As of July 26, 1992, Title I has affected all employers with 25 or more employees and as of July 26, 1994, it has affected employers with 15 or more employees. The effective date of Titles II and III is July 26, 1992, and the other Titles became effective July 26, 1994.

The ADA is very broad and inclusionary in its provisions. It encompasses many areas of intervention appropriate for occupational therapists. To understand how far-reaching the provisions are, it is important to understand the various terms used in the law. The U.S. Equal Employment Opportunity Commission (EEOC) has clearly defined and described the employment provisions in the Technical Assistance Manual of the Employment Provisions (Title I) of the Americans with Disabilities Act.[14] Any occupational therapy clinician or consultant interested in providing services in regard to this portion of the ADA should obtain and become very familiar with this publication and associated documents and resources.

DEFINITIONS

It is important to understand terms used in the law. A person with a disability is defined as someone who has a physical or mental impairment that "substantially limits" one or more "major life activities"; has a record of such an impairment; or is regarded as having such an impairment. A person's impairment is determined without regard to any medication or assistive device that he or she may use.[2]

According to the ADA, an impairment is a physiologic or mental disorder; simple physical characteristics such as eye color, handedness, or height or weight within a normal range are not impairments. A physical condition that is not the result of a physiologic disorder, such as pregnancy, is not an impairment. Similarly, personality traits such as poor judgment or quick temper are not impairments. Environmental, cultural, or economic disadvantages such as lack of education or a prison record also are not impairments.[2] An illustrative example given by the EEOC is that dyslexia, a specific learning disability, is an impairment whereas inability to read because of dropping out of school is not considered an impairment.

An impairment is a disability only if it substantially limits one or more major life activities. That is, the person must be unable to perform or be significantly limited in the ability to perform an activity compared to an average person in the general population. Major life activities are activities that an average person can perform with little or no difficulty. Examples of major life activities include the following: walking, speaking, breathing, performing manual tasks, seeing, hearing, learning, caring for oneself, working, sitting, standing, lifting, and reading.

There are three factors to be considered in determining whether an impairment constitutes substantial limitation. The nature and severity of the limitation and the length or expected length of the limitation are considered. The permanence or long-term or expected impact is also considered. It is important to consider all of these factors because simply identifying the name of the condition or the diagnosis does not indicate whether it is sufficiently limiting to the life of an individual. If an individual has two or more impairments, neither of which substantially limits a major life activity, there may be substantial limitation when taken together; thus the individual would be protected under the ADA.

A few other classes of individuals are covered by the provisions of the Act. Persons who have successfully completed or are participating in a drug rehabilitation program or have otherwise been successfully rehabilitated and are no longer engaged in illegal use of drugs are covered on the basis of past addiction.

Persons who have a record of a disability or who are regarded as having a disability are protected by the ADA whether or not they are currently limited in a major life activity.[2] This definition brings up a host of possible scenarios. The law protects people with a history of cancer, heart disease, mental illness, or other conditions, whose illnesses are cured, controlled, or in remission. It also protects people who have been misclassified or misdiagnosed as having a disability. Perception of disability also entitles a person to protection. Facial scars, for instance, may create the perception of disability and concern about acceptance by coworkers or customers. The intent is to protect people from discrimination based on myths, stereotypes, and fears about disability.

TITLE I: EMPLOYMENT PROVISIONS OF THE ADA

A goal of legislators in drafting the bill was to ensure equal access of qualified individuals to the rights and privileges of employment. Title I specifically states that it is against the law to discriminate against qualified job applicants or employees on the basis of disability. These protections cover the job application process, testing, hiring, job assignment, advancement, discharge, compensation, job training, disciplinary actions, leave, benefits, and several other aspects of employment.

As defined by the ADA, a qualified individual with a disability is an individual with a disability who meets the skill, experience, education, and other job-related requirements of a position held or desired and who, with or without reasonable accommodation, can perform the essential functions of the job.[2,14]

For an individual to be deemed substantially limited in working, he or she need not be totally unable to work. Persons are generally not considered substantially limited if they are merely unable to perform a particular job for one employer or are unable to perform a very specialized job in a narrow field. To qualify for protection under the ADA they must be significantly restricted in the ability to perform either a class of jobs or a broad range of jobs in various classes, compared to average persons with similar training, skills, and abilities.

PERSONS NOT COVERED BY TITLE I OF THE ADA

Persons with temporary illness such as influenza or impairments such as broken bones are not considered impaired unless normal healing does not occur and permanent disability or significant limitation in a major life activity results.

Current illegal drug use does not qualify a person for protection under the ADA. Homosexuality and bisexuality are not covered disabilities. The Act also specifically states that the following are not covered disabilities: transvestism, transsexualism, pedophilia, exhibitionism, voyeurism, gender identity disorders, compulsive gambling, kleptomania, and pyromania.

SPECIFIC PROVISIONS OF TITLE I

The primary intent of the ADA is to allow qualified persons with disability to participate in the work force to the same degree as those without disability. It is not a preference law nor is it a quota law. Qualified persons with disability must have equal access to employment opportunities provided they are able to perform the "essential functions of a job with or without reasonable accommodation."[2]

By definition a person with a disability cannot perform tasks in the same manner as people without a disability; they need some type of accommodation. The ADA requires "reasonable accommodation" meaning that the accommodation is effective for accomplishment of the task.[2] These accommodations can take many forms such as restructuring the job, altering the work schedule, providing a signing interpreter, providing assistive aids or equipment, widening doors, and a host of other modifications.

The obligation of the employer does not extend to providing items that may be for the personal benefit of the individual, on or off the job. The ADA further states that these accommodations must not pose an "undue hardship" for the employer;[2] that is, the employer is not required to provide an accommodation that poses substantial difficulty or expense. Such a hardship can exist because an accommodation is unduly costly, extensive, substantial or disruptive, or fundamentally alters the nature of operation of the business. A night club, for instance, would not be required to accommodate a visually impaired employee by raising the light level because to do so would fundamentally alter the nature of the business.

Several more concepts must be understood to appreciate the impact of this Act. Besides the undue hardship exception, an employer is also not required to accommodate an applicant or employee if doing so would pose a "direct threat" to the health and safety of the individual or others in the workplace if the threat cannot be eliminated or reduced by reasonable accommodation. There must be "a significant risk of substantial harm" according to EEOC regulations.

Determination of direct threat consists of an individual assessment of the person's present ability to perform the essential functions of the job safely. Four factors must be considered in making this determination: (1) the duration of the risk; (2) the nature and severity of the potential harm; (3) the likelihood that the potential harm will occur; and (4) the imminence of the potential harm. It is not acceptable, for instance, to deny employment to a person who uses a wheelchair, citing concern for fire evacuation safety, if there has never been a fire in the building. The law states that these considerations must rely on objective, factual evidence and not on subjective perceptions, irrational fears, patronizing attitudes, or stereotypes.[2] For individuals with physical disabilities or dysfunctions, the employer must first identify the specific aspect of the disability that poses the direct threat.

Once the risk is identified the employer must then evaluate whether the risk poses significant risk of substantial harm. For individuals with mental or emotional disabilities the employer must identify the specific behaviors on the part of the individual that pose the direct threat. There is the obvious intent in the regulations that persons with disability not be denied employment because of risks that are not truly significant and threatening. Occupational therapists are always concerned about the safety and health of persons with disabilities. Diligent care must be taken by therapists to ensure that the individual is not in any way unfairly barred from employment because of well-meaning but overly protective concern for their safety.

The requirement to accommodate reasonably applies again to this area. An employer must consider whether a reasonable accommodation is possible to reduce sufficiently or to eliminate the potential risk of harm. If no accommodation is possible, the employer is not required to hire the individual. For example, an employer is not required to hire an individual with narcolepsy, who unexpectedly loses consciousness, for a carpentry job an essential function of which requires use of power saws and other dangerous equipment.

ESSENTIAL FUNCTIONS

The concept of "essential functions" is new to many employers who may be accustomed to providing job descriptions that focus more on describing the means to accomplishing the end product. In a 1981 case filed under the Rehabilitation Act, the Postal Service required each employee to be able to use both arms when performing the job of distribution clerk. One employee with limited mobility of one arm demonstrated that he was able to perform the essential function of lifting and moving mail, though with one arm rather than two. In this case the court found that the essential function was lifting and moving mail, not using two arms, thus the employee was determined to be a qualified individual with a disability.[1]

In general, the term *essential function* means the fundamental job duties of the employment position the person holds or desires. In determining the essential functions of a job the employer must consider all relevant evidence. This evidence includes the following: (1) the employer's judgment as to which functions are essential; (2) a written job description prepared before advertising or interviewing applicants for a job; (3) the amount of time spent performing the function; (4) the consequences of not requiring a person to perform the function; (5) the terms of collective bargaining agreements; and (6) work experience of people who have performed and currently perform similar jobs.

A function cannot be deemed essential if it is in reality marginal or peripheral. For instance, a secretary may be requested to drive to the post office to buy stamps, but in reality this task may be an incidental one that could be performed by any of several employees and is not essential to the position of secretary. The example of an airline pilot is often used to illustrate the wisdom of considering all relevant evidence and not just certain points such as the amount of time spent performing the function. An airline pilot may spend only 5 percent of the work shift landing and taking off, but, this function is certainly essential for pilots. Likewise, a firefighter may only occasionally carry an unconscious person from a burning building but the consequences of not requiring performance of this function would be serious.

OTHER PROVISIONS OF TITLE I OF THE ADA

Employers are permitted to perform physical agility tests, medical examinations, aptitude and ability qualification tests, and tests for illegal drug use. It is vitally important to be aware that certain restrictions apply to the administration of tests and examinations. There must be no disparate impact; that is, there must be no discrimination because the test screens out or tends to screen out persons with disabilities.[2] It is not permissible, for instance, to give a written test to a person with the specific learning disability dyslexia unless reading is an essential function of the job.

If testing is required for employment, all persons being considered for the job category must be tested in the same manner. It is not permissible to require a medical examination or screening of physical ability only for persons with disabilities; all persons in the job category must be tested equally. It must also be remembered that reasonable accommodation is required in the testing process and testing environment if notice of the need for accommodation is received before test administration.

It is also not permissible to require testing or examination before a conditional offer of employment. Nor can the employer ask questions about disability before a conditional offer of employment. Within the prescribed boundaries, the offer of employment can be rescinded upon results of the examination or inquiry. Aside from testing, the employer is permitted to ask the applicant to describe or demonstrate how a job-related function would be performed with or without accommodation.

Physical agility tests are not considered medical tests; thus they may be given at any point in the application or employment process. If, however, a determination of employment is based on results of these tests, they must be job-related and consistent with business necessity.

OPPORTUNITIES FOR OCCUPATIONAL THERAPISTS TO ASSIST EMPLOYERS

Given the broad provisions of Title I of the ADA, it is apparent that employers, physicians, workers' compensation insurance carriers, and other parties involved in employment of persons with disabilities may need special expertise to fulfill their obligations lawfully. One important mandate is that the employer show good-faith efforts to comply with the law. Many employers are lacking the in-house knowledge and resources to meet this obligation. The unique training of occupational therapists, especially pertaining to functional performance, adaptation, daily life activities and knowledge of community resources, equips them well to provide assistance. Several specific areas for involvement by clinicians are inherent in the provisions of this law and are suggested by "The 12 Steps to ADA Compliance"[8] (Box 29-1).

Occupational therapists must prepare themselves to provide services and consultation in the area of ADA compliance. Thorough knowledge of the law, its interpretation, and implications must precede their involvement and offering of any services. Armed with this requisite knowledge and additional expertise in the world of work and employment practices, occupational therapists can be important resources to employers in many phases of compliance with the law. By looking at the tasks in the 12-step process, it is possible to envision many opportunities for assisting employers to meet their legal and human resources obligations while satisfying their business needs.

Determination of Essential Functions

Employers are usually accustomed to thinking about their jobs in terms of the means to accomplish production of products or delivery of services. The ADA requires them to examine the precise functional physical activities required to perform these tasks. It is the right and responsibility of the employer to determine which functions of their jobs are essential, though assistance to understand the precise physical nature of the essential functions may not have been part of their thinking and may be more accurately determined by an occupational therapist. To determine the physical demands of essential functions, a job analysis is performed. The reader is referred to Chapter 30 of this text for techniques for performing a job analysis. It should be noted that a job analysis for ADA purposes must concentrate on the precise nature of physical activities, such as weights of loads handled, hand functions, duration of effort and number of repetitions of physical movements, etc.

BOX 29-1

THE 12 STEPS TO ADA COMPLIANCE

1. Identify the essential functions of each job.
2. Examine employment applications for discriminatory language or questions concerning medical conditions or history.
3. Prepare a job description before advertising or interviewing for a position.
4. Review interview procedures for discriminatory language, questions, or behaviors.
5. Develop methods and resources for investigating reasonable accomodations.
6. Train interviewers and supervisors about reasonable accommodations requirements for new hires and returning employees.
7. Make sure qualification, skill, and medical tests are valid, job-related, and nondiscriminatory and can be modified to accommodate individuals with disabilities.
8. Develop postoffer screening programs that do not discriminate, are consistent with business necessity, and are job-related.
9. Prepare a system for keeping medical records confidential.
10. Train employees and supervisors in how to work with individuals with disabilities.
11. Do an audit of facilities to be certain they are accessible to individuals with disabilities.
12. Make sure all facilities, including break rooms, vending machines, etc. are accessible and integrated for disabled and nondisabled workers.

Isom R, Boyle K, Smith P: ADA compliance system, Athens, Ga, 1993, Elliot & Fitzpatrick. Reprinted with permission.

The difference between the process used in production of a product and the physical activity required for that production process is an important distinction to understand. For instance, while a job function may require loading boxes of machine parts into a truck, it may not, in fact, require manually lifting the box with two hands, carrying the box using its two handles, and climbing into the truck. In other words, it should not be assumed that manual lifting, using the handles, and climbing are essential functions. By contrast, in the case of a secretary, using the hands to type on a computer keyboard may well be an essential function. Each job needs to be analyzed separately to determine these factors accurately.

A job description prepared for the purpose of announcing an employment opportunity should contain information about the functional physical abilities required to perform the essential functions of the job. An employee or applicant with a disability can then review the job description and determine whether a reasonable accommodation may be required and may request such an accommodation. As described previously, the occupational therapist may assist in development of this analysis.

Employers may tend to think that all functions of their jobs are essential when in reality some functions can be distributed among other workers, can be eliminated or combined, or are really marginal functions and are not actually essential. This situation presents another opportunity for an occupational therapist to make a meaningful contribution by assisting employers to understand the true nature of their jobs from the standpoint of their physical and mental demands.

Eliminating Discriminatory Questions, Language, and Behaviors

Human resources personnel and hiring managers may not be familiar with preferred terminology with respect to persons with disabilities and may not necessarily be sensitive to issues of nondiscriminatory language. The therapist may be able diplomatically to assist the employer in purging employment applications, interview procedures, and other employment practices of discriminatory language, both overt and subtle. All employment documents should be free of negative wording such as the following: confined to a wheelchair, wheelchair-bound, victim of, suffering from, afflicted with, and crippled.

The ADA encourages self-identification by persons with disabilities, which often creates an opportunity for occupational therapists to train hiring personnel so they learn to appreciate and internalize the need for nondiscriminatory behaviors and procedures. Persons unaccustomed to interacting with individuals with disabilities may benefit from various training techniques such as role playing, mock interviewing, and provision of information about various disabilities and their sequelae. They need to know, for instance, that HIV and AIDS are not contracted by casual contact and that to deny equal employment opportunities to qualified persons with these disorders constitutes illegal discrimination.

A handbook of basic tips and suggestions for communicating with persons with hearing impairments may be developed and distributed to managers and coworkers. General principles should include reminding coworkers and managers to talk directly to the person with the disability and maintain eye contact, even when an attendant or interpreter is present. Managers and coworkers should be reminded that communication skills of persons with speech and hearing impairments may be weak, but that this weakness is not an accurate measure of intelligence or self-confidence. They should also be advised to keep their voices at a normal volume, not raised or exaggerated, when speaking to these individuals.

Language used in training materials should be free of jargon. Information should be presented with the intent to inform objectively rather than to depict persons with disabilities as deserving of pity or conversely as fortunate and "chosen."

If employees participate in an empathy experience such as using a wheelchair, they learn to appreciate the difficulties of performing otherwise routine tasks. They should be advised to ask first before providing help such as pushing a wheelchair or taking an arm.

Community resources and social service agencies can be tapped for information and referral. Disability advocacy groups in the community may be pleased to come to the work site and address groups of employees. Special interest organizations such as the Arthritis Foundation, Cancer Society, Heart Association, and many others can usually provide pamphlets and speakers for presentation of educational programs.

Integration of employees can be fostered by forming work groups to promote contact between workers with disabilities and their coworkers. It may be helpful to assign tasks to a work group rather than to an individual to encourage mainstreaming and to foster reduction of social isolation, which frequently occurs for persons with disabilities.[1] Removing the mystique of disability and promoting comfort in the interview situation and everyday working environment can be especially beneficial for all involved.

Reasonable Accommodation Investigation

The ADA requires that persons with disabilities must be accommodated to ensure their equal opportunity to be considered for a job, to enable them to perform the essential functions of a job, and to participate in all privileges of employment.[2] Specific regulations of the EEOC require a systematic investigation of reasonable accommodations to enable persons with disabilities to perform the essential functions of the job.[14] The investigation is to be conducted on an individual basis and should include the participation of the person with disability, using a problem-solving approach. The ADA mandates provision of an effective accommodation, not necessarily the best solution, but one that will enable a qualified employee to perform essential functions to meet employer standards of production, quality, and safety.[2]

The EEOC has given several examples, not an exhaustive list, of possible accommodations.[14] Providing physical access to the work site is a fairly obvious accommodation. The employer should remove structural barriers to any areas where the employee will perform the essential functions of the job as well as to adjacent areas such as rest rooms, break rooms, lunch rooms, recreational spaces, and any other areas an employee may expect to use. More suggestions about barrier removal for physical access are given later in this chapter as they pertain to Title III of the ADA.

In developing reasonable accommodation strategies it is useful to approach possible solutions in terms of a hierarchy. The simplest and most cost-effective should be considered initially. For instance, investigate whether there is a way to modify how the function is performed, which at the same time satisfies employer business needs. Energy conservation techniques may be appropriate for many people and should usually be incorporated. If these very simple interventions are not sufficient it may be necessary to consider modification of tools or purchase of equipment and aids, preferably commercially available rather than custom-made to save costs. If these administrative and ergonomic solutions are not adequate, it may be necessary to consider custom-made devices and assistive technology. Employers may have the perception that the latter options are the only ones available to them because they are not knowledgeable about other creative solutions.

Job restructuring is another reasonable accommodation that may be considered. This approach is described as examining a job analysis and rearranging its contents in terms of tasks performed. This step may involve combining several tasks the disabled individual is able to perform and/or removing tasks that cannot be performed and transferring them to another employee who can perform them. Perhaps the job can be modified so that the hours of work are flexible to allow for needed breaks in the day, or the job may be changed to part-time. All of these changes are considered possible and desirable accommodations in the view of the EEOC.

Another accommodation might be reassigning a person with a disability to a vacant position. The ADA does not require the employer to create a position; there is, however, the requirement to consider placement of the person in a vacant position if one is available. The occupational therapist may assist the employer in identifying appropriate vacant positions within the company and evaluating the functional abilities of candidates to perform the essential functions of the available positions.

Modifying equipment, providing assistive aids, and training in adaptive methods can also constitute reasonable accommodation. Products designed for other purposes can be combined in creative and new ways. The Job Accommodation Network (JAN) is a service of the President's Committee on Employment of People with Disabilities. JAN provides free telephone information about resources and reasonable accommodations. By sending follow-up questionnaires to callers who have used the JAN services, they have been able to compile data about the costs of accommodations. They have determined that two thirds of accommodations cost less than $500. Fifteen percent have no cost at all. In a 1982 study for the Department of Labor by Berkeley Planning Associates, it was found that half of all accommodations cost nothing, and more than two thirds cost less than $100.[9] Many products, readily available for consumer use, are extremely useful for persons with disabilities. For example, telephones with oversize buttons are thought of as decorative and trendy, but they are also very useful for persons with visual or motor impairments.

It is sometimes necessary to consider designing and fabricating custom devices. Occupational therapists are becoming increasingly proficient in locating and applying assistive technology. Detailed information about assistive technology can be found in Chapter 28. It must be remembered that Title I of the ADA pertains to employment issues; thus the concern of the clinician is confined to assistive technology for job performance rather than for other areas of functioning such as personal care. The employer's responsibility does not usually extend to durable medical equipment such as wheelchairs. Ethical dilemmas may arise for occupational therapists about employee needs for such personal care equipment and concerns for independence and self-esteem; however, it is wise for the occupational therapist who is consulting in this area of practice to maintain focus on the rights and responsibilities of the employer as well as those of the person with disability.[13]

Persons with psychiatric disabilities may need any of these types of accommodations and/or other types of accommodations to enable them to be successfully employed. Interpersonal communication may be an area of functioning that is especially difficult. It may be helpful to train supervisors to provide written instructions or feedback for the person who becomes anxious and confused when given verbal instructions. Added time structure and organization may be helpful. Removing distraction may be useful and readily achievable by positioning room dividers or facing work stations away from open areas. Extra support and reassurance may be necessary for the person reentering the work force following psychiatric hospitalization.

Medical Inquiries, Examinations, and Post-Offer Screenings

When an employee is ready to return to work after an injury or illness, the employer may require passage of a job-related examination (sometimes referred to as a fitness-for-duty exam) as a condition of returning to work. The examination must evaluate only the ability to perform the essential functions of the job with or without reasonable accommodation.

The employer may also require passage of an examination by job applicants; however, different regulations apply in the case of an applicant compared to a returning employee. An applicant for a job may be required to participate in an examination only after a conditional offer of employment has been made. These specific postoffer examinations are also frequently called preemployment screenings or exams. Such an applicant examination/screening of physical ability does not have to be job-related. If, however, a person with a disability is screened out, the reason for disqualification must be job-related and of business necessity. The job-related screening activity must be a valid and legitimate measure of qualification for a specific job. If a test or activity does not relate to the essential functions of the specific job, it is not consistent with business necessity. All persons applying for the job must be examined irrespective of disability. An employer may give follow-up tests or examinations where the initial examination indicates a problem that may affect job performance and further information is needed.[6]

The postoffer screening should be preceded by a thorough job analysis to ensure that the screening is based on the physical requirements to perform the essential functions of the job. The screening protocol should be closely linked to the specific job and include the physical requirements of each function; the frequency with which each function is performed; the use of customary tools, protective clothing, or equipment such as helmet or gloves; and should replicate the work environment as much as possible. The reader is referred to Chapter 30 of this text for information about developing a similar protocol referred to as a Work Tolerance Screening. Depending on employer needs and funding mechanisms, a screening may be performed in a clinical setting or at the work site. The length of time required may be very brief especially if only a select number of essential functions are included in the protocol, which may be the case if only certain functions are apt to present substantial challenge in terms of physical functional performance. It is important to remember that a screening is a measure of current performance and does not predict risk of future injury or evaluate ability to perform over time.

Confidentiality of Record Keeping

The ADA requires that all information gathered during any type of medical inquiry or examination must be kept on forms separate from all other personnel records. The records are to be maintained separately and treated as confidential medical records. The information is to be used for the purpose of making reasonable accommodations and to ensure safety of the worker. The records may be made available only to those persons who have a legitimate need to know, such as the medical department at the place of employment, the supervisors and managers who must be advised of work restrictions, and accommodations for the employee and government officials investigating compliance with the ADA.

TITLE II OF THE ADA: PUBLIC SERVICES

This section of the law pertains to all state and local government activities, services, and programs, including courts, police and fire departments, town meetings, and employment offices.[2] Unlike section 504 of the Rehabilitation Act of 1973, which covers only programs receiving federal financial assistance, Title II extends to all the activities of state and local governments whether or not they receive federal funds. This title prohibits state and local governments from denying participation in any service, program, or activity on the basis of disability. All programs, services, and activities must be integrated and must not have unnecessary eligibility standards or rules that deny participation by persons with disabilities.

New construction and alterations to existing facilities must be accessible to ensure access. New buses and rail vehicles must also be accessible. Effective communication must be ensured.[2] Occupational therapists may have opportunities in this area similar to those afforded by Title III. A more complete explanation of potential opportunities is discussed later in this chapter.

TITLE III: PUBLIC ACCOMMODATIONS

Title III covers all public accommodations such as restaurants, hotels, theaters, retail stores, museums, libraries, parks, private schools, day care centers, social service agencies, health care service providers, and other facilities used by the public. It requires that existing facilities must remove structural barriers where such removal is "readily achievable," which has been defined as "easily accomplishable and able to be carried out without too much difficulty or expense."[2] Barriers must be removed to allow access to the premises and use of the facilities, including the following: parking areas, walks, ramps, entrances, display racks, signage, doors, alarms, restrooms, toilet stalls, grab bars, and others features. If barrier removal is not readily achievable other methods of providing access may be substituted. Examples include providing curb service or a drive-up window, providing home delivery, having employees retrieve items that are beyond reach, and moving certain activities to accessible areas of the facility.

Title III also mandates access to communication. Persons with disabilities must be given the opportunity to see, hear, and understand what is occurring in the environment and program.[2]

Facilities remodeled after January 26, 1992, must be readily accessible and usable by persons with disabilities to the "maximum extent feasible." Specific requirements apply to "key conveniences." These are listed as the path of travel to the altered area (for example, curb cuts, ramps, doors, elevators), rest rooms, telephones, and drinking fountains. These key conveniences must be accessible to the maximum extent feasible unless the cost and scope is "disproportionate to the cost of the overall alteration."[2]

New facilities must be "readily accessible to and usable by" persons with disabilities regardless of cost. Certain implementation dates and exceptions apply to new construction. The reader is referred to the Americans with Disabilities Act Accessible Guidelines for Buildings and Facilities for detailed information about compliance.[2]

OPPORTUNITIES FOR OCCUPATIONAL THERAPIST REGARDING ACCESSIBILITY AND PUBLIC SERVICES

Title II and Title III mandates create numerous opportunities for occupational therapists to be of assistance. Whereas Title II allows persons with disabilities to reach their destinations, Title III allows them to participate fully once they arrive. Various references have been developed and are being developed to provide specific guidelines regarding accessibility.[11,12,14]

General principles of accessibility are part of the basic training of occupational therapists. The process of determining appropriate solutions begins with an analysis of the tasks to be performed or accessibility that is desired, often referred to as an accessibility audit. An audit of the facilities may have been performed previously and should be obtained if available, or an audit should be performed if not already done. This information forms the basis of the services and recommendations to be provided.

The physical activities required for access should be clearly established. The means of travel, strength requirements, and dexterity demands, etc. should be determined. Next is an analysis of the person with disability and his or her capabilities and limitations with respect to the task. It should be remembered that persons with disabilities are truly the experts when it comes to questions about their own needs, capabilities, and possible solutions. All of the provisions of the ADA pertaining to confidentiality must be kept in mind when making these inquiries.

When approaching this analysis of accessibility, it is helpful to think in terms of the sequential steps taken by an individual when seeking access to a facility or service. Transportation to the setting may be via public transportation, which also must be in compliance with the ADA. Access and egress from the transportation vehicle are the initial tasks. Upon arriving at the facility there is entrance to the facility. If arriving by private vehicle there is a drop-off spot or a parking area. The facility is entered and once inside there may be a receptionist or building directory or simply corridors, elevator, or stairs.

All of the activities and movements in and about the facility should be determined and noted in this systematic manner so that any barriers become evident. It is very useful to be accompanied on this excursion by the person with disability as well as persons familiar with the facility and the access alternatives that may be feasible. Perhaps another route is more suitable or a different entrance door is more easily used. It must be kept in mind that facilities for persons with disabilities must be enabling and not discriminatory or segregated. A freight elevator on the loading dock is not usually considered to be a suitable entrance for a person who uses a wheelchair.

General principles about accessibility have been developed by various organizations and regulatory agencies. These standards are reviewed and revised periodically; thus the reader is referred to current local sources such as the building department of the city or county. If local regulations are more stringent than the ADA, the local regulations take precedence.

Some general sequential guidelines are presented here as a basis for beginning to think about opportunities for occupational therapists.

Step 1: Building Access

Parking spaces or a drop-off zone should be located near the building entrance and connected by walkways to an accessible building entrance. Handicapped parking spaces should be designated and reserved. Parking spaces should be 12 feet wide and have an access aisle for loading/unloading. Curb cuts should be textured and should meet the street surface with as little lip as possible. Walkways and ramps should be sloped at no more than 2° to the side (cross slope) and 5° in rise and have a nonslip surface. A handrail should be provided on at least one side; railing on both sides is preferred. The rail should extend beyond the top and bottom of the ramp.

Ramps to doorways should have a 5 foot level surface at top and bottom. Entrance doors should have at least 32 inches of clear opening and should be power-operated or should be easy to grasp and easy to push or pull open. Doors in series should have adequate space between them to permit door swing into the space. Revolving doors and turnstiles should not be considered as accessible entrances. Any entrance doors that are not accessible should have appropriate directional signs to the nearest accessible entrance.[10]

Step 2: Building Interiors

All essential areas should be accessible without having to leave the building or negotiate steps. Corridors should be at least 48 inches wide and be free of obstructions such as drinking fountains, supporting columns, telephones, and decorative plants. Floors should have a nonslip hard surface or low pile carpet. If public telephones are provided, at least one should be mounted not more than 48 inches high. Drinking fountains, if available, should be no more than 36 inches high to the level of water flow. The path of travel in all areas such as between desks should be adequate in width.

Identifying signs and labels should be of sufficient size and color contrast for easy viewing. Tactile letters and numbers and Braille letters are advisable as is an auditory signal in elevators to identify floor level. Elevator controls should be at a maximum height of 60 inches. Interior doors to public areas should have at least 30 inches of clear opening. Stairs, if present, should have ample lighting and should not have abrupt or open risers that may catch toes or braces.[10]

Step 3: Rest Rooms

Rest rooms present special challenges in terms of providing for safety given that they are often small. In general, each building should have a minimum of one rest room for women and one for men that is accessible to persons using wheelchairs. All doors and passages should be wide enough to permit a wheelchair to make any required turns. Toilet stalls should be of sufficient width to permit a front or side transfer. Handrails should be appropriately located and capable of supporting a 250-pound load. Dispensers, hand dryers, and other fixed items should not impede movement and should be positioned for easy reach, generally not higher than 48 inches. Mirrors should be full length or tilted downward. Sinks should have easy-to-operate handles and clearance underneath the fixture. Drains and hot water pipes should be insulated to prevent burns.[10]

Step 4: Other Considerations

All areas of facilities used by the public should be free of barriers to physical movement and impediments to hearing, seeing, and understanding the business being conducted. Unique or unusual environments require careful inspection and questioning. For instance, if voice communications must occur through an opening in a glass security window, is there some way to augment communication for the user who is seated or very short in stature? Is there appropriate provision for persons using crutches or walkers to enjoy a sporting event from the grandstand?

It is important to consider energy expenditure of persons with disabilities as well as the needs of elderly persons who may have decreased endurance. The opportunity to sit and rest may be essential to participating in activities.[3]

All of these issues of access and accommodation require expert and sensitive advice from trained professionals such as occupational therapists. Low cost modifications can often be recommended for upgrading existing facilities. Advice may also be given during the design phase of new construction. The reader is encouraged to seek out recent guidelines and local government publications concerning regulations and building codes for minimal requirements. Technical advances such as voice-synthesized direction signs and traffic signals, infrared sensors in buildings, and other devices are being developed and are becoming increasingly prevalent.

TITLE IV: TELECOMMUNICATIONS; TITLE V: MISCELLANEOUS

Title IV requires that all intrastate and interstate telephone companies establish relay systems for use by hearing-impaired and speech-impaired persons 24 hours per day. These services must be available at no additional cost. This title also requires that television public service announcements produced or funded by the federal government must include closed captioning. Title V concerns applicable rules and regulations of implementation of the ADA.

SUMMARY

In summary, it is apparent that the ADA mandates a broad range of services to ensure equal opportunities for persons with disabilities. Its various titles, particularly the portions pertaining to employment and to access to public services and facilities, encourage participation in society by the estimated 43 million persons with disabilities in the United States. As employers, public agencies, and services strive to comply with the provisions of the ADA, there are many exciting opportunities created for knowledgeable occupational therapists.

Basic training of the therapist must be augmented with thorough study of the law and its regulations and interpretations. To this base of knowledge should be added experience with persons with all types of qualifying disabilities and expertise in accommodations to compensate for the impairments that may be associated with these disabilities. Finally, the therapist must have an understanding of the business and human resources needs of employers. Armed with this knowledge and experience, it is difficult to imagine professionals more uniquely qualified to provide consulting and direct services to aid in compliance with the ADA.

REVIEW QUESTIONS

1. Does the ADA pertain to small employers or only to very large employers?
2. What qualifies a person for protection under the ADA?
3. What is meant by *substantially limits* a person?
4. What are the major life activities to which the law refers?
5. Can a person be prevented from participating in a job if the supervisor has any concern about his or her ability to safely perform the job?
6. What six categories of evidence should be considered in determining essential functions of a job?
7. How can a person with a specific learning disability be tested for ability to perform the essential functions of a job?
8. How can occupational therapists assist employers to develop employment application forms and interview questions that comply with the ADA?
9. What are some of the ways qualified persons with disabilities can be accommodated if they are unable to perform an essential function of a job?
10. Must all job applicants or only applicants with disabilities be required to pass a screening of physical ability before they begin a new job?
11. Does public access to buildings apply only to government facilities or does it also apply to buildings owned by private parties?
12. Access is required to what parts of the building?
13. Are telecommunications companies required to provide any particular services according to the ADA? If so, what are they?

REFERENCES

1. American Management Association: Special report: ADA in action, *HR Focus, Special Report,* 1992.
2. Americans With Disabilities Act of 1990 (PL 101-336), 42 U.S.C. 12101, *Federal Register,* vol. 56:144, 35543-35691.
3. Bachelder JM, Hilton CL: Implications of the Americans with disabilities act of 1990 for elderly persons, *Am J Occup Ther* 48:73, 1994.
4. Carbine M, Schwartz G: *Strategies for managing disability costs,* Washington DC, 1987, Washington Business Group on Health.
5. Civil Rights Act of 1991 (PL 101-166), 42 U.S.C. 2000 e Note, *Congressional Record,* Vol. 137:191.
6. Ellexson M: ADA compliance: to screen or not to screen?, *Work Programs Special Interest Section Newsletter, Am Occup Ther Assoc* 8:1, 1994.
7. International Center for the Disabled: *ICD survey of disabled Americans: bringing disabled Americans into the mainstream,* New York, 1986, International Center for the Disabled.
8. Isom R, Boyle K, Smith P: *ADA compliance system,* Athens, Ga, 1993, Elliot & Fitzpatrick.
9. Job Accommodation Network: *The truth about accommodations,* Morgantown, WV, 1994, Job Accommodation Network.
10. National Rehabilitation Association: *Revised manual for accessibility,* Alexandria, Va, 1988, The Association.
11. National Rehabilitation Hospital-ADA Compliance Program: *Answers to questions commonly asked by hospitals and health care providers: ADA,* Washington DC, 1993, National Rehabilitation Hospital.

12. President's Committee on Employment of People with Disabilities: *ADA and the health professions,* Washington DC, 1993, Government Printing Office.

13. Rein J: Reasonable accommodation in the workplace, *Work Programs Special Interest Section Newsletter, Am Occup Ther Assoc* 6:2, 1992.

14. U.S. Equal Employment Opportunities Commission: *Technical assistance manual of the employment provisions of the Americans with disabilities act,* Washington DC, 1992, Equal Employment Opportunities Commission.

CHAPTER 30

Work Evaluation and Work Hardening

Cynthia M. Burt, Patricia Smith

In American society, feelings of personal identity and self worth are closely tied to a person's role as a competitive wage earner. Abrupt loss of the worker role because of injury frequently leads to forced role reversal within the family, life style changes caused by economic hardship, forced inactivity and dependence, depression, and maladaptive psychosocial responses. When recovery from injury is prolonged or compounded by poor coping techniques, the worker may slip into a mire of discouragement, lowered self-esteem, and lost confidence. Chronic pain syndromes and a host of other disabling cycles can result, ultimately leading to low motivation for return to work.

Industrial injuries have reached astronomical proportions in terms of monetary costs and lost productivity. Paramount among work-related injuries are low back injuries, followed by injuries to the upper extremities. Although 90% of persons with acute episodes of low back pain recover within 3 months, the remainder develop chronic conditions lasting for many months or even years. The economic and social costs of these chronic conditions are high to both the worker and the employer. As a result, employers and their industrial insurance carriers (Workers' Compensation Insurance Programs) are continually looking for measures to control costs and improve employee productivity.

During the last two decades, there has been an increasing incidence of chronic musculoskeletal disorders with cumulative trauma etiology. These injuries have not been adequately treated with a traditional medical model, which generally focuses on acute trauma intervention. As the need for treatment of injured workers with chronic disorders has grown, work hardening programs have been developed to fill this service gap.

Work hardening is defined by the Commission on Accreditation of Rehabilitation Facilities as "a highly structured, goal oriented, individualized treatment program designed to maximize a person's ability to return to work".[41] It is interdisciplinary in nature and comprehensive in scope. Work hardening uses work, defined as real or simulated job tasks, as the treatment modality. These tasks may be combined with injury-specific, progressive strengthening and flexibility training, as well as emotional support and encouragement to develop behaviors necessary for successful return to competitive employment.

Since the mid 1970s, work hardening has emerged as an effective industrial injury management service. Although considered a new service, work hardening has a long history, with deep roots in occupational therapy theory and practice.[29] Formal involvement of occupational therapy in the vocational rehabilitation movement can be traced to the federal Vocational Rehabilitation Act of 1923, which required inclusion of occupational therapy in general hospitals serving persons with industrial accidents and illnesses. Amendments to the Act in 1954 increased the prominence of the profession in the vocational rehabilitation field through provisions for establishment of prevocational services within facilities. The role of occupational therapy was further enhanced with amendments in 1978 to the Vocational Rehabilitation Act.[19]

HISTORY OF OCCUPATIONAL THERAPY INVOLVEMENT

Work therapy, as work hardening was often called, dates far back in occupational therapy literature. In the 1800s, tuberculosis patients were prescribed graded exercise and work tolerance activities as part of a medical regimen of good food and fresh air. Activities such as woodworking and clerical tasks of a progressively demanding nature were added to the treatment protocol in the final stages. These activities were designed to prepare the patient for return to work and to estimate resistance to breakdown from physical effort and emotional upsets.[40]

In 1919 Barton stated that the purpose of work was to divert the mind, to exercise some part of the anatomy, and to relieve the monotony and boredom of illness. Work did not, he suggested, have to be of practical value beyond its immediate purpose. World War I reconstruction workers, the first occupational therapists, taught crafts in military hospitals as "work cure." Crafts were regarded as therapeutic modalities, and were used to foster a sense of intrinsic productivity and fulfillment.[19] In the early 1920s, programs of "habit training" were described, with the goal of developing work habits that had been impaired by disease or accident.

The psychiatric literature of the 1940s described work hardening as a program to prepare the patient for return to competitive life after the sheltered environment of the hospital. Realistic work environments were used, including the hospital laundry, barber shop, and carpentry shop. The patient was also observed for personality traits such as cooperation and friendliness, characteristics felt to be important for harmonious working.[33]

The physical disability literature of the same era also stressed real work experiences designed to make the worker aware of the relationship of a work hardening program to productive employment. Work speed was variable, but quality standards were not altered during the treatment program.[40]

In the 1950s, a program at Massachusetts General Hospital was described that focused on the objective evaluation of progress. A graded resistive exercise component was used with strength measured objectively in pounds throughout the program. This approach made it possible to track and document improvements. The principles of objective and quantified outcome measures were incorporated for the first time.[46]

Lillian Wegg, a leader in the field of work hardening and work therapy during the late 1950s, described a multi-disciplinary program composed of an occupational therapist, vocational counselor, physiatrist, and industrial engineer. Work hardening activities included use of work samples (in early stages of development at that time), work tests, and job simulations. At program completion, a list of recommendations was given, including assistive equipment, length of work day, and job classifications that should be considered for placement.[47] Several years later, Wegg revised the program and elaborated on program components. Work hardening had moved away from a medical model to a vocational model. A physician's prescription was no longer required for referral. Work hardening was regarded as a vocationally oriented program with the purpose of developing work habits and improving work assets that had been identified as deficient in the evaluation process.[48] Florence Cromwell, another leader of the time, emphasized the evaluation of work habits, intellectual and attitudinal factors, and work quality issues such as neatness and safety as components of vocational retraining programs.[10]

In other programs of the era, an emphasis on real work was maintained. Patients produced items for sale, working in hospital or community settings to build a sense of self worth, repertoires of appropriate work habits, and physical work tolerances.

Chronic pain, particularly low back pain, became a major focus of therapeutic intervention for efficient return to work in the 1970s and 1980s. Programs adopted a multidisciplinary approach incorporating medicine, therapy, psychology, vocational counseling, and rehabilitation engineering.[12,13,14] Behavioral factors received greater attention. Abnormal illness behaviors, unwillingness to take responsibility, depression, excessive anger, and lack of maximum and consistent effort were found to be inappropriate in terms of the requirements of competitive employment.[31]

In the 1980s, there was a return to the techniques of work therapy and work cure of previous decades. More commonly called work simulation, the activities of real or simulated work activity were embraced. Technological developments provided more objective information through use of computerized equipment that precisely measured effort, force, endurance and other factors. Therapists became skilled in combining realistic work activities with high tech equipment to measure and analyze results.[5]

The Commission on Accreditation of Rehabilitation Facilities (CARF) drafted work hardening standards requiring an interdisciplinary approach in 1989.[41] The standards were updated in 1992 with retention of the interdisciplinary requirement.[42]

CURRENT MODELS OF WORK HARDENING PRACTICE

The worker role has been and continues to be the major focus of intervention in the occupational therapy profession.

To the occupational therapy practitioner, any activity that contributes to the goods and services of society, whether paid or unpaid, is considered a work activity. Engaging in work is a productive activity and a medium and goal of occupational therapy.[9]

In an historical perspective, Robert Bing reiterated that work must be purposeful and have meaning for the individual and society. A social context is suggested when the outcome, or product, is of value to someone else.[5]

Work hardening program models currently used by occupational therapists clearly draw on concepts from past experiences, while adding present day technology as well as models of occupational and career development, medical intervention models, and ergonomic and anthropomorphic principles.[40] Only in the last few decades of the profession's formal existence has there emerged a sound theory that explains and applies the beliefs about work professed by its early founders.[11] The occupational therapy process incorporates a continuum of services. These services are designed to prepare the worker for return to the preinjury job or provide retraining or job modification if necessary. Reemployment at the highest possible level of independent functioning is the ultimate goal.

The basic principles and responsibilities of occupational therapy practice in provision of work hardening services were summarized by the American Occupational Therapy Association (AOTA) in the Work Hardening Guidelines in 1986.[2] These guidelines provided the basic structure for services provided in a variety of settings, encompassing several theoretical models and frames of reference represented in occupational therapy practice. In 1992, the Work Practice Statement was developed by AOTA to further clarify the role of occupational therapy in the rehabilitation process of injured workers.[2]

Work hardening is a multidisciplinary, comprehensive program combining work simulation with strengthening and behavioral components. Work conditioning, rather than work hardening, is offered by some programs. In contrast to work hardening, work conditioning concentrates on the physical components of flexibility, strength, coordination, and endurance for return to work. The behavioral and vocational components of the return-to-work process are not integrated in this approach.[17]

Occupational therapy intervention through work hardening services can occur at any of several points in the return-to-work process. Services may begin during the medical phase of treatment. Work hardening services in this early intervention model are guided by the physician and are usually provided on a prescription basis. In the earliest stages, work hardening may be provided simultaneously with traditional physical therapy services. In the absence of substantial lingering or permanent disability, there is the expectation that the worker will return to customary work roles as soon as sufficient medical and functional recovery has occurred. The goals of work hardening in the early intervention model are closely tied to the requirements of the preinjury job.

When return to the original job and original employer is not feasible either because of medical preclusions or other factors, the worker enters the vocational rehabilitation phase. The goals of work hardening remain the same in this late intervention model; rapid and safe return to employment. However, the program must consider and allow for additional difficulties and constraints. Among these are the worker's fears and anxieties about a forced career change, unrealistic expectations of the vocational rehabilitation/legal system, and other real and imagined barriers and disappointments experienced by the displaced worker.

The clinician should be aware of other possible intervening variables that may challenge successful return to work at any stage in the rehabilitation process. Among these are several socioeconomic issues.

The demographics of the work place have been changing over the last two decades. The American work force is becoming older with more females entering the market. Age and gender have been correlated with dynamic balance skills, ability to climb, and ability to lift. Older workers and female workers are generally less skilled than younger workers and male workers.[21] Implications are that older workers, female workers, and particularly older, female workers may be at high risk of injury. Once injured, these individuals may be more challenging to rehabilitate as well as more susceptible to reinjury.

Secondary gains have been correlated with delayed recovery. These can include sympathy or attention from others, avoidance of responsibility, and opportunity for financial gain.[22,23]

Role changes within the family structure may be incentives for family members or others to reinforce the injured worker's sick role.[31] A newly employed wife might like her new role as breadwinner and reinforce her husband's sick role. A father may suddenly have time to spend with his family and avoid returning to work.

Injured workers with pending litigation improve at a slower rate than nonlitigated workers, until litigation is settled.[16] Financial opportunities including unemployment benefits, welfare benefits, and workers' compensation can all adversely influence return to work. Therapists should be aware of these secondary reinforcers and address issues with the worker if they occur.

The employer's attitudes regarding the return to work of an injured worker can affect the rehabilitation plan. Fear of reinjury and reduced productivity are often verbalized as concerns employers have regarding reemploying an injured worker.[31] Employer/employee relations have also been reported to be related to disability claims and eventual return to work. Employers who reported unsatisfactory supervisors had higher incidence of injuries than employees reporting a good relationship with their managers.[49]

Cultural norms and personal attitudes towards work can be critical factors in successful work injury rehabilitation. What work means to a person within his or her culture can be crucial in returning to work.

Alcohol and drug abuse are frequently reported in workers with painful injuries. Abuse can be premorbid, related to attempts to control pain, or result from attempts to reduce or avoid stress. Abuse can affect outcome and should be considered within the treatment plan.

Pain is an inherent part of all musculoskeletal injuries. The therapist must be aware of the physiological and psychological implications of pain as they relate to the recovery process. These implications frequently occur in the presence of chronic pain, which is defined as pain lasting longer than six months.[22,23,31] Prolonged chronic pain can result in psychological disturbances including insomnia, anxiety, depression, and feelings of helplessness.[28] Psychosocial problems including difficulties with relationships, alcohol and drug abuse, weight fluctuations, and sexual dysfunction can result.[22] Pain behaviors including verbal complaints, postural bracing, grimacing, rubbing and holding affected body parts, and rigid guarded movements are frequently displayed to communicate that pain is being experienced by the worker.[5,7]

THE WORK HARDENING PROCESS

The goals of work hardening should be individually designed to maximize employability through achievement of a level of productivity acceptable in the labor market. There are several objectives within the overall goal of preparing the worker for return to work. These are (1) attaining optimal physical tolerances and abilities, (2) reducing fear and increasing confidence for resumption of productive work, (3) developing appropriate worker behaviors, (4) maximizing cognitive and psychosocial functioning, and (5) identifying problems that may require placement in an alternative job.

Work hardening is a multifaceted process. Whenever possible, development of an individualized work hardening program should begin with a specific job analysis to determine critical job demands. An assessment of the worker's physical, sensorimotor, cognitive, and psychosocial skills and abilities should be completed next. Information from the job analysis and the assessment of the worker should then be consolidated to develop an individualized work hardening program. This program must be designed to develop the tolerances required for completing critical job demands so the worker can return to competitive employment.

STEP 1: JOB ANALYSIS

To plan a program for an injured worker that is meaningful, relevant, and measurable, the worker's job requirements must be understood. Because design of program activities is based on job demands, it is necessary to have an accurate description of all job requirements. The job analysis should include detailed information about the demands placed on the worker for the following: walking, balancing, climbing, standing, sitting, crouching, bending, lifting, carrying, pushing/pulling, reaching, handling, and fingering. Sensory components including vision, hearing, and smell should also be considered along with environmental conditions including noise, cold, and vibration. Unique psychological demands such as the ability to deal with irate customers and tolerate distracting environments could also be important considerations if determined to be critical job functions.

Evaluation of critical job functions must include identification of all factors that could result in risk of cumulative trauma disorders. These include frequency, force, duration, posture, and exposure to vibration and cold.

The occupational therapist may not always be the professional who completes the job analysis. The job may have been previously analyzed by the employer, insurance carrier, rehabilitation nurse or counselor, or other professional involved in the case. If using a previously completed job analysis, the therapist should review the primary job functions with the employer and employee to verify current validity.

When an adequate job analysis is unavailable, an onsite visit should be made to observe job tasks and the work environment. Occupational therapists are qualified by their basic training to perform these on-site evaluations of physical and cognitive demands. However, medical/legal documentation requirements usually necessitate additional experience and training. Several government publications can serve as references to assist in development of a document that can be used in the medical/legal arena. These include the *Dictionary of Occupational Titles* (Ed. 4, 1991),[24,43] *Handbook for Analyzing Jobs,*[24,43] and *A Guide to Job Analysis.*[20] A sample job analysis form is shown in Fig. 30-1.

STEP 2: ESTABLISHING WORK TOLERANCE BASELINE

Determination of the worker's current level of functioning is as important as the job analysis in individual program planning. Assessment of functional status is undertaken through a screening of all pertinent physical, cognitive, and behavioral factors. A factor is pertinent if it is a requirement of the job and is subject to impairment as a result of the injury. Relevant conditions such as dia-

JOB ANALYSIS

Job Title______ Employee______
Location______
Work Hours______ to______ Days______ Overtime Per Wk______
General Job Description:

Equipment, tools, work aids:

Primary job functions:

Time spent:
Standing______ hrs Sitting______ hrs Inside______ hrs Outside______ hrs

ACTIVITY	YES	NO	REPETITIVE (Frequency)	CONTINUOUS (# Hours)	COMMENTS
Stoop/Bend					
Squat/Crouch					
Kneel					
Climb					
Crawl					
Reach Overhead					
Manipulate/Finger					
Grasp					

LIFT/CARRY	HRS/REPS/POSITION	LIFT/CARRY	HRS/REPS/POSITION
0-10 lbs		11-20 lbs	
21-50 lbs		Over 50 lbs	

Environmental Conditions: (check if present)
Cold______ Dampness______ Heat______ Dust/Fumes______ Noise______
Psychological Requirements:

Analyst______ Date______

FIG. 30-1 Sample job analysis form.

betes, hearing loss, and hypertension, which may not be sequelae of the work injury, should also be considered because of potential impact on job performance and need for possible job modification.

The determination of the work tolerance baseline can be completed using a variety of assessment instruments. Some of these are commercially available whereas others are developed by individual therapists or facilities. This assessment of baseline has been called by many names including functional capacity evaluation, physical capacity evaluation, work tolerance screening, or work capacity evaluation. Whatever the name, the purpose of the evaluation is to determine the extent of the worker's physical and mental ability to perform specific job tasks.

The Commission on Accreditation of Rehabilitation Facilities has listed components that should be included in the evaluation process.[41] These are as follows: musculoskeletal status, cardiovascular status, cognitive status, behavioral and attitudinal status, functional work capacity, and vocational status. The Work Practice Statement of the AOTA expands these components to include consideration of the injured worker's age, interests, values, culture, and motivation for change.[9] A typical functional capacity evaluation should include the following:

Medical history

The medical history should include past conditions such as cardiac status, diabetes, etc., that are relevant for the activities to be completed by the worker during work hardening treatment. Orthopedic conditions such as previous fractures, soft tissue problems, etc. should also be included. Psychological conditions and treatment must be considered as they relate to performance issues. Any available medical records should be reviewed including information concerning the current injury and medical treatment. Work restrictions must be obtained from the referring agency and noted.

Worker interview

An initial interview is useful to determine the worker's perception of the injury. This interview provides the evaluator with insight into the worker's attitude, potential fear of reinjury, motivation, acceptance or nonacceptance of responsibility for rehabilitation, as well as other potential impediments to successful recovery. Program goals and rules should be established at this time with the worker as an active participant.

Job description with critical work demands

The job analysis should identify critical work demands. If a job analysis is unavailable, the worker is asked to describe job functions. This information should be validated with the employer if possible. Generic job descriptions with physical work demands can be obtained from the *Dictionary of Occupational Titles*[24,43] as a last resort to assist in determining critical job demands.

Pain assessment

The worker should be asked to describe areas of pain, including a description of the type, quality and intensity. Frequency of pain as well as activities that increase or reduce pain should be reported. Techniques used for pain control including modalities and medications are important. Many pain questionnaires and charts are available for clinical use. These include topographical pain representations or "pain drawings," analog pain scales, and pain rating scales such as the McGill-Melzack Pain Questionnaire.[18,30]

Physical assessment

The physical assessment is developed to determine the worker's abilities and limitations to perform critical work demands as described in the job analysis. These can include functional range of motion, strength, endurance, sensation, coordination and dexterity among others. The assessment of a sedentary office worker would be very different from that of an airline baggage handler. The evaluator should individualize the physical assessment by comparing physical functions of the worker to critical work demands and noting any discrepancies. Because many injured workers are involved in litigation, it is important to use standardized evaluation tools whenever possible.

Body flexibility is evaluated to determine functional range of motion. This rating includes trunk, lower and upper extremity flexibility. Postural strength should also be considered. The Krause-Weber Test[26] is a standardized test to measure postural strength. The VALPAR Work Sample #9 (Whole Body Range of Motion)[45] is frequently used to measure the individual's gross body movements as they relate to the functional ability to perform work tasks.

Strength can be evaluated using a variety of standardized and functional tests. Dynamometers and pinch gauges are used to measure hand strength. The Baltimore Therapeutic Equipment (BTE) Quest System and Work Simulator,[3] Cybex II,[15] Lido WorkSet,[27] ERGOS,[51] WEST 2, and WEST 4[50] are among several commercially available devices used to measure strength. Endurance can be evaluated with devices such as the Upper Body Ergometer,[15] Fitron/Lifecycle,[15] and treadmill. Endurance tolerance is also observed throughout the evaluation as related to completion of job tasks.

Sensation evaluation is vital for workers with hand injuries. The Semmes-Weinstein Monofilament Test (Von-Frey Monofilaments) is used to determine tactile discrimination.[36] Additional considerations should include edema and coordination. The Schultz Upper Extremity Evaluation is a comprehensive test of hand function used by many clinicians.[37,44]

Coordination and dexterity tests are used to determine the worker's ability to complete physical work tasks such as handling, manipulating, and fingering.

Commonly used tests include the Crawford Small Parts Dexterity Test,[35] Bennett Hand-Tool Dexterity Test,[35] Purdue Pegboard,[38] and the Minnesota Rate of Manipulation Test.[1] Work samples such as the VALPAR #1 Small Tools Mechanical, VALPAR #4 Upper Extremity Range of Motion, and VALPAR #8 Simulated Assembly,[45] the BTE Bolt Box,[3] and the WEST 7 Bus Bench[50] can also be used to measure upper extremity coordination and dexterity.

Lifting/carrying ability. Lifting and carrying tasks are inherent in most jobs. The worker's ability to lift on a frequent and infrequent basis is determined by work simulation. During the functional capacity evaluation, maximum lifting tolerance on a one-time basis is most frequently assessed. It is imperative to monitor body mechanics of the worker during this assessment to avoid reinjury. Work samples such as the WEST 2A,[50] VALPAR Work Sample #9 (Whole Body Range of Motion),[45] and WEST 3 (Comprehensive Weight System)[50] can assess lifting/carrying abilities.

Pushing/pulling. Pushing and pulling abilities can be determined through the use of a Chatillon force gauge.[8] Pushing and pulling tasks must simulate actual work conditions (for example, friction against surfaces, height of handles, inclination of surface). The Blankenship sled[6] is an example of a commercially available device useful for both evaluation and treatment.

Stooping / bending / kneeling / crawling. Stooping, bending, and kneeling can be assessed by observing the patient completing simulated work tasks or samples such as the VALPAR #9 (Whole Body Range of Motion)[45] or the WEST 2A.[50] Workers with knee and back injuries often have impairments in the ability to crawl. The evaluator should design a work task to simulate the work environment to observe this physical demand if inherent to required work demands.

Sitting/standing. The functional abilities to sit and stand should be observed by the therapist throughout the functional capacity evaluation. The initial interview and dexterity tests provide the evaluator with opportunities to observe the worker while concentrating on functional tasks or interacting with others. Actual tolerances should be compared to reported tolerances.

Work task simulation

Critical work demands of the worker's job should be evaluated. Work demands could include use of tools, materials handling, or activities that require repetitive movement or maintenance of prolonged postures. Potential problem areas should be prioritized during the evaluation.

In addition to the primary physical demands described above, the evaluator should evaluate any other job demands identified by the job analysis. These could include environmental factors such as vibration, cold, and noise.

Cardiovascular function must be measured during the functional capacity evaluation. This check could be completed as a pre and post measure during the endurance testing using a treadmill or the Upper Extremity Ergometer.[15]

Work samples are the primary modality for work evaluation. These samples can evaluate single worker traits or clusters of traits. Many of the WEST[50] and VALPAR[45] samples measure clusters of traits, such as strength, endurance, and range of motion that are inherent in a job. Therapists must use their skills of task analysis to determine specific problem areas when evaluating a worker completing a cluster trait work sample.

A variety of clinic-made devices exist that simulate work demands. These include bird cages, boxes, sleds, and pipe tree assemblies.

There are commercially available functional capacity evaluations used in many clinics. These include programs designed by Matheson,[50] Blankenship,[6] and Isernhagen.[21] Proprietary systems including both equipment and training are also available and include the Functional Capacities Assessment by Polinsky Medical Rehabilitation Center[34] and the KEY Functional Assessment.[25] A comprehensive review of work assessments and evaluations has been compiled by Jacobs in the Second Edition of Occupational Therapy, Work-Related Programs and Assessments.[23]

The final step in the evaluation process is to identify problems that interfere with work performance and make recommendations to address deficits. Issues related to identified pain behaviors, poor materials handling ability, and poor posture and body mechanics should be identified as they relate to completion of functional tasks. Recommendations for referral to a work hardening program can be made if indicated.

The evaluation of physical function and work tolerances is usually a preliminary step to a work hardening program. The functional capacity evaluation can also be used as a stand-alone service, however, to assist the physician in setting work restrictions or determining readiness for release from medical treatment. The worker is evaluated for the ability to perform the activities addressed in the job analysis (e.g., reaching, lifting, and carrying) that are critical to the job for which the worker hopes to qualify. Emphasis is placed on tasks and functions that are most likely to be impaired by the worker's injury or disability (Fig. 30-2). For example, evaluation of a worker with a low back injury would focus on lifting, standing, carrying, and climbing abilities if relevant for the worker's job. Grip and pinch strength would not be critical areas to evaluate, because they are not normally affected by lumbar dysfunction. If any restrictions have been placed on the worker by the treating physician, they must be followed at all times to avoid possible reinjury.

Work evaluations are most commonly three to five hours in duration and are generally completed on the

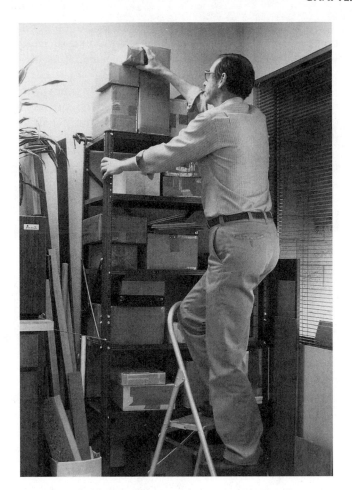

FIG. 30-2   Reaching and climbing.

first or second day of treatment. In some cases, baseline values may have already been established by another professional or estimated by the physician. The work hardening therapist should verify this information with a brief screening assessment to identify any changes that may have occurred, especially if time has lapsed since measurements of function were made. Deconditioning with resultant functional losses can occur very rapidly if there are delays or intervening medical treatment or complications.

Assessment of other factors such as worker behaviors, safety awareness, and stressors may be extended over a longer time to permit sufficient observation and evaluation. The purpose of the initial screening is to determine baseline function and establish areas of deficit that are amenable to treatment and improvement through the work hardening process.

STEP 3: INDIVIDUAL WORK HARDENING PLAN

After functional abilities are defined and requirements of the desired job are determined, an individualized work hardening plan is developed. This plan must specifically identify how the goals of the worker's program will be met. The plan should function as an agreement between the worker and the therapist. As such, it must be developed with the cooperation and collaboration of the injured worker. Areas of deficit and outcomes must be mutually agreed upon if the program is to be successful. A typical work hardening plan could include the following goals:

Increase duration of daily participation

Depending on tolerances determined through the functional capacity evaluation, the worker's program begins at a comfortable level, for example, two hours per day. As ability improves, the hours of participation are incrementally increased.

Increase physical tolerances identified as deficient for critical work demands

Work activities requiring identified tolerances are introduced in graded fashion. Activities should be increased one at a time to avoid confusion about which tolerances have been increased. These work activities should, as much as possible, replicate the actual tasks required for the worker's job.

Improve body mechanics and postures

The worker is trained through didactic instruction and other methods with new learning practiced and reinforced in all phases of the program.

Develop pain management strategies

The worker is encouraged to explore strategies for managing pain so that functional performance is ensured. Energy conservation principles are introduced as appropriate. Pain behaviors should be addressed with feedback given to the worker. The treating physician may be consulted regarding altering the medication regime or substituting other pain control methods.

Develop problem-solving skills for self-management at the work site

Injured workers often have poor judgment and lack ability to set reasonable limits. They must learn to ask for assistance when indicated.[4] The ability to recognize and set safe limits within individual tolerance levels must also be demonstrated by the worker to avoid reinjury.

Facilitate appropriate worker behaviors

Punctuality and attendance issues should be addressed as needed. Often the worker has been off the job for a long time and has adopted maladaptive patterns such as sleeping late. Appropriate interaction skills with supervisors and peers must be developed if deficient. Attention is given to task completion, quality standards, and productivity.

IMPLEMENTING THE WORK HARDENING PLAN

At this point, information from the job analysis and the functional capacity evaluation should have been used to develop an individualized work hardening plan. The goals and interests of the worker and questions of the referring agency are part of the plan. Actual or simulated work tasks are the treatment modalities of choice. The selection of work tasks and activities is based on the worker's particular job demands and functional limitations as established in the functional capacity evaluation.

It is not always possible to duplicate all tasks of a job in the work hardening setting. In this case, activities are chosen that require similar physical and cognitive levels of function. For example, if it is not feasible for a worker to replace automobile mufflers, it may be possible to design an activity requiring tool use in a prolonged overhead reaching position. Individual program design is limited only by the therapist's creativity and resources at hand. Activities are selected to be compatible with the worker's beginning level of function, progressing in graded increments until reaching the level required for work reentry.

While facilitating efficient progression towards goals, the therapist must ensure a safe environment. Workers must increase their capabilities, and at the same time, develop skills to reduce discomfort or maintain symp-

toms at manageable levels. Although it may not be possible to eliminate all residual physical symptoms associated with the injury, the worker must still be capable of productive efforts within competitive levels.

A work hardening program must include training in proper body mechanics and materials handling techniques to protect the worker from further injury. Education for back protection, pacing, and safety principles must be taught in a manner consistent with the worker's level of education and background. The principles taught must be applied to the person's job demands and practiced consistently while performing job tasks. Skills must become automatic and integrated into all daily life tasks (Fig. 30-3).

Fear of movement because of pain can lead to dysfunctional pain behaviors such as bracing, guarding, rigidity, and other abnormal postures. These abnormal postures can lead to increased muscle tension, which is a normal physiologic response to pain and pain memories. The resulting tension leads to increases in pain, which leads to more tension and becomes a cycle that is difficult to interrupt. Potential for development of chronic pain syndromes is increased if this cycle is not broken.

THE WORK HARDENING MILIEU

Work hardening programs can be found in a variety of settings ranging from hospital-based programs to industrial settings. These include outpatient facilities, workshops, private practices, rehabilitation centers, and industrial medical programs. Regardless of setting, a work hardening facility must replicate a realistic work environment with actual and simulated work tasks provided. The use of work that is relevant and meaningful is vital in helping the injured worker understand and accept his or her abilities and limitations (Fig. 30-4).

Work schedules and environmental conditions should be replicated in a work hardening program. A typical program simulates the actual work schedule of the worker including work breaks, meal breaks, and split shifts if appropriate. The work milieu consideration should include environmental aspects such as working indoors versus outdoors, dust, and noise. Work hardening is a group process with a number of workers present who may be experiencing similar difficulties and fears. The desire to be competitive with one's peers can be invaluable in facilitating the rehabilitation process. An atmosphere of peer understanding and support can also be beneficial to the worker. These features should be fostered by the therapist. The therapist should also offer necessary support, while making suggestions for compensatory techniques, providing adaptive tools, and reinforcing new learning and skills.

Work hardening programs typically range from two to six weeks in duration. Successful completion has been most strongly related to length of disability before pro-

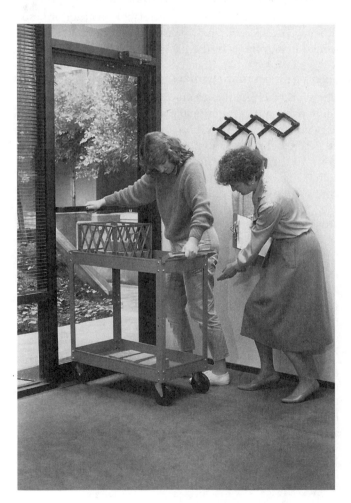

FIG. 30-3   Training in proper body mechanics.

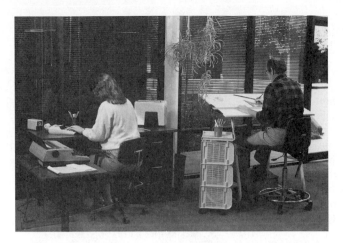

FIG. 30-4 Work is performed in realistic work stations.

gram initiation.[32] Severity of injury, stage of medical recovery, motivation, and degree of discrepancy between current functional capabilities and necessary levels of function are important predictors of program success. Progress should be continual throughout the duration of the program. Services are usually terminated when goals are substantially met to permit a return to work, when improvement has reached a plateau, or when sufficient progress is not demonstrated and does not appear to be reasonably attainable. If reasonable and measurable improvements are not demonstrated, discontinuation of the program or referral to other services that may be more beneficial should be considered. Program personnel must be diligent in avoiding unnecessary costs and delays. Pressure to achieve rapid results is part of the growing climate of accountability and cost containment that is evident in all areas of health care.

REPORTING RESULTS

In an arena of increasing litigation, work hardening professionals must be skilled at completing objective, quantifiable, and defensible reports. In accordance with facility protocols and accrediting requirements, program results should be reported at agreed upon intervals and include goals and progress. Case conferences should be held periodically to discuss progress and concerns. Timely submission of these reports is imperative. These reports are often reviewed by individuals who are not medically trained. Language used must be clear, concise, and free of jargon.[39]

At program termination, a final report is submitted that includes recommendations based on information gathered in the work hardening process. Adaptive equipment, modified techniques, and any other reasonable accommodations recommended should be included. For example, use of a specific tool handle design might be recommended to avoid overuse and improve productivity.

Occupational therapists have unique training and experience in physical, cognitive, and behavioral sciences that gives them the ability to play a vital role in this dynamic area of practice. The profession's focus on holistic concepts, task analysis, and use of activities as therapy explains its long history and pivotal role in work programs.

CASE STUDY

KL, a 36-year-old man, was injured in a fall from a ladder while working as a carpenter. He sustained a lumbar strain superimposed on degenerative disc disease. He was referred for work hardening to improve his ability to tolerate full time participation in a computer repair training program scheduled to begin in 3 weeks. A job analysis of a computer repairer was provided by the training school.

During the functional capacity evaluation, KL demonstrated ability to lift 15 pounds in a full range of body postures. He was able to carry this weight at waist level using both hands and place it on a table. He sat comfortably for only a few minutes and performed all movements stiffly and slowly while rigidly holding his body erect.

His individual work hardening plan addressed his goals of gradually increasing tolerances for lifting and working with tools at a workbench while seated and while standing.

Additional goals concerned improving his pattern of spontaneous movement without unnecessary bracing or fear of reinjury. Specific tasks were assigned to simulate his training requirements for working continuously with small tools and parts at workbench level. Twice daily stretching and conditioning activities were assigned to promote more natural movements. He was given frequent coaching and support to promote proper body mechanics while reducing his anxiety about anticipated pain.

KL made steady gains toward meeting all of his goals while maintaining his commitment to enter training. His work hardening program was concluded after 3 weeks so that he could enter training. After the program conclusion, he continued to be active by attending an evening swimming program at a local spa and walking each day to maintain flexibility and a feeling of well-being.

REVIEW QUESTIONS

1. Identify three prominent leaders of the occupational therapy profession advocating a role in work activities.
2. When did the profession first use work as a treatment modality?
3. Why is a job analysis a necessary component of the work hardening process?
4. What relationship do the critical job demands have to the functional capacity evaluation and the work hardening plan?
5. Name four intervening variables that may challenge successful return to work.
6. Name the three steps in the work hardening process.
7. Why is it important for work hardening to use a real-work approach and have a work-like environment?
8. How frequently should the worker be reassessed for physical tolerances and limitations?
9. What should the therapist do to provide a safe working environment for the recovering injured worker?
10. What factors are considered when making a decision to adjust or terminate a work hardening program?

REFERENCES

1. American Guidance Service, Inc., Publisher's Building, Circle Pines, Minn 55014.
2. American Occupational Therapy Association: *Work hardening guidelines,* Rockville, Md, 1992, The Association.
3. Baltimore Therapeutic Equipment Company, 7455-L New Ridge Road, Hanover, MD 21076. (800) 331-8845.
4. Bettencourt CM, Carlstrom P: Using work simulations to treat adults with back injuries, *Am J Occup Ther* 40(1):12, 1986.
5. Bing R: Work is a four-letter word: a historical perspective. In Hertfelder S, Gwin C, editors: *Work in progress: occupational therapy in work programs,* Rockville, Md, 1989, American Occupational Therapy Association.
6. Blankenship Corporation, P.O. Box 5084, Macon, GA 31208-5084. (800) 248-8846.
7. Caruso LA, Chan DE: Evaluation and management of the patient with acute back pain, *Am J Occup Ther* 40:347, 1986.
8. Chatillon, John and Sons, Inc., Force Measurement Division, 7609 Business Park Drive, Greensboro, NC 27409. (919) 668-0841.
9. Commission on Practice: *Occupational therapy services in work practice: official statement, Am Occup Ther Assoc,* 1992.
10. Cromwell F: A procedure for pre-vocational evaluation, *Am J Occup Ther* 13:1, 1959.
11. Cromwell F: Work-related programming in occupational therapy: its roots, course and prognosis. In Cromwell F, editor: *Occupational therapy in health care,* New York, 1985, Haworth Press.
12. Curry R: Understanding patients with chronic pain in work hardening programs, *Work Programs Special Interest Section Newsletter, Am Occup Ther Assoc* 3:1, 1989.
13. Curry R: Understanding patients with chronic pain in work hardening programs, *Work Programs Special Interest Section Newsletter, Am Occup Ther Assoc* 3:3, 1989.
14. Curry R: Understanding patients with chronic pain in work hardening programs, *Work Programs Special Interest Section Newsletter, Am Occup Ther Assoc* 4:1, 1990.
15. Cybex, P.O. Box 9003, Ronkokoma, NY 11779-0903. (800) 645-5392, in NY (516) 585-9000.
16. Deyo RA: The role of the primary care physician in reducing work absenteeism and costs due to back pain, *O Med: State of the Art Reviews* 3:17, 1988.
17. Fisher T: Work conditioning is not work hardening, *Special Interest Section Newsletter, Am Occup Ther Assoc* 7:3, 1993.
18. Flower A and associates: An occupational therapy program for chronic back pain, *Am J Occup Ther* 35:243, 1981.
19. Harvey-Krefting L: The concept of work in occupational therapy: a historical review, *Am J Occup Ther* 39:301, 1985.
20. Heck C: Job site analysis for work capacity programming, *Physical Disabilities Special Interest Section Newsletter, Am Occup Ther Assoc* 10:2, 1987.
21. Isernhagen SJ: *Work injury: management and prevention,* Rockville, Md, 1988, Aspen.
22. Jacobs K: *Occupational therapy: work related programs & assessment,* Boston, 1985, Little, Brown.
23. Jacobs K: *Occupational therapy: work related programs & assessments,* ed 2. Boston, 1991, Little, Brown.
24. Jist Works, Inc., 720 North Parke Avenue, Indianapolis, IN 46202-3431. (800) 648-5478.
25. KEY Functional Assessment, Inc., 1010 Park Avenue, Minneapolis, MN 55404. (800) 333-3KEY.
26. Kraus H: *Backache, stress and tension: cause, prevention and treatment,* New York, 1965, Simon & Schuster.
27. Loredan Biomedical Inc., 3650 Industrial Blvd., West Sacramento, CA 95691. (800) SAY-LIDO.
28. Loeser JD, Egan KJ: *Managing the chronic pain patient,* New York, 1989, Raven Press.
29. Matheson L and associates: Work hardening: occupational therapy in industrial rehabilitation, *Am J Occup Ther* 39:314, 1985.
30. Melzack R: The McGill pain questionnaire: major properties and scoring method, *Pain* 1:277, 1975.
31. Ogden-Niemeyer LO, Jacobs,K: *Work hardening: state of the art,* Thorofare, NJ, 1989, Slack.
32. Ogden-Niemeyer LO and associates: Work hardening: past, present, and future: the work programs special interest section national work-hardening outcome study, *Am J Occup Ther* 48:327, 1994.

33. Phelan LB: Role of manual arts therapy in a neuropsychiatric hospital, *J Rehabil* 14:3, 1949.

34. Polinsky Medical Rehabilitation Center, 530 East Second Street, Duluth, MN 55805.

35. Psychological Corporation, P.O. Box 9954, San Antonio, TX 78204-0954. (800) 228-0752.

36. Research Designs, 7520 Hilcroft, Houston, TX 77081 (713) 995-8591.

37. Schultz KS: The Schultz structured interview for assessing upper extremity pain, *Occu Ther in Health Care* 1:69, 1984.

38. Science Research Associates, Inc., 259 East Erie Street, Chicago, Il 60611.

39. Smith PC, Bohmfalk JS: *Work related programs in occupational therapy*, New York, 1985, Haworth Press.

40. Smith PC, McFarlane B: *A work hardening model for the 80's: proceedings of the national forum on issues in vocational assessment*, Menomonie, Wisc, 1984, Materials Development Center.

41. Commission on Accreditation of Rehabilitation Facilities: *Standards manual for organizations serving people with disabilities*, Tucson, Ariz, 1989.

42. Commission on Accreditation of Rehabilitation Facilities: *Standards manual for organizations serving people with disabilities*, Tucson, Ariz, 1992.

43. Superintendent of Documents, United States Government Printing Office, Washington, D.C. 20402.

44. Upper Extremity Technology, 2001 Blake Avenue, 2-A, Glenwood Springs, CO 81601. (800) 736-1894.

45. VALPAR Corporation, 3801 East 34th Street, Suite 105, Tucson, AZ 85713.

46. Watkins AL: Prevocational evaluation and rehabilitation in a general hospital, *JAMA* 171:4, 1959.

47. Wegg L: Role of the occupational therapist in vocational rehabilitation, *Am J Occup Ther* 11:4, 1957.

48. Wegg L: Essentials of work evaluation, *Am J Occup Ther* 14:65, 1960.

49. Wood DJ: Design and evaluation of a back injury prevention program within a geriatric hospital, *Spine* 12:77, 1987.

50. Work Evaluations Systems Technology, P.O. Box 2477, Fort Bragg, CA, 95437. 707 964-7377.

51. Work Recovery, Inc. 2341 South Friebus Avenue, Suite 14, Tucson, AZ 85713. (800) 332-ERGO.

PART IV

Treatment Applications

Upper Extremity Amputations and Prosthetics

Lynda M. Rock, Diane J. Atkins

Section 1   Amputations and body-powered prostheses

Lynda M. Rock

Limb loss can result from disease, injury, or congenital causes. Individuals born with congenital limb deficiencies or whose amputations occur very early in life usually grow and develop sensorimotor skills and self-images without the limb. The individual who experiences an amputation in adolescence or adulthood is confronted with the task of adjusting to the loss of a well-integrated part of the body scheme and self-image. These two types of patient populations present different problems for the rehabilitation worker.[18] This chapter is limited to the discussion of the adult with an acquired upper extremity (UE) amputation.

An UE amputation is a traumatic event for both the individual and the family. A successful rehabilitation program requires the coordinated effort of a rehabilitation team, which may include the individual, physician, occupational therapist, physical therapist, prosthetist, psychologist, nurse, social worker, and vocational counselor.[18]

The occupational therapist's primary responsibility in the rehabilitation program is the formulation and execution of the preprosthetic program and prosthetic training. During the preprosthetic phase, the treatment plan includes preparing the limb for a prosthesis; during the prosthetic phase, treatment includes increasing prosthesis wearing tolerance and functional use. The rehabilita-

tion program includes an individualized treatment plan that assists the person in the physical and psychological adjustments. This program is designed so that he or she may learn to accept his or her new body image and also function as independently as possible.[3,18]

The rehabilitation of a individual with an UE amputation involves knowledge in areas such as wound care, strengthening, prosthetic components, and adaptive methods for the completion of independent living skills (ILS). Each person is unique and has his or her own strengths and weaknesses. Working with a person with an amputation can be challenging because there are many treatment areas and goals to accomplish. With a creative approach to therapy and team interaction, however, the experience can be rewarding and enjoyable. As is true when treating many kinds of disability, the more one works in a particular area the easier it becomes.

CAUSE AND INCIDENCE

The majority of amputations result from the following: trauma; peripheral vascular disease (PVD); peripheral vasospastic diseases; chronic infections; chemical, thermal, or electrical injuries; and malignant tumors. Elective amputations may occur as a result of a severe or complete brachial plexus injury.[6]

It is estimated that annually 40,000 Americans lose a limb. Approximately 30% of those lose a hand or arm. The incidence of amputation remains fairly constant between the ages of 1 and 15. From 15 to 54 years of age, however, there is a gradual increase in incidence because of work-related injuries and highway accidents. Approximately 75% of UE amputations in adults is caused by trauma.[11,12]

SURGICAL MANAGEMENT

The surgeon is an important team member. Before surgery, the surgeon should consult with the team to maximize the functional outcome. The surgeon attempts to preserve as much length as possible and provide a residual limb that has good skin coverage and vascularization. During and after surgery the primary goal is to form a residual limb that (1) maintains maximal function of the remaining tissue and (2) allows maximal use of the prosthesis.[3,11,18] Blood vessels and nerves are severed and allowed to retract so that residual limb pain is minimized during prosthetic use. Bone beveling is a surgical procedure that smoothes the rough edges and prevents spur development of the remaining bone. Muscles are sutured to the bones distally by a surgical process called myodesis. The muscles involved in the function of the amputated limb are correspondingly affected by the loss.[15]

A closed or open surgical procedure may be performed. The open method allows drainage and minimizes the possibility of infection. The closed method reduces the period of hospitalization but also reduces free drainage and increases the risk of infection. In either case the residual limb that results should be strong and resilient. It must be possible to fit the prosthesis to the residual limb snugly and comfortably, because the wearer will exert considerable pressure on the residual limb when using the prosthesis.[18]

PROSTHETIC CANDIDATES

Information regarding prostheses and the rehabilitation program should be provided before the amputation if possible because afterward pain medication and anxiety may interfere with the person's ability to process new information. Team discussion including the individual is vital in determining whether to generate a prosthetic prescription, and if so, which components to include, or alternatively, if a prosthesis is inappropriate. The person's age, medical status, amputation level, skin coverage, skin condition, cognitive status, and desire for a prosthesis are important factors in making the decision.[11]

PSYCHOLOGICAL ADJUSTMENT
REACTIONS TO AMPUTATION

Profound psychological shock is likely to accompany amputation, particularly for those who experience a sudden trauma that causes or necessitates amputation. Reac-

tions to amputation may be less severe in individuals who have had a chance to adjust before the surgery.[7,10,11]

The reaction to amputation is determined by the person's personality, age, cultural background, and his or her psychological, social, economic, and vocational resources. Ultimately, the individual must come to terms with the consequences of limb loss and perceived diminished attractiveness. The person confronts discomfort, inconvenience, economic expense, loss of function, increased energy expenditure, and possible curtailment of favorite activities. He or she may need to change occupations, deal with social discrimination, and cope with resultant medical problems.[7]

Cultural factors are important in the reaction to amputation. In some social, cultural, or religious groups, the amputation may be considered a means of punishment or atonement. Such beliefs and society's aversion to amputation can cause the person to adopt the same viewpoint. Such attitudes can result in self-hatred and self-deprecation, which may affect the person's reactions and adjustment to the disability.[7]

It is not uncommon for the person to feel a wide range of emotions in response to amputation. Older persons may demonstrate postoperative confusion, whereas younger persons may have a sense of mutilation, emasculation, or castration.[7,10]

When the person views the residual limb for the first time, he or she may experience substantial shock. Subsequent reactions may include fear of the future, panic, rage, and anger. Grief, self-pity, anxiety, despair, frustration, and suicidal impulses can also occur.[7]

Depression and a sense of futility are considered a normal part of the adjustment process unless these symptoms are severe and prolonged. The person's previous personality and the team's management of the rehabilitation affect the severity and duration of the reactions and ultimately the adjustment to the amputation and prosthetic use. Medication may also be necessary to reduce depression.[7]

FACILITATING ADJUSTMENT

The individual needs reassurance during the preoperative, postoperative, and rehabilitation phases of care.[10] In any phase the person may have hostile reactions directed towards self and the medical team. Often such hostility may be masked by overt solicitousness and friendliness. Caregivers should not react with hostility, but should make allowances for such behavior. Positive reinforcement through involvement in the rehabilitation process and contact with people having similar amputations aids in solving the problems of returning to former life roles.

Adjustment to the amputation directly affects the individual's adjustment to the prosthesis. Loss of a body part necessitates a revision and acceptance of the body image. Difficulties with the acceptance of the change in body image may cause difficulties in prosthetic training.[18] Because the prosthesis substitutes for the missing limb, it can assist with reintegration of the body image.[7] Fostering acceptance of the UE prosthesis is a primary way to promote the person's adjustment. Establishing a training program that presents the prosthesis in a manner that meets the person's needs and goals has a beneficial effect in integrating the prosthesis into the body scheme. The prosthesis must become part of the self before it can be used most effectively. The prosthesis contributes to a normal appearance helping the person identify with able-bodied individuals.[7,18]

The person may experience fear about returning to family, social, vocational, and sexual roles. Frequent discussions of fears and resolving real or imagined problems, if possible with a similar, successfully rehabilitated person, are important to facilitate adjustment.[7]

Following a mourning period the person may minimize the significance of the amputation and actually joke about it. When this phase of adjustment has subsided, the person begins seriously to consider the future. At this point the therapist can discuss with the individual social, vocational, and educational plans.[7]

LEVELS OF AMPUTATION AND FUNCTIONAL LOSSES IN THE UPPER EXTREMITY

The higher the level of amputation, the greater the functional loss of the arm, thus requiring a more complex prosthesis and more extensive training in its operation and use (Fig. 31-1).[18] Table 31-1 provides an outline of progressively higher UE amputations, associated loss of function, and appropriate components required for a functional body-powered prosthesis.[13,18]

COMPONENT PARTS OF THE UE BODY-POWERED PROSTHESIS

Various prosthetic components are available for each level of amputation (Fig. 31-2). Each prosthesis is prescribed according to the patient's needs and lifestyle and is custom-made and individually fitted. The prosthesis can be either functional or passive. It is important to remember, however, that passive does not mean nonfunctional because the prosthesis provides postural balance and can act as an assist to secure items for the functional limb.

The first five prosthetic components described below are common to all body-powered prostheses prescribed for wrist disarticulations and higher levels. They are the socket, harness, cable, terminal device (TD), and wrist unit. Many people with UE amputations wear a prosthetic sock between the residual limb and the prosthesis.[18]

Prosthetic sock

A prosthetic sock of knit wool, cotton, or Orlon-Lycra is worn between the prosthesis and the limb (Fig. 31-3). It absorbs perspiration and protects against irritation that could result from direct contact of the skin with the socket. It compensates for volume change in the residual limb and contributes to fit and comfort in the socket.[18,21]

Socket

The socket is the fundamental component to which the remaining components are attached. A cast molding of the residual limb is used to construct the socket to opti-

TABLE 31-1	Amputation Levels, Functional Losses, and Suggested Prosthetic Components	
LEVEL OF AMPUTATION	**LOSS OF FUNCTION**	**SUGGESTED FUNCTIONAL PROSTHETIC COMPONENTS**
Partial hand	Some or all grip functions	Dependent on cosmesis and functional loss
Wrist disarticulation	Hand and wrist function; about 50% of pronation and supination	Harness, control cable, socket, flexible elbow hinges and triceps pad, oval wrist unit, and TD
Long BE	Hand and wrist function; most pronation and supination	Same as for wrist disarticulation but circular wrist unit
Short BE	Hand and wrist function; all pronation and supination; impaired elbow flexion and extension	Harness, control cable, socket, rigid elbow hinges, and biceps half cuff, wrist unit, and TD
Elbow disarticulation	Hand and wrist function; all pronation and supination; elbow flexion and extension	Harness, dual-control cables, socket, externally locking elbow, forearm shell, wrist unit, and TD
Long AE	Hand and wrist function; all pronation and supination; elbow flexion and extension	Harness, dual-control cables, socket, internally locking elbow, lift assist, turntable, forearm shell, wrist unit, and TD
Short AE	All of the above; shoulder internal and external rotation	Same as for long AE, but socket may partially cover shoulder, restricting its function
Shoulder disarticulation	Loss of all arm and hand functions	Same as for long AE, but socket covers shoulder; chest strap; shoulder unit; upper arm shell; chin-operated nudge control for elbow unit
Forequarter	Loss of all arm and hand functions; partial or complete loss of clavicle and scapula	May be same as above but with lightweight materials. When minimal function is attainable, however, endoskeletal cosmetic prosthesis may be preferred
Bilateral amputation	Dependent on levels of amputation	Appropriate to level of amputation, plus wrist flexion unit and cable-operated wrist rotator

BE, Below elbow; *AE,* Above elbow; *SD,* Shoulder disarticulation.

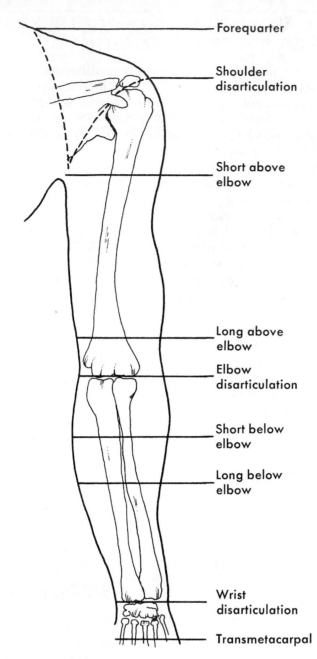

FIG. 31-1 Levels of UE amputation.

mize fit, comfort, and function. It fits snugly over the limb and extends as far as the wrist unit on a below-elbow (BE) prosthesis, or to the elbow unit on an above-elbow (AE) prosthesis. It should cover enough of the residual limb to be stable, but not so much that it unnecessarily restricts movement.

The limb's length determines whether the socket is of single- or double-wall construction. Most sockets have a double wall. The outer wall provides a structurally cosmetic surface. The inner wall maintains total contact on the residual limb's skin surface to distribute the socket pressure evenly. Uneven pressure distribution may lead to skin problems. When the residual limb's diameter and length is sufficient to provide the cosmetic surface, such

as the elbow disarticulation and long BE, the single-wall socket is used.[18,20]

Harness and control system

The prosthetic control system functions through the interaction of a Dacron harness and stainless steel cable. The figure-of-eight harness is commonly used, although others are available. The harness is worn across the back and shoulders or around the chest and fastens to the socket to secure the prosthesis. The higher the level of amputation the more complex the harnessing system. Loss of muscle power and ROM may necessitate variations in the harness design. A properly fitted harness is important for both comfort and function.[16,18,20]

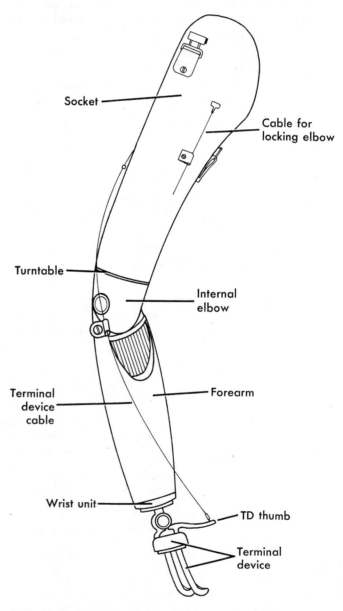

FIG. 31-2 Component parts of standard above-elbow (AE) prosthesis. (Adapted from Santschi W, editor: *Manual of upper extermity prosthetics,* ed 2, Los Angeles, 1958, University of California Press.)

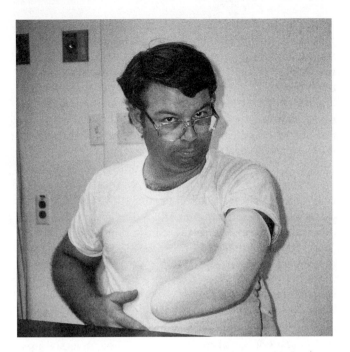

FIG. 31-3 Prosthetic sock worn under the prosthesis.

A flexible stainless steel cable, contained in a Teflon housing, attaches to the harness on one end via a T bar or hanger fitting and attaches to a functional component of the prosthesis on the other. A BE prosthesis uses one cable to operate the TD connected by a ball swivel. An AE prosthesis uses a second cable to lock and unlock the elbow unit. Specific upper body movements create tension on the cables, thereby operating the prosthesis. A properly fitted control system maximizes prosthetic control while minimizing body movements and exertion.[1,16,20]

Terminal device

The TD is the most distal component, which functions to grasp and hold an object. When choosing the most appropriate TD for a prosthesis, team members consider the person's age and life roles.

Two styles of TDs are commonly prescribed: the hook and the hand. Many TDs and prosthetic hands have the same shaft size at their base, which allows them to be interchangeable. They may be either a voluntary opening (VO) or voluntary closing (VC) design.[13]

The VO TD opens when the wearer exerts tension on the control cable which connects to the "thumb" of the TD. When tension is released, rubber bands or springs close the fingers of the TD. The holding force of the TD is determined by the number of rubber bands or springs.

VC TDs close by tension applied to the control cable. The tension may also lock the TD and maintain the grasp on the object. The VC TD automatically opens by spring operation when the cable is relaxed. The VO TD is prescribed more frequently because it is mechanically simpler and is available in a wider variety of sizes and styles than the VC TDs.[1,20]

VO TDs have several options to better suit the wearer's lifestyle. The options listed below depend on the desired durability, weight, or grip of the TD.

Stainless steel TDs are prescribed for activities requiring a durable TD such as yard work or construction. Aluminum TDs are recommended for lighter work and to reduce the total weight of the prosthesis for a person with a higher level amputation.

Most terminal devices have either a neoprene lining or a serrated grid between their fingers. The neoprene lining increases the holding friction and minimizes damage when holding objects. Neoprene is a high-density rubber, which wears out faster than the stainless steel grid and disintegrates if it comes in excessive contact with some chemical solutions. The TD must be sent back to the manufacturer for neoprene replacement.

A variation of the standard VO TD is the heavy-duty model (Fig. 31-4). This model is made of stainless steel

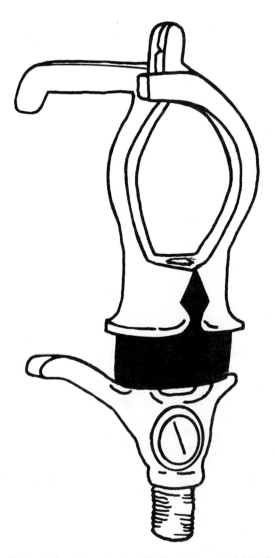

FIG. 31-4 Heavy-duty hook, TD Dorrance model 7, heavy-duty stainless steel.

and has a serrated grid between its fingers. The heavy duty model is designed to hold tools, nails, and long-handled instruments such as a broom or shovel.

A prosthetic hand is also available as a TD. It attaches to the wrist unit and is either passive or cable-operated. The passive hand has cosmetic and lightweight appeal, but is also functional because it is used to push, pull, and stabilize objects.

The functional prosthetic hand is activated by the same control cable that operates the hook. It comes in VO and VC styles. Like the hook style TD, the VO hand is preferred and prescribed more than the VC hand. A flesh-colored rubber glove fits over the prosthetic hand for protection and a cosmetic appearance.[18]

The person's life style and activities determine the most appropriate TDs. It is important to provide the wearer with the following information regarding the differences between hook- and hand-style TDs. The hook TD is lighter and provides better visibility when grasping objects. It is more durable and functional than prosthetic hands. The hook VO TDs are mechanically simpler than both the VC TDs and functional prosthetic hands. Prosthetic hands provide a more cosmetic appearance than the TDs. The cosmetic glove that covers the hand is easily stained, however, wears out quickly, and disintegrates if it comes in contact with certain cleaning solutions and chemicals.

Wrist unit[1,13,18,20,21]

The wrist unit connects the TD to the forearm socket and serves as the unit to interchange and to pronate and supinate the TD for prepositioning purposes. The rotation occurs either by the sound hand, by pushing the TD against an object or a surface, or by stabilizing the TD between the knees and using the arm to rotate it. In bilateral cases TD rotation in the wrist unit may be accomplished by cable operation. There are four basic types of wrist units selected according to their ability to meet the person's needs in daily living and vocational activities. They are the friction-held unit, the locking unit, the wrist flexion unit, and the oval unit.

The friction-held wrist units hold the TD in place by friction provided by a rubber washer or setscrews. Tightening them increases the friction. There is sufficient friction to hold the TD against moderate loads. The friction-held units are mechanically simple but not as strong as the locking unit.

The locking wrist unit allows the TD to be manually positioned and locked into place. The quick-disconnect locking wrist unit is one example. An adapter is permanently attached to the base of the TD. The unit has a button on its side that locks, unlocks, and ejects the TD. Inserting the TD into the wrist unit locks it into place. Another style TD with the same adapter type on its base may be locked into place. The friction and locking wrist units allow the TD to be rotated up and down, but not flexed in towards the body.

The wrist flexion unit allows the TD to be manually flexed and locked into position. It is generally used on the dominant side of a person with bilateral amputations for facilitating midline activities close to the body such as dressing and toileting.[1,13,18,20,21]

The oval unit, which conforms to the shape of the wrist, is used on the wrist disarticulation prosthesis. It is thinner than the other wrist units so the prosthesis may more closely match the length of the sound arm.

The socket, harness, control system, terminal device, and wrist unit are components common to all body-powered prostheses. The remaining body-powered prosthetic components maximize function at specific levels of amputation. They are the elbow hinges for BE prostheses, elbow units for AE prostheses, and shoulder units designed for shoulder prostheses.

Below elbow hinges

A BE prosthesis employs two hinges, one on each side of the elbow, which attach to the socket below the elbow and to a pad or cuff above the elbow. The hinges stabilize and align the BE prosthesis on the residual limb. When properly aligned, the hinges help distribute the stress of the prosthesis on the limb.

Two hinge styles, flexible and rigid, are available for a BE prosthesis. Flexible hinges are used on wrist amputation and long BE prostheses. They are usually made of Dacron and connect the socket to a triceps pad positioned over the triceps muscle. The flexibility permits some forearm rotation, thus decreasing the need to rotate the TD manually in the wrist.

Medium to short BE prostheses have a socket that covers most of the residual limb below the elbow and rigid hinges to provide stability. Rigid hinges are usually steel and attach to a laminated Dacron biceps half-cuff positioned behind the arm, which is sturdier and provides more support than the triceps pad. Team members consider the amount of residual function and the limb's length when choosing the appropriate style hinge for the BE prosthesis.[13]

Elbow units for AE prostheses

A prosthetic elbow unit is prescribed for the person who has had an amputation through the level of the elbow or higher. The elbow unit allows 5 to 135° of elbow flexion and locks in various positions. The two main types of elbow units are the internally and externally locking units. The more durable internally locking unit is prescribed for a person who has had an amputation two inches or more above the elbow. The unit connects the AE socket to the prosthetic forearm. The locking mechanism is contained within the unit and attaches to a control cable. A lift assist, which consists of a tightly coiled spring attached to the elbow unit and forearm shell, helps reduce the amount of energy required to lift the forearm shell. The lift assist also allows a slight bounce in the forearm when walking with the elbow

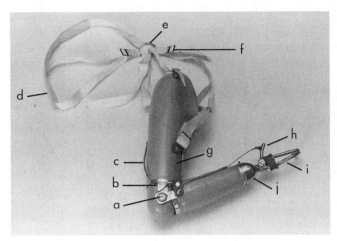
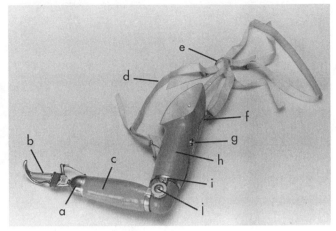

A   **B**

FIG. 31-5 **A,** Lateral side of AE prosthesis, *a,* Elbow unit; *b,* turntable; *c,* control cable; *d,* adjustable axilla loop; *e,* harness ring; *f,* figure-of-eight harness; *g,* elbow lock cable; *h,* TD thumb; *i,* hook TD; *j,* wrist flexion unit. **B,** Medial side of AE prosthesis. *a,* wrist unit; *b,* hook TD; *c,* forearm; *d,* harness; *e,* harness ring; *f,* control cable; *g,* baseplate and retainer; *h,* socket; *i,* turntable; *j,* spring-loading device.

unlocked, which increases the appearance of a natural arm swing.

A friction-held turntable positioned on top of the elbow unit allows the prosthetic forearm to be rotated manually toward or away from the body. Fig. 31-5 shows the lateral and medial aspect of an AE prosthesis. The internally locking unit is about two inches in length and therefore does not fit on a person who has had an amputation close to the elbow.

Correspondingly the externally locking elbow unit is prescribed for a person who has an elbow disarticulation or an amputation within 2 inches above the elbow. It consists of a pair of hinges positioned on either side of the prosthesis and attaches the socket to the forearm. The cable attaches to one of the hinges, which locks and unlocks the unit.

Shoulder units

A person with an amputation at the shoulder requires a prosthesis with a shoulder unit in addition to the TD, wrist unit, forearm shell, elbow unit, socket, harness, and cables. Because of the high level of amputation, however, shoulder and back movements are not sufficient to use a cable-operated shoulder unit. Thus, most shoulder units are manually operated and friction held. The TD and elbow units may still be cable-operated.

Two shoulder unit styles that are often prescribed are the flexion-abduction unit and the locking shoulder joint. The flexion-abduction (or double-axis) unit provides manual prosthetic positioning in flexion and abduction and is friction-held. The locking unit allows the prosthesis to be locked in various degrees of shoulder flexion. This feature is helpful because the prosthesis is heavy, and the friction style may not be strong enough.

Shoulder forequarter considerations

In a forequarter amputation all or a portion of the scapula and clavicle are removed with the arm. If standard prosthetic components were used, the prosthesis might be too heavy for practical use. Therefore, an endoskeletal prosthesis made from lightweight materials such as aluminum and dense foam is often prescribed to decrease its weight. The system provides its own style of prosthetic joints, which will not withstand heavy-duty usage. Many of the TDs discussed earlier may be used on the endoskeletal system.

THE UE PREPROSTHETIC PROGRAM

The preprosthetic program begins when the decision to perform an amputation is made or when a person is evaluated following a traumatic amputation.[11] Education regarding prostheses, relaxation techniques, and general strengthening may in some cases begin before the surgical amputation. During the period between the amputation and the fitting of the prosthesis the individual participates in a program designed to (1) prepare the residual limb for a prosthesis, (2) facilitate adjustment to the loss, and (3) achieve maximal independence in self-care.[14,20] It is important for the team to assist the person in securing the financial resources necessary to complete rehabilitation and obtain a prosthesis if desired.

PREPROSTHETIC EVALUATIONS

To establish an individualized treatment plan, a thorough evaluation must be completed. The evaluation includes the following:

- past medical history
- family, work, and avocational history

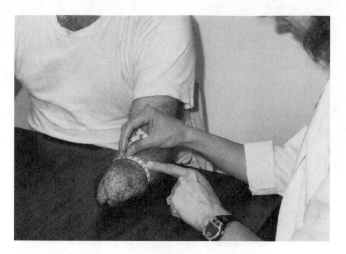

FIG. 31-6 Measuring residual limb circumference.

- passive and active ROM measurements
- manual muscle testing
- sensory testing
- condition of the opposite arm
- residual limb length and circumference measurements
- documentation of residual limb and upper body skin condition
- independent living skills (ILS) status

A statement of the person's goals is important to orient the treatment towards meeting them and to determine the person's understanding of the program and the prosthesis.[3]

A tape measure is used to record residual limb length and circumference. Care must be taken to measure the limb's circumference at the same place each time. A drawing of the residual limb with the different levels that were measured marked off in inches or centimeters will help the therapist chart progress (Fig. 31-6).

PREPROSTHETIC TREATMENT

The treatment plan is based on evaluation results. Most plans include the following:
- wound care
- desensitization techniques
- wrapping the residual limb to shrink and shape it and document circumference changes
- education regarding proper skin hygiene
- education regarding care of insensate skin
- maintaining passive and active ROM
- increasing upper body strength and endurance
- improving ILS status
- education regarding prosthetic components and prosthetic prescription

Depending on the level of amputation, medical condition, and ILS status the decision is made whether to complete the preprosthetic program on an inpatient or outpatient basis. In most cases in which the person has had a unilateral amputation, therapy may be completed on an outpatient basis. A person with bilateral amputations may need to be admitted to the facility because of the amount of therapy and assistance he or she will require. The team closely monitors the residual limb and reports problems to the physician. If the person is followed on an outpatient basis, frequent clinic visits are required to monitor progress.

Wound Healing

When the surgical dressing is removed the residual limb is massaged to discourage scar adhesions, increase circulation, aid in desensitization, and reduce swelling. It also helps the person overcome fear of handling the residual limb. Massage over the incision site begins after the incision has healed.[3] Initially, deep massage over healed areas is performed, followed by lighter pressures as tolerated by the person.

Desensitization

The residual limb may be hypersensitive after surgery and require a technique known as desensitization. Massage is one method of desensitization. Other methods include tapping, vibration, constant pressure, and the application of various textures to the limb, such as terry cloth and cotton. When the therapist performs the techniques, he or she teaches them to the person and family members or caregivers to perform on a home program basis.[3,9]

Wrapping

Shrinking and shaping the residual limb is necessary to form a tapered limb that will tolerate a prosthesis. Compression aids in the shrinking and shaping process, using either an elastic Ace bandage, tubular bandage, or a shrinker sock applied to the residual limb. A figure-of-eight method (Fig. 31-7) is used when an elastic bandage is applied to the limb, not a circumferential method in which the bandage is wrapped around the limb spirally. Care must be taken to apply the bandage smoothly, evenly, and not too tightly from the distal to the proximal end of the residual limb. A limb that is wrapped incorrectly may not be able to be fitted with a prosthesis or may take longer to shrink and shape. A BE limb should be wrapped up to or above the elbow. An AE limb should be wrapped up to or above the shoulder. Short AE amputations usually require wrapping around the chest to help stabilize the wrap.[18,20] The elastic bandage should be changed several times a day and the skin checked between wrappings. Several bandages are required to allow the limb to be wrapped in a clean bandage at all times except when bathing. The wraps should be washed often with a mild soap, rinsed well, and allowed to dry thoroughly lying flat. To prolong the bandages' life, they should not be wrung out after washing.[3]

Circumference Measurements

The residual limb's circumference measurements are taken often and in the same area to determine when the person is ready to be casted for a prosthesis. The thera-

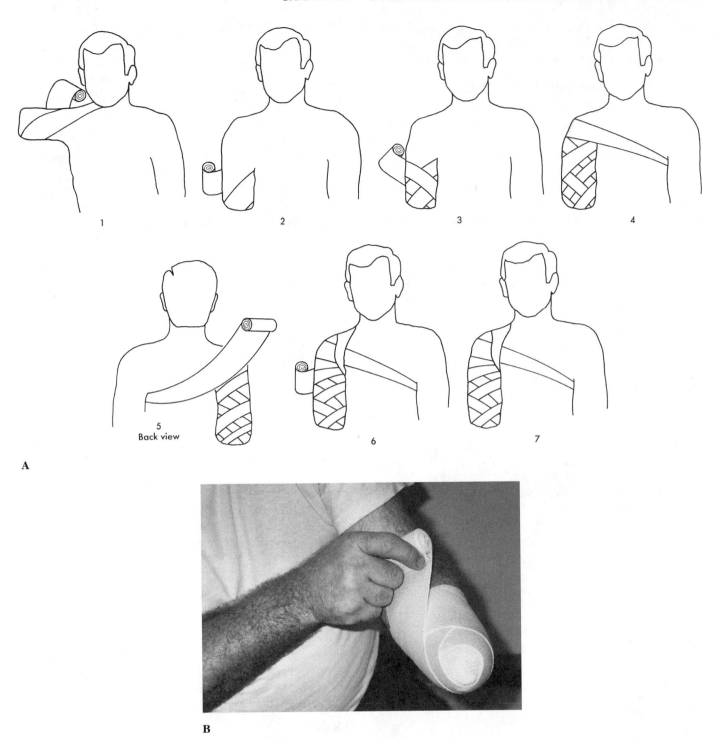

FIG. 31-7   Residual limb bandaging. **A,** Step-by-step procedure. **B,** Bandaging in progress.

pist uses a tape measure to establish baseline and subsequent measurements (Fig. 31-6). When the edema is gone and the circumference measurements have stabilized, the limb is ready to be casted.

Skin Hygiene

Instruction in proper residual limb hygiene is also an important aspect in the preprosthetic program. The limb should be washed daily using a mild soap, rinsed thor-

oughly, and gently patted dry. The limb should dry completely before reapplying the wrap.[2]

Insensate Skin

The person with an UE amputation requires instruction regarding the care and safety of a residual limb that lacks all or partial sensation. The person should learn to inspect the limb when removing the wrap and washing the limb. Problems should be reported to the therapist or physician. The person should also learn to track a sensory impaired limb when completing activities and not to use it for sensory input, such as testing water temperature.

UE ROM, Strength, and Endurance

Following medical approval the person begins exercises designed to encourage residual limb usage, maintain ROM, and strengthen upper body muscles. Depending on the level of amputation the therapist instructs the person to complete specific exercises that mimic and strengthen the movements required to operate the prosthesis. The therapist manually positions and holds the residual limb and asks the person to resist the hold. In the case of a BE amputation, it is important to strengthen the muscles of the shoulder, elbow, and scapula. Pronation and supination movements are also important for long BE amputations. AE amputation strengthening includes a movement combining shoulder depression, extension, and abduction. Chest expansion is important for higher level amputations and when the harness wraps around the chest. A tape measure positioned around the chest helps to document increased chest expansion. A home program should be provided containing exercises for general strengthening as well as the specific movements taught during therapy (Fig. 31-8).

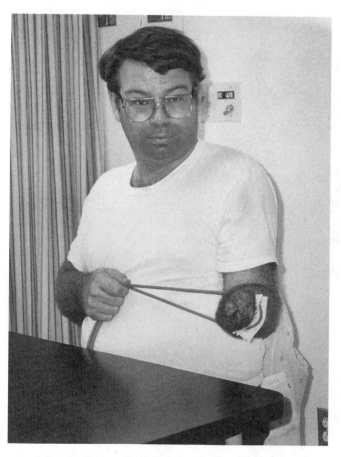

FIG. 31-8 Home program of UE strengthening to prepare arm for prosthesis. Thera-tubing being used for resistive exercise.

Independent Living Skills Status

During the preprosthetic period the person with a unilateral amputation should be encouraged to use the sound arm to perform ILS. If the dominant arm was amputated, special training may be required for the nondominant limb to assume the dominant role. Practice in writing and activities requiring dexterity and coordination may be helpful in the retraining process.[14,18,20] Most individuals change dominance to the sound extremity automatically.

In the case of a bilateral amputation, adaptive equipment should be introduced as soon as possible to increase the person's level of independence. The equipment may include a utensil cuff secured by elastic or Velcro to the residual limb to aid in eating, writing, and hygiene; a dressing tree to improve dressing skills; and loops added to items such as socks and towels. The person with a bilateral amputation can also learn to complete activities using foot skills.

PROSTHETIC INFORMATION AND PRESCRIPTION

During the preprosthetic period the person should receive information about the prosthesis, its benefits, and limitations. The therapist needs to be aware of what the amputation and the prosthesis may mean to the person. In selecting prosthetic components and presenting the prosthesis, it is important to consider whether the person's primary need is function or cosmesis.

There are several ways to introduce prosthetic componets to the person. They include an introduction to a person with a similar amputation, slides, video, showing a prosthesis, and scheduling a trip to the prosthetist.

SPECIAL CONSIDERATIONS AND PROBLEMS

Several factors and potential problems can affect the outcome of the person's rehabilitation. They include the following: residual limb length, skin coverage, rate of healing, range of motion, hypersensitivity, pain, infection, and allergic reactions to the prosthesis.

SKIN

Residual limb skin complications account for most postsurgical problems. These complications occur in either the preprosthetic or postprosthetic phase. Delayed healing and extensive skin grafting are complications in the preprosthetic phase. Skin breakdown, ulcers, infected sebaceous cysts, and allergic reactions to the prosthesis relate to the postprosthetic phase. Residual limb edema can occur in either phase.

Preprosthetic Phase

Delayed healing of the incision site is one of the earliest preprosthetic complications resulting in postponed prosthetic fitting. Necrotic areas may develop requiring surgical intervention.[4]

To achieve a residual limb length suitable for prosthetic use, the surgeon may perform extensive skin grafting. If the skin graft adheres to bone, the area may ulcerate and require medical attention.[4] Daily massage by the person and/or therapist decreases the likelihood of skin grafts adhering to bone and the attendant complications.

Immediately following surgery the residual limb is normally edematous as a result of fluid that collects within the soft tissues, especially in its distal portion. Compression wrapping or a rigid dressing helps decrease the edema.[5,8,11]

Postprosthetic Phase

During the postprosthetic phase, skin breakdown may be caused by an ill-fitting socket, wrinkles in the prosthetic sock, or scar adhesions.[9] Residual limb ulceration is associated with ischemia and pressure exerted by the prosthesis on the limb. The patient should be seen by the physician and the prosthesis not worn until the area heals. The prosthetist should also examine the prosthesis to determine if the socket requires adjustment. If these problems persist, surgical revision of the limb may be needed before rehabilitation can continue.[15]

The residual limb is predisposed to the development of sebaceous cysts caused by the torque forces between the socket and the residual limb. Treatment includes the application of moist heat. When the cyst becomes infected, drainage ensues and enucleation of the cyst wall may be required.

The development of residual limb edema during the postprosthetic phase is usually indicative of an ill-fitting socket. Proximal tightness of the socket may result in distal edema, which may require a new, well-fitted socket.[4]

SENSORY PROBLEMS

The loss of sensory feedback from the amputated limb is a major problem that confronts the person. Residual limb hyperesthesia, neuromas, and phantom sensation or pain are problems that may interfere with the functional use of the arm either with or without the prosthesis.

Residual limb hyperesthesia, or an overly sensitive limb, limits functional use and causes discomfort. Desensitization consists of tapping and massage, which helps decrease the discomfort.[3,9] Sympathetic nerve blocks may be used to manage residual limb hypersensitivity medically.[17]

A neuroma is a small ball of nerve tissue that develops when growing axons attempt to reach the distal end of the residual limb. All cut nerves form neuromas. As the axons grow they turn back on themselves, thus producing a ball of nerve tissue. If the neuroma adheres to scar tissue or skin subject to repetitive pressure it can be painful when pressed. Diagnosis is made by palpating the

neuroma.[5] Most neuromas occur 1 to 2 inches (2.5 cm to 5.0 cm) proximal to the residual limb end and are not troublesome.[4] Treatment includes local anesthetic injections or ultrasound. Both treatments should be followed by massage and stretching. Surgical intervention may be necessary. In addition, the residual limb socket may be fabricated or modified to accommodate the neuroma.[3,19,20]

After an amputation people commonly experience phantom sensations. It is the sensation of the presence of the amputated limb or a portion of it. Phantom sensations may occur for life or may eventually disappear. They do not usually interfere with prosthetic use. Desensitization, supportive counseling, and early use of the residual limb with a temporary or permanent prosthesis are effective measures for dealing with phantom sensations.[18] In many cases it is best not to dwell on discussion of phantom sensation but rather to focus on prosthetic training and the return to a former lifestyle.

A phenomenon that can prohibit good use of the prosthesis is phantom pain. In this condition the amputated limb is not only perceived as present but is also cramping, burning, or aching.[19,20] There is no strict treatment protocol for phantom pain. Isometric exercises begun five to seven days following the amputation and performed several times throughout the day may help control phantom pain. Biofeedback, transcutaneous electrical nerve stimulation (TENS), ultrasound, progressive relaxation exercises, and controlled breathing exercises may assist in reducing phantom pain. Activities such as rubbing, tapping, and/or applying pressure and heat may be beneficial. The physician may treat the pain either by prescribing amitriptyline (Elavil) at bedtime, by injecting anesthetics into the tender area, or performing sympathetic nerve blocks. Surgical revision of the residual limb is sometimes necessary to alleviate the pain.[3,19] The appearance of phantom pain or overdue concern with phantom sensation requires the intervention of the team. The therapist can allay the patient's fears about these phenomena by offering support, information, and reassurance.

The residual limb may have absent or impaired areas of sensation that require special attention and education when wearing the prosthesis. The person must rely on visual and proprioceptive feedback because sensation is functionally lost when the prosthesis is on the residual limb. The person must adjust to new sensations such as the pressure of the residual limb inside the socket and the feel of the harness system.[18]

BONE PROBLEMS

The formation of bone spurs is another complication that may occur during the preprosthetic phase. Because most bone spurs are not palpable, an x-ray film is needed to confirm their presence or absence. Bone spurs that cause pain or result in persistent drainage require surgical excision.

THE PROSTHETIC PROGRAM

The amount of training each person needs depends on how fast he or she is able to understand the body mechanics required to operate the prosthesis, the person's problem-solving skills, motivation, the carry-over between activities and the cuing needed to include the prosthesis in an activity. When a long period has elapsed between the amputation and receiving the prosthesis, the person may require more cuing because he or she has become adept at one-handed activities. Some individuals will arrive at therapy already able to operate the prosthesis whereas others will require extensive hands-on training.

It is recommended that the prosthetist and therapist coordinate the final fitting of the prosthesis and the initial training session. The therapist may arrange to be present for the final fitting. Communication between the wearer, therapist, and prosthetist is essential to ensure that the prosthesis fits and functions optimally. The therapist should be aware of a possible need for prosthesis adjustment and consult with the prosthetist if this need becomes evident.

The prosthesis will not be as functional as a normal arm, and training should stress that the prosthesis is more like an assist or helper than an arm. If presented in this manner, the wearer may have an easier time accepting the prosthesis.

COMMON CONSIDERATIONS IN TRAINING

The prosthetic training program begins after the final fitting of the prosthesis. Although a treatment plan includes the person's prosthetic goals, some information and initial training points are common to all prosthetic training programs. The common points include the following:

- residual limb and prosthetic sock hygiene
- prosthetic terminology and function
- care of the prosthesis
- prosthetic wearing schedule
- prosthetic checkout
- controls training
- functional training
- driving
- home program
- follow-up appointments

The prosthetic checkout, controls training, and functional training are individualized according to the level of amputation.

Residual Limb and Prosthetic Sock Hygiene

The person is instructed in residual limb hygiene and care of the prosthetic sock in the early phase of prosthetic training. The residual limb and armpit should be inspected, washed, and patted dry, and deodorant applied daily. If the person chooses to wear a prosthetic sock, it is recommended that he or she own several. This

way a clean one may be worn daily to decrease chances of skin problems. The socks should be washed, gently squeezed, and placed on a flat surface to dry in their original dimensions. An undergarment is often recommended to wear under the harness because it will absorb perspiration and protect the axillae and back from irritation. Prosthetic socks and undergarments may need to be changed twice a day in hot weather.[20,21]

Prosthetic Terminology and Function

The wearer should learn the terminology and function of each prosthetic component. This task is important so that the person can communicate with the rehabilitation team, using terminology understood by all, regarding difficulties with or repairs needed to the prosthesis.[2,20,21]

Care of the Prosthesis

Instructions regarding care of the prosthesis are provided and reviewed. The socket should be cleaned daily using a soft cloth and mild soap and rinsed thoroughly with warm water. Cleaning is recommended at night to allow the prosthesis to dry completely. Wearing the prosthesis when the socket is wet may lead to skin problems. Components should be cleaned and maintained according to the manufacturer's or prosthetist's specifications. Daily inspection of the prosthesis will help prevent unnecessary problems.[2]

Prosthetic Wearing Schedule

A prosthetic wearing schedule is provided and reviewed during the first training session. Initially the person wears the prosthesis 15 to 30 minutes three times a day. The skin must be closely monitored and wearing time advanced only if the skin remains in good condition. If there are no skin problems, the three scheduled wearing periods may be increased by 30 minutes each day. By the end of the first week the person should be wearing the prosthesis all day. If skin problems occur the therapist, prosthetist, or physician must be notified. The prosthesis should not be worn until the skin problem has cleared. It may be necessary to restart the initial wearing schedule to decrease the chance of more skin problems.[2]

As the person's wearing tolerance increases, the number of rubber bands on the TD can be increased. Each rubber band added to the TD increases the pinch force by approximately one pound. It is best to wait several days after adding one rubber band before adding another to allow the residual limb's skin and strength to acclimate. If adding a rubber band substantially increases limb pain or skin irritation, it should be removed until the pain diminishes and skin tolerance increases.

CHECKOUT OF THE PROSTHESIS

When the prosthesis is received, it is checked by team members to ensure that it meets prescription requirements, is functioning efficiently, and is mechanically sound. The prosthesis is checked for fit and function against specific mechanical standards developed from actual tests on prostheses worn by individuals. These are the following: comparative range of motion with the prosthesis on and off; control system function and efficiency; TD opening in various positions; amount of socket slippage on the residual limb under various degrees of load or tension; compression fit and comfort; and force required to flex the forearm.[1,16,20] Communication between the wearer, therapist, and prosthetist is essential to ensure an efficiently operating and comfortable prosthesis. The following methods and standards for the prosthesis checkout were adapted primarily from Wellerson.[20] Step-by-step instructions for the prosthetic checkout are available in Wellerson and Santschi.[16,20]

Checkout of BE Prosthesis

The therapist measures elbow flexion with the prosthesis on and off the wearer. The ROM should not differ by more than 10° except if there are joint or muscle limitations. Pronation and supination of a wrist disarticulation or long BE residual limb with the prosthesis on should not be less than 50% of the rotation possible without the prosthesis.

With elbow flexed at 90°, the person should be able to open the TD fully. The TD is also opened near the mouth (elbow fully flexed) and again near the fly of the trousers (elbow extended). From 70% to 100% of TD opening should be achieved in these two positions.

Checkout of AE and Shoulder Prosthesis

With the AE prosthesis on and the elbow locked the person is instructed to move the residual limb (humerus) into shoulder flexion, extension, abduction, and internal and external rotation. The ROM of each of these is measured. Minimal standards for shoulder ROM with the prosthesis on are as follows: 90° flexion, 30° extension, 90° abduction, and 45° rotations. The previous part of the checkout is not applicable for the shoulder prosthesis.

With the elbow unlocked, the person is instructed to flex the shoulder slowly, which flexes the mechanical elbow. The elbow ROM should be about 10°-135°. The therapist measures the amount of shoulder flexion, which should not exceed 45°, required to fully flex the mechanical elbow. The person should also be able to abduct the prosthesis to 60° without the elbow locking.

The person flexes the forearm to 90°, locks the elbow, and then activates the TD. Full TD opening should be attained in this position. The TD is then opened in full elbow flexion with elbow locked (TD at mouth, Fig. 31-9) and extension with elbow locked (TD at fly of trousers). At least 50% of full TD opening should be obtained.

With the elbow unlocked the person is asked to walk and practice swinging the prosthesis without locking the elbow. This action mimics a normal arm swing during gait.

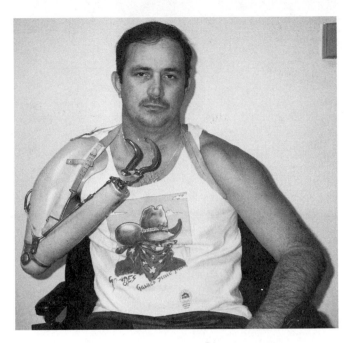

FIG. 31-9   AE prosthesis checkout: opening TD at mouth with elbow locked in full flexion.

The person flexes the elbow to 90° and locks the elbow, and then is instructed to abduct the residual limb to 60°, and then rotate the humerus. The person should be able to control the prosthesis during this motion. The socket should neither slip around the residual limb nor should the person experience pain or discomfort during these maneuvers. When the prosthesis is removed, the residual limb should not appear discolored or irritated.

The prosthesis checkout also includes a technical inspection of the prosthesis to determine correct length, fit, and mechanical function of all parts. Various forms have been devised to record all information for the complete checkout of the prosthesis. The initial checkout is done before prosthetic training begins, and the final checkout is done following prosthetic revisions and adjustments and either during or following training.[2,16]

CONTROLS TRAINING

Controls training is best accomplished in front of a mirror to help the person learn the minimal motions necessary to operate the prosthesis while maintaining proper body mechanics (Fig. 31-10). Joint protection, energy conservation, and work simplification techniques should also be stressed. The therapist may need to provide physical cues such as laying a hand on the shoulder to relax it or guiding the prosthesis and shoulder "down, out, and away" to operate the elbow mechanism.

Each prosthetic component should be reviewed separately and understood before combining them into purposeful activities. Some movements such as elbow flexion and TD opening are cable-operated. Other movements such as TD or elbow rotations are passively positioned using the sound hand or an item in the environ-

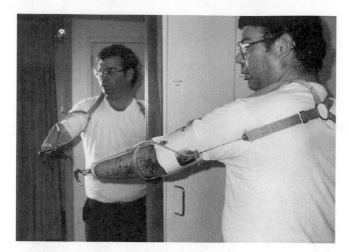

FIG. 31-10 Controls training in front of mirror.

ment such as a table. Emphasizing external assists from the environment is an important part of the training process.

Donning and Doffing the Prosthesis

There are two common methods of donning and doffing the prosthesis. They are the coat method and the sweater method. Either method can be used with unilateral or bilateral amputations. The decision depends on which method is easier for the wearer. Whichever the method, the harness and cables must not be kinked or twisted around the prosthesis before starting. When the prosthesis is removed, it should be placed on a surface ready for the person to don again.

The coat method

There are two variants of the coat method. These are equivalent to placing one arm in the coat sleeve and manipulating the coat to a position where the other arm can reach the sleeve. In the first method the person places the prosthesis on a table or bed and pushes the residual limb between the control cable and the Y strap from the medial side into the socket. By raising the residual limb or leaning sideways, the harness is placed across the shoulder on the amputated side and dangles down the back. The sound hand reaches around the back and slips into the axilla loop. The person then slips into the harness as if putting on a coat. The shoulders are shrugged to shift the harness forward and into the correct position.

The second method works by placing the axilla loop of the harness on the sound arm first. For example, if the person has an AE amputation it may be easier to lock the elbow at 90°, position the axilla loop on the sound arm above the elbow, grasp the prosthetic forearm, and raise the prosthesis over the head allowing the harness to position itself across the back. Then by raising the residual limb the person positions it in the socket (Fig. 31-11).

To remove the prosthesis, the person uses the TD to slip the axilla loop off the sound side and then slips the

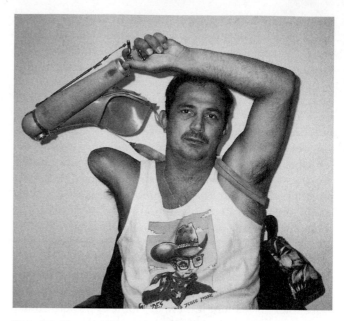

FIG. 31-11 Coat method of donning prosthesis.

shoulder strap off the amputated side. The harness is then slipped off like a coat.[1,16,20]

The person with bilateral amputations can use the coat method by placing the prostheses face up on a surface, placing the longer residual limb into the socket, and elevating the prosthesis allowing the other prosthesis to hang across the back. The person then leans to the side and places the shorter limb in the prosthesis.[16,21]

To remove the prostheses, the person shrugs the harness off the shoulders and removes the prosthesis from the shorter side first. Before removing the prosthesis on the longer side, the person should position the prostheses somewhere convenient for the next donning.

The sweater method

The sweater method (Fig. 31-12) is equivalent to entering both sleeves at the same time and then raising both arms up and out to don the sweater. To apply a unilateral prosthesis using the sweater method the person places the prosthesis on a surface face up, positions the residual limb in the socket under the Y strap, and places the opposite arm in the harness. The person then raises both arms above the head allowing the axilla loop to slide down to the axilla and the harness to be properly positioned across the back and on the shoulders. To remove the prosthesis, the person raises both arms above the head and grasps and removes the prosthesis with the sound arm while allowing the axilla loop to slide off the arm.[16]

A person with a bilateral amputation dons the prostheses using the sweater method by placing them on a surface face up. Then, with the longer limb stabilizing the socket, the shorter residual limb is positioned under the harness and in the socket. The longer limb is then positioned similarly under the harness in the socket, and

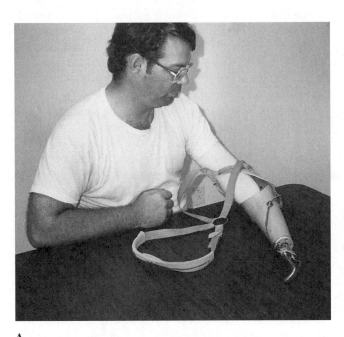

A

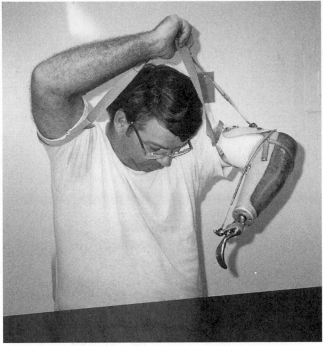

B

FIG. 31-12   Sweater method of donning prosthesis.

the arms are raised allowing the harness to flip over the head and across the back and shoulders. The prostheses are removed by shrugging the shoulders to bring the harness up, grasping it with the TD, and pulling it over the head while allowing the residual limbs to come out of their sockets.

Controls Training for the Unilateral BE Prosthesis

TD control. Scapula abduction and glenohumeral flexion are the motions necessary to open and close the TD. The person is instructed to operate the TD first by flexing the humerus on the amputated side, then by scapula abduction while the humerus remains at the body's side. The therapist instructs the person to operate the TD with the arm in various positions in space such as overhead and leaning over towards the floor.[21]

Pronation/supination. If the residual limb was long enough for flexible hinges to be prescribed on the prosthesis, pronation and supination should be practiced. The therapist asks the person to stabilize the elbow at 90° and to pronate and supinate the forearm. If rigid hinges were prescribed, the TD is manually rotated in the wrist unit to achieve pronation and supination. Manual TD rotation is accomplished by using the opposite hand or stabilizing the TD between the knees and turning the forearm or shoulder.

Exchanging TDs. The person learns to exchange the TD in the wrist unit, if more than one TD is prescribed. Cable slack is needed to release the cable from the TD.

To obtain enough slack in the cable it may be necessary to place an item between the fingers of the hook or hand. The TD is then removed according to the wrist unit prescribed. When the TD has been removed, another TD style may then be positioned in the wrist unit and the cable attached to it.

To complete BE controls training, the therapist instructs the person to repeat the motions required to position and operate the TD until they are performed in one continuous smooth and natural sequence in both sitting and standing positions.[20] Once controls training is completed, functional training may begin to improve the person's bilateral and ILS activities.

Controls Training for the Unilateral AE Prosthesis

Most AE prostheses operate through the use of a dual-control cable system. That is, when tension is applied on the cable attached to the elbow unit it locks and unlocks. When the elbow unit is unlocked, tension on the second cable attached to the TD raises the prosthetic forearm. A spring assist helps reduce the amount of effort required to raise the forearm, and gravity assists in lowering it. When the elbow unit is locked, tension on the second cable can also be used to operate the TD. The person learns to operate each component separately.

Internal/external rotation. Many internally locking elbow units have a manually operated turntable located between the elbow unit and the socket that allows forearm internal and external rotation. The person operates the turntable, first with the elbow at 90°, by manually rotating the forearm medially (toward the body) or laterally (away from the body).

Elbow flexion/extension. Flexion and extension of the mechanical elbow is the next step in the training process. The therapist should protect the person's face when teaching elbow flexion control. This precaution is important because initially the person may have poor control over elbow flexion, which could result in the TD hitting the face.[1]

The therapist makes sure that the elbow unit is unlocked and asks the person to flex the humerus slowly and abduct the scapula to accomplish elbow flexion and slowly extend the shoulder to achieve elbow extension. This movement is repeated until the person gains sufficient control to accomplish elbow flexion and extension smoothly and easily.[1,21]

Elbow locking. The elbow unit operation has an audible two-click cycle. Both clicks must be heard each time the unit is locked or unlocked. The same body movement both locks and unlocks the unit. The person is instructed to operate the elbow unit by moving the shoulder into a combination of hyperextension, abduction, and scapula depression. This movement places tension on the cable that attaches the harness to the elbow unit and may be difficult to master. The reminder of "down, out, and away" may be repeated until the person develops a proprioceptive memory. The person is then asked to practice locking and unlocking the elbow in various ranges of elbow flexion and extension (Fig. 31-13).[1,2,21]

TD control. The same motions of shoulder flexion and scapula abduction that flex the forearm with the elbow unlocked also control the TD when the elbow is locked.

The person is instructed to lock the elbow, first at 90°, and perform the motions to operate the TD. Care must be taken not to unlock the elbow by placing tension on the cable that operates the elbow unit. The sequence of elbow positioning, elbow locking, TD operation, elbow unlocking, elbow repositioning, and locking is repeated at various points in the elbow range of motion from full extension to full flexion.[1,21]

The person then learns how to rotate the TD manually in the wrist unit and to exchange TDs in the same manner as described previously for the BE prostheiss. Once the AE prosthesis controls are performed in a smooth manner, functional training begins.

Controls Training for the Shoulder Disarticulation Prosthesis

A prosthesis prescribed for the person with a shoulder disarticulation may have different components and methods of operation than the AE prosthesis. The prosthesis may have a manually operated, friction-held shoulder unit that the person prepositions using the sound arm or a table's edge. A chin-operated nudge control may be used to operate the elbow unit because the person does not have the shoulder movements needed to lock and unlock the elbow (Fig. 31-14). A cable connects the nudge control to the elbow unit. The person still learns the two-click cycle and dual-cable system of operation described previously for the AE prosthesis. The elbow turntable is also available for a shoulder prosthesis.

A chest harness may be needed to secure the prosthesis on the person. It can also assist TD operation by using chest expansion to increase tension on the TD cable. Shoulder flexion and scapula abduction on the opposite side also assist in TD operation. Wrist operation is the same as explained for the BE prosthesis.

Controls Training for Bilateral Prostheses

A person with bilateral amputations usually receives two prostheses that are attached to one harness (Fig. 31-15).

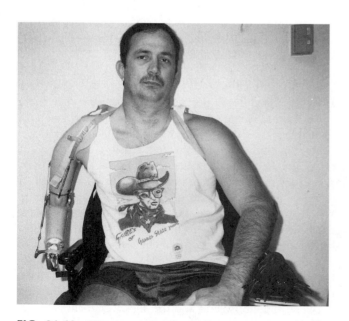

FIG. 31-13   "Down, out, and away" movement used to unlock the elbow unit.

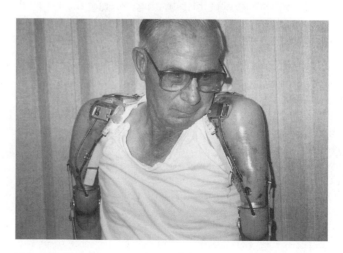

FIG. 31-14   Nudge control used to operate the elbow unit for shoulder disarticulation prosthesis.

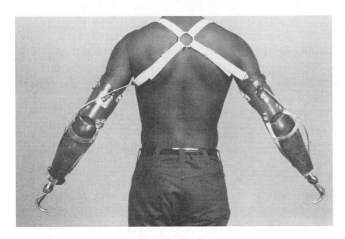

FIG. 31-15   Single harness for bilateral prostheses.

Operating one of the prostheses may transmit tension through the harness to the other prosthesis, causing it to operate as well. The person must learn to operate each prosthetic component without affecting the components on either side. This skill is called separation of controls and may require extensive practice to master. Each prosthesis operates according to the level of amputation as described in the previous sections with special attention given to relaxing the opposite side (Fig. 31-16).

Two components not generally used on unilateral prostheses may be prescribed on bilateral ones to improve the person's independence. These are the wrist flexion unit and a cable-operated wrist rotation unit. The wrist flexion unit assists completion of midline activities and is prescribed either for both prostheses or for the dominant side. The ability to achieve midline is important to complete many activities such as dressing, grooming, and eating. The flexion unit is operated by depressing the unit's control button and creating tension on the TD cable. The button can be depressed by the opposite TD, a surface edge, the knee, or other surface. The TD cable must be medial to the flexion axis of the unit to pull the TD into flexion. A spring in the flexion unit repositions the TD in extension when the button is depressed and slack is provided in the TD cable.

There are several ways to achieve wrist rotation. One is by using the wrist units mentioned earlier and rotating the TD by placing it between the knees or by pulling on the thumb of one hook with the other. Another method to achieve wrist rotation is by a button on the medial side of the forearm, which controls a cable attached inside the forearm to a wrist-locking device. The wrist is locked and unlocked by pressing the button against the side of the body. When unlocked, tension on the TD cable rotates the TD to the desired position.

After the person understands how the components operate, he or she gains control of the prostheses by practicing passing items such as a ruler or a piece of paper back and forth between the TDs without dropping them. Another activity that assists the person to learn separation of controls involves holding an object in one prosthesis without dropping it while completing an activity with the other prosthesis (Fig. 31-16).

FUNCTIONAL TRAINING WITH PROSTHESES

Functional or use training begins after the person understands how to operate and control the prosthetic components. Repetition is important for the person to gain an understanding of how to preposition the prosthesis and the objects and how to use the environment to help preposition them. Also covered are prehension training and methods to complete ILS, including prevocational, avocational, and driving skills. The program trains the person to use all TDs prescribed in a meaningful manner such as using the heavy-duty TD with tools and the hand to eat. For details the therapist is referred to Santschi's work on prosthetic training.[16]

Prepositioning

The first stage in functional training involves prepositioning the prosthetic units in their optimum position to grasp an object or perform a given activity. All prosthetic components must be prepositioned in a proximal to distal order. Thus, the person with the BE prosthesis rotates the TD into the desired degree of pronation or supination to accomplish an activity. With an AE prosthesis the person flexes and locks the elbow and rotates the turntable before prepositioning the TD. The person with a shoulder disarticulation prepositions the shoulder unit before the elbow and wrist components. The person with bilateral prostheses must still preposition all components in

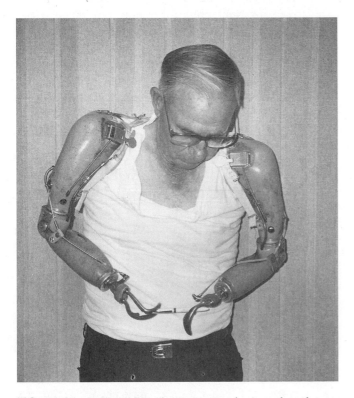

FIG. 31-16   Passing a pen from one prosthesis to the other to practice separation of controls.

the same fashion. The goal of prepositioning is to allow the person to approach the object or activity as one would with a normal hand and thereby avoid awkward body movements used to compensate for poor prepositioning.[16]

Prehension Training

Along with prepositioning, prehension training begins, first using large, hard objects such as blocks, cans, and jars, and progressing to soft, then to crushable objects, such as rubber balls, sponges, paper boxes, cones, and paper cups. These objects should be placed in positions that require elbow and TD prepositioning and TD operation at various heights. The hook TD has a nonmovable finger and a movable one. If a hook is used to pick up objects, the person is taught to stabilize the item with the nonmovable finger and then release the tension on the movable finger to secure the object. Prehension training should be completed using all prescribed TDs.[20,21]

A training board consisting of common household hardware (e.g. door knobs, spigot, light switch) or actual hardware found in the training facility may be used as the next step in functional training. Items such as a pencil sharpener, lock and key, jar and lid, and bottle opener should be used to challenge the person.[1,20] Remember, however, that initially there are only two or three rubber bands on the TD, which limits its grip strength. In bilateral activities the person should be encouraged to use a problem-solving approach to determine the best position and appropriate use for the prosthesis and the sound arm. The prosthesis should be regarded as an assistive device and not as the dominant arm.[20]

Independent Living Skills

Functional training should progress to performing necessary ILS. Activities should be introduced in a simple-to-complex order. The therapist should also ask the person what areas are important for him or her to be able to accomplish. The person is encouraged to analyze and perform the activities of personal hygiene and grooming, dressing, feeding, home management, communication, avocation, and vocation as independently as possible. The therapist may help the person analyze and accomplish a task or help achieve it by means of adaptive equipment or by encouraging repetitious practice to reach maximum speed and skill. The sound arm or longer prosthesis should complete most of the work while the opposite side acts as a stabilizer,[20] as discussed in greater detail in section 2 of this chapter.

Work-Related Activities

Prevocational evaluation may be included in the rehabilitation program. The therapist assesses the person's potential for returning to a former occupation or a possible change of vocation. A work site visit may be necessary to make reccomendations that would enable the person to return to work in a safe and efficient environment. It may also be necessary to restrict work activities such as the amount of weight the person may lift and carry and working on ladders. Initially the person may be able to work only part-time to gradually improve work endurance. Training and education for new jobs may be necessary. Home management skills and child care should be included as part of the person's assessment when appropriate.[18]

Driving Training

The ability to drive increases independence and may enhance vocational opportunities. The person should be referred to an adaptive driving program where he or she can be evaluated and trained using assistive devices such as the Northrop driving ring or a steering knob (Fig. 31-17). The controls of the car, such as the ignition switch and turn signals, can be modified to improve safety and comfort. The amount of training and extent of modifications will vary depending on the level of amputation.

The occupational therapist is responsible for assessing predriving skills. A predriving evaluation may include an assessment of visual acuity, traffic signal recognition, color vision, glare recovery, night vision, peripheral vision, depth perception, reaction time, and UE function. When necessary additional cognitive, visual, and perceptual skills are evaluated. See Chapter 26 for more information on driving.

Upon completion of the predriving evaluation, the therapist is responsible for making driving recommendations. These may include treatment for deficits, referral to a driver education center for training, and installation of assistive devices. The therapist's evaluation should include a statement regarding the person's potential for safe driving. If the person is unable to drive, alternative methods of transportation should be explored.

In some states, people are required to report any change in physical health status to the motor vehicle department and to their insurance company. Failure to do so may result in an uninsured driver.

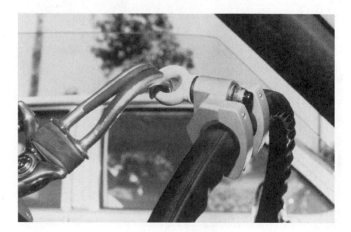

FIG. 31-17 Steering knob used for driving with a prosthesis.

Leisure Interests

The rehabilitation program should include information and/or training regarding leisure interests. With the person's and the rehabilitation team's joint effort and motivation, the person should be able to return to a meaningful and productive life. A wide variety of specialized prosthetic devices is available for all kinds of sports and recreational hobbies. Therapeutic Recreational Systems (TRS)* provides a catalog of prosthetic devices designed to improve the person's ability to participate in activities such as photography, ball games, and skiing.[2]

DURATION OF TRAINING

The average adult with a unilateral BE amputation who is otherwise healthy and well-adjusted will require approximately 5 hours of training to master control and use of the prosthesis for daily living. The person with a unilateral AE amputation under the same conditions will require approximately 10 hours of training. About 12 hours

---

* 2860 Pennsylvania Ave., Boulder, CO 80303.

will be required for bilateral BE prosthetic training whereas about 20 hours are required for bilateral AE prosthetic training. The initial training session should be about 1 hour long, and subsequent sessions increase in duration commensurate with increased prosthetic tolerance and physical endurance.[2,11,20]

SUMMARY

Acquired UE amputations can occur as a result of trauma, infections, neoplasms, and vascular diseases. Occupational therapists play an important role in the rehabilitation by addressing residual limb conditioning and care, preprosthetic exercise, and prosthetic training. The desired outcomes of occupational therapy intervention are independent management of ILS and resumption of work and leisure roles.

Working with an individual with an amputation can be a real challenge. Careful assessment of the person's needs, a creative approach to therapeutic intervention, and close communication with the team can make the challenge rewarding and successful.

Section 2 Electric-powered prostheses

Diane J. Atkins

Electric upper extremity prostheses have opened a new world of freedom and function for persons with upper extremity amputations. The advent of electronic microminiaturization has allowed the development of prosthetic devices with totally self-contained services of power, motor units, and electrodes.[4] Powered prostheses have existed for decades, but it was not until the 1960s that myoelectrically controlled prostheses were clinically introduced. The activities of the Otto Bock Company, in Duderstadt, Germany, began this process, as they aimed at developing an electro-mechanically driven prosthetic hand that would match both the technical and cosmetic demands of a human hand.[6]

The clinical use of these devices began in Europe because of government-supported health care systems and a large patient population of persons with congenital (postthalidomide) amputations. By the late 1970s and early 1980s, North America had an increasing but limited experience with myoelectric prostheses.[3] Today, when

funding permits, hundreds of myoelectric prostheses are prescribed for children and adults throughout the United States.

The term *myoelectric prosthesis* is often used interchangeably with *electric prosthesis*. A myoelectric prosthesis uses muscle surface electricity to control the prosthetic hand function. The muscle membrane generates an electric potential at the time of contraction. The myoelectric signal is sensed, amplified, and processed by a control unit that generates a motor that in turn drives a terminal device.[3] This terminal device is often an electromechanical hand.

A myoelectric prosthesis requires no cables for control, and most patients with below-elbow amputation should not require any straps or harnesses for suspension. These prostheses are generally suspended at the condyles of the elbow. The most common condition for which these prostheses are prescribed is a BE amputation where a natural, functional elbow is retained. Myo-

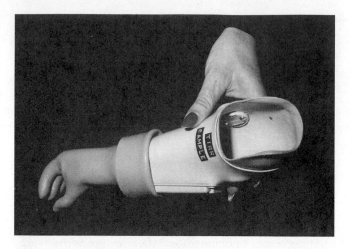

FIG. 31-18 Surface electrodes, recessed within wall of myoelectric socket, detect muscle contractions.

electric controls require minimal physical effort for operation and rarely require adjustment.

The muscle groups in the below-elbow area are used according to their physiologic function, that is, the wrist extensor muscles for hand opening and the wrist flexor muscles for hand closing. Muscular contractions are detected by surface electrodes recessed within the wall of the prosthetic socket (Fig. 31-18).

Before prescribing a myoelectric prosthesis, it is critically necessary that the patient is strong enough and able to contract each individual muscle group separately. The surface electric signals are amplified by a miniature electrode and led to the relay system. The relay is responsible for the energy supply to the battery-operated motor in the electric hand. When the alternating contractions of extensor and flexor muscles take place, the direction of the current changes in the electric motor, and the hand opens and closes accordingly.[6] The batteries are energy-storing devices and are rechargeable in a charging unit. The unit is plugged into an outlet and generally charged overnight (Fig. 31-19).

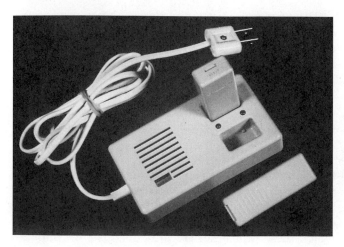

FIG. 31-19 Battery of myoelectric arm is inserted in battery charger and charged overnight.

There are many schools of thought regarding the advantages and disadvantages of myoelectric prostheses. The list in Box 31-1 describes some of these points that differentiate it from a body-powered, cable-controlled, hook-type terminal device.

Although the myoelectric hand is the most commonly prescribed electric terminal device, a specially designed gripping device, or Greifer, is also recommended at times. The Greifer was designed by the Otto Bock Company in Germany and provides a universal working tool designed to handle various specialized tasks. It can be used for heavy work in industry or farming and provides quick handling and precise manipulation of small objects. Features of the Greifer include a 38-lb. grasp as well as parallel gripping surfaces and a flexion joint for dorsal and volar flexion[6] (Fig. 31-20).

For amputation levels above the elbow, the complexity of function, and the power level required to accomplish functional movement, increases considerably. At the same time, the capability of the patient to operate a prosthesis by harnessing body movement via straps and cables, in the traditional body-power manner, decreases considerably.[7] The task of training a patient with an above elbow or shoulder disarticulation how to operate and function with a body-powered prosthesis is substantially more challenging.

Some rehabilitation professionals who work with patients who have UE amputation feel that electric components may be the only appropriate alternative for high level unilateral or high level bilateral amputations. Conversely, some rehabilitation professionals believe that body-powered prostheses remain the most functional and appropriate type of prosthesis for the majority of patients, despite the level of amputation.

The purpose of this section is to highlight the following: (1) preprosthetic training, (2) muscle-site control training, (3) the early basics of prosthetic training, and (4) functional use training. Although there are many methods of activating an electric elbow or hand (e.g., switch, touch, servo, proportional), the author will address "myo" (muscle contraction) control only, which to date remains the most common method of controlling electric components. Additionally, the main focus of this section will be the adult with a unilateral below-elbow amputation.

Children with upper extremity limb loss are managed quite differently from adults, and it is beyond the scope of this text to explain the principles in this unique population. Training an individual with bilateral limb loss requires extensive rehabilitation experience and background as well, and it is not recommended for the therapist with little or no previous exposure to the rehabilitation of patients with amputations. Individuals with bilateral limb loss should be referred to a "center of excellence" where rehabilitation of persons with amputations is an ongoing specialty area of treatment.

B O X   3 1 - 1

ADVANTAGES

1. Improved cosmesis
2. Increased grip force (approximately 25 lbs. in an adult myoelectric hand)
3. Minimal or no harnessing
4. Ability to use overhead
5. Minimal effort needed to control
6. Control more closely corresponds to human physiologic control

DISADVANTAGES

1. Cost of prosthesis
2. Frequency of maintenance and repair
3. Fragile nature of glove and frequent replacements necessary
4. Lack of sensory feedback (a body-powered prosthesis has some sense of proprioceptive feedback)
5. Slowness in responsiveness of electric hand
6. Increased weight

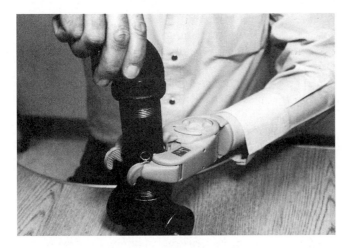

FIG. 31-20 Myoelectric Greifer is designed as universal working tool with parallel gripping force of up to 38 pounds.

PREPROSTHETIC THERAPY PROGRAM

Awareness of postoperative and subsequent preprosthetic principles of care is crucial to the successful management of the individual who has sustained traumatic limb loss. The patient has little control over what is happening and must depend upon the health care team to provide the best treatment possible.[2]

The crucial points and treatment goals of a postoperative program include the following:

1. promote wound healing
2. control incisional and phantom pain
3. maintain joint range of motion (to prevent contractures)
4. explore patient's and family's feelings about change in body
5. obtain adequate financial sponsorship for prosthesis and training.[5]

These goals should be addressed by the rehabilitation team, which should include the physician, nurse, oc-cupational or physical therapist, social worker, and patient.

When the sutures are removed, the preprosthetic program can begin. This program has been extensively discussed in Section 1 of this chapter and should include the following goals:

1. residual limb shrinkage and shaping
2. residual limb desensitization
3. maintenance of normal joint range of motion
4. increasing muscle strength
5. instruction in proper hygiene of limb
6. maximizing independence
7. myoelectric site testing and training (if myoelectric prosthesis is prescribed)
8. orientation to prosthetic options
9. exploration of patient goals regarding the future.

The reader is referred to the text *Comprehensive Management of the Upper Limb Amputee,*[2] Chapter 2, for additional clarification of these goals if necessary. For the patient receiving a myoelectric prosthesis, this sec-

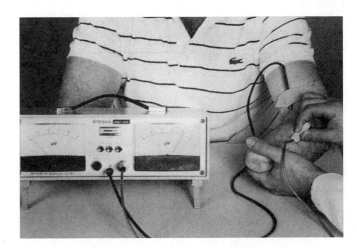

FIG. 31-21 Otto Bock myotester determines magnitude of muscle contraction.

tion will focus on a discussion of goal No. 7, myoelectric site testing and training.

A myoelectric prosthesis functions by detecting electromyographic (EMG) signals produced by muscles. Physical examination of the forearm can often detect sufficient wrist extensor and wrist flexor contractions in the person with a BE amputation and sufficient biceps and triceps contraction in the person with an AE amputation. Often, however, these signals are weak, and the therapist and prosthetist require a biofeedback system or myotester (Fig. 31-21, see p. 587).

MUSCLE SITE CONTROL TRAINING

Locating appropriate muscle sites superficially is the most important aspect of the successful operation of a myoelectric prosthesis. The muscle groups selected should approximate normal movements as much as possible. The following muscle groups are generally used during muscle-site selection:

- Persons with BE amputation use wrist extensors and flexors for terminal device (i.e., hand) opening and closing.
- Persons with AE amputation use biceps for elbow flexion and extension and triceps for terminal device opening and closing.
- Persons with shoulder disarticulation and forequarter amputation may use the deltoid, trapezius, latissimus, or pectoralis muscle for control.

It is important to note that the more proximal the level of amputation, the more difficult it becomes for the prosthetist to fit the individual and for the therapist to train that individual.

For the patient to understand the desired muscle contraction, the therapist instructs the patient to imitate the desired movement on both sides. The therapist should ask the patient to raise the sound hand at the wrist (wrist extension), and imagine that motion with the phantom hand on the amputated side (Fig. 31-22). Often a therapist can palpate the wrist flexors and extensors on the residual limb during this exercise. The patient should be instructed to contract and relax each muscle group separately and on command. For this step a myoelectric tester is particularly useful because it indicates the magnitude of the EMG signal. Once the maximum response is found, its location should be marked on the skin. This process is often done with a prosthetist to select the most appropriate muscle site.

When measuring surface potentials with the electrodes and a myotester, it is important that all electrodes have good contact with the skin and are aligned along the general direction of the muscle fibers. Moistening the skin slightly with water may improve the EMG signal by lowering skin resistance. EMG testing is begun with the most distal portion of the remnant muscles.

The myoelectric tester can be used to train the mus-

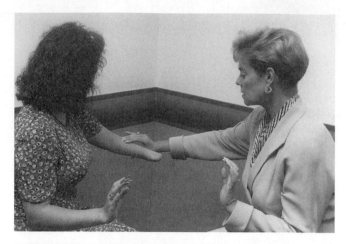

FIG. 31-22 Therapist instructs patient to imitate desired muscle contraction on both sides.

cles with both visual and auditory feedback. The goals at this point are to increase muscle strength and to isolate muscle contractions. As confidence and accuracy improve, the visual or auditory feedback should be removed. This task teaches the patient to internalize the feeling of each control movement. The advantage of creating this internalized awareness of proper muscle control is done so that control and strengthening practice can be continued between treatment sessions without the feedback equipment.[8]

It is essential that the individual with an amputation receive adequate training and practice in initiating these muscle contractions before receiving the myoelectric prosthesis. Anxiety and frustration often accompany the training of an individual to use a myoelectric prosthesis. The therapist also needs to recognize muscle fatigue, which is frequently a side effect in this process, and time must be given to allow that muscle to relax during the treatment session. The patient's success and effectiveness in using the prosthesis is closely related to the quality of the preprosthetic training.

EARLY BASICS OF PROSTHETIC TRAINING

An extremely important aspect of a prosthetic training program is to orient the patient realistically as to what the prosthesis can and cannot do. If the individual has an unrealistic expectation about the usefulness of the prosthesis as a replacement arm, he or she may be dissatisfied with the ultimate functioning of the prosthesis and may reject it altogether. It is imperative that the therapist be honest and positive about the function of the prosthesis. If he or she believes in and understands the functional potential and limitations of the prosthesis, success can be more realistically achieved.[1]

INITIAL VISITS

Training with a prosthesis should begin as soon as the prosthesis is received, preferably the same day. An excellent resource in the training process of a patient with a myoelectric hand is covered in the text *Comprehensive Management of the Upper Limb Amputee,* Chapter 7, Adult Myoelectric Upper Limb Prosthetic Training.[1]

It is important during the initial visits to review the following: orientation to prosthetic terminology, independence in donning and doffing, orientation to a prosthetic wearing schedule, and care of the residual limb and prosthesis.

Orientation to prosthetic terminology

Considering that this prosthesis is now a natural extension of the individual's body, it is particularly important to know the function and names of the major parts such as the electrodes, battery, glove, and electric hand. The initial visit is an appropriate time to introduce the battery charging procedure and the proper use of the battery packs to the patient. Instruction manuals are often included from the manufacturer and should be shared as well.

Independence in donning and doffing the prosthesis

Donning the prosthesis should be performed with the electronics in the OFF position to avoid any uncontrolled movements. At times a residual limb pull sock may be required for donning the prosthesis to accomplish close contact with the limb, particularly for very short residual limbs. The prosthetic arm should be stored in the OFF position with the batteries removed. The hand should be fully opened for storage to keep the thumb web space stretched.

Orientation to a prosthetic wearing schedule

This information is important to review during the first visit. Initial wearing periods should be no longer that 15 to 30 minutes. This limit is particularly important if scarring or insensate areas are present on the residual limb. If redness persists for more than 20 minutes in a particular area, the patient should return to the prosthetist for adjustments. If no skin problems exist, the wearing periods can be increased in 30-minute increments three times a day. By the end of the week, full-time wearing should be achieved.

Care of the residual limb and prosthesis

Appropriate care of the skin is vitally important. The residual limb should be washed daily with mild soap and lukewarm water. It should be rinsed thoroughly and dried using patting motions with a towel so as not to irritate sensitive or scar tissue.

The prosthesis may be cleaned with soap and water by using a damp cloth. Rubbing alcohol may be used to clean the inside of the socket if an odor develops. The cosmetic gloves stain easily, so special attention should be paid to avoiding ink, newsprint, mustard, grease, and dirt. A glove-cleansing cream can be obtained from the prosthetist that will remove general soil but not stains. The average life of a glove is approximately 6 months. The prosthesis should never be immersed in water because it will seriously damage the internal electronic components.

FUNCTIONAL USE TRAINING
TEACHING APPROACH, GRASP, AND RELEASE

Simple approach, grasp, and release activities are often accomplished with a formboard on which objects of various shapes, sizes, and densities are displayed (Fig. 31-23). It is important for the individual first to visualize how the object should be approached and grasped, and then to preposition the myoelectric hand. Prepositioning involves placing the terminal device in the optimum position for a specific activity. In approaching a glass, the hand should face in toward the midline to grasp the glass as a normal hand (Fig. 31-24). To approach a glass or cup, the fingers of the hand should not be positioned downward, because a normal hand does not approach a glass in this position.

Often the patient adjusts his body, using compensatory body motions, rather than adjusting or prepositioning the hand first. This action is important to avoid because it appears awkward and often becomes a habit. The patient also should make certain the angle of elbow flexion is appropriate if the person has lost the arm above the elbow and uses a body-powered or electric elbow. A mirror can be effective in assisting the patient to see the way the body is positioned and visualize how the sound arm would approach a particular object or activity. It is often necessary to remind the patient to maintain an upright posture and avoid extraneous body movements.

Another important aspect of training an individual to grasp an object is to master the control of the gripping force of the terminal device. This skill involves close visual attention to grade the muscle contraction for a specific result in the myoelectric hand. Styrofoam packaging bubbles work well for developing this skill. The individual must learn how to pick up the styrofoam without crushing it. Too strong a grasp crushes the object being held (Fig. 31-25). Good grasp control through training with styrofoam, cotton balls, or sponges will help develop the control needed to handle paper cups, eggs, potato chips, sandwiches, or even to hold someone's hand.[8] Release is accomplished by visualizing a wrist extension contraction, or hand up or hand open. This response should become quite automatic if good preprosthetic training of the muscles has occurred.

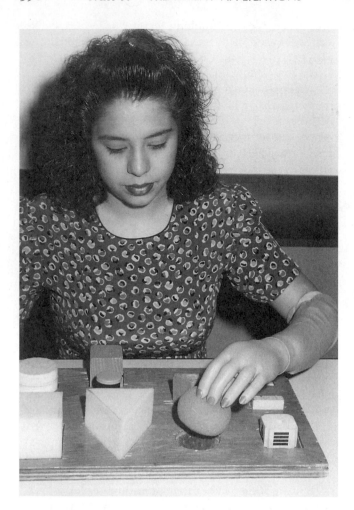

FIG. 31-23 Formboard provides useful tool in practicing approach, grasp, and release of objects of various sizes, shape, and densities.

Eventually the effort to perform specific movements will take less cognitive effort; the movements soon become automatic. Functional use activities can now be introduced into the therapy program.

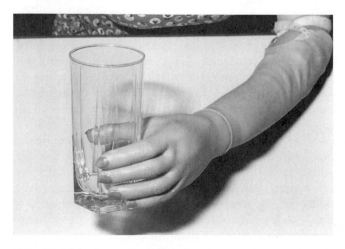

FIG. 31-24 When approaching glass, hand is prepositioned in midline to grasp glass as normal hand.

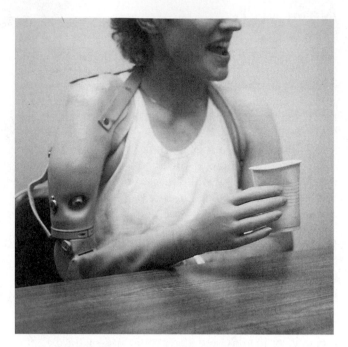

FIG. 31-25 Above-elbow amputee demonstrates how excessive grasp crushes object (plastic cup) being held.

ACTIVITIES OF DAILY LIVING

It is important to keep in mind that the prosthesis is used as a functional assist in the majority of bilateral activities. Therefore, most activities of daily living (ADL) will be accomplished with the sound arm and hand. Other than perhaps for practice, it is not appropriate to train a person with a unilateral amputation to eat holding a spoon, write, or brush his teeth using the myoelectric hand. In almost all cases the sound hand becomes the dominant extremity and performs those types of tasks. Occasionally if the right arm is the dominant arm and is amputated, and the individual is fitted with a myoelectric hand in a timely manner, he or she may prefer to use the myoelectric hand for some of these activities. The critically important component of sensory feedback is often the determining factor in deciding which hand to use. A person with amputation almost always chooses to perform most activities with a hand that has feeling. A myoelectric hand has no sensory feedback.

It is important to review a list of bilateral ADL tasks with the patient to determine which tasks are the most important to accomplish. These are the activities to focus upon, stressing throughout the activity that the myoelectric hand is used as an assist and stabilizer. The bilateral activities listed on Table 31-2 are good examples to review and practice.

With practice, these activities and many others will continue to improve and become automatic in their completion. It is extremely important to reinforce and emphasize the fact that bathing, grooming, and hygiene skills involving water must be done wihout a myoelectric hand because of the damaging effects of water on the

TABLE 31-2   Roles of Myoelectric Hand and Sound Hand in Bilateral ADL

ACTIVITY	MYOELECTRIC HAND	SOUND HAND
1. Cutting meat	Hold fork with prongs facing downward; hold knife as grip strength increases	Hold knife Hold fork
2. Opening a jar (Fig. 31-26)	Hold the jar	Turn the lid
3. Opening a tube of toothpaste	Hold the tube	Turn the cap
4. Stirring something in a bowl	Hold the bowl with a strong grip	Hold the mixing spoon or fork
5. Cutting fruit or vegetables (Fig. 31-27)	Hold the fruit or vegetable firmly	Hold the knife to cut
6. Using scissors to cut paper	Hold the paper to be cut	Use scissors in normal fashion
7. Buckling a belt	Hold the buckle end of belt to keep stable	Manipulate long end of belt into buckle
8. Zipping a jacket from bottom up	Hold anchor tab	Manipulate pull tab at base and pull upward
9. Applying socks	Hold one side of socks	Hold other side of socks and pull upward
10. Opening an umbrella (Fig. 31-28)	Hold base knob of umbrella	Open as normal

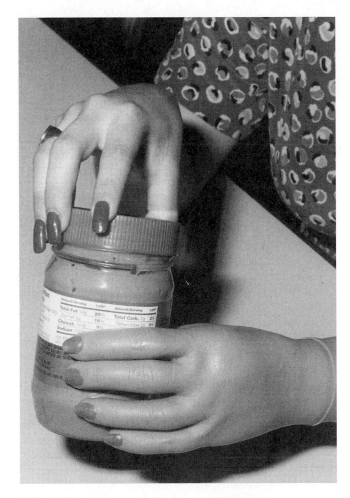

FIG. 31-26   Opening jar is accomplished with myoelectric hand holding jar and sound hand turning lid.

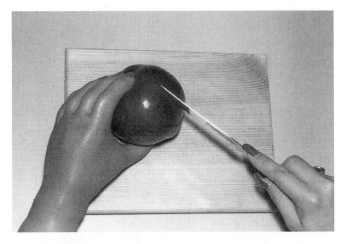

FIG. 31-27   Cutting apple is accomplished with myoelectric hand holding apple while sound hand holds knife to cut.

electric motor and battery. Additionally, it is important to advise myoelectric users against excess vibration, sand, dirt, and the extremes of heat and cold. These, too, can seriously impair the electronic components.

VOCATIONAL AND LEISURE ACTIVITIES

As training proceeds and a sense of self-acceptance and comfort with the amputation is experienced, a therapist

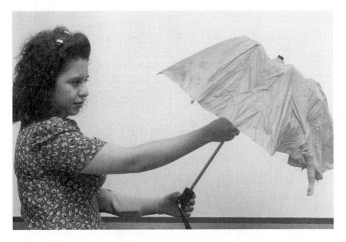

FIG. 31-28   Opening umbrella is accomplished by holding base knob of umbrella with myoelectric hand and using sound hand to open as normal.

should broach the subject of return to work. If possible, the various job requirements can be discussed and then practiced in a simulated step-by-step process. Ideally, an on-site visit could be made by the therapist, and several requirements of the job could be practiced. If changes and adjustments to the work environment are necessary, the therapist could advise in these modifications.

Recreational activities are also critically important to discuss at this time, for these activities contribute not only to physical well-being but also to important psychological well-being. The terminal devices for recreational activities are not myoelectric. As discussed in Section I, Therapeutic Recreation Systems (TRS) has some excellent TD adaptation components, including an Amputee Golf Grip (Fig. 31-29) and a Super Sports terminal device (Fig. 31-30).

HOME INSTRUCTIONS

At the conclusion of training, home instructions that include a wearing schedule and care instructions should be reviewed with the patient and the family. A follow-up appointment should also be given at this time, as well as a list of the rehabilitation team members and their telephone numbers, which will enable the patient to contact the appropriate person when problems arise.

SUMMARY

The rehabilitation process of a person with upper limb loss can be a challenging and rewarding process. In the

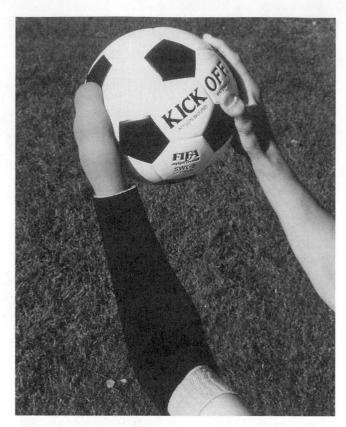

FIG. 31-30 Super Sports terminal device is highly flexible, strong, prosthetic sports accessory for volleyball, soccer, football, floor exercise gymnastics, or any activity in which shock absorption, safety, and bilateral control are important.

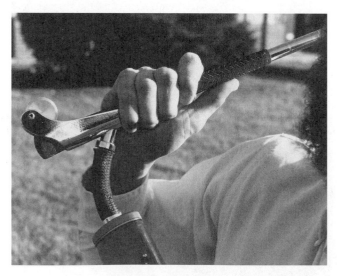

FIG. 31-29 Amputee Golf Grip is high-performance prosthetic golf accessory that allows for smooth swings and complete follow-through.

instances of above elbow, shoulder disarticulation, and bilateral limb loss, significant training and expertise on the part of the therapist is essential.

The potential of the indivudals with amputation is limitless and often they are able to accomplish activities one never would have expected. The success of their rehabilitation does not rest solely on the quality of training to use a prosthesis. Success is closely intertwined with the quality of their medical management, the quality of the prosthesis, their functional training, and the conscientious follow-up of that individual once the rehabilitation phase is complete. Follow-up is critically important and often overlooked. Perhaps the most important aspect of a successful rehabilitation program however, is the motivation and the desire of the person with amputation to become more independent. As a team member, this aspect is a pivotal ingredient to cultivate and reinforce. The impact a therapist makes during this important process will remain with the patient for life.

SAMPLE TREATMENT PLAN

CASE STUDY

Mr. K is 41 years old. He has lived in poverty all of his life. He is intellectually limited, which may be a result of poor education. Mr. K recently sustained an AE amputation of the nondominant left upper extremity as the result of a traumatic injury. The residual limb is well healed, and there is good shrinkage. There are no medical complications. Mr. K is receiving state aid, and a prosthesis and vocational training have been authorized for him. He has worked as a janitor and as a field hand picking vegetables in the past. He reads the basic vocabulary necessary for everyday life at home and in the street (for example, signs and newspaper headlines). When employed Mr. K is a steady and hard worker. He is married and has four children, all living at home. His interests are watching television, playing cards, and gardening.

The client is accepting the prosthesis and is no longer depressed about the loss of his arm. Strength in the musculature of the residual limb is good to normal. He was referred to occupational therapy for prosthetic training and vocational evaluation.

Personal data

Name: Mr. K
Age: 41
Diagnosis: Traumatic injury to left arm
Disability: Long left AE amputation
Treatment aims as stated in referral: Prosthetic training and vocational evaluation

Other services

Medical: Surgery, medical management, prescribe prosthesis and OT
Social service: Patient and family adjustment, exploration of available financial support
Vocational counseling: Interview, test potential for employment

Frame of reference/treatment approaches

Occupational performance
Biomechanical and rehabilitative approaches

OT EVALUATION

Performance components

Sensorimotor
   Strength: Manual muscle test to muscles of residual limb and the sound RUE
   Active and passive ROM: Left shoulder, test
   Physical endurance: Observe
   Manual dexterity, unilateral: Observe
   Speed of movement and motor planning skill: Observe
   Sensation (touch, pain, temperature) of residual limb: Test
   Residual limb pain: Observe
Cognitive
   Judgment: Observe
   Problem-solving skills: Observe
   Language skills: Observe

Psychosocial
   Adjustment to disability: Observe
   Dyadic and group interaction skills: Observe

Performance areas

Potential work skills: Observe, test
Work habits and attitudes: Observe
Self-care independence: Test, observe
Independent travel: Observe or test
Leisure interests/activities: Interview

EVALUATION SUMMARY

Muscle test of residual limb musculature revealed grades of N (5) in shoulder flexors, extensors, and abductors. Grades of G (4) were noted for shoulder rotators and adductors. Active and passive ROM for all shoulder motions are within normal limits. Sensory modalities of touch, pain, and temperature are intact. There is no pain in the residual limb. Physical endurance for light and moderate activity is adequate for a full day's work. Mr. K needs some additional practice in one-handed skills to improve right-handed manual dexterity, and the need for assistive devices will be ex-

plored. Mr. K's reading skills are limited, and he cannot follow written directions. He needs assistance with problem solving but succeeds with some verbal guidance. The patient tends to be quiet, cooperative, and compliant. He socializes when drawn into group interaction but is somewhat hesitant and shy in interactions with the therapist. He appears to be well-motivated for the prosthesis and for return to employment.

Mr. K is performing most self-care activities independently, using the sound right arm, except for bilateral activi-

EVALUATION SUMMARY—cont'd

ties such as cutting meat, buttoning the shirt, applying deodorant, carrying large objects, and tying shoes. He needs some assistance in analyzing methods for one-handed performance.

There is good potential for performance of unskilled work similar to that done in the past. Janitorial or assembly work and simple use of tools will be part of the last phase of the prosthetic use training program.

Assets

Good use of right arm
Motivated to use prosthesis

Motivated to return to work
Cooperative
Family support
Positive adjustment to limb loss

Problem list

1. Muscle weakness
2. Inability to use AE prosthesis
3. ADL dependence
4. Limited literacy and problem-solving skills
5. Loss of role as family provider

PROBLEM 1: MUSCLE WEAKNESS

Objective

Strength of shoulder rotators and adductors will increase from good to normal

Method

Progressive resistive exercise (PRE) to shoulder adductors, using Thera-Band[R] in a home program; PRE to shoulder rotators, using weighted cuffs on residual limb; client holds limb in 90° shoulder flexion, then 90° shoulder adduction and rotates shoulder internally and externally. Manual resistance exercise to combined shoulder depression, extension, and abduction in preparation for prosthesis controls training

Gradation

Increase resistance by adding weight; increase number of repetitions from 10 to 30 per day

PROBLEM 2: INABILITY TO USE AE PROSTHESIS

Objectives

To know the names of functions of all the parts of the prosthesis by the end of the first week of training
To put on and remove the prosthesis smoothly and efficiently within 5 minutes
To achieve proficiency in controls of AE prosthesis so that each control motion is performed when needed with little or no hesitation

Method

Review names and functions as parts of prosthesis; review repetitively. Repetitive application and removal of prosthesis for practice. Practice in elbow flexion control, elbow locking, elbow and wrist rotation, and TD opening and closing; practice in performing these tasks in sequence

Gradation

Decrease repetitions
Decrease amount of supervision, direction, and assistance
Increase time spent in training sessions and wearing

PROBLEM 3: ADL DEPENDENCE

Objective

Achieve proficiency in care of residual limb so that care is performed independently on a daily basis at home without cuing

Method

Washing and drying residual limb; application and removal of prosthetic socks; washing out socks; daily change of socks

Gradation

Decrease amount of direction and assistance as proficiency is achieved

SAMPLE TREATMENT PLAN – cont'd

PROBLEMS 2, 4: INABILITY TO USE PROSTHESIS, LIMITED PROBLEM-SOLVING SKILLS

Objective

To preposition the TD when using practice objects so that he can preposition the TD and pick up 75% of the objects with little or no hesitation

Method

Grasp and release of objects of various weights, textures, sizes, and shapes in a variety of positions, for example, cans, jars, wood cylinders, blocks, pencils, doorknob, and cabinet handles

Gradation

Hard to soft objects; large to small objects; progress from table surface to grasp and release at side, overhead, and on floor

PROBLEMS 3, 4: ADL DEPENDENCE, LIMITED PROBLEM-SOLVING SKILLS

Objective

Achieve moderate skill in performance of bilateral ADL so that he is performing 75% of these activities independently at home

Method

Fasten trousers; handle wallet; tie shoes; clean fingernails; apply deodorant; tie necktie; button shirt; use phone; cut food. Cue patient to analyze best use for prosthesis as an assist and best role for sound arm in each activity

Gradation

Simple to complex activities client is expected to perform; decrease amount of supervision and assistance

PROBLEMS 4, 5: LOSS OF VOCATIONAL ROLE, LIMITED PROBLEM-SOLVING SKILLS

Objective

Evaluate potential for employment so that specific information about potential work skills, work habits and attitudes, and work tolerance can be conveyed to the vocational counselor.

Method

Janitorial work—floor cleaning, emptying trash
Assembly jobs—electronic parts assembly

Use of hand tools in light woodwork, such as sawing, hammering, drilling, using a screwdriver, planing, and sanding. Cue patient to analyze best use for prosthesis and sound arm in bilateral work activities.

Gradation

Increase complexity, speed, and durtation at work tasks; increase amount of manipulation required of prosthesis; decrease amount of instruction and supervision.

REVIEW QUESTIONS

1. Define the following abbreviations: AE, TD, and BE.
2. Which arm function is lost and which functions are maintained in a long BE amputation?
3. Name two common medical problems that can interfere with prosthetic training. How is each solved?
4. What is the purpose of the pre-prosthetic program?
5. Describe activities and exercises suitable for the preprosthetic period.
6. List the five major steps in the prosthetic training program.
7. What is the sequence of training in learning controls of the AE prosthesis?
8. What is the sequence of training in learning the use of the BE prosthesis?
9. What motion of the arm accomplishes elbow locking on the AE prosthesis?
10. Before the TD on an AE prosthesis can be operated, what must the user do?
11. What motions accomplish TD opening?

12. How is the TD prepositioned by the prosthesis user?
13. Name the two types of TDs. Which is more frequently prescribed and used?
14. How is functional training graded?
15. What is the source of power that activates the electric-powered prosthesis?
16. What are some advantages of the electric-powered prosthesis over the body-powered prosthesis?
17. What are some of its disadvantages?
18. What is a Griefer and how is it used?
19. What is meant by muscle-site control training?
20. Describe how the therapist trains the patient to control muscle contraction for prosthesis operation.
21. Describe the relative roles of a prosthesis and a sound arm/hand in the following activities: cutting meat; opening a jar; using scissors; buckling a belt; using an eggbeater; hammering a nail.

REFERENCES

SECTION 1: AMPUTATIONS AND BODY-POWERED PROSTHESES

1. Anderson MH, Bechtol CO, Sollars RE: *Clinical prosthetics for physicians and therapists,* Springfield, Ill, 1959, Charles C Thomas.
2. Atkins DJ: Adult upper limb prosthetic training. In Atkins DJ, Meier RH, editors: *Comprehensive management of the upper-limb amputee,* New York, 1989, Springer-Verlag.
3. Atkins DJ: Postoperative and preprosthetic therapy programs. In Atkins DJ, Meier RH, editors: *Comprehensive management of the upper-limb amputee,* New York, 1989, Springer-Verlag.
4. Banerjee SJ: *Rehabilitation management of amputees,* Baltimore, 1982, Williams & Wilkins.
5. Bennett JB, Alexander CB:
Amputation levels and surgical techniques. In Atkins DJ, Meier RH, editors: *Comprehensive management of the upper-limb amputee,* New York, 1989, Springer-Verlag.
6. Bennett JB, Gartsman GM: Surgical options for brachial plexus and stroke patients. In Atkins DJ, Meier RH, editors: *Comprehensive management of the upper-limb amputee,* New York, 1989, Springer-Verlag.
7. Friedman LW: *The psychological rehabilitation of the amputee,* Springfield, Ill, 1978, Charles C Thomas.
8. Hill SL: Interventions for the elderly amputee, *Rehabil Nurs* 10:23, 1985.
9. Hirschberg G, Lewis L, Thomas D: *Rehabilitation,* Philadelphia, 1964, JB Lippincott.
10. Larson CB, Gould M: *Orthopedic nursing,* ed 8, St Louis, 1974, CV Mosby.
11. Leonard JA, Meier RH: Prosthetics. In DeLisa JA, editor: *Rehabilitation medicine principles and practice,* Philadelphia, 1988, JB Lippincott.
12. Meier RH, Atkins DJ: Preface. In Atkins DJ, Meier RH, editors: *Comprehensive management of the upper-limb amputee,* New York, 1989, Springer-Verlag.
13. Muilenburg AL, LeBlanc MA: Body-powered upper-limb components. In Atkins DJ, Meier RH, editors: *Comprehensive management of the upper-limb amputee,* New York, 1989, Springer-Verlag.
14. Olivett BL: Management and prosthetic training of the adult amputee. In Hunter JM and associates, editors: *Rehabilitation of the hand,* St Louis, 1984, CV Mosby.
15. O'Sullivan S, Cullen K, Schmitz T: *Physical rehabilitation: evaluation and treatment procedures,* Philadelphia, 1981, FA Davis.
16. Santschi WR, editor: *Manual of upper extremity prosthetics,* ed 2, Los Angeles, 1958, University of California Press.
17. Shands A, Raney R, Brashear H: *Handbook of orthopaedic surgery,* ed 8, St Louis, 1971, CV Mosby.
18. Spencer EA: Amputation and prosthetic replacement. In Hopkins HL, Smith HD, editors: *Willard and Spackman's occupational therapy,* ed 8, Philadelphia, 1993, JB Lippincott.
19. Walsh NE, Dumitru D, Ramamurthy S, Schoenfeld LS: Treatment of the patient with chronic pain. In DeLisa JA, editor: *Rehabilitation medicine principles and practice,* Philadelphia, 1988, JB Lippincott.
20. Wellerson TL: *A manual for occupational therapists on the rehabilitation of upper extremity amputees,* Dubuque, Iowa, 1958, Wm C Brown.
21. Wright G: *Controls training for the upper extremity amputee* (film), San José, Calif, Instructional Resources Center, San José State University.

RECOMMENDED VIEWING

Art Heinze: *The Use of Upper Extremity Prostheses,* 1988. Dynamic Rehab Videos and Rentals, 307 Spruce Ave. South, Thief River Falls, MN 56701.

REFERENCES

SECTION 2: ELECTRIC-POWERED PROSTHESES

1. Atkins DJ: Adult myoelectric upper-limb prosthetic training. In Atkins DJ, Meier RH, editors: *Comprehensive management of the upper limb amputee,* New York, 1989, Springer-Verlag.
2. Atkins DJ: Postoperative and preprosthetic therapy programs. In Atkins DJ, Meier RH, editors: *Comprehensive management of the upper limb amputee,* New York, 1989, Springer-Verlag.
3. Dalsey R and associates: Myoelectric prosthetic replacement in the upper extremity amputee, *Orthopedic Review* 18(6):697, 1989.

4. Jacobsen SC and associates: Development of the Utah artificial arm, *IEEE Trans Biomed Eng* 29(4):249, 1982.

5. Meier RH: Amputations and prosthetic fitting. In Fisher S: *Comprehensive rehabilitation of burns,* Baltimore, 1984, Williams & Wilkens.

6. Nader M, Ing EH: The artificial substitution of missing hands with myoelectric prostheses, *Clinical Orthopedics and Related Research* 258:9, 1990.

7. Scott RN, Parker PA: Myoelectric prostheses: state of the art, *J Med Eng Tech* 12(4):143, 1988.

8. Spiegal SR: Adult myoelectric upper-limb prosthetic training. In Atkins DJ, Meier RH, editors: *Comprehensive management of the upper limb amputee,* New York, 1989, Springer-Verlag.

Lower Extremity Amputations and Prosthetics

Sharon Pasquinelli

mputations may result from diseases such as peripheral vascular disease (PVD) and peripheral vasospastic diseases, chronic infections such as gas gangrene and osteomyelitis, and malignant tumors. They may also result from external causes such as trauma and chemical, thermal, or electrical injuries. The most common cause of lower extremity (LE) amputations in adults is peripheral vascular disease, especially diabetes.[3,23]

It is estimated that 1 American in every 300 to 400 has had a major amputation.[7,20] Most of these are LE amputations which occur three times as frequently as those of the upper extremity.[3,30] While the incidence of amputation remains fairly constant between the ages of 1 and 15, from 15 to 54 years of age there is a gradual increase in incidence because of work-related injuries and highway accidents. Above age 55, there is a sharp increase in the incidence of LE amputation, which is indicative of the relatively large number of older patients with PVD.[3]

SURGICAL MANAGEMENT

During surgery, the physician attempts to preserve as much soft tissue as possible. A primary surgical goal is to form the residual limb in a manner that maintains function of the remaining tissues and allows use of a prosthesis.[22,23] Blood vessels and nerves are severed and allowed to retract so that residual limb pain is minimized during prosthetic use. Muscles are sutured to the bones distally by a surgical process called myodesis.[16] In any amputation the muscles involved in the function of the amputated part are affected by the loss.

A closed or open surgical procedure may be performed. The open method allows drainage and minimizes the possibility of infection. The closed method reduces the period of hospitalization but also reduces free drainage and thereby increases the risk of infection. In either case, the remaining limb must be strong and resilient to fit the prosthesis socket snugly and comfortably and to ensure that body weight may be exerted on the residual limb when using the prosthesis.[22]

POSTSURGICAL CONSIDERATIONS AND PROBLEMS

Several factors and potential problems can affect the outcome of rehabilitation. Length of the residual limb, skin integrity, edema, sensation, rate of healing, infections, and allergic reactions to the prosthesis are among the physical factors that affect rehabilitation potential.

SKIN PROBLEMS

Skin complications account for the major portion of postsurgical problems in persons with LE amputation. These complications can be present in either the preprosthetic or the postprosthetic phase of rehabilitation. Delayed healing and extensive skin grafting are potential complications during the preprosthetic phase. Skin breakdown, ulcers, "corns," and infected sebaceous cysts occur in the postprosthetic phase. Edema can develop in either phase.

Preprosthetic Phase

Delayed healing of the incision site is one of the earliest preprosthetic complications. This complication is most common among patients who have PVD and compromised circulation. As a result, prosthetic fitting is postponed. In severe cases, necrotic areas may develop. If the necrotic area is less than ½ inch (1.3 cm) wide, surgical intervention is not usually necessary. For wider necrotic areas, surgical closure is indicated.[3]

Immediately following surgery the residual limb is normally edematous as a result of the fluid that has collected within the soft tissues. Swelling is usually most prominent in the distal portion of the residual limb.[10]

In order to achieve a limb length suitable for prosthetic use, the surgeon may perform extensive skin grafting. The grafted area can pose a problem in prosthetic use, as adherent grafted skin may not withstand the pressure exerted by the prosthesis. If the skin graft adheres to a bone in a weight-bearing area, the grafted area may ulcerate and require surgical revision.[3] Daily massages by the patient and therapist decrease the adherence of grafts to underlying bones.

Postprosthetic Phase

During the postprosthetic phase skin breakdown may be caused by an ill-fitting socket or by wrinkles in the prosthetic sock. Ulceration of the residual limb is associated with ischemia and pressure exerted by the prosthesis.[16] The ulcer is treated by rest, elevation, and hot compresses.[21] If these problems persist, surgical revision of the amputation to a more viable tissue level is needed before further rehabilitation can occur.[16]

Some patients may develop "corns" on the residual limb similar to those that appear on the foot. These areas may be resected or pared down to minimize discomfort.

Persons with above-knee amputation (AKA) are predisposed to the development of sebaceous skin cysts.[8] These cysts are caused by the forces between the socket and the limb. If the cyst becomes infected, drainage ensues, and enucleation of the cyst wall may be required.

The development of edema during the postprosthetic phase is usually indicative of an ill-fitting socket. Proximal tightness of the socket may result in distal edema. A new, properly-fitted socket is the solution.[3]

SENSORY PROBLEMS

The loss of sensory feedback from the residual limb is a major problem following amputation.[23] The patient must rely on visual and proprioceptive feedback to control prosthetic use and function. Sensation in the residual limb is functionally lost when the prosthesis is applied. An ill-fitting socket, or a limb that is not well formed at the distal end, can cause pain and discomfort when the prosthesis is worn. In addition to the loss of normal sensation, the individual must become accustomed to new sensations. The pressure of the residual limb inside the socket and the feel of the harnessing system must be accommodated.[22] Hyperesthesia, neuromas, and phantom sensation or pain are problems that may interfere with use of the prosthesis.

Hyperesthesia of the residual limb limits functional use. The limb is desensitized by tapping and gentle massage.[11] Sympathetic nerve blocks are sometimes used to manage hypersensitivity medically.[21]

A neuroma, a small ball of nerve tissue, is caused by excessive growth of axons towards the distal portion of the residual limb. As these axons grow into soft tissue, they may turn back on themselves, thus producing a ball of nerve tissue. Most neuromas occur 1 to 2 inches (2.5 cm to 5.1 cm) proximal to the end of the residual limb and therefore are not problematic. However, subcutaneous neuromas cause pain when they are pressed or moved.[3] Treatment options include surgical excision and ultrasound. Additionally, the prosthesis socket may be fabricated to accommodate the neuroma.[25]

Following surgery, phantom sensation, the sensation of the presence of the amputated limb or a portion of it, is a common experience. The phantom sensation may be present for life or may eventually disappear. Phantom sensation does not usually interfere with prosthetic use. A much less common phenomenon that can prohibit use of the prosthesis is phantom pain, wherein the amputated limb is perceived as present and is painful as well.[25] Surgical revision of the limb is sometimes necessary to alleviate the discomfort. Phantom sensations occur most frequently in crush injuries and are usually felt as distal parts, that is, a hand or foot, rather than the entire extremity. Supportive counseling and early use of a temporary or permanent prosthesis are effective measures for dealing with phantom sensations.[22] The therapist can allay the patient's fears about these phenomena by offering information, support, and reassurance. The appearance of phantom pain or overconcern with phantom sensation may require the intervention of a psychiatrist who may work with the patient or consult with the occupational therapist.[25]

BONE AND JOINT PROBLEMS

Joint contractures are common postsurgical problems among patients with LE amputation.[3] The person with an AKA typically develops an external rotation, abduction, and flexion contracture of the affected hip. The person with below-knee amputation (BKA) develops an external rotation, abduction, and flexion contracture of the hip and a flexion deformity of the knee.[16]

The formation of bone spurs is another complication that may occur during the preprosthetic phase. Because most bone spurs are not palpable, an x-ray film is needed to confirm their presence. Large bone spurs that cause pain or result in persistent residual limb drainage require surgical excision. Bone beveling is a surgical procedure that removes rough edges of the bone and prevents further spur formation.

PSYCHOSOCIAL SKILLS
REACTIONS TO AMPUTATION

Amputation is likely to be accompanied by a profound sense of loss. Reactions are usually less severe in patients who have been well prepared for surgery and more severe in persons who have experienced sudden traumatic injuries that necessitate amputation.[7,15]

In accordance with the occupational performance model, the reaction to amputation is considered within the individual's physical, social, and cultural environments and within the temporal aspects of age, life cycle, and disability status.[2,5] Ultimately, the patient must come to terms with the loss of the limb. The patient is confronted with discomfort, inconvenience, expenses, loss of function, increased energy expenditure, and possible curtailment of leisure activities. It may be necessary to change vocations and cope with further medical problems.[7]

Sociocultural factors are important in the reaction to amputation. If the society in which the individual lives tends to have aversive reactions to amputation, the patient is likely to hold these same feelings. Such attitudes can result in self-hatred and self-deprecation. In some social, cultural, or religious groups, the amputation may be considered a means of punishment or atonement for sin. Such beliefs will affect the patient's reactions and adjustment to the disability.[7,8]

It is not uncommon for the individual to feel self-pity, anxiety, shock, grief, depression, anger, frustration, and a sense of futility in response to amputation. Older persons may demonstrate postoperative confusion, whereas younger persons may have a sense of mutilation or emasculation.[7,8,15]

Unless it is severe and prolonged, depression is considered a normal part of the grieving process after amputation. The preexisting personality of the patient determines the severity and duration of the reactions and ultimately the adjustment to the amputation and to prosthetic use.[7,8]

FACILITATING ADJUSTMENT

After an amputation, the patient will need a lot of reassurance during all phases of care.[15] In the acute postoperative phase, the individual may have hostile reactions that can be directed to the self and the medical team. The patient's hostility may be masked by solicitousness and friendliness. Involvement in the rehabilitation process and with other similar patients enhances the return to former occupational roles. Depression can be reduced with an activity program and, if necessary, medication.[7]

Adjustment to the prosthesis depends upon the adjustment to the amputation. Loss of a body part requires that the patient develop and accept a new body image.[22] The prosthesis can assist with reintegration of the body image, because its presence replaces the missing part, obscures the amputation, and enhances a "normal" appearance.[7] Such adjustment will have a beneficial effect on prosthetic training, because the patient must integrate the prosthesis into the body scheme. The prosthesis must become part of the self before it can be used effectively. Difficulties with acceptance of the patient's resultant body image may cause difficulties in prosthetic training.[22]

Fears about returning to family, social, vocational, and sexual roles are common. Frequent discussion of the fears and active participation in problem-solving activities helps to facilitate adjustment. The availability of a peer, or a support group, may help to decrease fear and encourage emotional expression.[1,7]

Following a mourning period, the patient may minimize the significance of the amputation and actually joke about it. When this phase of adjustment has subsided, the patient begins seriously to consider the future. At this point social, vocational, and educational planning should be stressed.[7]

LEVELS OF AMPUTATION AND FUNCTIONAL LOSSES IN THE LE

Hemipelvectomy and hip disarticulation amputations result in loss of the entire lower extremity; thus hip, knee, ankle, and foot functions are lost.[3] Above knee amputations (AKA) and knee disarticulation result in loss of knee, ankle, and foot motions. The residual limb of a person with an AKA may vary in length from 10 to 12 inches (25.4 cm to 30.5 cm) below the greater trochanter. For someone with a below-knee amputation (BKA), it is approximately 4 to 6 inches (10.1 cm to 15.2 cm) in length from the tibial plateau.[16,22] Some classification systems further delineate between upper ⅓, middle ⅓, and lower ⅓ above-knee (AK) and below-knee (BK) amputations respectively[16] (Fig. 32-1). The Syme's am-

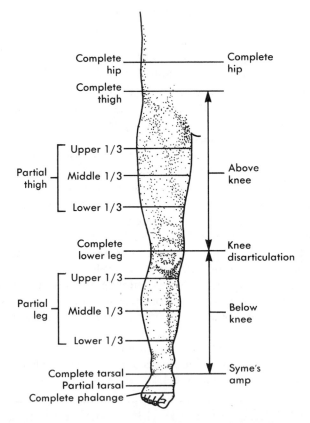

FIG. 32-1 Levels of extremity amputation. Comparison of systems for classifying acquired amputations of the lower limb and functional loss at each level. *Left,* System established by the Task Force on Standardization of Prosthetic-Orthotic Terminology. *Right,* Older system. (From O'Sullivan SB, Cullen K, Schmitz T: *Physical rehabilitation: evaluation and treatment procedures,* Philadelphia, 1981, FA Davis.)

putation is equivalent to an ankle disarticulation with removal of the medial and lateral malleoli and the last inch of the tibia. These patients lose ankle and foot functions. Transtarsal amputations are avoided. In a transmetatarsal amputation, the foot is severed through the metatarsal bones and ankle function remains intact.[3] Loss of the small toes does not result in functional impairment. Loss of the great toe, however, prevents toe-off during ambulation.[24]

ACCESSORIES AND COMPONENT PARTS OF THE LE PROSTHESIS

The major components of an LE prosthesis may include a suspension device, a socket, an artificial knee joint, a shin, an ankle joint, and an articulated foot.[19] The specific type and construction of prosthesis selected depend on the level of amputation and on the individual's needs. Some of the commonly used prostheses are described briefly below.

The Canadian-type hip disarticulation prosthesis meets the needs of the patient with hemipelvectomy or hip disarticulation. This prosthesis is suspended from the pelvis and is equipped with hip and knee joints, a shaft, and a solid ankle cushioned heel (SACH) foot. Pelvic movements provide energy for prosthetic use.[24]

The patient with an AKA benefits from either a suction socket or a conventional above-knee prosthesis. The conventional socket prosthesis is held in place by a silesian bandage or a pelvic belt.[11,17,21] As its name implies, the suction socket is held in place by suction (negative air pressure). Both these prostheses have a quadrilateral-shaped socket, a knee joint that permits flexion and extension, a shank, and a SACH foot.

Patients with a BKA use either the patella tendon-bearing (PTB) prosthesis or the standard BK prosthesis. The PTB prosthesis has a soft socket for the BK residual limb. It is composed of a strap around the thigh just above the patella[11,17] for suspension, a shank, and the ankle/foot assembly.[12] The standard BK prosthesis consists of a thigh corset, lateral hinges for a knee joint, a shin piece, and the ankle/foot assembly.

The person with a Syme's amputation uses the Canadian-type Syme prosthesis or "plastic Syme." This prosthesis consists of a total-contact plastic socket and SACH foot; there is no ankle joint.[24]

Transmetatarsal and toe amputations do not require prostheses. These patients need a shoe- or toe-filler, for which wool is often used.[3,24]

MANAGEMENT OF LE AMPUTATION
THE REHABILITATION TEAM

Rehabilitation of the patient with an LE amputation is best accomplished by a team approach.[7,8,9,17] Following surgery, the patient may be transferred to a rehabilitation facility. The rehabilitation team includes the physician, nurse, occupational therapist, physical therapist, prosthetist, and social worker. In some facilities the health care team also includes a vocational counselor, psychologist, discharge planner, dietitian, and recreation therapist.[21]

The physician is responsible for overseeing the patient's medical care. This includes reviewing the patient's past medical history, performing a physical examination, making a complete diagnosis of the patient's past and present medical conditions, providing an account of the surgical procedure, and ordering medications, laboratory tests, and therapies.

In general, the nursing staff is responsible for administering medications, monitoring vital signs, caring for the patient during hospitalization, and offering psychological support. The nursing staff assists in wound care, such as daily dressing changes, inspection of the surgical site, and prevention of contractures and decubiti. As the patient progresses, the nursing staff encourages the patient to perform activities that have been learned in therapy.

The physical therapist is responsible for evaluating range of motion (ROM), strength, sensation, coordination, balance, pain, gait, and the condition of the residual limb. Depending on the evaluation results, a treatment program may include therapeutic exercise, limb and wound care, pain management, and gait training. The physical therapist may assist in prosthetic selection and recommend the appropriate device for use during ambulation. As the patient progresses in pregait and gait activities, instruction in stair climbing, outdoor ambulation, and floor transfers may be introduced.

The prosthetist specializes in fabricating artificial limbs. Based on the individual's needs, the prosthetist advises on the selection of the prosthesis and its component parts. "The prosthetist should be able to design innovative prosthetic systems for difficult and unusual cases."[3]

The social worker interviews the patient and the patient's family members to assess the patient's social environment and the patient's psychological functioning since the onset of the disability. Recommendations regarding family problems, housing, and finances are provided. The social worker may also be involved with third-party payers, other sources of financing the patient's care, and discharge planning.

Occupational therapy may be initiated in the preoperative or postoperative phases of care. Preoperative visits provide a means of introducing the patient to the proposed postoperative regimen and rehabilitation care plan.[6,16,24] Preoperative training includes a baseline evaluation, exercises to improve cardiovascular endurance and muscle strength, and instruction in postoperative positioning techniques. Phantom pain and the methods employed to minimize these sensations should be discussed.[6,24] Postoperative occupational therapy begins before the patient is fitted for a prosthesis.

OCCUPATIONAL THERAPY INTERVENTION

The first step in the occupational therapy process is assessment.[18] The assessment determines the patient's functional status in the areas of occupational performance, occupational performance components, and occupational performance contexts.[2] Performance areas are broad categories of human activity that typify daily life, such as activities of daily living (ADL), work and productive activities, and play or leisure.[2,18] Occupational performance components relevant to the patient include specific skills from the sensory, motor, neuromuscular, cognitive, psychosocial, and social areas. These skills are used as a foundation to perform occupations.[2,5]

History. Before the initial occupational therapy evaluation, a review of the patient's medical chart is completed to assist the therapist in establishing a treatment plan. Important medical history includes the following: (1) date and level of amputation, (2) etiology, (3) disease processes that may be associated with the amputation, (4) presence of amputation-associated symptoms, (5) medications, and (6) past medical history.[3]

OCCUPATIONAL PERFORMANCE COMPONENTS
Soft Tissue Integrity

Prevention of soft tissue contractures is an immediate postoperative concern.[6] Positioning techniques are used to prevent abduction, flexion, and external rotation of the hip, and flexion of the knee.[11,16,24] To prevent hip flexion contractures, patients are instructed in lying prone and are encouraged to sleep and rest in the prone position. A positioning schedule is established in collaboration with the patient and is communicated to the rest of the team. Positions that encourage knee and hip flexion, such as prolonged sitting in a bed or chair, are avoided. In supine or sitting positions, pillows should not be placed beneath the knee in a BKA, under the residual limb in an AKA, or between the legs because these positions encourage knee flexion, hip flexion, and hip external rotation, respectively.[8]

The patient with a BKA benefits from the use of a support for the residual limb in the wheelchair (also called a stumpboard) (Fig. 32-2) or knee extension splint. The support and splint protect the wound and keep the knee of the affected extremity passively extended. A calf pad on an elevated wheelchair leg rest may be used temporarily.

To prevent decubiti, the patient is instructed in pressure relief and skin inspection techniques. For wheelchair-bound patients, pressure should be relieved every fifteen minutes, which can be accomplished by weight shift pressure relief techniques or wheelchair push-ups. While in bed, prone-lying, side-lying, and supine posi-

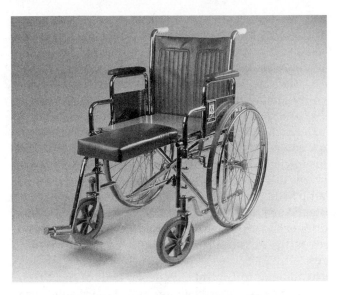

FIG. 32-2   A support for the residual limb in the wheelchair (also called a stump board) maintains knee extension and prevents flexion deformity. It is fastened to the wheelchair at the back with a strap, which goes under the seat.

tions are alternated every two hours. Skin inspection techniques, using a long-handled mirror, are conducted one to two times per day.

Edema Reduction

Although edema is a normal part of the postsurgical process, an early rehabilitation goal is to reduce edema. If edema persists, it can cause secondary complications such as pain, contractures, and soft tissue adhesions. Following surgery, the most commonly used edema reduction technique is elevation. Elevation, with precautions against creating hip flexion contractures, is part of the positioning program. As the wound heals, further edema reduction techniques such as Ace bandage wrapping, or shrinker sock, and the use of a temporary prosthesis or pylon may be used.

The occupational therapist incorporates Ace bandage wrapping techniques or the use of a shrinker sock into the patient's dressing program. There are several methods of wrapping the limb. Most methods are based on similar principles, which include diagonal bandaging, application of firm, even pressure distally, which decreases as the bandage is applied proximally, and reapplication of the bandage as ordered. The advantages of wrapping are that it allows for patients contouring and frequent checking of the wound. The disadvantages are that improper wrapping may result in a poorly shaped residual limb and impairment of blood supply to its distal portion.[20] Additionally, some patients have difficulty managing this technique independently.

Because of these disadvantages of wrapping, clinicians may choose to use a shrinker sock.[20] The primary advantage of shrinker socks is that they are easily applied and removed. The shrinker sock is donned as follows:

1. The sock is turned so that the bulky seam at the end is on the outside.
2. The top is turned so that it is folded back on itself about two thirds of the way.
3. The end of the sock is stretched so that it fits smoothly on the end of the residual limb.
4. The sock is gently pulled up over the limb.[4]

The therapist instructs the patient to don and doff the sock and periodically to check its fit. There are two reasons to check the sock: to prevent sock wrinkles and to prevent the top rim of the sock from rolling over into an elastic band. The latter will impair circulation and cause distal edema; the former may irritate the skin and cause skin breakdown. The major disadvantage of the shrinker sock is that it is available in only a limited number of sizes.

In addition to controlling edema, both of these techniques prevent hemorrhage, promote limb shaping, provide a sense of security, assist in desensitization, and aid in venous return. Ace bandages and shrinker socks should be washed frequently, rinsed thoroughly, and dried on a flat surface. Over time, both Ace bandages and socks lose their elasticity and need to be replaced.[17]

Physical Endurance and Muscle Strength

On initial evaluation the patient's strength may well be within the good-to-normal range. Because of the deconditioning effects of bed rest and surgery, however, patients with LE amputation require a therapeutic exercise program to regain the strength and endurance needed for performing occupations. Therapeutic exercise programs serve the multiple goals of strengthening specific muscle groups, conditioning the cardiovascular system, and increasing endurance. Scapular depressors, elbow extensors, and wrist extensors are specifically exercised because these muscles are needed for sit-to-stand activities during transfers and ambulation. Trunk exercises are incorporated into the program to assist in transferring, bathing, and LE dressing. Patients with PVD require close monitoring while exercising to avoid undue fatigue.

Some examples of grading activities for endurance include increasing the number of repetitions of an exercise or activity within the same time allotment, increasing the total time the patient performs the activity, or increasing the distance the patient propels a wheelchair. Wheelchair mobility activities can be graded from level to uneven surfaces as a means of simultaneously providing upper extremity exercise, endurance, and wheelchair mobility training.

Activity Tolerance

The ability to sustain a purposeful activity over time is observed and graded. For example, following initial wheelchair positioning, increasing sitting tolerance is a therapeutic goal. Standing tolerance may be increased during hygiene and grooming tasks and meal preparation activities.

Postural Control

Patients with either BKA or AKA need a firm sitting surface for pelvic support. As a result of prolonged use, wheelchairs develop a hammock-type seat that may cause poor sitting postures. Observation of the patient's posture often reveals a posterior pelvic tilt and incorrect limb and spinal alignment, which may lead to long-term complications. A solid seat insert solves these problems and prevents secondary low back pain. Patients with hemipelvectomy or hip disarticulation benefit from the use of a hemipelvectomy wheelchair cushion.

Because the patient's center of gravity in a sitting position is shifted posteriorly, a wheelchair designed to accommodate the amputation is needed. The wheelchair is constructed so that the axis of the rear wheels is set back 1⅞ inches (4.7 cm) from that of a standard wheelchair. This axis compensates for weight shift caused by limb loss, maintains proper chair balance, and prevents the chair from tipping backward. Antitipping devices for wheelchairs are also available. If such a wheelchair is not available, an adapter may be mounted to a standard wheelchair to offset the rear wheels by 2 inches (5.1 cm). Another option is temporarily to substitute a semireclining or reclining wheelchair, because the axes on these wheelchairs are also set back 2 inches (5.1 cm) from a standard wheelchair.[26] When used by patients with LE amputation, the primary disadvantage of reclining wheelchairs is the added weight (approximately 6 to 10 pounds, 2.7 to 4.5 kg) and back height, which make wheelchair mobility activities more demanding.

Good dynamic sitting and standing balance is a basic need of the patient and a prerequisite to occupational performance. The patient who lacks good balance will have difficulty with activities such as bending over to bathe the LEs, pulling up pants, reaching into a cupboard, and retrieving an object from the floor. These activities tax the patient's ability by demanding that postural adjustments be made to regain equilibrium. Balance activities that involve reaching in all directions may be graded by increasing the reaching radius or increasing the weight of the item being pursued.

Pain Management

Successful pain management begins with a thorough physical and psychosocial evaluation. The physical examination includes inspecting the residual limb for poorly healed areas, neuromas, bone fragments, edema, and abscesses or infection. The psychosocial assessment includes questions regarding the patient's family background, level of education, cooperativeness, legal problems, description of pain, attitude toward health care, and the family's attitude toward the patient's condition.[3]

There is no strict treatment protocol for patients with phantom limb pain.[3] The physician may treat the pain by injecting anesthetics into the tender area or by using sympathetic nerve blocks. In the acute phase, medication, positioning techniques, edema reduction techniques, and desensitization techniques are used to decrease pain. Many patients find that desensitization activities such as rubbing, tapping, and/or applying pressure and heat or cold provide relief. Biofeedback, transcutaneous electrical nerve stimulation (TENS), ultrasound, progressive relaxation exercises, and controlled breathing exercises may assist in reducing chronic pain in the residual limb.

OCCUPATIONAL PERFORMANCE AREAS

ACTIVITIES OF DAILY LIVING
Bed Mobility

The patient is taught bed mobility activities so that it is possible to move independently in bed without the assistance of an overhead trapeze bar, bed rails, or an electric hospital bed. Rolling from side to side, scooting up and down, and bridging activities are achieved by flexing the hip and knee of the unaffected leg and pushing the foot down into the bed. The upper extremities naturally assist in rolling, scooting, and bridging activities. To sit at the edge of the bed, the patient rolls to side-lying, slides the LEs off the bed, and, using upper extremity strength, pushes to an upright sitting position.

Wheelchair Mobility and Parts Management

Following surgery, the patient's primary mode of mobility is the wheelchair. Wheelchair propulsion is practiced on level and uneven surfaces, indoors and outdoors, and eventually on ramps and curbs. To propel straight forward the patient places both hands on the hand rims and pushes forward with equal force. If one arm exerts more effort than the other, the wheelchair will not roll straight. To make a right turn the patient pulls backward on the right hand rim and pushes forward with the left arm. To make a left turn the opposite actions are performed. The unaffected LE provides control and guides the wheelchair direction.[27] To use a wheelchair safely, the patient is instructed in operation of the wheelchair components. This training may include locking and unlocking the brakes, removing and replacing armrests and legrests, elevating and lowering legrests, and folding the wheelchair for transport.

Community Mobility

A patient with good bilateral upper extremity strength and endurance can be instructed to manage ramps independently. As the patient propels up a ramp, the upper body leans slightly forward to compensate for the gravitational forces that pull backward on the patient and wheelchair. During instruction, the occupational therapist stands behind the patient to prevent loss of steering control and/or tipping over backward.

If the patient must regularly negotiate ramps, a "grade-aid" may be mounted on the wheelchair. The grade-aid prevents backward rolling on an incline. To descend a ramp the patient leans slightly backward and controls speed by gripping the hand rims. The wheel brakes are *not* used to slow the descent because of the potential for accidental locking. Such an abrupt stop could pitch the wheelchair forward or cause it to veer to one side and tip over sideways.[26]

Transfer Training

Persons with unilateral LE amputation use the stand-pivot transfer technique. Stand-pivot transfers of 90° to the uninvolved side are the safest and easiest to perform. Stand-pivot transfers of 180° to either side and 90° stand-pivot transfers to the affected side are practiced for restrictive environments. When transferring to the toilet and bathtub, the patient may benefit from adaptive bathroom equipment such as toilet rails and tub seats.

Those with a bilateral LE amputation use the sliding board or push-up-and-over transfer technique. Another technique is available for those individuals who have a zippered-back or detachable-back wheelchair. These wheelchair accessories allow for transfers to and from the rear of the wheelchair. The patient reverses in, locks the brakes, detaches or unzips the back, and slides backward onto the surface. The patient slides forward to return to the wheelchair.

As the patient progresses in gait training, the occupational therapist incorporates ambulating transfers into the treatment plan. The ambulation aid and techniques used are discussed with the physical therapist. Generally, to make the transition from a sitting to standing position, the individual scoots forward in the chair, places the feet about shoulder distance apart, and uses upper extremity strength to push up to a standing position. Good standing balance is achieved before reaching for the ambulation aid. From standing to sitting positions, the patient is taught to feel the chair with the back of the legs, reach backward with both hands to the arms of the chair or the sitting surface, and then sit down.

Residual Limb Hygiene

After the wound is healed and the sutures are removed, daily hygiene is initiated. The purpose of good hygiene is to prevent irritation and infection. The following hygiene principles are taught until the patient incorporates them into the daily routine independently.

1. The residual limb is washed daily with warm water and mild soap. Thorough cleansing prevents a buildup of salt deposits, skin flakes, and debris. Use of a medicated soap, such as pHisoHex, decreases bacteria count.
2. Rinsing with clean water and thorough towel drying are essential. Soap residue and dampness irritate the skin and facilitate bacterial growth.
3. Skin folds are cleansed with a cotton swab.
4. The patient is instructed in skin inspection techniques. Using a long-handled mirror the patient

checks for skin breakdown, blisters, sores, reddened areas, and skin separations or ulcerations. If any of these conditions are observed, the doctor is notified immediately.

5. Application of oils, creams, or alcohol is not recommended. Oils and creams soften the skin, making it difficult to tolerate the prosthesis. Alcohol dries the skin and may cause skin sloughing and breakdown.

Because of the increased demand placed on the unaffected leg, skin inspection techniques and hygiene principles are equally important in maintaining skin integrity of the remaining leg. To prevent skin breakdown and absorb perspiration, a well-fitted shoe and wool sock are recommended. Because elderly patients and those with diabetes may have impaired vision, poor eye-hand coordination, and reduced sensation in the foot, callous removal and toenail trimming should be performed by a podiatrist. Thick toenails should be soaked and then cut straight across.

These hygiene principles and skin inspection techniques must be performed indefinitely and on a daily basis for both lower extremities. When the patient is independent in these activities, hygiene should be carried out in the evening. Evening care is preferred so that the residual limb is not softened before daily prosthetic use.

Bathing

Bathing or showering involves obtaining and using supplies, cleaning oneself, rinsing and drying, transferring to and from the shower or tub, and balance activities to reach the faucets and all body parts. Knowledge of the patient's bathroom floor plan and the type of shower or tub unit assists the therapist in selecting the safest type of transfer technique to perform at home.

Dressing

On evaluation, most patients are independent in all areas of dressing except for hiking pants, donning shoes and socks, tying shoelaces, and donning and doffing the prosthesis. Impaired dynamic standing balance initially interferes with the ability to stand independently and pull up the pants in persons with unilateral amputation. LE dressing training may be graded from donning pants in bed to sitting and standing positions. When dressing in bed, patients roll or bridge to pull up their pants. Thus, bed mobility activities and LE dressing techniques may be integrated into one treatment session. In a similar manner, LE dressing in sitting and standing positions provides an opportunity simultaneously to treat dynamic sitting and standing balance.

Problems with donning and doffing shoes and socks, managing zippers, tying shoelaces, and fastening buttons as a result of deficits in balance, vision, fine motor coordination, manipulation, and dexterity skills may be due to diabetes or advanced age. In such cases, it is appropriate to evaluate and treat these performance problems.

Patients with an AKA don the prosthesis in a standing position. The residual limb is pushed into the socket while the prosthesis is steadied against a firm object. The adductor longus tendon fits into the adductor longus tendon groove and the ischial tuberosity rests on the ischial shelf. The patient must exert weight into the prosthesis while fastening the suspension apparatus to prevent hip internal rotation and a concomitant gait deviation.[3] If the patient has difficulty with sock wrinkling, the sock may be placed in the socket before donning the prosthesis.

The patient with a BKA dons the prosthesis in a sitting position. Initially the leg is flexed at the knee. After the limb enters the socket, the knee is extended. To align the limb and socket properly, the patient stands and exerts weight on the prosthesis.

Sexual Expression

There is a lack of literature regarding sexual adjustment following LE amputation. One study found a statistically significant decrease in frequency of sexual intercourse following amputation. The decreased frequency was greater for males than for females. Men cited less interest as the reason for decreased frequency, and women reported fear of injury. None of the respondents cited "uncomfortable position" as a reason for the decline in frequency. Of the 60 respondents, only 15 discussed sexuality with a health care professional. The authors of this study concluded that there is a risk of sexual dysfunction following amputation and that sexual counseling should be included in the rehabilitation process.[19] (See Chapter 17.)

WORK AND PRODUCTIVE ACTIVITIES
Home Management

Home management activities such as clothing care, cleaning, meal preparation and cleanup, shopping, household maintenance, and safety procedures may pose challenges for the person with a LE amputation. Patients are instructed in home management activities with an emphasis on cognitive skills such as safety judgment, problem solving, and generalization of learning.

Energy Conservation and Work Simplification

More energy is expended by persons with an amputation during ADL than by other individuals of the same sex, age, and stature.[3] Energy expenditure increases with age and obesity.[12] Several studies suggest that there is a statistically significant correlation between residual limb length and energy demands.[3] Those with a BKA average a 10% increase in energy expenditure, whereas those with an AKA average a 40% increase. For these reasons patients benefit from instruction in work simplification and energy conservation techniques.

Transportation

The ability to drive a car increases independence and enhances vocational opportunities. Hand controls and adaptive devices are commercially available for persons with LE amputations. These controls are mounted near the steering wheel in such a manner that they do not impede use of the car by other drivers. Hand control systems, which substitute for the inability to use standard floor-mounted pedals, are classified into three types: pull-push, right angle–push, and twist-push. (See Chapter 26, Section 2.)

Safe driving requires that the appropriate adaptive equipment is used. Few individuals with BKA have adequate kinesthetic awareness to use standard gas pedals, clutches, and floor-mounted parking brakes. If the sensory feedback is not adequate, the person with a left BKA needs adaptive equipment such as a left hand–operated clutch and a hand parking brake. The person with a right BKA requires a left-foot accelerator. Those with AKAs use the same types of adaptive equipment used by individuals with below knee amputation because kinesthetic feedback is usually not adequate for driving without adaptive devices.

Although the occupational therapist may not be responsible for conducting an on-the-road driving test, the therapist does assess predriving skills. A predriving evaluation includes an assessment of visual acuity, traffic signal recognition, color vision, glare recovery, night vision, peripheral vision, depth perception, reaction time, upper extremity function, transferring to and from the car, and wheelchair management. When necessary, additional cognitive, visual, and perceptual skills are evaluated.

Upon completion of the predriving evaluation the therapist is responsible for making driving recommendations. These may include occupational therapy intervention to remedy deficits, referral to a driver education center for driving training and installation of adaptive devices, and a statement regarding the patient's potential to return to safe driving. If the patient is unable to resume driving, the ability to use public transportation is included in the treatment plan.

In some states, patients are required to report an amputation to the motor vehicle department and to the insurance company. Failure to do so may result in lack of insurance coverage even when premiums have been paid in full.

Vocational Activities

Following a comprehensive rehabilitation program, persons with unilateral BKA usually return to their former jobs. A person with a unilateral AKA may have difficulty performing a job that requires carrying heavy objects and/or standing and walking for extended periods of time. Those who have sustained bilateral LE amputations, on the other hand, need to be employed in a wheelchair-accessible environment and where they can be seated most of the day.[24]

Prevocational and vocational evaluations assist in determining whether the patient will be able to return to the former job or whether job retraining is needed. These assessments may include evaluation of physical capacities, work habits, and behaviors needed to perform the job. Performance of real or simulated job tasks may be included. Training may include job site modification and occupational therapy intervention to remediate the deficits noted upon evaluation. (See Chapters 29 and 30.)

LEISURE ACTIVITIES

Two surveys of the recreational activities engaged in by persons with amputation revealed that approximately 60% of the respondents were active in sports. Fishing and swimming were the most common leisure activities. Sports requiring running, jumping, and walking long distances caused discomfort and were least frequently enjoyed. Factors limiting recreational activities included excessive perspiration of the residual limb, pain, lack of physical endurance and muscle strength, skin problems, and edema.[13,14]

Recreational LE prostheses are available for golfing, swimming, and skiing. Golfers may consider installing a rotator inside the prosthesis. Swimmers often use a waterproof prosthesis. Those with unilateral LE amputation participate in cross-country skiing without the use of a special prosthesis, because the gliding action of the skis allows them to cover a greater distance than they can negotiate when walking. Persons with unilateral BKA who downhill ski use a specially designed prosthesis that permits knee flexion. They ski on the unaffected leg and attach outrigger miniature skis to their ski poles. This approach is called the track three method.[3,14]

DISCHARGE PLANNING

The occupational therapy intervention process ends when the patient is discharged from the hospital or health care facility. To ease the transition from hospital to home, the patient, family, and other care givers participate in discharge planning activities. These activities include family training and provision of a home exercise program and necessary equipment. A home evaluation may be completed in anticipation of discharge.

Family Training

Depending on the level of independence achieved by the patient, the family may need training in some occupations. Frequently family members require training in transfer techniques, wheelchair mobility, wheelchair parts management, and loading the wheelchair into the car. These techniques are taught with an emphasis on safety and proper body mechanics. Following instruction and demonstration, family members and the patient are given the opportunity to perform these activities with the occupational therapist's guidance. If the patient is nonambulatory, instruction is included in community wheelchair mobility skills such as up and down stairs, ramps, curbs, and on and off elevators.

Home Program

A home exercise program is developed to maintain the skills acquired during rehabilitation, to prevent regression, and to facilitate further progress. Before discharge, the patient receives a written copy of the home program and instruction in performing the activities listed. The home program may include exercise, proper positioning techniques, ADL techniques, energy conservation principles, safety measures, instructions in care of the residual limb, and wheelchair maintenance.

Wheelchairs and Cushions

Wheelchairs are ordered for the nonambulatory patient and the ambulatory patient who needs assistance with long-distance community mobility. In selecting a wheelchair, consideration is given to the patient's size, weight, age, prognosis, and proposed wheelchair use. Lightweight and standard weight wheelchairs designed to accommodate amputation are available. If a standard wheelchair is used, adapters are needed to maintain proper chair balance. Wraparound armrests, detachable desk arms, swing-away elevating legrests, pneumatic tires, zipper backs, detachable backs, grade-aids, and reduced widths are some of the wheelchair options available to meet individual needs.[27]

Patients whose unilateral LE amputation is a result of PVD have a 33% chance of having bilateral LE amputation within 5 years.[9] If these individuals choose to purchase a wheelchair, detachable armrests should be ordered to allow for potential consequences of PVD, which may necessitate sliding board transfers in the future. Wheelchair cushions are available for those individuals who spend prolonged time sitting in the wheelchair. The cushions are designed to minimize pressure on bony prominences. Several varieties are available including foam, gel, or air-filled interiors. A wheelchair cushion pressure evaluation may be indicated before ordering the cushion.

Bathroom Equipment

Most persons with LE amputation find that the use of adaptive bathroom equipment provides increased safety in bathing and toileting. Proper use of bath and shower benches assists the patient to bathe independently. Without a bath bench, it is necessary either to transfer to the bottom of the tub or to stand while bathing. A survey of 130 individuals with amputation found that 55% of the respondents had difficulty bathing. These patients had not received occupational therapy.[13]

Grab bars may be affixed to walls or clasped on the side of the tub to aid with transfers and with dynamic balance activities performed while bathing. Soap dishes and towel racks cannot substitute for grab bars because they are not designed to hold body weight and are easily detached from the wall. A raised toilet seat and/or a toilet versa frame facilitate independent toilet transfers. If the bathroom is inaccessible, a commode chair and alternate bathing arrangements are indicated.

Physical Environment

An evaluation of the patient's physical environment assists the occupational therapist in determining whether or not structural modifications are required at home or at work. If stairs render the environment inaccessible, a ramp is needed. The preferred gradient is 1 foot (30 cm) of length for each inch (2.5 cm) of rise. The ramp width needs to allow for unobstructed wheelchair maneuvering. Ramp landings approximately 2 feet × 5 feet (6.1 cm × 152 cm) are needed to accommodate wheelchairs and doorways.[3]

The physical environment influences wheelchair width and the types of transfers used. To pass through a doorway, a standard wheelchair needs a minimal clearance of 2 feet 6 inches (76 cm). To self-propel a wheelchair in a hallway, a minimum of 3 feet 2 inches (97 cm) is needed. Minor modifications can be made to improve safety including the removal of scatter rugs, electrical cords, and casters on furniture. Wooden bed or chair blocks can be made to increase their stability and height thereby easing transfers.[3]

SUMMARY

Acquired LE amputations can occur as a result of trauma, infection, neoplasms, electrical or thermal injuries, and vascular diseases. Occupational therapists play an important role in the rehabilitation of the person with LE amputation. The purpose of occupational therapy intervention is to promote function in the occupational performance areas of ADL, work, and play or leisure. Evaluation of occupational performance areas and performance components provides a baseline for intervention.

In rehabilitation for LE amputation, the performance components addressed are derived from the sensorimotor, cognitive, and social areas. Therapeutic activities are analyzed, graded, and incorporated into the treatment plan for eventual resumption of occupational roles.

SAMPLE TREATMENT PLAN

This sample treatment plan is limited to a discussion of four problems and suggested modes of treatment that occur during the acute phase of rehabilitation. It serves as an introduction to occupational therapy intervention and is not designed to be a comprehensive program.

CASE STUDY

History
Mr. M is 48 years of age. He was admitted to the acute hospital for a left knee disarticulation. Significant past medical history includes: right below-knee amputation (approximately one year previous to this admission), insulin-dependent diabetes mellitus (IDDM), and end-stage renal disease (ESRD). Patient presently receives renal dialysis three times per week.

Sociocultural environment
Mr. M lives alone, is unemployed, and receives state aid. He is engaged to marry in approximately 18 months. His fiancée currently assists with home management activities such as cleaning, shopping, transportation, and household maintenance. He is responsible for meal preparation activities during the day. He does not drive.

Physical environment
Patient resides in a single-level home where there are no stairs. The bathroom is wheelchair-accessible and equipped with a commode and shower stall with a glass door. There is no adaptive bathroom equipment. The patient currently owns a lightweight wheelchair, front-wheeled walker, and a wheelchair cushion.

Personal data
Name: CM
Age: 48
Diagnosis: Left knee disarticulation; status post right BKA.
Treatment aims as stated in referral: OT evaluation and treatment

OTHER SERVICES
Medical
Physical therapy
Social work

Frame of reference
Occupational performance

Treatment approaches
Biomechanical and rehabilitative

OT EVALUATION

Performance components
Sensorimotor
  Pain: *Test and observe*
  Fine motor coordination, manipulation, and dexterity: Test and observe
  Activity tolerance: *Observe*
  Range of motion: *Test*
  Muscle strength: *Test*
  Physical endurance: *Observe*
  Postural control: *Test and observe*
  Soft tissue integrity: *Observe*
Cognitive/Cognitive Integration
  Orientation: *Test and observe*
  Memory: *Test*
  Problem solving: *Test and observe*
    Safety judgment: *Test and observe*
    Generalization of learning: *Test and observe*
    Body image: *Test and observe*
Psychosocial/Psychological
    Self-concept: *Observe*
    Affect: *Observe*
    Coping skills: *Observe*
    Social support: *Interview and observe*
    Interpersonal relationships: *Interview and observe*

Performance areas
  ADL: *Observe and test*
  Productive or work: *Observe and test*
  Leisure: *Observe and test*

SAMPLE TREATMENT PLAN – cont'd

EVALUATION SUMMARY

This 48-year-old male is pleasant, cooperative, and motivated for therapy. Before admission he was independent in ADL and light meal preparation activities. This evaluation reveals normal muscle strength. Presently, assistance is needed with all self-care activities.

Assets

Good bilateral upper extremity strength
Motivated to return to independent living

Problem list

1. Poor activity tolerance and physical endurance
2. At risk for contractures of the residual limb and skin breakdown
3. Severe pain and edema in left residual limb
4. Discharge plans are undetermined

PROBLEM 1: POOR ACTIVITY TOLERANCE AND PHYSICAL ENDURANCE

Objective

Increase activity tolerance and physical endurance in preparation for discharge

Method

Recommend to physician that bed rest orders be discontinued and to change activity orders to "out of bed as tolerated"
Establish PRE program
Practice wheelchair mobility activities

Gradation

Increase resistance of weights
Increase repetitions
Increase wheelchair mobility distance
Increase duration of therapy
Increase wheelchair sitting tolerance
Increase time patient is able to hold a wheelchair push-up

PROBLEM 2: AT RISK FOR CONTRACTURES OF THE RESIDUAL LIMB AND SKIN BREAKDOWN

Objective

Prevent contractures and skin breakdown

Method

Instruct patient in prone-lying position in bed
Adapt wheelchair
Fabricate knee extension splint
Establish positioning schedule
Instruct patient in pressure relief techniques in bed and in wheelchair
Instruct patient in skin inspection techniques

Gradation

Increase time in prone-lying
Increase time splint is used
Increase time patient holds wheelchair push-up
Decrease therapist assistance in pressure relief and skin inspection techniques

PROBLEM 3: SEVERE PAIN AND EDEMA IN LEFT RESIDUAL LIMB LIMIT PARTICIPATION IN THERAPY

Objective

Reduce pain and edema to allow full participation in therapy.

Method

Instruct patient in limb wrapping and desensitization techniques
Elevate limb in bed and in wheelchair

Gradation

Decrease assistance in wrapping residual limb
Grade desensitization techniques from light touch to firm pressure, tapping and rubbing
Increase duration of therapy

SAMPLE TREATMENT PLAN – cont'd

PROBLEM 4: UNDETERMINED DISCHARGE PLANS

Objective
Identify appropriate discharge site.

Determine appropriate discharge placement
Recommend discharge site to appropriate team members

Method
Consult with patient, fiancée, and other members of team

RECOMMENDATIONS
Initiate diabetic teaching
Psychology consult

Transfer patient to a rehabilitation facility

REVIEW QUESTIONS

1. Define the following abbreviations: AKA, IDDM, and PVD.
2. Which leg functions are lost and which functions are maintained in a BKA?
3. Name two common postsurgical problems that can interfere with rehabilitation of the person with LE amputation. How is each resolved?
4. What are the purposes of preoperative therapy?
5. What is the most common cause of LE amputation?
6. Describe the desired bed and wheelchair positions for the person with AKA following surgery.
7. List three methods for reducing edema in the residual limb.
8. What methods can be used to teach donning pants?
9. State two reasons why the patient should lie prone.
10. What is the purpose of a therapeutic exercise program?
11. What additional problems might one expect to observe in an older person or one with diabetes who has had an amputation?
12. What type of wheelchair is needed for someone with an LE amputation? Why?
13. List the immediate postoperative concerns. How do occupational therapists address these concerns?
14. What types of transfers are included in the treatment plan?
15. How can bed mobility activities, upper extremity exercise, postural control activities, and dressing techniques be incorporated in a single treatment session?
16. List several ways to grade wheelchair mobility activities.
17. Describe two methods of limb wrapping. What are the advantages and disadvantages of each technique?
18. Describe some of the home adaptations that can be made to increase safety and independence for the patient with an LE amputation.
19. What is the role of the occupational therapist in the predriving or driving evaluation?
20. What types of discharge equipment are ordered or recommended by the occupational therapist?

REFERENCES

1. American Amputee Foundation: *National Amputee Resource Directory*, P.O. Box 55218, Hillcrest Station, Little Rock, AR 77225.
2. American Occupational Therapy Association: Uniform terminology for occupational therapy, ed 3, *Am J Occup Ther* 48(11):1047-10154, 1994.
3. Banerjee SJ: *Rehabilitation management of amputees*, Baltimore, 1982, Williams & Wilkins.
4. Borcich D, Beukma L, and Olves T: *Amputee care: a handout for patients with below knee amputations*, Stanford, CA, 1986, Department of Physical and Occupational Therapy, Stanford University Hospital. (Unpublished.)
5. Christiansen C, Baum C, editors: *Occupational therapy overcoming human performance deficits*, Thorofare, NJ, 1991, Slack Inc.
6. Engstrand JL: Rehabilitation of the patient with a lower extremity amputation, *Nurs Clin North Am* 11:4, 1976.
7. Friedman LW: *The psychological rehabilitation of the amputee*, Springfield, IL, 1978, Charles C Thomas.
8. Friedman LW: Rehabilitation of the amputee. In Goodgold J, editor: *Rehabilitation medicine*, St Louis, 1988, CV Mosby.
9. Goldberg RT: New trends in the rehabilitation of lower extremity amputees, *Rehabil Lit* 45:2, 1984.

10. Hill SL: Interventions for the elderly amputee, *Rehabil Nurs* 10:23, 1985.
11. Hirschberg G, Lewis L, Thomas D: *Rehabilitation*, Philadelphia, 1964, JB Lippincott.
12. Kathrins RJ: Lower extremity amputations. In Logigian MK, editor: *Adult rehabilitation: a team approach for therapists,* Boston, 1982, Little, Brown.
13. Kegel B, Carpenter ML, Burgess EM: Functional capabilities of lower extremity amputees, *Arch Phys Med Rehabil* 59:109, March 1978.
14. Kegel B, Webster J, Burgess EM: Recreational activities of lower extremity amputees: a survey, *Arch Phys Med Rehabil* 61:258, June 1980.
15. Larson CB, Gould M: *Orthopedic nursing,* ed 8, St Louis, 1974, CV Mosby.
16. O'Sullivan S, Cullen K, Schmitz T: *Physical rehabilitation: evaluation and treatment procedures,* Philadelphia, 1981, FA Davis.
17. Palmer ML, Toms JE: *Manual for functional training,* ed 3, Philadelphia, 1982, FA Davis.
18. Reed KL, Sanderson SN: *Concepts of occupational therapy,* ed 3, Baltimore, 1992, Williams & Wilkins.
19. Reinstein L, Ashley J, Miller KH: Sexual adjustment after lower extremity amputation, *Arch Phys Med Rehabil* 59:501, November 1978.
20. Rusk H, Taylor E: *Rehabilitation medicine: a textbook of physical medicine and rehabilitation,* ed 2, St Louis, 1964, CV Mosby.
21. Shands A, Raney R, Brashear H: *Handbook of orthopaedic surgery,* ed 8, St Louis, 1971, CV Mosby.
22. Spencer EA: Amputations. In Hopkins HL, Smith HD, editors: *Willard and Spackman's occupational therapy,* ed 5, Philadelphia, 1978, JB Lippincott.
23. Spencer EA: Functional restoration: section 3, amputations and prosthetic replacement. In Hopkins HL, Smith HD, editors: *Willard and Spackman's occupational therapy,* ed 8, Philadelphia, 1993, JB Lippincott.
24. Stoner EK: Management of the lower extremity amputee. In Kottke FJ, Stillwell GK, Lehmann JF: *Krusen's handbook of physical medicine and rehabilitation,* ed 3, Philadelphia, 1982, WB Saunders.
25. Wellerson TL: *A manual for occupational therapists on the rehabilitation of upper extremity amputees,* Dubuque, Iowa, 1958, Wm C Brown.
26. *Wheelchair catalog,* Camarillo, Calif, 1980, Everest & Jennings.
27. *Wheelchair prescription booklet no. 3: safety and handling,* Camarillo, Calif, 1983, Everest & Jennings.

Burns and Burn Rehabilitation

Cheryl Leman Jordan, Rebekah Reishus Allely

It has been estimated that each year 2 million people in the United States sustain a burn injury; approximately 200,000 are hospitalized.[23] Since the early 1970s, advances in the medical, surgical, and rehabilitation management of burn survivors have expanded the focus of burn care professionals from patient survival to include the quality of life following a burn injury. Although functional recovery may be a long and arduous process, most burn survivors can expect to return as close as possible to their preinjury level of function. From the time the burn victim is admitted to the hospital through the outpatient phase of care, a multidisciplinary team approach is necessary to manage the medical, functional, and psychosocial problems encountered during burn recovery.

THE SKIN

The skin is the largest organ of the body and primarily serves as an environmental barrier. Included in its functions are sensation, thermoregulation, protection from chemical or bacterial invasion and ultraviolet rays, and prevention of loss of body fluids. Anatomically the skin consists of two layers: (1) the epidermis, a nonvascular layer made up of epidermal cells, and (2) the dermis, a network of capillaries, sweat glands, sebaceous glands, nerve endings, and hair follicles[16] (Fig. 33-1). When the skin is damaged a myriad of systemic, physiological, and functional problems can occur. In a burn injury the skin and possibly the underlying structures are damaged, causing a destruction of the environmental barrier. It is one of the most severe forms of trauma to the body, and it can be a life-threatening injury in severe cases.

BURN INJURY DESCRIPTION

Following a burn injury many factors must be taken into consideration in determining the severity of injury and its treatment needs. Functional recovery potential can also be predicted from an analysis of these factors. Primary considerations are the mechanism of injury, the extent and depth of the burn, specific body areas burned, other associated injuries such as inhalation injury, and the individual's age, past medical history, and preinjury health.

MECHANISM OF INJURY

Burns are categorized as thermal, chemical, and electrical. Thermal injuries can be caused by flame, steam, hot liquid, hot metals, and extreme cold.[16] The severity of the injury depends on the area exposed and the duration and intensity of thermal exposure. Superficial partial-thickness burns occur after a brief contact with hot liquids or flames. Deep partial-thickness burns are caused by longer exposure to intense heat, such as with hot water immersion scalds or contact of the skin with flaming materials. Full-thickness burns result from prolonged immersion or contact with flaming materials, contact with hot oil, tar, or chemical agents and electrical contact.

BURN DEPTH

The depth of burn is estimated from clinical observation of the appearance, sensitivity, and pliability of the wound.[60] A burn injury was traditionally classified as first, second, and third degree; now it is described as superficial, partial-thickness, or full-thickness injury (Table 33-1).

PERCENT TOTAL BODY SURFACE AREA INVOLVED

The extent of the burn is classified as a percentage of the total body surface area (%TBSA) burned. Two methods used to estimate burn size are the rule of nines and the Lund and Browder chart.[54] The rule of nines divides the body surface into areas of 9% or multiples of 9%, with the perineum making up the final 1%. Although simple, the rule of nines is relatively inaccurate (Fig. 33-2).

The Lund and Browder chart[40] provides a more accu-

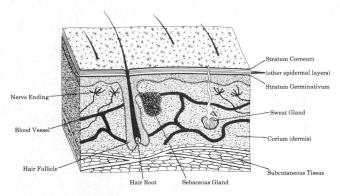

FIG. 33-1   Cross section of skin. (From Iles RL: *Wound care: the skin,* Marion Laboratories, 1988, p. 2, with permission.)

rate estimate of the body surface area involved and is used in most burn centers. This chart assigns a percent of surface area to body segments (Fig. 33-3). A patient's palm print, excluding the fingers, is approximately 1% of the TBSA, and may be used as a quick estimate of burn surface area involvement.

SEVERITY OF INJURY

The %TBSA and depth of burn are primary indicators of severity of injury; however, depending on the patient's age and preinjury health, small partial- or full-thickness burn wounds (<20% TBSA) can be a severe burn injury. A burn involving more than 20% of the body is frequently the determining factor for admission to a burn intensive care unit. An adult with a deep partial- and full-thickness burn of greater than 30% TBSA has a severe burn. The time involved in achieving wound closure may be protracted, and functional recovery will require intensive rehabilitation.

Burn involvement of certain body areas is also used to classify injury severity, although the %TBSA burn is limited. For example, deep partial- or full-thickness burns of the hands, face, or perineum are usually considered severe burns.[60]

MEDICAL MANAGEMENT
INITIAL CARE

A burn injury causes translocation of body fluids. Immediately following a burn injury, there is increased permeability of blood vessels, causing rapid leakage of protein-rich fluid into extravascular tissue, thus resulting in intravascular hypovolemia.[44] Burn shock can occur because of decreased plasma volume, blood volume, and cardiac output, all results of extensive intravascular fluid loss.[20] Fluid resuscitation, by using an intravenous fluid such as Lactated Ringer's solution, is essential to replace venous fluid and electrolytes. The fluid volume required is determined by various formulas, such as the Parkland and modified Brook formulas,[3] and is based on the extent of the burn and the weight of the patient. The rate of fluid infusion is monitored by pulse rate, urinary output, central venous pressure, and hematocrit.

The lymphatic system, which normally carries away excess fluid in the tissues, can become overloaded, causing subcutaneous edema. In the case of circumferential full-thickness burns, the edema can produce an increase in interstitial pressure sufficient to impair capillary filling of the distal portion of the extremity, causing limb ischemia.[16] Escharotomy, or incision of the eschar (necrotic tissue), is performed to relieve such pressure and is usually painless because of the destroyed nerve endings (Fig. 33-4). In deep wounds a fasciotomy or an incision down to the fascia is occasionally needed for adequate pressure relief.

Inhalation injury is a common secondary diagnosis with thermal injury, especially in facial burns, and can cause mortality in burn patients. When there is objective evidence of inhalation injury, bronchoscopy, arterial blood gas, and chest x-ray examinations are used to confirm the diagnosis. Nasotracheal intubation and ventilatory support may be required along with vigorous respiratory therapy and nasotracheal suctioning. A tracheostomy is generally not performed unless medically necessary.[61]

TABLE 33-1	Burn Wound Characteristics		
BURN DEPTH	**HISTOLOGIC DEPTH**	**CLINICAL DESCRIPTION**	**HEALING**
Superficial (First degree)	Superficial epidermis	Dry, painful, erythema	3 to 7 days
Partial Thickness: (Second degree)			
Superficial	Epidermis	Large fluid-filled, blisters; red, weepy; pain	7 to 21 days, minimal or no scar, pigment changes
Deep	Epidermis and part of dermis	Mottled white and/or hemorraghic with or without pain	>21 days, may have scar and pigment changes
Full Thickness (Third degree)	Epidermis, dermis, may involve tendons and subcutaneous tissue	Dry, leathery, no blisters, charred, blood vessels visible, no pain	Grafting required, pigment changes, scarring, disfigurement

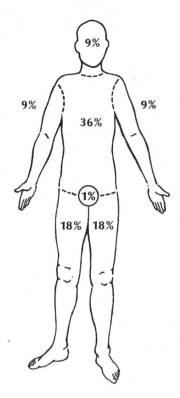

FIG. 33-2   Rule of nines.

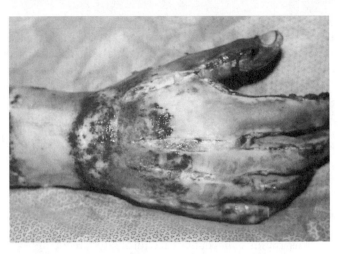

FIG. 33-4   Escharotomies on dorsum of hand with full thickness burn injury.

WOUND CARE

After fluid resuscitation has been started, attention is directed to wound care. Daily hydrotherapy is carried out in the Hubbard tank or tub to allow thorough cleansing of the wound and uninvolved areas. Various topical agents are available to treat burn injuries; their purpose is

to delay colonization and reduce bacterial counts in the wounds.[20] Burn wound colonization begins at the moment of injury; normal bacterial flora can be replaced by gram-negative organisms. Wound cultures and biopsies are performed when there are signs or symptoms of severe infection. Septic shock can occur, which is a state of circulatory collapse and a cardiovascular response to bacteria and their by-products (endotoxins). The syndrome is characterized by ischemia, diminished urine output, tachycardia, hypotension, tachypnea, hypothermia, disorientation, or coma.

Although all burn wounds are treated with some type of topical antibacterial agent, these agents do not substitute for surgical treatment if the need is indicated. When the depth and extent of the wound are known to require

AREA	ADULT	2°	3°	DONOR SITE	TOTAL
HEAD	7				
NECK	2				
ANTERIOR TRUNK	13				
POSTERIOR TRUNK	13				
RIGHT BUTTOCK	2.5				
LEFT BUTTOCK	2.5				
GENITALIA	1				
RIGHT UPPER ARM	4				
LEFT UPPER ARM	4				
RIGHT FOREARM	3				
LEFT FOREARM	3				
RIGHT HAND	2.5				
LEFT HAND	2.5				
RIGHT THIGH	9.5				
LEFT THIGH	9.5				
RIGHT LEG	7				
LEFT LEG	7				
RIGHT FOOT	3.5				
LEFT FOOT	3.5				
	TOTAL				

FIG. 33-3   Chart for calculating %TBSA. (Adaptation of Lund and Browder chart, from Burn Center at Washington Hospital Center, with permission.)

3 or more weeks for healing, surgery is generally needed to decrease burn morbidity and mortality. Surgical treatment for burns consists of excision (removal) of the burned tissue (eschar) and placement of skin grafts.

There are essentially three types of grafts: (1) xenograft, (2) homograft, and (3) autograft. A xenograft or heterograft is processed pigskin, and a homograft or allograft is processed cadaver skin. These are used as biological dressings to provide temporary wound coverage and pain relief. An autograft is a surgical transplantation of the person's own skin from an unburned area (donor site) and applied to the clean excised tissues of the burn wound (graft site). As the size of a survivable burn increases, available donor sites for autografting decrease. For this reason, alternatives to autografts are being explored. Examples of such alternatives are epidermal cultured skin substitutes[19] and cultured epidermal autograft (CEA).[5,11] When the wound is limited in size but the defect is so deep that tendon survival or graft adherence is extremely doubtful, microvascular skin flaps are used.

Adequate nutrition is essential during wound healing, because the metabolic rate of the burn patient is greatly increased and the protein, vitamin, mineral, and calorie needs are correspondingly increased.[20,41] Protein is essential for wound healing and must be provided in substantial amounts. Nutritional requirements are calculated based on the %TBSA and patient's admission weight. Calorie counts and the patient's weight are monitored daily to ensure adequate nutrition. If the patient is unable to meet individual requirements through diet, high-protein and calorie supplements are given either orally or through a nasogastric tube. Intravenous hyperalimentation is frequently necessary with severe burns of extensive %TBSA. As wound closure is achieved, nutritional demands decrease and the individual's eating habits must again be changed.

ASSOCIATED PROBLEMS
SCAR FORMATION

Hypertrophic scar and contracture frequently develop after burn wound healing. Most burn wounds have a hyperemic, flat appearance upon healing. As wound maturation advances, the wound's appearance may worsen as a result of scar formation. The quality of burn wound maturation can be affected by numerous factors, some of which occur during the early phases of burn care.[24,36] The time needed to achieve wound closure is a strong determinant. Bacterial infections in the wound increase the inflammatory response that can delay wound healing and also contribute to scar formation.[30]

Race and age as well as the location and depth of the burn wound have been reported anecdotally to influence hypertrophic scarring.[15,55] Hypertrophic scars are thick, rigid, red scars that become apparent 6 to 8 weeks after wound closure is achieved.[1] Histologically, these immature scars have increased vascularity, fibroblasts, myofi-

broblasts, fibroclasts, collagen fibers in whorls or nodules, and mast cells.[6,45] Biochemical investigations of hypertrophic scars have disclosed increased synthesis of collagen and connective tissue.

As hypertrophic scars mature, capillaries, fibroblasts, and myofibroblasts decrease significantly, with the collagen becoming arranged in parallel bands. The time needed for scars to mature differs markedly among individuals. Superficial burns that heal in less than 2 weeks generally will not form scar, whereas wounds that become hypertrophic may take up to 1 or 2 years to mature.[36]

The following is a summary of the characteristics of a hypertrophic scar:
1. Marked increase in vascularity. A scar that remains hyperemic at the end of 2 months following healing and becomes progressively firmer will become hypertrophic.
2. Marked increase in fibroblasts, myofibroblasts, collagen, and interstitial material. The contractile properties of fibroblasts, myofibroblasts, collagen, and interstitial material may exert sufficient force to cause contractures.
3. Voluntary muscle contraction. Most patients prefer to assume a flexed, adducted position for comfort, which permits the new collagen fibers in the wound to fuse together. The collagen becomes compact and piled up in whorls and nodules, which results in scar contracture.
4. Collagen linkage is less stable in new scars. New hypertrophic scar contracture is easily influenced by mechanical forces.

PSYCHOSOCIAL FACTORS

During hospitalization, the patient is often confronted with isolation, dependency, and pain. Because burn injuries and treatment procedures are often painful, narcotic analgesia is often liberally used.[33] Relaxation and imagery techniques are also employed to reduce stress and anxiety. The amount of narcotic analgesia given is gradually decreased as the wound heals, and patients usually require minimal pain medications on discharge.

Potential psychological reactions following a burn injury include the following: depression; withdrawal reactions to disfigurement; regression; anxiety and uncertainty about the ability to resume work, family, community, and leisure roles; and existential crisis.[17] Adjustment of the burn patient can be facilitated by providing emotional support, education, and helping the patient to develop coping mechanisms and self-direction. However, burn injuries can also result in positive changes including a reassessment of one's personal values and an appreciation of one's life. To determine how people will adjust psychologically to burn injury, consider the complex interaction between premorbid personality style, extent of injury, and social and environmental contexts.[43]

BURN REHABILITATION

THE TEAM AND PHASES OF RECOVERY

Successful care and rehabilitation of burn victims requires a multidisciplinary team approach.[3,50] This team approach begins immediately upon the patient's admission to the hospital and continues through and beyond hospitalization. The burn care team is composed of physicians, nurses, physical and occupational therapists, dietitians, social workers, respiratory therapists, art and play therapists, recreational therapists, clergy, and vocational counselors.[36,52]

Rehabilitation management of burn victims can be divided into three overlapping phases to aid in categorizing and determining effective treatment goals. These phases of recovery are as follows: (1) acute care, (2) surgical and postoperative, and (3) rehabilitation, inpatient and outpatient.[36]

The acute care phase is the first 72 hours following a major burn injury. When the burn is superficial partial thickness and heals per primam (primarily on its own) in less than two weeks, the time from injury until epithelial healing can also be considered acute care.[49] This phase is often the only burn care a person experiences if the wound is superficial.

The surgical and postoperative phase follows the acute phase and continues for varying lengths of time depending on the size of the burn injury. During this period vulnerability to wound infection, sepsis, and septic shock is especially great; medical treatment is focused on promoting healing and minimizing infection.

The final phase can extend for an indeterminate length of time. This phase is the postgrafting period when the patient is medically stable. The rehabilitation phase covers both inpatient and outpatient care. It is affected by the quality of wound healing, scar formation, and need for rehabilitation. It is the most challenging phase of all for burn patients and their families.

GOALS OF REHABILITATION

The entire burn team is involved in some aspect of burn rehabilitation, whether for verbal support during patient self-feeding or just reinforcing the importance of motion. The long-term goals of occupational therapy are fairly synonymous with the long-term goals of the burn team. This fact is easily understood considering the innate functional, cosmetic, and psychosocial consequences with a severe burn injury. Although specific goals may be the responsibility of various team members, everyone is focused on the same outcome. Role delineation between occupational and physical therapy differs by burn care facility; therefore, it is essential that the two disciplines work closely together and communicate frequently so patients benefit from the skills and viewpoints of both disciplines. Treatment goals will be presented as goals of rehabilitation. Inherent in this concept is the close communication and cooperation of burn team members.

Acute Care Phase

During the acute care phase, medical management is of utmost importance for survival of the patient, and the goal of occupational therapy is primarily preventive. As the patient recovers and wound closure progresses, the nature of the activities with the patient also changes, with treatment being directed at restoring function. Initially, however, when the wounds are partial- or full-thickness, the acute care rehabilitation goals are as follows:

1. Prevent loss of joint and skin mobility.
2. Prevent loss of strength and endurance.
3. Control edema.
4. Promote self-care skills.
5. Begin orientation and patient education about therapy.

Surgical and Postoperative Phase

Rehabilitation goals during the surgical and postoperative phase are aimed at preserving or assisting function while supporting surgical objectives. Excision and grafting procedures require periods of immobilization of the area treated. The preferred position and length of immobilization vary by physician preference and burn center; however, the range is from 1 to 7 days.[9,21,26,39,53] During this phase the goals of rehabilitation are as follows:

1. Fabricate splints and establish positioning techniques to support the surgeon's postoperative care orders.
2. Provide adaptive equipment when needed to increase self-care.
3. Provide orientation activities when necessary.
4. Provide exercise for areas not immobilized to prevent thrombophlebitis and disuse atrophy.
5. Continue patient and family education.

Rehabilitation Phase

The third phase of recovery is the rehabilitation phase, which begins as wound closure occurs. Individuals with large %TBSA burns frequently enter this phase needing further surgery; however, the majority of their wounds are closed and wound maturation is commencing. The focus of care during this phase is maximal self-care independence and controlled scar maturation to prevent deformity and contracture formation. Patient and family education is especially important to develop competence with care in preparation for discharge.

The rehabilitation phase is the most challenging for everyone because it extends past hospital discharge until wound maturation is complete. Before discharge from the hospital, emphasis is on independence and education. Once the individual is home, psychological support and intervention are often needed to restore motivation and self-confidence. Support is needed to cope with the physical and psychological ramifications of a severe burn injury.

Wound maturation is said to take approximately one year following injury; however, it is important to remember that each patient may react differently. Some wounds may mature in less than a year while others may take up to 2 years.[50] The goals of rehabilitation for this phase are exhaustive, but understandably so considering the potentially disabling effects of burn scar.[36] Goals are as follows:

1. Teach independent self-care skills.
2. Provide education and practice of home care activities, including appropriate exercise, positioning, and skin care.
3. Restore muscle strength and endurance.
4. Improve joint mobility and coordination.
5. Fit splints, compression and vascular support garments, and pressure adapters for edema and scar maturation control.[36]
6. Support reacquisition of social and vocational skills.
7. Provide instruction on skin and scar care techniques.
8. Provide education and potential changes in sensation.
9. Control edema and minimize scar hypertrophy when needed.
10. Teach compensation techniques for limiting exposure to ultraviolet light, chemical irritants, friction, and extremes of weather and temperature.[49]
11. Implement a plan that supports resumption of school, work, and participation in recreational activities.

ROLE OF OCCUPATIONAL THERAPY
ASSESSMENT

Occupational therapy plays an important role in both short- and long-term patient outcomes following a burn injury. While medical issues are a primary concern during acute care, there is no substitute for early and consistent intervention by the occupational therapist. Whenever possible the occupational therapist should complete an initial patient evaluation within the first 24 to 48 hours following hospital admission. Burn cause, past medical history, and any secondary diagnoses are obtained from the medical chart. A visual assessment of the wounds is done to determine the extent and depth of injury, noting any critical areas involved. Patient interview is used to establish rapport and to obtain specific information such as hand dominance; any previous functional limitations; preinjury daily activities including job, school, and home responsibilities; and psychological status. In the case of a severe burn requiring patient intubation, this information should be obtained from immediate family members or significant others as soon as possible.

Function of the body areas involved is the primary concern; however, it is important to establish a baseline of overall physical function before treatment planning.[36] Involved and noninvolved areas should be evaluated for strength, joint mobility, and sensation. A goniometer should be used for evaluation of range of motion (ROM) to ensure accuracy in recorded measurements. Before a ROM evaluation, the therapist should explain the purpose and what is involved, including the types of movements and the number of repetitions. Continually talking to the patient and offering encouragement may help to decrease anxiety. Gently guiding the individual through a specific motion can aid in ensuring achievement of full range. If pain, edema, tight eschar, or bulky dressings limit full ROM, this fact should be documented. Although active ROM should be assessed whenever possible, passive ROM of all extremities should be evaluated when a patient is unresponsive.

If the individual had normal functional muscle strength before injury, an initial test of gross muscle strength may not be needed if the ROM assessment revealed adequate strength to work against gravity. If the burn was an electrical contact injury, if severe edema is present causing a possible compartment syndrome, or other musculoskeletal or neurological injuries are suspected, however, a manual muscle test of major muscle groups should be performed.[63] If the hand is not involved or the burn is superficial partial-thickness, a dynamometer and pinch gauge are used for grip and pinch strength evaluation.

Assessment of activities of daily living (ADL) is initially done by interview with the patient. If the burn injury is severe, the ADL evaluation is often postponed (no more than 7 days) until the patient is medically stable and able to participate with therapy. Individuals with less severe burns and who are not intubated may be evaluated for basic ADL, such as the ability to feed self, basic grooming skills, and donning/doffing of hospital gowns. It is important to note any compensatory actions or awkward movements used to complete the activity. Any abnormal patterns should be discussed to determine if they were present before the injury.

After completion of an initial assessment (Table 33-2), the treatment plan should be formulated. The need for splints or positioning equipment is identified, as are potential problem areas. The plan should be logical and in accordance with those of other team members. Two fundamental principles should be kept in mind when working in burn rehabilitation: (1) the main factor that can hinder postburn functional recovery is the formation of scar contractures, and (2) severe scars and contractures are often preventable.[47] Therefore, most burn rehabilitation treatment techniques and objectives are directed at prevention and restoration.

ACUTE CARE PHASE TREATMENTS

The objective in positioning is to limit edema formation and to maintain involved extremities in an antideformity position. This step is critical because the position of

TABLE 33-2	Burn Rehabilitation Evaluation Components	
INITIAL	**INPATIENT REHAB**	**OUTPATIENT REHAB**
Burn cause	Graft adherence	
%TBSA, depth of burn	Skin/Scar condition	Skin/Scar condition
Area(s) involved	Contracture concerns	Compression garment fit
Age, hand dominance	Edema (if present)	Volumetrics if needed
Functional Status	ADL performance level	ADL performance level
Occupation	Work skills	Work skills
ROM and strength	Active and passive ROM	Active and passive ROM
Mobility and endurance	Strength and endurance	Strength and endurance
Developmental level (child)	Developmental level (child)	Developmental level (child)
Psychological status	Psychological status	Psychological status
Social support	Social support	Social support
Leisure activities	Leisure activities	Leisure activities
	Compression garment needs	Compression garment needs
	Home management	Home management
		Home care understanding
		Return to work capacity
		Return to school potential

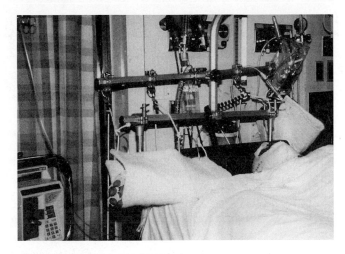

FIG. 33-5 Shoulder positioning using overhead traction and felt slings.

comfort for the patient is the position of contracture.[34,36] To use positioning techniques effectively, protective posturing should be understood. This posture generally consists of adduction and flexion of the upper extremities, flexion of the hips and knees, and plantar flexion of the ankles. Hands are held in a dysfunctional position with wrist flexion.

During the initial wound assessment, positioning needs are determined by (1) observing the surface areas burned, (2) considering the posture the individual will assume, and (3) determining if that posture would limit function if allowed. For example, if the burn injury involves the shoulder, chest, and axilla, the patient should be positioned in 90° of shoulder abduction using arm boards or overhead traction (Fig. 33-5). Achieving full shoulder abduction with frequent exercise and activity is also critical to preventing loss of abduction as wound healing progresses. Once positioning needs are determined, nursing should be advised to ensure continuity throughout the day.

During acute care, positioning is instituted primarily to limit edema formation.[46] Elevation of the extremity at or slightly above heart level can limit the severity of distal edema formation. As wound closure progresses, attention should be directed to more proximal body positioning concerns[36] (Table 33-3).

Initial splinting is used for three reasons, as follows: (1) to provide positioning assistance, (2) to limit edema

formation, and (3) to prevent pressure. Splints are not used as consistently during acute care as they were in the past. When a splint is used during the acute phase it is generally static in design and applied when at rest, with activity and exercise emphasized during the day. Volar hand splints are indicated if a burned hand is highly edematous or if active motion is limited. The volar burn hand splint is designed to provide approximately 30° wrist extension, 50 to 70° metacarpophalangeal (MCP) joint flexion, full interphalangeal (IP) joints extension, and the thumb abducted and extended[36] (Fig. 33-6).

The splint should be fitted considering any possible pressure points and ensuring correct positioning. A hand splint fabricated shortly after hospital admission requires daily assessment and alteration as edema changes. It is secured in place with a figure-eight wrap of gauze bandage and disposable elastic wraps. Straps are not used on acute burn splints because of infection control concerns and the potential consequence of distal edema.

When there is a partial- or full-thickness burn to the external ear(s), protection is required to prevent further damage caused by pressure from pillows, dressings, or endotracheal tube straps. This ear protection splint, referred to as headgear, is fitted upon admission and worn (with modification) until the external ear burns have healed. It consists of two thermoplastic ear cups that are secured in place by a three-point stabilizing strapping technique.[32]

Patients' ability to perform self-care is often limited because of their medical needs during acute care. If they are on a ventilator, they are dependent on nursing for their self-care. When medically cleared to eat, the occupational therapist must assess feeding skills. Dressings and edema may modify initial self-feeding motions. If necessary to support independence, adaptive equipment may be used for a short time. Temporary adaptive equipment may include built-up and extended handles on utensils and a plate guard. Grooming is another self-care activity that can be encouraged. Again, temporary adap-

TABLE 33-3	Antideformity Positioning for Specific Body Areas Following Burn Injury	
BODY AREA	**ANTIDEFORMITY POSITION**	**EQUIPMENT/TECHNIQUE**
Neck	Neutral/slight extension	No pillow: conformer, Watusi collar, triple-component neck splint
Chest/Abdomen	Trunk extension, shoulder retraction	Lower top of bed, towel roll beneath spine, clavicle straps
Axilla	Shoulder abduction 90 to 100°	Arm boards, airplane splint, clavicle straps, overhead traction
Elbow/Forearm	Elbow extension, forearm neutral	Pillows, arm boards, conformer splints, dynamic splints
Wrist/Hand	Wrist extension 30°, thumb abducted and extended, MCP flexion 50 to 70°, IP extension	Elevate with pillows, volar burn hand splint
Hip/Thigh	Neutral extension, hips 10 to 15° abduction	Trochanter rolls, pillow between knees, wedges
Knee/Lower leg	Knee extension; anterior burn: slight flexion	Knee conformer, casts, elevate when sitting, dynamic splints
Ankle/Foot	Neutral to 0 to 5° dorsiflexion	Custom splint, cast, AFO*
Ears/Face	Prevent pressure	No pillows; Headgear[32]

* Ankle-foot orthosis.

tations may be indicated to support independence. Withdrawing adaptations as soon as possible should be a goal of therapy. The therapist must convey to the patient that the goal for all ADL is independence with normal movement patterns, within a normal time frame.

Ambulation is initiated as soon as the patient is medically cleared to get out of bed and walk. If the patient has a lower extremity burn it is necessary to apply elastic wraps in a figure-eight pattern from the metatarsal heads (including the heel) to the groin. Dangling of feet or static standing are avoided to limit edema formation and unnecessary discomfort.

In addition to functional activities, active exercise is a primary component in every burn treatment plan. Exercise techniques employed during acute care are not unique for the injury[36] (Fig. 33-7). Active, active-assisted, or passive exercises are used depending on the patient's condition. The focus of exercise in acute care is to preserve ROM and functional strength and to decrease edema.

Strength and endurance activities are introduced into the acute care treatment program as appropriate. These activities range from simple active movement to resistive activities as tolerated. The purpose of resistive exercise is to counteract the deconditioning effects of hospitalization.[38] An old adage was that exercise following a severe burn injury could overstress an already hypermetabolic

patient. Research and experience have shown that graded progressive exercise is not deleterious in acute burn recovery.[27]

Although patient education is the responsibility of all burn team members, occupational therapy program success is dependent upon patients' understanding of their long-term needs and responsibilities. Initial educational objectives should focus on developing an understanding of (1) stages of burn recovery, (2) the need for and importance of independent activity and motion, and (3) pain and stress management techniques. These goals are necessary because motivation and compliance with treatments are essential for successful outcomes.[18]

SURGICAL AND POSTOPERATIVE PHASE TREATMENTS

Excision and grafting procedures require a period of postoperative immobilization to allow for adherence and vascularization of the grafts.[14] The occupational therapist must discuss postoperative positioning needs with the physician and nurses before surgery so splints and positioning devices are ready immediately after the surgical procedure. A wide variety of materials and protocols are available; all have the common purposes of immobilizing

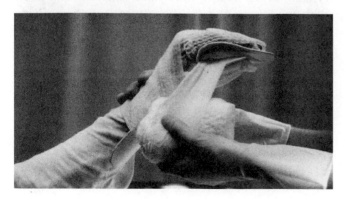

FIG. 33-6 Postburn hand splint. Note wrapping approach for thumb.

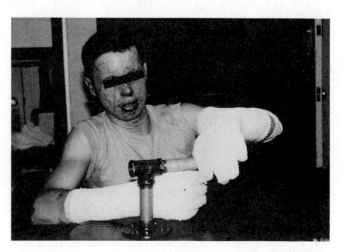

FIG. 33-7 Commonly used pipe tree is good activity for hand exercise following burn injury.

the grafted area, preventing edema, and assisting wound healing needs.[49]

Postoperative positioning techniques may use standard positioning techniques or may be unique, designed only for that surgical procedure. For example, when an axillary advancement flap is performed, the shoulder is abducted only 45° degrees. Gaining knowledge of the procedure performed and determining potential postoperative complications, such as suture line stress, enables the therapist to institute effective positioning procedures.

Although postoperative immobilization is frequently achieved through the use of bulky restrictive dressings and standard positioning equipment, splints are often needed to secure the position. Most splints are regularly made using plaster bandages or thermoplastics (Fig. 33-8). If a wet dressing will cover the graft site, a perforated or open-weave splinting material may be preferred to permit continuous drainage and to prevent graft maceration.[14] There are instances where movement of adjacent joints may disrupt graft adherence even though the graft does not cover the joint surface. In these cases, the splint design should incorporate immobilization of those joints in a functional position. A postoperative thermoplastic splint generally can be made by using a drape and trim technique.[14] Most postoperative splints are for temporary use and are discontinued once graft adherence is ensured.

Throughout the surgical phase of care, active and resistive exercise to the uninvolved extremities should be continued when possible to maintain ROM and strength. Immediately following excision and grafting procedures, exercises for adjacent body areas are discontinued for a short time. Although the time varies among burn centers, the average is 3 to 5 days, with 7 to 10 days for cultured epithelium grafts.[9,18,26] Exercises can be resumed as soon as graft adherence is obvious. Before resuming exercises, the occupational therapist should view the grafts and ad-

jacent areas to determine graft integrity and whether there are any exposed tendons.

Gentle active ROM is the treatment choice to avoid shearing of the new grafts. If the patient had good ROM before surgery and was immobilized for only 3 to 5 days, good ROM should be expected within 3 days following resumption of activity. Active exercise of a body area with a donor site is generally permitted after 2 to 3 days if there is no excessive bleeding. Lower extremity donor sites are treated similarly to lower extremity burns; therefore elevation and wrapping with elastic bandage are standard treatment.

Ambulation following lower extremity excision and grafting is usually not resumed until 5 to 7 days after surgery. With the physician's consent, the patient is then encouraged and assisted to ambulate for short distances and then slowly increase the distance. Before ambulation, double elastic bandage wraps are applied over a fluff gauze dressing to prevent graft shearing or vascular pooling. Wrapping with an elastic bandage, elevation, and avoidance of static stance are particularly important to protect lower extremity grafts. When the individual is able to walk, exercise on a stationary cycle ergometer is beneficial for increasing endurance.

Environmental stimulation, self-care, and leisure activities should be continued and increased if possible, commensurately with the patient's physical abilities and tolerance level. Self-care is often difficult during this phase owing to the immobilization positions necessary to ensure graft adherence. Creative ADL adaptations are frequently needed to allow patients some control of their care and environment during this time. Although only temporary, simple techniques such as prism glasses for those supine in bed, or universal cuffs and extended-handle utensils aid in preserving a feeling of self-worth and orientation. Continued verbal support and burn care education are also essential.

REHABILITATION PHASE TREATMENTS

During the inpatient rehabilitation phase, a thorough occupational therapy evaluation should emphasize assessment of performance skills. Active and passive ROM measurements should be taken, noting any beginning contractures. Muscle strength can be measured by the manual muscle test; however, this test should be done with caution when applying resistance on newly healed skin. Other components of the evaluation should include the following: muscular and cardiorespiratory endurance, performance of self-care and home management activities, skin and scar condition, presence of edema, and the need for compression garments (Table 33-2).

Treatment goals during inpatient rehabilitation are to (1) increase ROM, strength, and endurance; (2) achieve independence with self care; (3) familiarize the patient with the care necessary for discharge from the hospital; (4) aid psychological adjustment, and (5) begin skin conditioning and education. Although these goals are con-

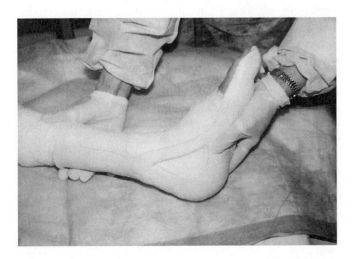

FIG. 33-8 Thermoplastic total-contact ankle dorsiflexion splint.

tinued and progressively increased through the outpatient rehabilitation phase, many other goals are added as the individual faces reintegration into the home and community.

The rehabilitation phase begins when a patient with a major burn injury is finally moved from the intensive care unit to a rehabilitation or step-down unit in the hospital and continues after the patient is discharged from the hospital. Being transferred from an intensive care unit, which implies that most of the wounds are closed, increases patient independence and ability to participate in therapy. Patients are encouraged to assume a more active role in establishing treatment goals. Discussions of work, recreation, and self-care skills are necessary to focus patients on returning to normal daily activities. A variety of rehabilitation equipment is introduced as methods to assist with increasing range, strength, and endurance.

Scar formation begins as wound closure occurs and results in patients frequently reporting increased tightness in joint movements or an inability to perform certain functional activities. To counteract the effects of scar maturation, numerous treatment techniques are advocated; skin conditioning (i.e., scar massage, lubrication, and interim garments), stretching before activity, and exercise are just a few examples.

Skin conditioning activities are used to improve skin tolerances for touch and shearing forces of garments, to decrease hypersensitivity, and to lubricate dry, newly healed skin. These activities are recommended for any individual whose burns healed per primam and those that required surgery to obtain timely wound closure. Lubrication and massage, using a nonwater-based cream, should be performed 3 to 4 times a day, or whenever the skin feels exceptionally dry, tight, or itchy. This action provides needed lubrication for skin that is dry because of damaged sweat and sebaceous glands; the massage is crucial for desensitizing grafted or newly healed skin. Instructions should be to massage using a rotary motion, gradually applying more pressure as tolerated over time.

Intermediate pressure garments are very beneficial for desensitization, general skin conditioning, edema control, and beginning scar management. The type of interim garment or bandage applied is dependent on how much pressure and shear force the individual can initially tolerate, and then is changed as tolerance gradually increases. Bandages and garments can be crudely graded in terms of pressure and shear force exerted by the consistency of the material and the technique used in application.[8] Elastic bandage wraps, self-adherent elastic wraps, tubular elastic support bandages, presized elastic pressure garments, and spandex garments custom-made by the therapist are commonly employed[2,42] (Fig. 33-9). Tubular elastic bandages, presized elastic garments and custom-made spandex gloves can be worn over minimal dressings and are routinely applied 5 to 7 days following removal of the postoperative dressing.

When patients have small open areas requiring mini-

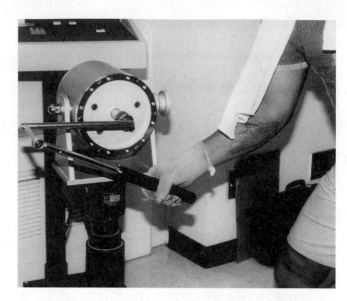

FIG. 33-9 Presized intermediate glove is worn all the time, including during exercise and activity, to condition skin and control edema.

mal wound care, a nylon can be used over the dressing to ease donning of tubular bandages while ensuring dressing placement underneath. Intermediate garments are worn consistently day and night, taken off only for bathing and massage. Independent donning and doffing of interim garments encourages active participation in self-care.

Every therapy session should begin by lubricating and massaging healed areas to prepare the dry or tight skin for increased motion. Patients should learn to perform their own skin care and be encouraged to do so independently before attending therapy. Once the scar/skin is lubricated, stretching is performed to increase flexibility and fluidity of movement.[37] Slow, sustained stretch is desired avoiding forceful dynamic stretch, with attention given to the position of adjacent joints during the stretching motion. Stretching in front of a full-length mirror is helpful for correcting abnormal postures.

Active ROM, strengthening, and endurance activities should follow stretching exercises. During the rehabilitation phase more complex motions must be emphasized. Flexibility motions that require movement of several joints simultaneously are complex motions. An activity that requires hand manipulation skills while reaching overhead is an example of a complex motion for a burn injury that involved the shoulder, elbow, and hand. For individuals recovering from severe hand burns, various treatment activities may include exercise putty, hand manipulation boards, the BTE work simulator,[4] Valpar Work Samples[58] and other fine motor activities. Strengthening activities may include use of cuff weights or dumbbells, the WEST II,[62] or the BTE work simulator[4] (Fig. 33-9). The Valpar Full Body ROM Sample provides full body range as well as finger manipulation.[58]

Following severe hand burns, hand edema can occur because of decreased hand function, dependent positioning without adequate external compression, or circumferential scarring to the upper extermity with associated lymphatic damage. Dependent edema is also frequently observed in the lower extremities following healing of full-thickness burns. When edema is present, motion is limited and painful, the skin is prone to damage from shearing forces, and if allowed to remain it may lead to fibrosis.[38] Self-adherent elastic bandage material (Coban) is often used as compression dressing. Before applying the self-adherent wrap, circumferential and volumetric measurements are recommended to monitor treatment effect (Fig. 33-10).

To treat hand edema, elevation, progressive compression, and activity are recommended. A compression wrap, using a self-adherent bandage (Coban), is applied in a spiral fashion overlapping the previous turn by one-half on each digit and continuing in this manner across the hand and onto the wrist. Strips are also applied to each web space (Fig. 33-11). The wrapped hand should then be used for ADL and other functional motions and elevated just above heart level when resting. For lower extremity edema, double elastic wraps, elevation when

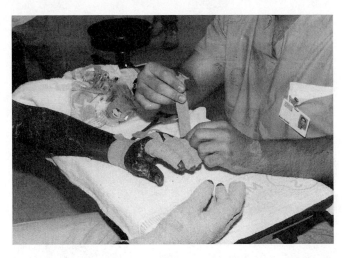

FIG. 33-11 Self-adherent elastic wrap (Coban) applied to hand to provide external compression for treatment of edema.

not ambulating, avoidance of static standing, and active ankle exercises (e.g., pumping) should be encouraged. Intermittent compression pump therapy is often used to treat chronic edema of the extremities.[28]

As patients near discharge from the hospital, stressing independent self-care is extremely important. Eating, dressing, grooming, and bathing skills should be emphasized as part of the normal daily routine. When problems occur, the therapist must determine if the dysfunction originates from a physical limitation, scar contracture, pain, edema, or an assumed abnormal postural reaction. Identification of abnormal movements assists patients in understanding their needs and allows an opportunity for relearning normal movement patterns. Practicing ADL with personal supplies from home can foster a positive attitude toward hospital discharge and feelings about personal abilities. Major burn injuries may require adaptations to support independence initially. Assessing the need for adaptive self-care should differentiate between a scar limitation that can be rehabilitated or a more permanent disabling result.

In addition to self-care, any training needs for effective home management should be identified. Experience has proven that fears of hot water, the stove, or an iron can hinder functional recovery. For those individuals injured during a home activity, counseling, support, and practice of the skills or activity in the clinic should be organized. Prevention techniques can be taught as part of the home program but also are part of the treatment program.[64]

Splinting at this stage is used to (1) limit or reverse potentially disabling or disfiguring contracture formations, (2) increase ROM, (3) distribute pressure over problem areas, or (4) assist function (Fig. 33-12). Static and dynamic splints and casts[7,31,48] may be used depending on the need. Regardless of the purpose of the splint, every effort should be made to ensure that its purpose is easily understood and it is simple to apply. Nighttime

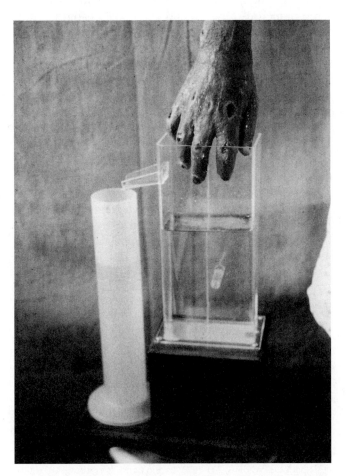

FIG. 33-10 Comparison of sequential volumetric measurements of hand edma identifies treatment effect.

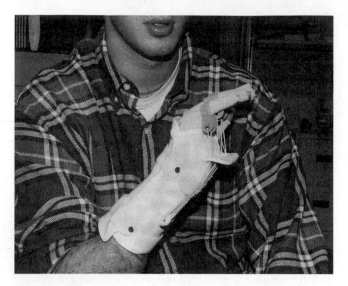

FIG. 33-12 Bivalved dynamic MCP flexion splint. Presized intermediate glove is worn for skin conditioning and edema control.

splinting allows functional use of the extremity during the day, but provides contracture treatment while at rest.

Patient and family education becomes extremely important during this phase to aid the transition from hospital to home. Increased understanding is needed in the following areas: (1) wound healing, (2) the effect of scar contracture, (3) the importance of preserving independence in ADL, (4) the need for continued activity and exercise, and (5) scar management techniques and principles. Before discharge from the hospital, the patient and family should receive thorough home care education[29,33] (Table 33-4). Only with a detailed understanding of home care techniques and potential outcomes can patients be expected to assume responsibility for their own care and recovery.[64]

OUTPATIENT REHABILITATION

Assessment procedures expand during burn recovery. Range of motion, strength, endurance, ADL, and skin and scar status must be assessed frequently to ensure early identification of specific problem areas. In addition to these physical components, the effectiveness of com-

pression garments, the fit and need for certain splints, home care activities, emotional responses, and coping skills should be constantly monitored.

Physical tolerance and work skills assessment are indicated when patients are ready for return to work or vocational rehabilitation. Driving evaluation and prevocational assessment, using simulated work activities or work sample testing, may also be needed for the more severely injured burn survivor. Vocational counseling and exploration should be undertaken in the later stages of recovery if residual dysfunction necessitates a change in former vocational role.

An underlying objective of most burn rehabilitation techniques is the prevention or treatment of hypertrophic scars and scar contractures. To treat scar problems effectively, scar characteristics must be monitored to recognize when maturation occurs. Active scars have been described as red, raised, and rigid.[29] As they mature their color, contour, and texture improve; the scar becomes less vascular in color, more pliable, and smoother. The time since injury is one evaluation measurement. A rating scale has been designed that allows for serial assessment of scar pigment, vascularity, pliability, and height.[56] Although the ratings are somewhat subjective, the scale is a useful clinical tool.

During outpatient rehabilitation, patients may undergo numerous physical and emotional changes. Once discharged from the hospital, they are faced with the overwhelming task of becoming responsible and self-reliant while dealing with discomforting scarring. They may not participate fully with therapy or adequately follow through with home care activities because of the physical and emotional effects of the injury.[30] Noncompliance, apathy, avoidance of pain, scar tightness, and sensitivity all contribute to dysfunction after injury.

In addition to standard treatments such as counseling, support, and imagery techniques, attending a burn support group can help with adjustment. Experience has shown that burn patients at different stages of recovery tend to provide positive support to each other. Group discussions can facilitate understanding what they have been through and what they have to do.[30]

The wearing of intermediate pressure garments prepares the skin for fitting of custom-made compression garments. Compression garment wearing is indicated for all donor sites, graft sites, and burn wounds that take more than 2 to 3 weeks to heal spontaneously.[10,12,39] The occupational therapist is often responsible for the measurement, ordering, and fitting of the custom-made garments.* All custom-made garments need to be measured and ordered following the special instructions of each company.

TABLE 33-4	Home Program Outline*
ITEM	**INFORMATION NEEDED**
1. Wound care	Dressing technique, precautions
2. Skin/Scar care	Lubricant frequency, sun protection
3. Self-care (ADL)	Importance, equipment needed
4. Splint and Orthotics	Schedule, problem identification
5. Pressure garments	Purpose, washing, ordering
6. Exercises	Frequency, techniques for specific areas

*Information should be presented in many ways to reinforce learning, for example, verbally, in writing, and/or by video.

* Custom-made garments are available from the following: Jobst Institute, Charlotte, NC (800) 221-7573; Barton Carey, Perrysburg, OH (800) 421-0444; Bio-Concepts, Phoenix, AZ (800) 421-5647; Medical-Z, Seattle, WA (800) 368-7478.

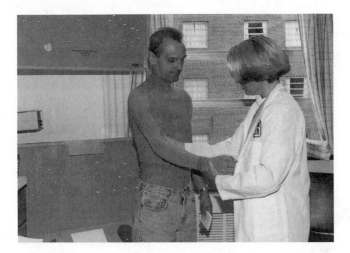

FIG. 33-13 Fit of custom-made compression garments must be frequently assessed to ensure adequate compression for scar management.

Ideally, patients should be fitted with custom-made compression garments no later than 3 weeks after wound healing. Otherwise the wearing of interim garments is continued until custom garments can be applied. Custom-made compression garments are constructed to provide gradient pressure, starting with 35 mm Hg pressure distally. They must be worn 23 hours a day, being removed only for bathing, massage, or changing into a clean garment (Fig. 33-13). Face masks need to be removed for meals many times. In most cases, patients are able to return to work and previous activities without interference from the garments.

Pressure should be applied to the burned area for approximately 12 months or until scar and wound maturation is complete. Donor sites sometimes need conditioning activities and compression garments for approximately 2 months. It is recommended that a minimum of two garments be ordered at one time to allow for laundering. Because of the resilient construction of the fabric, patients should be instructed to hand wash the garments with pure soap and allow them to air-dry. Use of washing machines, dryers, and direct heat should be avoided to prolong the life of the garments. If they are properly cared for, the garments will last approximately 2½ months before a new set is needed. Some individuals who have returned to work may need more than 2 sets of garments at a time; children may need replacements more frequently as a result of their growth and active lifestyle.

To be effective, compression garments must exert equal pressure over the entire area. Because of body contours, bony prominences, and postural adjustments, flexible inserts or pressure adapters are frequently applied to distribute the pressure of the garment more evenly. Areas commonly needing pressure adapters are the supraclavicular region of the chest, between and under the breasts on women, the nasolabial folds, upper and lower lip areas, and the web spaces on the hands.

Pressure inserts were originally made from thermoplastics but skin reactions limited their use. Inserts or adapters are now made from a variety of materials; the choice is based on the area to be treated and need for flexibility when applied. When one is applied, its fit should be monitored at regular intervals. During the early phases of healing when scar remodeling is possible, pressure adapters need to be replaced frequently to maintain exact contouring. Silicone gel, Silastic elastomer, Otoform-K, and Plastazote are used for hand scars; Aquaplast and Silastic elastomer are used on face scars; closed cell foams, prosthetic foam elastomer, Elastogel pads, and Plastazote are used for other body areas.*

In addition to skin and scar management, the outpatient plan must be directed at augmenting the home care plan while also emphasizing resumption of normal life including return to work, school, and leisure activities. Scar contracture is often the primary cause of dysfunction (Fig. 33-14). Activities performed in therapy should emphasize strength, endurance, and function ROM to counteract the effects of scarring and preserve functional abilities.

Inpatient rehabilitation techniques, equipment, and therapeutic activities are also appropriate for outpatient therapy except their intensity must be progressively increased. Grading exercise and activity frequency, intensity, and duration is necessary to successfully regain or improve an individual's strength, endurance, and functional skills. Sequencing the order of treatment activities is necessary to prevent injury and to minimize patient discomfort. That is, skin lubrication, massage, and

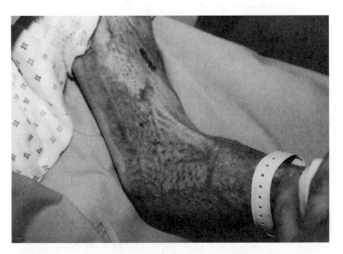

FIG. 33-14 Example of scar contracture of antecubital skin of elbow. Note taut, shortened skin when elbow is extended.

---

* Vendors of materials used for pressure inserts include the following: Alimed, Dedham, MA (800) 225-2610; North Coast Medical Inc., San José, CA (800) 821-9319; Smith & Nephew Roylan, Menomonee Falls, WI (800) 558-8633.

stretching should precede progressive strengthening exercises and activities.[37] As soon as possible, outpatients should learn how to prepare for exercise and activity by doing their own skin lubrication, massage, and stretching. This approach will maximize actual therapy time and may develop habits that will improve compliance with home activities.

Return to school or work becomes a primary objective during outpatient rehabilitation. Many recovering burn survivors are capable of resuming normal daily routines before their wound maturation is complete. That is, some individuals will still be wearing compression garments and inserts and needing to do more skin care than others when they are in school or at work. Return to school and association with friends can be a difficult process for children who have cosmetic disfigurement or functional loss or restrictions. Many burn centers have developed school reentry programs to educate teachers and students about burn injuries and what the child has been through, and to explain the purpose of compression garments, splints, exercise, and care of the skin. The goal of the programs is to prevent restrictions to the child's activities and to ease the transition in returning to school.

Preparing a burn patient for return to work does not have to be a long-term process. Burn rehabilitation and work skills training have many similarities; therefore, it is possible to design treatment activities that simulate not only functional activities but also various work skills. Often identified as work tolerances, strength, endurance, and flexibility are obvious goals of burn rehabilitation.[35] Physical demands of jobs, as described in the *Dictionary of Occupational Titles*,[57] are also components of functional skills; lifting, stooping, pushing, pulling, handling, and manipulating are a few examples. A job analysis interview, as part of the activity needs analysis, will provide the type of information needed to integrate activities into the treatment plan that should not only improve functional ability but also provide beginning work conditioning.

Preparing an individual for return to work postburn, however, also requires attention to two other types of tolerance, skin and temperature. Skin conditioning activities and exercises while wearing garments will improve skin tolerance for friction and shear force demands (Fig. 33-15). Education about the body's response to temperature variations after burn and precautions about how to deal with extremes of temperature are the only ways to address temperature tolerance abnormalities.

The outpatient therapy program should be reevaluated periodically to determine if the frequency of treatment, program progression, and return to work or school status has changed.[37] When patients have resumed their preinjury activities, outpatient therapy may be discontinued. Because burn scar maturation may take up to 18 months following injury, some schedule of follow-up

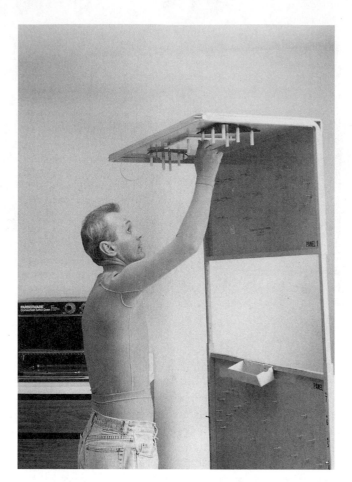

FIG. 33-15 Combined ROM and skin conditioning activity. Use of Valpar Whole Body ROM for UE exercise while wearing compression garments.

care, every 2 to 3 months, is needed until the wearing of compression garments is discontinued.

BURN-RELATED COMPLICATIONS
HETEROTOPIC OSSIFICATION

Heterotopic ossification (HO) is new bone formation in tissues that normally do not ossify.[59] Although HO is frequently found in the posterior aspect of the elbow, it may occur in other joint areas such as the shoulder, wrist, hand, hip, knee, and ankle. It occurs either in the soft tissue around the joint, in the joint capsule and ligaments, or more commonly is known to form a bony bridge across the joint.[25] Signs that HO may be present usually appear during the latter stages of hospitalization with the patient experiencing increased pain at a point in the ROM. The pain is fairly localized and severe; ROM losses are usually rapid. Inflammatory signs, such as redness or swelling, are not easily discernible within healing burn wounds. Once HO has developed, frequent active ROM exercise to the joint should be carried out within the pain-free range to maintain joint motion.[13] Use of splints and forceful passive stretching to the involved joint should be discontinued. The condition may resolve itself with time or surgical intervention may be required.

NEUROMUSCULAR COMPLICATIONS

Peripheral neuropathic conditions are the most common neurological disorder observed in burn patients. They usually occur in burns greater than 20% TBSA, with the exception of high-voltage electrical burns of lesser surface area.[22] Peripheral nerve damage may be caused by infections, metabolic abnormalities, or neurotoxicities. A peripheral neuropathic condition is generally demonstrated with symmetrical distal weakness with or without sensory symptoms. Most conditions improve with time; however, patients often complain of easy fatigability and decreased endurance for months after.[22]

In addition to peripheral neuropathic conditions, localized compression or stretch injuries to nerves are also encountered during burn recovery. Various causes of a localized nerve injury include improper or prolonged positioning in bed or on the operating room table, tourniquet injury, and extreme edema. Common injury sites are the brachial plexus and ulnar and peroneal nerves. Prolonged frog-leg positioning can cause a stretch injury, whereas prolonged side-lying can cause a compression injury to the peroneal nerve.[22] The ulnar nerve is subject to a compression injury with the elbows flexed and forearms pronated. The brachial plexus is subject to stretch or compression injury dependent on the shoulder positioning technique used. Therapists should be aware of the causes for various nerve injuries to implement more effective prevention and intervention techniques.

FACIAL DISFIGUREMENT

A facial burn can be devastating both physically and psychologically. Hypertrophic scar not only distorts the smooth contours of the cheeks and forehead, but it also can alter the nasal contours, eyelids, lips, and oral commissures. Psychologically, this disfigurement can affect an individual's self-image. Much of our communication involves the face either while making eye contact or through nonverbal facial expressions.

There are two main treatment choices for controlling hypertrophic facial scar. A custom-made elastic face mask can be worn, using silicone or elastomer inserts to provide more effective contouring and pressure distribution when needed. The other option is a rigid, total-contact transparent facial orthosis.[51] The therapist can visually evaluate the amount of pressure exerted on the scars and can make more precise adjustments using a rigid facial orthosis. Fabrication of the transparent, rigid orthosis is an involved process consisting of taking a negative impression of the patient's face, making a positive plaster mold of the impression, heating and stretching the plastic over the mold, finishing the edges, applying elastic straps, and fitting it to the patient.[30] Frequent al-

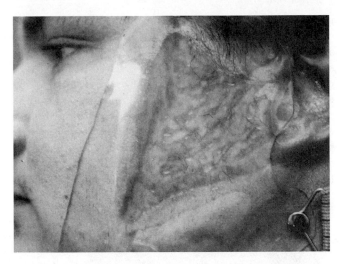

FIG. 33-16   Close-up view of transparent rigid facial orthosis. Mold and mask are adjusted to increase pressure on scarred areas (note blanching of cheek midsection). Orthosis is held in place by elastic straps.

terations are necessary to achieve and maintain adequate blanching of all facial scars (Fig. 33-16).

Patients are instructed to wear the face mask at all times except while eating or bathing. Appropriate skin care education is also important. Massage with lotion twice a day will aid scar desensitization and provide necessary lubrication. Facial exercises are also performed at least twice a day. Many patients prefer to wear the transparent mask during the day and an elastic mask at night for sleeping. Individuals wearing either type of mask often report feelings of self-consciousness, a heightened awareness of being looked at, and a fear of going out in public. To successfully manage these social and personal issues, supportive intervention is required from the family, therapist, and social worker. Compliance is critical in controlling facial scar and disfigurement. The therapist must provide encouragement and continual support to ensure perseverance with wearing a facial orthosis, despite the social barrier it can cause.

SUMMARY

A thermal injury can be one of the most devastating physical and psychological injuries a person can suffer if appropriate treatment is not received in a timely and comprehensive manner. Successful burn care requires a coordinated, multidisciplinary team approach from the date of the patient's admission to the hospital until wound maturation is complete. The occupational therapist is an integral member of the burn team, providing treatment that promotes recovery of functional skills. Treatment activities include positioning, exercise, ADL, splints, skin conditioning, external compression techniques, and patient and family education.

Advancements in medical and surgical burn care have

made it possible to expect not only self-care independence, but also early return to school, work, and leisure activities. Although functional recovery is possible, pain, scar contracture, disfigurement, and adverse psychological reactions (noncompliance, apathy, and depression) can contribute to dysfunction postinjury. In addition to progressive physical rehabilitation, patient education is necessary. A comprehensive patient education program should incorporate information about the physical, psychological, and social components of burn injury to facilitate the patient cooperation and adjustment to the in-

jury. Frequent assessment of the patient's physical abilities, emotional status, and social needs is also important to ensure effective treatment programming.

A concept that should be observed in all burn care is treatment of the whole person. Although this concept is apparent with large, severe burn injuries, it is also important to remember when treating small (less than 20% TBSA) burn injuries. A saying in the burn care field that exemplifies this point is, "There is no such thing as a small burn, unless it is on someone else."

SAMPLE TREATMENT PLAN

CASE STUDY

JM was a 36-year-old male who was injured when a carburetor backfired while he was trying to prime it to start the car. His burn surface area involvement was 20% TBSA, primarily deep partial-thickness with a few areas of full-thickness burn. Body surface areas involved included the right hand and upper extremity (UE), right anterior axillary fold, the superior aspect of the chest, neck, and face. No inhalation injury was noted upon admission to the hospital. Past medical history was unremarkable.

JM recently was married; he and his wife were in the process of renovating a house they just purchased. He was employed by the state Department of Transportation, and was responsible for computer design, drafting and on-site management of bridge construction. Although his wife works, his income was needed to support the purchase of

the new home. His recreational hobbies included spectator sports, motorcycle riding and repair, and home renovations. He was right-hand dominant and had a college degree.

JM was admitted to the intensive care unit of the burn center. Occupational therapy was requested for evaluation and treatment. The basic goal of the burn team was to return JM to his preinjury level of function as soon as possible.

Escharotomies were performed to the right hand upon admission to the intensive care unit. Initial nursing care included hydrotherapy and twice-a-day dressing changes using silver sulfadiazine cream. JM underwent two surgical procedures for burn wound excision and grafting on postburn days 4 and 11. Donor sites were on the thighs. He was discharged to home on day 21 postinjury.

TREATMENT PLAN

Personal data
Name: Mr. JM
Age: 36
Diagnosis: Partial-thickness and full-thickness burn, 20% TBSA, involving right arm and hand, right anterior axillary fold, chest, neck, and face.
Disability: Potential contracture and dysfunction of hand; potential contracture of elbow and axilla; potential hypertrophic scarring of hand, arm, and face.
Treatment aims stated in referral: Evaluation and treatment; restore patient to preinjury level of function.

Other services
Physician: Wound and medical assessment; prescribe medication; perform debridement or escharotomy as needed; supervise rehabilitation therapies; grafting
Nursing: Nursing care; positioning; administer medications; change dressings; carry out ADL
Physical therapist: Prevent contractures through ROM and strengthening exercises; hydrotherapy procedures

Psychologist: Evaluate psychological status; counsel; consultant to staff
Social worker: Explore financial problems; counsel patient and family
Family: Provide support, acceptance, encouragement, and assistance
Vocational counselor: Explore feasibility of return to same or similar job; explore job alternatives, if needed
Recreational therapist: Mental stimulation; activities for enjoyment and diversion; function of affected and unaffected parts
Dietitian: Assess and monitor calorie and protein requirements and intake; provide supplemental diet as needed

Frame of reference
Human occupation

Treatment approach
Biomechanical

SAMPLE TREATMENT PLAN – cont'd

OT EVALUATION

Acute care phase

Active and passive ROM: Test
Muscle strength: Observe for function; gross muscle testing
ADL: Observe
Need for splints and positioning: Observe burn areas to determine need
Psychological status: Observe, interview, and consult with psychologist
Assistive devices: Observe, assess need

Surgical/postoperative phase

Potential for deformity: Observe
Need for positioning and splints: Observe, assess ROM, consult with physician
Assistive devices for ADL: Observe ADL (feeding) to determine needs.
Strength and ROM: Test

Rehabilitation phase

ADL: Assess performance

Active and passive ROM: Test
Muscle strength: Functional muscle test
Hand function: Test
Wound maturation: Assess color, contour, texture; assess need for pressure adapters and garments
Psychosocial adjustment: Observe, interview
Knowledge of burn wound, wound care, home program: Observe, interview

Outpatient phase

ADL: Assess skill performance
ROM and strength: Test
Hand function: Test
Scar maturation: Observe
Physical endurance: Test, observe
Vocational evaluation: Test, observe

EVALUATION SUMMARY

(See problem list by phase of recovery for more in-depth summary.)

Acute care phase

Active ROM limited to 0 to 150° of shoulder flexion and abduction; elbow flexion: 10 to 90°.
Functional strength: Good (4)
ADL: Needs minimal adaptations for eating because of edema; needs minimal assistance for bathing back.
Hand function: AROM*: MCPs 0 to 45°; PIPs† 15 to 30°; DIP‡ 0
Splinting needs: Hand volar pan splints
Positioning: Shoulder abduction to 90°; elbow extension; forearm in neutral; hands slightly elevated; no pillow because of face burns

Surgical/postoperative phase

Positioning: Same as for acute care phase

* Active ROM.
† Proximal IPs.
‡ Distal IP.
§ Passive ROM.

Splints: Use only at night
AROM: Shoulder flexion and abduction 0 to 165°
Hand ROM: Limited, with edema

Rehabilitation phase

AROM and PROM§ of UEs: Slight limitations
Endurance: Decreased from previous test
Hand function: Grip and pinch strength decreased
ADL: Awkward performance

ASSETS

Good health, preinjury
Supportive wife
New home
Many leisure interests
Good potential for returning to same employment
Good intelligence and cognitive functioning

S A M P L E   T R E A T M E N T   P L A N – cont'd

ACUTE CARE PHASE

Problem List

1. Limited active ROM and ADL because of hand and arm edema
2. Hand edema causes decreased AROM of fingers, decreased grasp
3. Anxiety about being hospitalized and facial burns
4. Potential for hypertrophic scarring on hand, arm, and face determined from observed burn depth; potential scarring and contractures of face and neck
5. Decreased strength and endurance
6. No understanding about burn care or postburn outcomes

PROBLEMS 1, 2

Objective

Hand edema will be decreased to increase grasp and ADL performance

Method

Volar hand splint fabricated for night positioning using elastic wraps for application; active ROM; ADL and functional use. Initial positioning of right arm and hand on two pillows, with elbow flexion to no more than 30° when at rest and the hand elevated to just above heart level; no pillow behind head

Gradation

Decrease use of splint as edema decreases and ROM increases

Objective

Increase AROM of fingers

Methods

Hand exercises; ADL and functional activities

Gradation

Increase active use; ROM exercises and functional activities

PROBLEM 4, 5

Objective

Preserve functional strength, endurance, and AROM

Methods

Ambulation or cycle ergometer twice daily (BID), ROM exercises BID to right upper extremity, free-weight exercise to uninvolved extremity and involved extremity as tolerated;

neck and facial exercises

Gradation

Increase time spent on exercise, ambulation, and cycle as endurance improves. Introduce self-care activities and whole-body activities as tolerated.

PROBLEM 1, 2, 6

Objective

Increase patient understanding of the functional importance for exercise and independent self-care

Method

Support independent feeding by wrapping foam around

utensil handle to increase grasp: monitor functional use of involved extremity

Gradation

Progress to independent use of utensils without adaptations

PROBLEM 6

Objection

Increase understanding of wound healing concepts

Method

Patient education about the need for activity, exercise, and

independent ADL, beginning education about wound healing and scar formation

Gradation

Increase instruction as appropriate

SAMPLE TREATMENT PLAN—cont'd

PROBLEM 3

Objective
Decrease anxiety and depression

Method
Emotional support to decrease anxiety in all phases of treat-

ment

Gradation
Increase or decrease support as needed for emotional state

SURGICAL/POSTOPERATIVE PHASE
PROBLEM LIST

1. Immobilization of right upper extremity for 3 days post-operatively
2. Possible loss of strength and ROM from immobilization
3. Possible need for adaptations to support independent

feeding
4. Potential for thrombophlebitis
5. Patient anxiety; lack of understanding of burn care and burn rehabilitation outcomes

PROBLEM 1

Objective
Maintain postoperative immobilization for 3 days, as per medical direction

Method
Provide hand splint for postoperative immobilization

Gradation
Decrease immobilization per physician's orders and increase mobility as medically allowed

PROBLEM 2

Objective
Prevent loss of strength and ROM

Method
ROM exercises to left UE and lower extremity; active ROM to injured extremity following removal of postoperative

dressings; continued neck and facial exercises

Gradation
Gentle active ROM initially; in 3 to 4 days progress to active-assisted exercises if needed. By 5 days, stretch can be applied. Increase repetitions and frequency as tolerated

PROBLEM 3

Objective
Maintain ability to feed self independently

Method
Issue plate guard and adapted utensils for eating

Gradation
Decrease use of assistive devices as soon as function increases

PROBLEM 4

Objective
Prevent thrombophlebitis

Method
Ambulation when cleared by physician, leg with donor sites should be wrapped from foot to thigh using elastic bandages. Active ankle exercise (pumping) for leg with donor

site

Gradation
Start with bedside activities; in 2 days ambulate short distances; progressively increase distance, surfaces (e.g., floor, stairs), and frequency

SAMPLE TREATMENT PLAN – cont'd

PROBLEM 5

Objective

Increase patient's understanding of burn care and burn rehabilitation outcomes

Method

Patient education about wound healing, scar formation, and need for activity; psychological support provided in all treatment activities.

Gradation

Increase information given; observe ability to understand through activities performed in rehabilitation and functional use of extremities

---

REHABILITATION PHASE

Problem list

1. Right hand weakness possibly caused by hypersensitivity, edema
2. Awkward use of right upper extremity for functional activities
3. Anxiety about face wounds, questions about beard growth potential
4. Complaints of stiffness with ROM exercises of right UE
5. Blistering on healed donor site
6. Tendency to lean head to the right to avoid stretch to healing wounds on neck: turns upper body to look to the right
7. Beginning wound maturation of grafted areas on right UE and hand
8. Concerns about going home

PROBLEM 1

Objective

Decrease edema to increase right UE function

Method

Volumetric measurement, then self-adhesive elastic wrap (Coban) to right hand preexercise, functional activities using right hand with wrap on, rewrap hand after skin care for three days then progress to intermediate compression glove, then to a custom-made compression garment.

Application of tubular elastic bandage to right UE, followed by fitting of custom-made garment. Continue to monitor face wounds for possible scar treatment needs

Gradation

Compression wraps progressing from Ace bandage to Coban, to intermediate garments, and finally to custom-made garments. Increase repetitions and resistance of hand activities and exercise.

PROBLEMS 1, 2, 4

Objective

Restore normal, fluid functional motions with the upper extremities

Method

Active and resistive ROM exercises and functional activities using weights; emphasize right UE but also total body conditioning with focus also on tool usage and lifting, fine motor activities with right hand

Gradation

Increase resistance, time spent in exercise and activity as strength, endurance, and normal movement patterns improve; that is, change frequency, intensity, and duration of activities used.

Objective

Increase flexibility for independent ADL

Method

Massage and slow, sustained stretches of right axilla with shoulder abduction and flexion emphasized, also stretch to right elbow in extension

Gradation

Increase motions, repetitions, and frequency of stretching and exercise

Objective

Increase functional strength and endurance for normal daily activities

Method

Cycle ergometer at progressively increased cadence and work levels; active and resistive isotonic exercise using weights and functional activities

Gradation

Increase frequency, intensity, and duration

SAMPLE TREATMENT PLAN – cont'd

PROBLEMS 5, 7

Objective
Improve skin tolerance for shear forces

Method
Skin conditioning to right UE: lubrication and massage; ac-tivity and exercise wearing compression garments

Gradation
Progress to independent patient performances of activities BID while also increasing pressure massage as tolerated

PROBLEMS 3, 8

Objective
Increase patient competencies in home care activities

Method
Beginning home care education—teach skin care, home exercises, instruct on ways to manage time to ensure all activities get completed at home: education about protec-tion of face and healing wounds from ultraviolet rays

Gradation
Provide patient education throughout hospitalization as appropriate to stages of recovery and functional problems developing. Focus on all areas of ADL with patient

PROBLEMS 5, 6, 8

Objective
Increased patient understanding of face scar care and home care responsibilities

Methods
Measure for custom-made compression garments; order glove, jacket with long right sleeve and short left sleeve, turtleneck collar on jacket, modified face mask with small area open in center of face (burns limited to cheeks and just outside of right eye). Elastic bandage wraps to donor sites when up and moving around; try to fit tubular elastic bandage when blisters are dry. Recommend burn support group participation, continue supportive discussions

Gradation
Decrease wear of compression garments, face mask, and elastic wraps as scar matures

OUTPATIENT REHABILITATION

Problem list
1. Minimal but obvious raising of facial skin on right cheek
2. Limited opposition with right thumb caused by thumb web contracture
3. Slight limitation in right elbow extension, ROM measure 20 to 130°
4. Healed wounds demonstrating active scar formation by the color, contour, and texture (i.e., the right arm is highly vascular in appearance, skin feels taut, slight ridging noted on forearm and at wrist)
5. Expresses feeling fatigued all the time
6. Expresses need to return to work as soon as possible

PROBLEM 1

Objective
Control wound maturation of the face, minimize scarring

Method
Recommend rigid transparent facial orthosis for face, explain that the design of the orthosis will be a lower half face mask; suggest elastic mask for night wear only; after discussion, fabricate and fit rigid orthosis

Gradation
Frequent adjustments to rigid face mask to increase pressure on any raised scars; adjust fit as scars mature

PROBLEM 2

Objective
Increase ROM of thumb web space

Method
Thumb ROM exercises and activities; scar massage; fabri-cate a Plastazote insert for wear under the glove during the day and an elastomer insert in the evening or when not working (different materials used to allow greater hand flexibility during the day for computer and drafting tool use)

SAMPLE TREATMENT PLAN—cont'd

PROBLEMS 2, 5

Objective
Increase hand function and hand scar control

Method
No later than 7 to 10 days after hospital discharge, fit with custom-made compression garments, instruct on 23 hours a day wearing; order three or more gloves in preparation for return to work; hand rehabilitation activities

Gradation
Decrease use of garments as scar matures and web space ROM is achieved and maintained. Progressively increase the resistance and complexity of hand activities

PROBLEM 3

Objective
Increase right UE ROM and flexibility

Method
Fit with dynamic elbow extension splint for use at night to help stretch the antecubital scar contracture that is developing; evaluate ROM periodically to determine when to discontinue the splint. Strengthening exercises for right hand and arm—exercise equipment that stress functional motions with increasing resistance

Gradation
Decrease and discontinue use of splint as contracture is reduced; increase exercise and functional activities as hand and arm function improves

PROBLEM 5

Objective
Improve scar management

Method
Pressure adapter for forearm ridging—fit with an Elastogel pad on areas on forearm where there is slight ridging, recommend holding pad in place with a nylon whose end can be held in the hand while the custom-made jacket is being applied. Lubricate and massage right arm scars before exercise, have JM demonstrate home technique

Gradation
Change pads as needed; progress to more rigid materials if needed; decrease massage by therapist as patient improves in self-care and self-massage

Objective
Improve understanding and demonstration of appropriate skin care including how to avoid sun exposure

Method
Patient education about work outside—avoid sun exposure, dress appropriately for temperatures being aware that perspiration abilities may be slightly increased in left UE to compensate for decrease on right

Gradation
As scar matures, slowly increase exposure using sun screen lotions and sun protection

PROBLEM 6

Objective
Increase endurance and patient motivation for performing daily activities

Method
Emphasize home care education about exercise and stress frequent neck exercises and right arm exercises during the day; discuss ways to incorporate exercise into work schedule when returned to work

Gradation
Increase independent personal care activities when in rehabilitation; increase independence with exercises

SAMPLE TREATMENT PLAN – cont'd

PROBLEM 7

Objective
Return to work and leisure activities

Method
JM should be able to be cleared for return to work with the restrictions of having to wear compression garments, avoidance of sun exposure until facial scars mature, and no exposure to extremes of temperature until wounds mature

Endurance testing revealed no limitation in cardiopulmonary function; recommend resuming more personally enjoyable activities and also make referral for supportive counseling

FOLLOW-UP CARE

JM should be followed in the burn clinic where evaluation by the occupational therapist is part of the clinic protocol. Follow-up visits should first be two weeks following hospital discharge, then once a month up to a year or until scar maturation is complete. Occupational therapy visits should be once every two to three weeks to monitor pressure adapters fit, rigid facial orthosis fit, compression garment wear, and for scar evaluation. This check should be done for a minimum of two months, but can be longer if needed. If scar activity seems to be stabilized, the occupational therapy visits can be once a month with the scheduled clinic time, until the patient is discharged from all follow-up care.

REVIEW QUESTIONS

1. What are the two layers of the skin? In which layer are the sebaceous glands?
2. Which factors are considered in determining burn severity?
3. What is an escharotomy?
4. Describe two factors that can affect the quality of burn wound healing and lead to scar formation.
5. When ROM is evaluated during acute care, which factors may limit full ROM?
6. What are the two basic principles underlying most burn rehabilitation treatment techniques?
7. Why may a patient need temporary adaptations for self-care during the acute care?
8. What is the primary objective for positioning during acute care?
9. Why are patients immobilized postoperatively?
10. On the average, how soon after grafting can gentle, active ROM be resumed?
11. How soon postoperatively should an intermediate garment or dressing be applied?
12. What are the two options for facial scar treatment?
13. Why are skin conditioning activities used in burn rehabilitation? What are examples of skin conditioning techniques?
14. When a splint is ordered, what is the preferred wearing schedule? Why?
15. What is the primary cause of dysfunction following a burn injury?
16. Which points should be covered in a home program?
17. What are possible causes of limitations in ADL during the rehabilitation phase?
18. Should exercise be performed during the surgical/postoperative phase of care?
19. Are splints always used during the acute care phase?
20. When should patient education about burn injury and rehabilitation begin?

REFERENCES

1. Abston S: Scar reaction after thermal injury and prevention of scars and contractures. In Boswick JA, editor: *The art and science of burn care,* Rockville, Md, 1987, Aspen.
2. Apfel LM and associates: Computer-drafted pressure support gloves, *J Burn Care Rehabil* 9:165-168, 1988.
3. Artz CP, Moncrief JA, Pruitt BA: *Burns: a team approach,* Philadelphia, 1979, WB Saunders.
4. Baltimore Therapeutic Equipment Co., 1201 Bernard Dr., Baltimore, MD, 21223.
5. Bariollo DJ, Nangle ME, Farrell K: Preliminary experience with cultured epidermal autograft in a community hospital burn unit, *J Burn Care Rehabil* 13(1):158-165, 1992.
6. Baur PS and associates: Wound contractions, scar contractures and myofibroblasts: a classical case study, *J Trauma* 18:8-21, 1978.
7. Bennett GB and associates: Serial casting: a method for treating burn contracture, *J Burn Care Rehabil* 10:543-545, 1989.
8. Bruster J, Pullium G: Gradient pressure, *Am J Occup Ther* 37:485, 1983.
9. Burnsworth B, Krob MJ, Langer-Schnepp M: Immediate ambulation of patients with lower extremity grafts, *J Burn Care Rehabil* 12:33-36, 1991.

10. Carr-Collins JA: Pressure techniques for the prevention of hypertrophic scar. In Salisbury RE, editor: *Clinics in plastic surgery: burn rehabilitation and reconstruction*, Philadelphia, 1992, WB Saunders.

11. Clark JA, Burt AM, Eldad A: Culture epithelium as a skin substitute, *Burns* 13:173-180, 1987.

12. Covey MH: Occupational therapy. In Boswick JA, editor: *The art and science of burn care*, Rockville, Md, 1987, Aspen.

13. Crawford CM and associates: Heterotopic ossification: are range of motion exercises contraindicated? *J Burn Care Rehabil* 7:323-325, 1986.

14. Daugherty MB, Carr-Collins JA: Splinting techniques for the burn patient. In Richard RL, Staley MJ, editors: *Burn care and rehabilitation principles and practice*, Philadelphia, 1994, FA Davis.

15. Dietch EA and associates: Hypertrophic burn scars: analysis of variables, *J Trauma* 23:895-898, 1983.

16. Dyer C: Burn care in the emergent period, *J Emerg Nurs* 6:9, 1980.

17. Fleet J: The psychological effects of burn injuries: a literature review, *British J of Occup Ther* 55:198-201, 1992.

18. Giuliani CA, Perry GA: Factors to consider in the rehabilitaiton aspect of burn care, *Phys Ther* 65(5):619-623, 1985.

19. Hansbrough JF: Current status of skin replacements for coverage of extensive burn wounds, *J Trauma* 30(suppl 12):s155-162, 1990.

20. Hartford C: Surgical management. In Fisher S, Helm P: *Comprehensive rehabilitation of burns*, Baltimore, 1984, Williams & Wilkins.

21. Heimbach DM, Engrav LH: *Surgical management of the burn wound*, New York, 1984, Raven Press.

22. Helm PA: Neuromuscular considerations. In Fisher SV, Helm PA, editors: *Comprehensive rehabilitation of burns*, Baltimore, 1984, Williams & Wilkins.

23. Helm PA: Burn rehabilitation: dimensions of the problem. In Salisbury RE: *Clinics in plastic surgery*, Philadelphia, 1992, WB Saunders.

24. Helm PA, Fisher SV: Rehabilitation of the patient with burns. In Delisa J, Currie D, Gans B, editors: *Rehabilitation medicine principles and practice*, Philadelphia, 1988, JB Lippincott.

25. Hoffer MM, Brody G, Ferlic F: Excision of heterotopic ossification about elbows in patients with thermal injury, *J Trauma* 18:667-670, 1978.

26. Howell JW: Management of the acutely burned hand for the nonspecialized clinician, *Phys Ther* 12:1077-1089, 1989.

27. Humphrey C, Richard RL, Staley MJ: Soft tissue management and exercise. In Richard RL, Staley MJ, editors: *Burn care and rehabilitation principles and practice*, Philadelphia, 1994, FA Davis.

28. Hunter JM, Mackin EJ: Management of edema. In Hunter JM, Schneider LH, Mackin EJ, Callahan AD, editors: *Rehabilitation of the hand*, St Louis, 1990, CV Mosby.

29. Johnson CL: Physical therapists as scar modifiers, *Phys Ther* 64:1381-1387, 1984.

30. Jordan CL, Allely RA, Gallagher J: Self-care strategies following severe burns. In Christiansen C, editor: *Ways of living: self-care strategies for special needs*, Rockville, Md, 1994, American Occupational Therapy Association.

31. Jordan MH and associates: Dynamic plaster casting for burn scar contracture, *Proc American Burn Association* 16:17, 1984.

32. Jordan MH and associates: A pressure prevention device for burned ears, *J Burn Care Rehabil* 13(1):673-677, 1992.

33. Kaplan SH: Patient education techniques used at burn centers, *Am J Occup Ther* 39:655, 1985.

34. Larson DL and associates: Techniques for decreasing scar formation and contracture in the burned patient, *J Trauma* 11:807-822, 1971.

35. Leman CH: An approach to work hardening in burn rehabilitation, *Top Acute Care Trauma Rehabil* 1:62-73, 1987.

36. Leman CJ: Burn rehabilitaiton. In Hopkins HL, Smith HD, editors: *Willard and Spackman's Occupational Therapy*, ed 8, Philadelphia, 1993, JB Lippincott.

37. Leman CJ, Ricks N: Discharge planning and follow-up burn care. In Richard RL, Staley MJ, editors: *Burn care and rehabilitation principles and practice*, Philadelphia, 1994, FA Davis.

38. Leman CJ and associates: Exercise physiology in the acute burn patient: do we really know what we're doing?, *Proc American Burn Assoc* 24:91, 1992.

39. Linares HA: Hypertropic healing: controversies and etiopathogenic review. In Carvajal HF, Parks DH, editors: *Burn in children: Pediatric burn management*, Chicago, 1988, Yearbook Medical Publishers.

40. Lund C, Browder N: The estimation of area of burns, *Surg Gynecol Obstet* 79:352-355, 1944.

41. Mahon LM, Neufeld N: The effect of informational feedback on food intake of adult burn patients, *J App Behav Anal* 17:392, 1984.

42. Miles WK, Grigsby L: Remodeling of scar tissue in the burned hand. In Hunter JM, Schneider LH, Mackin EJ, Callahan AD, editors: *Rehabilitation of the hand*, St Louis, 1990, CV Mosby.

43. Moss BF, Everett JJ, Patterson DR: Psychologic support and pain management of the burn patient. In Richard RL, Staley MJ, editors: *Burn care and rehabilitaiton principles and practice*, Philadelphia, 1994, FA Davis.

44. Nolan WB: Acute management of thermal injury. *Ann Plast Surg* 7:3, 1981.

45. Peacock EE Jr: *Wound repair*, ed 3, Philadelphia, 1984, WB Saunders.

46. Pullium G: Splinting and positioning. In Fisher SV, Helm PA, editors: *Comprehensive rehabilitation of burns*, Baltimore, 1984, Williams & Wilkins.

47. Richard RL, Staley MJ: Burn patient evaluation and treatment planning. In Richard RL, Staley MJ, editors: *Burn care and rehabilitation principles and practice,* Philadelphia, 1994, FA Davis.

48. Ricks N, Meager D: The benefits of plaster casting for lower extremity burns after grafting in children, *J Burn Care Rehabil* 13:465-468, 1992.

49. Rivers EA: Rehabilitation management of the burn patient, *Advances in Clin Rehabil* 1:180, 1978.

50. Rivers EA, Fisher SV: Rehabilitation for burn patients. In Kottke FJ, Lehmann JF, editors: *Krusen's handbook of phyiscal medicine and rehabilitation,* ed 4, Philadelphia, 1990, WB Saunders.

51. Rivers E, Strate R, Solem L: The transparent face mask, *Am J Occup Ther* 33:108-113, 1979.

52. Salisbury RE, Petro JA: Rehabilitation of burn patients. In Boswick JA, editor: *The art and science of burn care,* Rockville, Md, 1987, Aspen.

53. Schmitt MA, French L, Kalil ET: How soon is safe? Ambulation of the patient with burns after lower-extremity skin grafting, *J Burn Care Rehabil* 13:89, 1992.

54. Solem L: Classification. In Fisher S, Helm P: *Comprehensive rehabilitation of burns,* Baltimore, 1984, Williams & Wilkins.

55. Staley MJ, Richard RL: Scar management. In Richard RL, Staley MJ, *Burn care and rehabilitation principles and practice,* Philadelphia, 1994, FA Davis.

56. Sullivan T and associates: Rating the burn scar, *J Burn Care Rehabil* 11:256-258, 1990.

57. U.S. Department of Labor, *Dictionary of Occupational Titles,* ed 4, Washington, D.C., 1977, U.S. Government Printing Office.

58. Valpar Component Work Samples, Valpar International Corporation, P.O. Box 5767, Tucson, AZ

59. Varghese G: Musculoskeletal conditions. In Fisher SV, Helm PA, editors: *Comprehensive rehabilitation of burns,* Baltimore, 1984, Williams & Wilkins.

60. Wachtel T: Epidemiology, classification, initial care, and administrative considerations for critically burned patients. In Wachtel T: *Critical care clinics,* Philadelphia, 1985, WB Saunders.

61. Weil R and associates: Smoke inhalation injury, *Ann Plast Surg* 4:2, 1980.

62. Work Evaluation Systems Technology (WEST), PO Box 2477, Fort Bragg, CA 95437.

63. Wright PC: Fundamentals of acute burn care and phyiscal therapy management, *Phys Ther* 64:1217-1231, 1984.

64. Yurko L, Fratianne R: Evaluation of burn discharge teaching, *J Burn Care Rehabil* 9:643-644, 1988.

Rheumatoid Arthritis

Jocelyn M. Hittle, Lorraine Williams Pedretti, Mary C. Kasch

Rheumatoid arthritis (RA) is a chronic systemic autoimmune disorder that can affect the lungs, cardiovascular system, and eyes in some patients. The primary clinical feature is chronic symmetrical erosive synovitis of the joints, particularly the peripheral joints.[7,16,21] The disease may range from mild to severe and can result in joint deformity and joint destruction of varying degrees.[16]

Rheumatoid arthritis occurs most frequently in persons between the ages of 20 and 40[7] and about three times more frequently in women than in men. Although it can occur from infancy to old age,[7,16,21] its prevalence increases with age in the adult onset group.[33] The cause of the disease is unknown; however, it is thought to result from a combination of agents acting upon an individual who may be genetically predisposed to developing the disease.[21,33]

DIAGNOSIS

Definitive diagnosis may not be possible at initial onset because of the large number of connective tissue disorders that present with similar symptoms. In most cases, it may take weeks or even months for the constellation of symptoms to develop that may eventually lead to a diagnosis of RA.[21] In 1987 the American Rheumatism Association revised its criteria for classification of RA. The new method requires that the patient show 4 of 7 criteria that are clinical manifestations of the disease for a diagnosis of RA to be made[33] (Table 34-1). One criterion is the presence of rheumatoid factors in the blood. Rheumatoid factors are autoantibodies that are present in a number of diseases but also appear in 75 to 90% of patients with RA. These patients are said to have seropositive RA. The presence of rheumatoid factors in the blood correlate with increased severity of symptoms and increased involvement of systemic symptoms.[33]

PATHOLOGY AND PATHOGENESIS

Rheumatoid arthritis affects the synovial or diarthrodial joints. In a normal synovial joint, the joint surfaces of the bones are covered with smooth, avascular articular cartilage, which serves to reduce friction and assist with shock absorption. The maintenance of healthy cartilage is dependent on active motion and the compression and decompression associated with normal movement.[25,39] The joint is surrounded and supported by a joint capsule, which, depending on functional demands, may vary from very thin to thick ligamentous tissue. Extracapsular structures such as ligaments, tendons, and muscles also contribute to joint stability. The synovium covers all noncartilaginous joint surfaces inside the capsule. The lining of the synovium is normally 1 to 3 cells thick and is supplied by the vascular, lymphatic, and nervous systems. The fluid secreted by this lining (called synovial fluid) lubricates, adds to joint stability, and provides nutrition to the joint.[33,39]

The initial and precipitating event in the development of rheumatoid arthritis is thought to be the transport of an activating agent to synovial cells in the joint via the bloodstream. This agent either activates or injures the epithelial cells of the synovium, which respond with an inflammatory or immune response. Once this response occurs, it tends to be self-perpetuating.[39]

Inflammation is a process of swelling and cell recruitment, which in RA may vary in its severity. In some cases inflammation may become chronic, however, leading to hypertrophy or thickening of the synovium through the activity of fibroblasts and abnormal vascular proliferation. The lining layer of the synovium may proliferate to become 5 to 10 cells thick and there may be tumorlike growth of the tissue, which invades the joint cavity and surrounding structures. This abnormal tissue, called pannus, is accompanied by enzymes such as collagenase that destroy the tissue and lead to erosions of bone and cartilage and destruction of soft tissue, resulting in joint deformity and disability.[33]

COURSE OF RA

The onset of rheumatoid arthritis is usually gradual or insidious, although it may be abrupt. It is characterized by bilateral, symmetrical involvement of many large

TABLE 34-1   The American Rheumatism Association 1987 Revised Criteria For The Classification Of Rheumatoid Arthritis

CRITERIA	DEFINITION
1. Morning stiffness	Morning stiffness in and around the joints, lasting at least 1 hour before maximal improvement
2. Arthritis of 3 or more joint areas	At least 3 joint areas simultaneously have had soft tissue swelling or fluid (not bony overgrowth alone) observed by a physician. The 14 possible areas are right or left PIP, MCP, wrist, elbow, knee, ankle, and MTP joints
3. Arthritis of hand joints	At least 1 area swollen (as defined above) in a wrist, MCP, or PIP joint
4. Symmetric arthritis	Simultaneous involvement of the same joint areas (as defined in 2) on both sides of the body (bilateral involvement of PIPs, MCPs, or MTPs is acceptable without absolute symmetry)
5. Rheumatoid nodules	Subcutaneous nodules over bony prominences, extensor surfaces, or in juxtaarticular regions, observed by a physician
6. Serum rheumatoid factor	Demonstration of abnormal amounts of serum rheumatoid factor by any method for which the result has been positive in <5% of normal control subjects
7. Radiographic changes	Radiographic changes typical of rheumatoid arthritis on posteroanterior hand and wrist radiographs that must include erosions or unequivocal bony decalcification localized in or most marked adjacent to the involved joints (osteoarthritis changes alone do not qualify)

From *Primer on the rheumatic diseases,* tenth edition, copyright 1993. Used by permission of the Arthritis Foundation.
For classification purposes, a patient shall be said to have rheumatoid arthritis if he/she has satisfied at least 4 of these 7 criteria. Criteria 1 through 4 must have been present for at least 6 weeks. Patients with 2 clinical diagnoses are not excluded. Designation as classic, definite, or probable rheumatoid arthritis is *not* to be made.

joints as well as the small joints of the hands and feet.[1,21] The joints are typically painful, stiff, tender, hot, and occasionally, red.

Muscles that act on the involved joints may decrease in strength and size fairly early in the course of the disease because of disuse. Reflex inhibition of muscle action because of pain may also cause shortening of flexors and weakening of extensors.[21] Range of motion (ROM) is limited because of edema and pain in the early stages and later may be due to destructive changes in the joint.[1]

The systemic manifestations should not be overlooked. Signs, which may be present in varying degrees, include fever, weight loss, weakness, fatigue, and general stiffness.[1]

Morning stiffness is a common feature of rheumatoid arthritis. Noting the duration of stiffness after prolonged sleep is helpful in documenting the progress of the disease because the duration tends to decrease with decreasing inflammation.[33]

There may be an apparent depression and lack of motivation that may be related to the fatigue and organic symptoms and should be differentiated from the same symptoms that can be psychogenic.[21]

The course of the disease is unpredictable. Some individuals experience a single, brief episode, and others experience multiple episodes of varying severity. A small percentage of patients experience a gradual and continuous progression to severe joint deformity and dysfunction.[1]

The course is usually characterized by exacerbations and remissions. The patient's level of function and independence can fluctuate from independent to completely dependent, varying with the stage and severity of the disease process.[16,21]

DRUG THERAPY

Traditionally the approach to medical management of RA has followed the pyramid model with well established and less toxic treatment methods forming the foundation of treatment, or the base of the pyramid[33] (Fig. 34-1). These methods include rest, education, and what are referred to as first line medications. If these methods are

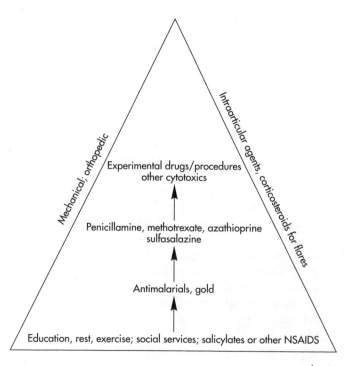

FIG. 34-1 Treatment pyramid for arthritis. (From the *Primer on the rheumatic diseases* tenth edition, copyright 1993. Used by permission of the Arthritis Foundation.)

not effective in preventing disease progression, treatment progresses up the pyramid to agents that can be more toxic to the patient. At the apex of the pyramid are the more experimental and cytotoxic medications, which are generally reserved for those patients who have severe disease not responding to other medication. Supportive measures such as therapy and cortisone injections form the sides of the pyramid.[33]

The medications used in the treatment of RA are divided into two groups. The first group, or first line drugs, are fast-acting drugs such as nonsteroidal antiinflammatory drugs (NSAIDs), intraarticular corticosteroid injections, and aspirin, which can suppress inflammation but not alter the progression of the disease. These drugs cannot prevent joint destruction.[33] Because they are less toxic, they are often prescribed at the initial diagnosis of RA. NSAIDs are frequently used instead of aspirin because administration is easier and improved compliance may result.[13]

The second group of drugs include disease-modifying antirheumatic drugs (DMARDs), which may actually have an effect on the course of the disease although this possibility is still in question. The drugs in this group include gold salts, penicillamine, hydroxychloroquinine, and methotrexate among others. All of these medications require careful medical monitoring because of potentially serious side effects. Frequent blood and urine tests may be required to rule out adverse effects. DMARDs and cytotoxic agents are slow acting with two to three months of drug therapy required before their full benefit is realized. During this time, first line drugs to control synovitis and the addition of steroids may improve the patient's functional status. It is also important that supportive measures such as joint protection, energy conservation, and splinting be employed until synovitis is controlled.

Corticosteroids are very strong medications with potentially serious side effects, so they are reserved for those patients who would become severely disabled without them. They may be used in low dosage with relatively few side effects, however, and when used as an adjunct to other drug therapy, may make a substantial difference in those patients whose disease is not adequately controlled by other medications alone.[23]

The methods of using drugs in treatment are constantly being examined. There are advocates for inverting the pyramid and using DMARDs early in the disease to prevent joint damage and also to use these drugs in combination. Researchers continue to evaluate the traditional and newer treatment approaches.[11,15,19]

PSYCHOLOGICAL FACTORS

The so-called rheumatoid personality is undoubtedly a myth arising from research done in the 1950s and 1960s. Its validity has since been questioned. These reports suggested that persons with rheumatoid arthritis show characteristics of rigidity, hostility, and a variety of other personal variables. These conclusions have since been shown to be drawn from inadequate data.[31]

Personality factors seen in patients with rheumatoid arthritis are found in persons with other chronic disorders and in the healthy population. The psychological factors are probably a response to chronic disease rather than a predisposing cause.[21] The patient may have suffered a serious change in physical function and life roles, and even appearance may be altered by deformity and drug side effects. These changes evoke an adjustment process akin to the grief process after a death. The patient may respond to the disability with depression, denial, a need to control the environment, and dependency.[21]

Some aspects of the illness that may contribute to the psychological state include constant pain and fear of pain; changed body image and perception of self as a sick person; continuous uncertainty about the course and prognosis of the disease because of remissions and flares; sexual dysfunction because of the pain or deformity; and altered social, family, vocational, and leisure roles.

Rehabilitation workers need to be aware of the patient's response to disability and the adjustment that is in progress. All the factors and the behaviors just cited will have an influence on rehabilitation. The interaction of personnel with the patient can facilitate the development of healthy coping mechanisms and acceptance of disability. The reader is referred to Melvin[21] for a more detailed discussion of this subject.

APPLYING PRINCIPLES OF REHABILITATION TO OCCUPATIONAL THERAPY

Rehabilitation of the patient with rheumatoid arthritis is somewhat different from that of a patient with an acute or traumatic condition.[21] Because of the chronic and progressive nature of the disease, rehabilitation intervention may be required periodically for months or even years depending on the course of the disease and the individual patient.

The goals of the basic treatment regime are to decrease inflammation and pain, preserve function, and prevent deformity. The treatment methods used include systemic, emotional, and joint rest; drug therapy; and appropriate exercise[7] and activity. In some instances surgery is required.[12]

Joint rest in nonweight-bearing positions and prone lying to prevent hip and knee flexion contractures are part of the program of rest. Splints are used to provide temporary rest of individual joints.[12]

The amount of rest required varies with the patient. In some instances complete bed rest is necessary, whereas in others the patient may continue with normal daily living, incorporating 2 hours of rest into the daily schedule.[7]

It is of primary importance in the treatment program to preserve function of the hips, knees, elbows, and MP joints. Therefore exercise to other joints must not interfere with functions of these joints or be done at their expense. Complete joint rest is applicable to acutely involved joints only. Self-care activities are permitted to pain tolerance, even in acute arthritis.

INDICATIONS FOR EXERCISE

The concomitant use of the appropriate therapeutic exercise along with rest in proper balance is basic to the management of rheumatoid arthritis. The objectives of the exercise program are to preserve joint integrity, muscle strength, and endurance. Active-assisted exercises are useful and can be performed within limits of pain tolerance from the outset in the treatment program. As disease activity subsides and tolerance for exercise increases, gradation of the program may be increased to include active and resistive exercises.[7]

Acute Stage

During the acute stage, involved joints are inflamed and swollen. There may be systemic signs and symptoms, and rest may be required. Splints, braces, and positioning are used to provide joint rest and prevent deformity.

Active or passive ROM is done only to the point of pain in the acute stage with no stretching at the end of the range. Usually 1 to 2 repetitions of full joint ROM per day is enough to preserve ROM, although because of stiffness it may take several repetitions before maximum joint range is achieved.[21]

Isometric exercise without added resistance (muscle setting) may be used to maintain muscle tone. During the acute stage, one isometric contraction per day is probably sufficient to preserve muscle strength.[21,37] Active exercises should be performed in a manner to prevent active stretching and joint stress. Pain or discomfort that results from exercise and lasts more than 1 hour indicates that the exercise was too stressful and should be decreased.[21]

Active resistive exercise, isometric exercise against added resistance, and stretching exercise are contraindicated during the acute stage of the disease.[42]

Subacute Stage

During the subacute stage of the disease, a few joints are actively involved and there may be mild systemic symptoms. Short periods of rest and splints for corrective or preventive purposes are used.

Gentle passive stretch and active isotonic exercise with minimal joint stress may be added to the passive or active ROM exercise program. Their purpose is to regain lost ROM in those joints that have become limited. A graded isometric strengthening program may be used to maintain or increase muscle strength and endurance.[42]

Chronic-Active and Chronic-Inactive Stages

During the chronic-active and chronic-inactive stages, stretch at the end of the ROM during exercise is recommended to increase ROM. Active ROM, isometric, and isometric resistive exercises may also be continued.

Isotonic resistive exercise has traditionally been thought to produce excessive and undesirable joint stress.[21,42] This fact is undoubtedly true for joints in the acute stage of the disease, when synovitis is present, or when there is instability of the joint from stretching or deformity. In some postsurgical cases or when weakness is present in a chronic patient with a stable inactive joint, however, an individually prescribed isotonic resistive exercise program may be appropriate.[21,24,37]

Home Program

A home exercise program that is designed for the particular patient should be carried out. It is best for the therapist to write out the directions for exercises for the patient to follow. The exercises should be done when the patient is feeling best, often after a warm shower or bath or in the afternoon when joint stiffness is at a minimum. Patients should be advised that taking pain medication in preparation for exercise or other physical activity is rarely recommended because of the need to use pain as a guideline for monitoring duration or intensity of the activity. Application of heat or cold for muscle relaxation and analgesic effect may benefit some patients.[7,20]

There is some conflict in the literature about the appropriateness of having patients with arthritis adhere to a prescribed exercise program over the long term versus incorporating the therapeutic activities and goals into the patient's normal ADL routine. This approach may best be decided on an individual basis with exercise to tolerance[12] as a guideline and keeping principles of joint protection and energy conservation in mind. For a patient recovering from an acute flare, an exercise program should be as efficient as possible so as not to take away valuable energy from one who may be barely able to cope with self-care.[26] For most patients, however, there comes a time when ADL will not be sufficient to enhance improved muscle tone, which aids in joint protection,[24] or to maximize general physical fitness.

In addition to well-accepted therapeutic exercise such as ROM and strengthening, there is evidence that patients with arthritis may benefit from general conditioning exercise and recreational exercise with appropriate modifications to protect involved joints.[2,3] Particularly low-intensity aerobic activities such as walking, swimming, and bicycle riding, or a well-designed low-impact aerobics class have been shown to not only improve exercise tolerance and aerobic capacity but to decrease fatigue and improve functional status as well.[10]

INDICATIONS FOR SPLINTING

Splints may be used to rest inflamed joints; provide stability and improve function; or in the case of dynamic splints, to correct position or deformity. Splints are frequently used for the wrist and fingers but may also be used for the cervical spine, elbows, knees, and ankles. All splinting must be preceded by careful evaluation and be applied with skill, because inappropriate application may be not only ineffective but damaging as well.[34]

It is important to remember that splinting one joint may increase stress to the joints proximal and distal to it. In particular, wrist splints may increase stress to MP joints.[21]

Some of the splints commonly used in treatment of the arthritic hand are summarized from Melvin.[21] These include the volar resting, wrist stabilization, protective MP, combined, and ulnar drift positioning splints.

Volar Resting Splint

The volar resting splint is indicated when there is acute synovitis of the wrist, fingers, and thumb. Its purpose is to rest involved joints and thus decrease inflammation and pain. It is also used when multiple joint contractures are beginning to develop for the purpose of maintaining proper positioning during sleep.

Wrist Stabilization Splint

A wrist stabilization splint immobilizes the wrist but allows motion of the MP joints. It is used when hand function is limited by wrist pain, to improve hand function and grip strength. It may be helpful when there is severe chronic wrist pain or inflammation to provide joint rest and protect extensor tendons from attenuation and rupture.

Protective MP Splint

The protective MP splint maintains the MP joints in normal alignment, allowing 0 to 25° of MP flexion. It is used to protect the MP joints from ulnar deviation and the forces of volar subluxation.

Combined Wrist Stabilization and Protective MP Splint

A combined wrist stabilization and protective MP splint is used when both the wrist and MP joints are involved for the purposes just described.

Ulnar Drift Positioning Splint

An ulnar drift positioning splint prevents ulnar drift and maintains normal alignment of MP joints during pinch and grasp activities.

Splints and other orthoses must be removed regularly for ROM exercises to the involved joints.

The reader is referred to *Rheumatic Disease in the Adult and Child: Occupational Therapy and Rehabilitation* by JL Melvin[21] for a full discussion and description of a wide variety of hand splints and their uses in the treatment of rheumatoid arthritis.

INDICATIONS FOR ACTIVITY

Treatment principles that apply to therapeutic exercise also apply to therapeutic activities. The activities selected should be nonresistive and provide opportunities for the maintenance or increase of ROM and strength. They should be meaningful and interesting to the patient. Joint protection principles, to be discussed subsequently, should be employed during leisure and work activities and activities of daily living (ADL).

Crafts and games as therapeutic modalities are not as frequently or effectively used as therapeutic exercise regimes. They can be of value and interest to some patients, however, and should not be overlooked as a purposeful application of therapeutic exercise procedures.[21]

Activities should be chosen with consideration of how all joints will be affected. For example, macramé on an incline board could be an appropriate activity to increase shoulder and elbow ROM, but would be contraindicated if there is hand involvement caused by metacarpophalangeal (MP) joint synovitis.

The use of crocheting, knitting, and similar traditional needlecrafts is controversial. In principle they are to be avoided because they involve the use of prolonged static contraction of hand muscles in the intrinsic-plus position for holding tools and material. They also facilitate MP ulnar drift and MP volar subluxation through the forces in the hand during the performance of the activity. Melvin points out that in general the only conditions in which knitting and crocheting can be harmful are when there are active MP synovitis, beginning swan-neck deformity caused in part by intrinsic tightness, and degenerative joint disease of the carpometacarpal (CMC) joint of the thumb.[21]

Adverse effects can be prevented by using an MP extension splint, performing intrinsic stretching exercises, and using a thumb CMC stabilization splint, depending on the specific potential problem. Frequent rest breaks during the activity or performing the activity for short, intermittent periods may also be helpful in preventing adverse effects. These considerations are important for those patients who would derive much pleasure and psychological benefit from these traditional and readily available leisure activities.[21]

ADL, including self-care and home management skills, is an important part of the rehabilitation program for the patient with rheumatoid arthritis. Self-care activities to pain and fatigue tolerance should be performed even during early acute stages of the disease episode. The number and types of activities are gradually increased as the patient's endurance and strength improve and pain and discomfort subside.[21]

These activities can be used to maintain or improve joint ROM, muscle strength, and physical endurance. Joint protection, work simplification, and energy conservation principles should be applied during the performance of these activities. The patient, with the aid and direction of the therapist, needs to work out a daily schedule of intermittent rest and activity that is suitable for the stage of the disease, activity tolerance, and any special systemic or joint problems that affect performance.

These principles apply to work activities. Because there are more women than men affected by arthritis, there has been an emphasis in the literature on home management activities, and joint protection principles related to these focused on the traditional role of woman as homemaker. The therapist must not lose sight of the facts that men also perform homemaking tasks and that a substantial percentage of women are employed outside of their homes. Therefore job analysis and application of joint protection and energy conservation principles may be an important part of the rehabilitation program for both men and women. Prevocational evaluation may be necessary if a job change is necessitated by the disability.

For juvenile rheumatoid arthritis, school and leisure activities need to be considered and appropriate pacing of activities employed.

ASSISTIVE EQUIPMENT

Assistive devices and equipment are used to reduce pain, decrease joint stress, and increase independence.

In general the purposes of various devices are to (1) facilitate grasp (built-up soft handles on tools); (2) compensate for lost ROM (dressing sticks or reachers); (3) facilitate ease of performance (lightweight equipment or electrical appliances); (4) stabilize materials or equipment (nonskid mats or suction brushes); (5) prevent deforming stresses (extended faucet handles or adapted key holder); (6) prevent prolonged static contraction (book stand or bowl holder); (7) compensate for weak or absent motor function (universal cuffs or stocking devices); and (8) prevent accidents (bathtub grab bars and nonskid mats for shower or bathtub).

Assistive devices may be used to substitute for lost range of motion, but should not be used for this purpose unless necessary because daily task completion through available range of motion is important to maintaining mobility. Because of the chronic nature of the disease, this concept should be taught to patients who may need to use devices to extend their reach during a flare, but should then use all available range of motion as inflammation subsides and mobility improves.

PRINCIPLES OF JOINT PROTECTION

The purpose of joint protection training is to instruct the patient in methods of reducing joint stress, decreasing pain, preserving joint structures, and conserving energy.[21]

The arthritic joint is predisposed to deterioration from abuse that can lead to reduced performance abilities.[6] Patients with rheumatoid arthritis need to employ joint protection principles in all of their daily activities when in active phase of the disease or where joint instability is present to maintain maximal function and prevent joint damage and deformity.

Maintain Muscle Strength and Joint ROM

During daily activities each joint should be used at its maximal ROM and strength consistent with the disease

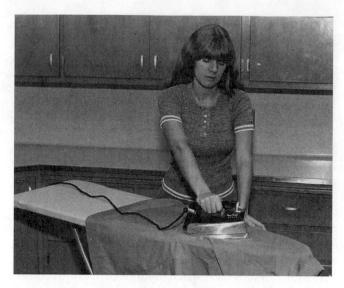

FIG. 34-2 During ironing, full extension at elbow can be practiced.

process. For example, long, sweeping, flowing strokes to maintain and increase ROM can be employed when ironing. The arms should be straightened as far as possible, especially on flat work (Fig. 34-2). When vacuuming or mopping the floor a long, forward stroke of the implement, then pulling it in close to the body so the arm is first fully straightened, then fully bent, will achieve full or nearly full range of elbow flexion and extension and shoulder motion. The use of dust mitts on both hands keeps fingers straight and prevents the static contraction and potentially deforming forces of holding a dust cloth. Light objects such as cereal, oats, or sugar can be kept on high shelves so that full ROM in the shoulder can be used with reaching.[17]

Avoid Positions of Deformity and Deforming Stresses

Positions that place internal forces (such as a tight grasp) and external forces (such as propping the chin on the side or back of the fingers) may contribute to deformity and should be avoided during daily activity. Some applications of this principle include always turning the fingers toward the thumb side, such as turning a doorknob toward the thumb or opening the door with the right hand and closing it with the left. Jars should be opened with the right hand and closed with the left (Fig. 34-3). Dishcloths or hand laundry can be placed over the faucet and squeezed between the palms or rolled in a towel to absorb water.[17]

Pressures along the thumb side of fingers should be avoided. These pressures contribute to ulnar deviation. This position of ulnar deviation decreases the use of the hands. Pressure can be prevented by (1) avoiding leaning chin on fingers or palm of hand; (2) picking up coffee cup with two hands instead of with index, middle finger, and thumb; (3) twisting a jar cap off and on with the palm of the hand and not with the fingers (Fig. 34-3); (4) in-

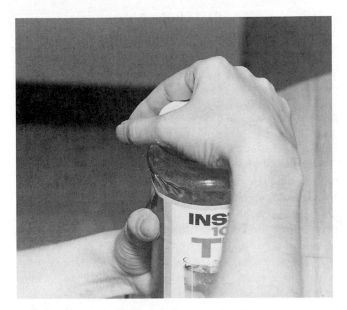

FIG. 34-3 Jar cap is twisted off, using palm of hand, and opened with right hand to prevent ulnar drift.

stalling lever extensions on faucet handles to avoid use of fingers to turn on and off; and (5) using electric can opener instead of hand-operated type, because this device requires sustained grasp of one hand and forced motion of the thumb and fingers of the other hand for operation.

Tight grasp should be avoided. This position increases the strength of the muscles that allow grasp and therefore contributes to ulnar deviation and dislocation of joints. This problem happens in activities such as carrying pails and baskets; using pliers, scissors, and screwdrivers; and holding spoons to stir or mix foods.

When standing up, the patient should be instructed to take the body weight through the wrist with fingers straight rather than on the fingers (Fig. 34-4). The palm of the hand, rather than the fingers, should be used when taking down or hanging clothes in the closet. The palm can be used to lift the hanger at the exposed area in its apex. This method is most useful for heavy coats and jackets.

Excessive and constant pressure against the pad of the thumb should be avoided. For example, pressure against the pad of the thumb to open a car door, sew through thick fabric, and rise to a standing position all contribute to dislocation of the thumb joints.[17]

Use Each Joint in Its Most Stable Anatomical and Functional Plans

The patient should be instructed in the use of good body mechanics for transitional movements. The patient should stand or position self directly in front of a drawer to open it and not pull while standing to one side. In reaching for objects on a shelf the patient should stand or position self directly in front of or under the shelf, not at the side. The wrist and fingers should always be used in good alignment.[21]

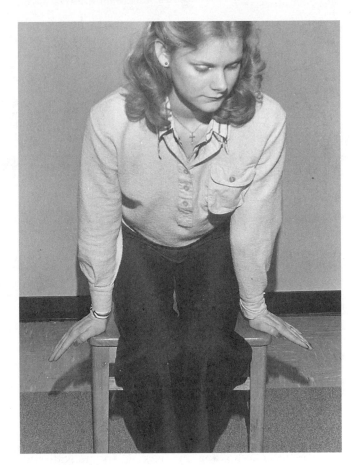

FIG. 34-4 Use of palms to push off chair helps to prevent dislocation of finger joints.

Use the Strongest Joints Available for the Activity

Applications of using the strongest joints include using the hips and knees, not the back, when lifting and using the entire body to move heavy things. Carts and chairs should be pushed from behind; use straps for opening and closing heavy doors and drawers; and roll objects on counters and floors rather than lifting them. If any objects must be lifted, they should be scooped up in both hands, palms upward. This technique can be used when handling baking pans and casseroles if long oven mits are used and in handling dishes, packages, books, and laundry.[17]

Avoid Using Muscles or Holding Joints in One Position for Any Undue Length of Time

Sustained muscle contraction is fatiguing and can contribute to joint subluxation and dislocation because fatigued muscles cannot provide support to weakened joints. Applications of this principle include (1) using a book stand instead of holding the book while reading; (2) when mixing, stabilizing the bowl with the palm of the hand and fingers against the body or wall or in an open drawer to avoid handling the bowl with the fingers

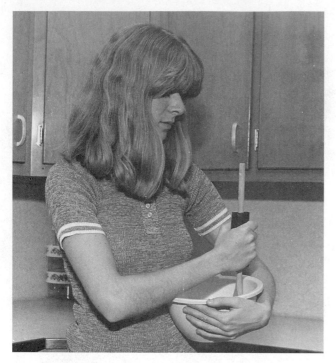

FIG. 34-5 Mixing bowl is stabilized with forearm. Spoon with soft, built-up handle is held so that pressure is toward radial side of hand.

and thumb; (3) holding the mixing spoon with the thumb side pointing upward, not with the thumb pointing downward, and using a built-up handle to decrease the force of grasp (Fig. 34-5); (4) using a brush to scour pans, not the fingertips; (5) using the palm of the hand or the bend in the elbow instead of fingers in carrying handbags and coats; (6) holding objects, such as a vegetable peeler or knife, parallel to MP joints and not across the palms.[17,21]

Never Begin an Activity That Cannot Be Stopped Immediately If It Proves To Be Too Taxing

In climbing up and down stairs, standing balance should be adequate to allow stopping and resting. In transferring from bed to wheelchair, a sliding board should be used for less stress and to allow for stopping if necessary. In getting in and out of a bathtub, graded platforms to ascend and descend gradually at individual speed and tolerance can be used. Planning rests during walks and when carrying objects will decrease fatigue.

Respect Pain

Some discomfort during treatment and activity may be tolerable and acceptable. If rest produces rapid relief, the level of activity need not necessarily be considered excessive.[6] Pain lasting 1 or more hours after activity, however, is a sign that the activity needs to be stopped or modified.[6,21] Pain can evoke protective muscle spasm and inhibit muscle contraction.

ENERGY CONSERVATION AND WORK SIMPLIFICATION

Because prevention of fatigue is an important consideration in the management of rheumatoid arthritis, methods of simplifying work to save energy should be employed. One of the most important means to this end is to determine and carry out an appropriate balance between rest and play. The recommended amount of rest is 10 to 12 hours of rest per day, including a 1- to 2-hour nap in the afternoon.

Short rest breaks of 5 to 10 minutes during daily activities can be very helpful in increasing overall endurance. In general, 5 to 10 minutes of rest to 20 minutes of activity is adequate. It may be difficult for the patient to accept the notion of these short rest breaks, because it is often the desire to get work or housekeeping over with as quickly as possible. However, intermittent rest can actually save energy for more enjoyable tasks.[21] Work can be planned for an entire week and month. Light and heavy tasks can be alternated and work paced throughout the week, instead of doing a lot of work in one day. Work should be planned so that it is efficient, that is, not requiring getting up and down and moving to and fro repeatedly.

Time management needs to be explored if rushing is a tendency of the patient. Rushing increases tension and fatigue. Most important, the patient should learn an energy-saving program and work schedule that prevent pushing to exhaustion.[17]

Other suggestions for conserving energy include the following: (1) avoid bending and stooping by using long-handle reachers and flexible-handle dust mops; (2) avoid long periods of standing during activities such as ironing and food preparation; rather, use a high stool; (3) avoid extra trips by using a utility cart to convey as many items as needed at once; and (4) relax homemaking standards by using prepackaged foods and by air-drying dishes, for example.

Work may be simplified by adjusting the work height for maximal comfort. The elbows should be flexed to 90°, and shoulders should be in a relaxed position. This position can be accomplished without expensive home modification by using an adjustable ironing board as a work surface, placing a board over an open drawer, or using a high stool with a backrest to work at counters. A rack may be placed in the sink bottom to elevate the dishpan and thus prevent stooping during dishwashing.

Work areas can be rearranged so that frequently used tools, equipment, and supplies are stored nearby and at easily reached levels. Counter tops may be used for convenient storage of small appliances. Commercial organizers, such as step shelves and revolving turntables, can make work easier.[17]

OCCUPATIONAL THERAPY FOR RHEUMATOID ARTHRITIS

The patient with rheumatoid arthritis should be seen for occupational therapy services shortly after the diagnosis of arthritis is made. It is often the case, however, that occupational therapy may not be initiated until many joints are involved, after surgery, or when the disease is severe enough to cause hospitalization or moderate-to-severe performance limitations.

EVALUATION
Medical History

An initial intake should include medical chart or record review if available. If not, a brief medical history should be taken from the patient because the therapist must be aware of all health problems. Current medications should also be noted. The patient's report of which joints are currently involved or have been involved in the past as well as any other systems affected should be recorded.

Observation

The occupational therapist should observe the appearance of joints for heat, redness, edema, deformity, deforming tendencies on motion, skin quality, and joint enlargement. In the early stages of the disease joints may appear puffy and soft. If the disease is active, joints may be red and hot.

ROM

The occupational therapy evaluation includes active and passive ROM measurements, which may take a considerable amount of time if there is discomfort or pain in the joints. It may be necessary to perform the measurements gradually over two or three treatment sessions. The therapist should be aware of how the joints feel, that is, stiff, unstable, or crepitant. A major discrepancy between active and passive ROM may be caused by pain secondary to inflammation in the joint or soft tissue, as well as from weakness[30] or tendon involvement.[4]

Strength

Testing of muscle strength may be done by group or individual muscle testing. The usual procedures for manual muscle testing need to be adapted for the patient who has arthritis. Resistance should be applied within the patient's pain-free ROM rather than at the end of the ROM, as is usual in manual muscle testing. It is not unusual for patients with arthritis to have pain in the last 30 to 40° of joint motion. Therefore if resistance is applied within the pain-free range, the inhibition of muscle strength by pain will be avoided.[21]

The use of the manual muscle test is controversial, because some physicians prohibit any resistance that can cause harm to diseased tissue and joints and place deforming forces on the joint.[41] Functional muscle or motion testing may be used if resistance is prohibited.

In both the ROM assessment and the muscle strength test, the therapist should make note of the time of day and the amount of antiinflammatory or analgesic medication taken. These medications can affect results of the evaluation.[21]

Hand Function

Hand function testing is important. Pinch and grip strength testing with instruments is not done in patients with joint involvement in the hand.[41] Grip and pinch can be tested, however, with an adapted blood pressure cuff and measured in millimeters of mercury.[21,30] A test of hand function that evaluates grasp and prehension patterns such as the Jebsen Test of Hand Function[14] or observation of hand use with common functional tasks should be done. Hands that have severe involvement and obvious deformity may, in fact, have very good function.

Sensation

Sensory evaluation is indicated if there is potential nerve compression caused by swelling. Modalities that should be tested are senses of touch, pain, temperature, and position. Paresthesias should be noted.

Endurance

The patient's physical endurance should be evaluated by observation and an assessment of the daily or weekly schedule. Specific lower extremity evaluation may be carried out by the occupational or physical therapist. The occupational therapist should observe the gait pattern and the mode of rising and sitting and the patient's posture during ambulation and when sitting. Safety for ambulation should be assessed because the patient may require an assistive device.

The therapist should observe for any obvious joint limitations and weakness in the lower extremities and have data from specific evaluation of ROM, strength, and deforming tendencies in the legs. These factors are important considerations in planning treatment, presenting joint protection and energy conservation techniques, and positioning to prevent loss of ROM in the lower extremities.

Specific lower extremity joint problems or problems with the feet may benefit from physical therapy or orthotic assessment. Note should also be made of footwear so that recommendations can be made to provide good support to arthritic feet.

Performance

Assessment of performance is a very important part of the occupational therapy program. Evaluation of ADL, including self-care, child care, home management, work activities, exercise behaviors, and leisure activities should be carried out by interview and observation. A home evaluation should be carried out to assist the patient in learning new methods and in making modifications to simplify work, save energy, and protect joints from undue stress. Job performance may be evaluated by observation in a real or simulated situation. The job tasks can be analyzed, and joint protection principles can be applied, if possible. Pacing of work responsibilities may be a consideration to incorporate the required rest periods into the working day.

TREATMENT OBJECTIVES

The general objectives of treatment for patients with rheumatoid arthritis are to (1) maintain or increase joint mobility; (2) maintain or increase muscle strength; (3) increase physical endurance; (4) prevent or correct deformities, if feasible; (5) minimize the effect of deformities; (6) maintain or increase ability to perform daily life tasks; (7) increase knowledge about the disease and the best methods of dealing with physical, performance, and psychosocial effects; and (8) aid with stress management and adjustment to physical disability.

TREATMENT METHODS

Methods used by occupational therapists to minimize the dysfunction that can result from rheumatoid arthritis include a variety of exercise, just described, tailored to the patient's needs and stage of the disease.

Training in ADL is an important aspect of the occupational therapy program for many patients. This training includes joint protection, energy conservation techniques, and use of assistive devices and special equipment. Self-care, child care, home management, and work activities may be included in the ADL training program. Joint protection principles and energy-saving techniques should be introduced gradually, and the number and complexity of procedures should be increased as the patient incorporates previously learned skills into daily life. For some patients arts and crafts games, as described earlier, can be a meaningful part of the treatment program. This approach will depend on the patient's needs, interests, and lifestyle and should be explored with the patient and not overlooked.

Splints to protect joints and prevent or retard the development of deformity are usually made by the occupational therapist. The therapist may recognize the need for splints and recommend them to the physician in some instances. Some splints that may be of benefit in the treatment of rheumatoid arthritis include the resting, cock-up, ulnar drift, MP extensor assist, flexor assist, CMC stabilization, and three-point finger extension splints.[21]

Psychosocial factors may be treated by exploring the patient's attitude toward the disability, the patient's goals, how the patient deals with pain and fear, and performance priorities and objectives. Activity groups, such as movement or exercise classes, home management classes, or arthritis education classes, can serve as mutual support and problem-solving groups. Occupational therapists may lead or participate with other rehabilitation specialists in such activity groups. Sexual counseling may be necessary to teach joint protection techniques during sexual activity and explore attitudes about body image, self-acceptance, and acceptance by the partner as a sexual being. Several excellent treatments of this subject are available.[5,32,35] (See Chapter 17.)

Education of the patient and family about the disease, potential disability, treatment, and home program to achieve maximal function is essential. Such education can be provided through classes and literature available from the Arthritis Foundation. Family roles may need to be changed or modified as a result of one member's physical dysfunction. Therefore it is important for families to understand and support the disabled member and to lend aid for tasks the patient cannot or should not do.[28,31]

The occupational therapist should assist in designing a home program for the patient. This program should include a suitable work and rest schedule, activities, and exercises that will maximize function and minimize deformity and dysfunction. The home program should be outlined for the patient in writing.

TREATMENT PRECAUTIONS

Fatigue should be avoided, and pain should be respected. It may be difficult for the patient to do things in the morning because of joint stiffness. A warm shower may be helpful to begin moving. Static, stressful, or resistive activities should be avoided. The use of a ball, putty, or clay for squeezing should be avoided, because these involve forceful flexion of the fingers, which can produce ulnar deviation, MP subluxation, and extensor tendon displacement.[9,21]

Heat may be beneficial to reduce pain and stiffness but may not be indicated in an acutely inflamed joint. Cold packs may be more beneficial during this stage; however, either modality can be used in the subacute phase based on the patient's response. Associated conditions such as vasculitis or Raynaud disease may make the use of heat and cold contraindicated.[22]

Resistive exercises for strengthening muscles do *not* improve joint stability and should not be used for this purpose. Joint instability is usually caused by ligamentous laxity, and resistive exercises can make this condition worse.

If sensation is impaired, the patient may not be aware of it, as the onset may be insidious and manifest itself subtly as gradual weakness and loss of hand function,[38] which may be attributed to other disease factors or hand deformity.[4] Because of possible involvement of the cervical spine in RA, it should be determined if any peripheral neuropathic condition is due to a cervical myelopathy or to a more distal lesion.[38] Appropriate protective mechanisms should be taught.

ASSESSMENT AND TREATMENT OF SPECIFIC JOINT PROBLEMS AND DEFORMITIES

Rheumatoid arthritis can result in tendon, muscle, and nerve dysfunction and a variety of joint deformities. All joints of the upper extremity should be evaluated. Tests for specific deformities or potential deformities of the hand should be administered as appropriate. The therapist might evaluate for possible carpal tunnel syndrome,

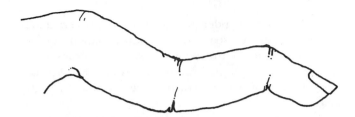

FIG. 34-6 Swan-neck deformity results in PIP hyperextension and DIP flexion.

swan-neck deformities (Fig. 34-6), boutonnière deformities (Fig. 34-7), flexor tendon nodules, ulnar drift (Fig. 34-8), MP subluxation (Fig. 34-9), wrist subluxation (Fig. 34-10), intrinsic and extrinsic muscle tightness, ruptured tendons, extensor tendon displacement, and laxity of the MP collateral ligaments.[4]

SHOULDER JOINT
Shoulder Synovitis

The shoulder is a complex joint, which owes its great mobility to a small amount of bony stability. Pain-free movement is the result of mobility at the glenohumeral, acromioclavicular, scapulothoracic, and sternoclavicular joints and to perfectly balanced and rhythmic contraction of many muscle groups. In addition to synovitis of the glenohumeral joint, there may be involvement of the bursae and tendons of the joint. Problems in these areas may result in a frozen shoulder, which causes major problems with ADL and in ambulation with crutches.

Intervention

Corticosteroid injection early is very effective in reducing pain and restricted motion. Aggressive active and passive ROM and isotonic exercise are imperative, especially preceded by hot packs. A joint protection program is strongly indicated. Slings are a hazard and should be avoided.

Surgical procedures used in severe problems may include bursectomy, synovectomy, acromioplasty, or total shoulder replacement.

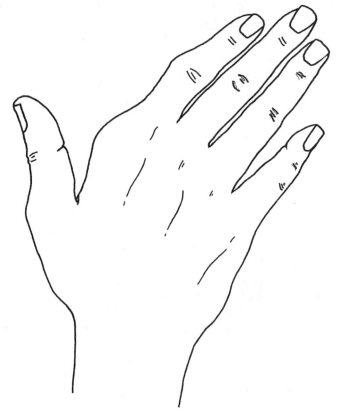

FIG. 34-8 MP joint ulnar drift.

ELBOW JOINT
Elbow Synovitis

The humeroulnar joint is a hinge joint, and synovitis results in loss of ROM. Disease of the radiohumeral joint can result in loss of pronation-supination at the elbow. Loss of flexion can result in contracture that prevents feeding and many other ADL. Loss of extension can result in contracture that decreases reach and makes ADL and crutch use difficult and some tasks impossible. Loss of pronation-supination severely compromises the use of the hands and wrists in ADL. A dominant arm with severe loss of extension and pronation makes writing and other activities extremely difficult. Both elbows with severely limited flexion seriously impair ADL and functional activities; both elbows with severely limited extension make transfers and crutch use extremely difficult.

The ulnar nerve may also become compressed at the elbow because of synovitis or surgery, and initial screening should include assessment of nerve function.

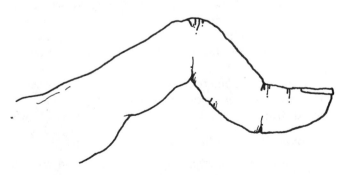

FIG. 34-7 Boutonnière deformity results in DIP hyperextension and PIP flexion.

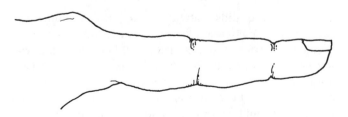

FIG. 34-9 MP palmar subluxation.

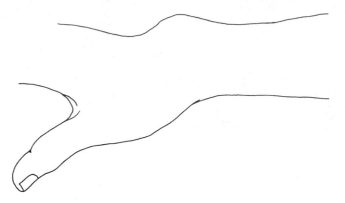

FIG. 34-10 Flexion subluxation of wrist.

Intervention

As with other joints, synovitis of the elbow is treated with rest, use of cold, and corticosteroid injection. With disease in the elbows, splints and slings limiting movement must be used judiciously. Splints are beneficial for providing rest or in the case of joint instability.[27]

Active and passive ROM exercises are strongly indicated daily for the elbow. Isometric exercise is indicated for strengthening only if isotonic exercise is too painful. Isotonic exercise is best given through proper ADL instruction. Sometimes surgery is aimed toward (1) improving extension at the expense of flexion in the dominant arm to permit crutch use and writing and (2) improving flexion at the expense of extension in the nondominant extremity for feeding and personal grooming.

Chronic synovitis may be treated with elbow synovectomy and resection of the radial head. An elbow arthroplasty can be indicated if there is intractable pain, joint destruction, or loss of self-care ability.[21,27]

WRIST JOINT
Wrist Subluxation

Subluxation of the wrist (Fig. 34-10) is a volar slippage of the carpal bones on the radius. It is caused by weakness of the supporting ligaments caused by chronic synovitis. To test for wrist subluxation, the therapist should palpate from the distal radius to the carpals on the dorsal side of the forearm. If there is subluxation, there will be a step. It may be merely palpable if mild, visible if moderate, and grossly malaligned if severe.[21]

Intervention

Wrist splinting adds stability (1) to improve function, (2) to relieve pain, and (3) to prevent tendon rupture of digital extensor tendons. A flexible splint during the day with rigid splinting at night may be the most appropriate approach. The patient who does not wear splints all the time should be taught to use the splint during those activities that will be particularly stressful to the structures of the wrist.[20]

Carpal Tunnel Syndrome

The carpal tunnel under the transverse flexor carpal ligament is a tightly closed space, and inflammation can lead to high pressure on the median nerve, which runs in the carpal tunnel. This pressure produces pain and sensory disturbances over the median nerve distribution in the hand.

Initial symptoms may be numbness and tingling in the thumb, index, and middle fingers. Median nerve motor weakness and atrophy of the opponens pollicis and abductor pollicis brevis may result in thenar atrophy. *If not already known by the physician, this condition should be promptly brought to his or her attention for treatment.* Untreated, median nerve compression can result and can progress to permanent loss of feeling in the hand and weak-to-lost thumb opposition, which are serious impairments to hand use.

Intervention

Until medically treated, heat and any exercises of the wrist other than active ROM are contraindicated. A cock-up splint with a neutral wrist position is worn at night and in some cases during the day as well. Techniques to reduce edema may be used, such as the use of cold packs, contrast baths, and elevation. ADL training to prevent aggravation of the problem is important, and some job tasks or household activities may need to be modified.[29] Patients should be instructed to use the wrist in neutral alignment during activities.

Corticosteroid injection may be beneficial, but none of these measures is effective, surgical release of the transverse carpal ligament is indicated.

Synovial Invasion of Extensor Tendons

Dorsal swelling can be seen and felt in cases of invasion of the extensor tendon sheaths. This swelling can lead to their weakness or rupture, resulting in weak to lost extension of the fingers at the MP, proximal interphalangeal (PIP), and distal interphalangeal (DIP) joints, flexion contractures, and loss of hand function, which is serious.

Intervention

As soon as discovered, surgical synovectomy can correct and prevent further problems. Tendon repair may be done if caught promptly. Active ROM exercises at the wrist and night splints for the wrist can preserve function before surgery but are not substitutes for surgery. Passive and active ROM of the MP, PIP, and DIP are indicated to prevent flexion contracture.

Isotonic and isometric exercise or resistive exercise of the wrist extensors is of no value and may produce further damage.

Synovial Invasion of Carpal Bones

Synovial invasion of the carpal bone results in erosion and destruction of the intercarpal ligaments and joints. It can result in progressive loss of wrist motion, contracture of the wrist in a nonfunctional position, or in flexion subluxation-dislocation of the wrist (Fig. 34-10).

Intervention

Loss of ROM can be minimized by active ROM exercise. Passive ROM should be gentle to avoid damaging ligaments. Using volar resting splints at night with the wrist in the position of function (neutral radioulnar position and slight wrist extension) can prevent contracture in nonfunctional positions. Surgery is not feasible except to fuse in more functional positions. Because surgery can offer wrist fusion only in the position of function, static wrist splints in the position of function produce the same result. Splints causing loss of pronation-supination are contraindicated. Active pronation-supination ROM exercise and gentle passive ROM are indicated several times a day with the wrist out of the splint to prevent this loss. Joint protection against forceful flexion is strongly indicated. Isometric strengthening of wrist extensors is indicated.

Isotonic and isotonic resistive exercise may lead to subluxation-dislocation.

Synovial Invasion of Radioulnar Joint

Synovitis of the radioulnar joint, causing erosion of joint cartilage, usually results in progressive loss of pronation and supination at the wrist, particularly if there is associated elbow disease. It can result in partial-to-complete loss of pronation and supination of the wrist with severe functional impairment.

Intervention

Surgical resection of the distal ulna can be done to restore lost pronation-supination. Active pronation-supination ROM exercises and passive ROM are indicated daily to prevent loss. Pronation-supination in ADL is encouraged.

Isotonic or resistive exercises are contraindicated.

HAND ASSESSMENT
Extrinsic Muscle Tightness

To test for tightness (contracture) or adherence of the extensor digitorum communis (EDS) tendon, the wrist is positioned at neutral. Then the MP joint is passively flexed to different positions, and simultaneously the PIP and DIP joints are flexed. The test is positive if the position of the proximal joint (MP) influences the degree of flexion possible at the distal joints (IPs). For example, when the MP joint is fully flexed, the PIP joint will lack full active or passive flexion. When the PIP joint is fully flexed, it will not be possible fully to flex the MP joint because the tendon does not have sufficient length to go over all the joints it crosses when they are all flexed.[8,21]

When performing this test, forceful flexion of the wrist and fingers should be avoided, and all joint movements should be done gently. If there is any attrition of the extensor tendons, forceful flexion of these joints could cause tendon rupture.[36]

Intrinsic Muscle Tightness

Intrinsic muscles become weak, scarred, and shortened when they are invaded by pannus during the rheumatoid disease process.[4,21] This condition can create an excessive pull on the PIP joint, causing hyperextension.[20] Whenever intrinsic muscle tightness is found, patients should be taught intrinsic muscle exercise.

When testing for intrinsic tightness, the test for extrinsic muscle tightness is applied first to prove that the extensor tendons do not have adhesions.[8,30] Then the MP joint is passively moved into full extension, and the PIP joint is flexed. Resistance to PIP flexion indicates intrinsic tightness. The PIP joint will not flex fully in this position if the intrinsic muscles are shortened. The reason is that the lumbricales act to extend the IP joints during MP flexion. By extending MP joints and flexing PIP joints, these muscles are fully stretched. If they have become shortened, there will be insufficient elasticity or length to achieve the test position. It is important to rule out intrinsic tightness when measuring PIP joint motion so that accurate joint mobility is recorded.

MP Joints of Second to Fifth Fingers
MP ulnar drift

In the normal hand, the MP ligaments, particularly when the MPs are flexed at 45°, give medial and lateral stability. Both the extensor and flexor tendons to the fingers are bowed to produce an ulnar drift tendency of the tendons at the MP joints during normal contraction. Forced contractions and especially forceful hand grips accentuate this tendency. With MP ligaments weakened, the normal forces result in ulnar drift. The fifth MP joint buttresses the remainder of fingers from static, postural ulnar drift, but when the fifth MP ligament loses stability, ulnar drift can occur with gravity and posture even at rest (Fig. 34-8).

The result is that the MP ligament damage is mild or if the stability of the fifth joint is preserved, the ulnar drift may occur only dynamically with finger extension-flexion. This condition gives weak pinch, which may result in thumb adduction and lateral pinch being substituted for true opposition. If the MP ligament damage is severe or if the stability of the fifth MP joint is lost, there will be ulnar drift even at rest, posturally, and the problem of opposition will be severe.

The dynamic and static ulnar drift plus lifting of the extensor hood by MP synovitis will result in dislocation of the extensor tendons from the extensor hood over the metacarpal heads into the space between the heads, leading to possible tendon injury and loss of ability completely to extend the MP joints. The lateral pinching of the thumb will result in radial subluxation and deformity of the IP joint of the thumb.

The therapist may test for the deformity by measuring the angle between the proximal phalanx and the MP joints during active extension. This measurement should be compared with the normal ROM. The index finger normally has 10 to 20° of ulnar deviation during active extension. The severity of the ulnar drift is described as follows:

Severity	Index Finger	Fingers 3 to 5
Mild	20 to 30°	0 to 10°
Moderate	30 to 50°	10 to 30°
Severe	50° or more	30° or more[21]

Intervention. Treatment consists of early synovectomy, which may prevent progressive MP ligament damage. Extensor tendons dislocated ulnarly may be able to be replaced surgically with excision of MP synovial tissue. Severe problems may require replacement of the MP joints, because the MP ligaments cannot be successfully repaired surgically. Daily passive ROM exercises of the MP joints are indicated only if daily active ROM does not produce full flexion and extension. A joint protection program is strongly indicated to prevent forceful flexion and extension in ADL. Dynamic ulnar deviation splints during the day coupled with static splints with the MPs in neutral deviation and 45° of flexion at night may halt progression of deformity and improve opposition.

Isotonic and isometric exercise or resistive exercise of the fingers will not help this deformity and may produce further MP ligament damage.

MP palmar subluxation-dislocation

Synovitis of the MPs results in MP ligament damage. Because finger flexors are much stronger and are used much more than extensors, palmar dislocation will result. Palmar dislocation is often associated with ulnar drift but may occur by itself. Loss of effective MP extension and shortening and weakening of the intrinsic muscles are the usual isolated problems. Complete dislocation can occur (Fig. 34-9). Functionally, the patient will have limited ability to open the hand or lay the hand flat, causing a problem for activities such as putting the hand into a pocket or glove.

The therapist can test for this deformity by palpating over the dorsum of the joint when it is at the 0° neutral position. If there is subluxation, a step can be felt between the metacarpal and the first phalanx. The deformity is described as mild if the step is palpable, but full extension is possible; as moderate if the step is visible, palpable, and there is a slight limitation of extension; and as severe if there is gross malalignment and definite limitation of ROM.[21]

Intervention. Early, complete surgical replacement or repair of the MP joints is the only effective treatment. Passive and active ROM exercises of the MPs to prevent loss of ROM are indicated. No exercises or splints are effective in correcting or treating this problem. A joint protection program is strongly indicated to prevent further progressive damage during ADL.

PIP and DIP Joints of Second to Fifth Fingers
Swan-neck deformity

Swan-neck deformity results in hyperextension of the PIP joint and incomplete extension or slight flexion of the DIP joint. There are several causes of swan-neck deformity. Three types are discussed here. It is important for the therapist and physician to know the underlying cause if appropriate treatment is to be instituted.

One type of swan-neck deformity is caused by initial involvement at the MP joint[21] and results in intrinsic muscle tightness.

Another type of swan-neck deformity is a result of initial involvement at the DIP joints[21] and rupture of the lateral slips of the extensor tendons (Fig. 34-11). To test for this type, the test for extrinsic tightness is applied first to prove that there is no adherence of the extensor tendon.[21] Then the MP joint is moved into extension, and the PIP joint is flexed to prove that there is no intrinsic tightness. Then the patient should extend the finger actively. If there is a rupture of the lateral slips of the extensor tendon, the DIP joint will drop into flexion because ruptured lateral slips of the EDC cannot function to extend the joint. The middle slip of the EDC, acting on the PIP joint, pulls too hard and hyperextends the joint when active extension is attempted, resulting in the swan-neck appearance.

A swan-neck deformity with initial involvement at the PIP joint is caused by chronic synovitis, which leads to stretching of supporting structures or rupture of the flexor digitorum superficialis (FDS) tendon[21] (Fig. 34-12). To test for this condition, the test for extrinsic tightness is applied as before. The MP joint is moved into hyperextension, and the PIP joint is flexed to rule out intrinsic tightness. The patient is then asked to flex the finger into the palm actively while the examiner holds the adjacent fingers in extension. If the FDS tendon is ruptured, it will not be possible to flex the PIP joint. The tendon rupture is a result of synovitis of the PIP joint with infiltration of the FDS tendon. Bony spurs producing tendon erosion may also cause the tendon to rupture.[21] With progression of a swan-neck deformity, the patient may lose active flexion, which will limit function.

Intervention. Direct surgery involving the lateral slips of the extensor tendons is rarely done because of poor

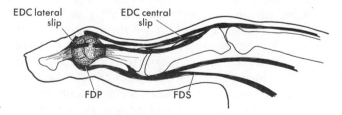

FIG. 34-11 Swan-neck deformity resulting from rupture of lateral slips of EDC tendon.

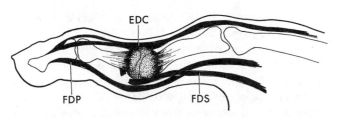

FIG. 34-12 Swan-neck deformity as a result of rupture of FDS tendon.

technical results. Sometimes synovectomy is indicated early to remove the invading synovium at the MP joints. Daily passive ROM and gentle stretching are indicated for the DIPs. Active ROM should be done daily to the MPs, PIPs, and DIPs to prevent contractures. A small, short splint may be applied to the PIPs during daily activity to prevent progressive hyperextension. A three-point finger splint is sometimes used to maintain range of PIP flexion and relieve stress to the volar aspect of the PIP joint resulting from severe hyperextension.[21]

This approach will provide improved function, because with severe deformity, the patient cannot overcome the hyperextended position and thus loses active flexion.

Isotonic and isometric resistive exercise to the finger extensors will not strengthen damaged tendons and may damage them further.

Boutonnière deformity

Boutonnière deformity can occur when synovitis at the wrist, MP, or PIP joints weakens or destroys the central slip of the extensor tendon, which inserts into the base of the middle phalanx. There is often associated PIP joint arthritis. The result is incomplete and weak-to-absent extension at the PIP joint when the lateral slips of the extensor tendon, which insert into the base of the distal phalanx, slip below the axis of the PIP joint becoming flexors of that joint and hyperextending the DIP joint where they insert (Fig. 34-13). The central slip of the extensor tendon is the major extensor of the finger, and if this problem is recent (days) and if *the physician does not know of it,* he or she should be informed immediately. Invariably a flexion contracture of the PIP joint and hyperextension of the DIP joint with loss of flexion range

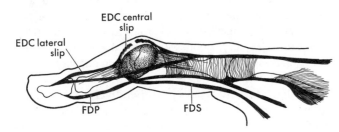

FIG. 34-13 Boutonnière deformity caused by rupture or lengthening of central slip of EDC tendon.

will ensue. Function of the finger will be seriously compromised because of inability to straighten the finger and loss of flexion at the tip for pinch or fisting.

Intervention. Direct surgery of the central slips is often done if caught early enough, but there may be severe damage to the extensor tendon by the synovium, which may require a tendon graft from another site or may be irreparable. Therefore the fourth and fifth fingers are rarely operated on, whereas the second and third fingers are operated on because of hand function priorities. Synovectomy will not restore tendon integrity but may be indicated to prevent the invasion of other tendons in proximity. Daily passive ROM is indicated for the MPs, PIPs, and DIPs to correct or prevent deformity. Active ROM exercises should be done daily to the MPs, PIPs, and DIPs to preserve joint ROM and muscle tone. Dynamic extension splints of the second and third fingers may be indicated to improve function and opposition.

Isotonic and isometric exercise or resistive exercise to the extensors will not help this deformity and may further damage tendons.

Trigger finger

Trigger finger deformity is caused by a nodule or thickening of the flexor tendons of the fingers or thumb as they pass through the digital pulleys. This condition is caused by a nodule on the FDS tendon or thickening of the synovium which blocks or makes difficult the slipping of the tendon through its sheath, preventing full extension of the PIP joint.[4,21] To test for this problem the examiner should ask the patient if the fingers ever catch or stay closed when attempts are made to open the hand. If the patient answers affirmatively, the examiner should determine if the condition occurs rarely, occasionally, or consistently; if there is any pain associated with it; and if it inhibits function.

The therapist should palpate for a nodule over the flexor pulleys. A click or crepitation may be palpated at the point where the nodule is pulled through the sheath. The palpation point is in the palm distal to the palmar creases at the base of the involved finger. The deformity is described as mild if there is inconsistent, painless triggering during active motion; as moderate if there is constant triggering during active motion or if it is intermittent but painful; and as severe if it prevents full active motion and is severely painful.[21]

Intervention. If persistent triggering occurs, it may result in lost range of motion or tendon rupture. Treatment includes hydrocortisone injection, tendon protection techniques, splinting, and the use of heat to improve tissue mobility and cold to decrease inflammation.[4] ADL evaluation and training as well as instruction in the use of heat and cold may be appropriate.

Thumb

Flexion of MP joint with hyperextension of the IP joint (type I deformity)

Chronic MP synovitis causes attenuation of the joint capsule, MP collateral ligaments, and the overlying extensor mechanism. Pain and distention of the joint capsule cause damage of the intrinsic muscles of the thumb, which may progress to MP palmar subluxation and ulnar-volar displacement of the extensor pollicis longus tendon. Once displaced this tendon acts as an MP flexor and with intrinsic muscle damage, causes hyperextension of the IP joint. The result is MP flexion and IP hyperextension.[21]

Flexion of the MP joint with IP hyperextension and carpometacarpal (CMC) involvement (type II deformity)

Type II deformity appears similar to type I deformity, but CMC joint damage and subluxation, a result of chronic synovitis of this joint, are the major factors. Once there is subluxation of the CMC joint, the adductor pollicis muscle pulls on the first metacarpal, which can result in a fixed adduction contracture with hyperextension of the distal phalanx.[21]

MP lateral instability and CMC joint adduction (type III deformity)

Type III deformity begins with MP joint synovitis resulting in stretching of the ligaments. As the MP joint shifts radially, the metacarpal adducts with gradual webspace contracture. There is no CMC joint involvement.

MP hyperextension and IP flexion (type IV deformity)

Type IV deformity is similar to type II but with no CMC involvement. The gradual progression of MP hyperextension leads to IP flexion.

Intervention. These problems may be treated surgically by extensor tendon repair, synovectomy, arthrodesis, or joint replacement. A joint protection program is indicated, and a CMC stabilization splint may be helpful to relieve pain and increase hand function.

SURGICAL INTERVENTION

Treatment of the patient with long-term rheumatoid arthritis will often include operative procedures to repair soft tissue or replace joints destroyed by the rheumatoid process.

Surgical procedures that may be of benefit to patients with rheumatoid arthritis include synovectomy, tendon repair and transplant, soft tissue reconstruction, joint replacement, bone resection, and joint fusion.[1,21]

Synovectomy, which is a surgical process of removing excessive synovium in an effort to control its proliferation, may be performed when the inflammation cannot be controlled by more conservative methods. It is most often delayed until soft tissue, such as finger extensors, appear to be jeopardized by the synovitis.

Resection implant arthroplasty is performed more successfully and more often since the development of high-grade Silastic spacers and joints. Early models of joints made out of metal and Silastic failed because of breakage of the implants from shearing forces applied during daily use. Current implant spacers are reinforced with Dacron and withstand normal hand usage more reliably than earlier models. Metal implants are generally no longer used in the fingers.

MP Joint Arthroplasty

Although implants exist to replace almost any joint affected by arthritis, resection arthroplasty of the MP joints is the most common rheumatoid surgery in the hand. Guidelines given for timing of treatment vary with the surgeon, the patient, and the expertise of the treating therapist. The program described in the paragraphs that follow was developed for the Swanson-type Silastic implant, but the general principles apply to other types of spacers as well.

Some joint replacements, such as the total hip replacement, are designed to work like the joint they replace. However, the MP joint arthroplasty uses a joint spacer that is not a joint but acts as an interface between the metacarpal bone and the proximal phalanx. The stems of the Swanson spacer are not fixed within the intermedullary canal but move with a piston action within the bone. This approach allows adequate excursion of the implant for finger flexion and extension and reduces stress on the implant.

During the healing phase following the MP arthroplasty the implants go through an encapsulation period. During this time the tissue surrounding the Silastic forms a capsule that supports the stems of the spacer. Collagen fibers are present microscopically on the fourth or fifth day and gradually change from the cellular formation into collagen fibers.[18] This process appears to be complete by the end of the sixth week. During the encapsulation period it is extremely important that the joints be held in the desired position of extension and slight radial deviation.

During surgery the head of the metacarpal is resected and cleaned. The proximal phalanx is prepared but usually not resected. The bone canals are also prepared, and the spacer carefully inserted. Soft tissue release of the ulnar intrinsic muscles, reconstruction of the radial intrinsic muscles, and reconstruction and alignment of the extensor hood may be performed during surgery.

The patient's hand is placed in a bulky dressing and immobilized for 3 to 6 days postoperatively. At that time a dynamic splint is applied, which places the fingers in a slight radial deviation at the MP joints while lightly supporting the fingers into full extension and allowing active flexion to 70°[40] (Fig. 34-14). A splint is worn 24 hours a day for the next 6 weeks. Some surgeons prefer a static

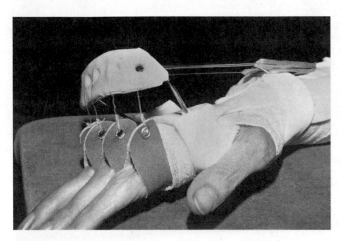

FIG. 34-14 Low-profile dynamic splint is used to assist MP joints into extension while maintaining about 15° of radial deviation following implant arthroplasty of MP joints. MP joints should not be pulled into hyperextension by splint.

splint, which maintains the fingers in the proper position while sleeping, and a dynamic splint during all waking hours. Frequent splint adjustments and goniometric measurements are necessary during this postoperative period to monitor joint position and excursion.

Starting with the application of the dynamic splint, passive ROM may be performed by the therapist on a daily basis to maintain 70° of pain-free passive flexion and full extension. Passive motion is applied gently with consideration to tissue reaction. Increased pain or edema indicates that the treatment is too aggressive. The patient is instructed to perform active ROM and light ADL only in the splint for the first 6 weeks to ensure that the fingers are not used in an ulnarly deviated position. Heavy activities are restricted.

During the 4- to 6-week period the patient may begin active flexion while wearing the splint under the supervision of the therapist. Care is taken that flexion occurs at the MP joints and not primarily at the IP joints. Individual

finger splints may be placed on the fingers to prevent IP flexion during active MP flexion. Also during this period flexion splinting may be begun if the patient has not regained a full 70° of flexion. The flexion cuff should allow for slight radial pull and should not be painful or cause swelling of the fingers.

Other exercises that should be stressed are radial walking of the fingers individually toward the thumb and active exercise of the extensors by placing the fingers in the intrinsic minus position (IP joints slightly flexed) while extending the MP joints.

Extension and flexion splints are adjusted for fit and wearing time based on goniometric measurements. Strength usually returns as the patient is allowed to use the hand for normal activities. Heavy resistive exercise is contraindicated.

Night splinting is continued for 12 to 14 weeks, although the patient may go without the splint during the day following the sixth week.

The principles of wound healing and encapsulation may be applied to joint implant arthroplasty of other joints. A balance of controlled splinting and active motion should be achieved following any joint arthroplasty.

SUMMARY

Rheumatoid arthritis is a chronic systemic disease that affects the joints. It is treated with drug therapy, rest, exercise, appropriate activity, and surgery. Potential joint deformity can be decreased or prevented with proper treatment. The occupational therapist has an important role to play in the treatment of rheumatoid arthritis. Teaching principles of joint protection and their application to self-care, home management, and leisure and work activities is an important function of occupational therapy. Provision of splints and a guided home exercise program are other important roles of the occupational therapy service. Early intervention is important for the best treatment outcomes.

 S A M P L E   T R E A T M E N T   P L A N

This treatment plan is not comprehensive. It deals with three of eight problems identified and two stages of the disease

process. The reader is encouraged to add objectives and methods to the plan to make it more complete.

CASE STUDY

Mrs. J is a 36-year-old woman with a diagnosis of rheumatoid arthritis. The onset was 3 years ago. She is a wife and the mother of an 8-year-old girl. She lives with her husband

and daughter in a three-bedroom, single-level tract home. Mrs J's primary role is that of homemaker. She has held a part-time job at a florist shop, however, doing wreath design

✓ SAMPLE TREATMENT PLAN – cont'd

and construction and flower arranging. She both enjoys this work and sees her salary as a necessary adjunct to the family income.

Mrs. J experiences intermittent acute disease episodes that have primarily involved the elbows, wrists, MP, and PIP joints bilaterally. There are slight losses of ROM and strength at all involved joints.

To date there is no permanent deformity, but ulnar deviation, MP subluxation, boutonnière deformity, wrist subluxation, and further limitation of ROM at all involved joints are possible deformities.

Medical management has been through rest and salicylates. Medical precautions are no strenuous activity, no resistive exercise or activity, and avoidance of fatigue.

She was referred to occupational therapy during the acute phase of her most recent episode for (1) prevention of deformity and loss of ROM and (2) maintenance of maximal function. She continued with occupational therapy services during the subacute period with the same goals.

TREATMENT PLAN

Personal data
Name: Mrs. J
Age: 36
Diagnosis: Rheumatoid arthritis

Disability: Limited ROM, decreased strength, potential deformity of elbows, wrists, MP and PIP joints bilaterally.
Treatment aims stated in the referral: Prevent deformity, prevent loss of ROM, maintain maximal function

OTHER SERVICES

Physician: Supervise medical management and rehabilitation therapies
Physical therapy: May be used for specific exercise program
Social services: Patient and family counseling, if needed; financial arrangements, if appropriate
Vocational counseling: Explore feasibility of return to same or

modified occupation in floral work

Frame of reference/treatment approach
Occupational performance
Biomechanical and rehabilitation approaches

OT EVALUATION

Performance components
Sensorimotor function
  Active and passive ROM: Test
  Muscle strength: Observe, test
  Endurance: Observe, interview
  Hand deformities: Observe, test MP stability
    Ulnar drift: (measure if present)
    Wrist subluxation
    MP subluxation
    Boutonnière deformity
    Swan-neck deformity
    Thumb deformities
  Hand function: Test
  Sensation: Test
  Carpal tunnel syndrome: Test
Cognitive functioning

Memory: Observe, interview
Motivation: Observe, interview
Functional language skills: Observe, interview comprehension of written/spoken
Psychosocial function
  Adjustment to disability: Observe, interview
  Interpersonal and coping skills: Observe
  Social skills

Performance areas
Family and community support: Interview
Self-care: Observe, interview
Home management: Observe, interview
Prevocational: Observe, interview
Play/Leisure: Observe, interview

SAMPLE TREATMENT PLAN – cont'd

EVALUATION SUMMARY

Weakness is noted particularly in wrist and finger extensors (F+) and to a lesser degree in flexor groups (G). Mild ROM limitations are present in elbows, wrists, and fingers with some MP instability noted (10° ulnar drift). No subluxation or other deformities were noted. Hand function testing revealed difficulty with fingertip prehension, and pinch and grip are good but not normal in strength. Forceful use of the thumb in opposition enhances ulnar drift and produces MP discomfort.

Sensation is intact, and cognitive state appears to be within normal limits.

The patient's family has noted that the patient demonstrates withdrawal from social situations during flares and has limited patience when fatigued and in pain. Her family appears to be supportive, and her daughter helps with household tasks. During inactive periods, she is independent for light housekeeping, self-care, and work. She fatigues after 2 hours of light-to-moderate activity and requires a 20-minute rest period. During flares she is severely limited in ADL, leaves home management tasks to her family, and is unable to work. She manages to do only light self-care activities independently.

Observation of the job by another worker and Mrs. J in simulated tasks revealed that some aspects of her job would contribute to development of deformity. Cutting and twisting floral wire, forcing stems and stem supports into Styrofoam, and binding wreaths were thought to be likely to enhance ulnar drift and MP subluxation because of the resistance and direction of joint forces. Wreath design and layout and fresh flower arrangement are possible alternatives, however. Mrs. J's employer is willing to retain her on a part-time basis to perform these duties.

Assets

No lower extremity involvement
Good preservation of function
Supportive and intact family unit
Potential job skills, flexible employer
Intelligence, motivation

Problem list

1. Muscle weakness
2. Limited ROM
3. Potential deformity
4. Fluctuating vocational role
5. Limited ADL independence
6. Fluctuating role as wife and mother
7. Tendency to social withdrawal
8. Limited endurance

ACUTE STAGE
PROBLEM 1: MUSCLE WEAKNESS

Objective

Muscle strength will be maintained

Method

Isometric exercise without added resistance to biceps, triceps, flexor and extensor carpi radialis and ulnaris, 1 to 3 repetitions once a day. Active ROM exercise to elbows and wrists, 2 to 3 repetitions once a day; and self-care to tolerance

Gradation

Increase number of exercise sessions or repetitions as synovitis and pain subside

PROBLEM 2: LIMITED ROM

Objective

ROM of affected joints will be maintained

Method

Active or active-assisted ROM exercises to elbow, MP and PIP flexion and extension, wrist flexion, extension, radial and ulnar deviation. Active ROM exercises may be carried out in a warm bath or shower or immediately following bathing.

Gradation

Grade to active exercise and add gentle active and passive stretching during subacute stage

S A M P L E   T R E A T M E N T   P L A N – c o n t ' d

PROBLEM 5: LIMITED ADL INDEPENDENCE

Objective
With adaptive aids and use of joint protection techniques the patient will perform self-care activities independently

Method
Therapist will provide instruction in joint protection and make specific recommendations for modifications to existing equipment (building up handles on toothbrush, hairbrush, eating utensils, etc.). Patient will be provided with necessary self-care adaptive equipment (buttonhook, washing mitt, etc.) and instruction in their use. Treatment sessions within the clinic will include dressing and grooming tasks to facilitate problem solving and permit patient to demonstrate competence in the use of adaptive equipment and techniques.

Gradation
As synovitis subsides patient will gradually be able to taper the use of adaptive equipment and to increase her activity level

SUBACUTE STAGE
PROBLEM 1: MUSCLE WEAKNESS

Objective
Strength of weakened muscles will increase by ½ grade as compared with the initial evaluation

Method
Patient's activity level in the home will increase to include light housekeeping activities (ironing, dust mopping, dishwashing). Patient will be given isometric exercise with resistance to elbow and wrist flexors and extensors, MP and PIP extensors, 3 to 10 repetitions 3 times daily.

Gradation
Increase the amount of physical activity as tolerated. Increase the number of exercise repetitions as tolerated

PROBLEM 2: LIMITED ROM

Objective
ROM of affected joints will be increased or maintained

Method
Active ROM exercise to elbow, wrist, MP, and PIP joints, gentle passive stretching to elbow flexion, and extension and PIP extension. Patient will be instructed to use full ROM for light resistance ADL such as dust mopping, folding linen, and ironing

Gradation
Increase resistance for stretching exercise as tolerated

REVIEW QUESTIONS

1. What is the outstanding clinical feature that produces joint limitation and deformity in arthritis?
2. What sex and age groups are most frequently affected by arthritis?
3. What is meant by *rheumatoid factor?*
4. List four systemic signs of rheumatoid arthritis.
5. What is the characteristic course of the disease?
6. Describe the appearance and mechanics of two common finger deformities that may affect the DIP and PIP joints in rheumatoid arthritis.
7. What deformities can result at the MP joints? How are they treated or prevented?
8. What are the major problems at the elbow and shoulder in arthritis? How can they be prevented?
9. What kinds of exercises are appropriate for arthritis patients in the acute stage of disease?
10. When is stretching exercise indicated?
11. When is joint rest indicated in treatment of arthritis?
12. Which joints should not be splinted in treatment of arthritis?
13. Which joints are frequently splinted in treatment of arthritis?
14. What is the role of the occupational therapist in splinting for arthritis?
15. List appropriate occupational therapy evaluation procedures for rheumatoid arthritis.
16. What are the general objectives of occupational therapy in treatment of arthritis?
17. What kinds of activities are contraindicated for the arthritis patient during the acute stage of the disease?
18. What kinds of activities are appropriate during the acute stage?

19. When the acute stage of the disease has abated, how can the patient's activity be graded?
20. Discuss some of the ways work can be simplified for the arthritis patient.
21. List some of the principles of joint protection directed toward maintaining ROM of the elbow and shoulder joints. Give some practical examples of methods of application of the principles to household tasks.
22. List five assistive devices for self-care or home management that could be useful to an arthritis patient, and give the rationale for each.

REFERENCES

1. Arthritis Foundation: *Arthritis manual for allied health professionals, The Professional Manual Subcommittee of the Education Committee, Allied Health Professions Section,* New York, 1973, The Foundation.
2. Banwell B: Physical therapy in arthritis management. In Ehrlich G, editor: *Rehabilitation management of rheumatic conditions,* ed 2, Baltimore, 1986, Williams & Wilkins.
3. Banwell B: Exercise behaviors. Presentation at the Arthritis Health Professions Association annual conference: State of the Art Exercise and Arthritis, Washington, DC, June, 1987.
4. Colditz J: Arthritis. In Malick M, Kasch M, editors: *Manual on management of specific hand problems,* Pittsburgh, 1984, AREN.
5. Comfort A: *Sexual consequences of disability,* Philadelphia, 1978, George F Stickley.
6. Cordery JC: Joint protection: a responsibility of the occupational therapist, *Am J Occup Ther* 19:285, 1965.
7. Engleman E, Shearn M: Arthritis and allied rheumatic disorders. In Krupp M, Chatton M, editors: *Current medical diagnosis and treatment,* Los Altos, Calif, 1980, Lange Medical Publications.
8. Flatt A: *The care of the arthritic hand,* ed 4, St Louis, 1983, CV Mosby.
9. Fries JF: *Arthritis: a comprehensive guide to understanding your arthritis,* Reading, Mass, 1986, Addison-Wesley.
10. Harcom TM and associates: Therapeutic value of graded aerobic exercise training in rheumatoid arthritis, *Arthritis and Rheumatism* 28:32, Jan, 1985.
11. Healy L: The current status of methotrexate use in rheumatic diseases, *Bull on the Rheum Dis* 36(4), Atlanta, 1986, The Arthritis Foundation.
12. Hollander J: Rheumatoid arthritis. In Riggs G, Gall E, editors: *Rheumatic diseases: rehabilitation and management,* Boston, 1984, Butterworth.
13. Huskisson E: Routine drug treatment of rheumatoid arthritis and other rheumatic diseases, *Clin Rheum Dis* 5:697, Aug, 1979.
14. Jebsen RH and associates: An objective and standardized test of hand function, *Arch Phys Med Rehabil* 50:311, 1969.
15. Klippel J: Winning the battle, losing the war? Another editorial about rheumatoid arthritis, *The Journal of Rheumatology* 17:9, Sept, 1990.
16. Larson CB, Gould M: *Orthopedic Nursing,* ed 8, St Louis, 1974, CV Mosby.
17. Lorig K, Fries JF: *The arthritis helpbook,* rev ed, Reading, Mass, 1986, Addison-Wesley.
18. Madden JW, DeVore G, Arem AJ: A rational postoperative management program of metacarpal joint implant arthroplasty, *J Hand Surg* 2:26, 1977.
19. McCarty D: Suppress rheumatoid inflammation early and leave the pyramid to the Egyptians, *The Journal of Rheumatology,* 17:9, Sept, 1990.
20. Melvin JL: Hand dysfunction associated with arthritis. In Riggs G, Gall E, editors: *Rheumatic diseases: rehabilitation and management,* Boston, 1984, Butterworth.
21. Melvin JL: *Rheumatic disease in the adult and child: occupational therapy and rehabilitation,* ed 3, Philadelphia, 1989, FA Davis.
22. Michlovitz SL: *Thermal agents in rehabilitation,* ed 2, Philadelphia, 1990, FA Davis.
23. Million R and associates: Long term study of management of rheumatoid arthritis, *Lancet* 1:812, April, 1984.
24. Minor M: Aerobics. Presentation at the Arthritis Professions Association annual conference: State of the Art Exercise and Arthritis, Washington, DC, June, 1987.
25. Minor M: Physical activity and management of arthritis, *Ann Behav Med* 13:3, 1991.
26. Moncur C: Attacking the sacred cows. Presentation at the Arthritis Health Professions Association annual conference: State of the Art Exercise and Arthritis, Washington, DC, June, 1987.
27. Morrey B: *The elbow and its disorders,* ed 2, Philadelphia, 1992, WB Saunders.
28. Navarro A: Rheumatic conditions causing hip pain. In Rigg G, Gall E, editors: *Rheumatic diseases: rehabiltation and management,* Boston, 1984, Butterworth.
29. RL Petzoldt Memorial Center for Hand Rehabilitation: *Carpal tunnel syndrome protocol,* RL Petzoldt Memorial Center for Hand Rehabilitation, 1987, San José, Calif, (unpublished).
30. Polley H, Hunder G: *Rheumatological interviewing and physical examination of the joints,* ed 2, Philadelphia, 1978, WB Saunders.
31. Potts MG: *Psychosocial aspects of rheumatic diseases: rehabiltation and management,* Boston, 1984, Butterworth.
32. Richards JS: Sex and arthritis, *Sexuality and Dis* 3:97, 1980.
33. Schumacher HR, editor: *Primer on the rheumatic diseases,* ed 10, Atlanta, 1993, Arthritis Foundation.
34. Seeger M: Splints, braces and casts. In Riggs G, Gall E, editors: *Rheumatic diseases: rehabilitation and management,* Boston, 1984, Butterworth.

35. Sidman JM: Sexual functioning and the physically disabled adult, *Am J Occup Ther* 31:81, 1977.

36. Simpson C: Exercise and arthritis. Presentation at the Northern California Chapter of the Arthritis Health Professionals, Arthritis Foundation, San Francisco, June, 1987.

37. Sliwa J: Occupational therapy assessment and management. In Ehrlich G, editor: *Rehabilitation management of rheumatic conditions,* ed 2, Baltimore, 1986, Williams & Wilkins.

38. Sturge RA: The remote effects of rheumatic disease on the hand and their management. In Wynn-Parry CB, editor: *Clinics in rheumatic diseases,* vol 10, London, 1984, WB Saunders.

39. Swanson A: Pathogenesis of arthritic lesions. In Hunter JM and associates: *Rehabilitation of the hand,* ed 3, St Louis, 1990, CV Mosby.

40. Swanson A, Swanson G, Leonard J, Boozer J: Postoperative rehabilitation programs in flexible implant arthroplasty of the digits. In Hunter JM and associates: *Rehabilitation of the hand,* ed 3, St Louis, 1990, CV Mosby.

41. Trombley CA: Arthritis. In Trombly CA, editor: *Occupational therapy for physical dysfunction,* ed 3, Baltimore, 1989, Williams & Wilkins.

42. Wickersham B: The exercise program. In Riggs G, Gall E, editors: *Rheumatic Diseases: rehabilitation and management,* Boston, 1984, Butterworth.

Hand Injuries

Mary C. Kasch

Treatment of the upper extremity is important to all occupational therapists who work with physically disabled persons. The incidence of upper extremity injuries is significant and accounts for about one third of all injuries. The nearly 16 million upper extremity injuries that occur annually in the United States result in 90 million days of restricted activity and 12 million visits to physicians. The upper extremities are involved in about one third of work-related farm injuries and one third of disabling industrial injuries. In addition, disease and congenital anomalies contribute to upper extremity dysfunction, and it is estimated that only about 15% of those suffering from severe cerebral vascular accident recover hand function.[55]

The hand is vital to human function and appearance. It flexes, extends, opposes, and grasps thousands of times daily, allowing the performance of necessary daily activities. The hand's sensibility allows feeling without looking and provides protection from injury. The hand touches, gives comfort, and expresses emotions. Loss of hand function through injury or disease thus affects much more than the mechanical tasks that the hand performs. Hand injury may jeopardize a family's livelihood and at the least affects every daily activity. The occupational therapist with training in physical and psychological assessment, prosthetic evaluation, fabrication of orthoses, assessment and training in the activities of daily living (ADL), and in functional restoration is uniquely qualified to treat upper extremity disorders.

Hand rehabilitation, or hand therapy, has grown as a specialty area of both physical therapy and occupational therapy. Many of the treatment techniques used with hand-injured patients have evolved from the application of therapy and knowledge of both specialties to be used by the hand therapist. It is not the purpose of this chapter to instruct the occupational therapy student in physical agent modalities. Rather, treatment techniques that have been found to be beneficial to hand injury patients are presented. It is assumed that these techniques will be provided by the therapist best trained to provide them. Hand rehabilitation requires advanced and specialized training by both physical and occupational therapists. A role delineation study of hand therapy that includes definition and scope of practice has been reported.[22] Treatment techniques, whether thermal modalities or specifically designed exercises, are used as a bridge to reach a further goal of returning to functional performance. Thus some modalities may be used as adjunctive or enabling modalities in preparation for functional use. It is within this context that treatment techniques will be presented in this chapter.

Treatment of the injured hand is a matter of timing and judgment. Following trauma or surgery a healing phase must occur in which the body performs its physiological function of wound healing. Following the initial healing phase when cellular restoration has been accomplished, the wound enters its restorative phase. It is in this phase that hand therapy is most beneficial. Early treatment that occurs in this restorative phase is ideal and in some cases essential for optimal results.

Although sample timetables may be presented, the therapist should always coordinate the application of any treatment with the referring physician. Surgical techniques may vary, and inappropriate treatment of the hand patient can result in failure of a surgical procedure. Communication between the surgeon, therapist, and patient is especially vital in this setting. A comfortable environment in which group interaction is possible may increase patient motivation and cooperation. The presence of the therapist as an instructor and evaluator is essential, but without the patient's cooperation limited gains will be achieved. Treating the psychological loss suffered by the patient with a hand injury is an integral part of the rehabilitative therapy as well.

Hand therapy is provided in a number of treatment settings, ranging from private therapy offices to outpatient rehabilitation clinics and hospitals. The source for reimbursement for services may be directly from the patient, through private medical insurance, workers' compensation insurance, or a variety of managed care programs. In the future, there may be a single payer system in the United States that covers individuals 24 hours a day, which would integrate workers' compensation into the plan.

Reimbursement patterns have altered the provision of services by limiting the number of visits authorized. Therapists are also being asked to provide outcome data that supports the need for services. Continuous quality improvement documentation is often required for participation in managed care programs. With fewer authorized visits, the therapist must be more adept at instructing the patient in self-management of the condition being treated. Occupational therapists should anticipate a greater need to justify treatment in the future as part of the national challenge to control medical costs. Aides, certified assistants and other support personnel will be used increasingly, but the quality of service provided must continue to meet all professional and ethical standards. This climate of change will present unique opportunities for the occupational therapist.

EXAMINATION AND EVALUATION

When approaching a patient who has a hand injury, the therapist must be able to evaluate the nature of the injury and the limitations it has produced. First the injured structures must be identified by consulting with the hand surgeon, reviewing operative reports and x-ray films, and discussing the injury with the patient. Evaluation of bone, tendon, and nerve function must be ascertained using standardized evaluation techniques whenever possible.

The patient's age, occupation, and hand dominance should be taken into account in the initial evaluation. The type and extent of medical and surgical treatment that has been received and the length of time since such treatment are important in determining a treatment plan. Any further surgery or conservative treatment that is planned should also be noted. The treatment plan should have the written approval of the referring physician.

The purposes of hand evaluation are to identify (1) physical limitations, such as loss of range of motion (ROM), (2) functional limitations, such as inability to perform daily tasks, (3) substitution patterns to compensate for loss of sensibility or motor function, and (4) established deformities, such as joint contracture.

The movement of the arm and hand must be coordinated for maximum function. Shoulder motion is essential for positioning the hand and elbow for daily activities.[20]

The wrist is the key joint in the position of function.[15] Skilled hand performance depends on wrist stability. While a mobile wrist is preferable, function is possible as long as the wrist is positioned to maximize movement of the fingers. Function also depends on arm and shoulder stability and mobility for fixing or positioning the hand for functional use. The thumb is of greater importance than any other digit. Effective pinch is almost impossible without a thumb, and attempts will be made to salvage or reconstruct an injured thumb whenever possible.

Within the hand, the proximal interphalangeal (PIP) joint is critical for grasp and is considered to be the most important small joint.[15] Limitations in flexion or extension will result in significant functional impairment.

OBSERVATION AND TOPOGRAPHICAL EVALUATION

The occupational therapist should observe the appearance of the hand and arm. The position of the hand and arm at rest and the carrying posture can yield valuable information about the dysfunction. How the patient treats the disease or injury should be observed. Is it overprotected and carefully guarded or ignored? The skin condition of the hand and arm should be noted. Are there lacerations, sutures, or evidence of recent surgery? Is the skin dry or moist? Are there scales or crusts? Does the hand appear swollen? Does the hand have an odor? Palmar skin is less mobile than dorsal skin normally. The degree of mobility and elasticity and the adherence of scars is determined. Trophic changes in the skin should be observed. The vascular system is assessed by observing the skin color and temperature of the hand and evaluating for presence of edema. Are there contractures of the web spaces? The therapist should observe the relationship between hand and arm function as the patient moves about and performs test items or tasks.

The therapist should ask the patient to perform some simple bilateral ADL, such as buttoning a button, putting on a shirt, opening a jar, and threading a needle, and observe the amount of spontaneous movement and use of the affected hand and arm.

PHYSICAL EVALUATION

The effect of trauma or dysfunction on anatomical structures is the first consideration in evaluating hand function. The joints must be assessed for active and passive mobility, fixed deformities, and any tendency to assume a position of deformity. The ligaments must be evaluated for laxity or contracture and their ability to maintain joint stability. Tendons must be examined for integrity, contracture, or overstretching; muscles are tested for strength and function.

Soft Tissue Tightness

Joints may develop dysfunction following trauma, immobilization, or disuse. Mennell emphasizes the importance of the small, involuntary motions of the joint, which he refers to as "joint play."[80] Others[70] describe these as "accessory motions." Joint play or accessory motions are those movements that are nonvoluntary, physiologic, and can be performed only by someone else.[56] Examples of accessory motions are joint rotation and joint distraction. If accessory motions are limited and painful, the active motions of that joint cannot be normal. Therefore it is necessary to restore joint play through the use of joint mobilization techniques before attempting passive or active range of motion.[81]

Joint mobilization may date back to the fourth century BC, when Hypocrites first described the use of spinal traction.[56] In the 1930s an English physician, James Mennell, encouraged physicians to perform manipulation without anesthesia, a practice that is advocated today by James Cyriax, who explored the use of manipulation of the intervertebral discs. Current theorists include Cyriax, Robert Maigne, FM Kaltenborn, GD Maitland, Stanley Paris, and John Mennell, son of the late James Mennell. While physicians originally practiced manipulation, therapists have adapted the techniques, which are now called "joint mobilization."

The techniques used to assess joint play are also used in the treatment of joint dysfunction. During assessment the evaluator determines the range of accessory motion and the presence of pain by taking up the slack only in the joint. During treatment a high-velocity, low-amplitude thrust or graded oscillation is applied to regain motion and relieve pain.[70]

Guidelines must be followed in applying joint mobilization techniques, and they should not be attempted by the untrained or inexperienced practitioner. Postgraduate courses are offered in joint mobilization of the extremities, and the therapist must be familiar with the orthokinematics of each joint as well as with the techniques used.

Joint mobilization is generally indicated with restriction of accessory motions or the presence of pain due to tightness of the joint capsule, meniscus displacement, muscle guarding, ligamentous tightness, or adherence. It is contraindicated in the presence of infection, recent fracture, neoplasm, joint inflammation, rheumatoid arthritis, osteoporosis, degenerative joint disease, or many chronic diseases.[56]

Limitations in joint motion may also be caused by tightness of the extrinsic or intrinsic muscles and tendons. If the joint capsule is not tight and accessory motions are normal, the therapist should test for extrinsic and intrinsic tightness.

To test for extrinsic extensor tightness the metacarpo phalangeal (MP) joint is passively held in extension and the PIP joint is moved passively into flexion. Then the MP joint is flexed, and the PIP joint is again passively flexed. If the PIP joint can be flexed easily when the MP joint is extended but not when the MP joint is flexed, the extrinsic extensors are adherent.[3]

If there is extrinsic flexor tightness, the PIP and distal interphalangeal (DIP) joints will be positioned in flexion with the MP joints held in extension. It will not be possible to pull the fingers into complete extension. If the wrist is then held in flexion, the IP joints will extend more easily as a result of slack being placed on the flexor tendons.

Tightness of the intrinsic musculature is tested by passively holding the MP joint in extension and applying pressure just distal to the PIP joint. This action is repeated with the MP joint in flexion. If there is more resistance when the MP joint is extended, intrinsic tightness is indicated.[3]

If there is no difference in passive motion of the PIP joint when the MP joint is held in extension or flexion and there is limitation of PIP joint flexion in any position, tightness of the joint capsule is indicated. The therapist should assess the joint for capsular tightness if this step has not already been done.

Edema Assessment

Hand volume is measured to assess the presence of extracellular or intracellular edema. Volume measurement is generally used to determine the effect of treatment and activities. By measuring volume at different times of the day, the effects of rest versus activity may be measured as well as the effects of splinting or treatment designed to reduce edema.

A commercial volumeter[27] may be used to assess hand edema. The volumeter has been shown to be accurate to 10 ml[112] when used in the prescribed manner. Variables that have been shown to decrease the accuracy of the volumeter include (1) the use of a faucet or hose that introduces air into the tank during filling, (2) movement of the arm within the tank, (3) inconsistent pressure on the stop rod, and (4) the use of a volumeter in a variety of places. The same level surface should always be used.[44] The evaluation is performed as follows (Fig. 35-1):

1. A plastic volumeter is filled and allowed to empty into a large beaker until the water reaches spout level. The beaker is then emptied and dried thoroughly.
2. The patient is instructed to immerse the hand in the plastic volumeter, being careful to keep the hand in the midposition.
3. The hand is lowered until it rests gently between the middle and ring fingers on the dowel rod. It is important that the hand does not press onto the rod.
4. The hand remains still until no more water drips into the beaker.
5. The water is poured into a graduated cylinder. The cylinder is placed on a level surface, and a reading is made.

A method of assessing edema of an individual finger or joint is circumferential measurement using either a circumference tape[62] or jeweler's ring-size standards. Measurements should be made before and after treatment and especially following the application of thermal modalities or splinting. While patients often have subjective complaints relating to swelling, objective data of circumference or volume will help the therapist to assess the

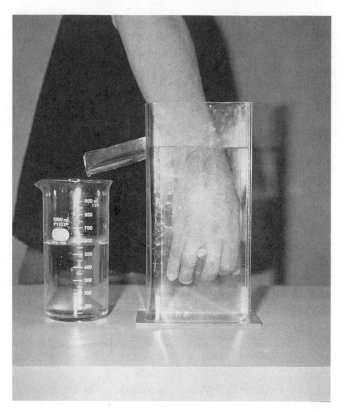

FIG. 35-1 Volumeter is used to measure volume of both hands for comparison. Increased volume indicates presence of edema.

response of the tissues to treatment and activity. Edema control techniques will be discussed later in this chapter.

Sensibility
Mapping

Sensibility testing can begin with sensory mapping of the entire volar surface of the hand.[18] The hand must be supported by the examiner's hand or be resting in a medium such as putty. Either the examiner or the patient can draw a probe, usually the eraser end of a pencil, lightly over the skin from the area of normal sensibility to the area of abnormal sensibility. The patient must immediately report the exact location where the sensation changes. This is done from proximal to distal and radial and ulnar to medial directions. The areas are carefully marked and transferred to a permanent record. Mapping should be repeated at monthly intervals during nerve regeneration.

Categories of tests

A variety of evaluations may be required to assess sensibility adequately. These tests can be divided into three categories: (1) modality tests for pain, heat, cold, and touch pressure; (2) functional tests to assess the quality of sensibility, or what Moberg described as "tactile

gnosis"; (3) objective tests that do not require active participation by the patient. Examples of functional tests are stationary and moving two-point discrimination and the Moberg Pick-up Test; objective tests include the wrinkle test, the Ninhydrin sweat test, and nerve-conduction studies.[18]

Sympathetic function

Recovery of sympathetic response (sweating, pain, and temperature discrimination) may occur early but does not correlate with functional recovery.[31] O'Rain[90] observed that denervated skin does not wrinkle. Therefore nerve function may be tested by immersing the hand in water for 5 minutes and noting the presence or absence of skin wrinkling. This test may be especially helpful in diagnosing a nerve lesion in young children. The ability to sweat is also lost with a nerve lesion. A ninhydrin test[84] evaluates sweating of the finger.

The wrinkle test and the ninhydrin test are objective tests of sympathetic function. Recovery of sweating has not been shown to correlate with the recovery of sensation, but the absence of sweating correlates with the lack of discriminatory sensation. Other signs of sympathetic dysfunction are smooth, shiny skin; nail changes; and "pencil-pointing" or tapering of the fingers.[111]

Nerve compression and nerve regeneration

Sensibility testing is done to assess the recovery of a nerve following laceration and repair, as well as to determine the presence of a nerve compression syndrome and the return of nerve function following surgical decompression, or the efficacy of conservative treatment to reduce compression. Therefore tests such as vibratory tests may be interpreted differently depending on the mechanism of nerve dysfunction. In the following section tests will be described and differences drawn as appropriate to assist the therapist in selecting the correct evaluation technique as well as in planning treatment based on the evaluative measures.

Tinel's sign and Phalen's maneuver

While these tests are not considered to be tests of sensibility, they are used to assess the rate of nerve recovery (Tinel's) and are considered provocative tests in nerve compression syndromes because they elicit the pathological response of the nerve when employed.

During the first 2 to 4 months following nerve suture, axons regenerate and travel through the hand at a rate of about 1 mm per day or 1 inch (2.54 cm) per month. Tinel's sign may be used to follow this regeneration.[61] The test is performed by tapping gently along the course of the nerve, starting distally and moving toward the nerve suture to elicit a tingling sensation in the fingertip. The point at which tapping begins to elicit a tingling sensation is noted and indicates the extent of sensory axon growth.

As regeneration occurs, hypesthesias develop. Although this hypersensitivity may be uncomfortable to the patient, it is a positive sign of nerve growth. A treatment program for desensitization of hypersensitive areas can be initiated as soon as the skin is healed and can tolerate gentle rubbing and immersion in textures. Desensitization is discussed further in the treatment section.

The examiner can also attempt to elicit Tinel's sign in nerve compression by percussing the median nerve at the level of the wrist carpal tunnel.[65] Tinel's sign is positive if there is tingling along the course of the nerve distally when percussed. Phalen's maneuver also produces the nerve paresthesias present in compression of the median nerve. The patient is asked to hold the wrist in a fully flexed position for 60 seconds. The response is considered positive if tingling occurs within this time.[65]

Vibration

Dellon advocated the use of 30-cycles-per-second (30-cps) and 256-cps tuning forks for assessing the return of vibratory sensation following nerve repair as regeneration occurs and as a guideline for initiating a sensory reeducation program.[32,33] He found that an orderly progression of sensory return occurred: pain, perception of 30-cps stimuli, moving touch, constant touch, and 256-cps stimuli. When using a tuning fork for testing, the hand should be supported by resting on a table. The examiner hits the tuning fork briskly and places the prong on the fingertip, moving it proximally until the vibration is perceived by the patient. The corresponding contralateral finger is then tested, and the patient is asked if the vibration is more, less, or the same. Vibration is considered altered if it is not the same on both digits.[30]

Lundborg[66] has described the use of commercial vibrometers to detect abnormal sensation. Gelberman[45] found that vibration and touch perception as measured by the Semmes-Weinstein monofilaments are altered before two-point discrimination because they measure a single nerve fiber innervating a group of receptor cells. Two-point discrimination is a test of innervation density that requires overlapping sensory units and cortical integration. Thus two-point discrimination is altered following nerve laceration and repair but remains normal if the nerve is compressed as long as there are links to the cortex. Bell[11] has also found normal two-point values in the presence of decreased sensory function.

Vibration and the Semmes-Weinstein test are more sensitive in picking up a gradual decrease in nerve function in the presence of nerve compression where the nerve circuitry is intact. They also correlate with decreases in the potential amplitude of sensory nerve action as measured by nerve conduction studies.[101] Therefore vibration, Semmes-Weinstein, and electrical testing are reliable and sensitive tests for early detection of carpal tunnel syndrome and other nerve compression syndromes. Vibration and Semmes-Weinstein can be performed in the clinic with no discomfort to the patient and are excellent screening tools when nerve compression is suspected.

Touch pressure

Moving touch is tested using the eraser end of a pencil. The eraser is placed in an area of normal sensibility and, pressing lightly, is moved to the distal fingertip. The patient notes when the perception of the stimulus changes. Light and heavy stimuli may be applied and noted.[31]

Constant touch is tested by pressing with the eraser end of a pencil, first in an area with normal sensibility and then moving distally. The patient responds when the stimulus is altered; again light and heavy stimuli may be applied.[31]

The Semmes-Weinstein monofilaments are the most accurate instrument for assessing cutaneous pressure thresholds.[9] The test is composed of 20 nylon monofilaments housed in plastic handheld rods. The diameter of the monofilaments increases and when applied correctly exert a force ranging from 4.5 mg to 447 g. Markings on the probes range from 1.65 to 6.65 but do not correspond to the grams of force of each rod. Normal fingertip sensibility has been found to correspond to the 2.44 and 2.83 probes.

The monofilaments must be applied perpendicularly to the skin and are applied just until the monofilament bends. The skin should not blanch when the monofilament is applied. Probes 1.65 through 2.83 are bounced three times. Probes marked 3.22 to 4.08 are applied three times with a bend in the filament, and probes marked 4.17 to 6.65 are applied once. The larger monofilaments do not bend, and therefore skin color most be observed to determine how firmly to apply the probe.

The examiner should begin with a probe in the normal range and progress through the rods in increasing diameters to find the patient's threshold for touch throughout the volar surface.[9] A grid should be used to record the responses so that varying areas of touch perception can be demonstrated. Two out of three correct responses are necessary for an area to be considered as having intact sensibility. It is preferable to place the monofilaments randomly rather than to concentrate on an area, to allow the nerves recovery time. When a filament is placed three times, it should be held for a second, rested for a second, and reapplied.

Results can be graded from normal light touch (probes 2.83 and above) to loss of protective sensation (probes 4.56 and below). Diminished light touch and diminished protective sensation are in the range reflected by the central probes.[11]

Two-point and moving two-point discrimination

Discrimination, the second level of sensibility assessment, requires the subject to distinguish between two direct stimuli. Static or stationary two-point discrimination measures the slowly adapting fibers. The two-point discrimination test, first described by Weber in 1853, was modified and popularized by Moberg,[83] who was interested in a tool that would assess the functional level of sensation. A variety of devices has been proposed to use in measuring two-point discrimination. The bent paper clip is inexpensive but often has burrs on the metal tip. Other devices include industrial calipers[21] and the Disk-Criminator.[36,68] A device with parallel prongs of variable distance and blunted ends should produce replicable results.

The test is performed as follows:[61]

1. The patient's vision is occluded.
2. An area of normal sensation is tested as a reference, using blunt calipers or a bent paper clip.
3. The calipers are set 10 mm apart and are randomly applied starting at the fingertip and moving proximally and longitudinally in line with the digital nerves, with one or two points touching. The skin should not be blanched by the caliper.
4. The distance is decreased until the patient no longer feels two distinct points, and that distance is measured.

Three to four seconds should be allowed between applications, and the patient should have four out of five correct responses.[11] Because this test indicates sensory function, it is usually administered at the tips of the fingers. It may be used proximally to test nerve regeneration. Normal two-point discrimination at the fingertip is 6 mm or less.[3]

Moving two-point discrimination measures the innervation density of the quickly adapting nerve fibers for touch. It is slightly more sensitive than stationary two-point discrimination.[63] The test is performed as follows:[31]

1. The patient's vision is occluded.
2. An area of normal sensation is tested as a reference, using blunt calipers or a bent paper clip.
3. The fingertip is supported by the examining table or the examiner's hand.
4. The caliper, separated 5 mm to 8 mm, is moved longitudinally from proximal to distal in a linear fashion along the surface of the fingertip. One and two points are randomly alternated. The patient must correctly identify the stimulus in seven out of eight responses before proceeding to a smaller value. The test is repeated down to a separation of 2 mm.

Two-point values increase with age in both sexes, with the smallest values occurring between the ages of 10 and 30. Females tend to have smaller values than men, and there is no significant difference between dominant and nondominant hands.[63]

Modified Moberg pick-up test

Recognition of common objects is the final level of sensory function. Moberg used the phrase *tactile gnosis* to describe the ability of the hand to perform complex functions by feel. Moberg described the Picking-Up Test in 1958,[83] and it was later modified by Dellon.[31] This test is used with either a median nerve injury or a combination of median and ulnar nerves. Clinically it has been observed that it takes twice as long to perform the tests with vision occluded than with vision. The test is performed as follows:

1. Nine or ten small objects (coins, paper clip, etc.) are placed on a table, and the patient is asked to place them one at a time in a small container as quickly as possible while looking at them. The patient is timed.
2. The test is repeated for the opposite hand with vision.
3. The test is repeated for each hand with vision occluded.
4. The patient is asked to identify each object one at a time with and then without vision.

It is important to observe any substitution patterns that may be used when the patient cannot see the objects.

GRIP AND PINCH STRENGTH

Upper extremity strength evaluation is usually performed following the healing phase of trauma. Strength testing is *not* indicated following recent trauma or surgery. Testing should not be performed until the patient has been cleared for full-resistive activities, usually 8 to 12 weeks following injury.

A standard adjustable-handle dynamometer is recommended for assessing grip strength (Fig. 35-2).

The subject should be seated with the shoulder adducted and neutrally rotated, the elbow flexed at 90°,[76] forearm in the neutral position, and the wrist between 0° and 30° extension and between 0° and 15° of ulnar deviation. Three trials are taken of each hand with the dynamometer handle set at the second position.[77] The dynamometer should be lightly held by the examiner to prevent accidental dropping of the instrument. A mean of the three trials should be reported. The noninjured hand is used for comparison. Normative data may be used to compare strength scores.[54,78] Variables such as age will affect the strength measurements.

Pinch strength should also be tested, using a pinch gauge. The pinch gauge by B & L Engineering has been found to be the most accurate.[77] Two-point pinch (thumb tip to index fingertip), lateral or key pinch (thumb pulp to lateral aspect of the middle phalanx of the index finger), and three-point pinch (thumb tip to tips of index and long fingers) should be evaluated. As with the grip dynamometer, three successive trials should be obtained and compared bilaterally[44] (Fig. 35-3).

Manual muscle testing is also used to evaluate upper extremity strength. Accurate asessment is especially important when preparing the patient for tendon transfers or other reconstructive surgery. The student who wishes

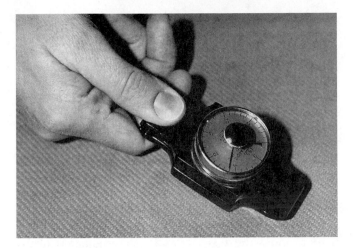

FIG. 35-3   Pinch gauge is used to evaluate pinch strength to variety of prehension patterns of pinch.

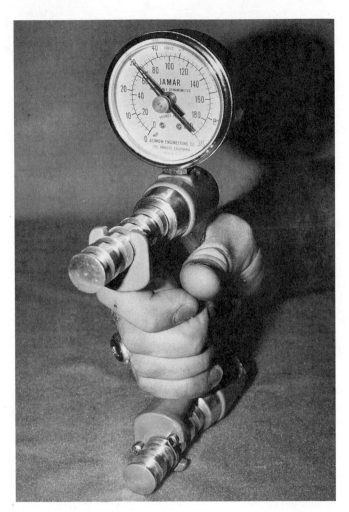

FIG. 35-2   Jamar dynamometer is used to evaluate grip strength in both hands.

to study kinesiology of the upper extremity is referred especially to Brand's work.[17]

Maximum voluntary effort during grip, pinch, or muscle testing will be affected by pain in the hand or extremity and it should be noted if the patient's ability to exert full force is limited by subjective complaints. Localization of the pain symptoms and consistency in noting pain will help the therapist to evaluate the role that pain is playing in the recovery from injury. Pain problems will be discussed in more detail later in this chapter.

FUNCTIONAL EVALUATION

Evaluation of hand function or performance is important because the physical evaluation does not measure the patient's ingenuity and ability to compensate for loss of strength, ROM sensation, or presence of deformities.[20]

The physical evaluation should precede the functional evaluation because awareness of physical dysfunction can result in a critical analysis of functional impairment and an understanding of why the patient functions as he or she does.[79]

The effect of the hand dysfunction on the use of the

hand in activities of daily living (ADL) should be observed by the occupational therapist. In addition, some type of a standardized performance evaluation, such as the Jebsen Test of Hand Function[49] or the Carroll Quantitative Test of Upper Extremity Function,[20] should be administered.

The Jebsen Test of Hand Function[49] was developed to provide objective measurements of standardized tasks with norms for patient comparison. It is a short test that is assembled by the administrator. It is easy to administer and inexpensive. The test consists of seven subtests, comprising (1) writing a short sentence, (2) turning over 3 × 5-inch cards, (3) picking up small objects and placing them in a container, (4) stacking checkers, (5) eating (simulated), (6) moving empty large cans, and (7) moving weighted large cans. Norms are provided for dominant and nondominant hands for each subtest and also are divided by sex and age. Instructions for assembling the test, as well as specific instructions for administering it, are provided by the authors.[49] This has been found to be a good test for overall hand function.

The Quantitative Test of Upper Extremity Function described by Carroll[20] was designed to measure ability to perform general arm and hand activities used in daily living. It is based on the assumption that complex upper extremity movements used to perform ordinary ADL can be reduced to specific patterns of grasp and prehension of the hand, supination and pronation of the forearm, flexion and extension of the elbow, and elevation of the arm.

The test consists of six parts, comprising (1) grasping and lifting four blocks of graduated sizes to assess grasp; (2) grasping and lifting two pipes of graduated sizes from a peg to test cylindrical grip; (3) grasping and placing a ball to test spherical grasp; (4) picking up and placing four marbles of graduated sizes to test fingertip prehension or pinch; (5) putting a small washer over a nail and putting an iron on a shelf to test placing; and (6) pouring water from pitcher to glass and glass to glass. In addition, to assess pronation, supination, and elevation of the arm, the subject places hand on top of head, behind head, and to mouth, and writes the name. The test uses simple, inexpensive, and easily acquired materials. Details of materials and their arrangement, test procedures, and scoring can be found in the original source.[20]

Other tests that are useful in the evaluation of hand dexterity are the Crawford Small Parts Dexterity Test,[26] the Bennett Hand Tool Dexterity Test,[12] the Purdue Pegboard Test,[104] and the Minnesota Manual Dexterity Test.[82] The VALPAR Corporation[108] has developed a number of standardized tests that measure an individual's ability to perform work-related tasks. They provide information about the test taker's results compared to industry performance standards. All of these tests include comparison with normal subjects working in a variety of industrial settings. This information can be used in predicting the likelihood of successful return to a specific job. These tests are especially useful when administering a work capacity evaluation. Tests may be purchased and come with instructions for administering the test and the standardized norms. Melvin lists a variety of additional hand function tests.[79]

CLINICAL TESTS FOR SPECIFIC DYSFUNCTION
Peripheral Neuropathic Conditions

Several quick clinical observations to detect dysfunction of peripheral nerves are available, based on the sensory and motor function of the individual nerve.

The ulnar nerve may be tested by asking the patient to pinch with the thumb and index finger and palpate the first dorsal inteosseous muscle. The radial nerve may be tested by asking the patient to extend the wrist and fingers. Median nerve function is tested by asking the patient to oppose the thumb to the fingers and flex the fingers.[23] The median nerve may be affected by carpal tunnel compression in conditions such as rheumatoid arthritis. Early signs of median nerve compression are sensory in nature and may be tested by performing Phalen's maneuver and percussing over the median nerve at the wrist to elicit Tinel's sign as described earlier in this chapter.

Patients may also develop compression syndromes of the ulnar and radial nerves which will be indicated by paresthesias along the course of those nerves. Tinel's sign may also be present. In patients with rheumatoid arthritis, it is important to test for nerve compression periodically, because synovial proliferation can cause compression in closed areas. Nerve compression must be relieved before motor fibers are damaged.

TREATMENT
FRACTURES

In treating a hand or wrist fracture the surgeon attempts to achieve good anatomical position through either a closed (nonoperative) or open (operative) reduction. Internal fixation with Kirschner wires, metallic plates, and/or screws may be used to maintain the desired position. External fixation may also be used with internal fixation. The hand is usually immobilized in wrist extension and MP joint flexion with extension of the distal joints whenever the injury allows this position.[115] Trauma to bone may also involve trauma to tendons and nerves in the adjacent area. Treatment must be geared toward the recovery of all injured structures, and this fact may influence treatment of the fracture.

Occupational therapy may be initiated during the period of immobilization, which is usually 3 to 5 weeks. Uninvolved fingers of the hand must be kept mobile through the use of active motion. Edema should be carefully monitored, and elevation is required whenever edema is present.

As soon as there is sufficient bone stability, the surgeon allows mobilization of the injured part. The surgeon should provide guidelines for the amount of resistance or force that may be applied to the fracture site. Activities that correct poor motor patterns and encourage use of the injured hand should be started as soon as the hand is pain-free. Early motion will prevent the adherence of tendons and reduce edema through stimulation of the lymphatic and blood vessels.

As soon as the brace or cast is removed, the patient's hand must be evaluated. If edema remains present, edema control techniques can be initiated using techniques described later in this chapter. A baseline ROM should be established, and the application of appropriate splints may begin. A splint may be used to correct a deformity that has resulted from immobilization, or it may be used to protect the finger from additional trauma to the fracture site. An example of this type of splinting would be the application of a Velcro "buddy" splint (Fig. 35-4) or a Bedford finger stall[72] (Fig. 35-5). A dorsal block

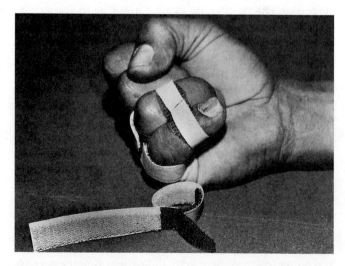

FIG. 35-4 Velcro "buddy" splint may be used to protect finger following fracture or to encourage movement of stiff finger. (Splint available from Smalley and Bates, Inc, 85 Park Avenue, Nutley, NJ.)

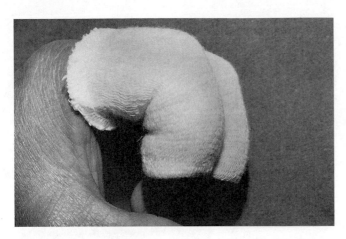

FIG. 35-5 Bedford finger stall may be used as "fellow traveler" to protect injured finger. Slight compression applied by stretch gauze may reduce edema, and pressure may alleviate pain. Finger stall can be worn for prolonged periods of time.

splint that limits full extension of the finger may be used following a fracture or dislocation of the PIP joint. A dynamic splint may be used to achieve full ROM or to prevent the development of further deformity at 6 to 8 weeks following fracture.

Intraarticular fractures may result in injury to the cartilage of the joint, resulting in additional pain and stiffness. An x-ray film examination will indicate if there has been damage to the joint surface, which might limit the treatment of the joint. Joint pain and stiffness following fracture without the presence of joint damage should be alleviated by a combination of thermal modalities, restoration of joint play, or joint mobilization and corrective and dynamic splinting followed by active use. Resistive exercise can be started when bony healing has been achieved.

Wrist fractures are common and may present special problems for the surgeon and therapist. Colles' fractures of the distal radius are the most common injury to the wrist[15] and may result in limitations in wrist flexion and extension, as well as pronation and supination resulting from the involvement of the radioulnar joint. Use of splints, active motion that emphasizes wrist movement, and joint mobilization may be beneficial. The weight well (Fig. 35-6) may be used to provide resistance to wrist motions.

The carpal scaphoid is the second most commonly injured bone in the wrist[15] and is often fractured when the hand is dorsiflexed at the time of injury. Fractures to the proximal portion of the scaphoid may result in nonunion because of poor blood supply to this area. Scaphoid fractures require a prolonged period of immobilization, sometimes up to several months in a cast, with resulting stiffness and pain. Care should be taken to mobilize noninvolved joints early.

Trauma to the carpal lunate may result in avascular

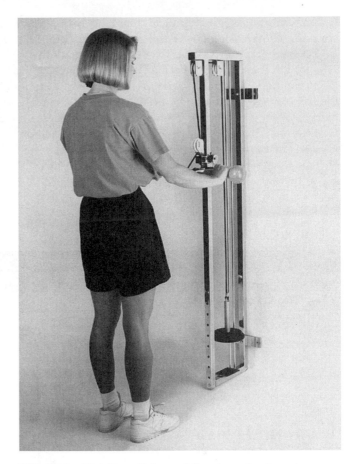

FIG. 35-6 Weight well is used for strengthening upper extremity with progressive resistance applied to weakened musculature and is also useful in retraining prehension of pinch and grip. (Photo courtesy of Karen Schultz Johnson)

necrosis of the lunate or Kienböck's disease,[15] which may result from a one-time accident or may be caused by repetitive trauma. Lunate fractures are usually immobilized for 6 weeks. Kienböck's disease may be treated with a bone graft, Silastic implant, or partial wrist fusion.

Stiffness and pain are common complications of fractures. The control of edema coupled with early motion and good patient instruction and support will minimize these complications, however.

NERVE INJURIES

Nerve injury may be classified into the following three categories:

1. Neurapraxia is contusion of the nerve without wallerian degeneration. The nerve recovers function without treatment within a few days or weeks.
2. Axonotmesis is an injury in which nerve fibers distal to the site of injury degenerate but the internal organization of the nerve remains intact. No surgical treatment is necessary, and recovery usually occurs within 6 months. The length of time may vary, depending on the level of injury.
3. Neurotmesis is a complete laceration of both nerve

and fibrous tissues. Surgical treatment is required. Microsurgical repair of the fascicles is common. Nerve grafting may be necessary in situations in which there is a gap between nerve endings.[89] Peripheral nerve injuries may occur as a result of disruption of the nerve by a fractured bone, laceration, or crush injury. Symptoms of nerve injuries include weakness or paralysis of muscles that are innervated by motor branches of the injured nerve and sensory loss to areas that are innervated by sensory branches of the injured nerve. Before evaluating the patient for nerve loss, the therapist must be familiar with the muscles and areas that

are innervated by the three major forearm nerves. A summary of upper extremity peripheral neuropathic conditions can be found in Table 35-1.

Radial Nerve

The radial nerve innervates the extensor-supinator group of muscles of the forearm, including the brachioradialis, extensor carpi radialis longus, extensor carpi radialis brevis, extensor digitorum communis, extensor digiti minimi, extensor indicis, extensor carpi ulnaris, supinator, abductor pollicis longus, extensor pollicis brevis, and extensor pollicis longus. The sensory distribution of

TABLE 35-1 Nerve Injuries of the Upper Extremity

NERVE	LOCATION	AFFECTED	TEST
Radial nerve (Posterior cord, fibers from C5, C6, C7, C8)	Upper arm	Triceps & all distal motors; sensory to superficial radial nerve (SRN)	MMT; sensory test
Radial nerve	Above elbow	Bracioradialis & all distal motors; sensory to SRN	MMT; sensory
Radial nerve	At elbow	Supinator, ECRL, ECRB & all distal motors; sensory to SRN	MMT; sensory
Posterior interosseous nerve	Forearm	ECU, ED, EDM, APL, EPL, EPB, EIP; no sensory	Wrist extension — if present, indicates PIN rather than high radial nerve
Radial nerve at ECRB, radial artery, arcade of Frohse, origin of supinator	Radial tunnel syndrome	Weakness of muscles innervated by PIN; no sensory loss	Palpate for pain over extensor mass; pain with wrist flexion and pronation, pain with wrist ext. and supination; pain with resisted middle finger extension
Median nerve (Lateral from C5, C6, C7 Medial cord from C8, T1)	High lesions (elbow and above)	Paralysis/weakness of FCR, PL, all FDS, FDP I & II; FPL, pronator teres & quad., opponens pollicis, APB, FPB (radial head), lumbricals I & II; sensory cutaneous branch of median nerve	MMT; sensory
Median nerve	Low (at wrist)	Weakness of thenars only	Inability to flex thumbtip and index fingertip to palm; inability to oppose thumb, poor dexterity
Median nerve under fibrous band in PT, beneath heads of pronator, arch of FDS, origin of FCR	Pronator syndrome	Weakness in thenars, but *not* muscles innervated by AIN; sensory in median n. distribution in hand	Provocative tests to isolate compression site
Median nerve under origin of PT, FDS to middle	Anterior interosseous nerve syndrome	Pure motor, no sensory; forearm pain precedes paralysis; weakness of FPL, FDP I & II, PQ	Inability to flex IP joint of thumb and DIP of index; increased pain with resisted pronation; pain with forearm pressure
Median nerve at wrist	Carpal tunnel syndrome	Weakness of med. intrinsics; sensory	Provocative tests; Tinel's; sensory
Ulnar nerve at elbow (Branch of medial cord from C7, C8, T1)	Cubital tunnel syndrome	Weakness/Paralysis of FCU, FDP III & IV, ulnar intrinsics; numbness in palmar cutaneous and dorsal cutaneous distribution; loss of grip & pinch strength	Pain with elbow flexion/extension
Ulnar nerve at wrist	Compression at canal of Guyon	Weakness and pain in ulnar intrinsics	Reproduced by pressure at site

MMT, Manual Muscle Test

the radial nerve is a strip of the posterior upper arm and the forearm; dorsum of the thumb; and index and middle fingers and radial half of the ring finger to the PIP joints. Sensory loss of the radial nerve does not usually result in dysfunction.

Clinical signs of a high-level radial nerve injury (above the supinator) are pronation of the forearm, wrist flexion, and the thumb held in palmar abduction resulting from the unopposed action of the flexor pollicis brevis and the abductor pollicis brevis.[91] Injury to the posterior interosseous nerve spares the extensor carpi radialis longus and brevis. Posterior interosseus nerve syndrome includes normal sensation and wrist extension with loss of finger and thumb extension. Clinical signs of low-level radial nerve injury include incomplete extension of the MP joints of the fingers and thumb. The interossei extend the interphalangeal (IP) joints of the fingers, but the MP joints rest in about 30° of flexion.

A dorsal splint that provides wrist extension, MP extension, and thumb extension should be provided to protect the extensor tendons from overstretching during the healing phase and to position the hand for functional use (Fig. 35-7). A dynamic splint is commonly provided.

Median Nerve

The median nerve innervates the flexors of the forearm and hand and is often called the "eyes" of the hands because of its importance in sensory innervation of the volar surface of the hands. Median nerve loss may result from lacerations as well as from compression syndromes of the wrist, such as the carpal tunnel syndrome.

Motor distribution of the median nerve is to the pronator teres, palmaris longus, flexor carpi radialis, flexor digitorum profundus to the index and long fingers, flexor digitorum superficialis, flexor pollicis longus, pronator quadratus, abductor pollicis brevis, opponens pollicis, superficial head of the flexor pollicis brevis, and first and second lumbricals.

Sensory distribution of the median nerve is to the volar surface of the thumb, index, and middle fingers; radial half of the ring finger and dorsal surface of the index and middle fingers; and radial half of the ring finger distal to the PIP joints.

Clinical signs of a high-level median nerve injury are ulnar flexion of the wrist caused by loss of the flexor carpi radialis, loss of palmar abduction, and opposition of the thumb. Active pronation is absent, but the patient may appear to pronate with the assistance of gravity. In a wrist-level median nerve injury the thenar eminence appears flat and there is a loss of thumb flexion, palmar abduction, and opposition.[91]

The sensory loss associated with median nerve injury is particularly disabling because there is no sensation to the volar aspects of the thumb and index and long fingers and the radial side of the ring finger. The patient when blindfolded substitutes pinch to the ring and small fingers to compensate for this loss. An injury in the forearm that involves the anterior interosseous nerve does not result in sensory loss. Motor loss includes paralysis of the flexor pollicis longus, the flexor digitorum profundus of the index and long fingers, and the pronator quadratus. The pronator teres is not affected. Pinch is affected.

Splints that position the thumb in palmar *abduction and slight opposition* increase functional use of the hand (Fig. 35-8). If clawing of the index and long fingers is present, a splint should be fabricated to prevent hyperextension of the MP joints. Patients report that they avoid use of the hand with a median nerve injury because of lack of sensation rather than because of muscle paralysis. Nevertheless, the weakened or paralyzed muscles should be protected.

Ulnar Nerve

The ulnar nerve in the forearm innervates only the flexor carpi ulnaris and the median half of the flexor digitorum profundus. It travels down the volar forearm through the canal of Guyon, innervating the intrinsic muscles of the

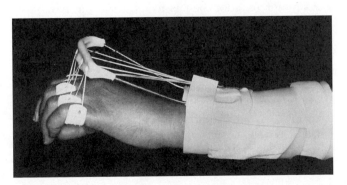

FIG. 35-7 Low-profile radial nerve splint is carefully balanced to pull MP joints into extension when wrist is flexed and allows the MP joints to fall into slight flexion when wrist is extended, thus preserving normal balance between two joints and preserving joint contracture. (Splint, courtesy of Judy C Colditz, Raleigh Hand Rehabilitation Center.)

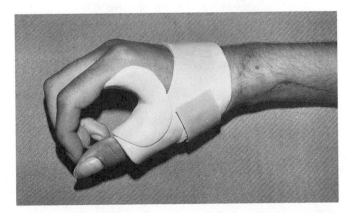

FIG. 35-8 Thumb stabilization splint may be used with median nerve injury to protect thumb and to improve functioning by placing thumb in position of pinch. Normal pinch cannot be achieved with median nerve injury because of paralysis of thumb musculature.

hand, including the palmaris brevis, abductor digiti minimi, opponens digiti minimi, flexor digiti minimi, dorsal and volar interossei, third and fourth lumbricals, and medial head of the flexor pollicis brevis. The sensory distribution of the ulnar nerve is the dorsal and volar surfaces of the little finger ray and the ulnar half of the dorsal and volar surface of the ring finger ray.

A high-level ulnar nerve injury results in hyperextension of the MP joints of the ring and small fingers (also called clawing) resulting from overaction of the extensor digitorum communis that is not held in check by the third and fourth lumbricals.[91] The IP joints of the ring and small fingers do not demonstrate a great flexion deformity because of the paralysis of the flexor digitorum profundus. The hypothenar muscles and interossei are absent. The wrist assumes a position of radial extension caused by the loss of the flexor carpi ulnaris. In a low-level ulnar nerve injury the ring and small fingers claw at the MP joints and the IP joints exhibit a greater tendency toward flexion because the flexor digitorum profundus is present. Wrist extension is normal.

Clinical signs of a high-level ulnar nerve injury may include clawhand with a loss of the hypothenar and the interosseous muscles. In a low-level ulnar nerve injury the flexor digitorum profundus and flexor carpi ulnaris are present and unopposed by the intrinsic muscles. When attempting lateral or key pinch the IP joint of the thumb flexes instead of extending because of paralysis of the intrinsic muscles, known as Froment's sign. Long-standing compression of the ulnar nerve in the canal of Guyon results in a flattening of the hypothenar area and conspicuous atrophy of the first dorsal interosseous muscle.[15]

With a low-level ulnar nerve injury a small splint may be provided to prevent hyperextension of the small and ring fingers without limiting full flexion at the MP joints. Stabilization of the MP joints will allow the extensor digitorum communis to extend the IP joints fully (Fig. 35-9).

Sensory loss of the ulnar nerve results in frequent injury to the ulnar side of the hand, especially burns. Patients must be instructed in visual protection of the anesthetic area.

Postoperative Management Following Nerve Repair

Following nerve repair the hand is placed in a position that minimizes tension on the nerve. For example, following repair of the median nerve, the wrist is immobilized in a flexed position. Immobilization usually lasts for 2 to 3 weeks, after which protective stretching of the joints may begin. The therapist must exercise great care not to put excessive traction on the newly repaired nerve.

Correction of a contracture may take 4 to 6 weeks. Active exercise is the preferred method of gaining full extension, although a light dynamic splint may be applied with the surgeon's supervision. Splinting to assist

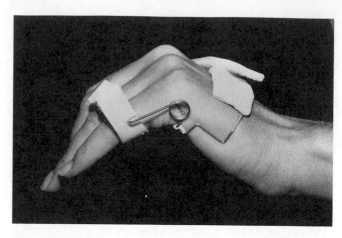

FIG. 35-9 Dynamic ulnar nerve splint blocks hyperextension of MP joints that occurs with paralysis of ulnar intrinsic muscles and allows MP flexion, which maintains normal ROM of MP joints. (Splint courtesy of Mary Dimick, University of California —San Diego Hand Rehabilitation Center.)

or substitute for weakened musculature may be necessary for an extended period during nerve regeneration. Splints should be removed as soon as possible to allow for active exercise of the weakened muscles. It is important to instruct the patient in correct patterns of motion, however, so that substitution is minimized.

Initially treatment is directed toward the prevention of deformity and correction of poor positioning during the acute and regenerative stages. Patients must be instructed in visual protection of the anesthetic area. ADL should be evaluated, and new methods or devices may be needed for independence. Use of the hand in the patient's work should be evaluated, and the patient should be returned to employment with any necessary job modifications or adaptations of equipment as soon as possible.

Careful muscle, sensory, and functional testing should be done frequently. As the nerve regenerates, splints may be changed or eliminated. Exercises and activities should be revised to reflect the patient's new gains, and adapted equipment should be discarded as soon as possible.

As motor function begins to return to the paralyzed muscles, a careful program of specific exercises should be devised to facilitate the return. Proprioceptive neuromuscular facilitation techniques, such as hold-relax, contract-relax, quick stretch, and icing may assist a fair-strength muscle and increase ROM. Neuromuscular electrical stimulation (NMES)[12] can also provide an external stimulus to help strengthen the newly innervated muscle. When the muscle has reached a good rating, functional activities should be used to complete the return to normal strength.

Sensory reeducation

Evaluation of sensibility has been described in some detail earlier in this chapter. This information should be used to prepare a program of sensory reeducation following nerve repair.

When a nerve is repaired, regeneration is not perfect and results in fewer and smaller nerve fibers and receptors distal to the repair. The goal of sensory reeducation is to maximize the functional level of sensation or tactile gnosis.

Parry first described sensory reeducation in 1966,[91] and Dellon reported a highly structured sensory reeducation program in 1974.[33] Dellon divided his program into early and late phase training, based on vibratory sensation for early phase and perception of moving and constant touch sensation for late phase reeducation. Localization of stimuli and recognition of objects was used by both Parry and Dellon. Higher cortical integration was achieved by focusing attention on the stimuli through visual clues and by employing memory when vision was occluded. The patients were taught to compensate for sensory deficits by improving specific skills and generalizing them to other sensory stimuli. Daily repetition appears to be a necessary component of reeducation.

Callahan[18] has outlined a program of protective sensory reeducation and discriminative sensory reeducation if protective sensation is present and there has been a return of touch sensation to the fingertips. Waylett-Rendall[111] has also described a sensory reeducation program utilizing crafts and functional activities as well as desensitization techniques. All programs emphasize a variety of stimuli used in a repetitive manner to bombard the sensory receptors. A sequence of eyes-closed, eyes-open, eyes-closed is used to provide feedback during the training process. Sessions are limited in length to avoid fatigue and frustration. Objects must not be potentially harmful to the insensate areas, to avoid further trauma. A home program should be provided to reinforce learning that occurs in the clinical setting.

Researchers[18,30,111] have found that sensory reeducation can result in improved functional sensibility in motivated patients. Objective measurement of sensation following reeducation must be performed and then compared with initial testing accurately to assess the success of the program.

Tendon transfers

If, following a minimal period of 1 year after nerve repair, a motor nerve has not reinnervated its muscle, the surgeon may consider tendon transfers to restore a needed motion. The rules of tendon transfer are to evaluate (1) what is absent, (2) what is needed for function and (3) what is available to transfer.[94] Some muscles, such as the extensor carpi radialis longus and the sublimis to the ring finger, are commonly used for transfers because their motions are easily substituted by the extensor carpi radialis brevis and flexor digitorum profundus to the ring finger, respectively. The surgeon may request assistance in evaluating motor status from the therapist to determine the best motor transfer.

Therapy before tendon transfer is essential if the motor being used is not of normal strength. A muscle loses a grade of strength when transferred, and a strengthening program of progressive resistive exercises, NMES, and isolated motion will help ensure success of the transfer.

Following transfer, many patients require instruction to perceive the correct muscle during active use of the transfer. Use of biofeedback, careful instruction, and supervised activity to note any substitution patterns during active use usually help the patient to use the transfer correctly. Therapy must be initiated before the patient has time to develop incorrect use patterns. NMES may be used to isolate the muscle and to strengthen it postoperatively.

TENDON INJURIES
Flexor Tendons

Injuries to tendons may be isolated or may occur in conjunction with other injuries, especially fractures or crushes. Flexor tendons injured in the area between the distal palmar crease and the insertion of the flexor digitorum superficialis are considered the most difficult to treat, because the tendons lie in their sheaths in this area beneath the fibrous pulley system and any scarring causes adhesions. This area is often referred to as zone 2 or "no-man's-land."

Primary repair of the flexor tendons within zone 2 is most frequently attempted following a clean laceration. Several methods of postoperative management have been proposed with the common goal to promote gliding of the tendons and to minimize the formation of scar adhesions.

Controlled mobilization of acute flexor tendon injuries: Louisville technique

Dr. Harold Kleinert of the University of Louisville School of Medicine was an early advocate of rubberband traction following repair of flexor tendons in zone 2. This technique is often referred to as the Kleinert technique. The doctor and therapist do not actively participate in moving the tendon or finger when this protocol is followed as outlined by Kutz.[58]

Following surgical repair, rubberbands are attached to the nails of the involved fingers using a suture through the nail or with a hook held in place with cyanoacrylate glue. A dorsal blocking splint is fabricated out of low-temperature thermoplastic material, with the MP joints held in about 60° of flexion. The splint is constructed so that the IP joints are able to extend fully to the splint. The rubberbands are passed through a safety pin in the palm and are attached to the distal strap of the splint. The rubberbands should be placed in sufficient tension to hold the PIP joints in 40° to 60° of flexion without tension on the rubberbands. The patient must be able to fully extend the IP joints actively within the splint or joint contractures will develop (Fig. 35-10).

The patient wears this splint 24 hours a day for 3 weeks and is instructed to actively extend the fingers

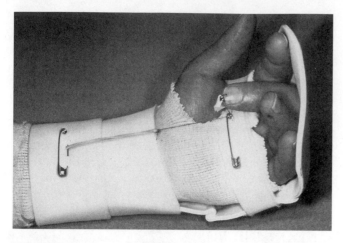

FIG. 35-10 Following flexor tendon repair, wrist is placed in 30° flexion with traction applied from the nail through a safety pin pulley in the palm and attached to proximal strap of splint. MP joints should be maintained in about 70° flexion, allowing full passive IP joint flexion and active extension.

several times a day in the splint, allowing the rubberbands to pull the fingers into flexion. This movement of the tendon through the tendon sheath and pulley system minimizes scar adhesions while enhancing tendon nutrition and blood flow.

The dorsal blocking splint is removed at 3 weeks and the rubberband is attached to a wristband, which is worn for 1 to 5 additional weeks, depending on the judgment of the surgeon.

The primary disadvantage of this technique is that contractures of the PIP joints frequently occur as a result of too much tension on the rubberband or incomplete IP extension within the splint. Dynamic extension splinting of the PIP joint can be started at 5 to 6 weeks if a flexion contracture is present. To be successful, this technique requires a motivated patient who thoroughly understands the program.

Controlled passive motion: Duran and Houser technique

Duran and Houser[38] suggested the use of controlled passive motion to achieve optimal results following primary repair, allowing 3 to 5 mm of tendon excursion. They found this amount to be sufficient to prevent adherence of the repaired tendons. On the third postoperative day the patient begins a twice-daily exercise regimen of passive flexion and extension of 6 to 8 motions for each tendon. Care is taken to keep the wrist flexed and the MPs in 70° of flexion during passive exercise. Between exercise periods the hand is wrapped in a stockinette. At 4 1/2 weeks the protective dorsal splint is removed and the rubberband traction is attached to a wristband. Active extension and passive flexion are done for 1 additional week and gradually increased over the next several weeks.

Immobilization technique

A third postoperative program is complete immobilization for 3 1/2 weeks following tendon repair. Immobilization has not resulted in consistently good results and may lead to a great incidence of tendon rupture following repair because a tendon gains tensile strength when submitted to gentle tension at the repair site.[100]

Postacute flexor tendon rehabilitation

When active flexion is begun out of the splint following any of the postoperative management techniques described previously, the patient should be instructed in exercises to facilitate differential tendon gliding.[114] Wehbe[113] recommends three positions—hook, straight fist, and fist—to maximize isolated gliding of the flexor digitorum superficialis and the flexor digitorum profundus tendons, as well as stretching of the intrinsic musculature and gliding of the extensor mechanism. Tendon gliding exercises should be done for 10 repetitions of each position, 2 to 3 times a day.

Isolated exercises to assist tendon gliding may also be performed using a blocking splint[40] (Fig. 35-11) or the opposite hand (Fig. 35-12). The MP joints should be held in extension during blocking so the intrinsic muscles that act on it cannot overcome the power of the repaired flexor tendons. Care should be taken not to hyperextend the PIP joint and overstretch the repaired tendons.

After 6 to 8 weeks passive extension may be started and splinting may be necessary to correct a flexion contracture at the PIP joint. A cylindrical plaster splint may be fabricated to apply constant static pressure on the contracture as described by Bell[10] (Fig. 35-13). Static splinting may be especially effective with a flexion contracture greater than 25°. A finger gutter splint may be made using 1/16-inch (0.16-cm) thermoplastic material for static extension at night, which will help maintain extension gains made during the day. Gentle dynamic

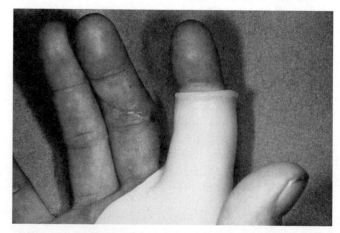

FIG. 35-11 Blocking splint can be used to isolate tendon pull-through and joint ROM by blocking out proximal joints. This splint is being used to facilitate motion at DIP joint following repair of FDP tendon.

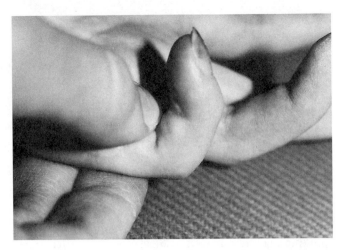

FIG. 35-12   Manual blocking of MP joint during flexion of PIP joint.

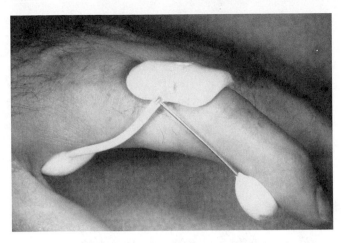

FIG. 35-14   This finger splint is used to increase extension of PIP joint. Splint available from LMB Hand Rehabilitation Products, Inc, PO Box 1181, San Luis Obispo, CA 93406.

traction may be applied using a commercial splint such as an LMB finger extension splint[62] (Fig. 35-14) or one that is fabricated by the therapist (Fig. 35-15). Dynamic flexion splinting may be necessary if the patient has difficulty regaining passive flexion.

At about 8 weeks the patient may begin light resistive exercises and activities. The hand can now be used for light ADL, but the patient should continue to avoid heavy lifting with or excessive resistance to the affected hand. Sports activities should be discouraged. Activities such as clay work, woodworking, and macrame are excellent, however. Full resistance and normal work activities can be started at 3 months following surgery.

When evaluating a hand that has sustained a tendon injury, passive versus active limitations of joint motion must be evaluated. Limitations in active motion may indicate joint stiffness, muscle weakness, or scar adhesions.[92]

If passive motion is greater than active motion, the therapist should consider that tendons may be caught in the scar tissue. The therapist should be able to determine if a tendon is adhering and causing a flexion contracture or if the tendon is free but the joint itself is stiff. Treatment should be based on this type of evaluation.

ROM, strength, function, and sensibility testing (if digital nerves were also injured) should be performed frequently with splints and activities geared to progress. Although performance of ADL is generally not a problem, the therapist should ask the patient about any problems he or she may have or anticipate. Disuse and neglect of a finger, especially the index finger, are common and should be prevented.

Gains in flexion and extension may continue to be recorded for 6 months postoperatively. A finger with

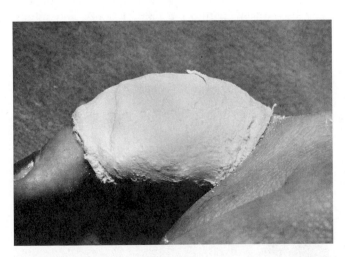

FIG. 35-13   Plaster cylindrical splint is used to apply static stretch of PIP joint contracture. It is not removed by patient and must be replaced frequently by therapist with careful monitoring of skin condition.

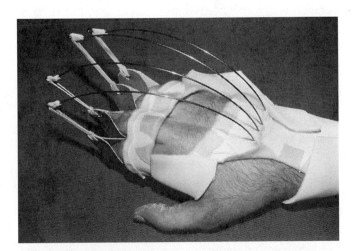

FIG. 35-15   Dynamic outrigger splint using spring-steel outriggers with a lumbrical block can be used to assist PIP joint extension, stretch against scar adhesions of extrinsic flexors, or reduce PIP joint contractures. Proper fit and tension of rubber bands must be assessed frequently by therapist.

limber joints and minimal scarring preoperatively will function better after repair than one that is stiff and scarred and has trophic skin changes.[16] It is important therefore that all joints, skin, and scars be supple and movable before reconstructive surgery is attempted. A functional to excellent result is obtained if the combined loss of extension is less than 40° in the PIP and DIP joints of the index and middle fingers and is less than 60° in the ring and little fingers[83] and if the finger can flex to the palm.[16]

If the tendon is damaged as a result of a crush injury or the laceration cannot be cleaned up enough to allow for a primary repair, staged flexor tendon reconstruction may be done. At the first operation a Silastic rod is inserted beneath the pulley system and attached to the distal phalanx. Other reconstructive procedures, such as pulley reconstruction, are performed at the same time. A mesothelial cell-lined pseudosheath is formed about the rod and a fluid similar to synovial fluid is formed in the postoperative recovery phase.[60] The second stage is performed about 4 months later when the digit can be moved passively to the palm. A tendon graft is inserted and the Silastic rod removed. The postoperative program is carried out in the same manner as for a primary tendon repair.[67]

Following a two-stage tendon reconstruction or primary repair, a tenolysis may be performed if there is a substantial difference between the active and passive motion. Tenolysis is usually not performed for 6 months to 1 year after tendon repair. At the time of tenolysis surgery, scar adhesions are removed from the tendon and gliding of the tendons is assessed. Patients are often asked to move their fingers in the operating room at the time of lysis to determine the extent of scar removal. Active motion is begun within the first 24 hours using bupivacaine hydrochloride (Marcaine) blocks[95] or transcutaneous electrical nerve stimulation (TENS)[19] to control pain.

LaSalle and Strickland[60] have recommended a system for evaluating the results of tenolysis surgery by comparing the preoperative passive IP joint motion with the postoperative IP joint motion. Based on this comparison LaSalle and Strickland found that in one group of patients undergoing tenolysis, 40% had an improvement in motion of 50% or better compared with their preoperative status.

Extensor Tendons

Dorsal scar adherence is the most difficult problem following injury to the extensor tendons because of the tendency of the dorsal extensor hood to become adherent to the underlying structures and thus limit its normal excursion during flexion and extension.

Extensor tendons in zones V, VI, and VII (proximal to the MP joints) become adherent because they are encased in paratenon and synovial sheaths and respond to injury in a way similar to flexor tendons, resulting in either incomplete extension, also known as extensor lag, or incomplete flexion resulting from loss of gliding of the extensor tendon.

Evans[42,43] studied the normal excursion of the extensor digitorum communis in zones V, VI, and VII to suggest guidelines for early passive motion of extensor tendons. She concluded that 5 mm of tendon glide following repair was safe and effective in limiting tendon adhesions and designed a postoperative splint that allows slight active flexion while providing passive extension.[43] The splint is worn for 3 weeks, with the initiation of active motion between the third and fourth weeks. A removeable volar splint is used between exercise periods to protect the tendon for 2 additional weeks. Dynamic flexion splinting may be started at 6 weeks postoperative to regain flexion if needed.

Injuries to extensor tendons proximal to the MP joint may be immobilized for 3 weeks. After this period the finger may be placed in a removable volar splint that is worn between exercise periods for an additional 2 weeks. Progressive ROM is begun at 3 weeks, and if full flexion is not regained rapidly, dynamic flexion may be started at 6 weeks.

Extensor tendon injuries that occur distal to the MP joint require a longer period of immobilization, usually 6 weeks. A progressive exercise program is then initiated with dynamic splinting during the day and a static night splint to maintain extension.

Dynamic splints may include a PIP-DIP splint first described by Hollis and now available commercially[62] (Fig. 35-16), a web strap made of lamp wick or elastic, a fingernail hook with rubber band traction, a traction glove, or another splint.

If a lysis of scar tissue is required because of persistent scar adhesion, the surgeon may place a thin sheet of Silastic between the tendon and bone at the time of surgery to reduce further scar adherence. The patient begins exercising within the first 24 hours, and splints are applied as needed. Active exercise is essential, and

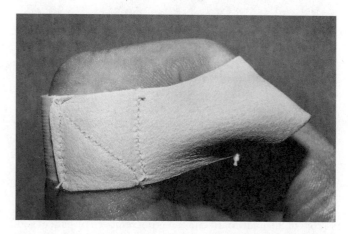

FIG. 35-16 PIP-DIP splint may be used to increase flexion of both PIP and DIP joints. Tension can be adjusted with Velcro closure. Wearing time should be determined by therapist.

the patient must be carefully instructed in a home program. The patient is encouraged to use the hand for all activities except those requiring heavy resistance. After 4 to 6 weeks the Silastic sheet is removed and ROM should be maintained.

Total Active Motion and Total Passive Motion

Total active motion (TAM) and total passive motion (TPM) is a method of recording joint ROM that is used to compare tendon excursion (active) and joint mobility (passive). It is the measure of flexion minus extensor lag of three joints. TAM and TPM have been recommended for use in reporting joint motion by The American Society for Surgery of the Hand.[3]

TAM is computed by adding the sum of the angles formed by the MP, PIP, and DIP joints in flexion minus incomplete active extension at each of the three joints. For example, MP joint flexion is 85° with full extension, PIP is 100° and lacks 15° extension, and DIP is 65° with full extension; therefore

$$TAM = 85 + 100 + 65 - 15 = 235°$$

TAM should be measured while making a fist. It is used for a single digit and should be compared with the same digit of the opposite hand or subsequent measurements of the same digit. It should not be used to compute a percentage of loss of impairment. TPM is calculated in the same manner but measures only passive motion.

EDEMA

Edema is a normal consequence of trauma but must be quickly and aggressively treated to prevent permanent stiffness and disability. Within hours of trauma, vasodilation and local edema occur with an increase in white blood cells to the damaged area.[69] The inflammatory response to the injury results in a decrease in bacteria to control infection.

Early control of edema should be achieved through elevation, massage, compression, and active ROM. The patient is instructed at the time of injury to keep the hand elevated, and a compressive dressing is used to reduce early swelling. Pitting edema is present early and can be recognized as a bloated swelling that "pits" when pressed. Pitting may be more pronounced on the dorsal surface where the venous and lymphatic systems provide return of fluid to the heart. Active motion is especially important to produce retrograde venous and lymphatic flow.

If the swelling continues, a serofibrinous exudate invades the area. Fibrin is deposited in the spaces surrounding the joints, tendons, and ligaments, resulting in reduced mobility, flattening of the arches of the hand, tissue atrophy, and further disuse.[69] Normal gliding of the tissues is eliminated, and a stiff, often painful hand is the result. Scar adhesions form and further limit tissue mobility. If untreated, these losses may become permanent.

Early recognition of persistent edema through volume and circumference measurement is important. It may be necessary to use several of the suggested edema control techniques.

Elevation

Early elevation with the hand above the heart is essential. Slings tend to reduce blood flow and should be avoided. Resting the hand on pillows while seated or lying down is effective. Resting the hand on top of the head or using devices that elevate the hand with the elbow in extension have been suggested. Suspension slings may be purchased or fabricated.

The patient should use the hand for ADL within the limitations of resistance prescribed by the physician. Light ADL that can be accomplished while the hand is in the dressing are permitted.

Contrast Baths

Alternating soaks of cold and warm water that is 66° and 96° F (18.9° and 35.6° C) have been recommended as a method preferred over warm water soaks or whirlpool baths. The contrast baths can be done for 20 minutes, alternating the hand between cool water for 1 minute and warm water for 1 minute, starting and ending with cool water. A sponge can be placed in each tub so that the hand is moved during the soaking period. The tubs should be placed as high as possible to provide elevation of the extremity. The alternating warm and cool water cause vasodilation and vasoconstriction, resulting in a pumping action on the edema. Combined with elevation and active motion, edema may be reduced and pain is often alleviated by this technique.

Retrograde Massage

A retrograde massage may be done by the therapist, but it should be taught to the patient so that it can be done frequently through the day. The massage assists in blood and lymph flow. It should be started distally and stroked proximally with the extremity in elevation.[29] Active motion should follow the massage but muscle fatigue should be avoided.

Pressure Wraps

Wrapping with Coban elastic wrap[37] may be employed to reduce edema (Fig. 35-17). Starting distally, the finger is wrapped snugly with Coban. Each involved finger should be wrapped distally to proximally until the wrap is proximal to the edema. The wrap remains in place for 5 minutes and then is removed. Active exercise may be done while the finger is wrapped or immediately following. Measurements should be taken before and after treatment to document an increase in ROM and a decrease in edema. The wrapping may be repeated 3 times a day.

Light compression may be applied throughout the day with a light Coban wrap, an Isotoner glove,[48] or a custom-made garment by Jobst[50] (Fig. 35-18) or Bio-

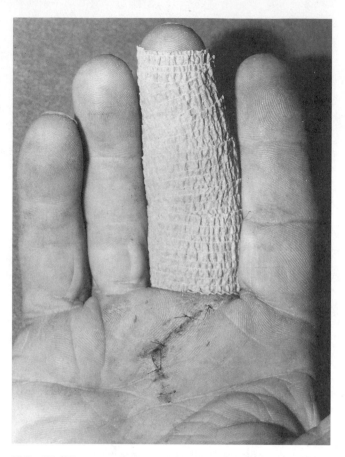

FIG. 35-17 One-inch Coban is wrapped with minimal pressure from distal end to proximal crease of digit. Patient is instructed to be aware of vascular compression or tingling. Coban may be worn several hours a day to reduce edema. Product available from Medical Products Division/3M, St. Paul, Minn.

Concepts.[14] The compression should not be constricting and should be discontinued if ischemia results.

Various pressure wraps are used by hand centers. Tubular gauze, Digi-sleeves,[3,35] and Bedford finger stalls provide compression to a specific finger. No one method

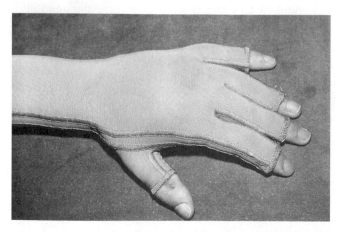

FIG. 35-18 Custom-fit Jobst garment may be used to reduce edema and to reduce and prevent hypertrophic scar formation following burns or trauma. Inserts may be used with garment to increase pressure over natural curves, such as dorsum of wrist.

is superior to another. A combination of techniques used at different stages of healing and according to patient comfort may be the most effective.

Active ROM

Normal blood flow is dependent on muscle activity. Active motion does not mean wiggling the fingers but rather maximum available ROM done firmly. Casts and splints must allow mobility of uninjured parts while protecting newly injured structures. The shoulder and elbow should be moved several times a day. The importance of active ROM for edema control, tendon gliding, and tissue nutrition cannot be overemphasized.

WOUND HEALING AND SCAR REMODELING

The first phase of wound healing, the acute inflammatory phase, is initiated within hours when the tissues are disrupted through injury or surgery, causing vasodilation and local edema as well as migration of white blood cells and phagocytic cells to the area. The phagocytes remove tissue fragments and foreign bodies and are critical to healing. The inflammatory process can subside or persist indefinitely depending on the degree of bacterial contamination.[69]

Fibroblasts in combination with associated capillaries begin to invade the wound within the first 72 hours and gradually replace the phagocytes, leading to the second phase: the collagen or granulation phase, between the fifth and fourteenth days. Collagen fiber formation follows the invasion by fibroblasts, so that by the end of the second week the wound is rich with fibroblasts, a capillary network, and early collagen fibers. This increased vascularization results in the erythema of the new scar.

During the third to sixth weeks fibroblasts are slowly replaced with scar collagen fibers and the wound becomes stronger and more able to withstand progressive stresses leading to the last phase of scar maturation. Strength continues to increase for 3 months or longer. The collagen metabolizes and synthesizes during this period, so that new collagen replaces old while the wound remains relatively stable. Covalent bonding between collagen molecules leads to dense scar adhesions and the formation of whorl-like patterns of collagen deposits, which may be altered as the scar architecture and collagen fiber organization within the wound changes over time.[37]

Myofibroblasts, which are fibroblasts with properties similar to smooth muscle cells, are contractile and cause a shortening of the wound.

Tissues that have restored gliding have different scar architecture from those that do not develop the ability to glide. With gliding the scar resembles the state of the tissues before injury, whereas the nongliding scar remains fixed on surrounding structures. Controlled tension on the scar has been shown to facilitate remodeling.

Scar formation is also influenced by age and the quantity of scar deposited.[69]

Wound Care and Dressings

There are many dressings that can be placed on a wound, including gauze that has been impregnated with petroleum, such as Xeroform gauze or Adaptic. Ointments such as Polysporin are also commonly applied. N-Terface[84] is a dry mesh fabric that looks and feels like interfacing that is used in sewing. Because it is nonadherent, it can be used directly over wounds and will not stick to them. Sterile dressings can be applied directly over the N-Terface[87] without ointments or gels. Spenco Second Skin[99] is an inert gel sheeting made from 96% water and 4% polyethylene oxide. It removes friction between two moving surfaces and is said to clean wounds by absorbing secretions. It comes in sterile and nonsterile packs and is encased in a light plastic covering. It is especially effective with abrasions or areas of skin loss because it is cool and reduces itching. It can be used after burns.

Spenco Dermal Pads[99] are artificial, fat pads that can be used to prevent pressure sores or can be cut to size to use around an existing pressure sore or wound to allow it to heal. Dermal pads are 1/8-inch thick (0.32-cm) and will adhere to the skin when the protective film is removed. The pad can be held in place with a dressing or with a pressure garment. It also can be washed without reducing its adherence. Dermal pads can be cut and placed around a healing wound to protect it under a splint or dressing. They are generally not needed after the wound is healed.

The wound can be cleaned with a solution of hydrogen peroxide and sterile saline, with dead tissue then being gently removed with sterile swabs. Sterile saline solution can be used to soak off adherent bandages rather than pulling them off the patient. The therapist should pour a very small amount of saline on the area that is sticking, wait a few moments, and gently pry the dressing off. Dead skin can be debrided using iris scissors and pickups. Betadine-impregnated scrub sponges may be used for cleaning and desensitization of the wound once it is healed and the stitches have been removed. The patient also can do this procedure at home. Sterile whirlpool may also be used for debridement especially if the wound is infected.

Pressure

A hypertrophic scar or a scar that is randomly laid down and thickened is reduced by the application of pressure, often by means of pressure garments.[14,50] Use of an insert of neoprene[86] fabric, or molds made from Silastic elastomer,[71,96] under the pressure garment increases the conformity of the garment. Pressure should be applied for most of the 24-hour period, and with a hypertrophic burn scar this treatment should continue for a period of 6 months to 1 year following the injury. Other forms of pressure outlined in the section on edema control may also be used.

Massage

Gentle-to-firm massage of the scarred area using a thick ointment, such as lanolin or Corrective Concepts Cream,[25] rapidly softens scar tissue and should be followed immediately with active hand use so that tendons glide against the softened scar.[29] Vibration to the area with a small, low-intensity vibrator will have a similar effect.[51] Active exercise using facilitation techniques and against resistance, or functional activity should follow vibration. Massage and vibration may be started at 4 weeks postinjury.

Thermal heat in the form of paraffin dips, hot packs, or Fluidotherapy immediately followed by stretching while the tissue cools provides stretch to the scar tissue. Wrapping the scarred or stiff digit into flexion with Coban during the application of heat often increases mobility in the area. Heat should not be used with insensate areas or if swelling persists.[52]

Active ROM and Electrical Stimulation

Active ROM provides an internal stretch against resistant scar, and its use cannot be overemphasized. If the patient is unable to achieve active motion because of scar adhesions or weakness, use of a battery-operated NMES may augment the motion.[116] Stimulation may be done by the patient for several hours at home and has been shown to increase ROM and tendon excursion.[85]

High-voltage direct current is used by many hand therapists as a treatment to increase motor activity and may be used for scar remodeling.[1] Ultrasound phonophoresis treatments are often prescribed but may be more effective if done within the first few months following trauma. A continuous passive motion (CPM) device may be used at home to maintain passive ROM and promote tendon gliding. It should be used for several hours a day for maximum benefit.

PAIN SYNDROMES

Pain is the subjective manifestation of trauma transmitted by the sympathetic nervous system, which may interfere with normal functioning. Because pain leads to overprotection of the affected part and disuse of the extremity, it should be treated early.

Desensitization

Stimulation of the large afferent A nerve fibers leads to a reduction of pain by decreasing summation in the slowly-adapting, small, unmyelineated C fibers, which carry pain sensation. The A axons can be stimulated mechanically with pressure, rubbing, vibration, TENS, percussion, and active motion. Desensitization techniques are based on the amplification of inhibitory mechanisms.

Yerxa has described a desensitization program that "employs short periods of contact with three sensory modalities: dowel textures, immersion or contact particles, and vibration."[118] This program allows the patient to rank 10 dowel textures and 10 immersion textures on the degree of irritation produced by the stimulus. Treatment begins with a stimulus that is irritating but tolerable. The stimulus is applied for 10 minutes 3 or 4 times a day. The vibration hierarchy is predetermined and is based on cps of vibration, the placement of the vibrator, and the duration of the treatment. Complete instructions for assembling the Downey Hand Center desensitization kit can be found in the literature in the references. The Downey Hand Center Hand Sensitivity Test can be used to establish a desensitization treatment program and to measure progress in decreasing hypersensitivity.[6,118]

Neuromas

Neuromas are a complication of nerve suture or amputation. A traumatic neuroma is an unorganized mass of nerve fibers, which results from accidental or surgical cutting of the nerve. A neuroma in continuity occurs on a nerve that is intact.[103] Neuromas may be clinically identified by a specific, sharp pain. Stimulation of a neuroma usually causes the patient to pull the hand away quickly; many patients report a burning pain that radiates up the forearm. Neuromas are disabling because any stimulation causes intense pain, and the patient avoids the sensitive area.

A generalized desensitization program may not work because the patient never develops a tolerance for stimulation of the neuroma. Injection of cortisone acetate may help break up the neuroma, making desensitization techniques more effective. Surgical excision of the neuroma or burying the nerve endings deeper may be necessary.

Reflex Sympathetic Dystrophy

Reflex sympathetic dystrophy (RSD) describes a disabling reaction to pain that is "generated by an abnormal sympathetic reflex."[59,88] The hallmarks of RSD are pain; edema; blotchy-looking, shiny skin; and coolness of the hand. There may be excessive sweating or dryness. The degree of trauma does not correlate with the severity of the pain and may occur following any injury. RSD appears to be triggered by a cycle of vasospasm and vasodilation following an injury. Abnormal edema and constrictive dressings or casts may be a factor in initiating the vasospasm. A vasospasm "causes tissue anoxia and edema and therefore more pain, which continues the abnormal cycle."[13,88] Circulation is decreased, which causes the extremity to become cool and pale.

Fibrosis following tissue anoxia and protein-rich exudates results in joint stiffness. The patient may cradle the hand and prefers to keep it wrapped. There may be an exaggerated reaction to touch, especially light touch. Osteoporosis may be apparent on x-ray films by 8 weeks after trauma following active use of the hand. Burning pain, associated with causalgia (a severe form of RSD), is a symptom that may be alleviated by interruption of the sympathetic nerve pathways.

There are three stages of RSD. Stage I may last up to three months; it is characterized by pain, pitting edema, and discoloration. Stage II may last an additional six months. Pain, brawny edema, stiffness, redness, heat, and bony demineralization are usually found in this stage. The hand usually has a glossy appearance. Stage III may last up to several years or indefinitely. Pain usually peaks and decreases over time. Thickening around the joints occurs, and fixed contractures may be present. If there is swelling, it is hard and not responsive to techniques such as elevation. The hand may be pale, dry and cool. There may be substantial dysfunction of the limb.

RSD is treated by decreasing sympathetic stimulation. It is most responsive in Stage I. The first goal of treatment is reduction of the pain and hypersensitivity to light touch. This goal may be accomplished with application of warm (not hot) moist heat, Fluidotherapy, gentle handling of the hand, acupressure, desensitization, and TENS before active range of motion. Treatment that increases pain (such as passive range of motion) should be avoided. Many patients respond well to gentle retrograde massage, which reduces the edema and reintroduces touching of the hand. Stellate ganglion blocks to eliminate the pain are effective early. They should be coordinated with therapy so the patient can perform active range of motion and functional activities during the pain-free period following the blocks.

A variety of drugs may be used including sympatholytic drugs,[59] which reduce the vasoconstrictive action of the peripheral vessels. Calcium channel blockers are also effective. Carefully monitored use of narcotics may interrupt the pain cycle and allow active use of the hand. A stress-loading program that has been used effectively to reduce symptoms of RSD has been described.[110] It can easily be adapted for home use.

Edema control techniques should be started immediately. Elevation, the Jobst intermittent compression pump, contrast baths, and high-voltage direct current in water have been found to be effective. Biofeedback training for relaxation may help muscle spasms and ischemia as well as reduce anxiety.

RSD frequently triggers shoulder pain and stiffness, resulting in shoulder-hand syndrome or a "frozen" shoulder. Therefore active range of motion and functional activities should include the entire upper quadrant. Use of skateboard exercises are helpful in the early stages for active-assisted exercise of the shoulder. Splints that reduce joint stiffness should be used as tolerated.

A tendency to develop RSD should be suspected in any patient who seems to complain excessively about pain, appears anxious, and complains of profuse sweating and temperature changes in the hand. Patients tend to overprotect the hand. Early intervention with a structured therapy program of functioinal activities, group interaction, and exercises that include the hand and shoulder may prevent the occurrence of a fully developed RSD. This problem is best recognized early and treated with tempered aggressiveness and empathy.

Transcutaneous Electrical Nerve Stimulation (TENS)

TENS is a treatment technique that is thought to stimulate the afferent A nerve fibers in the high-frequency mode and stimulate the release of morphine-like neural hormones, the enkephalins, in the low-frequency mode. Its efficacy as a treatment for pain control is well documented in medical literature. As with other electrical modalities that may be used by hand therapists, TENS should be correlated with functional use of the hand.

TENS should be used for treatment periods not to exceed 60 minutes at a time to achieve pain control.[53] A TENS diary should be used to record level of pain on a scale of 1 to 10 before and after treatment, as well as activities that exacerbate the pain. Use of TENS may be tapered down as the pain-free periods increase to avoid overuse. Treatment can be continued as long as necessary to provide pain control.

JOINT STIFFNESS

Joint stiffness has been discussed in other sections of this chapter because it is seen following almost any hand trauma or disease. In the acute phase it may also result from "internal splinting" done unconsciously by the patient to avoid pain. It may be prevented by early mobilization, pain control, reduction of edema, active and passive ROM, and appropriate splinting techniques. Grade I and II joint mobilization is especially helpful in preparing for passive and active motion and for pain relief.

Treatment of established joint stiffness is more difficult. Thermal modalities, joint mobilization, ultrasound and electrical stimulation, dynamic splinting, serial casting, and active and passive motion in preparation for functional use should all be included in the treatment regimen.

CUMULATIVE TRAUMA DISORDERS

A number of terms are used throughout the world to describe injuries to the musculoskeletal system including overuse syndromes, repetitive strain injuries, cervical-brachial disorders, repetitive motion injuries and, in the United States, cumulative trauma disorders (CTDs). The incidence of CTDs in the United States is on the rise with 281,800 cases reported in private industry in 1992.[21,97] Between 1981 and 1992, CTDs increased from 18% to 62% of all worker's compensation claims filed.

The term *cumulative trauma disorder* should be viewed as a description of the mechanism of injury and not a diagnosis. Even when the presenting symptoms are confusing, attempts to define a specific diagnosis are necessary because "each disorder has a different cause, treatment, and prognosis."[93] Diagnoses associated with cumulative trauma usually fall into one of three categories: (1) tendinitis (such as lateral epicondylitis or de Quervain's tenosynovitis); (2) nerve compression syndromes (such as carpal tunnel syndrome or cubital tunnel syndrome); or (3) myofascial pain.

Cumulative trauma occurs when force is applied to the same muscle or muscle group, causing an inflammatory response in the tendon, muscle, or nerve.[93] Muscle fatigue is an important aspect of cumulative trauma. Excessive use of the muscle or body system (overuse or overexertion) is experienced as a muscle cramp. Acute overuse is relieved by rest, but chronic fatigue is not relieved by rest. The amount of fatigue is related to the amount of force and the duration of force application.

Fatigue occurs more quickly with high force. If force is maintained, repetitions must be reduced to allow recovery. Therefore, if the force is decreased while repetitions are maintained and recovery time is adequate, harm is less likely to occur. The combination of repetitions without adequate recovery time and high force establishes an environment that is likely to lead to injury.

Treatment may be divided into phases. Acute phase treatment is geared toward decreasing the inflammation through dynamic rest. Splints are used for immobilization. Splinting alone may relieve symptoms; splinting is often combined with cortisone injections to reduce inflammation. Icing, contrast baths, ultrasound phonophoresis, and interferential and high-voltage electrical stimulation have all been found to be effective in reducing pain and decreasing inflammation. Nonsteroidal antiinflammatory drugs are also frequently used. When splints are used, they should be removed 3 times a day for stretching of the affected musculature (e.g., the extensor group with lateral epicondylitis) to maintain or increase muscle length and to avoid joint stiffness. Painful activities should be avoided during the dynamic rest phase. Vibration is contraindicated, because vibration may contribute to inflammatory problems.

As the acute symptoms decrease, the patient begins the exercise phase of treatment. After warming up the muscles by slow stretching, controlled progressive exercise is begun. Resistance should be given at the end of range when doing progressive resistive exercise. A tennis-elbow armband can be worn over the extensor muscle bellies to limit full excursion of the muscle during active use of the arm. Resistance should be increased slowly and should not cause an increase in pain.

Patients are instructed to continue stretching 3 times a day, especially before activity, for an indefinite time. Proper body mechanics are critical in the long-term control of inflammatory problems, so patients must become aware of what triggers their symptoms and learn early intervention if symptoms reappear. Icing, splints, stretching, and modified activities combined with correct body mechanics are usually effective. The key is that the patients learn self-management techniques and take an active role in their treatment.

Work-related risk factors for CTDs include the following:[4]
- repetition
- high force
- awkward joint posture
- direct pressure
- vibration
- prolonged static positioning

An evaluation of the job site, tools used, and hand position during work activities may be indicated with the patient whose symptoms are related to job demands. Modification of the equipment used and strengthening of the dominant muscle groups and their antagonist muscles may permit continued employment while controlling the inflammatory problem.

Tendinitis and tenosynovitis are frequently seen in cumulative trauma. The cycle of overuse leading to microtrauma, swelling, pain, and limitations in movement is followed by rest, disuse, and weakness. Normal activity is resumed and the cycle begins again.

Patients usually have a combination of localized pain, swelling, pain with resisted motion of the affected musculotendinis unit, limitations in motion, weakness and crepitation of the tendons. Symptoms are reproduced with activity or work simulation. Although isometric grip strength may be normal, wrist and forearm strength is often decreased and out of balance. Dynamic grip strength may be more limited because tendon gliding is more likely to increase inflammation and pain. Muscle imbalance leads to positioning and substitution patterns that may lead to worsening or spreading of symptoms.

Nerve compression syndromes, especially carpal tunnel syndrome, are frequently seen.[64] Symptoms of carpal tunnel syndrome are caused by pressure on the median nerve as it travels beneath the transverse carpal ligament at the volar surface of the wrist.[45] The syndrome is associated with increased pressure in the carpal canal because of trauma, edema, retention of fluids as a result of pregnancy, flexor tenosynovitis, repetitive wrist motions, or static loading of the wrist.

Symptoms are night pain that is severe enough to waken the patient; tingling in the thumb and index and long fingers; and, if advanced, wasting of the thenar musculature caused by pressure on the motor branch of the nerve. Early carpal tunnel syndrome may be recognized by a thorough nerve evaluation.

Conservative treatment is usually attempted first and includes splinting the wrist in no more than 20° exten-sion, contrast baths to reduce edema, wearing Isotoner gloves, and activity analysis. A custom fabricated semi-flexible splint (Fig. 35-19), or a neoprene splint rather than a completely rigid splint, may be used to provide support while allowing a small amount of flexion and extension for greater functional use in carpal tunnel syndrome.

Ultrasound phonophoresis may be used to reduce inflammation, and icing techniques are beneficial. Specific strengthening exercises of the wrist, fingers, and thumb should be given when the pain and inflammation have been controlled.

Myofascial pain and fibrositis are also conditions of pain elicited by activation of trigger points within the muscles and resulting in pain referred to a distal area; they are frequently encountered conditions. Travell[105] has studied myofascial pain and mapped out the traditional trigger points and their referral patterns. Poor posture and positioning of the body out of normal alignment are often the mechanism of injury in myofascial pain, so careful examination of the patient and his or her normal daily activities is indicated. The therapist should observe the patient performing the activity rather than rely on a verbal description.

Myofascial pain should be considered in cases where direct treatment of the painful area does not relieve the pain. Evaluation for trigger points must be done meticulously, and mapping of the trigger points and the referral areas must be documented. Because the pain is referred, the trigger point must be treated, not the referral area. The treatments used for other inflammatory problems, such as ice and ultrasound phonophoresis, can be used. In addition, there are specific treatments for the trigger points, such as friction massage and TENS, which may relieve the pain. Activity analysis is an essential part of treatment to relieve the stresses on the affected tissues.

STRENGTHENING ACTIVITIES

Acute care is followed by a gradual return of motion, sensibility, and preparation to return to normal ADL.

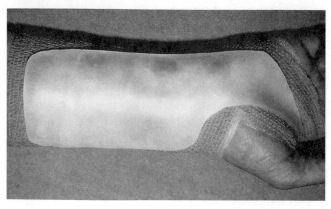

A

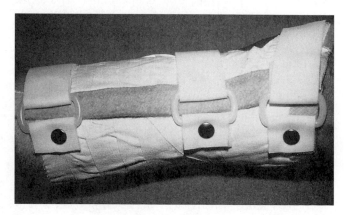

B

FIG. 35-19 Semiflexible splint. **A,** Constructed using Coban wrap and thermoplastic insert. **B,** Finished with coach tape and straps. Detailed instructions for this splint are available from RL Petzoldt Memorial Center for Hand Rehabilitation, 4155 Moorpark Ave., #21, San José, CA 95117.

Strengthening the injured and neglected extremity is usually not accomplished by the patient at home, because he or she is often fearful of further injury and pain. Because every hand clinic has its own armamentarium of strengthening exercises and media, only a few suggestions are provided here.

Computerized Evaluation and Exercise Equipment

Baltimore Therapeutic Equipment (BTE) has made available the BTE work simulator[28] (Fig. 35-20), an electromechanical device that has more than 20 interchangeable tool handles and can be used for both work evaluation and upper extremity strengthening. Resistance can vary from no resistance to complete static resistance, with tool height and angle also adjustable. When used for strengthening, the resistance is usually set low and gradually increased, with concurrent increases in length of exercise. The BTE work simulator allows for close simulation of real-world tasks that are easily translatable into physical demands common to manual work.

Other computerized evaluation equipment includes the EVAL system,[41] which allows the therapist to record the results of evaluation and prints a report. Percentage of impairment can also be determined electronically. The Dexter Evaluation and Therapy System[34] can be used to evaluate the patient, record, and report the results of evaluation. It also allows the therapist to establish an ex-

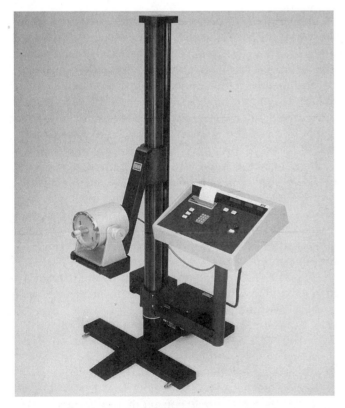

FIG. 35-20 BTE Work Simulator is electromechanical device used to simulate real-life tasks for upper extremity evaluation and strengthening. Patient's progress is monitored through computerized print-out, and program can be modified to increase resistance and endurance.

ercise program, record the results of each therapy session, and compare changes in the individual's strength or range of motion.

Portable systems are also being developed that allow the therapist to record daily treatment and download the information into a computerized network. Outcome data from many sources can then be compared. The advancement of technology in rehabilitation will allow greater efficiency of the therapist while capturing important information that is not available through traditional means.

Weight Well

The weight well[5] was developed at the Downey Community Hospital Hand Center in Downey, California, and is available commercially.[106] Rods with a variety of handle shapes are placed through holes in the box and have weights suspended. The rods are turned against resistance throughout the ROM to encourage full grasp and release of the injured hand, wrist flexion and extension, pinch, and pronation and supination patterns. The weight well can be graded for resistance and repetitions and is an excellent tool for progressive resistive exercise.

Theraband

Theraband[102] is a 6-inch-wide (15.2-cm) rubber sheet that is available by the yard and is color coded by degrees of resistance. It can be cut into any length required and used for resistive exercise for the upper extremity. Use of Theraband is limited only by the therapist's imagination; and it can be adapted to diagonal patterns of motion, wrist exercises, follow-up treatment of tennis elbow, and other uses. The Theraband can be combined with dowel rods and other equipment to provide resistance throughout the ROM. It is inexpensive and easy to incorporate into a home treatment program.

Hand-Strengthening Equipment

Hand grips of graded resistance are available from rehabilitation supply companies and sporting goods stores. They can be purchased with various resistance levels and can be used for progressive resistive hand exercises.

The therapist is cautioned against using overly resistive spring-loaded grippers often sold in sporting goods stores. These devices may be beneficial to the seasoned athlete but are usually too resistive for the recently injured.

Therapy putty can be purchased in bulk, and the amount given to the patient is geared to hand size and strength. Putty is also available in grades of resistance. It can be adapted to most finger motions and is easily incorporated into a home program.

Household items such as spring-type clothespins have been used to increase strength of grasp and pinch. Imaginative use of common objects should present a challenge to the hand therapist.

FUNCTIONAL ACTIVITIES

Functional activities are an integral part of rehabilitation of the hand. Functional activities may include crafts, games, dexterity activities, ADL, and work samples. Many of the treatment techniques described previously are employed to condition the hand for normal use.

Activities should be started as soon as possible at whatever level the patient can perform them with adaptations to compensate for limited ROM and strength. They should be used in conjunction with other treatments. The occupational therapist must continually assess the patient's functional capacities and initiate changes in the treatment program to incorporate activities as soon as possible in the restorative phase.

Vocational and avocational goals should be established at the time of initial evaluation and taken into account when planning treatment. The needs of a brick mason may be quite different from those of a mother with small children, and the environmental needs of the patient must not be neglected.

Crafts should be graded from light resistance to heavy resistance and from gross dexterity to fine dexterity. Crafts that have been found to work extremely well with hand injuries include macramé, turkish knot weaving, clay, leather, and woodworking.

All of these crafts can be adapted and graded to the patient's capabilities and have been found to have a high level of patient acceptance. When integrated into a program of total hand rehabilitation, they are viewed as another milestone of achievement and not as a diversion to fill up empty hours. For example, the pride of accomplishment for a patient who sustained a Volkmann's contracture caused by ischemia and who completed her first project in nearly four years is evidence that crafts belong in hand rehabilitation.

Activities that do not have an end product but provide practice in dexterity and ADL skills also fit into the category of functional activities. Developmental games and activities that require pinch or grasp and release may be graded and timed to increase difficulty. ADL boards that have a variety of opening and closing devices provide practice for use of the hand at home and increase self-confidence. String and finger games are challenging coordination activities that can be done in pairs and are fun to do.

Many times a hobby can be adapted for use in the clinic. Fly-tying is a difficult dexterity activity but one that will be enjoyed by an avid fisherman. Golf clubs and fishing poles can be adapted in the clinic to allow early return to a favorite form of relaxation.

Humor and patient interaction with the therapists and the other patients are factors that are vital but intangible benefits of treatment. Treatment should be planned to promote both.

PHYSICAL CAPACITY EVALUATION

The ultimate goal of therapy for an injured worker is to return to full employment. Many weeks or months may have elapsed between the time of the injury and the point at which the physician feels a return to work is appropriate from a medical standpoint. Despite the fact that x-ray film examinations may show full healing and restored ROM, many patients do not feel they have the strength, dexterity, or endurance to return to their former jobs. Pain may continue to be a limiting factor, especially with heavy activities. Light duty or part-time positions may not be available; and the physician, therapist, industrial insurance carrier, and most of all, the patient are frustrated by the lack of an objective method of evaluating an individual's physical capacity for work. Occupational therapists with training in evaluation, kinesiology, and adaptation of environmental factors coupled with a functional approach to the patient may play a key role in physical capacity evaluation.

A renewed interest in evaluation of prevocational factors has brought the profession of occupational therapy full circle. Although one of the cornerstones of the profession in its early years, prevocational evaluation has been neglected in many centers during the last two decades. Since the early 1980s, however, occupational therapists have rediscovered a need that the profession is in a unique position to provide. The term *prevocational evaluation* ambiguously implied that occupational therapists were involved in assessing the vocational needs of patients they treated. The terms *physical capacity evaluation* (PCE) and *work tolerance screening* (WTS), however, more clearly describe the process of measuring an individual's ability to perform the physical demands of work.

The results of this evaluation allow the therapist, worker, physician, and vocational counselor to establish a specific attainable employment goal using reliable data. This approach relieves the physician of the responsibility of returning the patient to work without objective information about the patient's ability to do a job. It also allows the patient to test his or her own abilities and may result in increased self-confidence about returning to work.

Many techniques for performing a physical capacity evaluation have been proposed.[8,47,74,75] Some basic steps may be followed regardless of the specific technique adopted. The patient should be evaluated for grip and pinch strength, sensation, and ROM. Edema and pain must also be assessed and reassessed during the course of the evaluation.

The GULHEMP (general physique, upper extremity, lower extremity, hearing, eyesight, mentality, and personality) Work Capacity Evaluation Worksheet[74] may be used as a general method of determining functional abilities. The GULHEMP Physical Development Analysis Worksheet[74] may be used to evaluate the job.

Job analysis may also be provided by a rehabilitation counselor and through information provided by the patient. The therapist should consult the *Dictionary of Occupational Titles* (DOT)[107] to obtain information about the worker traits required for the expected job. This dictionary contains 12,900 job descriptions and 20,000 job titles. If sufficient information about the job is not available through these methods, an on-site job analysis by the therapist may be necessary. Once the physical demand characteristics of work have been documented, it is possible to evaluate the patient's ability to perform them.

Baxter[8] has described a physical capacity evaluation adapted for upper extremity injuries based on the physical capacity requirements found in the *Dictionary of Occupational Titles.* Following evaluation the therapist may recommend a work therapy program.[7] Work therapy can include simulated job tasks to increase job performance.

Matheson[74,75] has written several manuals and articles that describe Work Capacity Evaluation (WCE). This 8- to 10-day work assessment includes evaluation of the patient's feasibility for employment (worker characteristics, such as safety and dependability), employability, work tolerances (such as strength, endurance, and the effect of pain on work performance), the physical demand characteristics of the job, and the worker's ability to "dependably sustain performance in response to broadly defined work demands."[74]

Tests with well-accepted reliability, such as the Purdue Pegboard Test,[104] the Crawford Small Parts Dexterity Test,[26] the Minnesota Manual Dexterity Test,[82] and the Jebsen Hand Dexterity Test,[49] may be administered as a screening process. These tests will give the therapist valuable information through observation whether the normal tables are used or the test is adapted to an individual worker.

Many evaluation tests and job simulation devices are available and should be reviewed before establishing a physical capacity evaluation program. To choose appropriate work samples the job market in a specific area should be determined. This can be done by consulting with vocational schools, rehabilitation counselors, and employment agencies in the area.

Work samples, available through Jewish Employment and Vocational Service,[109] Singer,[98] VALPAR,[108] and Work Evaluation Systems Technology (WEST)[117] may be used to test specific skills. Job samples may also be developed by the therapist using information on jobs in the local area. Discarded electronic assembly boards, a lawn mower motor, automobile engine, or other items from the local hardware store may provide valuable information about the worker's ability.

Work simulation using job samples or the BTE work simulator assess the worker's specific physical capacities as well as endurance and symptoms that become cumulative with prolonged use of the injured part (called symptom response to activity or SRA). Monitoring the client's SRA may prevent loss of time and money expended in training for an inappropriate vocational goal. King has written about the analysis of test results to determine the consistency of effort and veracity of evaluation findings, which assists in identifying patients who may be magnifying their symptoms.[57]

A combination of "normed" tests, job samples, job

simulation, and work capacity evaluation devices may provide the therapist with the best information about a worker's physical capacity. For more information about vocational evaluation and rehabilitation, the therapist should write to the Materials Development Center at the University of Wisconsin-Stout in Menomonie, Wisconsin.[73]

Work Hardening

Work hardening is the progressive use of simulated work samples to increase endurance, strength, productivity, and often feasibility. Work hardening may be performed for a period of weeks, and the progressive ongoing nature of the work usually results in improvements in physical capacity. It is an important contribution to return to work.

Because PCE is also performed over time, it may be difficult to identify the difference between PCE and work hardening. A PCE is generally done when the patient has stopped improving with traditional therapy methods and may have been released from acute medical care. The patient may be unable to return to his or her former employment or it may be questionable if the patient would be able to do the former work. A PCE may be initiated by a physician, rehabilitation counselor, insurance adjustor, or attorney.

Work hardening may be initiated earlier in the rehabilitation process, perhaps by the treating physician or therapist who recognizes that an individual may have difficulty returning to the former employment. It is performed before the end of medical care and may serve as a final checkout before discontinuing treatment.

Standards for work hardening services have been developed by the Commission on Accreditation of Rehabilitation Facilities (CARF)[24] to ensure that injured workers are offered quality programs that are maximally effective in successfully returning them to gainful employment. The Employment and Rehabilitation Institute of California (ERIC)[39] has many publications and resources available to therapists interested in establishing work capacity evaluation, work tolerance screening, or work hardening services. A publications and equipment listing is available on request.

It is important to stress that PCE and work hardening are adjuncts to the vocational rehabilitation process. Occupational therapists are trained to observe behavior and have the skills necessary to translate that observation into useful data. PCE and work hardening should not be a process that is in competition with the work of rehabilitation or vocational counselors but rather one that provides critical information about a worker's physical functioning and may serve as a program to foster reentry into the job market.

CONSULTATION WITH INDUSTRY

Occupational therapists may be asked to visit the job site to make recommendations for ergonomic adaptations including tool modification, ergonomic furniture and accessories, and training workers in proper postioning to reduce the incidence of CTDs. Prevention substantially reduces the costs to industry, which presents occupational therapists with a unique opportunity to apply their training in activity analysis and adaptation of the environment in a new setting. The Americans with Disabilities Act (ADA) mandates reasonable accommodations for workers with disabilities. Many occupational therapists have become active in helping companies comply with the requirements of the ADA. The American Occupational Therapy Association is an excellent resource for more information about how therapists can be involved in these efforts in their communities.[2]

SUMMARY

This chapter on hand injuries provides an overview of treatment of the upper extremity. Evaluation procedures are discussed, as well as the basic treatment techniques. Management of both acute injuries and cumulative trauma have been included, as has information on strengthening and programs for industrial injuries. References for additional study have been provided.

Most occupational therapists should be familiar with the basic treatment approaches because they work with patients who have some limitation in the upper extremities. Specialization in hand therapy requires both academic study and clinical experience. Therapists who have specialized in this area of practice and who meet minimum requirements may choose to take the Hand Therapy Certification Examination and become Certified Hand Therapists. Both levels of expertise are needed in the profession.

 S A M P L E   T R E A T M E N T   P L A N

This sample treatment plan is not comprehensive. It deals with three of four identified problems. The reader is encouraged to add objectives and methods to complete the treatment plan.

CASE STUDY

Mr. D is a 69-year-old right-handed retired sales manager with an 8- to 10-year history of Dupuytren's contracture of both hands, the right being more involved than the left. He stated that the long, ring, and small fingers on his right hand became contracted 4 to 5 years ago and the contractures gradually progressed until the fingers were nearly in the palm. The ring and small fingers on the left hand have recently begun contracting. [Study hints: What are the characteristics of Dupuytren's contracture? Is there a known cause? Would it have been possible to prevent the progression of contractures in the right hand? Would treatment to the left hand help now?]

Two weeks before referral to occupational therapy, Mr. D had release and reconstruction of the contractures in the right palm including a Z-plasty that was left partially open at the time of surgery for drainage. [Study hints: What is a Z-plasty and how does it differ from a linear incision? What are the benefits of this procedure for allowing skin closure versus a skin graft?] At the time of referral the surgeon noted that Mr. D also has underlying osteoarthritis of the small joints of his hands.

Mr. D has been retired for six years. He lives with his wife in their own home. They have three grown children and seven grandchildren whom they see frequently. Mr. D is independent in all his self-care activities. He enjoys fishing, golf, and cooking and likes to "putter" around the house. He does not smoke and drinks moderately. [Study hint: Does alcohol consumption have any correlation to Dupuytren's disease?] He is alert, pleasant, and cooperative.

TREATMENT PLAN

Personal data

Name: JD
Age: 69
Diagnosis: Dupuytren's contracture, both hands, with underlying osteoarthritis; status—postrelease after reconstruction of contractures with Z-plasty.
Disability: Unable fully to extend or flex fingers following surgery performed 2 weeks before referral.
Treatment aims stated in referral: Increase active and passive ROM; scar remodeling, static night splint and dynamic daytime splint; evaluate for compression garment. Frequency of 2 to 3 times per week for 4 weeks. [Note: This patient is insured by Medicare and has a $1900 limit for outpatient occupational therapy as well as secondary insurance that may or may not pay for additional therapy if needed. Some secondary or supplemental insurances pay only the 20% not paid by Medicare, and others pay for services not covered by Medicare. How will that affect the services provided to him in your outpatient clinic?]

SAMPLE TREATMENT PLAN — cont'd

Other services

Physician: Performed surgery; prescribes medication and treatment; supervises rehabilitation

Frame of reference

Occupational performance

Treatment approaches

Biomechanical and rehabilitative

OT EVALUATION

Performance components

Sensorimotor functioning
 Muscle strength: Test
 Passive and active ROM: Test
 Joint mobility: Test
 Scar adhesions: Observe and palpate
 Edema: Test
 Sensation: Test
Cognitive functioning

 Ability to follow directions: Observe
Psychosocial functioning
 Chemical dependency: Observe behavior
 Coping skills: Observe
 Interpersonal skills: Observe

Performance areas

 Self-care: Interview
 Home management: Interview

EVALUATION SUMMARY

Motor function (ROM)

Mr. D had normal strength within a limited ROM at his initial evaluation. Passive and active motion of the thumb, index, and long fingers were within normal limits. ROM of the ring and small fingers was as follows:

DIGIT	PASSIVE	ACTIVE
Ring finger		
MP joint	22/75	30/75
PIP joint	30/80	33/85
DIP joint	0/45	0/34
Small finger		
MP joint	0/72	0/70
PIP joint	32/75	35/74
DIP joint	0/45	5/40

Joint Mobility: Joint accessory motion was limited [Study hint: How is the treatment plan influenced by the presence of active joint inflammation caused by osteoarthritis in this patient?]
Scar adhesions: The surgical scar was dense and contractile in the palm and the volar surface of the ring and small fingers

Edema: Finger circumference was measured as well as hand volume to test for edema; circumferential measurements:

Ring finger	
Proximal phalanx	7.0 cm
PIP joint	7.4 cm
Middle phalanx	6.5 cm
Small finger	
Proximal phalanx	6.7 cm
PIP joint	6.7 cm
Middle phalanx	5.8 cm
Volume	
Right	595 ml
Left	530 ml

[Study hint: how could handsize be measured if the wound had not healed?]
Sensory: Sensation tested in the diminished light-touch range on the ring and small fingers using the Semmes-Weinstein monofilaments.

SUMMARY

Mr. D was highly motivated to have full use of his hand and was able to explain his home program to the therapist. His daughter is an RN and had helped him to understand the disease process and what to expect from therapy. He has coped well with the disease in the past and has adapted as needed to remain independent in all his activities, except for golf which is difficult because it has been hard to hold the club correctly. His use of alcohol is a general lifestyle coping mechanism that has not been exacerbated by his surgery. It did not interfere with his performance in OT.

Assets

Highly motivated and cooperative
Early postoperative referral allows scar remodeling
Scar and joints responded well to initial treatment
Good adherence to home treatment program

Problem list

1. Limited active and passive ROM
2. Dense scar tissue
3. Edema
4. Decreased functional use of right hand

SAMPLE TREATMENT PLAN–cont'd

PROBLEMS 1, 2: LIMITED ROM AND DENSE SCAR TISSUE

Objective
Increase passive extension of ring and small PIP joints to 0° extension

Method
A removable static night extension splint was fabricated out of low-temperature thermoplastic material in maximum extension and lined with a Silastic elastomer mold; the patient was instructed to wear splint while sleeping and to bring it to therapy with him.

Gradation
The splint was adjusted in greater extension as often as possible.

As the scar softened, new molds were made.

PROBLEM 1: LIMITED ROM

Objective
Increase passive extension of ring and small PIP joints to 0° extension

Method
The patient was fitted with two LMB finger extension splints and instructed to wear them each 3 times a day for 30 minutes; because of pain and edema, tension on the spring wire was decreased

Gradation
Tension was increased on the splints as patient was able to tolerate it; if these splints had caused an increase in joint inflammation, a different splint would have been substituted

---

PROBLEM 3: EDEMA

Objective
Decrease edema by 5 to 10 ml per week

Method
Mr. D was instructed in retrograde massage and given an Isotoner glove to wear when not exercising or wearing a splint [Patients often wear gloves under their Silastic molds if they have both. Be sure they understand that the mold must come in direct contact with the skin to be effective.]

Gradation
If the Isotoner was not effective, a custom garment could be ordered; a sequential intermittent compression device might also be used at home several times a day or in the clinic; the patient must also continue to elevate the hand

Edema responds best to a variety of methods employed either at the same time or interchangeably, rather than reliance on one method alone

---

REVIEW QUESTIONS

1. Discuss three approaches to postoperative care of flexor tendon injuries and compare how the differences between the methods would influence the initiation of occupational therapy.
2. To what does joint dysfunction refer? What are its causes?
3. List three treatment techniques that might be used in treatment of a pain syndrome.
4. Discuss the three classifications of nerve injury.
5. Define the area referred to as "no-man's land." What distinguishes injury to this area?
6. What techniques are employed to evaluate the physical demand characteristics of work?
7. List three methods of applying pressure to a hypertrophic scar.
8. What functional activities could be used for restoration of hand function following laceration and repair of the extrinsic finger flexors?
9. How does physical capacity evaluation differ from prevocational evaluation and vocational assessment?
10. List five components of hand evaluation.
11. List three objectives of splinting as they relate to injury of the radial, median, and ulnar nerves.
12. Describe the test for intrinsic and extrinsic muscle tightness.
13. What are the characteristics of a reflex sympathetic dystrophy? What are the treatment goals?
14. List four commonly used dexterity tests.
15. Define *work hardening*. How can work hardening be incorporated into occupational therapy?
16. How is the presence of edema evaluated? List three methods used to reduce edema.

17. What are the primary work-related risk factors associated with cumulative trauma? How can the occupational therapist intervene to prevent the development of cumulative trauma?
18. What is the goal of sensory reeducation following nerve repair? List the hierarchy of nerve function return as it relates to sensory reeducation.

REFERENCES

1. Alon G: *High voltage stimulation,* Chattanooga, Tenn, 1984, Chattanooga.
2. American Occupational Therapy Association, ADA Network, Practice Division, 4720 Montgomery Lane, PO Box 31220, Bethesda, MD 20824-1220.
3. American Society for Surgery of the Hand: *The hand examination and diagnosis,* ed 3, New York, 1990, Churchill Livingstone.
4. Armstrong TJ: Cumulative trauma disorders of the upper limb and identification of work-related factors. In Millender LH, Louis DS, Simmons BP, editors: *Occupational disorders of the upper extremity,* New York, 1992, Churchill Livingstone.
5. Barber LM: Occupational therapy for the treatment of reflex sympathetic dystrophy and post-traumatic hypersensitivity of the injured hand. In Fredericks S, Brody GS, editors: *Symposium on the neurologic aspects of plastic surgery,* St Louis, 1978, CV Mosby.
6. Barber LM: Desensitization of the traumatized hand. In Hunter JM and associates, editors: *Rehabilitation of the hand,* ed 3, St Louis, 1990, CV Mosby.
7. Baxter-Petralia PL, Bruening LA, Blackmore SM: The work tolerance program of the Hand Rehabilitation Center in Philadelphia. In Hunter JM and associates, editors: *Rehabilitation of the Hand,* St Louis, 1984, CV Mosby.
8. Baxter-Petralia PL, Bruening LA, Blackmore SM, McEntee PM: Physical capacity evaluation. In Hunter JM and associates, editors: *Rehabilitation of the hand,* ed 3, St Louis, 1990, CV Mosby.
9. Bell-Krotoski JA: Light touch-deep pressure testing using Semmes-Weinstein monofilaments. In Hunter JM and associates, editors: *Rehabilitation of the hand,* ed 3, St Louis, 1990, CV Mosby.
10. Bell-Krotoski JA: Plaster cylinder casting for contractures of the interphalangeal joints. In Hunter JM and associates, editors: *Rehabilitation of the hand,* ed 3, St Louis, 1990, CV Mosby.
11. Bell-Krotoski JA: Sensibility testing: state of the art. In Hunter JM and associates, editors: *Rehabilitation of the hand,* ed 3, St Louis, 1990, CV Mosby.
12. Bennett GK: *Hand-tool dexterity test,* New York, 1981, Harcourt Brace, Jovanovich.
13. Benton LA, and associates: *Functional electrical stimulation: a practical clinical guide,* ed 2, Downey, Calif. 1981, Rancho Los Amigos Hospital.
14. Bio-Concepts, 2422 E. University Drive, Phoenix, AZ 85034.
15. Boyes JH: *Bunnell's surgery of the hand,* ed 5, Philadelphia, 1970, JB Lippincott.
16. Boyes JH, Stark HH: Flexor-tendon grafts in the fingers and thumb, *J Bone Joint Surg* 53A:1332, 1971.
17. Brand PW, Hollister A: *Clinical mechanics of the hand,* ed 2, St Louis, 1993, Mosby-Year Book.
18. Callahan AD: Methods of compensation and reeducation for sensory dysfunction. In Hunter JM and associates, editors: *Rehabilitation of the hand,* ed 3, St Louis, 1990, CV Mosby.
19. Cannon NM and associates: Control of immediate postoperative pain following tenolysis and capsulectomies of the hand with TENS, *J Hand Surg* 8:625, 1983.
20. Carroll D: A quantitative test of upper extremity function, *J Chronic Dis* 18:479, 1965.
21. Central Tool Company of Germany. (Available from Anthony Products, 7311 E. 43rd St, Indianapolis, IN 46226.)
22. Chai SH, Dimick MP, Kasch MC: A role delineation study of hand therapy, *J Hand Ther* 1:7, 1987.
23. Chusid JG: *Correlative neuroanatomy and functional neurology,* ed 19, Los Altos, Calif. 1985, Lange Medical Publications.
24. Commission on Accreditation of Rehabilitation Facilities (CARF), 2500 N. Pantano Rd., Tucson, AZ 85715.
25. Corrective Concepts, 3045 Park Lane, Suite 1084, Dallas, TX 75220.
26. Crawford JE, Crawford DM: *Crawford small parts dexterity test manual,* New York, 1981, Harcourt, Brace, Jovanovich.
27. Creelman G: Volumeters Unlimited, Idyllwild, Calif.
28. Curtis RM, Engalitcheff J: A work simulator for rehabilitating the upper extremity: preliminary report, *J Hand Surg* 6:499, 1981.
29. Cyriax JH: Clinical applications of massage. In Basmajian JV: *Manipulation, traction and massage,* ed 3, Baltimore, 1985, Williams & Wilkins.
30. Dellon AL: Clinical use of vibratory stimuli to evaluate peripheral nerve injury and compression neuropathy, *Plast Reconstr Surg* 65:466, 1980.
31. Dellon AL: *Evaluation of sensibility and reeducation of sensation in the hand,* Baltimore, 1981, Williams & Wilkins.
32. Dellon AL: The vibrometer, *Plast Reconstr Surg* 71:427, 1983.
33. Dellon AL, Curtis RM, Edgerton MT: Reeducation of sensation in the hand after nerve injury and repair, *Plast Reconstr Surg* 53:297, 1974.
34. Dexter Evaluation and Therapy System. (Available from Smith & Nephew Rolyan, One Quality Drive, PO Box 578, Germantown, WI 53022.)

35. Digi-Sleeve. (Available from North Coast Medical, 187 Stauffer Blvd., San José, CA 95125.)

36. Disk-Criminator. (Available from Smith & Nephew Rolyan, Inc., One Quality Drive, PO Box 578, Germantown, WI 53022.)

37. Donatelli R, Owens-Burkhart H: Effects of immobilization on the extensibility of periarticular connective tissue, *J Orth & Sports Phys Ther* 3:67, 1981.

38. Duran RJ and associates: Management of flexor tendon lacerations in zone 2 using controlled passive motion postoperatively. In Hunter JM and associates, editors: *Rehabilitation of the hand*, ed 3, St Louis, 1990, CV Mosby.

39. Employment and Rehabilitation Institute of California (ERIC), 1160 N Gilbert St., Anaheim, CA, 92801.

40. English CB, Rehm RA, Petzoldt RL: Blocking splints to assist finger exercise, *Am J Occup Ther* 36:259, 1983.

41. EVAL Computerized System. (Available from Greenleaf Medical Systems, 2248 Park Blvd., Palo Alto, CA 94306.)

42. Evans RB: Therapeutic management of extensor tendon injuries. In *Hand clinics,* vol 1(2), Philadelphia, 1986, WB Saunders.

43. Evans RB, Burkhalter WE: A study of the dynamic anatomy of extensor tendons and implications for treatment, *J Hand Surg* 11A:774, 1986.

44. Fess EE, Moran CA: *Clinical assessment recommendations,* Indianapolis, 1981, American Society of Hand Therapists.

45. Gelberman RH and associates: The carpal tunnel syndrome, *J Bone Joint Surg* 63A:380, 1981.

46. Gelberman RH and associates: Sensibility testing in peripheral-nerve compression syndromes, *J Bone Joint Surg* 65A:632, 1983.

47. Harrand G: *The Harrand guide for developing physical capacity evaluations,* Menomonie, Wisc. 1982, Stout Vocational Rehabilitation Institute.

48. Isotoner gloves by Aris. (Available from North Coast Medical, 187 Stauffer Blvd., San José, CA 95125.)

49. Jebsen RH and associates: An objective and standardized test of hand function, *Arch Phys Med Rehabil* 50:311, 1969.

50. Jobst Institute, Inc, PO Box 653, Toledo, OH 43694.

51. Kamenetz HL: Mechanical devices of massage. In Basmajian JV: *Manipulation, traction and massage,* ed 3, Baltimore, 1985, Williams & Wilkins.

52. Kasch MC: Clinical management of scar tissue, *O.T. in Health Care* 4(3/4):37, 1987.

53. Kasch MC, Hester LA: Low-frequency TENS and the release of endorphins, *J Hand Surg* 8:626, 1983.

54. Kellor M and associates: *Technical manual of hand strength and dexterity test,* Minneapolis, 1971, Sister Kenney Rehabilitation Institute.

55. Kelsey JL and associates: *Upper extremity disorders: a survey of their frequency and cost in the United States,* St Louis, 1980, CV Mosby.

56. Kessler RM, Hertling D: Joint mobilization techniques. In Kessler RM, Hertling D: *Management of common musculoskeletal disorders,* New York, 1983, Harper & Row.

57. King JW, Berryhill BH: A comparison of two static grip testing methods and its clinical applications: a preliminary study, *J Hand Ther* 1:204, 1988.

58. Kutz JE: Controlled mobilization of acute flexor tendon injuries: Louisville technique. In Hunter JM, Schneider LH, Mackin EJ: *Tendon surgery in the hand,* St Louis, 1987, Times Mirror/Mosby College Publishing.

59. Lankford LL: Reflex sympathetic dystrophy. In Hunter JM and associates, editors: *Rehabilitation of the hand,* ed 3, St Louis, 1990, CV Mosby.

60. LaSalle WB, Strickland JW: An evaluation of the two-stage flexor tendon reconstruction technique, *J Hand Surg* 8:263, 1983.

61. Lister GL: *The hand: diagnosis and indications,* ed 3, New York, 1993, Churchill Livingstone.

62. LMB Hand Rehabilitation Products, Inc, San Luis Obispo, CA.

63. Louis DS and associates: Evaluation of normal values for stationary and moving two-point discrimination in the hand, *J Hand Surg* 99:552, 1984.

64. Lublin JS: Unions and firms focus on hand disorder that can be caused by repetitive tasks, *The Wall Street Journal,* January 14, 1983.

65. Lundborg G: *Nerve injury and repair,* New York, 1988, Churchill Livingstone.

66. Lundborg G and associates: Digital vibrogram: a new diagnostic tool for sensory testing in compression neuropathy, *J Hand Surg* 11A:693, 1986.

67. Mackin EJ, Maiorano L: Postoperative therapy following staged flexor tendon reconstruction. In Hunter JM and associates, editors: *Rehabilitation of the hand,* ed 1, St Louis, 1978, CV Mosby.

68. Mackinnon SE, Dellon AL: Two-point discrimination tester, *J Hand Surg* 10A:906, 1985.

69. Madden JW: Wound healing: the biological basis of hand surgery. In Hunter JM and associates, editors: *Rehabilitation of the hand,* ed 3, St Louis, 1990, CV Mosby.

70. Maitland GD: *Peripheral manipulation,* Boston, 1977, Butterworth.

71. Malick MH, Carr JA: Flexible elastomer molds in burn scar control, *Am J Occup Ther* 34:603, 1980.

72. Mark One Health Care Products, Inc, Philadelphia.

73. Materials Development Center, Stout Vocational Rehabilitation Institute, University of Wisconsin-Stout, Menomonie, WI.

74. Matheson LN: *Work capacity evaluation: a training manual for occupational therapists,* Trabuco Canyon, Calif. 1982, Rehabilitation Institute of Southern California.

75. Matheson LN, Ogden LD: *Work tolerance screening,* Trabuco Canyon, Calif, 1983, Rehabilitation Institute of Southern California.

76. Mathiowetz V, Rennells C, Donahoe L: Effect of elbow position on grip and key pinch strength, *J Hand Surg* 10A:694, 1985.

77. Mathiowetz V and associates: Reliability and validity of grip and pinch strength evaluations, *J Hand Surg* 9A:222, 1984.

78. Mathiowetz V and associates: Grip and pinch strength: normative data for adults, *Arch Phys Med Rehabil* 66:69, 1985.

79. Melvin JL: *Rheumatic disease occupational therapy and rehabilitation,* ed 3, Philadelphia, 1989, FA Davis.

80. Mennell JM: *Joint pain,* Boston, 1964, Little, Brown.

81. Mennell JM, Zohn DA: *Musculoskeletal pain diagnosis and physical treatment,* Boston, 1976, Little, Brown.

82. Minnesota Manual Dexterity Test. (Available from Lafayette Instrument Co, PO Box 5729, Lafayette, IN 47903.)

83. Moberg E: Objective methods of determining functional value of sensibility in the hand, *J Bone Joint Surg* 40A:454, 1958.

84. Moberg E: Aspects of the sensation in reconstructive surgery of the upper extremity, *J Bone Joint Surg* 46A:817, 1964.

85. Mullins, PT: Use of therapeutic modalities in upper extremity rehabilitation. In Hunter JM and associates, editors: *Rehabilitation of the hand,* ed 3, St Louis, 1990, CV Mosby.

86. Neoprene. (Available from Benik Corporation, 9465 Provost Road NW, Suite 204, Silverdale, WA 98383.)

87. N-Terface made by Winfield Laboratories. (Available from North Coast Medical, 187 Stauffer Blvd, San José, CA 95125.)

88. Omer GE: Management of pain syndromes in the upper extremity. In Hunter JM and associates, editors: *Rehabilitation of the hand,* ed 3, St Louis, 1990, CV Mosby.

89. Omer GE: Nerve response to injury and repair. In Hunter JM and associates, editors: *Rehabilitation of the hand,* ed 3, St Louis, 1990, CV Mosby.

90. O'Rain S: New and simple test of nerve function in the hand, *Br Med J* 3:615, 1973.

91. Parry CBW: *Rehabilitation of the hand,* ed 4, London, 1984, Butterworth.

92. Peacock EE, Madden JW, Trier WC: Postoperative recovery of flexor tendon function, *Am J Surg* 122:686, 1971.

93. Rempel DM: Work-related cumulative trauma disorders of the upper extremity, *JAMA* 267:838-842, 1992.

94. Schneider LH: Tendon transfers in the upper extremity. In Hunter JM and associates, editors: *Rehabilitation of the hand,* ed 3, St. Louis, 1990, CV Mosby.

95. Schneider LH, Hunter JM: Flexor tenolysis. In AAOS: *Symposium on tendon surgery in the hand,* St Louis, 1975, CV Mosby.

96. Silicone Elastomer. (Available from Smith & Nephew Rolyan, Inc, One Quality Drive, PO Box 578, Germantown, WI 53022.)

97. Silverstein S: Preventive medicine standards on cumulative trauma would cover every employee in the state, *L.A. Times,* January 13, 1994.

98. Singer Education Division, Career Systems, Rochester, NY.

99. Spenco Medical Corp, Box 8113, Waco, TX 76710.

100. Strickland JW, Glogovac SV: Digital function following flexor tendon repair in zone II: a comparison of immobilization and controlled passive motion techniques, *J Hand Surg* 5:537, 1980.

101. Szabo RM and associates: Vibratory sensory testing in acute peripheral nerve compression, *J Hand Surg* 9A:104, 1984.

102. Theraband: Smith & Nephew Rolyan, Inc, One Quality Drive, PO Box 578, Germantown, WI 33022.

103. Thomas CL, editor: *Taber's cyclopedic medical dictionary,* ed 14, Philadelphia, 1981, FA Davis.

104. Tiffin J: *Purdue pegboard examiner manual,* Chicago, 1968, Science Research Associates.

105. Travell JG, Simons DG: *Myofascial pain and dysfunction: the trigger point manual,* Baltimore, 1983, Williams & Wilkins.

106. UE Tech Weight Well. (Available from Upper Extremity Technology, 2001 Blake Ave 2A, Glenwood Springs, CO 81601.)

107. U.S. Department of Labor, Employment, and Training Administration: *Dictionary of occupational titles,* ed 4, Washington, DC, 1991, US Government Printing Office.

108. VALPAR Assessment Systems. (Available from VALPAR International Corp, PO BOX 5767, Tucson, AZ 85703.)

109. Vocational Research Institute, Jewish Employment and Vocational Service (JEVS), Philadelphia.

110. Watson HK, Carlson L: Treatment of reflex sympathetic dystrophy of the hand with an active "stress loading" program, *J Hand Surg* 12A:779, 1987.

111. Waylett-Rendall J: Sensibility evaluation and rehabilitation. In *Orthopedic Clinics of North America,* vol 19(1), Philadelphia, 1988, WB Saunders.

112. Waylett-Rendall J, Seibly D: A study of the accuracy of a commercially available volumeter, *J Hand Ther* 4:10, 1991.

113. Wehbé MA: Tendon gliding exercises, *Am J Occup Ther* 41:164, 1987.

114. Wehbé MA, Hunter JM: Flexor tendon gliding in the hand. Pt II. Differential gliding, *J Hand Surg* 10A:575, 1985.

115. Wilson RE, Carter MS: Management of hand fractures. In Hunter JM and associates, editors: *Rehabilitation of the hand,* ed 3, St Louis, 1990, CV Mosby.

116. Wolf SL: *Electrotherapy,* New York, 1981, Churchill Livingstone.

117. Work Evaluation Systems Technology (WEST), PO Box 2477, Fort Bragg, CA 95437.

118. Yerxa EJ and associates: Development of a hand sensitivity test for the hypersensitive hand, *Am J Occup Ther* 37:176, 1983.

Cardiac Dysfunction

Maureen Michele Matthews, Denise Foderaro,
Stephanie O'Leary

There has been a substantial decline in mortality from cardiovascular and vascular disease during the past 30 years. Coronary heart disease has decreased approximately 40% during that period.[15] Yet nearly a half million deaths from coronary heart disease were reported in the United States in 1991. Over six million people have a history of heart attack, angina pectoris (chest pain), or both. The National Institute of Health projects that about one and a half million Americans will have heart attacks this year and of those people one third will die.[6]

Despite these projected statistics, death rates related to coronary heart disease have been decreasing. As a result of improvement in modification of risk factors and in the treatment of patients with heart disease, survival rates are increasing. Rehabilitation of the coronary patient continues to be a problem of national concern.[40] Whereas accident victims need not fear recurrence of injury, patients with cardiac disease must attend to the continuing process of arteriosclerosis, which in many cases caused their injury.

Arteriosclerosis does not affect only the coronary circulation but often is manifest in the cerebral and peripheral circulation as well. It is not uncommon that a 65-year-old victim of a stroke also has a significant cardiac disease or that following a coronary episode a patient cannot engage in an aggressive conditioning program because of extensive peripheral vascular disease. These are the types of patients in general rehabilitation clinics who require special program modifications to accommodate their cardiovascular conditions and complications.

All occupational therapists working in the field of physical dysfunction must have a working knowledge of the cardiovascular system to provide safe, effective rehabilitation programs to all patients. The principles of exercise physiology and work simplification used in treating the patient with a cardiac condition apply to the occupational performance of self-care, work, and play/leisure abilities for all patients.

This chapter provides a basic review of cardiovascular anatomy, physiology, and pathophysiology. Its purpose is (1) to enable the therapist to obtain the necessary medical information through chart review and patient interview and (2) to identify and understand the appropriate precautions when treating both the less serious or "uncomplicated" cardiac problems and the more involved or "complicated" cardiac conditions. The area of cardiac care has special terminology. Terms and definitions are included in the body of the text.

With background knowledge in cardiovascular anatomy, physiology, and pathophysiology, the therapist can plan an appropriate activity progression guided by accurate and continuous vital sign monitoring. In this way the patient may attain a maximal yet safe level of independent function.

The occupational performance model is used in evaluation and treatment of the patient with a cardiac condition. Evaluation focuses on the performance components of sensorimotor, cognitive/cognitive integrative, and psychosocial functioning of the patient with cardiac dysfunction.[7] The patient's performance skills in the areas of self-care, work, and play/leisure are considered. During occupational therapy the patient will have the opportunity to learn and practice the tasks required for performance of role and developmental activities.

THE CARDIOVASCULAR SYSTEM
NORMAL CARDIOVASCULAR FUNCTION[8,30,31,34,48]

The cardiac cycle is an intricate interplay of events within the heart responsible for coordinating the direction and volume of blood flow. By this process the heart (1) delivers oxygen to vital organs and tissues of the body, (2) removes carbon dioxide and other by-products, and (3) regulates body core temperature to maintain hemostasis.

Anatomy and Circulation

The heart functions as a four-chambered pump.[41] The right side of the heart (right atrium and right ventricle) collects blood (venous return) and delivers it to the lungs

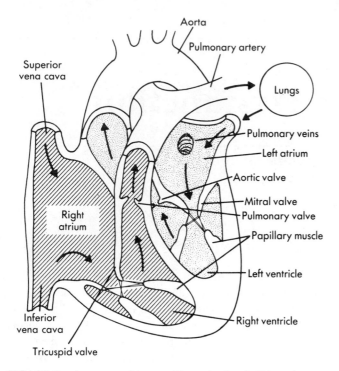

FIG. 36-1   Anatomy of heart. (From Andreoli KG and associates: *Comprehensive cardiac care: a text for nurses, physicians and other health practitioners,* St Louis, 1983, CV Mosby.)

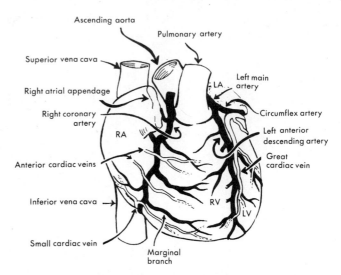

FIG. 36-2   Coronary circulation. (From Underhill SL and associates, editors: *Cardiac nursing,* Philadelphia, 1982, JB Lippincott.)

where it can be reoxygenated. The left side of the heart (left atrium and left ventricle) collects blood from the lungs and delivers it to the systemic circulation. Four heart valves assist in the passage and direction of blood flow within the heart (Fig. 36-1). The opening and closing of the valves depends on volume and pressure changes within the heart and on the papillary muscles. These muscles are connected to the inner myocardium and innervated by the conduction system. Although the heart muscle is always filled with blood, it receives its blood supply from the coronary circulation (Fig. 36-2).

The left main coronary artery and the right coronary artery are the major arteries that supply the outer layer of the heart muscle called the epicardium. These arteries divide further and extend into the myocardial wall called the endocardium. The small structure of these arteries predisposes them to atherosclerosis (arteriosclerosis of the coronary arteries), often referred to as coronary artery disease or CAD.

Cardiologists universally refer to these coronary arteries by abbreviations, such as LAD or left anterior descending coronary artery. The name of the artery describes the portion of the heart it supplies. A blockage in the LAD vessel interferes with blood supply to the left anterior aspect of the heart or the left ventricle. Because the left ventricle is responsible for pumping blood into the systemic circulation and to the brain, the consequences of LAD disease are often serious.

Innervation

Heart muscle, like skeletal muscle, requires nervous innervation to contract. A specialized nervous conduction network (Fig. 36-3) is responsible for causing myocardial contraction. This coordinated sequence of depolarization and contraction is initiated by the sinoatrial (SA) node or pacemaker of the heart. From the SA node the impulse makes its way to the ventricles through the atrioventricular (AV) node, bundle branches, and Purkinje fibers.

Because depolarization is the result of electrical cellular changes, this process can be studied and recorded graphically by the electrocardiogram (ECG, EKG).[26] Surface electrodes are placed on the limbs and chest to monitor the sequence, timing, and magnitude of the impulse as it travels through the conduction system (Fig.

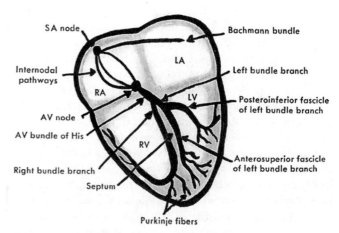

FIG. 36-3   Cardiac conduction. (Modified from Andreoli KG and associates: *Comprehensive cardiac care: a text for nurses, physicians, and other health practitioners,* St Louis, 1983, CV Mosby.)

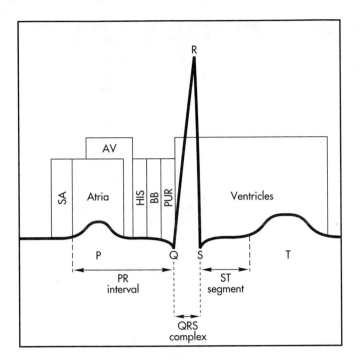

FIG. 36-4   Electrocardiography. (Modified from Andreoli KG and associates: *Comprehensive cardiac care: a text for nurses, physicians, and other health practitioners,* St Louis, 1983, CV Mosby.)

36-4). Each graphic segment, referred to as P, QRS, and T waves, corresponds to the wave of depolarization as it travels through the various chambers of the heart. For instance, the P wave represents electrical stimulation arising from depolarization in the atria. The QRS complex corresponds to the wave of depolarization as it travels through the bundle of His to the ventricles. The timing of depolarization can be studied by counting the blocks on EKG paper. If the PR interval or QRS complex is longer than normal, a conduction abnormality or "block" in the system can be suspected.

The SA node adjusts its rate to meet the demands of the body and working muscle. It is sensitive to vagal and sympathetic nervous input,[8] which explains why heart rate increases during anxiety and with exercise. This mechanism also explains why heart rate decreases with deep breathing, meditation, or other relaxation techniques. Thus the ability to monitor, influence, and modify heart rate is an important skill that can be learned by the patient with cardiovascular disease.

The Cardiac Cycle[17,23,31]

The cardiac cycle maintains and adjusts cardiac output. The cardiac cycle occurs in two phases: input (diastole) and output (systole). The following discussion is a review of the cardiac cycle.

Input (diastole)

During diastole the input valves (mitral and tricuspid) are open, and the output valves (aortic and pulmonary) are closed. This arrangement allows blood from the systemic pulmonary and coronary circulation passively to fill the ventricles. As ventricular volume increases, the pressure within the ventricles increases.

At this time the SA node initiates a wave of depolarization (P wave), which stimulates the atrial muscles to contract and "kick" their contents into the ventricles. The input valves close and the first heart sound is heard. The wave of depolarization (QRS wave) then stimulates the ventricles to contract. Pressure rises in the ventricles causing the output valves to open and allowing blood flow into the systemic and pulmonary circulation. The numerical value assigned to the pressure required to open the output valves is the diastolic pressure or lower number of a blood pressure reading.

Output (systole)

Once the aortic and pulmonary valves are open, the ventricles continue to contract and pressure continues to climb in the ventricles. The peak pressure generated by the ventricles ejecting blood is called the systolic blood pressure and is the upper number of the blood pressure reading. Once the ventricles empty, their volume and pressures decrease. When ventricular pressure falls, the output valves close and create the second heart sound. The total amount of blood ejected during one contraction is called stroke volume. The amount of blood ejected per minute is called cardiac output. The reader is referred to the references for more detailed information about the factors influencing the cardiac cycle and ultimate cardiac output.

PATHOPHYSIOLOGY
Ischemic Heart Disease

Ischemic heart disease is a chronic condition. Clinically an individual may remain symptom free for prolonged periods that alternate with acute symptomatic episodes including angina, acute myocardial infarction, possibly ending in death.[27]

The coronary circulation supplies oxygen to the heart muscle. An imbalance of oxygen supply and demand created by arteriosclerotic narrowing of the coronary arteries results in myocardial injury or myocardial infarction (death of tissue).

The consequences of ischemia include an excess accumulation in the myocardium of metabolic by-products. The presence of these metabolites may result in a decreased myocardial contractility, which can then decrease stroke volume.[35]

In addition, these circulating by-products predispose the myocardium to an increased occurrence of ectopic or irregular heart beats arising from irritable portions of the heart muscle. Depending on the origin and frequency of these ectopic beats, cardiac output may decrease and cardiac arrhythmias may develop. Angina pectoris or chest pain is a clinical manifestation of ischemia and includes the characteristics described in Table 36-1.

TABLE 36-1   Characteristics of Angina Pectoris and Myocardial Infarction

	CHARACTERISTICS OF ANGINA PECTORIS	CHARACTERISTICS OF MYOCARDIAL INFARCTION
Severity	Mild to moderate discomfort. The perception of the pain depends on the individual's age, culture, socialization, and previous experience. It is usually described as mild to moderate severity	Severe pain. A total loss of blood supply to a portion of the muscle results in severe pain and eventually necrotic tissue
Type and Description	Squeezing, tightness, aching, burning, choking. This sensation is often described not as pain but discomfort. A classic description is for patient to clench the fist over the sternum in an attempt to describe the pain	Oppressive pressure, choking, strangling, feeling of impending doom. The greater intensity of the pain is evidence of a more complete and prolonged loss of blood supply and oxygen to heart muscle
Location	Substernal: the heart occupies a central location in the chest	Substernal: pain can be misinterpreted because many people think that heart pain has to be in the left chest
Radiation	Radiation may occur to the neck, arms, jaw, and epigastric area. If radiation occurs, it is due to the shared nerve innervation in the thoracic area. Occasionally the pain does not radiate in the chest	Radiation to the neck, arms, jaw, and epigastric area. The extensive damage with infarction increases the number of pain nerve receptors stimulated; MI pain may be misinterpreted as indigestion
Duration	Brief, usually less than 20 minutes. The ischemia is transient, causing pain of brief duration	Prolonged, usually greater than 20 minutes. The extent of ischemia is great, causing the duration of pain to be lengthened
Precipitating Events	Emotions, exercise, extreme temperatures, heavy meals —these conditions increase the work of the heart, requiring an increased supply of blood and oxygen	Usually there may be precipitating factors; pain may occur at rest or during sleep. MI is the end result of the atherosclerotic process and is not affected by physical or emotional activity
Relief	Rest and/or nitroglycerin. Rest decreases the heart's work load and therefore the need for increased blood and oxygen supply. Nitroglycerin decreases the work of the heart by decreasing the resistance against which the heart has to pump	Pain is unrelieved by rest and nitroglycerin. Rest and nitroglycerin may decrease the intensity of the pain, but narcotics are usually required to eliminate it

Adapted and reproduced with permission from Cornett S, Watson J: *Cardiac rehabilitation: an interdisciplinary team approach*, New York, 1984, John Wiley & Sons.

Myocardial infarction (MI) occurs when severe ischemia lasts longer than 20 to 30 minutes. MIs can be either transmural, in which the whole thickness of the myocardium is involved, or nontransmural, in which a lesion is usually confined to the subendocardial layer of the myocardium. MIs are described by their location and size. An anterolateral MI affects both the anterior and lateral walls. Other types include septal, inferior, posterior, or any combination of these.

Nausea and vomiting are often associated with an acute MI. Other symptoms depend on the severity of MI (site and size) and the development of complications (congestive heart failure, arrhythmias, or cardiogenic shock). Additional characteristics of MI are compared with those of angina in Table 36-1. Those patients who develop complications are placed in a high-risk category, need close medical surveillance, and require slower progression in rehabilitation.

Congestive heart failure (CHF) can also be a manifestation of ischemia. When heart tissue is damaged, the heart's pumping function is impaired. If the left ventricle is not able to move blood out of the lungs, pulmonary venous congestion will result.[44] Should left heart failure continue, the system will back up further, causing the right ventricle to fail. The signs and symptoms of congestive heart failure are presented in Table 36-2.

Valvular Disease[30,53,55]

Valvular cardiac lesions can result from rheumatic fever and many nonrheumatic causes. Two different kinds of stress can be imposed on the heart by valvular lesions: pressure overload and volume overload.[30]

With age or in response to recurrent bacterial endocarditis, the valve leaflets may become fibrous and prevent the valves from closing. A backward flow or regurgitation occurs, creating a valve insufficiency and resulting in volume overload. Clinically, this regurgitation can be heard as a murmur. Mitral insufficiency, if severe, causes congestion in the pulmonary circulation with resultant shortness of breath and susceptibility to erratic heart rates, such as atrial fibrillation. Such heart rates interfere with ventricular filling and complete emptying. Blood tends to stagnate, and emboli are common complications. Valvular disease with resultant emboli is a common cause of cerebral vascular accident (CVA).

Aortic insufficiency and regurgitation may result in CHF or ischemia. Aortic stenosis (calcification) affects cardiac output. When aortic stenosis is present, the left ventricle hypertophies because of pressure overload in the heart.[30] Symptoms caused by a decreased cardiac output include arrhythmias as a result of decreased coronary circulation perfusion; cerebral insufficiency or confusion; syncope, or blacking out when exerting effort;

TABLE 36-2	Signs and Symptoms of Left and Right Heart Failure
SIGNS AND SYMPTOMS OF LEFT HEART FAILURE	**SIGNS AND SYMPTOMS OF RIGHT HEART FAILURE**

1. Dyspnea (shortness of breath)
  a. Exertional (with exercise)
  b. Orthopnea (in supine)
  c. Paroxysmal nocturnal dyspnea (sudden shortness of breath at night)
2. Rales, wheezes
3. Dry hacking cough
4. Weakness, fatigue
5. Poor exercise tolerance
6. Daytime oliguria, nocturia
7. Tachycardia, weak pulses
8. Behavioral changes
9. Chest pain
10. Pale or dusky, cool, moist skin
11. Changes in heart sounds (gallop rhythms)
	1. Weight gain
	2. Daytime oliguria (decreased urine output), nocturia (excessive urination at night)
	3. Dependent edema
	4. Jugular venous distention
	5. Hepatomegaly, right upper quandrant pain
	6. Anorexia, nausea
	7. Ascites (fluid in the peritonium)
	8. Changes in heart sounds (gallop rhythms)

Adapted and reproduced with permission from Cornett S, Watson J: *Cardiac rehabilitation: an interdisciplinary team approach,* New York, 1984, John Wiley & Sons.

and dizziness related to a drop in blood pressure. Aortic stenosis warrants close medical management. Depending on severity, exercise may be contraindicated and patients may require surgery, since these patients are at high risk for sudden death.

Cardiomyopathy[30,48,55]

Cardiomyopathy means disease of the heart muscle. Cardiomyopathy is applied to patients with congestive heart failure and similar findings in the absense of a common pathology (e.g., valvular disease).[30] The cellular mechanics (actin and myosin) responsible for muscle contraction have been altered, usually as the result of a virus or toxic substances, like alcohol, in the blood stream. There is a high incidence of cardiomyopathy among chronic alcoholics. Severe cases of cardiomyopathy, which cannot be medically controlled, produce a severely limited individual who is a prime candidate for occupational therapy intervention with energy conservation and equipment.

Risk Factors

The Framingham study[23] has correlated the presence of several risk factors to the progression of the arteriosclerotic process. The American Heart Association divides them into three categories: (1) risk factors that cannot be changed: heredity, male gender and age; (2) major risk factors that can be changed: cigarette smoke, high blood pressure, blood cholesterol levels, and physical inactiv-

ity; (3) contributing factors: diabetes, obesity, and stress.[19]

The Framingham study, a landmark study, inspired much research in an effort to understand the mechanisms responsible for arteriosclerosis. Medical science is now beginning to understand which factors control the development of arteriosclerosis. Much emphasis has been on prevention through exercise and diet. Consequently, much research has been performed on the cardiovascular benefits of aerobic conditioning at a target heart rate for a sustained 30- to 45-minute period.[9,24,27] Research shows that such conditioning alters metabolism and affects muscle mechanisms of oxygen transport and use, thus making the entire cardiovascular system a more efficient one.

Recent findings indicate that the heart will benefit from the cumulative effects of intermittent moderate spurts of activity. As little as one 15 minute exercise session per day can increase heart and lung strength. In July 1993 the American College of Sports Medicine along with the U.S. Centers for Disease Control changed its recommendations for aerobic exercise to: accumulative rather than sustained 30 minutes of unstructured, moderate activity on most, preferably all, days.[2,54]

Heart disease however is not solely the effect of arteriosclerosis. There are medical conditions and disabilities that have associated and secondary cardiac involvement. Some of these are as follows:[43]

Alcoholism
Anemia
Ankylosing spondylitis
Anorexia
Arteriosclerosis
Cerebrovascular disease
Cocaine use
Diabetes
Friedreich's ataxia
Gout
Hypertension
Marfan's syndrome
Obesity
Peripheral vascular disease
Progressive muscular dystrophy
Progressive systemic sclerosis (scleroderma)
Rheumatoid arthritis
Systemic lupus erythematosus
Patients in general rehabilitation clinics may require program modification and surveillance of vital signs because of these secondary diagnoses.

PATIENT MANAGEMENT
MEDICAL AND SURGICAL MANAGEMENT

The cardiologist's immediate concern is to preserve healthy heart tissue by controlling complications that may jeopardize healing and overall cardiac function. This goal is accomplished by a necessary period of bed rest

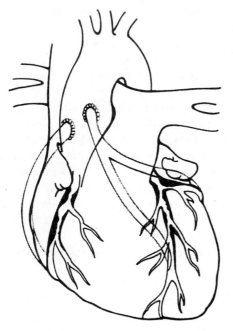

FIG. 36-5 Coronary artery bypass. (From *Heart facts,* 1986. Reproduced with permission. American Heart Association.)

during which the cardiac cycle is stabilized by medications.

Once the patient is stabilized at rest, medical surveillance continues through the cardiac program to ensure medical stability during activity. If patients demonstrate substantial CAD and are appropriate surgical candidates, coronary bypass surgery is performed. In this procedure a vein from another location (usually a leg) is placed in the heart to reroute blood around the occluded area to the myocardium (Fig. 36-5).

Other surgeries include valve replacement, aneurysm repairs, pacemaker inserts, and complete transplants. Techniques, like the percutaneous transluminal arterioplasty (PTCA), float a balloon-tipped catheter to the point of occlusion. The balloon is inflated, and the occlusion is compressed against the arterial wall.[58] This noninvasive technique avoids costly open-heart surgery.

PSYCHOSOCIAL ASPECTS

As with any physical disability, patients who experience a cardiac event progress through various stages of psychosocial reaction and adjustment. Anxiety produced by discomfort and fear of imminent death is often overwhelming. Patients may demonstrate their anxiety by asking many questions, acting out sexually, or pacing.

Anxiety places an increased physiological demand on the heart muscle at a time when it needs rest. It is most often noted during the first 48 hours of a patient's admission and at times of changing environments, such as transfers to step-down units and at discharge. Sedation may be used to alleviate anxiety; however, excessive sedation may produce medical problems and interfere with integrating the realities of the event, which is a necessary step toward successful rehabilitation.[14]

Anxiety is best alleviated through supportive and educational communication.[29] Once a patient verbalizes his or her feelings and learns of the nature of the condition and ways to control it, anxiety usually diminishes.

Early ambulation and resumption of self-care activities can also help alleviate the feelings of helplessness that are common with patients experiencing a recent cardiac event. In the event of dysfunction, the patient draws on coping and defense mechanisms to respond to major life events. Some previously used coping behaviors may not be available to the patient in the hospital (i.e., smoking, drinking, taking a walk). The occupational therapist must therefore assist the patient in establishing new, healthy coping patterns.

Denial is a mechanism used when an individual cannot cope with the surrounding events. Denial is common in coronary disease because of the vague characteristics of symptoms and the hidden nature of the disability. At times denial is considered a healthy response, and health professionals must be careful not to strip the patient of this coping mechanism by forcing the patient to face reality too quickly.[14] Careful monitoring of a patient's activities is important at this time to protect the patient from performing at unsafe, higher activity levels.

Depression is most commonly seen from the third to sixth day after MI[14] and may extend into the convalescent phase. A study of patients 6 months to 1 year following discharge found 88% of the patients reporting either anxiety or depression or both. The patients also reported that inactivity was the most frustrating experience following cardiac event.[18]

Family education is important. A patient's fears and feelings of inadequacy may be based on a misconception that may be reinforced from equally fearful and often noninformed family members.[12] Although initial efforts are made to alleviate stress, patients must eventually be educated to handle it, not circumvent it.[14] Relaxation programs,[1] assisted therapeutic introspection and examination of coping patterns, changes in life expectations and beliefs, and self-help groups[42] are methods to deal effectively with stress. "It is only when the patient has confronted stress successfully that he can resume a fully functioning way of life."[14]

The entire health team has the responsibility to prepare the cardiac patient to deal with a new life. The medical and psychological training of occupational therapists enables them to be an integral part of the rehabilitation team.

CARDIAC REHABILITATION

Early mobilization of patients after coronary incidence is now standard cardiological practice. This approach differs from management of the patient with cardiac disease in the 1950s and 1960s. At that time strict bed rest was prescribed for 6 to 8 weeks. Pathologic studies specified 6 weeks as required for the transformation of necrotic myocardium to form scar tissue.[57]

The 1960s marked the advent of coronary care units with better monitoring techniques for the patient with acute coronary distress. At this time Wenger implemented her hallmark 14-step, early mobilization, activity program at Grady Memorial Hospital.[16] Programs across the country demonstrated that progressive activity under supervised conditions prevented the negative effects of bed rest, shortened hospital stays, facilitated earlier return to work, and reduced the anxiety and depression that often led to the cardiac cripple mind-set.[57]

Following a cardiac event, current medical management of patients includes an acute recovery phase (1 to 3 days) to stabilize cardiac conditions. This phase is followed by a subacute recovery phase (called phase 1) of cardiac rehabilitation during which a course of progressive, low energy–expenditure hospital activity is prescribed.[15,49]

After the subacute recovery phase, patients usually undergo a predischarge graded exercise or treadmill test (GXT). By administering a symptom-limited GXT, a safe target heart rate (THR) and functional capacity are identified and can be used as guidelines during home, vocational, and exercise activity programs. Because phase I (inpatient) patients are discharged from the hospital as soon as they are medically stable, there is not sufficient time for substantial physiological improvement in exercise capacity to occur.[15] Patients continue the exercise program in phase 2, the outpatient phase of their convalescence in which the true benefits of cardiovascular conditioning occur.[24] The majority of patient education, risk factor modification, and lifestyle changes take place during this phase of rehabilitation.[15,50]

Individuals continue to advance to greater exercise intensities in phase 3 and 4 programs. They further develop their own knowledge and self-monitoring techniques so that medical surveillance needs to occur only on an intermittent basis.

Optimally, as the rehabilitative process of recovery is completed, the once anxious and functionally limited patient becomes an educated individual who continues risk factor modification and exercise as a way of life. The patient consequently attains maximal functional capacity and can resume an active role in society.

PROGRAM OBJECTIVES[49]
Phase 1—Inpatient Rehabilitation

The basic purposes of phase 1 rehabilitation are as follows:

1. to provide a program of monitored low-level physical activity including exercise and activities of daily living safely to maximize functional status
2. to decrease the effects of prolonged inactivity including the following: thromboembolism, atelectasis, orthostatic hypotension, hypovolemia, muscle atrophy, osteoporosis, and negative nitrogen and protein balance
3. to reinforce cardiac and postsurgical precautions
4. to identify medical problems via monitoring the patients during the various therapeutic regimes
5. to screen patients with a diagnosis of atypical chest pain for ischemia associated with activity
6. to promote optimal ADL function via instruction in energy conservation and graded activity during monitored self-care to Class III, IV cardiac patients (Classification are discussed later in this chapter.)
7. to assist in diagnostic work-up and establish appropriate exercise prescription and referral to outpatient rehabilitation program via graded exercise testing (GXT)
8. to manage patient anxiety and depression related to heart disease and return the patient to previous lifestyle
9. to provide an educational program for patients and families to include cardiovascular anatomy, pathophysiology, and coronary risk factors
10. to provide appropriate dietary modifications and education to patient and family
11. to provide coordinated discharge that identifies home health, outpatient, and equipment needs
12. to provide guidelines for home activities for early postdischarge period

Phase 2—Outpatient Rehabilitation

The following objectives form the basis for phase 2 rehabilitation:

1. to provide an individualized exercise prescription based on patient's past medical history and results of GXT, as well as to facilitate an independent home exercise program safely to maximize functional status
2. to provide ongoing monitored exercise
3. to initiate and/or continue patient surveillance concerning the effectiveness of therapeutic regimes
4. to provide simulated work evaluations and guidelines for return to work or avocational interests
5. to initiate and/or continue modification of risk factors
6. to initiate and/or continue diet education by means of regularly scheduled follow-up appointments with outpatient department
7. to provide appropriate referrals to community-based exercise program

TEAM APPROACH

Achieving such program objectives is a team endeavor and is not the sole responsibility of a single health profession.[22] In small community hospitals the cardiac rehabilitation team may include a physician and a nurse. In larger and more formalized rehabilitation programs other health professionals may be involved, including dietitians, exercise physiologists, occupational therapists, pharmacists, physical educators, physical therapists, psychologists, respiratory therapists, social workers, and vocational counselors.

The degree of the health professionals' involvement is largely dependent on (1) their availability, (2) their role as defined within the rehabilitation facility, (3) their specialty skills and experience in treating patients with cardiac disease, and (4) the financial resources available for the delivery of professional services. Whichever health professionals are involved, the most important members of the cardiac team are the patient and family.

PATIENT POPULATION

Following is a list of patients most often referred to medically supervised and monitored rehabilitation programs[49]:

 I. Patient population for cardiac rehabilitation
   A. Myocardial infarction
   B. Angina pectoris
   C. Cardiac surgery
   D. Congestive heart failure
   E. Cardiomyopathy
   F. Patients at high risk for development of coronary heart disease
   G. Valve disorders
   H. Cardiac arrhythmias
   I. Hypertension
   J. Atypical Chest Pain
 II. Patient population for general rehabilitation
   A. The 65-year-old patient with paraplegia, amputation, and/or CVA with substantial CAD and/or previous MI,
   B. The 70-year-old patient with a fractured hip and a history of CHF and chronic atrial fibrillation,
   C. The patient with muscular dystrophy or alcoholism and documented cardiac involvement,
   D. General rehabilitation patients at high risk for coronary incidence.

A monitored, graded activity progression is prescribed for all these patients; however, each condition varies, and activity progressions and modalities must reflect this variation. Therapists must be able to support their proposed rehabilitation programs and goals with sound physiological principles as documented in the literature discussing cardiac rehabilitation.

PROGRAM GUIDELINES

Graded activity is beneficial in minimizing the ill effects of bed rest and maximizing functional capacity. There are several conditions, however, for which exercise is absolutely contraindicated.[32,34] These conditions are the following:

1. unstable angina
2. resting diastolic blood pressure (DBP) 120 mm hg or resting systolic blood pressure (SBP) 200 mm hg
3. uncontrolled atrial or ventricular arrhythmias
4. second- or third-degree heart block

5. orthostatic SBP drop of 20 mm hg or more
6. recent embolism, either systemic or pulmonary
7. thrombophlebitis
8. dissecting aneurysm
9. fever greater than 100°F (38°C)
10. uncompensated heart failure
11. primary, active pericarditis
12. severe aortic stenosis
13. acute systemic illness
14. resting heart rate greater than 120 beats per minute in the patient with a recent MI
15. resting heart rate greater than 130 beats per minute for patients with recent bypass surgery, cardiomyopathy, CHF, or valve surgery

Patients must be medically stable before initiating or continuing with any progressive activity program. Special considerations, however, do exist when a patient may be relatively stable on an optimal medical regime. These specific conditions require a modified rehabilitation program with close medical supervision as follows:[29,49]

1. resting DBP over 100 mm hg or resting SBP over 180 mm Hg
2. hypotension
3. fixed rate pacemaker
4. intermittent claudication (cramps in legs)
5. any neuromuscular, musculoskeletal, or arthritic disorders that could prevent activity

THE ROLE OF OCCUPATIONAL THERAPY

During phase 1 of a cardiac rehabilitation program, the occupational therapist is primarily responsible for guiding the patient to achieve a safe yet maximal level of independent self-care. The process involves patient and family education and instruction in energy-conservation techniques to avoid stress to a healing myocardium. The occupational therapist's role is to evaluate the patient's technique of ADL performance and to identify ways to decrease the energy used so the patient can begin to perform the task without symptoms.

Adaptive aids and durable medical equipment are often necessary for these patients. Patient success with these simple activities, although using a varied technique, is of tremendous psychological benefit. Continued participation in their ADL gives them a sense of control and independence and thus alleviates the patient's and family member's fear and anxiety. As with any other patient evaluation and treatment there are special evaluation tools and techniques pertinent to patients with cardiac disease.

EVALUATION PROCEDURES
Chart Review

A thorough chart review is advised before meeting the patient. This approach implies that the therapist must be familiar with cardiac terminology and have a basic understanding of how a patient's clinical course and various test results affect program progression and treatment goals. Consultation with team members is important. The status of the phase 1 cardiac patient often changes rapidly. Current information may not yet be documented in the chart.

Patient Interview

Once a thorough chart review is completed, the therapist conducts an initial patient interview to obtain an activity history. Social, financial, architectural, psychological, cognitive/behavioral, vocational and/or avocational factors, and how they influence treatment planning may be further assessed. A sample evaluation as used at Santa Clara Valley Medical Center is shown in Fig. 36-6.

The initial patient interview is frequently the patient's first contact with a member of the cardiac rehabilitation team. Moreover, it often occurs at a particularly anxious time; for instance, the patient has just been informed of the MI, has just been weaned from the ventilator, or has just been moved to the transitional care unit. The patient/therapist relationship is established. The therapist must outline the terms and expectations of the relationship so that the patient (1) understands the importance of gradually increasing activity; (2) understands the logistics of the cardiac rehabilitation program (scheduling and

activity modalities); (3) begins to feel comfortable asking personal or repeated questions; and (4) begins to take an active part in the rehabilitation process, including reporting signs and symptoms experienced during activity.

Monitored Self-Care Evaluations

Self-care evaluations are most often performed in phase 1 of cardiac rehabilitation. They consist of ADL that require low energy expenditure and may include hygiene, grooming, simple bathing, dressing, and functional mobility tasks.[46]

The therapist chooses a combination of low-level self-care activities to both mobilize and evaluate the patient. The therapist's choice of activities is based on the patient's past medical and functional history, the patient's current clinical status and course of recovery, the therapist's knowledge of cardiovascular dynamics, and the metabolic energy costs of increasing activity.

For instance, a 74-year-old man is admitted to the hospital with a current bout of CHF. Before his admission to the hospital his activities were limited to independent seated bathing and dressing and walking for two blocks before experiencing shortness of breath. His hospital course is complicated by kidney problems. He has been resting in bed for 1 week, and his current hospital activity includes out-of-bed activity with assistance for short periods to use the commode.

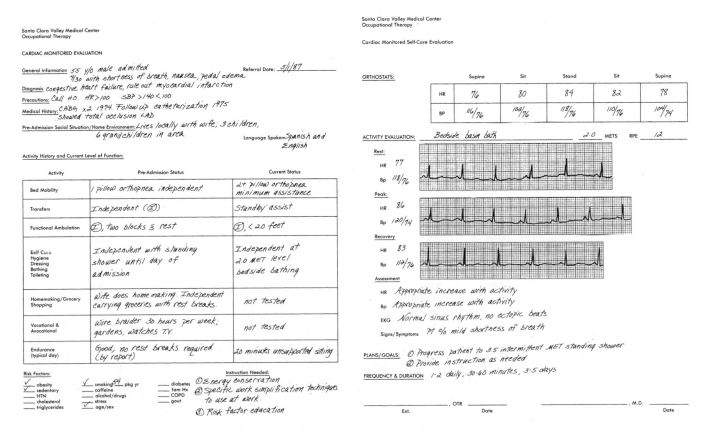

FIG. 36-6   Santa Clara Valley Medical Center Occupational Therapy Cardiac Evaluation Form. (Reproduced with permission, Santa Clara Valley Medical Center, OT Dept, San José, Calif, 1994.)

The initial self-care evaluation for this patient may consist of a 30- to 60-minute treatment session. The activity history and patient interview will continue while the therapist monitors the patient's orthostats. Orthostats are the measurements of baseline vital signs (heart rate, EKG, and BP) and symptoms as the patient moves from supine to sitting to standing. A substantial drop in blood pressure related to sitting or standing up is called orthostatic hypotension. Slow transitional movements, support stockings, and rhythmical extremity movements help to prevent this condition. Once it is established that the patient can tolerate positional changes with appropriate responses, the therapist can evaluate the patient during activity.

The therapist may encourage the patient to perform rhythmic ankle pumping to avoid venous pooling in the lower extremities and resultant dizziness. After a brief evaluation of the patient's lower extremity strength, the patient may then be asked to stand for a 1- to 2-minute period and perform bed-to-chair or bed-to-commode transfers. If the patient tolerates the transfer and clinically appears stable, the therapist may ask the patient to perform a simple hygiene or self-care task. Self-care performed seated in a chair with proper back support is less energy-consuming than performed seated at the edge of the bed, because less isometric trunk activity is required.[45]

The patient's vital signs and symptoms are recorded during the highest or peak level of activity and again 4 to 5 minutes after the activity is stopped (called the recovery phase). Patients sometimes experience inappropriate responses in recovery despite good performance of self-care activity. The patient will be asked to report his or her rate of perceived exertion (RPE), which is discussed later in this chapter. Evaluation results are discussed with the patient, and activity guidelines are established to provide structure and reassurance. Mutually agreed upon discharge goals may be established at this time.

Simulated Tasks Evaluation

Monitored task evaluations measure the cardiovascular response to a combination of lower and upper extremity work and variations in body position.[46] The tasks that are monitored simulate what the patient will actually be doing at home or at work to determine if this level of activity is safe to resume under nonmonitored circumstances. These tasks typically require more energy than that required during self-care and are therefore performed when the patient progresses to phase 2 or 3 of the cardiac rehabilitation program. Treadmill exercise tests are routinely used to evaluate a patient's functional capacity; however, the information obtained is based solely on lower extremity performance. Because upper extremity work elicits a different and more pronounced cardiovascular response,[9] simulated task evaluations can better evaluate a patient's response to specific vocational and leisure tasks.

A numerical scoring system of task analysis has been developed by Ogden.[45] She analyzes tasks by six variables: rate, resistance, muscle groups used, involvement of trunk muscles, arm position, and isometric work (straining). This system of analysis assists the therapist in evaluating which tasks demand the highest energy demand from the heart. Perhaps the application of this system is more useful to cardiac teaching and work simplification. Here the therapist reduces the energy demands of a task by altering the aforementioned variables. Other factors, such as environmental temperature, emotional stress related to the task, and length of time (sustained versus intermittent) the patient performs the task must be considered.

The need for a simulated task evaluation most often arises when the patient is ready to return to work. For instance, Mr. J, a 53-year-old cafeteria dishwasher, had a coronary artery bypass following his MI 2 months ago. He has been involved in an aggressive cardiac rehabilitation program consisting of walking, bicycling, and arm ergometry (arm crank) at a target heart rate of 120 beats per minute. He can now tolerate sustained, 30-minute activities that are 4 1/2 times the amount of energy he requires at rest. His treadmill test produced fatigue and a suboptimal blood pressure response.

The question arises whether Mr. J's current activity tolerance is sufficient for a safe return to work as a dishwasher. The therapist performs a chart review, patient interview, and job analysis that may include an interview with the patient's employer and an on-site observation to determine the energy demands of the job. The therapist finds that the job is full-time employment performed in three parts daily:

1. Dish tray assembly for 2 hours (sustained standing and light upper extremity activity)
2. General cleaning of work stations for 2 hours (intermittent activity with frequent bending and reaching)
3. Dishwashing for 3 hours (sustained standing with frequent stacking and lifting 5 to 10 pounds at once on an assembly line)

These tasks take place in a warm environment; the patient has no control over pace or rest period because of the fixed-rate assembly line and union regulations concerning breaks. The therapist designs a simulated task evaluation that takes place over 3 hours. The therapist evaluates cardiovascular responses to (1) sustained standing and light upper extremity activity, (2) intermittent activity with frequent bending and reaching, and (3) sustained standing with moderate upper extremity work at a fixed, moderate pace.

The therapist finds that the patient has considerable difficulty and demonstrates abnormal cardiovascular responses. The therapist discusses this response with the cardiologist, who implements a medication change and suggests a change in the patient's physical conditioning program so it is geared toward those tasks the patient must perform at work.

In this case the simulated task evaluation gave the cardiologist crucial information of functional performance that could not be obtained from a routine treadmill test.

Occupational therapists are becoming more involved with simulated work evaluations for patients with cardiac disease.[11] Further methods, studies, and applications of such evaluations should be developed.

EVALUATION TOOLS

Therapists assess a patient's cardiovascular response to activity by monitoring six parameters: heart rate, blood pressure, EKG readings, signs and symptoms of cardiac dysfunction, rate pressure product, and heart sounds. In some facilities therapists are not required to monitor EKG and heart sounds. These authors believe that, if therapists are treating a cardiac population, they would benefit from workshops to develop skills in basic EKG interpretation and in recognition of abnormal heart sounds. Monitoring skills and techniques should be objective, expedient, and accurate.

Heart Rate

"Normal" heart rates vary with age, sex, activity, attitude, temperature, health status, emotion, amount of coffee or tobacco intake, and electrolyte and fluid imbalances.[24] Basically, normal adult heart rate is 60 to 100 beats per minute. Abnormal heart rates are either too slow (called bradycardia: less than 60 beats per minute), too fast (called tachycardia: greater than 100 beats per minute), or irregular (called arrhythmias).

If the heart rate is bradycardic, the cardiac output may not be sufficient to meet the energy demands of the brain, systemic circulation, and working muscles. This condition results in fatigue; and if bradycardia is severe, dizziness, confusion, and syncope (loss of consciousness) can result. In highly trained athletes bradycardia is normal and reflects a highly efficient cardiovascular system. In other cases bradycardia that is symptom-free at 50 to 60 beats per minute may be desired to decrease the work of the myocardium. This response is often the result of medications, like propranolol (Inderal), in the beta blocker category. A sudden development of bradycardia, however, especially if associated with symptoms, warrants further medical work-up and could be indicative of severe cardiac conduction dysfunction, that is, heart blocks that may necessitate inserting a cardiac pacemaker.

Tachycardic heart rates (HR) may be caused by general deconditioning or conditions that alter stroke volume (SV), the amount of blood ejected with each heart beat. Tachycardia may be the heart's attempt to maintain cardiac output (CO) because CO = SV × HR. Heart rates greater than 110 do not allow adequate filling time in diastole, which further impinges on stroke volume. Furthermore, tachycardic heart rates increase myocardial oxygen demand. The increase may exceed available supply and cause myocardial ischemia.

Heart rate can be monitored by several methods as follows: palpation (feeling), auscultation (listening), and EKG monitoring (skin electrodes). Pulses can be palpated and counted at the radial, brachial, and carotid, sites. Therapists must exercise caution if monitoring carotid pulse, because this site is close to the carotid sinus that, if overstimulated, can cause bradycardia. If the pulse is regular, it is counted for 10 seconds and multiplied by 6, giving total beats per minute. Patients are routinely instructed in these techniques and precautions to begin self-monitoring.

Auscultation, or listening to the heart with a stethoscope to monitor heart rate, is recommended for patients with poor peripheral pulses or irregular heart beats. The stethoscope is placed over the apex of the heart (the fifth intercostal space at or just medial to the left midclavicular line).[10] This point of maximal impulse is referred to as PMI. Apical pulses, if irregular, should be counted for a full 60-second period for accuracy.

The EKG method of monitoring heart rate is a simple technique of reading heart rate from an accurate digital display. Heart rate can also be measured from EKG strips by counting blocks on the paper as they correlate to assigned heart rates[26] or by using a special rate ruler. Appropriate documentation of heart rate includes the number of beats per minute and a comment on regularity, such as "72 beats per minute and irregular."

Blood Pressure[4,17,30,44,53]

Blood pressure is simply the pressure of blood against the arteries created by the pumping of the heart and the peripheral resistance of flow. This pressure is responsible for driving the blood through the circulatory system to perfuse vital organs, tissues, and working muscle. The reader is referred to the discussion of the cardiac cycle. The diastolic blood pressure (lower number) is the amount of pressure generated by ventricular contraction, which is responsible for opening the aortic and pulmonary valves. Systolic blood pressure (upper number) is the peak pressure that the ventricles continue to generate over and above the point at which the valves open.

The amount of pressure generated from the time the valves open to peak pressure is the pressure available to move blood along the systemic circulation. This value is called pulse pressure. If this pulse pressure becomes less than 20 mm Hg (90/80), perfusion to the distal tissues may not be sufficient. In severe cases circulatory shock or collapse may occur with permanent damage related to the amount of time the vital organs and tissues do not receive oxygen.

Normal blood pressures increase with age.[24] Because arteriosclerosis and a decrease in the distensibility of the arteries is often associated with age, more pressure is required to propel blood through the system. Pressures become hypertensive if they are between 160/90 to 200/110 mm Hg or greater. A particularly high systolic blood pressure may generate too much pressure in the arteries and could result in an aneurysm or CVA. In addition, diastolic hypertensive states require that the ventricles perform increased and often sustained contractions that may result in myocardial hypertrophy (enlargement). In this case the heart needs even more oxygen as a result of the increase in muscle fibers. If the oxygen cannot be supplied to meet this demand, ischemia may result.

If systolic blood pressure is less than 90 mm Hg, hypotension or low blood pressure exists. Similarly, low blood pressure affects perfusion and the delivery of blood to vital organs and peripheral tissues. Hypotension may be associated with dizziness and light-headedness. In severe cases of hypotension caused by circulatory inadequacy, hands and feet may become cold, the patient's color may be dusky or pale, lips may be cyanotic or bluish, and the patient may become confused, indicating degrees of cerebral anoxia.

When patients are admitted to a medical service, physicians usually indicate vital sign precautions in the nursing orders. They are usually written as "Call H.O. (house officer or on-call physician) if SBP > 150 < 90; DBP > 90 < 50; HR > 120 < 50" (systolic blood pressure greater than 150 or less than 90; diastolic blood pressure greater than 90 or less than 50; heart rate greater than 120 or less than 50).

Blood pressure is monitored by two methods: invasive and noninvasive. Invasive techniques require that an arterial line be placed into the artery for direct blood pressure monitoring. This method is the most accurate and is the most often used in acute care for the hemodynamically unstable patient. It is not feasible in a rehabilitation setting. Most often therapists record blood pressure by the use of a sphygmomanometer or blood pressure cuff. Because this method is indirect, it is subject to sources of error, which the therapist must attempt to minimize.

An indirect measurement is one that uses and examines associated factors (cuff pressure) to derive and define the desired measurement (blood pressure).[53] More simply, if a given blood pressure is 120/80 mm Hg and the therapist pumps the cuff to 200 mm Hg, the brachial artery will be completely occluded, because cuff pressure (200) exceeds peak arterial pressure (120). If a stethoscope is placed over the artery at this time, no sounds will be heard, because there is no blood flow. Once the therapist gradually releases the cuff pressure to 120 mm Hg, the artery's peak pressure may be able to move some blood through a now partially occluded artery, and pulse sounds will be heard under the stethoscope.

The point at which the first two sounds are heard corresponds to the point where the arterial pressure exceeds the cuff pressure.[53] The therapist then reads the number on the dial as the systolic blood pressure. The systolic blood pressure is not the point where the needle or column of mercury visually bounces. Systolic blood pressure measurements are associated with auscultation or listening, not vision.

As the therapist continues to release pressure, the artery becomes less occluded, enabling greater blood flow and louder sounds under the stethoscope. Once the artery is not occluded and full blood flow is established, the sounds disappear (for example, 80 mm Hg). This point corresponds to diastolic blood pressure.

Sources of error can arise from faulty tools and techniques and errors in measurement.[38] The most common problems are noncalibrated meters and cracked or kinked tubing because of placement. All systems require calibration if the dial does not return to zero.

The relationship between the size of the cuff and circumference of the arm must be considered when choosing which cuff to use.[38] If a standard cuff is used on a very thin arm, the therapist will obtain a false, low pressure reading, whereas a standard cuff applied to an obese arm will result in a false, high reading. Alternate cuffs, for instance, pediatric or large adult cuffs, should be available in the clinic. Additional sources of error may include the following: placing the stethoscope underneath the cuff to hold it in place; varying the position of the arm during serial blood pressure monitoring; repeating inflation of the cuff to make sure measurement is correct; and deflating cuff too rapidly or slowly.[38]

Interpretation of blood pressure responses is based on accurate and expedient measurement. To ensure accuracy therapists are urged to use the same arm, position, evaluator, and equipment when measuring responses. In addition, therapists must be able to obtain a blood pressure response in 30 to 40 seconds. Once activity is stopped, blood pressure begins to recover and peak response will be missed.

EKG. Patients with cardiovascular disease are prone to arrhythmias, which, if frequent, can decrease cardiac output, cause symptoms, and affect overall cardiac function. If severe, they could be life-threatening. All therapists must be trained in cardiopulmonary resuscitation as a basic life-support measure. Therapists working with patients who have known or suspected heart disease must be able to recognize signs and symptoms related to cardiac dysfunction. Therapists not trained in EKG interpretation should note how irregular a pulse becomes (10 irregular beats per minute) during or after activity. Therapists using EKG during therapy should be familiar with monitoring equipment, including problems and artifacts (monitor interference). "They also should be capable of recognizing, at a minimum, the following EKG dysrhythmias:

1. sinus tachycardia
2. sinus bradycardia
3. premature atrial complexes
4. atrial tachycardia
5. atrial flutter
6. atrial fibrillation
7. junctional rhythms
8. atrioventricular blocks of all degrees
9. premature ventricular complexes
10. ventricular tachycardia
11. ventricular fibrillation
12. cardiac standstill or asystole."[4]

Changes in ST segments on the EKG should also be recognized, because these changes parallel cardiac ischemia and cardiac dysfunction. Because EKG interpretation is beyond the scope of this text, the reader is referred to

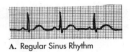

A. Regular Sinus Rhythm

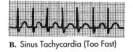

B. Sinus Tachycardia (Too Fast)

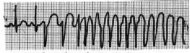

C. Ventricular Tachycardia (Too Fast)

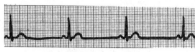

D. Sinus Bradycardia (Too Slow)

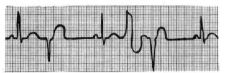

E. Multifocal Premature Ventricular Contractions (PVC) (Too Irregular)

FIG. 36-7 Sample EKG readings of cardiac arrythmias. **A,** Regular sinus rhythm. **B,** Sinus tachycardia (too fast). **C,** Ventricular tachycardia (too fast). **D,** Sinus bradycardia (too slow). **E,** Multifocal premature ventricular contractions (too irregular).

Dubin's *Rapid Interpretation of EKG.*[26] Sample strips are shown in Fig. 36-7 so that the reader may gain an understanding that any arrhythmia either too fast, too slow, or too irregular interferes with cardiac output and function.

Signs and Symptoms of Cardiac Dysfunction

The most important of all evaluation tools is the ability to observe and detect symptoms of cardiac dysfunction. Whenever patients become symptomatic or display signs of intolerance to an activity, the therapist should evaluate and record the event by noting the following:[51]

1. exact complaint
2. body location
3. quality
4. quantity
5. chronology
6. setting
7. aggravating or alleviating factors
8. associated symptoms

Angina

Many chest pains are not associated with ischemia. Angina pectoris induced by ischemia has specific hallmark characteristics (Table 36-1).[22] Patients should be asked to quantify the severity of the pain on an angina rating scale[10] with 10 being the worst pain felt. The surrounding activities that induce angina should be examined. Angina typically occurs during ambulation, shaving, bowel movement, stair climbing, observation of athletic events, arguing, or after a meal. Once these exacerbating factors are stopped, angina dissipates; prompt relief (3 minutes)

may occur with sublingual nitroglycerin tablets, a quick-acting vasodilator. Associated symptoms may include nausea, palpitations, and dizziness. Angina is not the only indication of ischemia. Some patients never experience angina with MI. Instead, weakness or dyspnea (shortness of breath) may be a symptom.

Dyspnea[10,51]

Dyspnea, difficulty in breathing, is a common symptom in heart disease and may be indicative of left ventricular failure (Table 36-2). When dyspnea is noted on exertion, the therapist must note the quantity of activity that produces this condition. Orthopnea is shortness of breath created by resting in the supine position. Because this position creates a greater venous return, stroke volume increases, demanding more work from the myocardium. Often a diseased myocardium is not capable of handling the demand, and shortness of breath or orthopnea will result. Two pillow orthopnea describes the propped-up position necessary to relieve this symptom.

Fatigue

Fatigue is often an initial sign of heart disease. When patients report fatigue, therapists must determine whether it is localized or generalized. Asking which muscles are fatigued will assist the patient in localizing it. If the patient has difficulty localizing the symptom and uses words like exhausted and drained and appears fatigued, the cause may be centralized, as in heart disease. One objective method of rating fatigue is the Borg rate of perceived exertion (RPE) scale[13] (Box 36-1). Patients experiencing centralized fatigue are asked to assign a number to their fatigue based on their perception of the difficulty of activity. Myocardial oxygen consumption studies have correlated RPE scores of greater than 15 RPE to 75% of maximal myocardial oxygen consumption.[13] RPE scores have been used during graded exercise tests and exercise training sessions, monitored self-care, and simulated task evaluations to guide the clinician in grading or stopping the activity.[49] In summary, whenever any sign or symptom is noted with activity, the therapist must accurately note its characteristics and associated factors for proper interpretation.[51]

Rate Pressure Product (Double Product)

Heart rate (HR) times systolic blood pressure (SBP) yields the rate pressure product (RPP). This usually five-digit number is reported with the last two digits dropped (for example, HR 95 × SBP 130 = 12350 = RPP 124). It is an excellent indicator of aerobic conditioning. As a patient becomes progressively more conditioned his RPP decreases for a given work load.[15]

Within a given evaluation session the RPP normally rises at peak work and returns toward baseline in recovery. Angina pectoris can be repeatedly generated at the same RPP during exercise testing, demonstrating the importance of measuring both heart rate and blood pressure during activity.

BOX 36-1

RATE OF PERCEIVED EXERTION

6		14	
7	Very, very light	15	Hard
8		16	
9	Very light	17	Very hard
10		18	
11	Fairly light	19	Very, very hard
12		20	
13	Somewhat hard		

From Borg G and associates: *Med Sci Sports Exerc* 14:376, 1982.

ASSESSMENT

If a patient has tolerated rehabilitation activities well, it implies that no adverse signs or symptoms were noted and that heart rate, blood pressure, and EKG responses were appropriate. Monitoring and assessing a response implies measuring and quantifying a change. Therefore therapists record each of these parameters before activity (resting phase), during activity (peak phase), and 4 to 5 minutes after the activity has stopped (recovery phase). To isolate the response to activity the therapist must monitor and record vital signs in the position of peak activity. For instance, if peak activity is performed while standing at the sink, baseline and recovery vital signs should be noted in the standing position.

Postural responses should also be noted, particularly because orthostatic hypotension is a common occurrence after immobility and is often a side effect of diuretic and antianginal medication regimens. Therapists must be able to assess patient responses so they may establish appropriate treatment progressions for patients. Table 36-3 lists appropriate (desired) and inappropriate cardiovascular responses to activity.[49]

In instances where significant maladaptive responses are noted, communication lines to the referring physician must be expedient. Emergency precautions and procedures[26,27] must be established in any program before placing any demand on patients with documented heart disease.

TREATMENT PROGRESSIONS
Graded Activities

Program progressions are guided by the patient's current clinical status, prognosis, and tolerance of current activities with appropriate cardiovascular responses. The rate of progression is further guided by the patient's past functional history and severity of coronary event. The physician synthesizes this information and ultimately categorizes the patient into one of four functional categories (Box 36-2).[43] Patients in Class I will obviously progress the most rapidly, depending on their continued demonstration to tolerate activities appropriately. Patients in Classes III and IV will progress slowly and may never achieve total independence in self-care.

Progressions are further guided by the energy costs of activities and the factors that influence them. Energy expenditure is measured by the amount of oxygen that is consumed. Years ago this value was expressed in calories

TABLE 36-3 Cardiovascular Responses to Activity

APPROPRIATE	INAPPROPRIATE
Heart rate: Increases with activity to a maximum of approximately 20 beats above resting rate	Heart rate: Excessive heart rate response to activity (> 20 beats above resting rate); resting tachycardia (> 120); bradycardic response to activity (pulse drops or fails to rise with increased work loads)
Blood pressure: Peak systolic blood pressure increases as work load increases	Blood pressure: Hypertensive responses (220/110 mm Hg maximum); postural hypotensive responses (> 10 to 20 mm Hg systolic blood pressure decrease); any drop in systolic blood pressure with activity; failure of systolic blood pressure to rise with activity
EKG readings: Absence of arrhythmias and segment changes	EKG readings: Any rapid arrhythmias or increase in ectopic activity; development of 2 or 3 degree heart blocks; ST segment depression (> 3 to 4 mm); any ST segment elevation
Symptoms: Absence of adverse symptoms	Symptoms: Excessive shortness of breath; angina and/or associated symptoms of nausea, sweating, and extreme fatigue (RPE > 15); cerebral symptoms (confusion or ataxia)

From Santa Clara Valley Center: *Cardiac rehabilitation program protocol*, San José, Calif, 1991, Unpublished.

BOX 36-2

FUNCTIONAL CLASSIFICATION OF CARDIAC DISEASE

Class I: Patients with cardiac disease but without resulting limitations of physical activity. Ordinary physical activity does not cause undue fatigue, palpitation, dyspnea, or anginal pain

Class II: Patients with cardiac disease resulting in slight limitation of physical activity. They are comfortable at rest. Ordinary physical activity results in fatigue, palpitation, dyspnea, or anginal pain

Class III: Patients with the cardiac disease resulting in marked limitation of physical activity. They are comfortable at rest. Less than ordinary physical activity causes fatigue, palpitation, dyspnea, or anginal pain

Class IV: Patients with cardiac disease resulting in inability to carry on any physical activity without discomfort. Symptoms of cardiac insufficiency or of the anginal syndrome may be present even at rest. If any physical activity is undertaken, discomfort is increased

From New York Heart Association, Inc: *Nomenclature and criteria for diagnosis of diseases of the heart and great vessels*, ed 8, Boston, 1979, Little, Brown.

---

but has been refined to METs. One MET (basal metabolic equivalent) is equal to the energy consumed when a patient is at rest in a semi-Fowler position (semireclined with extremities supported), which is equal to 3.5 ml O_2 per minute per kilogram of body weight. As soon as the patient sits up, walks, or performs activities, this metabolic demand and oxygen consumption increase. For instance, dressing requires 2 METs or twice the amount of energy required at rest. Several MET lists establish a comprehensive catalog of a variety of activities that require 1 to 9 METs. Table 36-4 is an energy-cost list for activities at the 3.0 MET level.

This method of grading activity, however, is a general guideline. Caution must be exercised when extrapolating the results of a treadmill test to apply to vocational and leisure tasks. For instance, because a patient achieves 5 METs on the treadmill does not necessarily mean that the patient can resume all activities listed at 5 METs on the energy-cost list. Hellerstein[33] found that the linear relationship between heart rate and oxygen use on a treadmill test may not remain linear during daily activ-

ity. Work-related factors such as emotion and use of small muscle groups produce a nonlinear relationship during vocational, leisure, and self-care activities. Astrand and Rodahl[9] reported consistently higher heart rates for all activities with the following conditions: hot environment, emotional stress, use of upper versus lower extremities, and use of isometric muscular efforts, especially during low to moderate levels of work (2 to 3 METs). Various factors, such as pace, position, muscles used, isometrics, techniques, and environmental factors, influence the energy cost of an activity.

Choosing very light-light[42] activities for a patient just recovering from an acute MI or cardiac surgery is essential. During a patient's acute recovery (phase 1) physicians wish to promote healing of the myocardium but also wish to avoid the deconditioning effects of inactivity. Physicians do not wish any activity to produce tachycardia or a heart rate response greater than 20 beats per minute above rest, because such myocardial work interferes with healing. Patients in phase 1 rehabilitation should not be permitted to perform tasks greater than 3.5

TABLE 36-4   Santa Clara Valley Medical Center's MET Levels of ADL and Vocational and Recreational Activities at the 3.0-MET Level

DAILY ACTIVITIES	METs	VOCATIONAL TASKS	METs
Walking 2 mph[37]	3.2	Light janitorial[28]	3.0
Bowel movement[21,37]	3.6	Bartending[28]	3.0
Warm shower[28,37]	3.5	Pressing[56]	3.6
Stairs (24 ft/min)[21,37]	3.5	Auto repair[28]	3.5
		Truck driving[52]	3-4
HOMEMAKING	**METs**	**RECREATION**	**METs**
Preparing meals[37]	3.0	Playing musical instrument[28]	3.0
Hand laundry[21]	3.5	Playing with children[39,56]	3.5
Mopping[21]	3.5	Golfing[28]	3.0
Ironing (standing)[21]	3.5	Cycling at 5 mph level[28]	3.0
Bed making[37]	3.9		
Window washing[28]	3-4		

STAGE	PHYSICAL THERAPY	OCCUPATIONAL THERAPY
TABLE 36-5	Santa Clara Valley Medical Center's Post MI and Post Open-Heart Surgery Phase 1 Rehabilitation Program*	

PHASE I—INPATIENT PROGRAM

STAGE	PHYSICAL THERAPY	OCCUPATIONAL THERAPY
1 in ICU or on ward 1.5 METs	Check and record heart rate, blood pressure, and EKG readings in supine, sitting, and standing positions (orthostats) In semi-Fowler position: 5-10 times active assistive exercise Teach breathing patterns with exercises Postoperative: deep breathing exercises Chest: physical therapy as indicated	General mobility (bed mobility transfers to commode and position changes) with energy-conservation techniques (environmental setups, equipment, and pacing) Sedentary leisure tasks with arms supported (reading, writing, and cards) OT may not treat in the ICU. OT usually starts in stage 3

2 in ICU or on ward 1.5 METs	Same as stage 1 except exercises are active
	Orthostats
	Ambulate: 50-100 ft, with assistance, as tolerated
		Stage 1 continued with focus on:
		  Unsupported sitting (5-30 min)
		  Standing tasks (seconds to 2 min)
		  Simple hygiene, semi-Fowler sitting position

3 On ward 1.5-2 METs	Orthostats
	In sitting position: 5-10 times active upper extremity (UE) and lower extremity (LE) exercise with coordinated breathing
	Ambulate: 100-200 ft, with monitoring (2-3 min)
		Unsupported sitting ½-1 hr
		  Standing tasks (3-5 min)
		  Bedside bathing (assist with feet and back)
		  Bathroom privileges
		  Light leisure tasks

4 2 METs	Orthostats
	In seated position: 5-10 times active UE and LE exercise with coordinated breathing
	Ambulate: 200-350 ft with monitoring (3-5 min)
		Standing tasks (5-8 min)
		  UE sustained activity (2-5 min)
		  Total body bathing at sink

5 2 METs	Orthostats
	Same as stage 4 except ambulate 350-700 ft with monitoring (5-10 min)
		Standing tasks (8-12 min)
		  UE sustained activity (5-30 min)
		  Total hygiene, bathing, and dressing at sink

6 2 METs	Orthostats Standing active UE and LE exercise (10-30 min) Ambulate: 700-1050 ft with monitoring (5-10 min) Stair climbing 1 flight monitored A predischarge GXT is recommended at this time	Standing tasks (10-30 min) with intermittent UE activity UE sustained activity (5-30 min) Total body mobility: bending for small object retrieval teaching Moderate leisure tasks
7 3-3.5 METs	Orthostats Same as stage 6, except ambulate 1050 feet for 10-20 minutes	Shower transfers Total showering task (hair washing, total body washing, drying, and dressing) Simple homemaking tasks Energy-conservation techniques with activity 3.5 METs (or greater as indicated by GXT) Home program with ADL guidelines and recommendations for equipment, as appropriate

From Santa Clara Valley Medical Center: *Cardiac rehabilitation program protocol,* San José, Calif. 1991, (Unpublished.)
* Education program to be performed by all team members per SCVMC *Cardiac Rehabilitation Education Manual.*

METs. Most self-care can be achieved within this very light-light work category.

Note that sexual activity is listed at 5 METs. Patients just recovering from heart attacks often have questions concerning safe sexual activity. Because sexual activity is intermittent and does not require prolonged, sustained high levels of rhythmical physical activity, physicians advise return to sexual activity if patients can tolerate walking up and down two flights of stairs without symptoms.[50] Therefore patients may be able to perform 5-MET-level activity as long as performance is intermittent and they can perform a lower level or 3.5-MET-level activity if performance is continuous or sustained. To ensure that patients gradually resume daily activities, a step-by-step program similar to the one used at Santa Clara Valley Medical Center is advised (Table 36-5).

In phase 1 the therapist gradually progresses the patient from simple bed mobility and commode transfers to independent dressing and showering, listed at 3.5 METs, under controlled environmental conditions. Myocardial healing and musculoskeletal and cardiac conditioning have occurred by 6 to 8 weeks after coronary event. At this time most patients can tolerate increased MET-level activities greater than 3.5 METs and are ready for simulated task evaluations.

ENERGY CONSERVATION

A balance of low-level activity and rest is essential to the healing myocardium, especially during phase 1 rehabilitation. Knowledge of how various activities evoke differing cardiovascular responses is the basis of energy conservation and work simplification principles.[3] Exercise physiology principles are included in many physiology texts,[9,24] but little is written concerning how these are applied to ADL, especially for the individual with severe cardiac disease.[47] For instance, UE work elicits a greater cardiovascular response than LE activity. Standing requires a greater cardiovascular positional adjustment and more energy than sitting. Any isometric muscular activity interferes with easy blood flow through the muscle and impinges a demand on the cardiovascular system, and Valsalva maneuvers (straining and breath holding) interfere with blood return to the heart and elicit large increases in blood pressure. In warm environments (for example, a hot shower or kitchen) the body has the added task of maintaining its core temperature and must direct blood to the periphery for cooling, which demands cardiovascular work and increased heart rate. Similarly, blood is shunted away from the muscles and to the stomach immediately after meals. Any activity immediately after a meal will elicit a higher heart rate and a higher myocardial oxygen demand.

Energy conservation addresses patterns of activities. For instance, Mrs. R can perform a standing shower (3.5 METs) with good cardiovascular responses and no symptoms. As she dries herself and then attempts to redress, however, she experiences increased heart rates and fatigue. Therefore a shower chair may be necessary, and a system of work and rest (such as work 5 minutes and rest 2 minutes) can be introduced. The therapist also notes that Mrs. R. has more energy in the evening and instructs the patient to perform her shower before retiring in the evening.

Patients need much guidance and education in this area. Once a patient understands the principles of work efficiency, anxiety is reduced and the patient feels in control of the events. For instance, Mr. J was extremely depressed because last evening he had chest pain during his shower; he now feels his cardiac condition is worse because this scenario never happened before. On further examination the therapist discovers that Mr. J had to run up and down the steps twice to get the phone before taking a shower. It is understandable that if he starts at a high heart rate, activity will certainly increase the rate further; in this case it was increased beyond Mr. J's angina threshold. Therapeutic intervention is to educate Mr. J in environmental and activity factors that increase heart rate and to instruct him in pulse monitoring. If Mr. J's pulse is greater than 90, he should wait to take a shower. Meditation or progressive relaxation 10 minutes before showering may be necessary so that showering begins at a heart rate of 70 beats per minute.

Patient education sheets can be used to instruct the patient in such principles. Furthermore a method of work simplification can be used to instruct patients in analyzing new tasks to be simplified at home or in their work environments.

Patient and Family Education

Patient and family education is of prime importance in cardiac rehabilitation. Topics covered include basic cardiac anatomy, basic exercise physiology, medications, pulse monitoring, diet and risk factor modification, energy conservation, and energy cost of activities.[42] The occupational therapist may be involved with instruction in several of these topics. Some occupational therapists coordinate cooking classes with the dietitian to address diet education and assess a patient's performance and use of energy conservation with kitchen tasks.

Patient and family education can be performed creatively in a variety of ways, such as direct instruction, experiential performance, demonstration, reinforcement, problem solving, and repeated practice. The reader is referred to the references that have evaluated the effectiveness of various presentation techniques geared toward patient education.[19,20,25,27,36]

Education of the patient's spouse does much to reduce stress on the family. Wives of survivors of sudden cardiac death experience a great deal of fear related to the near loss of their mate and possible recurrence. Furthermore, demands of the patient's disease process will necessitate changes in roles for family members.[36] A therapist sensitive to these issues will include family members in the educational process.

SUMMARY

This chapter is designed to enable the therapist to establish a background and theoretical foundation in cardiac rehabilitation. The therapist is then able to provide safe activities for the patient with a primary or secondary cardiac diagnosis.

To assist the therapist in synthesizing and applying the foregoing information a sample treatment plan is provided. The sample treatment plan is not comprehensive, and the reader therefore may wish to apply information from this chapter to develop a more complete plan.

SAMPLE TREATMENT PLAN

CASE STUDY

DD is a 64-year-old man admitted 4 days ago with a 5-hour history of bilateral arm pain and tightness in his throat associated with fatigue and shortness of breath.

Diagnostic work-up disclosed an acute anterolateral MI with subsequent complications of CHF and arrhythmias.

This patient is divorced and lives alone. He is a retired plumber and enjoys doing maintenance jobs around the house.

He was referred to occupational therapy for ADL evaluation and activity progression per cardiac protocol.

He was transferred out of the ICU and onto a general medicine floor today.

TREATMENT PLAN

Personal data

Name: DD
Age: 64
Diagnosis: Acute anterolateral MI (post day 4) with complications
Disability: Altered functional capacity
Treatment aims as stated in referral: achieve maximal, functional level of ADL without adverse cardiovascular symptoms

Other services

Physician: Supervision of patient's progress and effectiveness of current medical regime with increasing activity and program adjustments as indicated
Nursing: Provision of nursing and supportive care: reinforcement of ADL and ambulation programs in accordance with rehabilitation progress; provision of educational program with nursing emphasis on anatomy and physiology, medications, tests, and wound care
Social service: Assistance in family and social adjustment; exploration of financial resources for follow-up services and arrangement for equipment; outpatient and home health and/or homemaker services as needed
Physical therapy: Graded exercise program with focus on musculoskeletal conditioning progressing to cardiovascular conditioning program with various use of modalities (such as ambulation, arm ergometer, and calisthenics); formulation of home program; ordering of exercise equipment for program as necessary
Dietary service: Diet evaluation and modification with follow-up patient and family education as needed
Respiratory therapy
Community support groups (for example, Mended Hearts)

Frame of reference

Occupational performance

Treatment approach

Rehabilitative

OT EVALUATION

Performance components

Medical history and risk factors
Interview and chart review
Sensorimotor functioning
  Blood pressure, heart rate, EKG, and symptomatic responses to activity: Observe, test, chart review
  Functional capacity: Observe, interview, chart review, test
  Muscle test: Observe functional task performance
  ROM: Observe
  Balance: Observe, test
  Sensation (touch, proprioception, thermal): Observe
Cognitive/Cognitive Integration
  Safety awareness: Interview, observe
  Memory: Test, observe
  Insight into disability: Interview, observe

Psychosocial functioning
  Self-identity: Interview
  Coping skills: Interview, observe
  Adjustment to disability: Observe, interview
  Interpersonal skills: Observe and interview

Performance Areas

Self-care
  Dressing, bathing, transfers: Observe, test
Work-related skills
  Work habits and attitudes: Interview, observe
  Work tolerance: Interview, observe
  Home management: Interview
Play/leisure
  Past and present leisure interests/activities: Interview
  Modes of relaxation and handling stress: Interview, observe

EVALUATION SUMMARY

A chart review and interview reveal that Mr. D has positive risk factors for age, sex, borderline diabetes, smoking, and sedentary lifestyle. He has recurrent bouts of CHF caused by poor compliance with medications. A chart review of recent tests shows normal heart rhythm, enlarged lungs, a small infarct, and diffuse coronary heart disease.

Cardiac monitoring during self-care activities shows normal sinus heart rhythm with appropriate vital sign responses during seated basin bath at bedside. His functional capacity is at the 2.0-MET level.

By observation Mr. D has normal functional ROM, muscle strength, and balance. His endurance is limited to 15 minutes of unsupported sitting for eating. He transfers independently to the bedside commode.

Mr. D has strong denial of his disability resulting in poor safety judgment concerning his functional capacity and prognosis. He is sure he'll feel fine once he gets home where he can get a good night's rest. He would like to leave the transitional care unit for a cigarette, his usual method for handling stress.

Mr. D takes long, hot tub baths. He enjoys light housekeeping in his first-floor apartment, and likes to work straight through until he gets his chores done. He eats most of his meals out and uses the bus for transportation. He sends his laundry out and hires someone to help with the heavy cleaning once a month. He tends to keep to himself.

Assets

Potential for improved endurance
Good living situation
Presence of adults to assist with homemaking
Financial security

Problem list

1. Decreased functional capacity for self-care
2. Little knowledge of current condition and associated signs and symptoms
3. Positive risk factors of smoking and sedentary lifestyle
4. Limited knowledge/practice of energy-conservation techniques
5. History of poor compliance with medications
6. Diet consists of food with high fat, high sodium content.
7. Lives alone; socially isolated

PROBLEM 1: DECREASED FUNCTIONAL CAPACITY FOR SELF-CARE

Objective

Patient will be independent with seated shower at 3.0-MET level

Method

The patient will have daily practice in hygiene, dressing, and grooming with slow progression and close monitoring of blood pressure, heart rate, symptoms, and EKG; the patient will be instructed in energy-conservation techniques and provided with prescription for shower chair

Gradation

The patient will be progressed gradually according to MET-level program, beginning with bathing UEs and dressing independently in a bedside chair

He will progress to full body bathing at bedside, seated shaving, and independent dressing in a chair; if he has appropriate cardiovascular responses to activity, he will progress to seated bathing in the bathroom with standing for oral hygiene; if he continues to have appropriate responses, he will increase his activity level to standing bathing and hygiene (shaving and dental care) in the bathroom

Finally he will progress to a seated shower, shampoo, drying, and dressing

PROBLEM 3: POSITIVE HISTORY OF SMOKING

Objective

The patient will be able to describe on interview the physical effects of nicotine on the cardiovascular system plus the risks of smoking and identify and demonstrate three alternative behaviors to use instead of smoking

Method

The therapist and patient will view and discuss The American Heart Association slide show on smoking, then review and discuss the patient's patterns of smoking behavior; the patient will identify alternative behaviors learned from the slide show and discussion

An activity analysis on prior coping patterns that were successful for the patient when smoking was not acceptable may be completed

Gradation

The patient will demonstrate alternative behaviors (deep breathing, gum chewing); the slide show may be repeated, with pauses to discuss different points in the program to individualize the material

Begin with neutral questions, then move slowly to more personal questions as a trusting relationship is developed

S A M P L E   T R E A T M E N T   P L A N – c o n t ' d

PROBLEM 4: LIMITED KNOWLEDGE AND/OR PRACTICE OF ENERGY-CONSERVATION TECHNIQUE

Objective
The patient will be independent in energy-conservation and pacing techniques and will demonstrate these techniques during performance of the shower

Method
Demonstration of energy-efficient ADL techniques with daily practice; the patient will be trained in body mechanics, work simplification, and relaxation techniques through the use of a tape and slide show

    A written script that follows the slide show will be reviewed and discussed with patient; the patient will be reminded of environmental factors before each ADL treatment

Gradation
Initially the patient will have the entire treatment structured by the therapist (i.e., position, water temperature, duration of activity); as the patient begins to integrate information (as demonstrated during interview), allow the patient to set his own work pace and/or to set water temperature independently to assess his ability to put concepts into practice

REVIEW QUESTIONS

1. Describe the sequence of events (cardiac cycle) responsible for the heart's function as a systemic pump.
2. Name the symptoms and consequences encountered with prolonged cardiac ischemia.
3. Name the cardiac risk factors that can be controlled by medical and therapeutic intervention.
4. Which patients in general rehabilitation clinics may require special program modification as a result of secondary cardiac involvement?
5. Under what circumstances are exercise and activity absolutely contraindicated?
6. List the signs and symptoms of cardiac intolerance to activity.
7. Demonstrate and describe the method of taking an accurate blood pressure.
8. What are METs and how are they used in cardiac rehabilitation?
9. Design a cardiac rehabilitation activity program to be performed over 1 week for a 53-year-old man with cardiomyopathy. He has been described as a Class III cardiac case.
10. Name five factors that may alter the MET level and cardiovascular demand of an activity.
11. A patient with recent bypass surgery performs at a 3.5-MET level on a GXT the day before he goes home. Would you recommend that he take seated or standing showers? Why?

REFERENCES

1. Aiken LH, Henrichs TF: Systematic relaxation as a nursing intervention technique with open heart surgery patients, *Nurs Res* 20:212, 1971.
2. American College of Sports Medicine: *Exercise lite,* Indianapolis, 1993, American College of Sports Medicine.
3. American Heart Association: *The heart of the home,* Dallas, 1965, The Association.
4. American Heart Association: Cardio-pulmonary resuscitation: advanced life support, *JAMA* Suppl 224(5):453-509.
5. American Heart Association: *Recommendations for human blood pressure determination by sphygmomanometers,* Dallas, 1980, The Association Communications Division.
6. American Heart Association: *Fact sheet on heart attack, stroke and risk factors,* Dallas, 1993, The Association.
7. American Occupational Therapy Association: Uniform terminology for occupational therapy: third edition, *Am J Occup Ther* 48(11):1047, 1994
8. Andreoli KG and associates: *Comprehensive cardiac care: a text for nurses, physicians, and other health practitioners,* St Louis, 1983, CV Mosby.
9. Astrand PO, Rodahl K: *Textbook of work physiology,* New York, 1970, McGraw-Hill.
10. Bates B: *A guide to physical examination,* ed 2, Philadelphia, 1979, JB Lippincott Co.
11. Beauchamp N, Creighton C, Summers L: Cardiac work tolerance screening: a case study, *Occup Ther in Health Care* 1(2):99, 1984.
12. Bedsworth JA, Molen MT: Psychological stress in spouses of patients with myocardial infarction, *Heart Lung* 11:450, 1982.
13. Borg G and associates: RPE collection of papers presented at ACSM annual meeting, 1981, *Med Sci Sports Exerc* 14:376, 1982.

14. Bragg TL: Psychological response to myocardial infarction, *Nurs Forum* 14(4):383-395, 1975.

15. Brannon FJ and associates: *Cardiopulmonary rehabilitation: basic theory and application,* ed 2, Philadelphia, 1993, FA Davis.

16. Brock LL and associates: *Cardiac rehabilitation unit program guide,* Dallas, 1977, American Heart Association.

17. Burch GE, and De Pasquale NP: *Primer of clinical measurement of blood pressure,* St Louis, 1962, CV Mosby.

18. Cassem NH, Hackett TP: Psychological rehabilitation of myocardial infarction patients in the acute phase, *Heart Lung* 2:382, 1973.

19. Chandra N, Hazinski M: *Textbook of basic life suppport for healthcare providers,* Dallas, 1994, American Heart Association.

20. Chatham M, Knapp B: *Patient education handbook,* Bowie, Md, 1982, Robert J Brady.

21. Colorado Heart Association: *Exercise equivalents,* Denver, 1970, Cardiac Reconditioning and Work Evaluation Unit, Spalding Rehabilitation Center.

22. Cornett SJ, Watson JE: *Cardiac rehabilitation; an interdisciplinary team approach,* New York, 1984, John Wiley & Sons.

23. Dawber TR: *The Framingham study: the epidemiology of arteriosclerotic disease,* Cambridge, Mass, 1980, Harvard University Press.

24. de Vries HA: *Physiology of exercise,* Dubuque, Iowa, 1978, Wm C Brown.

25. Dracub K and associates: Management of heart failure II. Counseling, education, and lifestyle modifications , *JAMA* 272(18), 1994.

26. Dubin D: *Rapid interpretation of EKGs,* Tampa, Fla, 1974, COVER.

27. European Society of Cardiology: Long-term comprehensive care of cardiac patients, *Eur Heart Jour* 13(suppl C), 1992.

28. Fox SM, Naughton JP, Gorman PA: Physical activity and cardiovascular health: the exercise prescription, frequency and type of activity, *Mod Concepts Cardiovasc Dis* 41:6, 1972.

29. Gentry WD, Haney T: Emotional and behavioral reaction to acute myocardial infarction, *Heart Lung* 4:738, 1975.

30. Goldberger E: *Essential of clinical cardiology,* Philadelphia, 1990, JB Lippincott.

31. Halpenny CJ: The cardiac cycle. In Underhill SL and associates, editors: *Cardiac nursing,* Philadelphia, 1982, JB Lippincott.

32. Haskell WL: Design of a cardiac conditioning program. In Wenger N, editor: *Exercise and the heart,* Philadelphia, 1978, FA Davis.

33. Hellerstein HK: Rehabilitation of the cardiac patient, *JAMA* 164:225, 1957.

34. Kattus AA and associates: *Exercise testing and training of individuals with heart disease or at high risk for its development: a handbook for physicians,* Dallas, 1975, American Heart Association.

35. Katz A: Effects of ischemia and hypoxia upon the myocardium. In Russak H, Zohman B, editors: *Coronary heart disease,* Philadelphia, 1971, JB Lippincott.

36. King K: Emotional responses and experiences of wives of men who survive a sudden cardiac death event, *Cardiovascular Nursing* 28(3), 1992.

37. Kottke TE, Haney TH, Doucette MM: Rehabilitation of the patient with heart disease. In Kottke FJ, Lehmann JF: *Krusen's handbook of physical medicine and rehabilitation,* ed 4, Philadelphia, 1990, WB Saunders.

38. Lancour J: How to avoid pitfalls in measuring blood pressure, *Am J Nurs* 76:773, 1976.

39. Maloney FP, Moss K: *Energy requirements for selected activities,* Denver, 1974, Department of Physical Medicine, National Jewish Hospital, Unpublished.

40. May GS and associates: Secondary prevention after myocardial infarction: a review of long term trials, *Prog Card Dis* 24:331, 1982.

41. Milnor WR: The heart as a pump. In Mountcastle VB, editor: *Medical physiology,* vol 2, ed 14, St Louis, 1979, CV Mosby.

42. Newton K, Sivarajan E: Cardiac rehabilitation: life style adjustments. In Underhill SL and associates, editors: *Cardiac nursing,* Philadelphia, 1982, JB Lippincott.

43. New York Heart Association: *Nomenclature and criteria for diagnosis of disease of the heart and great vessels,* ed 8, Boston, 1979, Little Brown.

44. Niles N, Wills R: Heart failure. In Underhill SL and associates, editors: *Cardiac nursing,* Philadelphia, 1982, JB Lippincott.

45. Ogden LD: *Guidelines for analysis and testing of activities of daily living with cardiac patients,* Downey, Calif, 1981, Cardiac Rehabilitation Resources.

46. Ogden LD: *Procedure guidelines for monitored self-care evaluation and monitored task evaluation,* Downey, Calif, 1981, Cardiac Rehabilitation Resources.

47. O'Leary SS: *Monitored showers during inpatient rehabilitation following cardiac events,* master's thesis, San José, 1986, San José State University.

48. Rushmer RF: *Cardiovascular dynamics,* Philadelphia, 1976, WB Saunders.

49. Santa Clara Valley Medical Center: *Cardiac rehabilitation program protocol,* rev, San José, Calif, 1991, Unpublished.

50. Scalzi C, Burke L: Myocardial infarction: behavioral responses of patient and spouses. In Underhill SL and associates, editors: *Cardiac nursing,* Philadelphia, 1982, JB Lippincott.

51. Silverman M: *Examination of the heart: the clinical history,* Dallas, 1978, American Heart Association.

52. Sivarajan SE: Cardiac rehabilitation: activity and exercise programs. In Underhill SL and associates, editors: *Cardiac nursing,* Philadelphia, 1982, JB Lippincott.

53. Sokolow M, McIlroy MB: *Clinical cardiology,* Los Altos, Calif, 1977, Lange Medical Publications.

54. Stamford B: *Fitness without exercise,* 1990, Warner Books.

55. Trobaugh G: Cardiomyopathies. In Underhill SL and associates, editors: *Cardiac nursing,* Philadelphia, 1982, JB Lippincott.

56. University of Colorado Medical Center, Department of Physical Medicine and Rehabilitation: *Coronary Heart Disease Rehabilitation,* Denver, 1971 (pamphlet).

57. Wenger N: The physiological basis of early ambulation after myocardial infarction. In Wenger N, editor: *Exercise and the heart,* Philadelphia, 1978, FA Davis.

58. Wulff K, Hong P: Surgical intervention for coronary artery disease. In Underhill SL and associates, editors: *Cardiac nursing,* Philadelphia, 1982, JB Lippincott.

Low Back Pain

Joan Smithline

Low back pain (LBP) is a complex, multifaceted medical problem that represents an exciting challenge to the occupational therapist. LBP affects the physical, psychological, emotional, financial, and social aspects of a person's life.[1,10] The occupational therapist, well trained in the psychosocial and physical aspects of rehabilitation, is an important member of the health care team.

In the United States, approximately 24 billion dollars are spent each year on the direct and indirect costs of LBP.[4] "Back pain is second only to the common cold as a reason for Americans to visit their doctors."[9] LBP primarily affects adults aged 25 to 55 years, placing a significant burden on the work force.[4] In fact, LBP represents approximately 16% of all worker's compensation claims. Medical costs represent 32% of the total costs, and paid time for lost workdays represents 65% of the total costs.[16]

The goals for managing LBP are the prevention of prolonged disability and the speedy return to work. Occupational and physical therapists, working cooperatively with other members of the health care team, have vital roles in the rehabilitation process.

Diagnosis of LBP is difficult and presents an obstacle to successful treatment.[10] Other obstacles include frequent recurrence, wide variation in patient responses to specific pathological findings, and multiple causes of LBP in a patient.[12] LBP is often not the result of one single injury or event, but instead it results from the accumulation of stressful activities and positions over several hours, months, or even years. These activities include prolonged static postures such as slouched sitting and forward bending as well as repetitive tasks like pulling, lifting, and carrying. Poor posture and faulty body mechanics used during home and work activities contribute substantially to LBP.

The occupational therapist's role in the rehabilitation of the LBP patient may vary, depending on the division of responsibility at the particular health care facility. Patient education and training in functional activities while maintaining normal spinal alignment is a critical part of the rehabilitation program. Whether pain is acute or chronic, the patient with low back pain will respond best to a team approach with medical professionals who are knowledgeable, positive, and willing to work with the patient for a successful outcome.

SPINAL ANATOMY

To understand the medical and rehabilitation management of LBP, a brief review of lumbar anatomy is presented. A more in-depth study of spinal anatomy is recommended for those who will treat this population of patients.

VERTEBRAE

The spine is composed of 33 stacked spinal vertebrae, 24 of which are movable (7 cervical, 12 thoracic, and 5 lumbar). Below those are 5 that are fused together to form the sacrum, and 4 rudimentary fused vertebrae that form the coccyx. The vertebrae are arranged in an *S* curve balanced around the line of gravity. The lumbar vertebrae are the largest, reflecting the increasing load from head to pelvis. Each vertebra is made up of two parts: the vertebral body anteriorly, and the vertebral arch posteriorly. The vertebral bodies are kidney-shaped and separated by intervertebral discs.[8] The vertebral arch is made up of the pedicles, laminae, and seven bony transverse and articular processes.

The vertebral body and arch (Fig. 37-1) form an irregular ring called the vertebral foramen. The vertebral foramina of adjacent vertebrae form the spinal canal that encloses the spinal cord and its blood vessels. Facet joints made from the four articular processes above and below the transverse process guide and restrict the movements of the spine: flexion, extension, lateral flexion, and some rotation. The orientation of these facet joints allows considerable movement in trunk flexion and extension but limits lateral flexion and rotation. The transverse processes serve as the attachments for muscles and ligaments. At the junction of the vertebral body and arch, the vertebral notches of adjacent vertebrae form the intervertebral foramen where the spinal nerves exit.

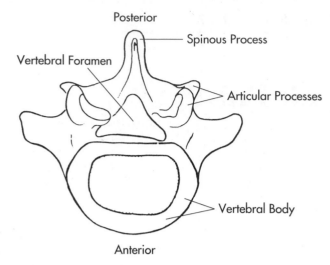

FIG. 37-1   Vertebral body and arch. (From Callahan P and associates: *Stanford Back School Manual,* Stanford, Calif, 1984, Dept. of OT/PT, Stanford University Hospital.).

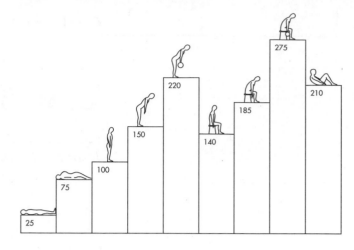

FIG. 37-2   Relative change in pressure in third lumbar disc with various postures and movements. (Adapted from Nachemson A: The lumbar spine: an orthopedic challenge, *Spine* 1(1):59, 1976.)

LIGAMENTS

Spinal ligaments function to restrain or align the vertebrae. The anterior longitudinal ligament (ALL), a thick, strong band of fibers, runs along the anterior surface of the vertebral bodies firmly attaching to the bodies and the intervertebral discs. The ALL limits extension of the vertebral column.

The posterior longitudinal ligament (PLL) runs along the posterior aspect of the vertebral bodies anterior to the spinal cord. In the lumbar region it narrows considerably contributing to the inherent structural weakness at the lower lumbar levels where there is the greatest amount of spinal movement. The PLL functions to limit spinal flexion.

The ligamenta flava connect the lamina of adjacent vertebrae and lie posterior to the spinal cord. These ligaments limit flexion of the spinal column, and their elastic quality assists the spine to return to upright from a flexed posture.[7]

INTERVERTEBRAL DISCS

Disorders of the intervertebral discs are common causes of LBP. The discs, interposed between adjacent surfaces of the vertebral bodies, are composed of two parts. The central portion or nucleus pulposus is a gelatinous substance and is surrounded by the annulus fibrosis, made up of concentric and oblique fibers that encase the nucleus. The nucleus is held under pressure in this casing. During vertebral column movements, the nucleus moves posteriorly with flexion, anteriorly with extension, and to the opposite side with lateral flexion. Rotation substantially increases disc pressure and stretches the annular fibers. Static or repetitive flexion forces the nucleus posteriorly and can more easily rupture through the annulus. The combination movement of flexion and rotation is even more stressful to the disc.[8]

The lumbar discs are the widest but suffer a substantial loss of height in the aging process, hence the loss of spinal flexibility and height with advancing age. The nucleus pulposus sits more posteriorly in the lumbar spine. The annulus is therefore narrower and offers less support. These anatomical factors make the lumbar discs more vulnerable to injury, which contributes to the high incidence of LBP. Once a load on the disc is removed, it regains its normal height. This process requires a finite amount of time and depends on the health and age of the disc. If the disc is loaded again without time to regain its height, premature aging and potential derangement can result.[8]

When the disc is young and healthy and there is violence to the spine, the bones give way first. After age 25, degenerative changes occur in the annulus fibrosis and the structure is weakened. Under these conditions, a minor strain can cause internal derangement of the disc, which causes severe pain and muscle spasm.[15] A study by Nachemson demonstrated stress to the L3 disc in various positions and postures (Fig. 37-2),[13] which correlates well with the common histories of patients with LBP as well as the anatomical considerations described previously.

NERVES

The lumbar nerves exit at the intervertebral foramen at the levels of their respective vertebrae, conveying sensation and motor control to and from the lower extremities. The three major nerves innervating lower extremity musculature are the femoral, obdurator, and sciatic nerves. The close relationship of the discs, ligaments, and facet joints to the nerves complicates the ability to diagnose LBP. Patients with LBP who develop lower extremity symptoms should seek medical attention. When pain and symptoms move distally, the spinal nerve root may be compromised, as in sciatica.

MUSCLES

The muscles of the spine function to move the vertebral column, but do little to keep it erect. This function is done by the hip and thigh muscles, primarily through the strong ligamentous support of the spine.[7] The muscles of the low back are divided into three groups: the postvertebral, prevertebral, and lateral trunk muscles. The postvertebral muscles act to extend the spinal column and limit flexion of the trunk, and they accentuate the lumbar lordosis. They are divided into deep, intermediate, and superficial muscles. The deeper they lie, the shorter their course. The deep muscles include the transversospinalis, interspinalis, spinalis, longissimus, and iliocostalis. At the intermediate level is only one muscle, the serratus posterior inferior. The superficial muscle is the latissimus dorsi. The paravertebral muscles are known as the abdominal muscles and include the rectus abdominus, internal and external obliques, and the transversus abdominus. They flex the spine, flatten the lumbar lordosis, and assist in rotating the spine. The lateral muscles of the trunk are the quadratus lumborum and the psoas. They flex the spine ipsilaterally and rotate it contralaterally, as well as accentuate the lumbar lordosis and flex the vertebral column when the pelvis is fixed.[8]

In summary, the spine is composed of a network of structures: the vertebrae, discs, ligaments, nerves, and muscles. The lumbar spine withstands the greatest kinetic strain and, because of the inherent structural weakness of the intervertebral discs and ligaments, is most vulnerable to injury.

REHABILITATION OF THE PATIENT WITH LBP

The 1990s have brought dramatic changes in health care delivery systems in the United States. In health maintenance organizations and managed care systems, the primary care physician (PCP) must screen all patients first, and insurance companies require prior authorization for medical care including physical therapy (PT) and occupational therapy (OT). Visits are limited and therapists must evaluate, plan treatment regimes, and establish functional outcomes in a limited time. Patients must demonstrate consistent compliance and motivation and take full responsibility for their medical care.

The PCP sees the patient with LBP first. The initial evaluation will vary, depending on the expertise of the PCP (e.g., internist, general practitioner, obstetrician/gynecologist, pediatrician). The examination should include a thorough medical history, both past and present; a review of the symptoms and functional limitations; observation of posture, gait, trunk mobility, strength, reflexes, and sensation; and palpation of the spine and surrounding soft tissues. A diagnosis is made and medication, usually nonsteroidal antiinflammatory drugs (NSAIDS), is prescribed along with rest and restrictions on activities. Unfortunately, pamphlets with instructions for exercise are sometimes given without additional direction. If substantial relief is not achieved in about a week, a course of PT and OT is prescribed if the physician is knowledgeable about rehabilitation.

CONSERVATIVE APPROACH
Evaluation
Physical therapy

Often the patient is first referred to PT to address the pain, muscle spasm, limited joint mobility, and postural defects. The physical therapy evaluation includes a subjective history including the following information: (1) mechanism of injury; (2) progression of symptoms; (3) recent treatment and results; (4) past medical history; (5) sleep disturbances, including sleep surface, positions, and pillows, (6) work postures; (7) ADL postures and the behavior of the symptoms during these postures and activities (Fig. 37-3); and (8) prior level of function in self-care, work, and leisure activities.

An objective examination follows including analysis of (1) static and dynamic posture; (2) gait; (3) active ROM of the spine; (4) active ROM of all extremities; (5) pelvic asymmetry; (6) tension signs, (7) strength, reflexes, and sensation; (8) lower extremity (LE) muscle flexibility and symmetry, (9) passive movement testing of the spinal segments; and (10) palpation of soft tissue restrictions along the spine and surrounding areas. Special tests are performed to help with differential diagnosis, especially to identify sacroiliac dysfunction and hip pathology.

Analysis of data will yield a treatment plan, which may include: (1) positioning for relief of muscle spasm and pain; (2) mobilization techniques to improve mobility of specific joints and soft tissues and relieve muscle spasm and pain; (3) muscle stretching to gain symmetry to all musculature, especially the LEs; (4) training in posture, body mechanics, strengthening, conditioning, and returning to recreational sports and activities. Training in a home program includes first aid tips for pain and muscle spasm relief, flexibility, mobility, symptom control, posture correction, strengthening, and general conditioning for optimal health and return to the preinjury level of function. The overall goals of PT are to provide symptom relief, to normalize joint and soft tissue mobility, and to establish an effective exercise regime to achieve the highest functional level for the patient.

Occupational therapy

The occupational therapist (OT) evaluates the patient through subjective history and observation, emphasizing ADL and work-related tasks. In a team approach, the subjective history obtained by the physical therapist can be shared with the occupational therapist. Then detailed information related to ADL and tolerance to activity can be ascertained. A physical assessment including strength, extremity and trunk mobility, general posture, and ambulation is performed.

A functional assessment of the patient's ADL is impor-

STANFORD HEALTH SERVICES
REHABILITATION SERVICES QUESTIONNAIRE

Name: _____ Age: _____ Date: _____

1. Pain Began: _____ How? _____
                    Month   Year

_____

2. Please draw a picture of your pain today.

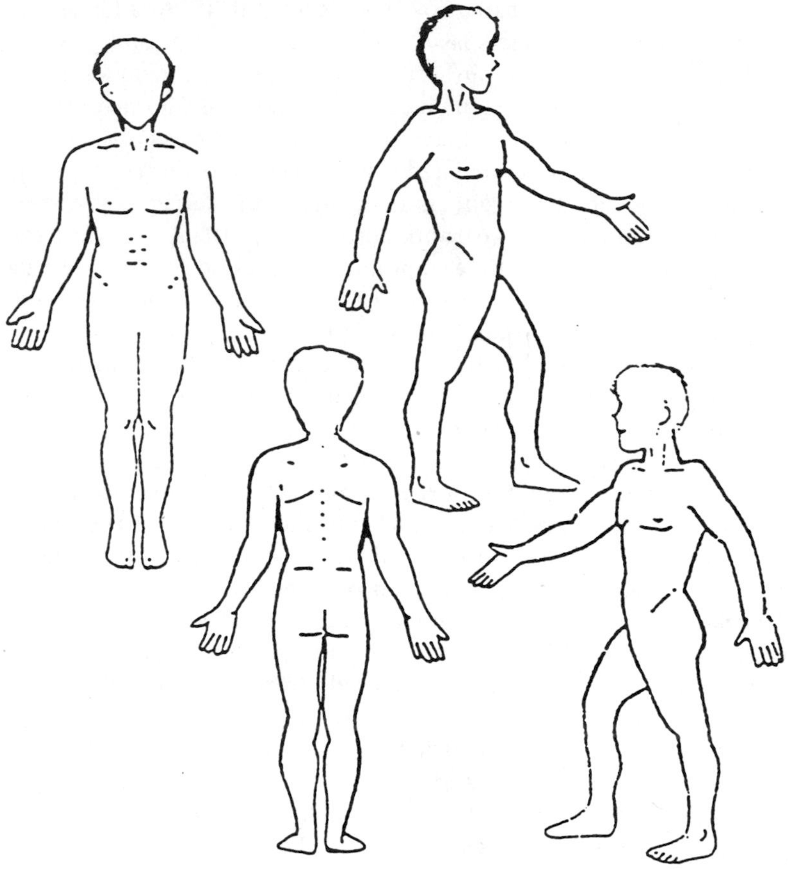

3. Rate your pain:
   0 = Painfree   10 = Severe/Disabling

   |----+----+----+----+----+----+----+----+----+----|
   0   5   10

4. Medications: _____

_____

5. Does rest help decrease your pain?
   yes_____   no _____

6. Please check if you have (or have had):
   ____ High blood pressure   ____ Bowel/Bladder
   ____ Respiratory   ____ Pregnancy
   ____ Heart disease   ____ Allergies
   ____ Diabetes   ____ Skin Disorders
   ____ Arthritis
   ____ Fractures (where?_____)
   ____ Cancer (where?_____)
   ____ Neurological disease

8. Please list surgeries/dates: _____

_____

_____

7. Please check if you have had:

√	Test	Results
	CT Scan	
	MRI	
	Myelogram	
	X-Rays	
	EMG/NCV	

9. Doctor's restrictions on activity – please list:

_____

_____

10. A. What is your occupation? _____
    B. Are you currently working? _____Yes _____No Last day worked: _____
    C. What percentage of your day do you sit? _____ Stand? _____

11. Please check if you have difficulty performing the following activities:
    ____ Dressing   ____ Childcare   ____ Gardening   ____ Housekeeping
    ____ Toileting   ____ Cooking   ____ Home or car repair   ____ Public transportation
    ____ Bathing   ____ Laundry   ____ Shopping   ____ Keyboard/typing
    ____ Eating   ____ Walking   ____ Telephone   ____ Driving car
    ____ Writing   ____ Other: _____

FIG. 37-3 *Rehabilitation Services Questionnaire.* (Reprinted with permission, J. Smithline, Stanford Health Services, Dept. Rehab Services, Stanford, Calif., 1993.

718

12.

My pain is	BETTER	WORSE	NO CHANGE	MAX. TIME (MINUTES)
Sitting (soft chair)				
Sitting (hard chair)				
Lying on my stomach				
Lying on my back				
Lying on my side				
Walking				
Standing				
Climbing stairs				
Coughing or sneezing				
Putting on my shoes				
Bending over				
Lifting				
First thing in the morning				
Middle of the day				
Before bedtime				

13. I wake up at night because of pain _____ 0, _____ 1-2, _____ 3 or more times a night.

14. Please check all treatments for pain that you have received and <u>circle</u> those that have helped the most.

√	TREATMENT	√	TREATMENT
	Medication		Chiropractic
	Bed rest		Acupressure
	Hospitalization, but no surgery		Acupuncture
	Injections		Other. Describe:
	Back manipulations		
	Corset or brace		
	Physical therapy, Where?		When?
	Name of P.T. or clinic:		Phone #

15. If you have had physical therapy, what did your treatment include? Please check all that apply:

√	TREATMENT	√	TREATMENT
	Hot packs		Ultrasound
	Ice packs		Massage
	Range of motion exercises		TENS (transcutaneous nerve stimulator)
	Strengthening exercises		Training in posture, body mechanics
	Spinal mobilization		Conditioning program
	Electrical stimulation		Home exercise program. Since:
	Traction (Sitting)		Other. Describe:
	Traction (Lying)		

16. Are you performing a home exercise program? _____ Yes _____ No   How often? _____ × week.

17. What are your leisure activities now? _____

_____

18. What activities (vocational, functional, recreational) do you want to return to? _____

_____

_____

19. If we could do <u>one</u> thing for you, what would it be? _____

FIG. 37-4   cont'd. For legend see opposite page.

tant. Actual observation of each task enables the OT to evaluate faulty postures and body mechanics. Often patients can verbalize the general principles for minimizing stress to the spine, but are not aware that they do not observe these principles in ADL. A kitchen, bedroom, and work simulation area greatly enhances the occupational therapist's ability for evaluation. Activities including dressing, toileting, hygiene and self-care, bed mobility, transfers (from bed, sofa, chair, bath, and shower), loading and unloading the dishwasher, meal preparation, oven use, refrigerator use, carrying and lifting from various heights, reaching, and simulated work activities can be observed and problems identified. Organization of the kitchen, home work environment, and arrangement of frequently used objects can be discussed and modified to minimize spinal stress.

Observation of spontaneous movements such as scratching the foot, sitting posture, and rising from a chair can also be observed and compared to simulated tasks performed when the patient knows he or she is being tested. Pain behaviors such as facial grimacing and audible grunts are noted. Specific lifting and carrying evaluations can be performed using work evaluation systems or simulations created in the OT clinic. The patient's functional capacity is quantified to establish a baseline for setting goals. Throughout the functional assessment the occupational therapist observes spinal posture, keeping in mind the anatomical constraints of the spinal structures. This approach enables the OT to design a specific treatment plan, which includes the following:

1. education in energy conservation and pacing skills to be used with all ADL and work-related tasks for symptom control
2. progressive repetitive tasks to build strength and endurance for specific activities, minimizing spinal stress
3. education in faulty body mechanics and poor postures with specific tasks and practice in correct techniques
4. training in use of assistive devices to increase independence in ADL when there is pain and limitation and to minimize recurrence of symptoms
5. training in simulated work tasks to minimize spinal stress and grading tolerance to these tasks

The overall goal of OT in treatment of patients with LBP is to achieve the highest level of functional independence in all ADL and leisure and work activities.

Treatment
Physical therapy

The first goal of PT is to help the patient find a pain-free position for rest. Each person is different but positions of comfort can often be found in prone, supine, and side-lying, using pillows and towel rolls to support the contours of the body and allow muscles to relax (Fig. 37-4). Resting should be performed as an exercise. Lying down for 10 to 20 minutes three or more times a day can decrease the stress to the spine and provide considerable

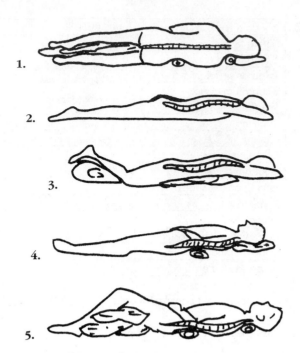

FIG. 37-4 Positions for rest using pillows and towel rolls to support body contours, allowing muscles to relax. (From Smithline J: *First aid tips for back pain,* Stanford, Calif, 1993, Stanford Health Services, Department of Rehab Services.)

pain relief. Bed rest is rarely prescribed now because of the threat of decreased muscle tone but if patients are unable to tolerate the upright position, lying down most of the day is indicated. Pain relief should occur in one to three days.

Patients with back pain should not exercise because this activity can aggravate the symptoms and prolong the disability. Once pain is controlled, exercise can be initiated. Exercises must be designed for the specific individual and should be performed slowly, gently, and progressively, as the symptoms allow. Exercise must be performed pain-free. Ice (or heat) can be used at home to relieve pain and decrease abnormal muscle tone while resting. Home remedies for ice or heat pack are detailed in Box 37-1. The side-lying and prone positions are most favored and allow ease in using ice or heat pack applications. Supine lying is least favored because of the direct pressure on the lumbar spine and the stress placed on the anatomical structures when the spine flattens to meet the supporting surface. Patients are cautioned against sitting in hot tubs or saunas.

Bed mobility can contribute to LBP if performed without elimination of torsion and flexion of the lumbar spine (Fig. 37-5). Lying down on the bed using a prone approach is also helpful. To do so, hands touch the bed while the leg closest to the bed is elevated to mattress level. The trunk is slowly lowered to the bed surface and the supporting leg is then lifted on to the bed. Spinal alignment is maintained during this maneuver.

Sitting, especially if prolonged, often aggravates LBP. Besides using correct posture, patients must learn to use

B O X   3 7 - 1

USE OF ICE OR HEAT TO REDUCE MUSCLE SPASM

USE ICE OR HEAT:

Ice or heat or both can be very helpful in reducing pain and muscle spasm. Ice is usually more effective than heat. Sometimes using heat for 10 minutes, then ice for 10 minutes works well. Below are some home preparation techniques.

REMEMBER:

1. Use ice or heat when resting, *not sleeping or sitting.*
2. Use no longer than 20 minutes.

3. Repeat 3 to 5 times per day as pain indicates.

ICE PACK PREPARATION:

Method 1

Place an unopened bag of frozen peas wrapped in a damp towel on the back. Use as directed above. Return peas to freezer. Use again and again. DO NOT EAT THE PEAS.

Method 2

Place cracked ice cubes in a Ziploc bag. Place on a damp towel on the back. Use as directed above. Return to the freezer. Recrack ice before next application.

HEAT PACK PREPARATION:

Method 1

Place damp towel in microwave to heat. Test temperature, then place on back. Use as directed above.

Method 2

Use heating pad set on LOW. Do *not* sleep on the heating pad. Do not sit in chair with heating pad. Use as directed above.

From Smithline J, *First aid tips for back pain,* Stanford, Calif, 1993, Stanford Health Services, Department of Rehab Services.

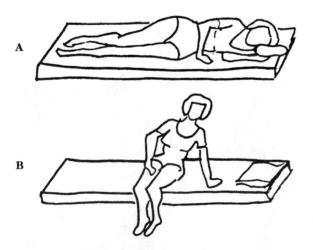

FIG. 37-5 Method for getting up from bed or couch to reduce stress on low back. **A,** Roll to side. **B,** Bend knees forward to bring feet off bed and push up to sitting, using arms and keeping back straight with normal curve. (From Smithline J: *First aid tips for back pain,* Stanford, Calif, 1993, Stanford Health Services, Department of Rehab Services.)

lumbar supports. These can be created by rolling up a towel to fit the lumbar curve (Fig. 37-6, see p. 722).

If the pain and muscle spasm continues, the therapist may use modalities such as ultrasound or electrical stimulation to normalize muscle tone and decrease pain. Pelvic traction can be helpful in relieving LE radicular symptoms, pain and paresthesias radiating into one or both lower extremities.

The physical therapist will perform a variety of manual therapy techniques including (1) joint mobilization to provide pain relief and reestablish normal physiologic and accessory ROM to the lumbar spinal segments; (2) soft tissue mobilization, including myofascial and massage techniques to alter soft tissue restrictions that contribute to pain and mobility limitations; (3) muscle stretching to achieve symmetry and normal length to LE muscles that directly affect spinal function. These muscles include the hamstrings, psoas, tensor fascia lata, piriformis, rectus femoris, gastrocnemius and soleus.

Once pain relief is achieved and symptoms are under control, aerobic and strength training can begin, but must be very conservative and graded very gently. Recurrence of LBP is frequent and often the result of advancing

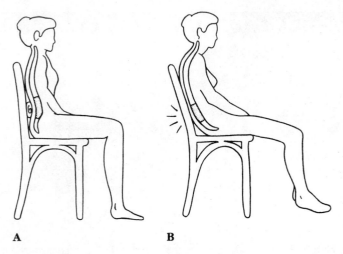

FIG. 37-6   Sitting postures. Most important is keeping normal curves in back, preferably by ensuring proper support, especially for low back. (From Callahan P and associates: *Stanford Back School Manual*, Stanford, Calif, 1984, Stanford Health Services, Dept of Rehabilitation Services.)

too rapidly with exercise or activity. Pool exercise is an excellent treatment alternative for patients in the acute stage. The buoyancy of the water and elimination of gravity on the weight-bearing joints allows ease of movement and a medium that enables pain-free exercise. Walking and specific exercise is more easily tolerated, and patient compliance is very good. Pool temperatures for ambulation and exercise should be 88 to 92° F. Swimming laps, if tolerated, can also be beneficial. Using aqua vests or flotation devices can allow vigorous aerobic activity to be performed without loading the spine vertically.

Teaching and modifying a home program will be ongoing during the course of treatment. With health insurance limitations, PT visits may be extended over time to allow musculoskeletal changes to take place, allowing for changes in the program with each visit. An average of three to six visits is commonly authorized by HMO and managed care programs. Some insurance benefits limit the duration of treatment to 60 days. These time constraints often make completion of a PT program and returning to work and regular activity difficult.

Occupational therapy

OT can begin as soon as the patient can tolerate activity in the upright position. Training in bed mobility and training in transfers to chair, toilet, bed, and car are also needed in the early stage. Communication with PT is important so that (1) both therapists teach posture and body mechanics with similar principles and (2) suggestions for spinal alignment are coordinated. The OT also addresses self-care, including hygiene, dressing, and meal preparation. Assistive devices are considered and ordered if necessary.

Functional training and practice with techniques will be more successful than just discussing them with the patient. Examples include sitting, lifting (Fig. 37-7), carrying, and standing. These activities are monitored to quantify progress. Work simplification and energy conservation skills are taught and applied to all functional activities.

Most important, the OT performs a functional capacity or work tolerance assessment. This information is vital to the physician, patient, and employer and is the foundation for the development of reasonable, achieva-

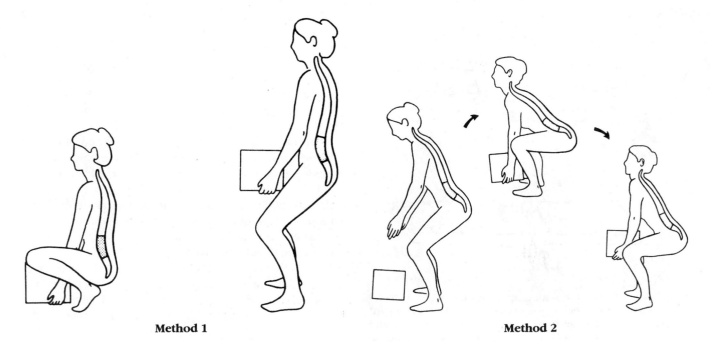

Method 1   **Method 2**

FIG. 37-7   Lifting methods that protect lumbar spine from injury. (From Callahan P and associates: *Stanford Back School Manual*, Stanford, Calif, 1984, Stanford Health Services, Dept of Rehabilitation Services.)

ble goals. Returning to work may mean part-time employment or activity-restricted work. This activity level can be determined by the OT through evaluation and observation of simulated work tasks. Troubleshooting is important before the patient attempts to return to work. This approach helps prevent exacerbation of symptoms or reinjury. Treatment frequency may increase as the patient improves. A work hardening program can be initiated and job simulation tasks practiced and timed (see Chapter 30).

Body mechanics training. Activities of daily living (ADL) require scrutiny to observe stresses on the lumbar spine. Keeping in mind the anatomical weakness in the lumbar disc and PLL, the OT needs to observe patients in all daily tasks, especially those that were reported to aggravate symptoms in the subjective assessment.

The following information is adapted from *Managing Low Back Pain.*[11] Numerous everyday activities are evaluated and faulty body mechanics are described as unbalanced. Stressful positions include prolonged static postures with a flexed lumbar spine, repetitive bending with a flexed spine, and lifting and carrying when the normal lumbar curve is not maintained. It is very important to avoid tasks or positions that do not allow a balanced posture. The patient should take a few seconds to approach each task in a way that minimizes stress to the back.

Bathroom activities. Forward bending places increased stress on structures in back and neck. To work

---

Forward bending places increased stress on the structures in the back and neck.

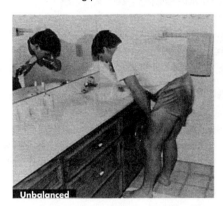 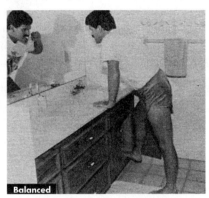 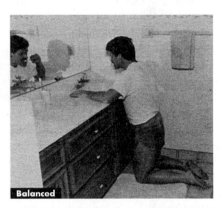

If you are going to work over the bathroom sink, place one hand on the counter to support your weight and bend at the hips, not the back. Elevate one foot and keep your head up and your back in a balanced position.

You can also try performing some of your sink activities in the kneeling position to reduce the temptation to bend forward. Use the counter for support when you come to standing.

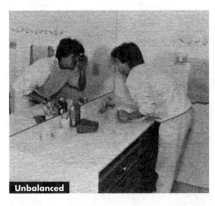 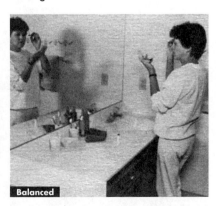 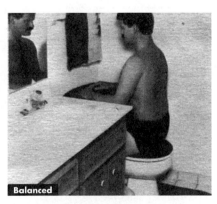

Using a hand-held mirror eliminates the need to bend over the sink.

During an acute episode of back pain you can minimize stress when using the toilet by facing the back of the toilet. This will prevent you from bending forward and will provide you with support when you come to standing.

Additional suggestions: Purchasing an accordion mounted mirror for shaving and applying make-up allows you to avoid the temptation to lean over the sink. Purchase a good shower caddy and place razor, toothbrush, tooth paste, and face cloth in the shower. Use a tub mirror (not glass) to avoid activities over a low sink.

FIG. 37-8 Bathroom activities. (From Melnik M, Saunders R, Saunders HD: *Managing back pain: daily activities guide for back pain patients.* Reprinted with permission, Educational Opportunities, H Duane Saunders, 4250 Norex Drive, Chaska, MN 55318.)

over the bathroom sink, the patient should place one hand on the counter to support weight and bend at the hips, not the back. The patient should elevate one foot and keep the head up and the back in a balanced position. The patient can also try performing some of the sink activities in the kneeling position to reduce the temptation to bend forward. The counter can be used for support when coming to standing (Fig. 37-8, **A**, see p. 723). Using a handheld mirror eliminates the need to bend over the sink. During an acute episode of back pain the patient minimizes stress when using the toilet by facing the back of the toilet to prevent bending forward and provide support when coming to standing (Fig. 37-8, **B**).

Additional suggestions include the following: (1) an accordion-mounted mirror for shaving and applying make-up prevents the temptation to lean over the sink; (2) a good shower caddy can hold razor, toothbrush, toothpaste, and facecloth in the shower; a tub mirror (not glass) can help the patient avoid activities over a low sink.

Bedmaking. When making the bed, the patient should not stand on one side and reach. The temptation to bend forward can be reduced by kneeling or climbing onto the bed, which encourages keeping the back in a balanced position. To perform the task while standing, the patient should walk around the bed to complete the far side. Using a lightweight comforter instead of a heavy bedspread decreases spinal stress (Fig. 37-9).

Kitchen activities. Commonly used items can be arranged between waist and shoulder height to reduce the need to bend over. To reach something from a lower level, the patient can drop down onto one knee, grab the object, put the object on the counter, and then use the support of a table, chair, or counter to assist in coming to standing. This support helps maintain the normal curves in the spine. If support is not available, the patient can place hands on thighs and push off with arms (Fig. 37-10, **A**).

To load the dishwasher, the patient should place the rinsed dishes on the counter near the dishwasher, go to one knee, and load the dishwasher from this position. This method helps avoid prolonged or repetitive forward bending and twisting movements. The process is reversed to unload the dishwasher. The patient should use support when coming to standing.

The following are additional suggestions: (1) remove silverware basket before loading and place it on the counter, fill with silverware while standing, then return basket to the dishwasher; (2) use top tray only to decrease need for bending (Fig. 37-10, **B**).

Laundry. When doing laundry, loads should be kept small and manageable. Several small loads place less stress on the back than one or two large ones. The patient should avoid bending forward into the machines and should not try to handle large bundles of clothes, particularly if they are wet. When loading or unloading a front-loading washer or dryer, the patient should drop to one knee to avoid any forward bending and twisting, and should use support when coming to standing (Fig. 37-11).

Home maintenance. *Participation in vacuuming, car maintenance, mowing, and shoveling is not*

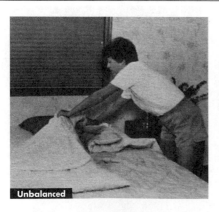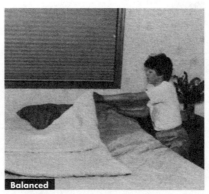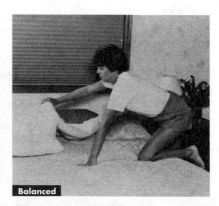

Unbalanced   Balanced   Balanced

When making the bed, do not stand on one side and reach. The temptation to bend forward can be reduced by kneeling or climbing onto the bed. This will encourage you to keep your back in a balanced position. If you are going to perform the task while standing, walk around the bed to complete the far side.

Additional suggestions: Use a light weight comforter instead of a heavy bedspread to decrease spinal stress.

FIG. 37-9   Making a bed. (From Melnik M, Saunders R, Saunders HD: *Managing back pain: daily activities guide for back pain patients.* Reprinted with permission, Educational Opportunities, H. Duane Saunders, 4250 Norex Drive, Chaska, MN 55318.)

It is very important to avoid tasks or positions which do not allow a balanced posture. Take a few seconds to approach each task in a way which will minimize the stress to your back.

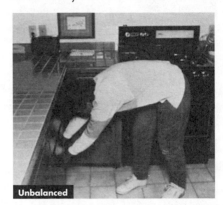
Unbalanced

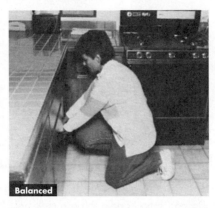
Balanced

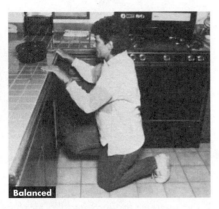
Balanced

Arrange commonly used items between waist and shoulder height to reduce the need to bend over. If you need to reach something from a lower level, drop down onto one knee, grab the object, put the object on the counter and then use the support of a table, chair or counter to assist you while you come to standing. This support will help you maintain the normal curves in your spine. If you do not have support available, place your hands on your thighs and push off with your arms.

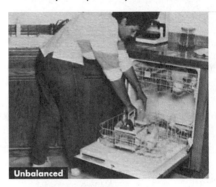
Unbalanced

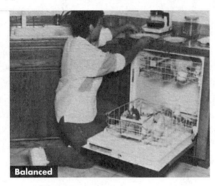
Balanced

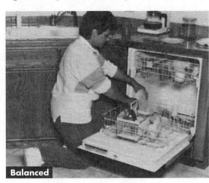
Balanced

To load the dishwasher, place the rinsed dishes on the counter near the dishwasher. Go to one knee and load the dishwasher from this position. This helps you avoid prolonged or repetitive forward bending and twisting movements. Reverse the process to unload the dishwasher. Use support when you come to standing.

Additional suggestions: Remove silverware basket before loading and place it on the counter. Fill with silverware while standing, then return the basket to the dishwasher. Use top tray only to decrease bending.

FIG. 37-10   Kitchen activities. (From Melnik M, Saunders R, Saunders HD: *Managing back pain: daily activities guide for back pain patients.* Reprinted with permission, Educational Opportunities, H. Duane Saunders, 4250 Norex Drive, Chaska, MN 55318.)

recommended during the early stages of recovery. These activities are presented to offer methods for preventing a recurrence of symptoms once the condition has stabilized.

Sweeping and vacuuming can be performed as if the vacuum or broom were attached to the body. The patient should move the feet and legs rather than reaching or bending forward and should avoid twisting. If it is necessary to vacuum or sweep under a table or chair, the patient should bend at the hips and knees and keep the back in a balanced position (Fig. 37-12). Lightweight electric brooms make the job much easier. The patient should beware of self-powered vacuum cleaners, which are very heavy.

Following are some additional recommendations for ADL. For gardening, the use of long-handled tools is helpful. Some shovels come with hand-controlled jaws to capture and hold the soil.

The home can be rearranged to meet the needs of the patient with low back pain. Some suggestions for the patient are as follows:

1. Place all frequently used items on shelves at waist to chest level.
2. Store refrigerator or freezer items most frequently used on top shelves of the compartment.
3. Keep a kneeling pad in the kitchen (or other rooms) and use it when using the oven, dish-

Keep loads small and manageable. Several small loads will place less stress on your back than one or two large ones.

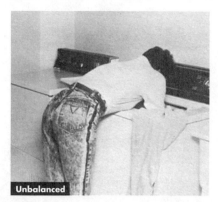 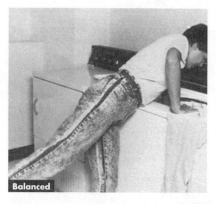 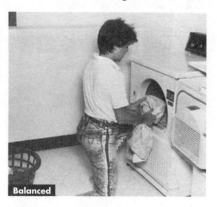

Avoid bending forward into the machines. Do not try to handle large bundles of clothes, particularly if they are wet. When loading or unloading a front-loading washer or dryer, drop to one knee to avoid any forward bending and twisting. Use support when coming to standing

FIG. 37-11 Doing laundry. (From Melnik M, Saunders R, Saunders HD: *Managing back pain: daily activities guide for back pain patients.* Reprinted with permission, Educational Opportunities, H. Duane Saunders, 4250 Norex Drive, Chaska, MN 55318.)

washer, lower shelves of the refrigerator or freezer and floor-level cupboards.

4. Have a wheeled cart available to conserve energy and avoid unnecessary lifting and carrying.
5. Ask packing clerks in the stores to pack bags lightly and ask for carry-out assistance.
6. Line the bottom of the car trunk with boxes, crates, or other means to raise the level of the floor, which

will reduce the necessity to lean far into the trunk to place or remove packages. Use the back seat of the car to hold groceries instead of the trunk.
7. Shop in stores that offer waist-high, shallow grocery carts.
8. If you find yourself in a stressful position, stand upright and realign the spine to its normal curves before resuming the same activity.

NOTE: Participation in the following activities (vacuuming, car maintenance, mowing and shoveling) is not recommended during the early stages of recovery. These activities are presented to offer methods for preventing a recurrence of your symptoms once your condition has stabilized.

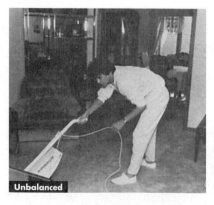 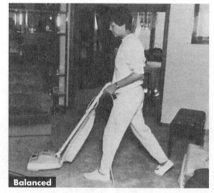 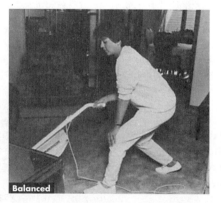

Perform the tasks as if the vacuum or broom were attached to your body. Move your feet and legs rather than reaching or bending forward. Avoid twisting. If you must vacuum or sweep under a table or chair, bend at your hips and knees and keep your back in a balanced position.

Additional suggestions: Light weight electric brooms make the job much easier. Beware of self-powered vacuum cleaners. They are very heavy!

FIG. 37-12 Sweeping/vacuuming. (From Melnik M, Saunders R, Saunders HD: *Managing back pain: daily activities guide for back pain patients.* Reprinted with permission, Educational Opportunities, H. Duane Saunders, 4250 Norex Drive, Chaska, MN 55318.)

MEDICAL MANAGEMENT OF LOW BACK PAIN

DIAGNOSTIC TESTS

If management of acute LBP is not successful with medication, rest, and rehabilitation, further diagnostic testing may be indicated. The PCP then refers the patient to a specialist, usually an orthopedist or neurosurgeon. Diagnostic tests, outlined below, are often ordered. These may include the following:

X-rays. Radiographic evaluation is used to rule out fractures, degenerative disease, possible metastatic disease, and structural abnormalities.

Magnetic resonance imaging (MRI). This technique visualizes bones and soft tissues using a magnetic field and radio waves. It is used to localize a problem area and confirm clinical impressions such as herniated discs or spinal stenosis. (A study using MRI showed 66% of people without complaints of LBP had abnormal findings at one or more vertebral levels).[9]

Computerized tomography (CT). This procedure, which uses cross-sectional X-ray films to define bony and soft tissue abnormalities, is used less often for spinal problems now because the MRI is superior at visualizing soft tissue abnormalities.

Discogram. Contrast material is injected into the intervertebral disc to see if symptoms are reproduced and clinical impressions are confirmed.

Myelogram. Iodinated contrast material is injected into the dural sac in order to outline spinal structures on X-ray film. Use has declined with the advent of the MRI and CT.

Bone scan. Radioactive material is injected intravenously and the body is scanned after several hours, making it possible to identify infections or tumors in the skeletal system.

Nerve conduction velocity (NCV)/electromyograph (EMG). These procedures use electric current to provide physiologic data about nerve root dysfunction and peripheral neuropathic conditions, often caused by disc herniation.[14]

INVASIVE, NONSURGICAL PROCEDURES

An option before surgery is an epidural corticosteroid injection. This outpatient procedure can be done in the hospital with local anesthesia. Relief can occur up to one week later, and the corticosteroid medication lasts up to three months. By then the patient has resumed activities and often continues to be functional. If partial relief is obtained, another injection may be performed from one to four weeks later.[5]

Another outpatient procedure performed with local anesthesia is the *percutaneous discectomy.* Specialized instrumentation is introduced that suctions out the damaged disc material. Very specific criteria are used to determine candidates for this procedure.[3]

SURGICAL PROCEDURES

Indications for surgery include bowel, bladder, and sexual dysfunction; saddle anesthesia; muscle weakness with progressive neurologic deficits; and significant pain with the presence of structural deformities. Common procedures include *laminotomy* and *discectomy* in which part of the lamina is excised to expose the nerve root and disc. The extruded material is removed, along with the fragmented part of the nucleus.[5]

In a *foraminotomy* small pieces of bone around the intervertebral foramen are excised to allow more room for the spinal nerve. This procedure is usually done in conjunction with a laminotomy. A *decompressive laminectomy* is the removal of the entire lamina and therefore the spinous process, to decompress the spinal canal. It is usually used for patients with spinal stenosis. A *posterolateral fusion* is performed when there is evidence of spinal instability. Autogenous iliac crest bone graft is used to stabilize the lumbar segments.[5]

Surgery for herniated disc(s) is controversial. Long-term outcome relative to pain and function is similar to that achieved with conservative care.[6]

REHABILITATION MANAGEMENT OF THE POSTSURGICAL PATIENT

The OT/PT team initiates treatment on the first postoperative day. Pain is often well controlled through the use of a patient-controlled analgesic device (PCA), allowing the patient to self-administer pain medication in premeasured doses, thus avoiding overdose. Postoperative bandages and surgical tape cover the sutures and help to prevent soft tissue stretching and unwanted pulling on the surgical site.

The goal of inpatient care is to achieve a safe discharge to home with or without supervision from a family member or health care attendant. OT focuses on functional training in dressing, bed mobility, self-care, transfers, standing tolerance, and other daily tasks. With little time for rehabilitation, adaptive equipment such as a commode and shower seat need to be rented in time for discharge to home. Education and training in posture and body mechanics are reviewed and practiced. The emphasis is on maintaining normal spinal alignment with ADL to minimize stress on the spine.

The length of stay in the hospital continues to be shortened. Patients with single-level laminotomies are often discharged in three days. Patients with multilevel procedures and fusions can stay five or six days because external stabilization devices sometimes need to be ordered and fitted before discharge.

Physical therapy works on strengthening, mobility,

and ambulation activities, as well as evaluation for ambulation aids such as a walker, cane, or other equipment for neurological deficits that are not resolved after surgery (e.g., ankle-foot orthosis). Functional training is also practiced and written exercise programs are reviewed and practiced. Home exercise programs usually include standing and bed exercises to improve extremity ROM and strength.

Both the occupational and physical therapist need to determine the need for further rehabilitation after discharge. Recommendations for home care and outpatient follow-up are made.

CHRONIC LOW BACK PAIN

Multidisciplinary pain service programs are challenged by the patients with chronic low back pain. A history of LBP from three months to fifty years is not uncommon. The primary role of occupational and physical therapy is to assess the musculoskeletal system and functional capabilities of the patient. Another important role is to evaluate previous rehabilitation experiences, treatment, and outcomes and advise the pain management team about present limitations and prognosis for positive change with further rehabilitation.

The physical therapist evaluates the asymmetries in muscle length, tone, and strength as well as joint mobility, asymmetry, or changes in soft tissues. Overall function, especially of gait, work-related tasks, ADL, recreation, and general fitness are also evaluated.

The occupational therapist evaluates strength and functional endurance for ADL and job requirements and assesses the psychological aspects and effects of the long-term disability. Occupational therapy uses functional capacity evaluations to set patient baselines, which are reported to the doctor. Thus, when medication trials are initiated their effectiveness can be measured after time frames determined by the physician.

Worker's compensation programs often invest the greatest amount of resources for treating chronic LBP, depending on financial issues, family situation, marital and family stress, and whether there is alcohol or drug dependency. These factors are evaluated because motivation, interest, and possible secondary gains from the disability directly affect the prognosis for successful treatment outcomes.

Many phases of the acute rehabilitation experience are used in working with chronic pain. Education in posture and body mechanics is still paramount. The exercise emphasis is directed toward conditioning and fitness because chronic pain leads to inactivity and general decline in physical fitness. Muscle stretching and mobility exercises are emphasized because of the severe joint restrictions seen in patients with chronic pain. Often the patient is referred to a ''back school'' program offered at the health care facility. The multidisciplinary approach to LBP requires good communication between the health professionals on the team for successful treatment outcomes.

SUMMARY

The patient with LBP is a challenge to the rehabilitation team. The occupational therapist, physical therapist, physician, psychologist, and rehabilitation counselor must work together to provide a multidisciplinary approach to this complex medical problem.

The OT has a vital role in educating and training the patient in posture, body mechanics, and energy conservation techniques. Patients are taught to change their faulty postures and behaviors at home, work, and play.

Understanding the anatomical weaknesses of the lumbar spine, especially with respect to discs and ligaments, enables the OT to educate patients in ways of moving that minimize spinal stress. This information is incorporated into each patient's daily activities for the rest of his or her life. Exacerbation of LBP is common. Patients often disregard safe techniques only to find the accumulation of stressors to the lumbar spine results in another episode of pain and disability.

The occupational therapist can use careful evaluation, functional practice, and psychological support to assist each patient to the highest level of function. Maintaining a positive attitude and planning realistic goals while encouraging the patient to take responsibility for his or her own rehabilitation are the ingredients to a successful recovery.

 SAMPLE TREATMENT PLAN

The following treatment plan is modeled after the program at Stanford Health Services in which back rehabilitation is a team effort between occupational and physical therapies. This treatment plan is merely an example and would not be suitable for any and every patient with low back pain. Each patient needs to be evaluated and have a treatment plan designed specifically to meet his or her needs.

S A M P L E   T R E A T M E N T   P L A N – c o n t ' d

CASE STUDY

Mr. M is a 29-year-old single man who was injured on the job 3 months ago. When he was lifting a 50-pound box, he lost his balance and felt a pull in his low back. Currently he continues to complain of pain in his right lower back and complains that he is unable to function and be as active as he was before his injury. His diagnosis is low back strain.

Mr. M is a picture framer and would like to return to work. He enjoys fishing, skiing, and basketball, and he wants to be able to engage in these sports again.

He was referred to an outpatient back rehabilitation program. The goals are to improve ROM, flexibility, strength, endurance, and body mechanics and to restore him to his maximal level of independence so that he can resume his former work and leisure roles.

TREATMENT PLAN

Personal data

Name: Mr. M
Age: 29
Diagnosis: Low back strain
Disability: Constant pain in lower right back; decreased functional capabilities
Treatment aims as stated in referral: Restoration to maximal functional independence through increased ROM and flexibility; improved strength and endurance; and participation in proper body mechanics in self-care, work, and leisure activities

Other services

Physician: Referral to rehabilitation, prescribe treatment and medication if necessary; supervise rehabilitation services
Physical therapy: Evaluate musculoskeletal abnormalities that affect LBP; evaluate physical potential of patient; strengthen lower extremities; increase endurance in conjunction with occupational therapy; plan treatment program to alter musculoskeletal abnormalities and help prevent further exacerbation
Social worker: Explore financial problems; provide support, education, and encouragement to family members as necessary
Family: Provide support and encouragement to the patient
Vocational rehabilitation: Explore feasibility of return to present occupation or explore new job possibilities and retraining

Frame of reference

Occupational performance

Treatment approaches

Biomechanical, rehabilitative, educational

OT EVALUATION

Performance components

Sensorimotor functioning
   Muscle strength: Test
   Passive and active ROM: Test
   Physical endurance: Test, observe upper extremity (UE) and LE
   Standing tolerance: Observe, interview
   Walking tolerance: Observe, interview
   Sitting tolerance: Observe, interview
   Lifting tolerance: Test, observe, interview
   Carrying tolerance: Test, observe, interview
   Functional movement patterns: Observe body mechanics
   Sensation (touch): Test
Cognitive functioning
   Judgment: Observe for correct use of body mechanics
   Safety awareness: Observe

Psychosocial/psychological functioning
   Adjustment to disability: Observe, interview
   Coping skills: Observe
   Social functioning: Interview, observe
   Interpersonal skills: Observe with family and peers

Performance areas

   Self-care: Observe, interview
   Work/work-related skills: Interview
   Work habits and attitudes: Interview, observe
   Potential work skills: Interview, possibly test; referral
   Work tolerance: Test if ordered or indicated; refer to appropriate agency
   Home management: Observe, interview
   Play/leisure: Interview

EVALUATION SUMMARY

Muscle testing revealed that strength was normal throughout except for right ankle dorsiflexion and right extensor hallucis longus; both were graded as Good (G)

Patient demonstrates limited ROM in trunk flexion, trunk extension, and lateral flexion; trunk mobility is limited 50% in all directions. He experiences an increase of pain with these motions. LE flexibility limited in hamstrings, rectus femoris, piriformis, greater on the right than the left. Abnormal tone noted in right paraspinous muscles from T10 to S1.

Further physical endurance skills were evaluated as follows:

Lifting: Patient is able to lift 10 lb (4.5 kg) from 0 to 36 inches (0 cm to 91.4 cm) and 36 to 72 in (91.4 to 182.9 cm) with only a pulling sensation.

Carrying: Patient is able to carry 10 lb (4.5 kg) for 5 minutes for 323 ft (98.4 m) with no complaints of pain

LE weights: Patient is able to extend both legs with 75-lb (34-kg) weights and hold a static quadriceps set for 10 seconds.

UE weights: Patient is able to flex elbow with 15-lb (6.8-kg) weight, and flex shoulder with 7-lb (6.8-kg) weights.

Treadmill: Patient able to walk 1.5 mph for 10 min with no aggravation of pain

Stationary bicycle: Patient is able to resist with 3.3 lb (1.5 kg) for 2 mi in 15 min but experienced right leg pain

Endurance walk: Patient is able to walk 1 mi (1609.35 m) in 30 min with some stopping because of pain.

Sensory testing reveals no deficits in LEs. Patient is independent but guarded in dressing and sink activities. He complains of pain when donning shoes and socks and demonstrated poor body mechanics with these activities. He has difficulty with sweeping, vacuuming, and mopping and used poor body mechanics. Outdoor tasks and driving are not attempted because they aggravate pain. He further dem-

onstrates improper body mechanics when sitting and when moving from a sitting to standing position. His standing posture demonstrates flattened lumbar lordosis with head forward.

The patient complains of constant burning pain in his right lower back. The pain is aggravated by prolonged standing and is relieved somewhat by lying down. The patient intermittently wears a back brace. He has attempted to return to work but has to take time off or quit because of pain. Patient lives with his wife and 6-year-old daughter in a modest two-bedroom suburban home. When not working he does daily chores and watches television. Patient expresses some anger at his insurance company. He is pleasant but withdrawn, and has lost social contact with many of his friends.

Assets

Expresses desire to get better
Expresses desire to return to work
No muscle atrophy or significant loss of strength
Limitation in ROM because of inactivity; no bony problems
Young, cooperative; appears motivated to follow treatment program
Supportive family

Problem List

1. Constant pain in right low back
2. Some limitation in ROM
3. Slight decrease in strength
4. Low lifting and carrying capabilities
5. Poor endurance
6. Use of improper body mechanics for ADL
7. Depression, withdrawal, low self-esteem
8. Change or loss in vocational role

PROBLEM 1: PAIN

Objective

Pain will be modulated or reduced so that patient can increase functional activities and return to work

Method

Teach rest positions 3 to 4 times a day to be performed as an exercise to provide pain relief and unload spine. Rest no

longer than 15 minutes. Use rest positions before and after ADL and household chores to improve endurance and decrease pain response

Gradation

Decrease rest as improvement occurs. Increase rest if symptoms persist or are exacerbated

SAMPLE TREATMENT PLAN – cont'd

PROBLEM 1, 2: PAIN, DECREASED ROM AND FLEXIBILITY

Objective

ROM will increase and pain will be reduced so that normal ROM is attained in the LEs

Method

Slow, gradual spinal mobility program in physical therapy with stretching program to lengthen hamstrings, rectus femoris, piriformis, and back extensors

OT

Teach patient to avoid activities that require prolonged periods of sitting. Teach body mechanics for ADL: self-care, kitchen, laundry tasks

Gradation

Introduce new techniques gradually. Repetitive practice of correct body mechanics for daily activities

PROBLEM 3: DECREASED STRENGTH

Objective

Increase general strength and endurance of both UEs and LEs to Normal (5)

Method

Functional training on the Baltimore Therapeutic Equip-

ment to simulate job tasks as a picture framer; lifting training using the WEST

Gradation

Add resistance and additional repetitions to all functional training tasks

PROBLEM 4: LOW LIFTING AND CARRYING CAPABILITY

Objective

Ability to lift weight with arms will increase from 10 lb (4.5 kg) to 15 lb (6.75 kg) and individual weight exercises will increase by 20%

Method

Functional training using the BTE or simulated tasks of lifting and carrying. Monitor pain behaviors and symptoms

Gradation

Progressive training, increasing weights and repetitions

PROBLEM 5: POOR ENDURANCE

Objective

General endurance will improve and work tolerance will increase to 4 hours

Method

Train in home program using ADL and leisure activities and ask patient to keep a graph of daily activity and time it takes

to perform tasks. Observe posture and body mechanics for each task and give feedback about the effectiveness of the techniques for reinjury prevention

Gradation

Gently increase time for each activity

PROBLEM 4, 6: LOW LIFTING AND CARRYING CAPABILITIES; IMPROPER BODY MECHANICS

Objective

Body mechanic techniques will improve so that proper body mechanics are used consistently in ADL and simulated work tasks

Method

Occupational therapist to teach principles of body mechanics and practical application of body mechanic principles by having patient try activities such as standing, sitting, lying, lifting, carrying, and reaching posture; and ADL such as dressing, hygiene, vacuuming, sweeping, and washing

windows. Patient to run through a "par course" of activities, such as carrying a bag of groceries, unloading the groceries on various shelf heights, sweeping a floor, and washing dishes

Gradation

In teaching posture techniques, start with standing posture; progress to sitting and lying; instruct in dynamic postures for lifting, carrying, and reaching. Start with demonstration, progress to patient participation; use as many real situations as possible

SAMPLE TREATMENT PLAN – cont'd

PROBLEM 7: DEPRESSION, WITHDRAWAL, LOW SELF-ESTEEM

Objective
Depression and low self-esteem will decrease and interaction with others will increase so that patient displays more interest in life tasks and displays a more positive attitude.

Method
Use a supportive, honest approach with patient; explain procedures carefully and thoroughly.

Workshop activities of woodworking, leather crafts, and mosaics to improve self-esteem; socialization and expression encouraged in group situations; observe sitting and standing tolerances during workshop activities.

Gradation
Simple, short-term crafts that the patient can accomplish easily and quickly; interact with other patients.

Progress to more difficult crafts, being sure to structure the activity for success.

Patient to perform activities in a group situation.

PROBLEM 8: CHANGE OR LOSS OF VOCATIONAL ROLE

Objective
Physical tolerances and capabilities will be documented to aid determination of feasibility of employment

Method
Give patient task, such as light woodwork during workshop time; patient to stand while working on project; observe patient and record amount of standing time tolerated.

While patient engages in a craft activity and is sitting, observe and record the amount of time patient is able to sit comfortably.

Provide patient with variety of lifting and carrying situations; for example, carry a weighted box for a set distance and lift a weighted box to various heights.

Patient to lift weighted tool box from floor to 36 inches (91.4 cm) and then to a shelf at 72 inches (183 cm).

Patient to carry a weighted tool box for a set time and distance.

Patient to lift and carry different sizes and shapes of wood or other objects, such as long but lightweight objects and bulky objects.

Gradation
Encourage patient to gradually increase standing time; patient to try using a footstool and varying work heights while standing.

Encourage patient gradually to increase sitting tolerance; patient to try different types of chairs, lumbar supports, work heights, and angles.

Patient to lift and carry to tolerance; amount of weight gradually increased as strength and endurance improve.

Patient to start lifting and carrying objects that are easily manageable; progress to more awkward sizes and shapes.

This treatment plan was adapted from the original by Sally Roozee, author of this chapter in the third edition (1990).

REVIEW QUESTIONS

1. List three causes of low back pain.
2. Name the major components of the spine.
3. Explain the movements of an intervertebral disk with spine flexion, extension, and lateral flexion.
4. List the four areas of assessment the therapist evaluates on an individual with low back pain.
5. What are some of the problems a person with chronic low back pain encounters?
6. List the major goals of postsurgical rehabilitation of the patient with low back pain.
7. Describe the progression of treatment for the patient with low back pain.
8. What is the foundation for good body mechanics?
9. List the general principles of proper body mechanics for ADL.
10. In a team environment what other disciplines might see or treat the person with low back pain?

REFERENCES

1. Bowman JM: The meaning of chronic low back pain, *American Association of Occupational Health Nursing (AAOHN) Journal,* 39(8):381-384, 1991.

2. Callahan P and associates: *Stanford back school manual,* Stanford, Calif, 1984, Stanford Health Services, Dept of Rehabilitation Services.
3. Davis G, Onik G, Helms C: Automated percutaneous discectomy, *Spine,* 16(3):359-363, 1991.
4. DeGirolamo G: Epidemiology and social costs of low back pain and fibromyalgia, *Clin J Pain,* 7(suppl 1):S1-7, 1991, (abstract).
5. Franklin TD: Personal communication, Dec. 10, 1994.
6. Frymoyer JW: Back pain and sciatica, *N Engl J Med,* 318:291, 1988.
7. Gardener W, Osborn W: *Structure of the human body,* Philadelphia, 1967, WB Saunders.
8. Kapandji IA: The physiology of the joints, vol 3: *The trunk and vertebral column,* New York, 1979, Churchill Livingstone.
9. Kolata G: Diagnosis of backache might need more spine, *San José Mercury News,* July 14, 1994.
10. Long DM: Failed back surgery syndrome, *Neurosurgery Clinics of North America,* 2(4):899-919, 1991.
11. Melnick MS, Saunders R, Saunders DH: *Managing back pain; daily activities guide for back pain patients,* Minneapolis, 1989, Educational Opportunities.
12. Moore S, Garg A: Ergonomics: low back pain and carpal tunnel and upper extremity disorder in the workplace; *Occupational Medicine, State of the Art Reviews* 7(4):593-594, 1992.
13. Nachemson AL: The lumbar spine: an orthopedic challenge, *Spine* 1(1):59, 1976.
14. Tollison C, Kriegel M: *Interdisciplinary rehabilitation of low back pain,* Baltimore, 1989, Williams & Wilkins.
15. Warwick P, Williams R: *Gray's anatomy,* ed 35 (British), Philadelphia, 1973, WB Saunders.
16. Webster BS, Snook SH: The cost of compensable low back pain, *J of Occupational Medicine,* 32(1):13, 1990.

Hip Fractures and Total Hip Replacement

Deborah Morawski, Karen Pitbladdo,
Elizabeth Maria Bianchi, Sheri L. Lieberman,
Jan Polon Novic, Helen Bobrove

The occupational therapist plays a key role in defining and remediating the many functional problems imposed by both acute and chronic orthopedic conditions, thus sharing in the goal of returning the orthopedic patient to optimal performance of safe and independent daily living activities.

This chapter discusses hip fractures and total hip replacement, their medical and surgical management, the psychological implications of hospitalization and disability, and the health care team approach in acute hospital and rehabilitation settings.

FRACTURES

It is important for the therapist working with orthopedic patients to have a good understanding of the site, type, and cause of the fracture before starting treatment. A basic understanding of fracture healing and medical management is also necessary to appreciate risks, precautions, and complications involved.

Fractures occur in bone when the bone's ability to absorb tension, compression, or shearing forces is exceeded. Fractures are classified according to the type of fracture sustained and the direction of the fracture line[5] (Fig. 38-1).

FRACTURE HEALING

Grossly, bone tissue occurs as cancellous or cortical. Cancellous or spongy bone surrounds spaces filled with bone marrow in the metaphysis of long bones and in the bodies of short bones and the flat bones of the pelvis and ribs. Cortical or compact bone is on the outer surface of the bone, giving it strength. It is covered with periosteum, and the inner surface is lined with endosteum.[5]

At the time of fracture, blood vessels are torn across the fracture site, causing bleeding then clotting; this situation is called a fracture hematoma. The repair cells or osteogenic cells form an internal and external callus from the endosteum and periosteum.[5] This callus begins to form from the time of injury, and its maturation rate is dependent upon the specific bone that is fractured. Primary woven bone is initially formed from osteoblasts and eventually matures through the action of osteoclasts and osteoblasts into compact or cortical bone. With maturation of the fracture comes bone stability, which is termed *union.*[5,12] Immobilization is required throughout this maturation period. In some cases, additional protection may be necessary to confirm maturation of the callus.

The fracture matures many months later when excess callus is reabsorbed and the bone returns to almost its normal diameter. Remodeling of bone occurs in response to physical stress according to a phenomenon known as Wolff's law.[12] Bone is deposited in sites where there is stress, such as weight bearing, and reabsorbed where there is little stress.

Cancellous bone is structurally different from cortical bone, so the healing process differs. The internal callus plays a greater role in forming primary woven bone; because of greater blood supply and larger surface area, healing occurs more rapidly.

As a result of the lack of blood supply, articular cartilage cannot regenerate into hyaline cartilage but instead forms fibrous tissue and fibrocartilage. This form of scar tissue cannot withstand normal wear-and-tear stresses. If the structural change is substantial, degenerative changes may develop.[5]

The time required for fracture healing varies with the age of the patient, site and configuration of the fracture, initial displacement of the bone, and the blood supply to the fragments. The fracture healing may be abnormal in one of three ways: (1) a bony deformity develops (called a malunion), (2) the healing process takes longer than

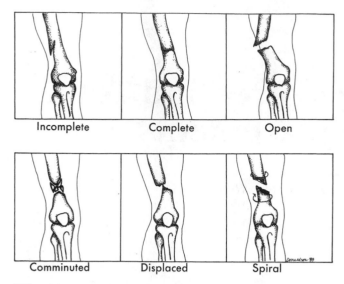

FIG. 38-1   Types of fractures. (Modified from Garland JJ: *Fundamentals of orthopaedics,* Philadelphia, 1979, WB Saunders.)

normal (called a delayed union), or (3) the fracture fails to heal (called a nonunion).

CAUSES OF FRACTURES

Trauma is the major cause of fractures. The force may be transmitted directly or through torsion. A forceful muscle contraction may also break a bone, as in certain patella fractures. Stress fractures occur when bone fatigues from repeated loading, as seen in some metatarsal fractures. Osteoporosis, a type of metabolic bony atrophy, is a common bone disease of people over 65 years of age. It involves mostly the vertebral bodies and cancellous metaphyses of the neck of the femur, humerus, and distal end of the radius. Because the bone becomes porous and thereby fragile, the affected bones are prone to fracture. A pathological fracture can occur because of a bone weakened by disease or tumor. This condition can occur in diseases, such as osteomyelitis and lytic tumors of bone caused by deposition of metastatic carcinoma.[5]

MEDICAL MANAGEMENT

The aims of fracture treatment are to relieve pain, maintain good position of the fracture, allow for bony union for fracture healing, and restore optimal function to the patient.[12] Occupational therapy plays a substantial role in the restoration of function of the patient; that role will be discussed later in this chapter.

Reduction of a fracture refers to restoring the fragments to normal alignment.[5] This process can be done by a closed procedure (manipulation) or by an open procedure (surgery). A closed reduction is performed by applying a force to the displaced bone opposite to the force that produced the fracture. Depending on the nature of the fracture, the reduction is maintained in a cast, brace, skin traction, skeletal traction, or skeletal fixation.

With open reduction, the fracture site is exposed sur-

gically so that the fragments can be aligned. The fragments are held in place with internal fixation by pins, screws, a plate, nails, or a rod. Further immobilization by a cast or a brace may be necessary. Usually an open reduction and internal fixation (ORIF) must be protected from excessive forces, so weight-bearing restrictions are indicated.[7]

In the hip fracture, the articular fragment of the hip may need to be removed and replaced by a prosthesis called an endoprosthesis. This approach is necessary when there are complications of avascular necrosis, nonunion, or degenerative joint disease. Often, following the fracture, soft tissue trauma, edema, and ecchymosis develops around the fracture site and can result in an increase of pain.[11]

HIP FRACTURES

A knowledge of hip anatomy is necessary to understand medical management of hip fractures. The hip is an enarthrodial or ball-and-socket joint formed by the head of the femur and the acetabulum.[6] The articular capsule of the hip joint refers to the dense connective tissue enclosing the joint, which provides stability and assists with hip motion. The capsule extends from the margins of the acetabulum downward anteriorly to the intertrochanteric ridge and posteriorly to the middle of the neck. The hip abductors (gluteus medius and gluteus minimus) and the external rotators (piriformis, gemellus, and iliopsoas obturators), attach to the greater trochanter; whereas the hip flexors (psoas major and iliacus) attach to the lesser trochanter. Blood supply to the femoral head is via the ligamentum teres, capsular vessels, and vessels from the femoral shaft (Fig. 38-2).

The levels of fracture lines are shown in Fig. 38-3. The names of the fractures generally reflect site and severity of injury. These terms are frequently indicators of which medical treatment will be used. For example, femoral neck fracture will be treated with femoral neck stabilization.

Femoral Neck Fractures

Femoral neck fractures are common in adults over 60 years old and occur more frequently in women. If the bone is osteoporotic, only slight trauma or rotational force causes the fracture.[3] Treatment of a displaced fracture in this area is complicated by poor blood supply; in addition, the osteoporotic bone is not suited to hold metallic fixation, and the thin periosteum limits fracture healing. The type of surgical treatment used is based on the amount of displacement and the circulation in the femoral head.

The age and health of the patient are considered in deciding on the surgical procedure. Generally hip pinning or use of a compression screw and plate is used when displacement is minimal to moderate and blood supply is intact. With a physician's approval, a patient is usually able to begin out-of-bed activities 2 to 4 days after

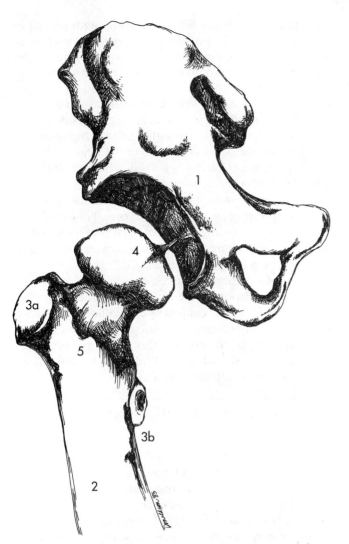

FIG. 38-2 Normal hip anatomy. *1,* Acetabulum; *2,* femur; *3a,* greater trochanter; *3b,* lesser trochanter; *4,* ligamentum teres; *5,* intertrochanteric crest. (Modified from Crouch JE: *Functional human anatomy,* ed 3, Philadelphia, 1978, Lea & Febiger; and Grant LC: *Grant's atlas of anatomy,* ed 6, Baltimore, 1972, Williams & Wilkins.)

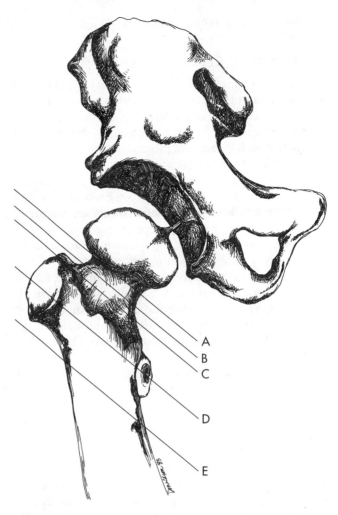

FIG. 38-3 Levels of femoral fracture. *A,* Subcapital; *B,* transcervical: *C,* basilar; *D,* intertrochanteric; *E,* subtrochanteric. (Modified from Crow I: Fracture of the hip: a self study, *ONA J* 5:12, 1978.)

Intertrochanteric Fractures

Intertrochanteric fractures between the greater and lesser trochanter are extracapsular, and the blood supply is not affected. Like femoral neck fractures, intertrochanteric fractures occur mostly in women but in a slightly older age group. The fracture usually is caused by direct trauma or force over the trochanter. ORIF (open reduction internal fixation) is the preferred treatment. A nail or compression screw with a sideplate is used. Sometimes as long as 4 to 6 months weight-bearing restrictions must be observed when a patient is ambulating. Again the patient is allowed out of bed 2 to 4 days after surgery pending the physician's approval.[7]

Subtrochanteric Fractures

Subtrochanteric fractures 1 to 2 inches (2.5 cm to 5.0 cm) below the lesser trochanter usually occur because of direct trauma. These fractures are most often in younger people less than 60 years old. Skeletal traction followed by an ORIF is the usual treatment. A nail with a long sideplate or an intramedullary rod is used, and the condi-

surgery. Per physician's orders, weight-bearing restrictions may need to be observed with the aid of crutches or a walker for at least 6 to 8 weeks while the fracture is healing. Limited weight bearing may be necessary beyond this time if precautions are not observed or delayed union occurs.[7]

With severe displacement or an avascular femoral head, the femoral head is excised and replaced by an endoprosthesis. This procedure is referred to as a bipolar arthroplasty.[11] Several types of metal prostheses can be used; each has its own shape and advantages. Weight-bearing restrictions are sometimes indicated. Because of the surgical procedure used, precautions for positioning the hip must be observed to avoid dislocation. The precautions vary according to the surgical approach used. Patients who have had a prosthesis implanted can usually begin out-of-bed activity, with a physician's approval, about 2 to 4 days after surgery.[7]

tion may possibly require further immobilization after surgery.

TOTAL JOINT REPLACEMENT

Restoration of joint motion and treatment of pain by total hip replacement is sometimes indicated in osteoarthritis, rheumatoid arthritis, and ankylosing spondylitis. Osteoarthritis or degenerative joint disease may develop spontaneously in middle age and progress as the normal aging process of joints is exaggerated. It may also develop as the result of trauma, congenital deformity, or a disease that damages articular cartilage. Weight-bearing joints, such as the hip, knee, and lumbar spine, are usually affected. There is a loss of cartilage centrally on the joint surface and formation of osteophytes on the acetabulum, peripherally, producing joint incongruity.

Pain arises from the bone, synovial membrane, fibrous capsule, and muscle spasm. When movement of the hip causes pain, the muscles are not used and shorten from disuse. The osteoarthritic hip may assume a flexed, adducted, and internally rotated position that also causes a painful limp.[8]

Ankylosing spondylitis, a chronic progressive polyarthritis, primarily involves the sacroiliac and spinal joints. The soft tissues eventually ossify, producing a bony ankylosis. The proximal joints of the extremities, particularly the hips, may be affected, which could also progress to bony ankylosis.[12]

Rheumatoid arthritis (covered in Chapter 34) is another type of arthritis that may involve the hip joint. Surgery is often performed early in the disease process to avoid fibrotic damage to joint and tendon structures.[12]

Total joint replacement or arthroplasty may be necessary in various types of arthritis. This surgery is designed to alleviate pain and regain joint motion. There are two components to a total hip replacement. A high-density polyethylene socket is fitted into the acetabulum and a metallic prosthesis replaces the femoral head and neck.

Methylmethacrylate or acrylic cement fixes the components to the bone. Various surgical approaches are used according to the surgical skill or technique of the orthopedist, severity of the joint involvement, and past surgery to the hip. With an anterolateral approach, the patient is unstable in external rotation, adduction, and extension of the operated hip and usually must observe precautions to prevent these movements for 6 to 12 weeks. If a posterolateral approach is used, the patient must be cautioned not to move the operated hip in specific ranges of flexion (usually 60° to 90°) and not to rotate internally or adduct the leg. Failure to maintain these precautions during muscle and soft tissue healing may result in hip dislocation. Most surgeons do not restrict weight-bearing postoperatively when cement fixation is used.

One of the major problems with total joint replacement is the loss of fixation at the prothesis interface. A recent development is the use of biological fixation. This procedure involves the use of bony ingrowth instead of cement to secure the prosthesis. The precautions following the surgery are those of the anterior or posterior hip replacements with an additional restriction on weight-bearing for 6 to 8 weeks. The restrictions on weight-bearing vary in terms of amount of pressure and length of time. A walking aid, usually a walker or crutches, is necessary for at least the first month while the hip is healing and muscles are becoming stronger. Patients with total joint replacements usually begin out-of-bed activity 1 to 3 days after surgery.[8]

It is important to be aware of complications or special procedures that occurred during surgery. For example, a trochanteric osteotomy may have been necessary. In this case, if the greater trochanter was removed and rewired down, active abduction is prohibited.[8]

Total joint surface replacements, which are rarely used, are a variation of the total hip replacement.[5] The surface of the femur is capped by a metallic shell, and the acetabular cavity receives a plastic cup. Both are held in place by methylmethacrylate. This technique preserves the femoral head and neck. With this technique, no weight-bearing restrictions apply.

PSYCHOLOGICAL FACTORS

Psychological issues are critical considerations in the overall treatment of the orthopedic patient. A large number of patients in this population are faced with either a chronic disability (such as rheumatoid arthritis), a life-threatening disease (such as cancer), or the aging process; therefore loss or potential loss of physical ability is a predominant problem faced by most of these patients. This process is stressful, requiring an enormous amount of physical and emotional energy.[10] An awareness of and a sensitivity toward the orthopedic patient is critical to the delivery of optimal patient care.

When dealing with this patient population, the therapist must realize that each patient's experience of loss will depend on intrinsic makeup (personality, physical diseases, specific changes, or experience of body dissolution) and the environmental factors affecting the patient (personal losses or gains, family dynamics, or the home environment).[10]

Those patients suffering from a chronic orthopedic disability often experience one or more of the following: body dissolution, deformity, disease of a body part, fear, anxiety, change in body image, decreased functional ability, and pain. The onset of these factors may occur at a relatively young age and often in rapid succession.

Orthopedic patients often consider themselves prisoners of their own bodies, left with accumulated layers of unresolved grief, fatigue, and a sense of emptiness.[3] Thus when treating a patient with a chronic orthopedic disability, it is important to address these issues and provide the support needed for the mourning and grieving process to take place. Without an opportunity to resolve these conflicts, the patient becomes depressed, filled with guilt and anxiety, and paralyzed with fear. These emotions inhibit the patient's progress and enhance the development of poor self-image. Therapists can help reintegrate some of these conflicts, which will give the patient a feeling of accomplishment and pride, enhancing the treatment process.

These considerations hold true for the elderly patient dealing with disability. In addition to the issues just discussed, however, the elderly also face psychological issues specific to the aging process. The elderly patient often experiences the need to reflect on and review past life experiences.[2]

A second important issue experienced by the elderly, disabled individual is dependency. With the onset of a disability late in life, the patient is forced to face the realities of the aging process and let go of years of independence and self-sufficiency.[10] For some this experience can be devastating, but others may use these negative changes to acquire benefits that are satisfying to them, such as the patients who remain in the hospital because they enjoy the extra attention or those who use their illness to manipulate their support systems and avoid taking responsibility for themselves and others.

A third psychosocial phenomenon experienced by the aged when hospitalized is relocation trauma, which presents itself through confusion, emotional lability, and disorientation. Older people, when removed from their familiar environment, often decompensate cognitively; therefore it is important that their new environment be made as familiar as possible. Decorating it with familiar objects from the patient's home and providing the patient with a calendar and current newspapers and magazines are often helpful in reducing this traumatic effect.

Learning to cope and adjust to the changes resulting from chronic disability or the aging process is a critical part of patient treatment. Therapists must realize that a great deal of a patient's functional independence has been relinquished as a result of disease or disability. For this reason it is critical that the psychosocial issues resulting from these losses be addressed while focusing on increasing a patient's functional level of independence.

REHABILITATION MEASURES[8,11]

Good communication and clear role delineation among members of the health care team are essential for an efficient and smooth therapy program. The health care team usually consists of a primary physician, nursing staff, a physical therapist, an occupational therapist, a nutritionist, a pharmacist, a discharge planner, and possibly a social worker. Regular team meetings to discuss each patient's ongoing treatment, progress, and discharge plans are necessary to coordinate individual treatment programs. Members from each service usually attend to provide information and consultation.

The role of the physician is to inform the team of the patient's medical status. Information includes previous medical history; diagnosis of the present problem; a complete account of the surgical procedure performed, which includes the type of appliance inserted, the anatomical approach, and any movement or weight-bearing precautions that could endanger the patient. The physician is also responsible for ordering specific medications and therapies. Any change or progression in therapy or changes in the patient's medication regime should be approved by the physician.

The nursing staff is responsible for the actual physical care of the patient during hospitalization. Responsibilities of the nurse include administering medications, assisting the patient with bathing and hygiene, and constant monitoring of vital signs and physical status. Each patient's blood pressure, pulse, and respiratory status are checked every 1 to 2 hours immediately after surgery.[8] During the rehabilitation phase, vital signs are usually checked once every 8 hours unless otherwise ordered by the physician.[8] Wound and skin care, such as the changing of dressings or the sterilization of wounds, are performed by the nurse.

The orthopedic nurse must have a thorough understanding of the surgical procedures and movement precautions for each patient. Proper positioning using pillows, wedges, and sometimes a ski box (described later) is carried out by the nurse, especially in the first few days following surgery. As the patient's therapy program progresses, the patient starts to take more responsibility for proper positioning and physical care. The nurse works closely with the physical and occupational therapists to help establish a self-care program that implements skills the patient has already learned in therapy.[8]

The physical therapist is responsible for evaluation and treatment in the areas of musculoskeletal status, sensation, pain, skin integrity, and mobility (especially gait). In many cases involving total hip replacements and surgical repair of hip fractures, physical therapy is initiated on the first day after surgery. The therapist obtains baseline information including range of motion (ROM), strength of all the extremities, muscle tone, mental status, and mobility, adhering to the prescribed precautions of protocol.[8,11]

A treatment program that includes therapeutic exercises, ROM activities, transfer training, and progressive gait activities is established. The physical therapist is responsible for recommending the appropriate assistive device to be used during ambulation. As the patient's ambulation status advances, instruction in stair climbing, managing curbs, and outside ambulation is given.[8,11]

The nutritionist consults with each patient to ensure that adequate and appropriate nutrition is received to aid the healing process. The pharmacist monitors the patient's drug therapy and provides information and assistance with pain management.[8]

The role of the discharge planner is to ensure that each patient is discharged to the appropriate living situation or facility. Usually the discharge planner is a registered nurse with a thorough knowledge of community resources and available nursing care facilities. With input from the health care team, the discharge planner makes the arrangements for ongoing therapy after hospitalization, for admission to a rehabilitation facility for further intensive therapy, or for nursing home care if necessary. The discharge planner works closely with the health care team and is instrumental in coordinating the program after the patient's discharge from the hospital.[8,11]

THE ROLE OF OCCUPATIONAL THERAPY

Following a total hip replacement or surgical repair of a fractured hip, occupational therapy is usually initiated 2 to 4 days after surgery when the patient is ready to start getting out of bed. The time varies depending on the age, general health, and surgical events or medical complications of the individual patient. Before any physical evaluation, it is important for the therapist to introduce and explain the role of occupational therapy, establish rapport, and then gather by interview any pertinent information regarding the patient's prior functional status, home environment, and living situation.

The goal of occupational therapy is for the patient to return home independent in activities of daily living (ADL) with all movement precautions observed during activities. It is the role of the occupational therapist to teach the patient ways and means of performing ADL safely.[8,11]

A baseline physical evaluation is necessary to determine whether any physical limitations not related to surgery might prevent functional independence. Upper extremity (UE) ROM, muscle strength, sensation, coordination, and mental status are assessed before a functional evaluation is made. It is also important to consider the patient's pain and fear at rest and during movement. Occupational therapy is then a progression of functional activities that simulate a normal, daily regime of activity in accordance with all the movement precautions.[8,11]

GUIDELINES FOR TRAINING[8,11]

Total Hip Replacement—Posterolateral Approach
(most frequently used approach)
Positions of hip stability: Flexion (within limitations of precautions), abduction, and external rotation
Positions of hip instability: Adduction, internal rotation, and flexion greater than limitations of precautions

Bed mobility
The supine position with the appropriate wedge or pillow in place is recommended. If a patient sleeps side-lying, it is recommended to sleep on the operated side if it is tolerable. When sleeping on the nonoperated side, the legs must be abducted with the wedge or larger pillows and the operated leg supported to prevent internal rotation. It is important to determine the type and height of the patient's bed at home.

Transfers
It is always helpful for the patient first to observe the proper technique for transfers.
Chair: A firmly based chair with armrests is recommended. The patient is instructed to extend the operated leg forward, reach back for the armrests, and sit slowly, being careful not to lean forward (Fig. 38-4). To stand, the patient extends the operated leg and pushes off from the armrests, being careful not to lean forward. Because of the hip flexion precaution, the patient should sit on the front part of the chair and lean back. Firm cushions or blankets can be used to increase the height of chairs, especially if the patient is tall. Low chairs, soft chairs, reclining chairs, and rocking chairs should be avoided.
Commode chair: Over-the-toilet commode chairs with armrests are to be used in the hospital and at home. The height and angle are adjusted so that the front legs are one notch lower than the back legs; thus, with the patient seated, the precautionary hip angle of flexion is not exceeded. The patient should wipe between the legs in a sitting position or from behind in a standing position with caution to avoid internal rotation of the hip. The patient is to stand up and step to turn to face the toilet to flush.
Shower stall: Nonskid strips or stickers are recommended in all shower stalls and tubs. To enter, the walker or crutches go first, then the operated leg followed by the nonoperated leg. A shower chair with adjustable legs or a stool and grab bars should be installed if balance is a problem or weight-bearing precautions are present.
Shower over tub (without shower doors): The patient is instructed to stand parallel to the tub facing the shower fixtures. Using the walker or crutches, the patient is to transfer in sideways by bending at the knees, not at the hips. For patients with weight-bearing precautions or poor balance, purchase of a tub bench may be considered, allowing the patient to sit on the edge of the bench and then swing the legs over the tub observing flexion precautions, or sponge bathing at the sink is advised.
Car: Bucket seats in small cars should be avoided. Bench-type seats are recommended. The patient is instructed to back up to the passenger seat, hold onto a stable part of the car, extend the operated leg, and slowly sit in the car. Remembering to lean back, the patient then slides the buttocks toward the driver's seat. The upper body and lower extremities then move as one unit to turn to face the forward direction. It is helpful to have the seat slid back and reclined to maintain the hip flexion precaution. Pillows in the seat may be necessary to increase the height of the seat. Prolonged sitting in the car should be avoided.

Lower body dressing
The patient is instructed to sit in a chair with arms or on the edge of the bed for dressing activities. The patient is instructed to avoid adduction and internal rotation or crossing the legs to dress. Crossing the operated extremity over the nonoperated extremity at either the ankles or knees is to be avoided. Assistive devices may be necessary to observe precautions (Fig. 38-5).

To maintain hip precautions, a reacher or dressing stick is used to aid in donning and removing pants and shoes. For pants, the operated leg is dressed first by using the reacher or dressing stick to bring the pants over the foot and up to the

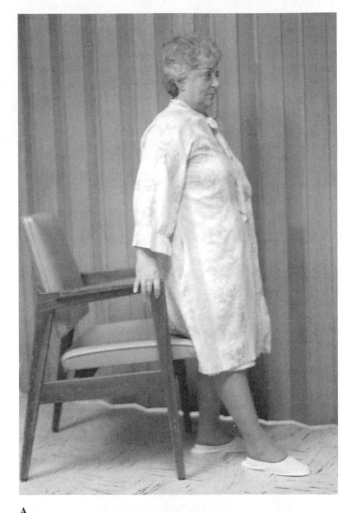

A

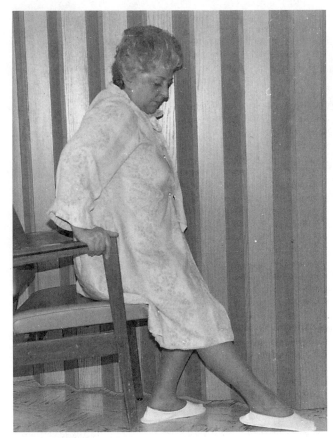

B

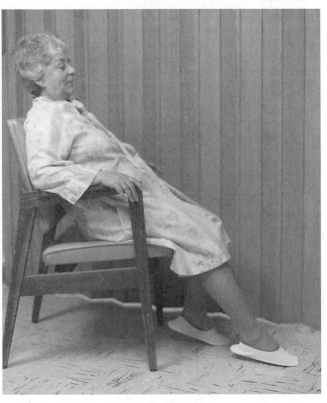

C

FIG. 38-4 Chair transfer technique. **A,** patient extends operated leg and reaches for arm rests. **B** and **C,** Bearing some weight on arms, patient sits down slowly, maintaining some extension of operated leg.

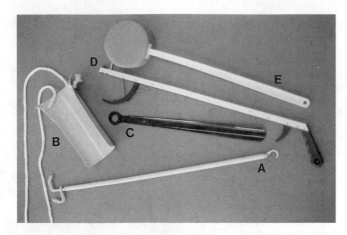

FIG. 38-5   Assistive devices for ADL. *A,* Dressing stick; *B,* sock aid; *C,* long-handled shoe horn; *D,* reacher; *E,* long-handled bath sponge.

knee. A sock aid is used to don socks or knee-high nylons and a reacher or dressing stick is used to doff. A reacher, elastic laces, and a long-handled shoehorn can also be provided.

Lower body bathing

Methods for transferring to and from shower or tub were described previously. Sponge bathing at the sink is indicated until showering is approved by the physician. Techniques to use for lower body bathing include the following: A long-handled bath sponge or back brush is used to reach the lower legs and feet safely; soap-on-a-rope is used to prevent the soap from dropping; and a towel is wrapped on a reacher to dry the lower legs.

Hair shampoo

Until the patient is able to shower, the patient is instructed to shampoo hair while standing or sitting on a stool at the kitchen or bathroom sink, observing hip precautions.

Homemaking

Heavy housework, such as vacuuming, lifting, and bed making, should be avoided. Kitchen activities are practiced with suggestions made to keep commonly used items at counter top level. Carrying items can be done by using aprons with large pockets, sliding items along the counter top, using a utility cart, attaching a small basket or bag to a walker, or wearing a fanny pack around the waist. Reachers are provided to grasp items in low cupboards or to pick up items on the floor.

Family orientation

A family member or friend should be present for at least one occupational therapy treatment session so that any questions can be answered. Appropriate supervision recommendations and instruction regarding activity precautions are given at this time. Instructional booklets on hip fractures and total hip surgery can be purchased from the American Occupational Therapy Association[1] and Krames Communications[9] to supplement the training.

Total Hip Replacement—Anterolateral Approach
Positions of hip stability: Flexion, abduction to neutral, and internal rotation
Positions of hip instability: Adduction, external rotation, and excessive hyperextension

Bed mobility

It is recommended that the patient lie in bed in the supine position. The appropriate wedge or pillow should be in place. If a patient sleeps side-lying on the nonoperated side, it is important to have a wedge or large pillow in place and to support the operated extremity to prevent adduction and external rotation. The patient is instructed in getting out of bed on both sides, although initially it may be easier to observe precautions by moving toward the nonoperated leg. Careful instruction is given to avoid adduction past midline and to maintain the operated extremity in internal rotation. It is important to determine the type and height of the patient's bed at home.

Transfers

It is always helpful for the patient first to observe the proper technique for transfers.
Chair: A firmly based chair with armrests is preferred. Before sitting, the patient is to extend the operated leg, reach back for the armrests, and then sit down slowly (Fig. 38-4). To stand from sitting the patient is instructed first to slide forward to the edge of the chair, then extend the operated leg and push off from the armrests. Low-seated or sling-seated chairs should be avoided.
Commode chair: An over-the-toilet commode chair is used initially while in the hospital. Usually by the time of discharge the patient has enough hip mobility to use a standard toilet seat safely. The patient is advised not to rotate the hip externally while wiping. To flush the toilet the patient should stand up and step to turn around to face the flusher.
Shower stall: Nonskid strips or stickers are recommended in all shower stalls and tubs. To transfer, walker or crutches go in first, then the operated leg followed by the nonoperated leg.
Shower over tub: The patient is instructed to stand parallel to the tub, facing the shower fixtures. Using a walker or crutches, the patient should transfer in sideways by bending one knee at a time over the tub. For patients with weight-bearing precautions or poor balance this transfer is not recommended. Purchase of a tub bench may be considered or the patient is advised to sponge bathe at the sink.
Car: A bench seat is recommended. The patient is instructed to back up to the passenger seat, sit down slowly with the operated leg extended, and then slide buttocks toward the driver's seat. The upper body and lower extremities move as one unit until the patient is squarely seated. Patients should avoid prolonged sitting in a car.

Lower body dressing

It is usually recommended to sit in a chair or on the side of the bed to dress. The patient is instructed to avoid externally rotating or crossing the legs to dress. Crossing the operated extremity over the nonoperated extremity at either the ankles or knees is to be avoided. Assistive devices may be necessary to observe precautions (Fig. 38-5). Refer to the section on lower body dressing for posterolateral approach.

Lower body bathing

If patient is unable to reach the lower legs or feet to wash or dry, refer to techniques stated in the section on lower body bathing of the posterolateral approach.

Hair shampoo

Same as for posterolateral approach.

Homemaking

Same as for posterolateral approach.

Family orientation

Same as for posterolateral approach.

Special Equipment

The occupational therapist should be familiar with the following equipment that is commonly used in the treatment of hip fracture and total hip replacement.

Nelson bed: An adjustable bed that allows for chair or 90° vertical tilt positions; may be used in some programs in the initial postoperative days to facilitate a change in the patient's position and allow a progressive tilting program before ambulation.

Hemovac: During surgery a plastic drainage tube is inserted at the surgical site to assist with drainage of blood postoperatively. The Hemovac has an area for collection of drainage and may be connected to a portable suction machine. The unit should *not* be disconnected for any activity, because disconnection may create a blockage in the system. The Hemovac is usually left in place for 2 days following surgery.

Abduction wedge: Large and small triangular wedges are used when the patient is supine to maintain the lower extremities (LEs) in the abducted position.

Ski box: This box is made of cardboard with foam padding inside and Velcro attachments to secure the leg in place. It is used to maintain the operated extremity in a position of neutral hip rotation. This device is no longer commonly used.[11]

Balanced suspension: This device is fabricated and set up by the physical therapist or cast room technician and physician and is usually used for about 3 days following surgery. Its purpose is to support the affected LE in the first few postoperative days. The patient's leg should *not* be taken out of the device for exercise until the device's use has been discontinued by the physician.

Reclining wheelchair: A wheelchair with an adjustable backrest that allows a reclining position; used for patients who have hip flexion precautions while sitting.

Commode chairs: The use of a commode chair instead of the regular toilet aids in safe transfers and allows the patient to observe necessary hip flexion precautions. The two front legs of the commode chair may be adjusted slightly lower than the back legs to increase the patient's ability to observe hip flexion limitations and decrease the risk of dislocation.

Assistive aids for ADL: Assistive aids are used to encourage independence while maintaining precautions against specific hip motions. These include a dressing stick, reacher, long-handled sponge, long handled shoehorn, elastic shoelaces, and sock aid (Fig. 38-5).

Sequential compression devices (SCDs): SCDs are used postoperatively to reduce the risk of deep vein thrombosis. They are inflatable, external leggings that provide intermittent pneumatic compression of the legs.[8]

Antiembolus hose: This device is thigh-high hosiery that is worn 24 hours a day and removed only during bathing. Its purpose is to assist circulation, prevent edema, and thus reduce the risk of deep vein thrombosis.[8]

Patient-controlled administration (PCA) IV: The amount of medication is predetermined and programmed by the physician and nursing to allow the patient to self-administer pain medication by pushing a button.

Incentive spirometer: Portable breathing apparatus to encourage deep breathing and prevent the development of postoperative pneumonia.

SUMMARY

The protocol for occupational therapy is determined by the surgical procedure performed and by the precautions prescribed by the physician. Patients who have weight-bearing precautions must observe them during all ADL. A simulation of the home environment or a home assessment is helpful to prepare the patient for potential problems that may arise after discharge. Areas to assess include the entry, stairs, bathroom, bedroom, sitting surfaces, and the kitchen. Recommendations to remove throw rugs and slippery floor coverings and obstacles are made because the patient will most likely be going home using an ambulatory assistive device. A kitchen stool or utility cart may be indicated. It is important to assess and instruct the patient and caregiver in ADL with adaptive equipment while observing any movement precautions.

Sexuality is often an area that is overlooked. Diagrams of positions that observe hip precautions can be provided with additional instruction regarding the method to get in and out of the recommended positions (see Chapter 17). Awareness of the psychosocial implications of hip fracture and total hip surgery can affect the success of therapy and is an important aspect to consider. Preoperative teaching programs are available at some facilities and are invaluable. The group class orients and familiarizes the patient to the hospital, nursing, physical therapy, occupational therapy, respiratory therapy, and discharge planning. Procedures and equipment, concerns regarding the hospitalization and discharge, and therapy are addressed. Participation in this type of class has been shown to relieve anxiety and fear, to empower the patient during the hospitalization, and to decrease the length of hospital stay.

SAMPLE TREATMENT PLAN

This sample treatment plan is not comprehensive. It deals with four of eight problems identified. The reader is encouraged to add objectives and methods to the plan, dealing with these and the other problems.

CASE STUDY

Mr. B is an 82-year-old man who has noticed increased right hip pain over the past year. He had a hip x-ray film examination 3 months ago, and a diagnosis of degenerative arthritis was confirmed. He has been admitted to the orthopedic unit of the hospital for elective right total joint replacement using the posterolateral approach.

Mr. B is a widower from Kentucky whose wife died shortly after they moved to California 6 months ago. Mr. B lives in his own cottage behind his son's home. Mr. B has been independent in meal preparation, self-care, and homemaking. He enjoys gardening, walking in the neighborhood, and visiting with his two grandchildren. His increased hip pain has limited his daily activity so that he must take frequent rests during the day and use a cane.

TREATMENT PLAN

Personal data

Name: Mr. B
Age: 82
Diagnosis: Degenerative arthritis affecting right hip; elective right total hip replacement
Disability: Limited LE ROM and ambulation
Precautions: Avoidance of right hip internal rotation, flexion greater than 90°, and adduction for 6 to 8 weeks after surgery; weight-bearing as tolerated
Treatment aims as stated in referral:
1. Orientation of patient to rehabilitation program
2. Evaluation of patient's function
3. Instruction of patient in maintaining hip precautions for ADL postoperatively.

Other services

Medical: Perform right total hip replacement surgery; prescribe rehabilitation therapies and medication
Nursing: Nursing care; positioning; supervise patient in activities and exercises following therapist's instruction of the patient
Physical therapy: LE ROM and strengthening exercises, transfer and gait training
Discharge planner: Arrange for home care follow-up
Family: Provide emotional support and physical assistance after discharge from hospital; encourage patient to observe precautions for hip movements at home

Frame of reference/treatment approach

Occupational performance/rehabilitative approach

OT EVALUATION

After surgery

Role of occupational therapy and rehabilitation program: Orient patient
Patient's goals from this surgery: Interview
General appearance: Observe ease of movement, personal hygiene, hospital equipment in use, and patient's position and expression
Mental and behavioral state: Observe
Communication, vision, and hearing: Observe
Sensation and pain: Test, observe
Strength of upper extremities and trunk: Test
Muscle tone: Test

Posture: Observe
Bulbar function: Screen
Perceptual and cognitive function: Test, observe
Avocational and vocational activities and endurance: Interview
Home layout and accessibility: Interview
Bed mobility: Demonstrate, interview
Transfers (bed, chair, toilet, shower, and car): Demonstrate or interview
Dressing: Interview
Personal hygiene: Interview

EVALUATION SUMMARY

After surgery. UE active ROM was limited to 160° of shoulder flexion bilaterally and strength was grades 4 to 5 (G to N).

The patient is very cooperative during treatment. He is tearful at times when he discusses the loss of his wife.

Mr. B requires assistive equipment for independence in self-care. Endurance is improved for homemaking, but assistance is still required for heavy household tasks because of hip precautions. After 8 weeks of recovery, he is expected to be independent in most household tasks and in all self-care without equipment.

For the first 8 weeks of recovery, Mr. B will be cautioned against activities such as gardening and heavy lifting, which may violate hip precautions. After 8 weeks, he will be al-

SAMPLE TREATMENT PLAN–cont'd

lowed to resume all of his leisure activities when less pain and increased endurance is expected.

Assets
Strives for independence
Good understanding of rehabilitation program
Supportive family
Good safety awareness and judgment

Problem list
1. Pain
2. Limited independence due to pain
3. Anxiety about surgery and dependence
4. Unable to ambulate without aids
5. ADL dependence
6. Limited leisure activities
7. Mild memory deficit
8. Limited endurance

PROBLEM 3: ANXIETY ABOUT SURGERY AND DEPENDENCE

Objective
Patient will understand hip precautions as related to functional activity and progression of rehabilitation following surgery

Method
Surgery and hip precautions are described to the patient

The occupational therapy program and progression of functional activities both in the hospital and at home are explained; a sound-slide module or written material may be used to help clarify explanations

PROBLEMS 4, 5: UNABLE TO AMBULATE WITHOUT AIDS, ADL DEPENDENCE

Objective
Patient will consistently demonstrate good safety skills during dressing, bathing, transfers, and ambulating with aids
    Patient utilizes assistive aids for self-care and observes hip precautions

Method
Correct use of assistive aids and transfer methods are demonstrated to the patient
    Patient practices with the assistive aids and transfer methods
    Patient ambulates safely with assistive aid during ADL

PROBLEMS 4, 6: UNABLE TO AMBULATE WITHOUT AIDS; LIMITED LEISURE ACTIVITIES

Objective
The patient will understand and demonstrate how he may modify gardening, visiting with grandchildren, and walking in the neighborhood to ensure observance of hip precautions and safety

Method
Patient participates in simulated gardening by bending, reaching, and carrying items in clinic
    Safety skills for ambulating with a walker or crutches around children are discussed and demonstrated; patient practices maneuvering in clinic obstacle course
    Therapist discusses the methods for pacing and awareness of safe surfaces for ambulating in neighborhood with the patient; patient practices pacing and maneuvering on various surfaces in hospital

Gradation
Patient solves problems through discussion, then in simulated situations

REVIEW QUESTIONS

1. Why is it critical for an occupational therapist to understand hip anatomy and treatment of hip fractures?
2. When reviewing the patient's medical history, what information should be obtained?
3. Define *clinical union.* How does it relate to weight-bearing and activity?
4. Identify four factors that influence fracture healing.
5. What is a pathological fracture, and in which diseases can it occur?
6. Describe the differences in approach and maintenance of closed and open reductions.
7. Femoral neck fractures are common in women older than 60 years of age. The type of surgical treatment used is based on the amount of displacement and what other factor?
8. Why would a compression screw and plate not be a surgical choice if there is poor blood supply to the femoral head?
9. Why are weight-bearing precautions observed with ORIF hip pinnings?
10. Which surgical procedure is generally used with a severely displaced femoral neck fracture or with an avascular femoral head?
11. Why must hip position precautions be observed during activity in patients with total hip replacements?
12. In which diagnostic groups other than fractures is there frequent indication for total joint replacement? What are the goals for this surgical approach in these diagnostic conditions?
13. Briefly describe the positions of instability in both the anterolateral and posterolateral approaches to hip replacement orthoplasty.
14. Briefly describe a total joint surface replacement and indications for its application.
15. Briefly describe a wedge and the indications for its use and application.
16. Following initial postoperative assessment, which functional activities are generally assessed in planning the initial treatment program?
17. Briefly describe the transfer method to a chair for a person after total hip replacement using posterolateral approach. What is the rationale applied here? What types of chairs should be avoided? Why?
18. Briefly describe a car transfer recommended for the patient with hip replacement orthoplasty using an anterolateral approach.
19. Which pieces of adaptive equipment might help a patient achieve independence in LE dressing following a posterolateral total hip replacement?
20. What suggestions could be made concerning carrying items when ambulation aids are necessary?

REFERENCES

1. American Occupational Therapy Association: *Daily activities after your hip surgery,* rev ed, Rockville, Md, 1990.
2. Butler RN: The life review: an interpretation of reminiscence in the aged. In Kastenbaum R, editor: *New thoughts on old age,* New York, 1964, Springer.
3. Butler RN: *Aging and mental health,* ed 3, St Louis, 1982, CV Mosby.
4. Crow I: Fractures of the hip: a self study, *ONA J* 5:12, 1978.
5. Garland JJ: *Fundamentals of orthopedics,* Philadelphia, 1979, WB Saunders.
6. Gray H: *Gray's anatomy,* Philadelphia, 1974, Running Press.
7. Hogshead HP: *Orthopaedics for the therapist,* Gainesville, 1973, University of Florida, unpublished.
8. Jones M, Lieberman S, Sitko S, Pitbladdo K: *The total hip replacement protocol,* Stanford, Calif, 1982 and 1986, Stanford University Hospital, Department of Physical and Occupational Therapy, unpublished.
9. Krames Communications: *After Total Hip Replacement* and *After a Hip Fracture,* San Bruno, Calif., 1989 (pamphlets).
10. Lewis SC: *The mature years: a geriatric occupational therapy text,* Thorofare, NJ, 1979, Charles B Slack.
11. Morawski D: *The total hip replacement protocol and hip fracture protocol,* Los Gatos, Calif, 1990, Community Hospital and Rehabilitation Center of Los Gatos-Saratoga, Department of Occupational Therapy, unpublished.
12. Salter RB: *Textbook of disorders and injuries of the musculoskeletal system,* Baltimore, 1970, Williams & Wilkins.

Motor Unit Dysfunction

Guy L. McCormack, Lorraine Williams Pedretti

The motor unit consists of four elements: (1) the cell body of the motor neuron in the anterior horn of the spinal cord, (2) the axon of the motor neuron that travels via spinal nerves and peripheral nerves to muscle, (3) the neuromuscular junction, and (4) the muscle fibers innervated by the neuron. The motor neurons in the anterior horn cells of the spinal cord mediate all voluntary movement and reflexes that subserve motor behavior. Muscle contraction is the output of the motor system. The pattern of recruitment and frequency of firing of various motor units determine variations in range, force, and type of movement. Thus, the motor unit is the elementary functional unit in the motor system.[34]

Diseases of the motor unit generally cause muscle weakness and atrophy of skeletal muscle and may be of neurogenic or myopathic cause. Those with a neurogenic basis are (1) the lower motor neuron disorders affecting the cell bodies and (2) peripheral neuropathies affecting peripheral nerves. Those with a myopathic basis affect the neuromuscular junction or the muscle itself.[34] Some of the motor unit disorders seen in clinical practice and their occupational therapy management are presented in this chapter.

NEUROGENIC DISORDERS

The lower motor neuron system includes the cell bodies in the anterior horn of the spinal cord and their axons, which pass by way of the spinal nerves and peripheral nerves to the neuromuscular junction. The nuclei of cranial nerves 3 through 10, located in the brain stem, and their axons are also part of the lower motor neuron system.[8,10] The motor fibers of the lower motor neurons are divided into the somatic and autonomic components. The somatic motor components include the alpha motor neurons, which innervate skeletal (extrafusal fibers) muscles, and gamma motor neurons, which innervate muscle spindles (intrafusal fibers). The autonomic component innervates the glands, smooth muscles, and heart musculature.[9,35] A lesion to any of these neurological structures consitutes neurogenic motor unit disease or a lower motor neuron (LMN) dysfunction.[9,34]

Lesions of lower motor neuron systems may be located in the anterior horn cells of the spinal cord, spinal nerves, peripheral nerves, and cranial nerves or their nuclei in the brain stem. Such lesions can result from (1) nerve root compression; (2) trauma: bone fractures and dislocations, lacerations, traction, penetrating wounds and friction; (3) toxins: lead, phosphorus, alcohol, benzene, and sulfonamides; (4) infections: poliomyelitis, Guillain-Barré syndrome; (5) neoplasms: neuromas and multiple neurofibromatosis; (6) vascular disorders: arteriosclerosis, diabetes mellitus, peripheral vascular anomalies, and polyarteritis nodosa; (7) degenerative diseases of the central nervous systems: amyotrophic lateral sclerosis; and (8) congenital malformations.[10,18,45,50]

POLIOMYELITIS

Because of the active immunization program (Salk and Sabin vaccines) in the United States since the mid 1950s, the disease has been essentially eradicated in the western hemisphere and new cases of poliomyelitis are rare.[45,53] Complacency about immunization has created some new cases, however. Adults who suffered poliomyelitis in early life in the United States, or those from countries that lacked the benefits of immunization and rehabilitation are referred to occupational therapy for vocational evaluation or improvement of the quality of life.[42,50]

Poliomyelitis is a contagious viral disease that affects the anterior horn cells of the gray matter of the spinal cord and the motor nuclei of the brain stem. The cervical and lumbar enlargements of the cord are affected most. Poliomyelitis results in a flaccid paralysis that may be local or widespread. The lower extremities, accessory muscles of respiration, and muscles that promote swallowing are primarily affected but there may be upper extremity involvement as well. Marked atrophy may be seen in the involved extremities, and deep tendon reflexes may be absent. Because poliomyelitis destroys the anterior horn cells, sensory roots are spared and sensation is intact. Contractures can occur very early in the course of the disease. In cases of local paralysis the asymmetry of muscles pulling on various joints may promote deformities, such as subluxation, scoliosis, and contractures. In severe cases osteoporosis (bone atrophy) may weaken the long weight-bearing bones and pathological fractures can occur.[26]

The medical treatment for poliomyelitis during the acute phase includes bed rest, positioning, and applications of warm packs to reduce pain and promote relaxation. Because there is no known cure for poliomyelitis, the disease must run its course. There is an incubation period of 1 to 3 weeks, and the recovery is dependent on the number of nerve cells destroyed. Paralysis may begin in 1 to 7 days after the initial symptoms. The medical aspects of rehabilitation may include reconstructive surgery, such as tendon transfer, arthrodesis, and surgical release of fascia, muscles, and tendons. Other medical procedures may include therapeutic stretching, casts, muscle reeducation, orthoses and bracing for standing or stability.[20]

Occupational Therapy Intervention

During the acute phase the patient receives symptomatic treatment and is confined to bed. Hot packs and positioning are used to relieve muscle spasm and to prevent contracture and deformity. The therapist can assist the nurse in providing good bed positioning to prevent contractures and protect weakened muscles. Because the poliomyelitis virus is infectious during this stage, isolation procedures should be carefully followed. The therapist should provide gentle passive range of motion (ROM) at the patient's physical tolerance level. Care should be taken not to grasp the involved muscle bellies, because they will be extremely tender and painful. The muscles may also be prone to spasm when painfully stimulated.[42]

Muscle fatigue, which can result in further weakness, should be avoided. If the patient has bulbar poliomyelitis, which affects the muscles of respiration, a respirator may be used or a tracheostomy performed to provide an airway. If the muscles necessary for swallowing are impaired, tube feeding may also be prescribed. The therapist should collaborate with the nursing staff when carrying out treatment to ensure proper functioning of the equipment necessary for the life support.[8,20,23,42]

The treatment program should include psychological support. The patient's fears and anxieties about the disabling effects of the disease should not be underestimated. The patient may need encouragement and positive experiences to promote an optimistic outlook during the rehabilitation process. The family may also need assistance in adjusting to the patient's disability.

As the rehabilitation process progresses, the precautions against physical and body fatigue continue. Assistive devices, splints, and mobile arm supports may be used to gain independence in daily activities. The long-

range rehabilitation program should follow a functional course of action. After the acute medical problems have subsided, the recovery stage may last as long as 2 years.[8] Because the damage to the anterior horn cells is permanent, the therapist should assist the patient in making the best possible use of whatever muscular function remains. Before treatment is started, an evaluation of the existing disability must be made. A thorough manual muscle test not only provides a baseline for muscle strength but detects joint deformities caused by contractured muscles, ligaments, tendons, and joint capsules. Manual muscle tests should be repeated monthly for the first 4 months and bimonthly for the next 4 months. After 8 months of therapeutic exercises the average patient has probably responded maximally.[6,18] In short, the therapeutic regime includes combinations of rest, movement, muscle reeducation, functional activities, and psychological support.

Movement for the patient who is recovering from acute poliomyelitis proceeds from passive to active ROM, depending on the patient's level of voluntary control. Muscle reeducation should be preceded by gentle stretching exercises. All active motions should be performed under careful supervision of the therapist. Compensatory movement should be avoided. A limited but correct movement is preferred to an ampler but incorrect movement. Active movements should be done in front of a mirror, which enables the patient to observe and correct motions accordingly.[20,23,41]

Muscle reeducation is accomplished in a graded fashion. At first the patient should learn "muscle-setting" exercises, that is, alternating contraction and relaxation of muscles without moving the joints. Isometric exercises and electromyographic (EMG) biofeedback may be beneficial. As the patient progresses, light resistance can be applied manually by the therapist before the use of resistance equipment. This approach allows the therapist to develop an empirical understanding of the patient's physical strengths and weaknesses.

Weakened muscles must be protected at all times. Muscles that cannot resist the forces of gravity are supported during exercise and rest periods. As a rule, resistive exercises are not attempted until the muscle is able to carry out a complete ROM against gravity. Weakened or flaccid muscles can be splinted at night to counteract the forces of gravity or the pull of the stronger antagonist muscles. During resistive exercises the therapist should stress correct body positioning, joint alignment, and energy conservation. Periods of rest should be included in the exercise program, as well as activities that incorporate the same movements and musculature.[14]

The goals for resistive exercises in the rehabilitation of the patient who has poliomyelitis are to strengthen undamaged muscles and give usefulness to the slightest contraction by integrating it into the global movement that permits the performance of a given activity. After the 8-month period if the muscle is unable to contract completely against gravity, it is doubtful that additional muscle strength will return. At this point the emphasis should be placed on maintenance of existing muscles and functional activities of daily living (ADL).

A self-care evaluation should be administered to achieve a baseline of function. Dressing activities may include donning and removing orthoses. Assistive devices should be tailored to the needs of the patient.[32] It may also be advantageous to begin activities for prevocational and vocational exploration. The patient's quality of life can be improved if he or she is employed and productive. The prognosis for successful rehabilitation depends on the personality of the patient and the perseverance of the therapist.

POSTPOLIO SYNDROME

Occupational therapists are seeing more patients with postpolio syndrome in rehabilitation centers. Patients who had polio earlier in life are experiencing the onset of additional weakness and other disabling symptoms years after the initial disease.[45,53] The number of such persons has increased, in part, because of the influx of immigrants from Southeast Asia and Latin America who suffered the original infection in their native lands.[15] It is estimated that there are more than 250,000 polio survivors in the United States. Of those, some 75,000 persons are experiencing symptoms of postpolio syndrome. Postpolio syndrome causes health and functional problems and patients who are affected are likely to be referred for occupational therapy services.[53]

The primary symptom of postpolio syndrome is progressive weakness.[15] There may be slowly progressive muscular weakness in muscles that were thought to be spared in the original illness as well as those previously affected. Pain, fatigue, cold intolerance, and new breathing difficulties may accompany the muscle weakness. Other symptoms include musculoskeletal problems such as joint, limb, or trunk deformities that can cause pain, decreased endurance, nerve entrapment, degenerative arthritis, falls, and unsteady gait.[53]

Fatigue is the most debilitating symptom because it limits activity, yet is not apparent to others. The fatigue may be severe and out of proportion to the apparent physical demands of the activity and can be overwhelming.[15,53] An increase in difficulties with ADL accompanies the symptoms. Problems with ambulation, transfers, using stairs, home management, driving, dressing, eating and swallowing, and bladder and bowel control may occur.[53]

The cause of postpolio syndrome is not fully understood. Motor unit dysfunction, musculoskeletal overuse, and musculoskeletal disuse are three factors, singly or in combination, thought to contribute to the onset of postpolio syndrome.[15] Several theories have been postulated about the cause of postpolio syndrome. These are that (1) it might be a form of amyotrophic lateral sclerosis; (2) there was reactivation of a dormant virus; (3) there

was a loss of anterior horn cells as a result of the normal aging process; and (4) immunologic factors were to blame. None of these causative factors has proved to be the explanation for the syndrome.[15,53]

Another theory is that postpolio syndrome is the result of motor neuron overwork. As a result of the original disease, many motor neurons died. Remaining healthy motor neurons sprouted, formed new neuromuscular junctions, and innervated orphaned muscle fibers in their regions. This process is called "reinnervation by terminal axon sprouting."[53] It results in a greater than normal responsibility for muscle fiber innervation by each surviving motor neuron, which eventually produces neuronal dysfunction. One hypothesis is that surviving motor neurons are impaired by the original infection and are unable to meet the metabolic demands of innervating the increased number of muscle fibers. The result is a dying back of overused axons with the resultant loss of muscle strength.[15,53]

Occupational Therapy Intervention

When a diagnosis of postpolio syndrome has been made, the affected person may be referred for rehabilitation services. The physical and occupational therapist are called upon to assess strength, range of motion, endurance, occupational performance, and psychosocial status. Gait and orthotic needs should be evaluated as well.[15]

The occupational therapist should begin by interviewing the patient to ascertain valued occupational roles and get an activity profile of daily life. The therapist should ask the patient which activities cause pain or fatigue, which activities have been curtailed or eliminated because of symptoms, when symptoms are most likely to occur (time, circumstances), and what kinds of aids, equipment, and human assistance are presently used. Manual muscle testing of the upper extremities may be indicated if there is weakness. It should be noted that postpolio muscles may actually function at levels of strength lower than estimated from scores on the manual muscle test and that upper extremity strength varies markedly throughout the range of motion.[53] Joint range of motion measurements are important if there are contractures and muscle imbalances.

An assessment of psychosocial status is necessary to select the best approach to the patient to facilitate rehabilitation efforts and adjustment to new limitations. Changes in physical capacities and curtailment of valued life skills confront the individual with psychologic issues of coping, adjustment, and adaptation. These changes may be as traumatic as they were at the time of the original illness. Feelings of denial, anger, frustration, and hopelessness must be dealt with in the occupational therapy intervention program.[15]

As a group, persons who originally had polio assumed that the disease was over, that disability was in the past, and that any residual weakness was static. They worked hard to overcome the effects of the initial paralysis and often performed well and achieved high levels of personal fulfillment. They were well integrated into society and so "disappeared" as a disabled group. The onset of new symptoms disrupts the performance and lifestyle achieved by years of hard work. There is the onset of new limitations, and old remedies do not work to ameliorate their effects. A personal history of success and overcoming early deficits combined with denial of new symptoms makes it difficult for the patient to confront the reality of the circumstances. As a result, it may be difficult for the therapist to facilitate changes in activity patterns and introduce needed equipment.[15]

Changes should be introduced gradually. Small changes may be more acceptable than major ones, even if the latter are obviously necessary.[15] The patient is confronted, for a second time, years after the disability was thought to be stabilized, with the notion of being "disabled" and limiting function and valued life activities. A supportive and realistic approach and patient education are key to lifestyle modification.[53]

The benefits of exercise are controversial. Exercise may aggravate pain. Overwork of muscles that have a decreased number of motor units may be damaging. Muscles weakened by disuse, however, may benefit from a nonfatiguing trial of gentle exercises for strengthening purposes. Strength may be maintained by performance of activities of daily living. Muscles being used for ADL should not be stressed further.[53] Patients should be encouraged to be active within limits of comfort and safety. A regular routine of activity or nonfatiguing exercise is important and affords the patient the feeling of doing something positive. Exercise programs must be carefully supervised, and long-term strengthening or maintenance exercise is recommended only in muscles that show no EMG evidence of prior polio involvement. Further weakness, discomfort, pain, muscle spasm, or chronic fatigue resulting from exercise are signs of excessive activity.[15,53]

Pain can be managed or alleviated by improving body mechanics, supporting weakened muscles, and promoting lifestyle modification. The occupational therapist can teach correct body mechanics in daily living tasks such as work and home management, ambulation, and transfers. Orthoses to support weakened muscles and lifestyle modification to reduce fatigue, stress, and activity that can cause overuse of muscles are indicated. Weight reduction is necessary for some patients.[15]

Perhaps the most important contribution of the occupational therapist is guiding and facilitating lifestyle modifications. Patients must avoid overuse of muscles. Evaluation and retraining in all aspects of ADL is important. Assistive devices for self-care and home managment may be indicted. Home and workplace modification can be important to prevent muscle overuse and decrease fatigue and potential deformity. Energy conservation and work simplifcation techniques should be taught. The patient and therapist should set priorities on occupational role performance. Energy conservation for the most valued activities may mean sacrificing less valued ones to be done by others or to be done with the assistance of equipment such as orthoses, assistive devices, or ambulation aids.[53]

Unless there is severe pulmonary or swallowing involvement in postpolio syndrome, the symptoms are not life-threatening. The symptoms can range from very mild weakness that is only slightly annoying to profound weakness that is severely incapacitating with risks of additional disabling problems such as fractures, osteoporosis, contractures, and depression. In general, however, it has been observed that improvement of symptoms and stabilization of function are experienced by patients who adjust their lifestyles by incorporating the recommendations that prevent muscle fatigue, improve body mechanics, and conserve energy.[15] Occupational therapy has an important role to play in achieving these goals.[53]

Guillain-Barré Syndrome

Guillain-Barré syndrome, also known as acute ideopathic neuropathy, infectious polyneuritis, and Landry's syndrome, is an acute inflammatory condition involving the spinal nerve roots, peripheral nerves, and, in some cases, selected cranial nerves. The Guillain-Barré syndrome often follows a viral illness, immunization, or surgery. It produces a hypersensitive response resulting in patchy demyelination of lower motor neuron pathways. The axons are generally spared, so recovery often follows a predictable course. In severe cases, however, Wallerian degeneration of the axon results in a slow recovery process. Guillain-Barré syndrome affects both sexes at any age.*

Clinically Guillain-Barré syndrome is characterized by a rapid onset. Initially there is no fever, but pain and tenderness of muscles, weakness, and decrease in deep tendon reflexes occur. As the disease progresses, it produces motor weakness or paralysis of the limbs, sensory loss, and muscle atrophy. The prognosis is varied. In severe cases cranial nerves 7, 9, and 10 may be involved and the patient may have difficulty speaking, swallowing, and breathing. If vital centers in the medulla are affected, the patient may experience respiratory failure and require tracheostomy or assisted ventilation. In most cases the patient recovers completely within a few weeks to a few months with relatively few residual effects.[18,45]

Occupational Therapy Intervention

Once the patient is medically stabilized, rehabilitation can be initiated. Treatment goals should be coordinated with the nurse, physical therapist, and other members of the team for a comprehensive rehabilitation program. The patient may be referred to occupational therapy while still totally paralyzed. During this initial phase of

---

* References 6, 8, 18, 36, 41, 42, 45, 50.

treatment, passive ROM, positioning, and splinting to prevent contracture and deformity and protect weak muscles are indicated. Passive activities such as watching television and light social activities such as visits from friends are encouraged. As improvement occurs and more active motion is possible, gentle, nonresistive activities and light ADL can be introduced to alleviate joint stiffness and muscle atrophy and prevent contractures. The occupational therapist should grade the activity program to the patient's physical tolerance level. *Fatigue should be avoided* and psychological support provided.[42]

The occupational therapy evaluation should include a test of strength, ROM measurement, and sensory tests. During the early stages of recovery the evaluation process itself may be fatiguing. It is often best to spread the evaluation over the course of a few days. The manual muscle test or functional motion test should not be done in one session. It is best to test a few muscles or motions at a time and allow the patient periods of rest.

Particular attention should be paid to the intrinsic muscles of the hands to determine residual weakness. If swallowing or speech is impaired an assessment of cranial nerve functions is indicated (see Chapter 11). Sensory testing should also be conducted because the sensory pathways are often affected. Sensory tests should include light touch, pressure, two-point discrimination, pain and temperature, proprioception, and stereognosis. Test findings should be recorded and deficits should be noted.

Passive ROM should begin with gentle movement of the proximal joints and should proceed only to the point of pain. As the patient's tolerance level increases, active ROM and light exercises may be introduced. The program should stress joint protection, and the therapist should look for muscle imbalance and substitution patterns. Progressive resistive exercises should be used conservatively. Throughout the course of recovery the therapist should guard against fatigue and irritation of the inflamed nerves. As the patient's strength and tolerance level increase, resistance can be gradually and moderately increased.

The therapist may also introduce sedentary or table top activities during the early stages of recovery. As the patient's strength increases, activities promoting more resistance, such as leather work, textiles, and ceramics, can be incorporated into the treatment regime. Grooming, self-care, and other ADL should be included as soon as the patient is capable of some independence and graded to include more activities as strength and endurance improve. Slings and mobile arm supports may be employed to alleviate muscle fatigue and gain independence. Activities should be varied between gross and fine and resistive and nonresistive to prevent undue fatigue.

Psychological support is important throughout the treatment program. The therapist should try to facilitate the feeling of self-worth, a positive attitude, and encour-

agement throughout the therapeutic process. Because the prognosis for recovery is good, the activities should be mentally stimulating and purposeful to the patient. The therapist should also respect the patient's level of pain tolerance during stretching and ROM exercises.[48]

PERIPHERAL NERVE INJURIES

GENERAL CHARACTERISTICS

Regardless of the origin of the injury, peripheral nerve lesions produce similar clinical manifestations. Seddon[37] described three categories of peripheral nerve injury: (1) neuropraxia, (2) neurotmesis, and (3) axonotmesis. Neuropraxia is a nerve lesion that is usually caused by orthopedic injuries resulting in compression, concussion, and traction injuries. Neuropraxis results in a block of neuronal transmission, usually in the larger myelinated nerve fibers. Although it produces muscle paralysis, there is usually some sparing of sensory modalities and an absence of peripheral nerve degeneration. Neuropraxia usually has a good prognosis for recovery if causal factors are removed.[5]

Neurotmesis is a complete severance of the nerve root or division of all the essential neuronal structures. This injury usually results from traumatic mechanisms such as severe traction forces or open lacerations. Axonotmesis represents disruption of nerve fibers (axons) causing peripheral (Wallerian) degeneration. Because the epineurium and surrounding connective tissues are preserved, spontaneous regeneration is likely to occur. Axonotmesis usually follows traction injuries, closed fractures or dislocations, or results from ischemia.[28,37]

The most obvious manifestation of peripheral nerve injury is muscle weakness or flaccid paralysis, depending on the extent of the nerve damage. Because of the loss of muscle innervation, atrophy follows and deep tendon reflexes are absent or depressed. Sensation along the cutaneous distribution of the nerve also is lost. Trophic changes, such as dry skin, hair loss, cyanosis, brittle fingernails, painless skin ulcerations, and slow wound healing in the area of involvement, may also be present as clinical signs. Occasionally minute muscle contractions called fasciculations may be seen on the surface of the skin overlying the denervated muscle belly. As a result of disturbances of sympathetic fibers of the autonomic nervous system, there is a loss of the ability to sweat above the denervated skin surfaces.

The patient may experience paresthesias, that is, sensations such as tingling, numbness, and burning or pain (causalgia), particularly at night. In addition, if the nerve damage was caused by trauma, edema is a prominent clinical manifestation. EMG examinations may reveal extremely small muscle contractions called fibrillations.*

Extensive peripheral nerve damage may produce de-

---

* References 3, 4, 8, 9, 13, 21.

formity if contractures, joint stiffness, and poor positioning are allowed to occur. Disfigurement of the hands is particularly noticeable and may produce some psychological complications. Other complications may include osteoporosis of bone and epidermal fibrosis of the joints. All of the clinical manifestations discussed may not be present. The clinical findings may vary with the underlying cause of the lesion.

The medical/surgical management of peripheral nerve lesions depends on the type of injury that has occurred. Lacerations may be treated with microsurgery to suture the severed nerve. Exploratory surgery (neurolysis) may be conducted to remove unwanted scar tissue from the site of the lesion. Nerve grafts and transplants are performed for severe traumatic injuries. Alcohol injections, vitamin B12, and phenol are used to alleviate the pain that might accompany peripheral neuropathy. For inflammatory processes high caloric diets with liberal use of vitamin B complex is the treatment of choice.[6,8,14]

Peripheral nerve regeneration begins about 1 month after the injury occurred. The rate of regeneration depends on the nature of the nerve lesion. If the nerve root has been cleanly severed and surgically repaired, the rate of regeneration ranges from ½ inch (1.3 cm) to 1 inch (2.5 cm) per month. Peripheral nerve injuries caused by burns, sepsis, or crushing present other complications to the healing process. Age is another factor: children usually have a faster rate of regeneration than adults.[29] In addition, proximal lesions regenerate faster than distal lesions and injuries to mixed nerves are slower to recover than single nerves.[5,27] Early medical treatment may require suturing the nerve and immobilizing the involved extremity to ensure good apposition of the severed nerves. In the past, full recovery of muscles was not probable because regenerated fibers lose about 20% of their original diameter and conduct impulses at a slower rate.[9,28] The introduction of microsurgery advancements has improved the regenerative process.

Because peripheral nerves have the capacity to regenerate, the course of recovery can be somewhat predictable. The clinical signs of regeneration do not always follow a specific sequence. The following clinical signs of nerve regeneration can be expected:

Skin appearance: As the edema subsides and collateral blood vessels develop, the circulatory system should become more normalized. The skin should improve in its color and texture.

Primitive protective sensations: The first signs of cutaneous sensation are usually the gross recognition of crude pain, temperature, pressure, and touch.

Paresthesias (Tinel's sign): Tapping or percussing from distal to proximal along the course of the damaged nerve route can be used to detect recovery. If the patient feels paresthesias (pins and needles) distal to the presumed site of lesion, regeneration is occurring, whereas a painful Tinel's sign at the lesion may indicate neuroma formation.[5,18]

Scattered points of sweating: As the parasympathetic fibers of the autonomic nervous system regenerate, the sweat glands recover their functions.

Discriminative sensations: The more refined sensations, such as the ability to identify and localize touch, joint movements (proprioception), recognition of objects in the three-dimensional form (stereognosis), speed of movement (kinesthesia), and two-point discrimination, should be returning at this point.

Muscle tone: As nerve fibers regenerate and reinnervate their respective musculature via their motor end plates, flaccidity decreases and muscle tone increases. An important principle is that paralyzed muscles must first sense pressure before tone and movement can be realized.

Voluntary muscle function: The patient is able to move the extremity first with gravity eliminated, and as strength increases, active movement of the extremity through full ROM is possible. At this point graded exercises can begin. Full recovery of muscle power is not probable because the possibility that thousands of regenerating fibers will find their previous connections is unlikely.*

For complete laceration of peripheral nerves, the two-point discrimination test and the wrinkle test are good methods of monitoring sensory return.[29] The two-point discrimination test provides a quantitative measure of sensation. The normal distance to discriminate one point from two points on the distal fingertip is 2 to 4 mm. A two-point discrimination of greater than 15 mm denotes tactile agnosia (absent sensation). This test can be done with the use of a high-quality caliper with blunted tips so that the pain sensation is not elicited. Light application of the calipers to the patient's skin in a random pattern can help the therapist map out the cutaneous, topographical areas that are innervated and denervated.

Another test that can be clinically significant is the wrinkle test. This test is performed by immersing the patient's hand in plain water at 108°F (42.2°C). The hand remains submerged for about 20 to 30 minutes until wrinkling occurs. At this point the patient's hand is dried, graded on a scale of 0 to 3, and photographed. The "0" on the scale represents an absence of wrinkling, whereas "3" represents normal wrinkling. The wrinkle test appears to provide an objective method of testing innervation of the hand with recent complete and partial peripheral nerve injuries. The actual physiologic mechanism that causes the wrinkling is not fully understood, and the test is not appropriate for patients with traumatic peripheral nerve compression injuries.[29] Nevertheless, the test can help in determining the rate of sensory regeneration and can provide a graphic record of denervated areas.

---

* References 3, 6, 8, 9, 21, 28.

SPECIFIC PERIPHERAL NERVE INJURIES
Brachial Plexus Injury

The nerve roots that innervate the upper extremity originate in the anterior rami between C4 and T1. This network of lower anterior cervical and upper dorsal spine nerves is collectively called the brachial plexus. This very important nerve complex can be palpated just behind the posterior border of the sternocleidomastoid as the head and neck are tilted to the opposite side.[6,8,20,40]

Lesions to the brachial plexus usually result from a variety of traumatic injuries. Most brachial plexus injuries in children are caused by birth trauma. Such injuries are called Erb's palsy and Klumpke's paralysis. Erb's palsy is indicative of lesions to the fifth and sixth brachial plexus roots. Paralysis and atrophy occur in the deltoid, brachialis, biceps, and brachioradialis muscles. Clinically the arm hangs limp, the hand rotates inward, and functional movement is extremely limited.

Klumpke's paralysis affects the more distal aspect of the upper extremity. The disorder results from injury to the eighth cervical and first thoracic brachial plexus roots. Consequently there is paralysis to the distal musculature of the wrist flexors and the intrinsic muscles of the hand.[6,8]

Long Thoracic Nerve Injury

The long thoracic nerve (C5-7) innervates the serratus anterior muscle, which anchors the apex of the scapula to the posterior of the rib cage. Although injury to this nerve is not common, it has been injured by carrying heavy weights on the shoulder, neck blows, and axillary wounds. The resulting clinical picture is winging of the scapula, difficulty flexing the outstretched arm above shoulder level and difficulty protracting the shoulder or performing scapula abduction and adduction.

Injuries involving the long thoracic nerve are usually treated by stabilizing the shoulder girdle to limit scapula motion. The therapist must avoid using activities that promote shoulder movements. If nerve regeneration is not complete, surgery may be indicated to relieve the excessive mobility of the scapula. After medical treatment the occupational therapist encourages maximal functional independence and teaches the patient to use long-handled devices to compensate for shoulder limitations.

Axillary Nerve Injury

The axillary nerve is composed from the C5-6 spinal nerves and derived from the posterior region of the brachial plexus. The motor branches of the axillary nerve innervate the superior aspect of the deltoid muscle and the teres minor muscle. Although the axillary nerve is rarely damaged by itself, it is often damaged along with traumatic lesions to the brachial plexus. As a result, the patient experiences weakness or paralysis of the deltoid muscle, which causes limitations in horizontal abduction and hyperesthesia on the lateral aspect of the shoulder.

In addition to the loss of muscle power, atrophy of the deltoid muscle produces asymmetry of the shoulders. If the nerve damage is permanent, a muscle transplantation may be required to provide some abduction of the arm.[6,8,36]

The occupational therapist should maintain ROM to prevent deformity and improve circulation. Passive abduction of the shoulder should be done daily. The teres minor and deltoid muscles should be protected from stretch during the manual ROM activities. The patient may be taught to use long-handled assistive devices to compensate for the abduction deficit. If a surgical transplant is performed, the therapist should be familiar with the surgical procedure and assist in muscle reeducation. An EMG biofeedback machine can be beneficial in providing the patient with visual and auditory incentives during muscle reeducation sessions.

The occupational therapist may also assist the patient in dressing activities. If the asymmetry of the shoulders presents a cosmetic problem when wearing shirts or jackets, a foam rubber or thermoplastic pad can be fabricated to fill in the space that was once occupied by the deltoid muscle. The patient should be encouraged to learn self-ranging techniques and implement an exercise program to maintain the integrity of the unimpaired muscles of the involved extremity.

Lesions of the radial, median, and ulnar nerves and cumulative trauma disorders affecting the hand are discussed in Chapter 35.

Volkmann's Contracture

A fracture of the lower end of the humerus (supracondylar region) may result in a diminished supply of well-oxygenated blood to the muscles of the forearm. This phenomenon can occur when the fracture has been tightly cast and bandaged. Edema sets in near the site of the injury and shuts down the blood supply to the muscle bellies because the site of injury cannot swell outward. Ischemia deprives tissues of oxygen and nourishment. The muscle can become necrotic, causing atrophy and contractures of the wrist, fingers, and forearm. The flexor digitorum profundus and flexor pollicis longus muscles are severely affected. The median nerve is often more impaired than the ulnar nerve.[8,20]

Shortly after a fracture of the humerus has been immobilized, the patient may have a cold, distal extremity with a smooth, glossy, or dusky appearance of the skin. If the therapist observes these symptoms and cannot detect a radial pulse, the physician should be informed immediately, and the cast should be removed. Early detection and prevention of this problem can eliminate a very severe deformity. If, for example, the ischemia lasts 6 hours, some contracture will follow. Ischemia lasting 48 hours or more results in a permanent deformity of the forearm. If mild ischemia has occurred, the physician may prescribe vigorous, active exercises to increase circulation, activate musculature, and prevent joint stiffness.[6]

TABLE 39-1 Clinical Manifestations of Peripheral Nerve Lesions

SPINAL NERVES	NERVE ROOTS	MOTOR DISTRIBUTION	CLINICAL MANIFESTATIONS
BRACHIAL PLEXUS			
C5-7	Long thoracic	Shoulder girdle, serratus anterior	Winged scapula
C5-6	Dorsal scapular	Rhomboid major and minor, levator, scapulae	Loss of scapular adduction and elevation
C7-8	Thoracodorsal	Latissimus dorsi	Loss of arm adduction and extension
C5-6	Suprascapular	Supraspinatus, infraspinatus	Weakened lateral rotation of humerus
C5-6	Subscapular	Subscapularis, teres major	Weakened medial rotation of humerus
C6-8, T1	Radial	All extensors of forearm, triceps	Wrist drop, extensor paralysis
C5-6	Axillary	Deltoid, teres minor	Loss of arm abduction, weakened lateral rotation of humerus
C5-6	Musculocutaneous	Biceps brachii, brachialis, coracobrachialis	Loss of forearm flexion and supination
C6-8, T1	Median	Flexors of hand and digits, opponens pollicis	Ape hand deformity, weakened grip, thenar atrophy, unopposed thumb
C8, T1	Ulnar	Flexor of hand and digits, opponens pollicis	Claw hand deformity, interosseus atrophy, loss of thumb adduction
LUMBOSACRAL PLEXUS			
L2-4	Femoral	Iliopsoas, quadriceps femoris	Loss of thigh flexion, leg extension
L2-4	Obturator	Adductors of thigh	Weakened or loss of thigh adduction
L4-5, S1-3	Sciatic	Hamstrings, all musculature below the knee	Loss of leg flexion, paralysis of all muscles of leg and foot
L4-5, S1-2	Common peroneal	Dorsiflexors of foot	Foot drop, steppage gait, loss of eversion
L4-5, S1-3	Tibial	Gastrocnemius, soleus, deep plantar flexors of foot	Loss of plantar flexion and inversion of foot

OCCUPATIONAL THERAPY INTERVENTION FOR PERIPHERAL NERVE INJURIES

The treatment goals for the various peripheral nerve injuries are similar. The aim is to assist the patient in regaining the maximal level of motor function and independence in performance areas. The therapist must know the anatomy and innervation of the affected part and evaluate the pattern of paralysis and its effects on the function of the part. Treatment is directed to the stage of recovery and the remediation and compensation for sensory, motor, and performance deficits. The rate of return and the residual impairments depend largely on the severity of the lesion and the quality of care during the rehabilitation process. Table 39-1 is a useful summary of the major nerve roots and clinical manifestation of their lesions.

The occupational therapist may be involved during the acute and rehabilitation phases of treatment. During the acute postoperative phase, treatment is aimed at preventing deformity. Initially static splints are used to immobilize the extremity and protect the site of injury.[41,46] (See Chapter 35 for more on postoperative management of peripheral nerve repair.) During this phase the reduction of edema may be important. Reduction of edema is achieved by elevating the extremity above the level of the heart, which decreases the hydrostatic pressure in the blood vessels and promotes venous and lymphatic drainage.

Manual massage while the extremity is elevated may also reduce edema. The massage should entail centripetal strokes gently to force the excess fluids toward the proximal aspects of the body. Care must be taken not to disturb the healing process of the site of injury. External elastic support can also be used to alleviate the edema, and passive ROM will assist in the prevention of edema, by promoting venous return.[49]

As the patient's muscle function returns, an appropriate exercise program can be established. Resistive activities, such as woodworking, ceramics, leather work, and copper tooling, may be used in conjunction with isometric and isotonic exercises when muscle function is adequate. The therapist should not overtax the returning musculature and should protect the weaker muscle groups from stretch and fatigue. The therapist may fabricate splints or slings for functional positioning and protection of weakened musculature from overstretching.

ADL assessment is necessary to identify difficulties with essential performance tasks. One-handed methods of dressing, eating, and hygiene activities may be necessary on a temporary or permanent basis. Assistive devices, such as long-handled reaching aids and one-handed kitchen tools, can be beneficial to increase independence.

Sensory reeducation is used to assist the patient in establishing appropriate responses to sensory stimuli. Sensory reeducation for peripheral nerve injuries is discussed in Chapters 13 and 35.

PERIPHERAL NERVE PAIN SYNDROMES

Pain is a common complication in peripheral nerve injuries.[7,52] For some patients the pain itself becomes an overwhelming disability. The types of pain that have been associated with peripheral nerve injuries are causalgia and neuroma pain.[37,43,52] Causalgia is pain of great intensity originating from peripheral lesions affecting the fibers of the autonomic nervous system.[13] The most common sites for peripheral nerve injuries producing causalgia are the brachial plexus, sciatic, tibial, median, and ulnar nerves.[5] Because the sympathetic and parasympathetic fibers travel in the walls of blood vessels until they reach their respective organs, the pain can radiate to quadrants of the body served by these major blood vessels.[12,27]

In the upper extremity, causalgia is described as an intense burning sensation so excruciating that the patient holds the affected limb immobile for fear of stimulating the pain. The affected limb becomes extremely sensitive to temperature change, wind, and even noise.[12,27] Causalgia is also exacerbated by emotional stress. Because of its origin in the sympathetic division of the autonomic nervous system, even mood changes alter the pain sensitivity levels.[12]

Neuromas are incompletely regenerated nerve endings and fibers at the site where the peripheral nerve was damaged. Neuromas are particularly problematic in nerve endings serving the fingers and in amputated limbs. Phantom limb pain is often the result of neuroma formation. Neuromas are exquisitely painful and tender when they develop in the extremities that bear weight or are easily traumatized. In some cases, surgical resection is necessary to remove neurons that adhere to fascia and subcutaneous tissue.

Occupational Therapy Intervention

Research on pain management has revealed that certain activities and noninvasive techniques can modulate pain perception.[22,43,44] A better understanding of pain control mechanisms and the discovery of endogenous opiate-like substances (endorphins, enkephalins, and substance P) in the body have provided therapists with new techniques for patients suffering from peripheral nerve pain.[1,7,22,30,39]

Pain stimuli travel from pain receptors (nociceptors) along ascending pathways to the thalamus to the cerebral cortex where the messages reach the conscious mind. The occupational therapist can modulate pain perception in several ways. The therapist must first evaluate the intensity, quality, and location of pain. This procedure can be done by having the patient mark the point of pain on an anatomical drawing and then estimate pain intensity on a numerical scale. The patient is asked to used terms such as sharp, dull, aching, throbbing, sore, or burning to describe the personal experience of pain. Factors that seem to contribute to pain should also be explored during the interview. These factors might include specific foods and drinks, positions, and activities.[22]

Several intervention techniques can alter pain messages or neuronal transmission within these pathways.

Peripheral pain emitting from neuromas can be alleviated by increased input to mechanoreceptors in the skin. This approach works because the sensory neurons transmitting pain messages must synapse in the dorsal horn of the spinal cord. The synapse to the secondary neurons in the dorsal gray matter is conducted through the release of substance P, one of the opiate-like neurotransmitters. Increased input to the mechanoreceptors in the skin inhibits the release of substance P.[30,43] The therapist can use several techniques to increase mechanoreceptor input. Graded light local percussion and therapeutic vibration over neuromas have been used to expedite this process.[1,24,25]

Transcutaneous electrical nerve stimulation (TENS) has been found to provide relief from pain related to neuromas, peripheral nerve injuries, residual limb pain, and phantom limb syndromes.[19,38] The occupational therapist who has been appropriately trained can use TENS when it is prescribed by a physician. Localized stimulation to acupoints and trigger points can also be used to modify neuroma pain.[39,43] Many patients obtain pain relief by protecting the tender regions of the body. The therapist can fabricate protective devices from splinting materials. Some patients find relief when the extremity is wrapped with a cloth material that has been soaked in water.[5]

Pain management for causalgia uses a different rationale and different neurophysiologic systems. Causalgia arises from the autonomic nervous system. Increased activity in the sympathetic division of the autonomic nervous system exacerbates causalgia. In addition, the neuronal connections to the limbic system suggest that emotions play an important role in causalgia.[5,12,27,30]

The neurophysiologic rationale for alleviating causalgia is very complex because it involves at least two distinct systems. Both systems originate in areas of the cortex. One system is more direct in that it projects to neurons in the reticular formation and to motor pathways terminating on excitatory and inhibitory neurons in the dorsal gray matter of the spinal cord. The other system includes neurons in the cortex projecting to cell bodies in the limbic system, which go on to transmit to the midbrain.[1,7,39,43]

The first cortical modulating system is very responsive to physical and emotional stress. Consequently, stress increases blood concentrations of catecholamines (dopamine, epinephrine, and norepinephrine) via the autonomic nervous system, which triggers the release of enkephalins that inhibit transmission of afferent interneurons in the dorsal gray matter. The second cortical modulating system, involving the limbic system and midbrain, responds by releasing endorphins to inhibit pain transmission.[1,7,39,43] The release of these endogenous opiates (enkephalin and endorphins) gives credence to the use of purposeful activities to modulate the perception of pain.

By involving the patient in successful and purposeful

activities the occupational therapist provides cognitive diversion from the pain experience. Engagement in purposeful activities can influence moods and emotions, an effect that in turn alters the perception of pain intensity and ultimately modifies the pain threshold.[16,22,27,43] The therapist can also use background music as a therapeutic modality. Concentration on music affects the cortical modulating system through connections with the limbic system. In addition, music can be used with earphones. While the patient is engaged in activities, it provides a control factor over the pain stimulus because the volume can be increased or decreased to accommodate the pain intensity.[22]

Because causalgia is related to tension and stress, the therapist can also employ relaxation techniques.[7,12] Deep breathing, progressive relaxation, and visualization techniques can promote a dominance of the parasympathetic system.[22,27,43] By eliciting the relaxation response, the patient's muscles relax, heart rate and respiration rate slow, and the patient experiences a sense of well-being. By learning relaxation techniques the patient can control emotional tension and depression, both contributors to causalgia and the perception of pain.[22]

DISEASE OF THE NEUROMUSCULAR JUNCTION
MYASTHENIA GRAVIS

Myasthenia gravis is a disease of chemical transmission at the nerve/muscle synapse or neuromuscular junction. It is caused by an autoimmune response in which antibodies are produced against nicotinic acetylcholine (ACh) receptors and interfere with synaptic transmission at the nerve/muscle junction. Because neurotransmission is defective, there is weakness of skeletal muscle.[33] Myasthenia gravis occurs at all ages but primarily affects younger women and older men.[18,45]

About 75% of patients with myasthenia gravis have enlarged thymus glands and some have tumors of the thymus gland. Removal of the thymus gland (thymectomy) reduces symptoms or causes remission in about 50% of patients, and this procedure has become standard therapy. Patients are also treated with anticholinesterase drugs, glucocorticoids, and other immunosuppressive pharmacologic agents.[33,51] Plasmapheresis, a procedure that entails filtering the blood to remove the IgG autoantibodies, is sometimes used for patients with severe disease who have failed to respond to other therapeutic measures. It is sometimes used before thymectomy in seriously ill patients.[2,17,18,45]

Myasthenia gravis is characterized by abnormal fatigue of voluntary muscle.[14] The disease can affect any of the striated skeletal muscles of the body but it has an affinity for the muscles of the eyelids and eyes and oropharyngeal muscles. Therefore the muscles most often affected are those that move the eyes, eyelids, tongue, jaw, and throat. The limb muscles may also be affected. The muscles that are used most often fatigue sooner.[14,33,51] Therefore the patient may have double vision, drooping of the eyelids, and difficulty with speech or swallowing as muscles fatigue. Patients with myasthenia gravis may experience life-threatening respiratory crises, which require hospitalization and use of a ventilator. The incidence of these crises has declined significantly in recent years, probably because of increased use of thymectomy.[33,51] The intensity of the disease fluctuates and its course is unpredictable.[51]

Spontaneous remissions occur frequently but relapse is usual.[8] Remissions or decrease in symptoms and improvement in strength and function can last for years. There may be exacerbations of unpredictable severity, however, induced by exertion, infection, or childbirth.[42] The prognosis for myasthenia gravis varies with each individual, but for most it is a progressively disabling disease and the patient may ultimately become bedridden with severe permanent paralysis. Death usually occurs as a result of respiratory complications.[8,42,45]

Occupational Therapy Intervention

The primary role of the occupational therapist is to help the patient regain muscle power and build endurance. It is important that the therapeutic program not cause fatigue. The therapist should monitor the patient's muscle strength on a regular basis. The therapist need not evaluate all of the muscles because the evaluation contributes to fatigue. Instead, the therapist can test the strength of a few muscles during each visit and keep a running record to note any important changes.

If the patient is taking oral cholinergic drugs, optimal strength is expected about 1 or 2 hours after the medication has been ingested.[2] Therefore the therapist should coordinate muscle testing with the drug treatment regime so the test results are not confounded by the medication. The therapist should also report to the physician any changes in the patient's physical appearance, such as ptosis of the eyelids, drooping facial muscles, or alterations of breathing or swallowing.

The therapist should provide gentle nonresistive activities that are intellectually and psychologically stimulating. The activities should be graded so they do not fatigue the patient. Overexertion must be avoided and respiratory problems prevented. The treatment plan should include energy conservation, work simplification, and necessary adaptive and assistive devices to reduce effort during daily activities. If appropriate, electronic communication devices can be installed in the patient's home so contact with community agencies can be maintained. In addition, the therapist may assist with home planning to determine architectural barriers, bathroom adaptations, and furniture rearrangements. Mobile arm supports and splints may be used to protect weakened musculature from overstretching and aid in positioning for function.[42]

The therapist should assist in educating the patient

about the disease. The patient should avoid emotional stress, overexertion, fatigue, and excessive heat or cold because they may exacerbate the symptoms of the disease. The therapist should also follow infection control procedures, because minor infections can also exacerbate the symptoms.

MYOPATHIC DISORDERS
THE MUSCULAR DYSTROPHIES

The muscular dystrophies are a group of uncommon inherited conditions. There are four major types of muscular dystrophy (MD).[34,51] They have in common the progressive degeneration of muscle fibers while the neuronal innervation to muscle and sensation remain intact. As the number of muscle fibers declines, each axon innervates fewer and fewer of them resulting in progressive weakness.[31]

Duchenne's muscular dystrophy. This type of MD affects males only, being inherited as an X-linked recessive trait. The disease begins at birth and is usually diagnosed between the ages of 18 to 36 months. It begins in the muscles of the pelvic girdle and legs, then spreads to the shoulder girdle. Calf muscles appear to be hypertrophic because of the infiltration of fat cells that accompanies degeneration of muscle fibers. The child has difficulty walking, has a waddling gait, and usually must use a wheelchair by age 12. Ultimately he becomes bedridden and usually death occurs by the age of 30.[34,42,51]

Facioscapulohumeral muscular dystrophy. This form of MD has its onset in adolescence and primarily affects the muscles of the face and shoulder girdle, hence its descriptive name. It progresses slowly and there is a normal life expectancy for its victims.[51] It is inherited through an autosomal dominant gene and affects both males and females equally.[34]

Myotonic muscular dystrophy. This type of MD not only causes weakness but has another component, myotonia (tonic spasm of muscles), which makes relaxation of muscle contraction difficult. It is inherited through an autosomal dominant gene and affects males and females. Its unique features, besides the myotonia, are that it involves the cranial muscles and that the limb weakness tends to be distal rather than proximal. Associated symptoms are cataracts, found in almost all patients, and testicular atrophy and baldness found in men. The disease may be mild or severe and can occur at any age.[34,51]

Limb-girdle dystrophy. This type of MD is probably a group of disorders that do not fit readily in the other types described. Affected persons differ in age of onset, extent of weakness, and familial inheritance patterns. It is inherited by an autosomal recessive gene.[34,51]

Occupational Therapy Intervention

Because this group of diseases is degenerative, decline of muscle function cannot be prevented. Medical management is largely supportive, and rehabilitation measures are vital in delaying deformity and achieving maximal function within the limits of the disease and its debilitating effects. The primary goal of occupational therapy is assisting the patient to attain maximal independence in ADL for a as long as possible. Self-care activities and assistive devices for independence and leisure activities are an important part of the treatment program.[42]

Wheelchair prescription and mobility training may be part of the occupational therapy program. Powered wheelchairs are necessary in some instances. The wheelchair may require a special seating system or supports to minimize scoliosis, hip and knee flexion contractures, and ankle plantar flexion deformity. A wheelchair lap board, suspension slings, or mobile arms supports are indicated to facilitate self-feeding, writing, reading, use of a computer and table top leisure activities when there is substantial shoulder girdle and upper limb weakness. Built up utensils may be helpful when grip strength declines.[42] Home and workplace modification may be necessary for some patients.[11]

Active exercise may be helpful but overexertion and fatigue must be avoided. For patients with respiratory involvement, exercise for breathing control may be administered by the physical therapist.[47]

Psychosocial problems and educational and vocational requirements also need attention by the occupational therapist. Deficits in cognitive function and verbal intelligence have been reported in some types of MD. Depression and other personality abnormalities may be concomitant problems.[11] Patient and family education is an important part of the occupational therapy program. A supportive approach to the patient and family is helpful as function changes and new mobility aids, assistive devices, and community resources become necessary.[42]

SUMMARY

This chapter reviewed some diseases of the motor unit, which comprises the lower motor neuron, neuromuscular junction, and muscle. Some of these conditions are reversible and others are degenerative. The role of the occupational therapist is to assess functional capabilities and provide positioning, exercise, pain management techniques, and orthoses, if indicated. ADL skills (including self-care, home management, mobility, and work-related tasks) and energy conservation, work simplification, and joint protection techniques are important elements of the occupational therapy intervention program. Assistive devices, communication aids, and mobility equipment and training in their use may be necessary. Psychosocial considerations and patient and family education are important aspects of the occupational therapy program.

SAMPLE TREATMENT PLAN

CASE STUDY

John is a 23-year-old man employed as a construction worker. He is a high school graduate, is married, and has two children. Recently while working he sustained a deep laceration of the right anterior forearm. This injury resulted in a severed ulnar nerve and partial damage to the median nerve. The patient has undergone microsurgery, and the severed nerves have been repaired with moderate success.

John is energetic and has difficulty adjusting to the hospital environment and to a sedentary existence.

He was referred to occupational therapy for services during the acute and rehabilitation phases of his treatment program. The goals are to prevent deformity, restore joint and muscle function to the maximal level possible, facilitate adjustment to hospital and disability, and evaluate potential for return to former employment.

TREATMENT PLAN

Personal data

Name: John
Age: 23
Diagnosis: Laceration to right forearm, peripheral nerve injury
Disability: Ulnar and median nerve dysfunction; moderate to severe motor paralysis
Treatment aims as stated in referral:
    To prevent deformity
    To restore joint and muscle function to maximal level possible
    To facilitate adjustment to hospital and disability
    To evaluate potential for return to employment

Other services

Medical-surgical: Surgery, medication, supervision of rehabilitation program

Nursing: Nursing care during acute phase of treatment, psychological support
Physical therapy: ROM, muscle reeducation, edema control
Social service: Financial arrangements, counseling to patient and family
Vocational rehabilitation counselor: Explore vocational potential, vocational counseling

Frame of reference

Occupational performance

Treatment approaches

Biomechanical and rehabilitative

OT EVALUATION

Sensation: Test (light touch, stereognosis, proprioception, two-point discrimination, pain)
Nerve regeneration: Wrinkle test
Muscle strength: Manual muscle test
ROM: Measure
Grip and pinch strength: Test with instruments

Hand evaluation: Observation, Jebsen-Taylor Test of Hand Function; tests of speed and dexterity
ADL: Observe performance
Psychosocial adjustment: Observe
Muscle function: EMG biofeedback evaluation to obtain quantitative information for baseline function

EVALUATION SUMMARY

Muscle testing revealed that the right upper extremity has considerable weakness in the distal musculature. Wrist flexors, finger adductors, finger abductors, and opposition of thumb are P (2). Muscles innervated by the radial nerve such as the wrist extensors are G (4) to N (5).

The joint motions are within normal limits, but some tightness is noted in the thumb and long finger flexors. Visual inspection shows some edema and marked muscle atrophy of the interossei (web space) and moderate atrophy of

the thenar muscles. The pattern of denervation has produced a muscle imbalance and the ape hand deformity.

Grip strength registers at 10 pounds (4.5 kg) in the right hand and 120 pounds (54 kg) in the left. Palmar pinch strength using lateral pinch is 4 pounds (1.8 kg) on the right and 24 pounds (10.8 kg) on the left.

The Jebsen Hand Function Test reveals below-standard norms for age in gross grasp, fine prehension, and manual dexterity on the right.

SAMPLE TREATMENT PLAN – cont'd

Sensory testing shows that light touch, proprioception, and two-point discrimination are absent in the ulnar aspect of the right hand. The medial aspect is impaired, especially in the thenar region. Stereognosis sensibility is impaired when comparing nickels with quarters and pennies with dimes. Superficial pain sensitivity (pinprick) is intact on medial anterior surface of the right hand and absent along ulnar nerve root distribution.

Tinel's sign is present distal to the laceration on the right forearm. The wrinkle test shows absence of wrinkling along the cutaneous sensory distribution of the ulnar nerve; some wrinkling is noted in the medial nerve root distribution. Photos of wrinkle distributions are included in record for visual inspection and documentation.

The accident does not appear to have had any effect on the patient's cognitive functions. He has performed within normal limits for a 23-year-old male of average intelligence. He exhibits normal long-term and short-term memory, good judgment, and problem-solving skills. He attended to cognitive perceptual tasks, followed directions effectively, and demonstrated the ability to concentrate for extended periods of time.

Psychosocial adjustment appears to be normal. John is married and has two children. His marriage appears to be stable, and his wife has been supportive. John has had difficulty adjusting to his hospitalization. He has a high level of energy and is accustomed to being active. At times he seems to be agitated, impatient, and mildly depressed because of his inactivity. The patient's leisure interests consisted of auto mechanics and playing handball and baseball. He also enjoyed home improvement projects such as painting, decorating, and light construction. John and his wife have many friends and engage in social activities on weekends.

The patient appears to have good vocational potential. He is very motivated for recovery and to return to his former occupation in the field of construction. Because he was injured while on the job, he is presently receiving worker's compensation and disability insurance for financial support. If residual weakness prevents his return to employment, further prevocational testing will be conducted to determine an alternative occupation.

In functional skills John is somewhat independent in most self-care activities. He has attempted to use one hand for personal hygiene skills. Assistive devices have been recommended to ease difficulty in cutting food, attaching buttons, and managing soap in the shower.

Assets

Very motivated
Good manual dexterity in uninvolved hand
Good strength in uninvolved hand
Good attention span and working tolerance
Independent in self-care
Family support
Good potential for reemployment
Age
Intelligence
Financial Support

Problem list

1. Muscle weakness and atrophy in right hand
2. Slight muscle imbalance
3. Sensory loss
4. Edema
5. Loss of ROM
6. Difficulty adjusting to inactivity
7. Decreased independence in personal hygiene activity
8. Decreased work capacity

PROBLEM 1: MUSCLE WEAKNESS

Objective
Strength of affected wrist flexors and hand muscles will increase from P to G

Method
Active exercise to wrist flexors, thumb flexors, finger abductors, and adductors; thumb abduction; opposition
   Construction of small jewelry box with mosaic tile top; ceramics—pinch pot or coil project; therapeutic putty exercises

Gradation
Increase resistance as F + muscle grades are attained; commence PRE program; increase time of activity; increase variety of activities

PROBLEM 2: MUSCLE IMBALANCE

Objective
Muscle imbalance at the wrist will be prevented and muscles will be maintained at normal length

Method
Static resting splint to maintain functional position of wrist and hand: to be worn at night and during periods of inactivity
   Teach gentle passive ROM 4 times a day for 15 minutes each session to stretch tight soft tissues

Gradation
Decrease use of static splint and manual stretching as hand function increases; integrate functional hand activities

PROBLEM 3: LOSS OF SENSATION

Objective

Sensation in hand will increase to normal limits

Method

Massage intrinsic muscles to maintain good circulation and elasticity of soft tissues; sensory stimulation and sensory reeducation to skin areas supplied by median and ulnar nerves

Gradation

Touch and tactile sensation are graded, beginning with crude touch and pinprick; increase discriminative touch stimuli to two-point discrimination less than 10 mm, stereognosis, and touch localization

PROBLEM 4: SLIGHT HAND EDEMA

Objective

Edema in the right hand will be reduced or remain minimal

Methods

Retrograde massage of hand from distal to proximal; application of vibratory stimuli to promote venous drainage; overhead sling attached to headboard of bed, which supports forearm and hand in elevated position; allow some movement to increase blood circulation

Gentle passive ROM exercises to thumb, fingers, and wrist after sufficient healing of nerve has occurred to allow some traction on the nerve; teach client ROM exercises and proper positioning of hand

Gradation

Decrease massage and manual stimulation of hand as it recovers normal circulation and skin color

Decrease then eliminate use of overhead sling when active rehabilitation program commences

PROBLEM 5: LOSS OF ACTIVE ROM

Objective

Increase joint mobility and ROM of hand and wrist

Method

Gentle passive ROM to all affected joints; 5 to 10 repetitions 3 times daily; immediately follow with active ROM of each joint or isolated active motion of affected joints and muscles to within practical limits

Gradation

Decrease passive exercise; increase active exercise as strength improves

Promote functional hand activities

PROBLEM 6: DIFFICULTY ADJUSTING TO HOSPITALIZATION AND INACTIVITY

Objective

Patient will be more relaxed and less depressed, resulting in tolerance for hospital routines and social interactions

Method

Isometric exercises for shoulder and elbow muscle groups; isometric resistive exercises for unaffected extremities; supportive approach to patient, positive reinforcement for participation in activities: puzzles, games (cards, checkers, chess, dominoes, Atari television sports games), reading (sports magazines)

Gradation

Decrease extrinsic motivation and initiation of activities; increase number of persons participating with patient

Elicit ideas on improving physical arrangement of clinic; draw up plans and material list

SAMPLE TREATMENT PLAN – cont'd

PROBLEM 7: DECREASED INDEPENDENCE IN PERSONAL HYGIENE ACTIVITIES

Objective
Given assistive device patient will perform personal hygiene and eating activities independently

Method
One-handed rocker knife, rubber placemat for stability of plate, suction soap holder to fix soap to wall, wash mitt, built-up handle on razor for shaving with right hand

Gradation
Decrease use of assistive devices as right hand function increases

---

PROBLEM 8: DECREASED WORK CAPACITY

Objective
Feasibility for return to employment or related job will be explored

Method
Construction of a large wood chest or bookshelf; patient is to plan and perform all operations; activities should be performed standing; purpose is to evaluate handling and use of hand tools, safety awareness, standing tolerance, and physical endurance

Engage patient in construction of closet or shelves for health care facility under direction of maintenance supervisor, as a job trial; aspects of the actual construction duties can be simulated in the clinic; weighted objects similar to construction materials will be lifted, carried, and manipulated and will be graded according to gained strength and endurance

Gradation
Increase weight of loads and requirements for bending, lifting, and carrying large objects

---

REVIEW QUESTIONS

1. List the components of the motor unit.
2. Describe the pathology and major clinical findings of poliomyelitis.
3. Describe the symptoms of post-polio syndrome.
4. What are the elements of the occupational therapy program for the patient with postpolio syndrome?
5. Compare and contrast poliomyelitis with Guillain-Barré syndrome.
6. Discuss treatment strategies for Guillain-Barré syndrome.
7. List at least six clinical manifestations of peripheral nerve injury.
8. Describe the sequential signs of recovery following peripheral nerve injury.
9. Describe some treatment strategies for peripheral nerve injuries.
10. List some contraindications when treating peripheral nerve injuries.
11. Differentiate between causalgia and neuroma.
12. Describe four noninvasive methods of modulating pain perception.
13. Describe the pathophysiology of myasthenia gravis.
14. Discuss the clinical signs of myasthenia gravis.
15. Describe the role of occupational therapy for patients who have myasthenia gravis.
16. What is the primary treatment precaution in myasthenia gravis?
17. Name and differentiate four types of muscular dystrophy. Which one primarily affects children?
18. What are the treatment goals for muscular dystrophy?

REFERENCES

1. Adler M: Endorphins, enkephalins and neurotransmitters, *Med Times* 110:32, 1982.
2. Barone D: Steroid treatment for experimental autoimmune myasthenia gravis, *Arch Neurol* 37:663, 1980.
3. Barr ML: *The human nervous system,* ed 2, New York, 1974, Harper & Row.
4. Bateman J: *Trauma to nerves in limbs,* Philadelphia, 1962, WB Saunders.

5. Birch R, Grant C: Peripheral nerve injuries: clinical. In Downie P, editor: *Cash's textbook of neurology for physiotherapists,* ed 4, Philadelphia, 1986, JB Lippincott.

6. Brashear RH, Raney RB: *Shands' handbook of orthopaedic surgery,* ed 9, St Louis, 1978, CV Mosby.

7. Brena SF, editor: *Chronic pain: America's hidden epidemic,* New York, 1978, Atheneum.

8. Chusid JG: *Correlative neuroanatomy and functional neurology,* ed 19, Los Altos, Calif, 1985, Lange Medical Publications.

9. Clark RG: *Clinical neuroanatomy and neurophysiology,* ed 5, Philadelphia, 1975, FA Davis.

10. deGroot, J: *Correlative neuroanatomy,* ed 21, Norwalk, Conn, 1991, Appleton & Lange.

11. Fowler WF, Goodgold J: Rehabilitation management of neuromuscular diseases. In Goodgold J: *Rehabilitation medicine,* St Louis, 1988, CV Mosby.

12. Gandhavadi B: Autonomic pain: features and methods of assessments, *Postgrad Med* 71:85, 1982.

13. Gardner E: *Fundamentals of neurology,* ed 6, Philadelphia, 1975, WB Saunders.

14. Gilroy J, Meyer J: *Medical neurology,* ed 3, New York, 1979, Macmillan.

15. Halstead LS: Late complications of poliomyelitis. In Goodgold J, editor: *Rehabilitation medicine,* St Louis, 1988, CV Mosby.

16. Heck SA: The effect of purposeful activity on pain tolerance, *Am J Occ Ther,* 42(9):577-581, 1988.

17. Kornfeld P: Plasmapheresis in refractory generalized myasthenia gravis, *Arch Neurol* 38:478, 1981.

18. Krupp MA, Chatton MJ: *Current medical diagnosis and treatment 1984,* Los Altos, Calif, 1984, Lange Medical Publications.

19. Lampe G: Introduction to the use of transcutaneous electrical nerve stimulation devices, *Phys Ther* 1:357, 1975.

20. Larson CB, Gould M: *Orthopedic nursing,* ed 9, St Louis, 1978, CV Mosby.

21. Laurence TN, Pugel AV: Peripheral nerve involvement in spinal cord injury: an electromyographic study, *Arch Phys Med Rehabil* 59:209, 1978.

22. McCormack GL: Pain management by occupational therapists, *Am J Occ Ther,* 42(9):582-590, 1988.

23. Melville ID: Clinical problems in motor neurone disease. In Obeham P, Rose FC, editors: *Progress in neurological research,* London, 1979, Pitman Publishing.

24. Melzack R: Prolonged relief from pain by brief, intense transcutaneous somatic stimulation, *Pain* 1:357, 1975.

25. Melzack R, Wall PD: Psychophysiology of pain, *Int Anesthesiol Clin* 8:3, 1970.

26. Morrison D, Pathier P, Horr K: *Sensory motor dysfunction and therapy in infancy and early childhood,* Springfield, Ill, 1955, Charles C Thomas.

27. Newberger P, Sallan S: Chronic pain: principles of management, *J Pediatr* 98:180, 1981.

28. Noback CR, Demares RJ: *The nervous system: introduction and review,* ed 2, New York, 1977, McGraw-Hill.

29. Phelps PE, Walker C: Comparison of the finger wrinkling test results to establish sensory tests in peripheral nerve injury, *Am J Occup Ther* 31:465, 1977.

30. Piercey MF, Folkers K: Sensory and motor functions of spinal cord substance P, *Sci* 214:1361, 1981.

31. Portney L: Electromyography and nerve conduction velocity tests. In O'Sullivan SB, Shmitz TJ: *Physical rehabilitation: assessment and treatment,* ed 2, Philadelphia, 1988, FA Davis.

32. Robinault I: *Functional aids for the multiply handicapped,* New York, 1973, Harper & Row.

33. Rowland LP: Diseases of chemical transmission at the nerve-muscle synapse: myasthenia gravis. In Kandel ER, Schwartz JH, Jessell TM: *Principles of neural science,* New York, 1991, Elsevier.

34. Rowland LP: Diseases of the motor unit. In Kandel ER, Schwartz JH, Jessell TM: *Principles of neural science,* New York, 1991, Elsevier.

35. Schmidt RF: *Fundamentals of neurophysiology,* ed 2, New York, 1978, Springer-Verlag.

36. Schumacher B, Allen HA: *Medical aspects of disabilities,* Chicago, 1976, Rehabilitation Institute.

37. Seddon HJ: *Surgical disorders of the peripheral nerves,* ed 2, Edinburgh, 1975, Churchill Livingstone.

38. Shealy C: Transcutaneous electrical nerve stimulation for control of pain, *Surg Neurol* 2:45, 1974.

39. Sjolund B, Erikson M: Electroacupuncture and endogenous morphines, *Lancet* 2:1985, 1976.

40. Smith B: *Differential diagnosis in neurology,* New York, 1979, Arco.

41. Spencer EA: Functional restoration, specific diagnoses. In Hopkins HL, Smith HD: *Willard and Spackman's occupational therapy,* ed 6, Philadelphia, 1983, JB Lippincott.

42. Spencer EA: Functional restoration, section 2. In Hopkins HL, Smith HD: *Willard and Spackman's occupational therapy,* ed 8, Philadelphia, 1993, JB Lippincott.

43. Swerdlow M: *The therapy of pain,* Philadelphia, 1981, JB Lippincott.

44. Tappan FM: *Healing massage techniques: a study of eastern and western methods,* Reston, Va, 1978, Reston.

45. Tierney LM, McPhee SJ, Papadakis MA: *Current medical diagnosis and treatment,* ed 33, Norwalk, Conn, 1994, Appleton & Lange.

46. Trombly CA, Scott AD: *Occupational therapy for physical dysfunction,* Baltimore, 1977, Williams & Wilkins.

47. Turner A: *The practice of occupational therapy,* ed 2, New York, 1987, Churchill Livingstone.

48. Van Dam A: Guillain-Barré syndrome: a unique perspective, *Occup Ther Forum* 2:6, 1987.
49. Vasudevan S, Melvin JL: Upper extremity edema control: rationale of the techniques, *Am J Occup Ther* 33:520, 1979.
50. Walter JB: *An introduction to the principles of disease,* Philadelphia, 1977, WB Saunders.
51. Walter JB: *An introduction to the principles of disease,* ed 3, Philadelphia, 1992, WB Saunders.
52. Wynn-Parry CB, Withrington R: Painful disorders of peripheral nerves, *Postgrad Med J* 60:869, 1984.
53. Young G: Occupational therapy and the postpolio syndrome, *Am J Occ Ther* 43(2):97-103, 1989.

Spinal Cord Injury

Carole Adler

R ehabilitation of the individual with a spinal cord injury (SCI) is a lifelong process that requires readjustment to nearly every aspect of life. Occupational therapists play an integral role in pursuing physical and psychosocial restoration as well as in enhancing functional performance to an optimal level of independence. Through analyzing, retraining, and adaptive techniques, occupational therapists provide their patients with the tools and resources to achieve their maximal physical and functional potential.

Spinal cord injuries have many causes. The most common are trauma from motor vehicle accidents, violent injuries such as gunshot and stab wounds, falls, sports accidents, and diving accidents.[4,12] Normal spinal cord function may also be disturbed by diseases, such as tumors, myelomeningocele, syringomyelia, multiple sclerosis, and amyotrophic lateral sclerosis. Some of the treatment principles outlined in this chapter may have application to these conditions, however, the emphasis will be on rehabilitation of the individual with a traumatic spinal cord injury.

RESULTS OF SPINAL CORD INJURY

Spinal cord injury results in quadriplegia or paraplegia. Quadriplegia is any degree of paralysis of the four limbs and trunk musculature. There may be partial upper extremity (UE) function, depending on the level of the cervical lesion. Paraplegia is paralysis of the lower extremities (LEs) with some involvement of the trunk depending on the level of the lesion.[4,12]

Spinal cord injuries are referred to in terms of the regions (cervical, thoracic, and lumbar) of the spinal cord in which they occur and the numerical order of the neurological segments. The level of spinal cord injury designates the last fully functioning neurological segment of the cord: for example, C6 refers to the sixth neurological segment of the cervical region of the spinal cord as the last fully intact neurological segment.[4,11] Complete lesions result in absence of motor or sensory function of the spinal cord below the level of the injury. Incomplete lesions may involve several neurological segments and

some spinal cord function may be partially or completely intact.[2,11] For example, C5-6 refers to C5 as being the last intact neurological level, and C6 as having incomplete innervation of musculature and absent neurological function below C6.

COMPLETE VERSUS INCOMPLETE CLASSIFICATIONS

The extent of neurological damage depends on the location and severity of the injury (Fig. 40-1). In a complete injury, total paralysis and loss of sensation result from a complete interruption of the ascending and descending nerve tracts below the level of the lesion. In an incomplete injury there is some degree of preservation of the sensory and/or motor nerves below the lesion.

The Frankel classification scale[3,4] has been replaced by the American Spinal Injury Association (ASIA) Impairment Scale[1]:

ASIA Impairment Scale Classification A indicates a complete lesion; there is no motor or sensory function preserved in the sacral segments S4-5.

ASIA classification B is an incomplete lesion in which only sensation is present below the neurological level, including the sacral segments S4-5.

ASIA classification C indicates an incomplete lesion with motor function below the neurological level and the majority of key muscles below the level having a grade less than 3.

ASIA classification D is an incomplete lesion with motor function preserved below the neurological level and the majority of key muscles below the level having a muscle grade of 3 or greater.

ASIA classification E indicates that motor and sensory functions are normal.[1]

Incomplete injuries are categorized according to the area of damage: central, lateral, anterior, or peripheral.

Central cord syndrome. Central cord syndrome results when there is more cellular destruction in the center of the cord than in the periphery. There is greater paralysis and sensory loss in the UEs because these nerve tracts are more centrally located than nerve tracts for the

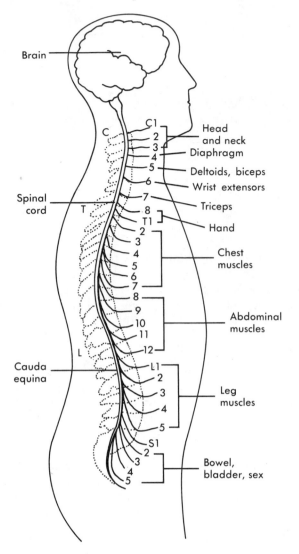

FIG. 40-1   Spinal nerves and major areas of body they supply. (From Paulson S, editor: *Santa Clara Valley Medical Center spinal cord injury home care manual,* ed 2, San José, Calif, 1994, Santa Clara Valley Medical Center.)

LEs. This syndrome is often seen in older people in whom arthritic changes have caused a narrowing of the spinal canal; in such cases cervical hyperextension without vertebral fracture may precipitate central cord damage.

Brown-Séquard syndrome (lateral damage). Brown-Séquard syndrome results when only one side of the cord is damaged, as in a stabbing or gunshot injury. Below the level of injury there is motor paralysis and loss of proprioception on the ipsilateral side and loss of pain, temperature, and touch sensation on the contralateral side.

Anterior spinal cord syndrome. Anterior spinal cord syndrome results from injury that damages the anterior spinal artery or the anterior aspect of the cord. There is paralysis and loss of pain, temperature, and touch sensation. Proprioception is preserved.

Cauda equina (peripherial). Cauda equina injuries involve peripheral nerves rather than the spinal cord directly. Because peripheral nerves possess a regenerating capacity that the cord does not, there is better prognosis for recovery. Patterns of sensory and motor deficits are highly variable and asymmetrical.*

After spinal cord injury the victim enters a stage of spinal shock that may last from 24 hours to 6 weeks. This period is one of areflexia, in which reflex activity ceases below the level of the injury.[11] The bladder and bowel are atonic or flaccid. Deep tendon reflexes are decreased, and sympathetic functions are disturbed. This disturbance results in decreased constriction of blood vessels, low blood pressure, slower heart rate, and absence of perspiration below the level of the injury.[10,14]

Because the spinal cord is usually not damaged below the level of the lesion, muscles that are innervated by the neurological segments below the level of injury usually develop spasticity because the monosynaptic reflex arc is intact but separated from higher inhibitory influences. Deep tendon reflexes become hyperactive, and clonus may be evident. Sensory loss continues, and the bladder and bowel usually become spastic ("upper motor neuron" bladder) in patients whose injuries are above T12. The bladder and bowel usually remain flaccid ("lower motor neuron" bladder) in lesions at L1 and below. Sympathetic functions become hyperactive. Spinal reflex activity (mass muscle spasms) usually becomes evident in the areas below the level of the lesion.[2,11,14]

PROGNOSIS FOR RECOVERY

Prognosis for substantial recovery of neuromuscular function after spinal cord injury depends on whether the lesion is complete or incomplete. In carefully assessed complete lesions in which there is no sensation or return of motor function below the level of lesion 24 to 48 hours after the injury, motor function is less likely to return. Partial to full return of function to one spinal nerve root level below the fracture can be gained, however, and may occur in the first 6 months after injury. In incomplete lesions progressive return of motor function is possible, yet it is difficult to determine exactly how much return and how quickly it will occur.[14] Frequently, the longer it takes for recovery to begin the less likely it is that it will occur.

MEDICAL AND SURGICAL MANAGEMENT OF THE PERSON WITH SPINAL CORD INJURY

After a traumatic event in which spinal cord injury is likely, the conscious victim should be carefully questioned about cutaneous numbness and skeletal muscle

---

* Reprinted in part with permission from Hanak M, Scott A: *Spinal cord injury, an illustrated guide for health care professionals,* New York, 1983, Springer-Verlag.

paralysis before being moved. Emergency medical technicians, paramedics, and air transport personnel are trained in spinal cord injury precautions and extrication techniques for moving a possible SCI victim from an accident site. Movement of the spine must be prevented during the transfer procedures. A firm stretcher or board to which the victim's head and back can be strapped should be procured before moving the victim. After transferring the victim to the stretcher or board, while maintaining axial traction on the neck and preventing any movement of the spine and neck, the victim is strapped to the board or stretcher and carefully transferred via air or ground transport to the nearest hospital emergency room. Careful examination, stabilization, and transportation of the patient may prevent a temporary or slight spinal cord injury from becoming more severe or permanent.

Initial care is directed toward preventing further damage to the spinal cord and reversing neurological damage if possible by stabilization or decompression of the injured neurological structures.[4,9,11] A careful neurological examination is carried out by the examining physician to aid in determining the site and type of injury. This procedure is done with the patient in a supine position with the neck and spine immobilized. A catheter is usually placed in the patient's bladder for drainage of urine. Anteroposterior and lateral x-ray films may be taken, with the patient's head, neck, or spine immobilized, to help determine the type of injury. A computerized axial tomography (CAT) scan or magnetic resonance imaging (MRI) may be required for further evaluation. In early medical treatment the goals are to restore normal alignment of the spine, maintain stabilization of the injured area, and decompress neurological structures that are under pressure.

Bony realignment and stabilization usually occur by placing the patient on a rotating kinetic bed (Fig. 40-2) that allows for skeletal traction and immobilization. The bed's constant rotation allows for continuous pressure

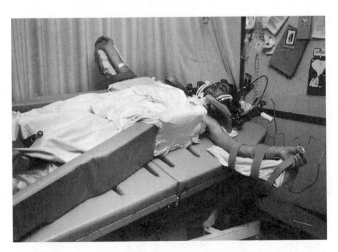

FIG. 40-2   Kinetic bed with arm positioner. (Designed and fabricated by Occupational Therapy Department, Santa Clara Valley Medical Center, San José, Calif.)

relief, mobilization of respiratory secretions, and easy access to the patient's entire body for bowel, bladder, and hygiene care. Open surgical reduction with wiring and spinal fusion may be indicated.

The goals of surgery are to decompress the spinal cord and achieve spinal stability and normal bony alignment.[4,11] Surgery, however, is not always necessary and the patient may be allowed to heal with adequate immobilization. As soon as possible a means of portable immobilization (usually a halo vest for cervical injuries (Fig. 40-3, *A*) and a thoracic brace or body jacket for thoracic injuries, Fig. 40-3, *B*) is provided. This approach enables the patient to be transferred to a standard hospital bed and subsequently to be up in a wheelchair and involved in an active therapy program in as little as 1 to 2 weeks after injury. Wheelchair use shortly after injury can substantially reduce the incidence and severity of further medical complications such as deep vein thrombosis, joint contractures, and the general deconditioning that can result from prolonged bed rest.

The benefits of early transport to a spinal cord injury center have been documented.[6] Patients treated initially in a spinal cord acute care unit as opposed to a general hospital had shorter acute care lengths of stay because patients in general hospitals tended to have a higher incidence of skin problems and spinal instability. It was found that spinal cord center patients made functional gains with greater efficiency.[15] Spinal cord centers are able to offer a complete multidisciplinary program executed by an experienced team of professionals who specialize in this unique and demanding disability.

COMPLICATIONS OF SPINAL CORD INJURY

Skin breakdown, pressure sores, or decubitus ulcers

Sensory loss facilitates the development of skin breakdown. The patient cannot feel the pressure and shearing of prolonged sitting or lying in one position or the presence of pain or heat against the body. Pressure causes loss of blood supply to the area, which can ultimately result in necrosis. Heat can quickly burn and destroy tissues. Shearing can destroy underlying tissue. Any combination of the above will hasten skin breakdown. The areas most likely to develop skin breakdown are bony prominences over the sacrum, ischium, trochanters, elbows, and heels; however, other bony prominences such as the iliac crest, scapula, knees, toes, and rib cage are also at risk.

It is important for all rehabilitation personnel to be aware of the signs of developing skin problems. At first the area reddens yet blanches when pressed. Later the reddened or abraded area does not blanch, which indicates that necrosis has begun. Finally a blister or ulceration appears in the area. If allowed to progress, a sore can become quite severe, destroying underlying tissues and going as deep as to the bone.

Skin breakdown can be prevented by relieving and eliminating pressure points and protecting vulnerable

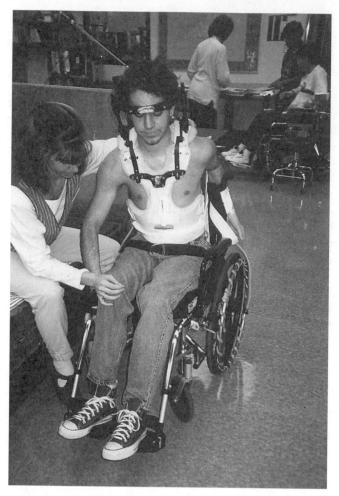

A

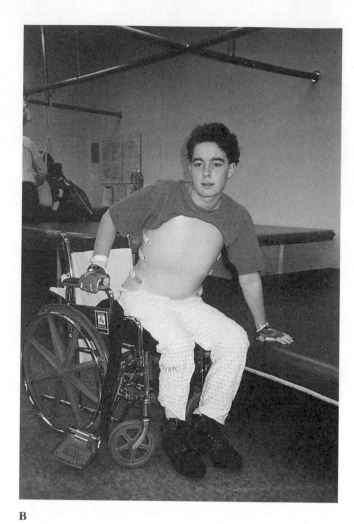

B

FIG. 40-3 **A,** Halo vest, neck immobilization device for patients with quadriplegia and high level paraplegia (T1 to T4). **B,** Body jacket, one type of immobilization device for paraplegia.

areas from excessive shearing, moisture and heat. Turning in bed on a routine basis, mattress overlays, protection of bony prominences with various types of padding, and performing weight shifts are some of the methods used to prevent pressure sores.

The use of hand splints, body jackets, and other orthoses can also cause skin breakdowns. The therapist must inspect the skin, and the patient must be taught to examine his or her skin compulsively, using a mirror or caregiver assistance to watch for signs of developing problems. Skin damage can develop within 30 minutes, so frequent weight shifting, repositioning, and vigilance are essential if skin breakdown is to be prevented.[11,14]

Decreased vital capacity

Decreased vital capacity is a problem in people who have sustained cervical and high thoracic lesions. Such individuals have markedly limited chest expansion and decreased ability to cough because of weakness or paralysis of the diaphragm and the intercostal and latissimus dorsi muscles, which can result in a tendency to respiratory

tract infections. The reduced vital capacity affects the overall endurance level for activity. This problem may be minimized by methods of assisted breathing and by vigorous respiratory and physical therapy. Strengthening of the sternocleidomastoids and the diaphragm along with manually assisted cough and deep breathing exercises are essential to maintain optimal vital capacity.[11,14]

Osteoporosis of disuse

Because of disuse of long bones, particularly of the lower extremities, osteoporosis is likely to develop in patients with spinal cord injuries. A year after the injury the osteoporosis may be sufficiently advanced for pathological fractures to occur. Pathological fractures usually occur in the supracondylar area of the femur, proximal tibia, distal tibia, intertrochanteric area of the femur, and neck of the femur. Pathological fractures are usually not seen in UEs. Daily standing on a tilt table or standing frame may slow the onset of osteoporosis[11,14]; however, a standing program must fit into the patient's daily ADL routine after discharge to be effective on an ongoing basis.

Orthostatic hypotension

Lack of muscle tone in the abdomen and LEs leads to pooling of blood in these areas with resultant decrease in blood pressure (hypotension). This problem occurs when the patient goes from supine to upright or changes body position too quickly. Symptoms are dizziness, nausea, and loss of consciousness.[4] The patient must be reclined quickly and if sitting in a wheelchair, should be tipped back with legs elevated until symptoms subside. With time this problem can diminish as sitting tolerance and level of activity increase; however, some people continue to experience hypotensive episodes. Abdominal binders, leg wraps, antiembolism stockings, and/or medications can aid in reducing symptoms.

Autonomic dysreflexia

Autonomic dysreflexia is a phenomenon seen in persons whose injuries are above the T4 to T6 level. It is caused by reflex action of the autonomic nervous system in response to some stimulus, such as a distended bladder, fecal mass, bladder irritation, rectal manipulation, thermal or pain stimuli, and visceral distention. The symptoms are immediate pounding headache, anxiety, perspiration, flushing, chills, nasal congestion, paroxysmal hypertension, and bradycardia.

Autonomic dysreflexia is a medical emergency and life threatening. The patient should not be left alone.[4,11,14] It is treated by placing the patient in an upright position and removing anything restrictive such as abdominal binders or elastic stockings to reduce blood pressure. The bladder should be drained or legbag tubing checked for obstruction. Blood pressure and other symptoms should be monitored until back to normal. The occupational therapist must be aware of symptoms and treatment because dysreflexia can occur at any time after the injury.

Spasticity

Spasticity is a nearly universal complication of spinal cord injury.[15] It is an involuntary muscle contraction below the level of injury that results from lack of inhibition from higher centers. Patterns of spasticity change over the first year, gradually increasing in the first 6 months and reaching a plateau about 1 year after the injury. A moderate amount of spasticity can be helpful in the overall rehabilitation of the patient with a spinal cord injury. It helps to maintain muscle bulk, assists in joint ROM, and can be used to assist during wheelchair and bed transfers and mobility. A sudden increase in spasticity can alert the patient to other medical problems, such as bladder infections, skin breakdown, or fever.

Severe spasticity can be very frustrating to both the patient and the therapist in that it can interfere with function. It may be treated more aggressively with a variety of medications. In select instances orthopedic procedures that involve cutting or lengthening involved muscles may benefit some patients. In severe cases, neurosurgical procedures such as nerve blocks or rhizotomies, the lesioning of spinal roots, have been performed.[4,11,14]

Heterotopic ossification

Heterotopic ossification (HO), also called *ectopic bone,* is bone that develops in abnormal anatomic locations.[15] It most often occurs in the muscles around the hip and knee but occasionally it can be noted also at the elbow and shoulder. The first symptoms are swelling, warmth, and decreased joint ROM. The onset of HO is usually 1 to 4 months after injury.

Treatment consists of medication and the maintenance of joint ROM during the early stage of active bone formation to preserve the functional ROM necessary for good wheelchair positioning, symmetrical position of pelvis, and maximal functional mobility. If HO progresses to the phase of substantially limiting hip flexion, pelvic obliquity while in the sitting position is likely to occur. This problem contributes to trunk deformities such as scoliosis and kyphosis with subsequent skin breakdown at the ischial tuberosities and sacrum.[4,11]

SEXUAL FUNCTION

The sexual drive and need for physical and emotional intimacy are not changed by spinal cord injury. There are, however, problems of mobility, dependency, and body image, plus complicating medical problems and the attitudes of partners and society that affect social and sexual roles, access, and interest. Sexuality is an important part of life, and rehabilitation is not complete until a person is comfortable with his or her sexual and social role.

Lack of sensation over one part of the body is accompanied by increased or altered sensation over other parts of the body. The sexual response of the body after spinal cord injury needs to be explored the same way a person learns what muscles are working and where he or she can feel.

In males erections and ejaculations are often affected by the spinal cord injury. This problem is variable, however, and needs to be evaluated individually. Independent of these individual differences are changes in function, and for reasons that are not well understood, the viability of sperm in SCI males is frequently decreased even when other function is near normal.

In females there is usually an interval of weeks to months after injury during which menstruation ceases. It will usually start again and return to normal in time. There may also be changes in lubrication of the vagina during sexual activity. In contrast to males, however, there is no change in female fertility. Females with SCI can conceive and give birth. Special attention must be given to the interaction of pregnancy and childbirth with spinal cord injury, especially in regard to blood clots, respiratory function, bladder infections, dysreflexia, and use of medications during pregnancy and breast-feeding.

To avoid pregnancy SCI women must take precautions, and the type of birth control used must be considered very carefully. Birth control pills are associated with blood clots, especially when combined with smoking, and probably should not be used. The intrauterine device (IUD) is not recommended even for able-bodied females. Diaphragms may be difficult to position properly when there is loss of sensation in the vagina or decreased hand function. Foams and suppositories are not very effective. The use of condoms by the male partner is probably the safest method.

Individuals with disability quickly sense the attitudes of professionals and caregivers toward their sexuality. Fortunately negative and uncomfortable attitudes are changing, and sexual counseling and education are a regular part of many rehabilitation programs for all types of physical disabilities. Some patients lack basic sex education. Others feel asexual because of their disabilities and are isolated from peers; thus they may feel uncomfortable with any type of sexual interaction. For these reasons sexual education and counseling must be geared to the needs of the individual patient and his or her significant other. In some instances social interaction skills need improvement before sexual activity can be considered, and occupational therapists play an important role in providing information and a forum to deal with these issues.* (See Chapter 17 for more information on sexuality with physical dysfunction.)

OCCUPATIONAL THERAPY INTERVENTION
EVALUATION

Assessment of the patient is an ongoing process that begins the day of admission and continues long after discharge on an outpatient follow-up basis. Depending on whether the patient is in an acute, inpatient rehabilitation, outpatient, or home setting, the occupational therapist should continually assess the patient's functional progress and appropriateness of treatment and equipment. An accurate and comprehensive formal initial evaluation is essential to determine baseline neurological, clinical, and functional status from which to formulate a treatment program and substantiate progress. Initial data gathering from the medical chart will provide personal information, a medical diagnosis, and a history of other pertinent medical information. Input from the multidisciplinary team will enhance the OT's ability to prognosticate optimal outcomes accurately.

Discharge planning begins during the initial evaluation; therefore the patient's social and vocational history as well as past and expected living situations are vital

information necessary to plan a treatment program that meets the patient's ongoing needs. It should also be noted that treatment should begin as soon as possible. It is possible quickly to gather enough information to begin addressing high priority areas such as splinting, positioning, and family training without having to wait for the evaluation to be completed.

Physical Status

Before evaluating the patient's physical status, very specific medical precautions should be obtained from the primary physician and consulting physicians. Skeletal instability and related injuries or medical complications will affect the way in which the patient is moved and the active or resistive movements allowed.

Passive range of motion (PROM) should be measured before manual muscle testing to determine available pain-free movement. This evaluation also identifies the presence of or potential for joint contractures, which could suggest the need for preventive or corrective splinting and positioning.

Shoulder pain, which ultimately causes decreased shoulder and scapular ROM, is extremely common in C4-7 quadriplegia. It can be caused by several factors such as scapular immobilization resulting from prolonged bed rest or nerve root compression subsequent to the injury. Shoulder pain should be thoroughly assessed and diagnosed so that proper treatment can occur before the onset of chronic discomfort and functional loss.

An accurate assessment of the patient's muscle strength is critical in determining a precise diagnosis of neurological level and to establish a baseline for physical recovery and functional progress. Because the occupational therapist's skills with activity analysis greatly enhance his or her effectiveness in treating the individual with SCI, a precise working knowledge of musculoskeletal anatomy and specific manual muscle testing techniques are essential. Using accepted muscle testing resources during testing is encouraged to ensure accurate technique while performing this complex evaluation. The muscle test should be repeated as often as necessary to provide an ongoing picture of the patient's strength and progress.

Sensation is evaluated for light touch, superficial pain (pinprick), and kinesthesia, which determines areas of absent, impaired, and intact sensation. These findings are useful in establishing the level of injury and in determining functional limitations (Fig. 40-4).[1]

If evaluating the patient in the acute stage, spasticity is rarely noted because the patient is still in spinal shock. When that subsides increased muscle tone may be present in response to stimuli. The therapist should then determine whether the spasticity interferes with or enhances function.

An evaluation of wrist and hand function determines the degree to which a patient can manipulate objects. This information is used to suggest the need for equip-

---

* Reprinted in part with permission from Paulson S, editor: *The spinal cord injury home care manual,* ed 3, San José, Calif, 1994, Santa Clara Valley Medical Center.

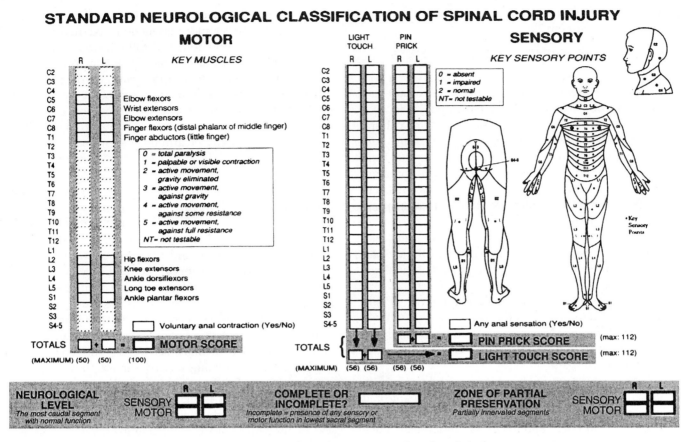

FIG. 40-4   Standard Neurological Classification of Spinal Cord Injury. (From American Spinal Injury Association (ASIA), 1992.)

ment such as positioning splints, universal cuffs, or, later, consideration of a tenodesis orthosis (wrist driven flexor hinge splint). Gross grasp and pinch measurements indicate functional abilities and may be used as an adjunct to manual muscle testing to provide objective measurements of baseline status and progress for those patients who have active hand musculature.[7]

Clinical observation is used to assess endurance, oral motor control, head and trunk control, LE functional muscle strength, and total body function. More specific assessment in any of these areas may be required depending on the individual.

As a result of recent documentation of an increased number of combined spinal cord injury/head injury diagnoses, a specific cognitive and perceptual evaluation may be necessary.[8] Assessing a patient's ability to initiate tasks, follow directions, carry over learning day to day and do problem solving contributes to the information base required for appropriate and realistic goal setting. Understanding the patient's learning style, coping skills, and communication style are essential elements as well.

Functional Status

Performing activities of daily living (ADL) is an important part of the occupational therapy evaluation. The purpose

is to determine present and potential levels of functional ability. If the patient is cleared of bedrest precautions, evaluation and simultaneous treatment should begin as soon as possible after injury. Light activities such as feeding, light hygiene at the sink, and object manipulation may be appropriate depending on the level of injury.

Direct interaction with the patient's family and friends provides valuable information regarding the patient's support systems while in the hospital and, more important, after discharge. This information will have impact on later caregiver training in areas in which the patient may require the assistance of others to accomplish self-care and mobility tasks.

In addition to physical and functional assessments, the occupational therapist has the opportunity to observe the patient's psychosocial adjustment to the disability and life in general through the nature of activities in which he or she participates.[11] This time is an important one for establishing rapport and mutual trust, which will facilitate participation and progress in later and more difficult phases of rehabilitation. An individual's motivation, determination, socioeconomic background, education, family support, acceptance of disability, problem-solving abilities, and financial resources can prove to be invaluable assets or limiting factors in determining the outcome of rehabilitation. A therapist must carefully observe the patient's status in each of these areas before determining the course of treatment.[7]

ESTABLISHING TREATMENT OBJECTIVES

It is important to establish treatment objectives in concert with the patient and with the rehabilitation team. The primary objectives of the rehabilitation team may not be those of the patient. Psychosocial factors, cultural factors, cognitive deficits, environmental limitations, and individual financial considerations must be identified and integrated into the development of a treatment program that will meet the unique needs of each individual. Every patient is different; therefore a variety of treatment approaches and alternatives may be necessary to address each factor that may affect goal achievement.[7] More participation can be expected if the patient's priorities are respected to the extent that they are achievable and realistic.

The general objectives of treatment for the person with spinal cord injury are as follows:

1. to maintain or increase joint ROM and prevent deformity via active and passive ROM, splinting and positioning
2. to increase strength of all innervated and partially innervated muscles through the use of enabling and purposeful activities
3. to increase physical endurance via functional activities
4. to develop the patient's maximal independence in all aspects of self-care, mobility, homemaking and parenting skills
5. to explore leisure interests and vocational potential
6. to aid in the psychosocial adjustment to disability
7. to evaluate, recommend, and train in the use and care of necessary durable medical and adaptive equipment
8. to ensure safe and independent home accessibility through home modification recommendations
9. to instruct the patient in communication skills necessary for training care givers to provide safe assistance.

The patient's length of stay in the inpatient rehabilitation program and the ability to participate in outpatient therapy determine the appropriateness and priority of the just-named activities.

TREATMENT METHODS
Acute Phase

During the acute or immobilized phase of the rehabilitation program the patient may be in traction or wearing a stabilization device such as a halo brace or body jacket. Medical precautions must be in force during this period. Flexion, extension, and rotary movements of the spine and neck are contraindicated.

Evaluation of total body positioning and hand splinting needs should be initiated at this time. In patients with quadriplegia, scapula elevation and elbow flexion as well as limited shoulder flexion and abduction while on bedrest cause potentially painful shoulders and ROM limita-

tions. Upper extremities should be intermittently positioned in 80° of shoulder abduction, external rotation with scapular depression, and full elbow extension to assist in alleviating this common problem. The forearm may be positioned in forearm pronation if the patient is at risk for supination contractures such as at the C5 level. At Santa Clara Valley Medical Center, a device was designed and fabricated by the Occupational Therapy Department to maintain the arm in an appropriate position while the patient is immobilized on a kinetic bed (Fig. 40-2).

Selection of appropriate splint style and its accurate fabrication and fit by the occupational therapist enhances patient acceptance and optimal functional gain. If musculature is not adequate to support wrist and hands properly for function and/or cosmesis, splints should be fabricated properly to support the wrist in extension and thumb in opposition and to maintain the thumb web space while allowing the fingers to flex naturally at the metacarpophalangeal (MP) and proximal interphalangeal (PIP) joints. Splints should be dorsal rather than ventral in design to allow maximal sensory feedback while the patient's hand is resting on any surface. If at least F+ (3+) strength of wrist extension is present, short opponens splints should be fabricated to maintain the web space and support the thumb in opposition. This splint can be used functionally while training the patient to use a tenodesis grasp.

Active and active-assisted ROM of all joints should be performed within strength, ability, and tolerance levels. Muscle reeducation techniques to wrists and elbows should be employed when indicated. Progressive resistive exercises to wrists may be carried out. The patient should be encouraged to engage in self-care activities such as feeding, writing, and hygiene if possible, using simple devices such as a universal cuff or a custom writing splint. Even though the patient may be immobilized in bed, discussion of anticipated durable medical equipment (DME), home modifications, and caregiver training should be initiated to allow sufficient time to prepare for discharge.

Active Phase

During the active or mobilization phase of the rehabilitation program, the patient can sit in a wheelchair and should begin developing upright tolerance. At this time a method of relieving sitting pressure should be initiated as a high priority for the purpose of preventing decubitis ulcers on the ischial, trochanteric, and sacral bony prominences. If the patient has quadriplegia yet has at least F+ (3+) shoulder and elbow strength bilaterally, pressure can be relieved on the buttocks by leaning forward over the feet. Simple cotton webbing loops are secured to the back frame of the wheelchair (Fig. 40-5). A person with low quadriplegia (C7) or one with paraplegia with intact UE musculature can perform a full depression weight shift off the arms or wheels of the wheelchair. Weight

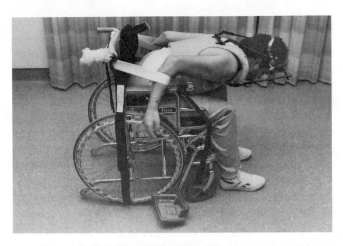

FIG. 40-5 Forward weight shift using loops attached to wheelchair frame. A patient with C6 quadriplegia with symmetrical grade 4 deltoids and biceps.

shifts should be performed at least every 30 minutes until skin tolerance is determined.

Active and passive ROM exercises should be continued regularly to prevent undesirable contractures. Splinting or casting of the elbows may be indicated to correct contractures that are developing. In patients who have wrist extension, which will be used to substitute for absent grasp through tenodesis action of the long finger flexors, it is desirable to develop some tightness in these tendons to give some additional tension to the tenodesis grasp. The desirable contracture is developed by ranging finger flexion with the wrist fully extended and finger extension with the wrist flexed, thus never allowing the flexors or extensors to be in full stretch over all of the joints that they cross[14] (Fig. 40-6).

Elbow contractures should never be allowed to develop. Full elbow extension is essential to allow prop-

ping to maintain balance during static sitting and to assist in transfers. With zero triceps strength a person with C6 quadriplegia can maintain forward sitting balance by shoulder depression and protraction, external rotation, and full wrist extension (Fig. 40-7).

Progressive resistive exercise and resistive activities can be applied to innervated and partially innervated muscles. Shoulder musculature should be exercised with emphasis on the latissimus dorsi (shoulder depressors), deltoids (shoulder flexors, abductors, and extensors), and the remainder of the shoulder girdle and scapular muscles for proximal stability. The triceps, pectoralis, and latissimus dorsi muscles are needed for transfers and for shifting weight when in the wheelchair. Wrist extensors should be strengthened to maximize natural tenodesis function, thereby maximizing the necessary prehension pattern in the hand for functional grasp and release.

The treatment program should be graded to increase the amount of resistance that can be tolerated during activity. As muscle power improves, increasing the amount of time in wheelchair activities will help the patient gain upright tolerance and endurance.

There are many assistive devices and equipment items that can be useful to the person with a spinal cord injury. It is important to note, however, that every attempt should be made to have the patient perform the task with no equipment or as little as possible. Modified techniques are available that enable an individual to perform efficiently without the need for costly or bulky equipment.

When appropriate the universal cuff for holding eating utensils, toothbrushes, pencils, and paintbrushes is a simple and versatile device that offers increased independence (see Fig. 26-12). A wrist cock-up splint to stabilize the wrist with attachment of the universal cuff can be useful for persons with little or no wrist extension. A

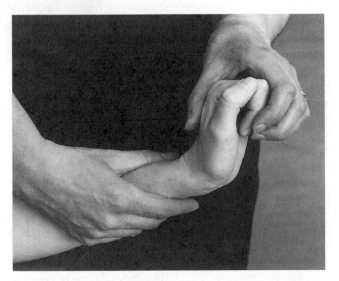

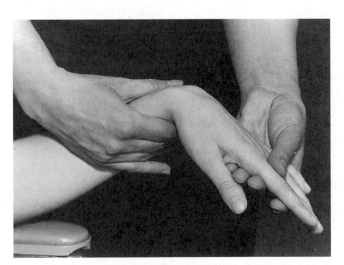

A   **B**

FIG. 40-6   **A,** Wrist is extended when fingers are passively flexed. **B,** Wrist is flexed when fingers are passively extended.

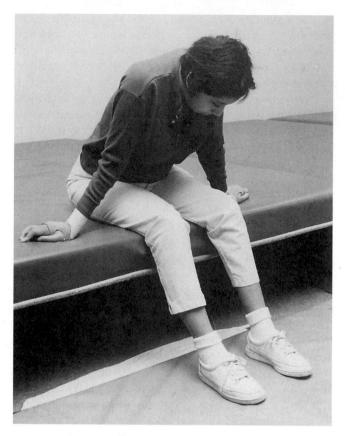

FIG. 40-7   A patient with C6 quadriplegia; forward sitting balance is maintained (without triceps) by locking elbows. A valuable skill for bed mobility and transfers.

plate guard, cup holder, extended straw with straw clip, and nonskid table mat can facilitate independent feeding (see Fig. 26-39). The wash mitt and soap holder or soap-on-a-rope can make bathing easier; however, the added difficulty of donning and doffing such equipment must be considered (see Fig. 26-14). Many people with quadriplegia can use a button hook to fasten clothing (see Fig. 26-8). A transfer board is an option for safe transfers. Through treatment, optimal muscle strength and coordination can occur, enabling the patient potentially to grow out of equipment that was initially provided.

The ADL program may be expanded to include independent feeding with devices; oral hygiene and upper body bathing; bowel and bladder care, such as digital stimulation and application of the urinary collection device; UE dressing; and transfers using the sliding board. Communication skills in writing and using the telephone, tape recorder, stereo equipment, and personal computer should be an important part of the treatment program. Training in the use of the mobile arm support (MAS) (see Chapter 19, section 2) wrist-hand orthosis (flexor hinge or tenodesis splint), and assistive devices is also part of the occupational therapy program.

The occupational therapist should continue to provide psychological support by allowing and encouraging the patient to express frustration, anger, fears, and con-

cerns.[12] The occupational therapy clinic in a spinal cord center can provide an atmosphere where patients can establish support groups with other inpatients and outpatients who can offer their experiences and problem-solving advice to those in earlier phases of their rehabilitation.

The assessment, ordering, and fitting of DME such as wheelchairs, seating and positioning equipment, mechanical lifts, beds, and bathing equipment are an extremely important part of the rehabilitation program. Such equipment should be specifically evaluated, however, and ordered only when definite goals and expectations are known. Frequently, equipment can impair function and cause further medical problems, such as skin breakdown or trunk deformity if a therapist has not thoroughly taken into account all functional, positioning, environmental, psychological, and financial considerations in evaluating the patient's equipment needs. The desired equipment, especially wheelchairs and positioning devices and bathing equipment, should be available for demonstration by the patient before final ordering.

It is imperative that the therapist involved in the evaluation and ordering of this costly and highly individualized equipment be familiar with what is currently on the market and be knowledgeable in ordering equipment that will provide the patient with optimal function and body positioning on a short- and long-term basis. A good working relationship with an experienced rehabilitation technology supplier (RTS), an equipment supplier specializing in custom rehabilitation equipment, is imperative. Advancements in technology and design have provided a wide variety of equipment from which to choose and working with another professional specializing in such equipment will help ensure correct selection and fit. See Chapter 27 for a more detailed discussion of wheelchairs, seating, and positioning equipment.

In addition to enhancing respiratory function by supporting the patient in an erect, well-aligned position, which maximizes sitting tolerance and optimizes upper-extremity function, wheelchair seating must also assist in the prevention of deformity and pressure sores. An appropriate and adequate wheelchair cushion helps to distribute sitting pressure, assist in the prevention of pressure sores, stabilize the pelvis as necessary for proper trunk alignment, and provide comfort. Whether it is the occupational therapist's or the physical therapist's role to evaluate and order the wheelchair and cushion, both should work closely together to ensure consistent training and use for the individual needs of each patient.

An increasing number of individuals with high-level SCI, C4 and above, are surviving and participating in active rehabilitation programs. Their treatment and equipment needs are unique and extremely specialized, ranging from mouthsticks and environmental control systems to ventilators and sophisticated electric wheelchairs and drive systems. (See Table 40-1, levels C1-3 and C3-4.) The use of experienced resources in determining appropriate

TABLE 40-1 Functional Outcomes Based on Level of Injury

NEUROLOGICAL LEVEL/MUSCLES INNERVATED*	MOVEMENTS POSSIBLE	PATTERN OF WEAKNESS	FUNCTIONAL CAPABILITIES AND LIMITATIONS

These guidelines were developed primarily from experience. The outcomes reflect the highest level of independence that may be expected of a complete injury given optimum circumstances. Let the reader be aware that these are meant as guidelines only and not as outcomes to be expected in all cases.

C1-3

Sternocleidomastoids Upper trapezius Levator scapulae	Neck control	Total paralysis of trunk, UEs, and LEs Dependence on respirator	Total ADL dependence Able to instruct others in care Can propel power wheelchair equipped with portable respirator and chin or breath controls Can operate communication devices and environmental control systems with mouthstick or pneumatic control Requires full-time attendant care

C3-4

~ Trapezius (superior, middle, and inferior) ~ Diaphragm (C3-5) Cervical and paraspinal muscles	Neck movements, scapula elevation Inspiration	Paralysis of trunk, UEs, and LEs Difficulty in breathing and coughing	Full time wheelchair user; can talk through all setups and train caregivers in care Respiratory assistance may be required full- or part-time Maximum assistance for skin inspection (patient cannot position mirrors but should inspect himself) Activities can be accomplished through use of mouthstick (e.g., typing, page turning, and manipulation of table top objects and games) Can operate power wheelchair with chin or breath Requires full-time attendant care

C5

All muscles of shoulder at least partially innervated except latissimus dorsi and coracobrachialis	Shoulder extension and horizontal abduction (weak)	Absence of elbow extension, pronation, and all wrist and hand movements	Unable to roll over or come to sitting position without hospital bed with rails Needs assistance in transfers
~ Partial deltoids	Shoulder flexion Shoulder abduction to 90°	Total paralysis of trunk and LEs	If good muscle power, may be able to perform UE dressing with minimum assist Dependent for skin inspection
~ Biceps brachii Brachialis Brachioradialis	Elbow flexion and supination		Independent indoors in wheelchair with handrim adaptations Power wheelchair for long distance and outdoors
Levator scapulae, diaphragm, and scaleni now fully innervated		Endurance low because of paralysis of intercostals and low respiratory reserve	With splints, adaptive equipment, and attendant setup can perform: eating, light hygiene, applying make-up, shaving, handwriting (sufficient for legal signature), telephoning, and typing
Rhomboids (major and minor	Scapular adduction and downward rotation (weak)		
Serratus anterior (C5-7)	Scapular abduction and upward rotation (weak)		Requires at least part-time attendant care; can instruct caregivers in all self-care, mobility, and functional setups
Teres major (5,6) Subscapularis (C5,6)	Shoulder internal rotation (weak)		Can direct bowel and bladder management
Pectoralis major (C5-8, T1)	Shoulder horizontal adduction (weak)		May drive a van with substantial adaptations
Infraspinatus Supraspinatus Teres minor (C5, 6)	Shoulder external rotation		

Carole Adler, OTR. Reprinted with permission.
* Each level includes the muscles and functions of the preceding levels.
~ Key muscles.

Continued

TABLE 40-1 Functional Outcomes Based on Level of Injury—cont'd

NEUROLOGICAL LEVEL/MUSCLES INNERVATED	MOVEMENTS POSSIBLE	PATTERN OF WEAKNESS	FUNCTIONAL CAPABILITIES AND LIMITATIONS
C6			
All partially innervated C5 muscles now fully innervated except serratus and pectoralis major	Full strength to shoulder flexion and extension, abduction and adduction, internal and external rotation, and elbow flexion	Absence of elbow extension and ulnar wrist extension	Able to perform many activities independently with equipment or natural tenodesis grasp
			Tenodesis splint or universal cuff for self-feeding with regular utensils; personal hygiene and grooming (oral and upper body); UE dressing; handwriting; typing; telephoning; light kitchen activities
			Roll from side to side in bed with aid of bed rails
			Can perform supine to side-lying to sit with minimum assistance
Partial but significant innervation to serratus anterior (C5-7)	Scapular abduction and upward rotation		Independent in propelling wheelchair on level terrain and minimum grade inclines with plastic- or foam-coated rims
Latissmus dorsi (C6-8)	Shoulder extension and internal rotation	Endurance may be low because of reduced vital capacity	
			Relieves pressure independently when sitting, using loops and forward weight shift
~ Pectoralis major (C5-8, T1)	Shoulder horizontal adduction and internal rotation	Absence of wrist flexion	Independent in managing communication devices with adapted equipment
Coracobrachialis (C6,7)	Shoulder flexion	Total paralysis of trunk and LEs	
Pronator teres (C6,7)	Forearm pronation		Assists in transfers by substituting shoulder adduction and rotation for elbow extension; may be independent with aid of transfer board
Supinator	Complete innervation for forearm supination		
~ Extensor carpi radialis longus and brevis (C6,7)	Radial wrist extension		Drives with adaptations
			Independent skin inspection with mirrors
			Able to assist caregiver in bladder care
			Requires adaptive equipment and assist for bathing and bowel care
			May require part-time attendant care
			May participate in sports (quad rugby, swimming)
C7-8			
Shoulder prime movers now fully innervated, as well as the rest of the partially innervated C6 muscles	Full strength of all shoulder movements, radial wrist flexors and extensors, and strong pronation	Lack of trunk muscles compromises full shoulder stability	Can perform transfers to and from bed and wheelchair independently
~ Triceps brachii	Elbow extension		
Extensor carpi ulnaris (C6-8)	Ulnar wrist extension		
~ Flexor carpi radialis	Radial wrist flexion		
~ Flexor digitorum superficialis and profundus (C7-8, T1)	PIP and DIP flexion	Limited grasp, release, and dexterity because of incomplete innervation of hand intrinsics	Can roll over, sit up, and move about in a standard bed
			Can dress independently and perform personal hygiene activities
			Independent with eating (usually with no assistive devices)
			Tenodesis splint may still be helpful for some patients because of weakness of grasp

Continued

TABLE 40-1   Functional Outcomes Based on Level of Injury—cont'd

NEUROLOGICAL LEVEL/MUSCLES INNERVATED	MOVEMENTS POSSIBLE	PATTERN OF WEAKNESS	FUNCTIONAL CAPABILITIES AND LIMITATIONS
~ Extensor digitorum communis (C6-8)	MP extension		Can propel manual wheelchair (may need friction tape on handrims for long distances; may need assistance on rough terrain) Drives with adaptations
Extensor pollicis longus and brevis Abductor pollicis longus	Thumb extension (MP and IP) Thumb abduction	Total paralysis of LEs Weakness of trunk control Limited endurance because of reduced respiratory reserve	Independent with bladder and bowel care Independent with skin inspection Light housework possible May participate in preparation for sexual activity (i.e., undressing, condom and diaphragm use)
C8-T1			
All muscles of UEs now fully innervated Pronator quadratus	Forearm pronation	Paralysis of LEs	Independent in bed activities, wheelchair transfers, self-care, and personal hygiene
Flexor carpi ulnaris	Ulnar wrist flexion	Weakness of trunk control	Can manage manual wheelchair on all surfaces
~ Lumbricales and ~ interossei dorsales and palmares	MP flexion	Endurance reduced because of low respiratory reserve	Can transfer from wheelchair to floor and return with standby assistance
~ Palmar interrossei	Finger adduction		Can get up and down from standing frame independently Independent bladder and bowel care and skin inspection
Flexor pollicis longus and brevis Adductor pollicis ~ Opponens digiti minimi ~ Opponens pollicis	Thumb flexion (MP, IP) Thumb adduction Opposition of fifth finger Thumb opposition		Independent in management of communication devices Drives with adaptations Light housekeeping can be done independently
T4-T9			
All muscles of upper extremities plus partial innervation of intercostal muscles and long muscles of the back (sacrospinalis and semispinalis)	All arm functions Partial trunk stability Endurance increased because of better respiration	Partial trunk paralysis and total paralysis of LEs	Independent in all self-care Independent manual wheelchair and transfers May use standing frame independently Drives car with adaptations Independent in light housekeeping
T10-L2			
Intercostal muscles fully innervated Abdominal muscles partially to fully innervated (rectus abdominis, internal and external obliques)	Partial to good trunk stability Increased physical endurance	Paralysis of LEs May have flaccid bowel, bladder, and sexual function	Independent in self-care, work, personal hygiene, sports, and housekeeping Ambulates with difficulty using braces and crutches, but a wheelchair is often chosen for speed, energy conservation, and sports Drives car with hand controls

Continued

TABLE 40-1 Functional Outcomes Based on Level of Injury—cont'd			
NEUROLOGICAL LEVEL/MUSCLES INNERVATED	**MOVEMENTS POSSIBLE**	**PATTERN OF WEAKNESS**	**FUNCTIONAL CAPABILITIES AND LIMITATIONS**
L3-L4 Low back muscles Hip flexors, adductors, quadriceps	Trunk control and stability Hip flexion Hip adduction Knee extension	Partial paralysis of lower extremities; hip extension, knee flexion, and ankle and foot movements	Independent in all activities outlined above Can ambulate independently with short leg braces, using crutches May still use a wheelchair for convenience, energy conservation, and sports
L5-S3 Hip extensors: gluteus maximus and hamstrings Hip abductors: gluteus medius and gluteus minimus Knee flexors: hamstrings, sartorius, and gracilis Ankle muscles: tibialis anterior, gastrocnemius, soleus, and peroneus longus Foot muscles	Partial to full control of LEs	Partial paralysis of LEs, most notable in distal segment	Independent in all activities May require limited bracing for ambulation May have volitional bowel, bladder, and sexual function May drive car without modifications

short- and long-term goals and equipment needs enhances the quality and functional ability of an otherwise quite dependent individual. Rehabilitation centers specializing in the care of ventilator-dependent patients should be sought for their expertise in addressing all aspects of care for this unique patient population.

When place of discharge is determined and the patient can tolerate leaving the hospital for a few hours, a home evaluation should be performed. The therapist, patient, and family members can then view and attempt activities in the home in anticipation of return to a safe and accessible environment. The therapist must be knowledgeable in safety and accessibility options for a variety of environments and often must advise architects or contractors to ensure that appropriate modifications are made. The therapist must be aware of accessibility requirements in the home as well as what is required in the workplace based on the Americans with Disabilities Act of 1990 (ADA), which outlines the accessibility requirements and rights of an individual with disability in the community and in the workplace (see Chapter 29).

Because of progressively shortened lengths of inpatient rehabilitation, the extended phase of treatment previously available as inpatient care may occur on an outpatient basis or via home therapy. Assessments such as adaptive driving, home management, leisure activities, or workshop skills using hand- or power-based tools are feasible and very appropriate treatment modalities employed to evaluate and increase UE strength, coordination, and trunk balance; however, they may not be a priority during inpatient hospitalization. Such activities

can improve socialization skills and assess problem-solving skills and potential work habits as well.

Occupational therapy services can offer valuable evaluation and exploration of the vocational potential of persons with SCI. By the sheer magnitude of the physical disability, vocational possibilities for individuals with high levels of spinal cord injury are limited. Many patients must change their vocation or alter former vocational goals. Low aptitude, poor motivation, and lack of interest and perseverance on the part of many patients make vocational rehabilitation challenging.

The occupational therapist can assess the patient's level of motivation, functional intelligence, aptitudes, attitudes, interests, and personal vocational aspirations during the process of the treatment program and through the use of ADL, craft, and work simulation activities. The occupational therapist can observe the patient's attention span, concentration, manual ability with splints and devices, accuracy, speed, perseverance, work habits, and work tolerance level. The OT can serve as a liaison between the client and the vocational rehabilitation counselor by offering valuable information from observations during activities. When suitable vocational objectives have been selected, they may be pursued in an educational setting or in a work setting usually out of the realm of OT.

AGING WITH SPINAL CORD INJURY

Following survival of acute spinal cord injury, the primary goal of rehabilitation has been defined in terms of independence. It is true that independence is good and dependence is not so good. Independence has therefore become the measure of quality of life for people with disabilities, an idea accepted and often perpetuated by professionals and survivors alike.[13]

Occupational therapists treating patients with spinal cord injuries have considerable responsibility in influencing the level of independence whether in the acute setting, during active rehabilitation, or in follow-up care throughout the life of a spinal cord-injured individual. Understanding the aging process both in the able-bodied and the disabled individual is necessary to provide appropriate options and foster attitudes that enhance the quality of the patient's life, at whatever age.

Physical aging is a natural, unpreventable process encountered by all humans. The signs of the process can occur at varying rates for each individual, and aging affects most systems of the body. In spinal cord-injured individuals, aging is usually accelerated by the secondary effects of the disability such as the presence of muscle imbalance, infections (both urinary and respiratory), deconditioning, pain, and joint degeneration secondary to overuse.[11]

One out of 4 SCI survivors is over 20 years postinjury.[11] For someone who acquired quadriplegia in his or her twenties, when the majority of spinal cord injuries occur, the degenerating conditions of normal aging become evident earlier than normal, usually before the forties.[4] Thus someone who was independent in transfers at home and loading a wheelchair in and out of the car may now require assistance getting in and out of bed; the person may have to trade the car for a van requiring costly modifications because his or her shoulders have given out.

It is important for the occupational therapist to be aware of why good trunk alignment and seating is essential from the onset so as to prevent fixed trunk and pelvic deformities such as kyphosis and scoliosis, which can lead to considerable skin problems and uncorrectable cosmetic deformities years later. In addition, it is necessary to be aware of the impact manual wheelchair propulsion can have on a weak shoulder complex in relation to the advantage of the cardiopulmonary conditioning that such an activity can provide.

When compounded by the increased fatigue and weakness often associated with normal aging, the functional status of the individual with SCI may be affected and a power wheelchair may be indicated. As the therapist responsible for these activities, many considerations must be weighed to make appropriate short- and long-term decisions. Contacting experienced resources who have a perspective of both acute and long-term injuries and issues can offer valuable insight into treatment decisions.

SUMMARY

Spinal cord injury can result in substantial paralysis of limbs and trunk. The degree of residual motor and sensory dyfunctions depends on the level of the lesion, whether the lesion was complete or incomplete, and the area of the spinal cord that was damaged.

Following a spinal cord injury, bony realignment and stabilization are established surgically or with braces. There are many possible complications of spinal cord injury including skin breakdown, decreased vital capacity, and autonomic dysreflexia, among others.

Occupational therapy is concerned with facilitating the patient's achievement of optimal independence and functioning. The occupational therapy program includes measures for physical restoration, self-care, independent living skills, and educational, work, and leisure activities. The psychosocial adjustment of the client is very important, and the occupational therapist offers emotional support toward this end in every phase of the rehabilitation program.

SAMPLE TREATMENT PLAN

The treatment plan deals with four of ten identified problems. The reader is encouraged to add objectives and methods for the remaining problems to make a more comprehensive treatment plan.

CASE STUDY

Mr. H is a 37-year-old male who sustained a cervical fracture in a diving accident. He suffered a C5-6 fracture dislocation, ASIA motor A, with resultant paralysis of hands, trunk, and LEs.

Before his injury he worked full-time as a policeman in a small town. He has been married for 13 years and has no children. His wife is an RN. Mr. H has led a very active lifestyle. His hobbies include raising horses, weight lifting, racquetball, and cycling. He has always been an extremely independent gentleman with a good sense of humor and

SAMPLE TREATMENT PLAN – cont'd

with a large circle of friends, mostly fellow police officers. His parents and two sisters live in a nearby town and visit frequently.

Immediately after his injury Mr. H was flown to a nearby community hospital, where after diagnosis his neck was surgically stabilized. A posterior fusion of C5 on C6 with laminar wiring was performed. A halo vest traction device was applied postsurgically, and he was subsequently transferred to a regional spinal cord injury center for further medical management and total spinal cord injury care. A referral for occupational therapy was received the day of admission, and a full evaluation was initiated.

TREATMENT PLAN

Personal data

Name: Mr. H
Age: 37
Diagnosis: C5-6 fracture dislocation resulting in C6 complete quadriplegia, ASIA motor A
Disability: Paralysis and sensory loss of hands, trunk, and LEs
Treatment aims stated in referral: Occupational therapy evaluation and treatment

Other services

Physician: Maintenance of general health, prescription of medication, coordination of rehabilitation team
Nurse: Administer medication, manage bowel and bladder program, assist in skin and self-care needs as necessary, follow through on ADL program as instructed by OT
Physical therapy: UE and LE ROM, strengthening of available musculature, standing program if indicated, increase vital capacity through breathing exercise program
Social service: Discharge and community resource planning, individual and family counseling
Psychological: Individual and family counseling
Recreation therapy: Develop leisure skills

Frame of reference

Occupational performance

Treatment approach

Biomechanical and rehabilitative

OT EVALUATION

Performance components

Sensorimotor functioning
   Muscle strength: Test
   Passive ROM: Test
   Physical endurance: Observe, interview
   Movement speed: Observe
   Coordination: Test, observe
   Functional movement: Test, observe
   Sensation (touch, pain, thermal, proprioception): Test
Cognitive/cognitive integrative functioning

Judgment: Observe
Safety awareness: Observe
Motivation: Observe, interview
Psychosocial functioning
   Coping skills: Observe
   Adjustment to disability: Observe, interview
   Interpersonal relationships: Observe

Performance areas

Self-care: Observe, interview
Home management: Observe, interview

EVALUATION SUMMARY

Patient's passive ROM (PROM) is within normal limits (WNL) in all joints of the UEs. Slight tightness at the MP and PIP joints will be encouraged to facilitate finger stability for natural tenodesis action. Specific manual testing revealed symmetry in all innervated UE muscle groups with the exception of elbow extension and wrist extension (Fig. 40-8).

Sensory tests performed were pain, light-touch, and kinesthesia, with the following findings:

Pain (pinprick)
L: C6 and above—intact; C7 and below—absent
R: C5 and above—intact; C6—impaired; C7 and below—absent

Light touch
L: C6 and above—intact; C7—impaired; C8 and below—absent

R: C6 and above—intact; C7 and below—absent
Kinesthesia
L: Wrist, elbow, shoulder—intact; radial fingers—impaired; ulnar fingers—absent
R: Wrist, elbow, shoulder—intact; radial and ulnar fingers—absent

Although physical endurance is low as observed in frequent rest periods during a 60-minute treatment session, the patient's wheelchair tolerance is 8 hours per day.

Sitting balance is fair on the mat or edge of bed. However, Mr. H requires a chest strap while pushing his wheelchair to maintain good sitting balance.

Coordination and muscle control are good in available musculature as evidenced by performance in table top and sink activities.

SAMPLE TREATMENT PLAN – cont'd

RIGHT CA	Region	EXAMINERS INITIALS / DATE	Root	Nerve	LEFT CA
	NECK	FLEXION			
		FLEXION/ROTATION: Sternocleidomastoid	C2-3,CRXI	Spinal Accessory	
		EXTENSION	C1-8	Dorsal Rami	
4	SCAPULA	ELEVATION: Upper Trapezius	C3-4	Spinal Accessory	4
3+		DEPRESSION: Lower Trapezius	C3-4	Spinal Accessory	3+
		ADDUCTION:			
3		Rhomboids	C5	Dorsal Scapular	3
3+		Middle Trapezius	C3-4	Spinal Accessory	3+
4		ABDUCTION: Serratus Anterior	C5-7	Long Thoracic	4
3+	SHOULDER	FLEXION: Anterior Deltoid	C5-6	Axillary	3+
		EXTENSION: Latiss/Teres Major	C5-7	Lower Subscapular/Thoracodorsal	3+
4		ABDUCTION: Middle Deltoid	C5-6	Axillary	3+
3+		HORIZONTAL ABDUCTION: Posterior or post. Deltoid	C5-6	Axillary	4
		HORIZONTAL ADDUCTION			
0		Pectoralis Major-Clavicular	C5-T1	Med. Lat. Ant. Thoracic	0
0		Pectoralis Major-Sternal	C5-T1	Med. Lat. Ant. Thoracic	0
4		EXTERNAL ROTATION: Inf. Sp/T Min	C5-6	Axillary/Subscap.	3+
3+		INTERNAL ROTATION: Subscap	C5-T1	Subscap./Thoracic	3+
	ELBOW	FLEXION:			
4		Biceps/Brachialis	C5-6	Musculocutaneous	4
4		Brachioradialis	C5-6	Radial	4
2−		EXTENSION: Triceps	C6-8	Radial	0
4		SUPINATION	C5-7	Radial	4
3		PRONATION: Pro. Teres/Pro Quad.	C6-T1	Median	3
	WRIST	FLEXION			
0		Flexor Carpi Radialis	C6-8	Median	
0		Flexor Carpi Ulnaris	C8-T1	Ulnar	0
		EXTENSION			
4 > ©*		Extensor Carpi Radial Longus/Brevis	C6-8	Radial	4
1		Extensor Carpi Ulnaris	C7-8	Radial	0
	FINGERS	FLEXION:			
0		Flexor Digitorum Superficialis	C7-T1	Median	0
0		Index			0
0		Long			0
0		Ring			0
0		Little			0
0		Flexor Digitorum Profundus			0
0		Index	C8-T1	Median	0
0		Long	C8-T1	Ulnar	0
0		Ring	C8-T1	Ulnar	0
0		Little	C8-T1	Ulnar	0
		Lumbricales			0
0		Index	C6-7	Median	0
0		Long	C6-7	Median	0
0		Ring	C8	Ulnar	0
0		Little	C8	Ulnar	0

*Grade 4 but slightly stronger than ©.

FIG. 40-8 Occupational therapy manual muscle evaluation.

LE spasticity is severe, requiring medication to regulate because it interferes with bed mobility and transfer progress.

Although finger function is absent bilaterally, Mr. H is able to pick up light objects of varied sizes and textures, using natural tenodesis grasp in both his dominant right and nondominant left hands.

Mr. H's judgment, safety awareness, and problem-solving abilities are good. He occasionally has difficulty in sequencing frustrating activities such as transferring from wheelchair to bed, however. His motivation varies daily in conjunction with the degree of despair he feels over his injury. His coping skills are generally very good in that his sense of humor and high level of intelligence help him through the bad days. He is having difficulty adjusting to his disability and accepting himself in a less physically capable and traditionally masculine role than before his injury. Ironically, he becomes very passive around his wife who assumes her nursing role when with him. On occasion Mr. H is easily angered and makes critical comments about himself and his body. In contrast, he is a great motivator with other patients, assuming more of a leadership role. Using appropriate humor, he takes charge of most group interactions. He has a large circle of close friends, several of whom drive 2 or more hours to visit.

Mr. H is independent in feeding with the exception of cutting meat. The only adaptive equipment he uses is a universal cuff. He requires minimal assistance for his hygiene setup at the sink. He requires moderate assistance with UE dressing secondary to the interference of the halo vest. He is dependent for LE dressing.

He currently requires moderate assistance of one person to perform sliding board transfers and wheelchair mobility to and from level surfaces; he requires maximal assistance on uneven surfaces.

He requires moderate to maximal assistance for bed mobility because of the halo vest, which is in place for approximately 3 months from the day of surgery.

Before his accident Mr. H had an excellent work record and habits. He continues to demonstrate these assets by his consistent timeliness and attendance in therapy sessions. His work potential is good as demonstrated by the clerical table top tasks he performs diligently although slowly. He will not, of course, be able to return to his prior job duties.

Mr. H has been unwilling to participate in community reintegration activities subsequent to feeling self-conscious in public; therefore his community mobility skills have not been assessed.

Light meal planning and preparation as well as some housekeeping skills will be assessed when the halo vest is removed.

Mr. H lives in a single story house that will require only bathroom modifications for safe accessibility. The majority of Mr. H's leisure activities were very active, and appropriate leisure interests after discharge will be assessed by recreation therapy.

Assets

Symmetrical UE strength
Strength of 3+ to 4 in innervated musculature
Relatively good coordination and dexterity in hand skills
Good living situation
Strong family and community support
Good coping skills

Good problem-solving skills
Marketable job skills
High level of education
Good potential for independent driving

Problem list

1. Poor prognosis for recovery
2. Paralysis of fingers, trunk, and LE
3. Sensation absent below C7 dermatome
4. Requires the assistance of one person for mobility when out of the wheelchair (bed mobility and transfers)
5. Requires the assistance of one person for dressing,

bathing, bowel and bladder program; dependent on wheelchair for all mobility
6. Potential for skin breakdown
7. Lack of assertiveness in directing wife in his care
8. Lack of knowledge regarding durable medical equipment
9. Requires the assistance of one person for kitchen and homemaking skills
10. Requires assistance for community mobility
11. Inability to return to former vocational and avocational activities

PROBLEM 4: DEPENDENT ON MODERATE PHYSICAL ASSISTANCE FOR TRANSFERS

Objective
Patient will require standby assistance only for all level surface transfers, including pretransfer and posttransfer setup

Method
Pretransfer and posttransfer setup: Patient backs wheelchair to bed and applies brakes and loosens chest and hip strap; he hooks arm behind push handle for balance and leans forward hooking hand and wrist under ipsilateral leg

Using wrist extension and elbow flexion to kick foot off footplate and onto opposite foot, patient then removes whole footrest using power from wrist extension; with one footplate off of chair, he then removes brake and positions wheelchair appropriately next to bed and relocks brake

Patient then repeats same sequence of movement, putting foot on floor; patient hooks other arm behind push handle and repeats sequence until both feet are on the floor

With modified depression, patient scoots buttocks forward in seat so as to clear wheel during transfer; he then places slide board under leg midway between knee and hip, angled toward opposite hip; patient then finds stable handholds, one on wheelchair and one on slide board, leans forward while maintaining balance with locked elbows (Fig. 40-7)

By using momentum of swinging head and shoulders away from slide board, patient slides across board, periodically adjusting feet with arms and repositioning UEs

Caregiver is in front of the patient within arm's length to provide assistance if necessary

Gradation
Therapist initially provides more assistance while patient moves through each step; gradually reduce amount of assistance and amount of time and energy required by patient

PROBLEM 6: POTENTIAL FOR SKIN BREAKDOWN

Objective
Patient will be independent in forward weight shifts using loops attached to back frame of wheelchair

Method
Using method just described for removing feet from footplates and putting flat on floor, patient then places both arms in loops (approximately 24 inch × 1 inch [61 cm × 2.5 cm] cotton webbing sewn into loops and screwed into top upholstery screws of back frame of wheelchair)

Patient pulls self forward using arms against armrests and slowly lowers self toward knees, using loops to control the speed in which he drops forward; patient lies completely across knees and remains down for 1 to 2 minutes to allow capillary blood flow to return over bony prominences of ischial tuberosities and sacrum

When ready to sit up, patient pulls symmetrically against loops, first using elbow flexion and then shoulder abduction and flexion to pull upper body upright, returning to a sitting position

Arms must then be removed from loops; patient must then place feet back on footplates by reversing procedure described previously; seatbelts must then be secured tightly and brakes released.

Gradation
Initially therapist sits in front of patient to provide assistance and security while patient is lowering self and pulling back to sitting

Gradually withdraw assistance as patient gains strength and confidence; time spent performing activity should decrease to no more than 5 minutes

SAMPLE TREATMENT PLAN – cont'd

PROBLEM 2: PARALYSIS OF FINGERS

Objective
Patient will increase wrist extension strength to at least grade 4, sufficient for successful natural tenodesis for grasping light objects and donning and doffing adaptive equipment and splints

Method
Patient is seated in wheelchair with arm supported on armrest; hand is hanging over end of armrest; patient self-ranges wrist by actively extending wrist through full ROM against gravity; this step is done before resistive exercise to ensure full active ROM; a wrist cuff and small weights are placed on the hand

Patient actively extends wrist through full available ROM 10 times; repeat repetitions 3 times

Weight is then decreased, and repetitions are repeated; therapist ensures that full ROM occurs upon each repetition; if not, then weight should be decreased

Weights are then removed and functional activities are then performed such as board games and object manipulation tasks using same motion

Gradation
Increase resistance; goal is reached at approximately 5 lb.
Increase repetitions; increase complexity and duration of subsequent functional activity

---

PROBLEM 7: LACK OF ASSERTIVENESS IN DIRECTING WIFE IN CARE

Objective
Patient will be independent in talking through, instructing, and critiquing wife in all aspects of his care when indicated

Method
Therapist instructs patient in the specific sequence of a dependent activity such as LE dressing; instruction includes predressing setup, such as bathing and legbag application. Patient then talks therapist through entire activity; therapist role-plays predictable responses of wife relating to body mechanics and other aspects of the procedure that may

prove difficult; therapist then arranges for wife to be present when patient can be successful

Patient then instructs wife in all aspects of the procedure and critiques the process; therapist observes entire process and intervenes when necessary

Gradation
Decrease therapist's physical and verbal cues and decrease amount of time taken to perform task

Decrease amount of stress on patient and wife so that process and interaction is positive and successful

---

REVIEW QUESTIONS

1. List three causes of spinal cord injury. Which is most common?
2. Describe the patterns of weakness in quadriplegia and paraplegia.
3. Describe the functional and prognostic differences between complete and incomplete lesions.
4. When reference is made to C5 in quadriplegia, what is meant in terms of level of injury and functioning muscle groups?
5. What are the characteristics of spinal shock?
6. What physical changes occur following the spinal shock phase?

7. What is the prognosis for recovery of motor function in complete lesions and incomplete lesions?
8. What are the purposes of surgery in management of spinal injury?
9. What are some medical complications, common to patients with spinal cord injuries, that can limit achievement of functional potential?
10. How should postural hypotension be treated?
11. How should autonomic dysreflexia be treated?
12. What is the role of the occupational therapist in the prevention of pressure sores?

13. Why is vital capacity affected in patients with spinal cord injuries?
14. What effect does reduced vital capacity have on the rehabilitation program?
15. Which level of injury has full innervation of rotator cuff musculature, biceps, and extensor carpi radialis and partial innervation of serratus anterior, latissimus dorsi, and pectoralis major?
16. What additional muscle power does the patient with C6 quadriplegia have over the patient with C5 quadriplegia? What is the major functional advantage of this additional muscle power?

17. What are the additional critical muscles that the patient with C7 quadriplegia has, as compared with the patient with C6 quadriplegia?
18. What additional functional independence can be achieved because of this additional muscle power?
19. What is the first spinal cord lesion level that has full innervation of UE musculature?
20. Which evaluation tools does the occupational therapist use to assess the patient with a spinal cord injury? What is the purpose of each?
21. List five goals of occupational therapy for the patient with a spinal cord injury.
22. How is wrist extension used to effect grasp by the patient with quadriplegia?
23. How does the patient with C6 quadriplegia substitute for the absence of elbow extensors?
24. What is the contracture that is encouraged in patients with spinal cord injuries? Why? How is it developed?
25. What is the splint that allows the C6 quadriplegic to achieve functional grasp?
26. What are some of the first self-care activities that the patient with a C6 spinal cord injury should be expected to accomplish?
27. List four assistive devices commonly used by persons with quadriplegia, and tell the purpose of each.
28. How can ordering an ill-fitting wheelchair affect the upper-extremity function and skin care of a C6 quadriplegic?
29. Describe the role of occupational therapy in the vocational evaluation of a patient with a spinal cord injury.
30. What are two considerations when prognosticating the future of a 25-year-old individual with T4 paraplegia?

REFERENCES

1. American Spinal Injury Association (ASIA): *Standards for neurological and functional classification of spinal cord injury,* Chicago, 1992, The Association.
2. Bromley I: *Tetraplegia and paraplegia: a guide for physiotherapists,* ed 3, New York, 1985, Churchill Livingstone.
3. Frankel H and associates: The value of postural reduction in the initial management of closed injuries to the spine with paraplegia and tetraplegia, *Paraplegia* 7:179, 1969.
4. Freed MM: Traumatic and congenital lesions of the spinal cord. In Kottke FJ, Lehmann JF, editors: *Krusen's handbook of physical medicine and rehabilitation,* Philadelphia, 1990, WB Saunders.
5. Hanak M, Scott A: *An illustrated guide for health care professionals,* New York, 1983, Springer-Verlag.
6. Heinemann AW and associates: Mobility for persons with spinal cord injury: an evaluation of two systems, *Arch Phys Med Rehabil* 68:90-93, 1987.
7. Hill JP, editor: *Spinal cord injury, a guide to functional outcomes in occupational therapy,* Rockville, Md, 1986, Aspen.
8. Institute for Medical Research, Santa Clara Valley Medical Center: *Severe head trauma, a comprehensive medical approach,* Project 13-9-59156/9, report to National Institute for Handicapped Research, Nov, 1982.
9. Malick MH, Meyer CMH: *Manual on the management of the quadriplegic upper extremity,* Pittsburgh, 1978, Harmarville Rehabilitation Center.
10. Paulson S, editor: *Santa Clara Valley Medical Center spinal cord injury home care manual,* ed 3, San José, Calif, 1994, Santa Clara Valley Medical Center.
11. Pierce DS, Nickel VH: *The total care of spinal cord injuries,* Boston, 1977, Little, Brown.
12. Spencer EA: Functional restoration. In Hopkins HL, Smith HD, editors: *Willard and Spackman's occupational therapy,* ed.8, Philadelphia, 1993, JB Lippincott.
13. Whiteneck and associates, editor, *Aging with spinal cord injury,* New York, 1993, Demos.
14. Wilson DJ, McKenzie MW, Barber LM: *Spinal cord injury: a treatment guide for occupational therapists,* rev ed, Thorofare, NJ, 1984, Slack.
15. Yarkony GM: *Spinal cord injury: medical management and rehabilitation,* Gaithersburg, Md, 1994, Aspen.

Cerebral Vascular Accident

*Lorraine Williams Pedretti, Jerilyn A. Smith,
Heidi McHugh Pendleton*

Cerebral vascular accident (CVA) or stroke is the most common disabling neurologic disease of adulthood.[33,61] It accounts for at least half the patients hospitalized with neurologic disease. An estimated 500,000 new strokes occur every year in the United States. The fatality rate of acute stroke victims is about 33%, making stroke the third leading cause of death in the United States, after heart disease and cancer. At least 50% of the survivors suffer permanent neurologic disability and one third of survivors undergo a second stroke, further compounding their disability. Because of the very limited success in the reversal of the effects of brain damage, prevention is the key to reducing mortality and morbidity resulting from CVA.[33]

Factors associated with a high risk for CVA are hypertension, coronary artery disease, carotid bruits, transient ischemic attacks (TIAs), congenital artery wall weakness, diabetes mellitus, hyperlipidemia, cigarette smoking, age and gender, race, heredity, alcohol consumption, polycythemia, obesity, and use of oral contraceptives.[27,33,56] Current stroke research emphasizes the effectiveness of surgery and drugs on reducing the effects of the CVA. Other preventive measures to reduce the risk are as follows: eliminate smoking, lower high blood pressure and high cholesterol levels, make use of anticoagulants and surgery, when indicated.

DEFINITION OF CVA

Cerebral vascular accident (CVA) is a complex dysfunction caused by a lesion in the brain. It results in an upper motor neuron dysfunction that produces hemiplegia or paralysis of one side of the body, including limbs and trunk, and sometimes the face and oral structures that are contralateral to the hemisphere of the brain that has the lesion. Thus a lesion in the left cerebral hemisphere, or left CVA, produces right hemiplegia, and vice versa. When referring to the patient's disability as right hemiplegia, the reference is to the paralyzed body side and not to the locus of the lesion.[56]

Accompanying the motor paralysis may be a variety of other dysfunctions. Some of these are sensory disturbances, perceptual dysfunctions, visual disturbances, personality and intellectual changes, and a complex range of speech and associated language disorders.[57,59]

CAUSES OF CVA

CVA, frequently called stroke, is caused by pathological conditions in the cerebral vasculature. A compromise in the blood supply to the brain caused by thrombus, embolus, or hemorrhage results in cerebral ischemia and ultimately, in secondary brain abnormality. The onset of CVA is often unanticipated and sudden.[57]

Cerebral anoxia and aneurysm also can result in hemiplegia.[10,14,56] Some of the treatment approaches outlined in this chapter may be applicable to hemiplegia that results from causes other than CVA or stroke, such as head injuries, neoplasms, and infectious diseases of the brain.[10]

Vascular disease of the brain can result in a completed CVA or cause transient ischemic attacks (TIAs). A TIA occurs as mild isolated or repetitive neurologic symptoms that develop suddenly, last from a few minutes to several hours, but not longer than 24 hours, and clear completely. The TIA is seen as a sign of impending CVA. Most TIAs occur in those with atherosclerotic disease. It is estimated that of those who experience TIAs and do not seek treatment, one third will sustain a completed stroke, another third will continue to have additional TIAs without stroke and one third will experience no further incidence.[50] If the TIA is caused by extracranial vascular disease, surgical intervention to restore vascular flow (carotid endarterectomy) may be effective in preventing the CVA and the resultant disability.[57]

EFFECTS OF CVA

The outcome of the CVA depends on which artery supplying the brain was involved in the vascular disease (Fig. 41-1).

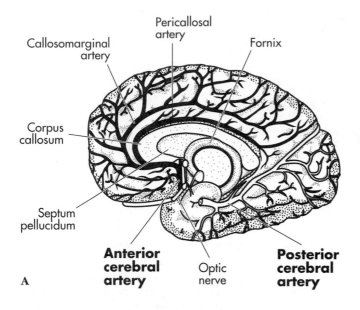

The Cerebral Hemispheres

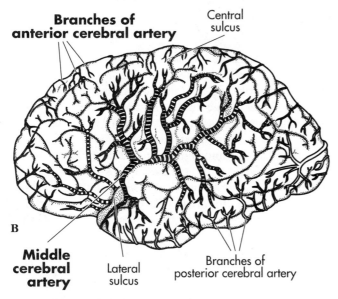

FIG. 41-1 Blood supply to brain. Middle cerebral, anterior cerebral, and posterior cerebral arteries supply blood to cerebral hemispheres. **A**, Medial surface. **B**, Lateral surface. (From Nolte J: *The human brain*, ed 3, St Louis, 1993, Mosby-Yearbook.)

MIDDLE CEREBRAL ARTERY

Involvement of the middle cerebral artery (MCA) is the most common cause of CVA.[12,32] Ischemia in the area supplied by the MCA results in contralateral hemiplegia with greater involvement of the arm, face, and tongue, sensory deficits, contralateral homonymous hemianopsia; and aphasia, if the lesion is in the dominant hemisphere. There is a pronounced deviation of the head and neck toward the side on which the lesion is located.[12,18,56,57] Perceptual deficits such as anosognosia, unilateral neglect, impaired vertical perception, visual spatial deficits, and perseveration are seen if the lesion is in the nondominant hemisphere.[7,17]

INTERNAL CAROTID ARTERY

Occlusion of the internal carotid artery, in the absence of adequate collateral circulation, results in contralateral hemiplegia, hemianesthesia, and homonymous hemianopsia.[17] Additionally, involvement of the dominant hemisphere is associated with aphasia, agraphia or dysgraphia, acalculia or dyscalculia, right-left confusion, and finger agnosia. Involvement of the nondominant hemisphere is associated with visual perceptual dysfunction, unilateral neglect, anosognosia, constructional or dressing apraxia, attention deficits, and loss of topographic memory. A tendency to tilt space in a counterclockwise direction is seen in some left hemiplegics, making ambulation and two-dimensional constructional tasks difficult.[57]

ANTERIOR CEREBRAL ARTERY

Occlusion of the anterior cerebral artery (ACA) produces contralateral lower extremity weakness that is more severe than that of the arm. Apraxia, mental changes, primitive reflexes, and bowel and bladder incontinence may be present. Total occlusion of the ACA results in contralateral hemiplegia with severe weakness of the face, tongue, and proximal arm muscles and marked spastic paralysis of the distal lower extremity. Cortical sensory loss is present in the lower extremity. Intellectual changes such as confusion, disorientation, abulia, whispering, slowness, distractibility, limited verbal output, perseveration, and amnesia may be seen.[17,57]

POSTERIOR CEREBRAL ARTERY

The scope of posterior cerebral artery (PCA) symptoms is potentially broad and varied because this artery supplies the upper brain stem region, as well as the temporal and occipital lobes. Possible results of posterior cerebral artery involvement depend on the arterial branches involved and the extent and area of cerebral compromise. Some possible outcomes are sensory and motor deficits, involuntary movement disorders (hemiballism, postural tremor, hemichorea, hemiataxia, intention tremor), memory loss, alexia, astereognosis, dysesthesia, akinesthesia, contralateral homonymous hemianopsia or quadrantopsia, anomia, topographic disorientation, and visual agnosia.[17,18,57]

CEREBELLAR ARTERY

Cerebellar artery occlusion results in ipsilateral ataxia, contralateral loss of pain and temperature sensitivity, ipsilateral facial analgesia, dysphagia and dysarthria caused by weakness of the ipsilateral muscles of the palate, nystagmus, and contralateral hemiparesis.[12,17,18]

VERTEBROBASILAR ARTERY SYSTEM

A CVA in the vertebrobasilar artery system affects brain stem functions. The outcome of the stroke is some combination of bilateral or crossed sensory and motor abnormalities, such as cerebellar dysfunction, loss of proprioception, hemiplegia, quadriplegia, and sensory disturbances, with unilateral or bilateral cranial nerve involvement of nerves III to XII.[57]

MEDICAL MANAGEMENT

Specific treatment of CVA depends on the type and location of the vascular lesion, the severity of the clinical deficit, concomitant medical and neurologic problems, availability of technology and personnel to administer special types of treatment, and the cooperation and reliability of the patient.

Early medical treatment includes maintenance of an open airway, hydration with intravenous fluids, and treatment of hypertension. Appropriate steps should be taken to evaluate and treat coexisting cardiac or other systemic diseases. Measures should be taken to prevent the development of deep venous thrombosis (DVT). DVT is the formation of emboli (blood clots) in the deep veins of the lower extremities, a common risk for all patients who experience prolonged periods of bed rest and immobility. The incidence of DVT in stroke ranges from 22% to 73%. Emboli that are released from deep veins and subsequently lodge in the lungs are referred to as pulmonary emboli. A pulmonary embolus is the most common cause of death in the first 30 days after the CVA.[11]

The physician oversees routine surveillance for thrombosis that includes daily evaluation of leg temperature, color, circumference, tenderness, and appearance. Preventive treatment for DVT can include medication, use of elastic stockings, use of reciprocal compression devices, and early mobilization of the patient.

The early poststroke course may be complicated by respiratory problems and pneumonia. The National Survey of Stroke reported that one third of all stroke patients studied had respiratory infections.[49] Symptoms are low grade fever and increased lethargy. Medical management includes the administration of fluids and antibiotics, aggressive pulmonary hygiene and mobilization of the patient. Ventilatory insufficiency is a major factor contributing to the high frequency of pneumonia. The hemiparesis of stroke involves muscles used in breathing. Exercise programs that include strengthening and endurance training of both inspiratory and expiratory muscles help to improve breathing and cough effectiveness and reduce the frequency of pneumonia.[11]

Cardiac disease is another frequently occurring condition that complicates the poststroke course. The stroke itself may cause the cardiac abnormality, or the patient may have had a preexisting cardiac condition. The former is treated as any new cardiac diagnosis (see Chapter 36). A preexisting cardiac condition is reevaluated and the treatment regime modified as appropriate. Monitoring of heart rate, blood pressure, and EKG during self-care evaluations is frequently indicated to determine cardiac response to activity.[43,44]

During the acute phase, bowel and bladder dysfunction is common. The physician is responsible for ordering a specific bowel program that includes a time schedule, adequate fluid intake, stool softeners, use of suppositories, oral laxatives, and medications or procedures to treat fecal impaction. A timed or scheduled toileting program is essential in treating urinary incontinence. Catharization may be necessary in stroke rehabilitation.

MOTOR DYSFUNCTION AFTER CVA
CHARACTERISTICS OF MOTOR DISTURBANCE AFTER CVA

After CVA, upper motor neuron paralysis follows a one-sided distribution and includes musculature of the trunk and limbs on the affected side. The muscles of the face and mouth also may be involved. The paralysis is usually characterized by increased muscle tone, called hypertonicity or spasticity. In some cases, hypotonicity or flaccidity may be apparent. Even in these instances some spasticity may be evoked in the finger and wrist flexors and the ankle extensors if prolonged and strong stretch stimuli are applied. In cases in which apparent flaccidity persists indefinitely, it is usually combined with severe sensory loss, making active motion impossible.[9]

Coordination or control of smooth, rhythmic movement is lost. Rather, the spasticity occurs in gross patterns of flexion and extension called synergies (Chapter 22). Synergies are released when cortical control of motion is interrupted. All muscles in the synergy are neurophysiologically linked, and when one of the movements is performed, some or all of the movement components are likely to occur simultaneously.[14,30]

Normal postural mechanisms are disturbed after CVA. Normal righting, equilibrium, and protective reactions (Chapter 10) are lost on the hemiplegic side. This condition affects the patient's ability to maintain and recover balance and make the normal postural adjustments that accompany movement and activity. Primitive reflexes (Chapter 10, 20) may be released so that changes of the position of the head and body in space have an abnormal influence on muscle tone.

Bobath described the loss of "adaptive changes of muscle tone as a protecition against the forces of gravity,"[9] referring to the ability to control slow, unresisted movements in the direction of gravity. For example, in lowering the upraised arm the antigravity muscles contract and hold while their antagonist muscles relax. The person with hemiplegia has lost this mechanism of automatic control on the affected side. He or she tends to compensate for the loss with the automatic reactions of the unaffected side. The patient does not initiate movement with the affected side, does not bear weight on the affected arm and hand, and bears little weight on the affected leg.

Because of the spasticity and release of abnormal synergistic movement patterns, loss of selective, discriminative, and isolated movement occurs after CVA. This loss is most apparent in the arm and hand, probably because of the nature of the normal function of this part. Selective movement is also lost in the leg and foot, however, and is evident (1) in the inability to dorsiflex the ankle and toes regardless of the position of the hip and knee or (2) in the inability to flex the knee while the hip is extended. In function this inability is evidenced by the gait pattern, which is usually performed with the leg held in stiff extension or in the extensor synergy pattern. The person with hemiplegia lacks ability to perform a wide variety of movement combinations to effect normal motor performance.[9]

Bobath outlined four major factors that interfere with normal motor performance in an adult hemiplegia: sensory disturbances, spasticity, disorder of the normal postural reflex mechanism, and loss of selective movement patterns.[9]

The degree of sensory involvement has a profound influence on the degree of spontaneous motor recovery and the results of treatment. Much movement is in response to sensory stimuli acting on the central nervous system (CNS) from the external and internal environments.[9,15] These sensory stimuli progress through the CNS and are integrated at the cortical level where they produce an effective, coordinated motor response to meet the demands of the environment. Sensations arising from the movement response serve to guide it through its course, determine its effectiveness, and give cues for the need for any revision of the movement response.[9]

Because of this critical sensory-motor relationship and interdependence, it is important to think of the sensorimotor cortex as one functional unit of the brain. The sensory disturbance in patients with hemiplegia aggravates the motor dysfunction even in the absence of severe spasticity. The patients lack the urge to move, probably in part because they cannot sense and interpret the environmental stimuli that normally evoke movement.[9]

RECOVERY PERIOD

Spontaneous recovery of voluntary motor function occurs primarily in the first 3 months after the onset of the CVA.[35] Motor recovery may continue up to 1 year and in rare instances somewhat longer. This fact does not imply that motor behavior cannot be influenced by appropriate therapy after a year. Improvement in functional performance may continue for years following stroke.

PROGNOSIS FOR FUNCTIONAL RECOVERY

The physician and therapist may wish to estimate the potential for recovery of function for purposes of planning rehabilitation goals. Factors associated with poor prognosis are coma at onset, poor cognitive functions, severe hemiparesis, prior history of CVA, and significant cardiovascular disease.[49] Following the initial period of acute illness, additional factors that adversely affect prognosis for functional recovery are prolonged hypotonia or severe hypertonicity, apraxia, severe sensory disturbances,[34] receptive aphasia, dementia, unilateral neglect, body scheme disturbance, disturbance of spatial percep-

tion, lack of motor return, and continued bowel and bladder incontinence.

Conversely, prognosis for functional recovery is good if the patient has early return of muscle tone and motor function (within 2 weeks), intact sensation and perception, good cognitive functioning, intact body scheme, minimal spasticity, absence of contractures, some spontaneous use of the arm in bilateral activities, and development of selective motion.[34]

CONCOMITANT DYSFUNCTIONS

In the rehabilitation program of patients with stroke, much emphasis is placed on treating the motor dysfunction, which is the part of the disability that can easily be seen and assessed. The disability is complicated, however, by many invisible problems, which have a significant impact on the patient's performance and prognosis for rehabilitation. If the therapist fails to recognize the problems concomitant with the motor disability, rehabilitation efforts result in frustration and failure for the patient and the therapist.[19] On the basis of a comprehensive evaluation, realistic rehabilitation goals and methods can be planned with the patient.

SENSORY DISTURBANCES

Disturbances in the senses of touch, pain, temperature, pressure, and vibration and proprioception may occur as a result of CVA.[34] Such disturbances prohibit the sensory feedback that is so important to the perceptual-motor functioning of the person and thus may be one cause of disuse of the affected extremities, even when motor recovery is apparently good.

With damage to the brain there is general impairment or absence of all sensory modalities in the involved segment (e.g. shoulder, forearm, and hand). Should sensation return, it usually occurs in a proximal to distal pattern. This pattern is unlike peripheral nerve or spinal cord injury damage in which involvement of isolated sensory modalities in delineated areas is characteristic. Return occurs hierarchically with pain and temperature returning first and stereognosis returning last, in the nerve's specific sensory distribution.[48]

Sensory evaluation should include light touch, superficial pain (sharp/dull), position sense (proprioception), and object identification (stereognosis). Information about sensation testing and sensory reeducation methods is included in Chapter 13.

PERCEPTUAL DYSFUNCTION

The ability to learn and make continuous adaptation to the ever-changing environment is dependent on intact perceptual processes. Perception is complex and involves processes of transforming, organizing, and structuring sensory information from the environment. Adaptation is dependent on intact perceptual processing. A patient who lacks adequate perceptual processing skills fails to adapt adequately to the tasks of daily living.[19]

Evaluation of visual perception and perceptual motor skills is discussed in Chapters 12 and 14. Some of the perceptual dysfunctions that commonly affect patients with hemiplegia are outlined below.

Body Scheme Disorders

Body scheme disorders are disturbances in the neurologic function that include knowledge of body construction, its anatomic elements, and spatial relationships. An intact body scheme includes the ability to visualize the body in movement and its parts in different positional relationships and the ability to differentiate right from left.[3] Body scheme disorders are found frequently enough in patients with hemiplegia to make routine evaluation for the presence of this dysfunction advisable.

Because knowledge of the body scheme is basic to all motor function, a disturbance in body scheme has a profound effect on the success of the patient's rehabilitation. Patients with body scheme disturbances have difficulty with activities of daily living (ADL), especially self-care and dressing activities that require a good knowledge of the body.[36] They may have difficulty following directions related to their own bodies.[5] They may be unable to localize body parts correctly, recognize right and left, and visualize and plan how to move their bodies to accomplish a certain activity.

Tactile Perception

Tactile perception is the ability to recognize, localize, and make discriminations about touch stimuli to the skin surface. It includes the ability to (1) recognize and localize light touch stimuli, (2) recognize two stimuli in close proximity (two-point discrimination), (3) recognize two simultaneous stimuli, and (4) identify common objects and geometric forms through manipulation without the aid of vision (stereognosis).[18]

The inability to perceive the tangible properties of an object tactually (astereognosis) interferes with perceptual-motor functioning in that the patient receives no sensory feedback about the objects he or she is manipulating unless vision is used to compensate for the sensory loss. This compensation is often ineffective, because it is difficult visually to supervise the hand performing an activity while trying to watch the activity and focus on its goal.

Apraxia

The disturbance in praxis, or the ability to plan motor acts, is often intimately associated with the body scheme disorder.[3,64] Apraxia is defined as an impairment of movement control that cannot be explained on the basis of disruptions to the sensorimotor systems, poor or absent comprehension of the task, intellectual deficit, inadequate attention, or poor cooperation by the patient.

Three types of apraxia have been identified. In *ideomotor apraxia*, the patient is unable to carry out a purposeful movement on command even though the concept of the task is understood and even though it may be possible to carry out the act automatically.[30,64] For example, when asked to pick up a cup and take a drink, the patient may be unable to do so. If he or she is thirsty and sees the cup, however, reaching out and drinking from the cup occurs automatically. If *ideational apraxia* is present as well, the patient is not able to carry out routine activities, such as combing hair automatically, or on command because the concept of the task is not understood.[64]

Constructional apraxia is difficulty or inability to produce two- or three-dimensional designs in copying, constructing, or drawing. Constructional apraxia is often related to body scheme problems and is associated with difficulties in ADL, particularly dressing.[62,64]

When apraxia is present, often the person cannot formulate a plan of movement to accomplish an act. He or she may be unable to imitate movements of the therapist in demonstrated instructions.

Visual Field Deficit and Homonymous Hemianopsia

Homonymous hemianopsia is blindness of the nasal half of one eye and the temporal half of the other eye.[18] The affected side of the vision corresponds to the paralyzed side of the body. A patient with left hemiplegia with left homonymous hemianopsia cannot see things in the left visual field unless the patient turns the head toward the affected side to compensate for the deficit. In practical activity, items placed on the left side may not be seen. Objects moving toward the patient from the left may be startling. The patient may bump into things on the left when walking. Some patients with hemiplegia compensate for this deficit automatically by turning their heads. Others need to be trained to turn the head, using the intact visual field to compensate for the visual loss.[59]

Unilateral Neglect

Unilateral neglect, also called unilateral inattention, is the inability to integrate and utilize perceptions from the hemiplegic side of the body or of space and is most frequently seen in persons with left hemiplegia. Homonymous hemianopsia can be a complicating factor, but unilateral neglect occurs in the absence of hemianopsia.[60,64] The cause of unilateral neglect is not exactly known. It has been attributed to body scheme disorder and to visual scanning disorders.[46,59,64]

Unilateral neglect poses serious problems in rehabilitation. It is associated with deficits in reading, writing, arithmetic, and self-care skills. Some studies have shown that the presence of unilateral neglect in patients with right hemisphere lesions is a predictor of poor outcome in recovery of performance skills in ADL.[60]

The patient with unilateral neglect ignores the affected limbs and the affected side of space. The patient may fail to shave the affected side of the face or to dress that side of the body. Food on the affected side of the tray may be ignored and the patient may read only one side of a page of printed material. Communication from the hemiplegic side may be ignored or poorly integrated.[64]

The degree of unilateral neglect may vary from mild to severe. Persons with mild neglect can be taught strategies for compensation such as verbally cuing themselves to attend to the affected side. Severe neglect poses a much more important safety risk and persons with persistent neglect may require continual supervision.

Visual Attention

The ability to attend visually to elements in the environment depends on visual fixation, a voluntary act for the normal adult. The normal adult is able to select objects in the environment that demand attention and to focus on them appropriately.[6,64] The process of selecting objects on which to focus attention involves visual search and scanning. Visual search is the process of scanning the environment to gather information for identification or to select elements that demand attention or response. Deficits in visual search and the oculomotor skills necessary for its performance are seen frequently in patients with CVA.[8] The patient with a visual attention deficit has difficulty shifting the gaze or attention and has slowed eye movements and loss of the visual fixation point.[52]

Spatial Relationships

The ability to recognize the relationship between one form and another and between form and self in spatial areas may be lost as a result of CVA.[25,64] Disturbances in the perception of visual-spatial relationships are particularly common among patients with right brain damage.[57] The result is difficulty with tasks such as drawing or constructing three-dimensional objects and designs. The patient with this deficit has difficulty or failure with tasks involving spatial analysis such as determining the distance between objects. For example, a person who is unable to judge the distance between the wheelchair and the bed is at risk for falling. The ability to follow a familiar route may be lost because of a lack of spatial orientation.[57] Dressing failures are common because understanding of space concepts such as over, under, through, and behind may be lost.[59]

The problem may be compounded by the patient's inability to perceive the shape and relationship of the clothing to his or her body. Tasks such as matching parts in a sewing or woodworking project are impossible, as are matching puzzle parts and block designs.

Figure-Ground Perception

Figure-ground perception is the recognition of forms hidden within a gestalt[25] and the ability to attend to a relevant visual stimulus while separating it from and ignoring background stimuli.[64] Some patients have difficulty distinguishing a figure from its background. The result is that they cannot always select and respond to the most relevant visual cue.[5] The patient may appear distractible but, in truth, he or she is responding to many irrelevant visual stimuli.[22,64] The patient may have difficulty selecting items from a drawer or refrigerator because he or she cannot perceive the desired object as separate from the surrounding objects that constitute its background.[59,64]

Visual Perception of Vertical

The perception of vertical lines and elements in the environment is essential to visual orientation in space. Patients with hemiplegia often have difficulty making visual judgments of what is vertical or horizontal. Patients with left hemiplegia tend to misjudge the vertical in a counterclockwise direction.[7,57] Because visual orientation to vertical is important to the optical righting reactions that help in the maintenance of upright posture, directional disturbances in perception of vertical and horizontal may interfere with balance and ambulation.[7]

Agnosia

Agnosia refers to the inability of the patient to recognize familiar objects in the environment. It may involve the following sensory perceptions: visual, tactile, auditory, and proprioceptive.

Visual agnosia is the inability to recognize objects, although vision is intact. Visual "stimuli pass through the eye and optic tracts normally, but are not interpreted correctly in the occipital cortex."[64] Patients may not recognize their family members by sight, but may be able to identify them by hearing their voices. Such patients may not recognize their own possessions.

Tactile agnosia or astereognosis is the inability to recognize familiar objects by touch or feel.

COGNITIVE DYSFUNCTIONS

Because CVA may interfere with integrative processes of the brain, and intelligence and cognitive abilities depend on the integrative functions of the brain, some patients with hemiplegia show impairment of specific cognitive abilities. This impairment may be demonstrated by an overall change in the areas of organization, mental abilities, knowing and understanding, judgment, awareness, and the ability to do abstract reasoning.[26,29] Evaluation of cognitive dysfunction is discussed in Chapter 15.

Memory

The reception, registration, integration, and retrieval of information may be disrupted in patients with CVA, at least in part, by factors such as language disorders, visual perceptual problems, alertness, motivation, and mental stamina, to name a few. Psychological reactions to stroke, such as anxiety and depression, can also affect memory adversely.[8]

Memory disturbance complicates rehabilitation efforts. The patient may have difficulty recalling persons, objects, and procedures learned. Retrieval of information may be reduced, and learning ability may be impaired. Day-to-day carry-over of learned techniques may be affected.

Patients with deficits in memory require much repetition of activity before the task is learned.[5] The therapist needs to discover each patient's best mode of learning and provide the necessary sensory and perceptual cues and methods of instruction to provide each patient with the optimal opportunity for learning.

Judgment

Poor judgment may be easily detected or may be masked by good social or verbal skills.[5] The patient may be unable to abstract the future and make judgments about the consequences of certain behaviors. The patient may not be able to judge, for example, that not locking his or her wheelchair may have grave consequences.

Abstract Thinking

Abstract thinking and reasoning also may be impaired. Patients are often concrete, dealing better with the realities of concrete objects and situations than with ideas and speculations about them. They may not be able to generalize learning from one situation or another and may be unable to comprehend abstract ideas.[28]

Sequencing

Sequencing involves the ability to plan, organize, and carry out the steps of a task. It includes temporal concepts such as first, second, and third and spatial ordering such as top, bottom, left to right, and around.[4] A disturbance in sequencing skills may affect the patient's ability to plan and initiate the steps of tasks and activities that require ordering of objects and steps for a procedure.

Initiation

Problems with initiation are characterized by difficulty or inability to do one or more of the following: plan, organize, begin, and carry out tasks involving more than one step. The patient may initially require step-by-step assistance to complete routine ADL tasks. Verbal and/or tactile cues may be necessary to provide the patient with information to initiate the activity. As initiation skills improve, cues can be decreased.

Impulsivity and Decreased Insight

The patient who has sustained a stroke often has poor insight into the limitations resulting from the disability. Physical dysfunction may be denied despite evidence to the contrary. Some patients appear to be unconcerned or indifferent to their deficits and may argue with those who attempt to point them out.[64] A result of this decreased insight is often impulsiveness and poor safety awareness. The patient is unable to make sound judgments about actions and is unable to see the cause-and-effect relationships of behavior. For example, an impulsive patient may attempt to try to get out of a wheelchair and into bed independently despite the fact that there is substantial paralysis and standing without assistance is not possible.

Problem Solving

Problem solving involves the integration of many cognitive functions. Attention to task, memory, organization, planning, and judgment all play important parts in the patient's ability to solve problems.[64] (See Chapter 15.)

PERSONALITY AND EMOTIONAL CHANGES
Depression

Depression is a common reaction to a catastrophic illness. The patient may feel inadequate in dealing with his or her problems and may be overwhelmed by them. The patient feels a loss of control over life and a sense of helplessness. He or she has experienced not only a loss of control but also a considerable loss of function and must mourn for the loss.[5,8]

Depression is one of the most underidentified and undertreated responses to stroke. Depression can develop, resolve, and reappear at any stage of the rehabilitation process. Early intervention is essential. There has been an increased awareness by physicians of the importance of identifying and treating the symptoms of depression.

Denial

Denial is a lack of acknowledgement of the stroke and its concomitant manifestations.[52] This phenomenon may be an adaptive response to the sudden and severe interruption in one's life. Continued denial, however, can prolong or prevent the patient's progress toward adjustment to disability.

Regression

Patients who exhibit regression may be reverting back to behaviors that were used successfully in the past to relieve anxiety. They may act towards those who are helping them as they did to their parents, lovers, and friends who met their needs during earlier phases of their lives. Such patients may appear less mature than they did before the stroke. Regression often resolves as the patient makes progress toward solving problems and achieving greater independence. This response is a fairly common one to illness and the concomitant losses.[5,8]

Perseveration

Perseveration is the meaningless, nonpurposeful repetition of an act.[18,45] The patient does not stop unless someone or something intervenes. It becomes particularly apparent during activities that are repetitive by nature, such as sanding wood, but can manifest itself in ADL bathing and grooming tasks.

Emotional Lability

The patient with CVA may lose the cortical control of emotional responses and thus may manifest loss of emotional control more easily than he or she did formerly. Emotional lability may exhibit itself in uncontrolled outbursts of laughing or crying that seem inappropriate. Emotionally charged situations of either a pleasant or unpleasant nature can provoke such responses. The patient is embarrassed by this behavior and requires the reassurance and understanding of family and rehabilitation workers.[5,8]

Motivation

Many patients with hemiplegia manifest an apparent decrease in intrinsic motivation, or the inner drive to act spontaneously. This deficit may be organic in origin or related to depression and should not be regarded as something that the patient can modify at will. This lack of motivation may cause rehabilitation workers and family members to overestimate the disability. It may cause them to regard the patient as stubborn or unwilling to try. It is important for those working with the patient to understand that the problem may be related to the patient's readiness to deal with the overwhelming ramifications of the disability and to the tremendous amount of energy it takes every day for these patients to put their all into everything they attempt to do.

Motivation can be enhanced by establishing treatment goals that are realistic and meaningful. The patient and therapist should plan and modify treatment goals together. The experience of success in the treatment program facilitates motivation. The therapist should explain the purposes of treatment so that the patient can understand the relevance of the treatment methods to goal attainment.[23]

Therapists must approach motivation problems with patience and perseverance. Patients need encouragement, reassurance, and praise for success.

Rigidity

Rigidity is an inability to be flexible or adapt to change. The patient feels most secure in a familiar and unchanging environment. This phenomenon manifests itself in inability to function with a changed time schedule, in disturbance at a change in personnel, and in a tenacity to old and familiar methods of performing familiar activities.[21]

Reduction in Behavioral and Evaluative Standards

The patient demonstrating a reduction in behavioral and evaluative standards may exhibit a reduced level of goal aspiration. He or she may seem satisfied with shoddy performance. His or her pride and perseverance in working toward goals may be poor. Inadequate performance and poor products may be acceptable to the patient in contrast to standards held before the illness occurred. This problem may be organic in origin but is enhanced by inactivity and the psychological trauma of the illness.[22]

Frustration Tolerance

Because of the numerous difficulties in performance posed by motor, sensory, perceptual, and cognitive impairments, the patient with CVA understandably experiences much stress and frustration. Excessive stress and frustration are experienced when the patient is confronted with tasks that are above the capacity for performance and success or lack meaning for the patient. It is important for the therapist to select relevant activities difficult enough to challenge the patient to improve function, yet not so difficult as to evoke undue stress or frustration. Also, the therapist should monitor the effect that any given treatment method has on the patient. It is important for the patient to experience success in the treatment program.

SPEECH AND LANGUAGE DISORDERS

CVA may result in a wide variety of speech disorders and language disorders that may vary from mild to severe. These dysfunctions occur most frequently in CVAs resulting from damage to the left hemisphere of the brain but also occur less frequently with damage to the right hemisphere. All persons with CVA should be evaluated by the speech pathologist for the presence of speech and language disorders. The speech pathologist can provide valuable information to other members of the rehabilitation team and the family regarding the best techniques to communicate with a particular patient. The occupational therapist should carry over the work of the speech therapist in the treatment sessions, as it is appropriate. Carryover may occur in reinforcing communication techniques the patient is learning, presenting instruction in ways the patient is able to understand and integrate.

When reading the descriptions of the specific speech and language dysfunctions that follow, it is important to remember that these dysfunctions can exist in mild to severe form and in combination.

Aphasia

Aphasia is a language disorder that results from neurologic impairment. It can affect auditory comprehension, reading comprehension (alexia), oral expression, written expression (agraphia) and ability to interpret gestures. Mathematical deficits (acalculia) can also be present in aphasia. There are several different types of aphasia.

Global aphasia. Global aphasia is characterized by a loss of all language skills. Oral expression is lost except for some persistent or recurrent utterance. Global aphasia is usually the result of involvement of the middle cerebral artery of the dominant cerebral hemisphere. The patient with global aphasia may be sensitive to gestures, vocal inflections, and facial expression. As a result the patient may appear to understand more than he or she actually does.[29]

Broca's aphasia. Broca's aphasia is characterized by speech apraxia and agrammatism. The apraxia is manifested by slow, labored speech with frequent misarticulations. Syntactical structure is simplified because of the agrammatism, sometimes referred to as telegraphic speech. There is good auditory comprehension except when speech is rapid, grammatically complex, or lengthy. Reading comprehension and writing may be severely affected, and deficits in monetary concepts and ability to do calculations are usually present.[29]

Wernicke's aphasia. Wernicke's aphasia is characterized by impaired auditory comprehension and feedback and fluent, well-articulated paraphasic speech. Paraphasic speech consists of word substitution errors. Speech may occur at an excessive rate and may be hyperfluent. The patient uses few substantive words and many function words. The speech is a running speech composed of English words in a meaningless sequence. Some patients produce neologisms (non-English nonsense words) interspersed with real words. Reading and writing comprehension is often limited and impairment of mathematical skills may occur.[29]

Anomic aphasia. Anomic aphasia is characterized by difficulties with word retrieval. Anomia or word finding difficulty occurs in all types of aphasia. However, patients in whom word finding difficulty is the primary or only symptom may be said to have anomic aphasia. The speech of these patients is fluent, grammatically correct, and well articulated, but there is significant difficulty with word finding. This problem can result in hesitant or slow speech and the substitution of descriptive phrases for actual names of things. Mild to severe deficits in reading comprehension and written expression occur and mild deficits in mathematical skills may be present.[29]

Dysarthria

Patients with dysarthria have an articulation disorder because of a dysfunction of the CNS mechanisms that control speech musculature in the absence of aphasia.[59] This disorder results in paralysis and incoordination of the organs of speech that make it sound thick, sluggish, and slurred.[10]

Communication with Aphasic Patients

Although the speech pathologist is responsible for the treatment of speech and language disorders, the occupational therapist can facilitate communication and meaningful interaction with aphasic patients.

Patients respond best to intelligent and empathetic understanding from professional staff and family members. Those communicating with the patient should adopt an attitude of patience, relaxation, and acceptance. When talking to the patient, simple, short, concrete sentences should be used. Instructions and explanations should be kept simple. The patient can be encouraged, but not pressured, to respond in any way possible. The use of gestures for communication should be encouraged. Having the patient demonstrate through

performance is the best way to ensure that instructions are understood.

Bizarre, inaccurate language and the use of profanity should be handled without amusement or anger. It is not necessary to raise the voice when speaking to aphasic patients. Hearing is usually not affected. Professional staff and family members should not talk about the patient in his or her presence. The patient can probably understand all or part of what is being said and should be included in conversations. Rapid, complicated speech with abstract and esoteric words should be avoided. Direct questions requiring one-word answers are useful.[31]

The occupational therapist can use routine ADL as opportunities to encourage speech. The patient needs to be reassured that the language disorder is part of the disability and is not a manifestation of mental illness.[31]

CONTRAST BETWEEN RIGHT AND LEFT BRAIN DAMAGE

There is an apparent difference between performance and learning in persons with right brain damage and those with left brain damage. The right cerebral hemisphere is concerned with the perception of the whole or Gestalt processing.[17] It is associated with perceptual skills such as the body scheme and visual spatial analysis. Therefore, right hemisphere lesions involving the parietal lobe result in body scheme disturbance, spatial perceptual disorders, and inattention to the left side.[1,59] Lesions of the right cerebral hemisphere result in difficulties with tasks of spatial analysis and spatial orientation and in dressing apraxia.[59,64]

There is a significant correlation between extremely poor performance on perceptual organization tasks and failures in dressing and grooming.[35] The patient with right brain dysfunction may retain good verbal skills, which may tend to mask the perceptual dysfunction and give the impression of good performance. The therapist needs to require performance evaluation of self-care skills and not rely on the interview as a means of determining the patient's ability to function.

The left cerebral hemisphere of most right-handed persons is primarily responsible for analytical processing of individual elements rather than perception of the whole. It is also responsible for temporal sequencing.[17] The control of language and complex voluntary movement resides primarily in the left hemisphere. Left hemisphere lesions result in varying degrees of aphasia.[1,59] The ability to deal with visual spatial tasks may be undisturbed, and the patient may benefit from demonstrated or pantomimed instructions rather than verbal ones. He or she is usually more successful in achieving self-care independence earlier than the patient with right brain damage.

Motor and functional goal attainment is dependent upon integration of perceptual, cognitive, and psychosocial skills. Rehabilitation goals cannot be based on motor evaluation alone. Rather, the total scope of the disability must be considered, including sensory, perceptual, cognitive, psychological, emotional, and intellectual capabilities. Equally important are the patient's social and family circumstances as well as the previous level of function. If the evaluation is incomplete or inadequate, appropriate goals cannot be set and the result is frustration and failure for patient, therapist, and family.

OCCUPATIONAL THERAPY INTERVENTION

The role of the occupational therapist in the treatment of CVA revolves around facilitating symmetric motor function, improving functional use of the affected side, integrating sensory and perceptual functions, and restoring the patient to his or her maximal level of independence.

Each patient must be evaluated for his or her residual abilities and disabilities. A treatment program must be tailored to the patient's particular needs, because the range and severity of possible motor, sensory, perceptual, and cognitive dysfunctions after CVA is wide. The selection of treatment objectives and treatment methods depends on many factors, such as stage of motor recovery, sensory perceptual status, cognitive functions, age, date of onset, concomitant illness, social and economic factors, and potential for further recovery.

The occupational therapist should be involved in the acute care of the patient and the early mobilization aspects of treatment. Subsequent occupational therapy may be a primary service in extended rehabilitation when the emphasis is on achieving self-care independence, independent living skills, and performance skills for work or leisure activities. Occupational therapy may be provided after discharge in the home setting or on an outpatient basis.

GOALS OF OCCUPATIONAL THERAPY

The overall goals of occupational therapy for the patient who has had a stroke include prevention of deformities, remediation of psychosocial dysfunction, achievement of maximal physical function, and facilitation of maximal independence in self-maintenance.[46] More specific goals are the following:

1. prevention of deformity caused by abnormal tone and poor positioning
2. inhibition of abnormal patterns of posture and movement
3. achievement of maximal active ROM, strength, and coordination of the affected extremities and body side
4. achievement of maximal voluntary bilateral and unilateral use of affected extremities in correct functional patterns
5. remediation of perceptual and cognitive dysfunction
6. achievement of maximal functional independence in self-care
7. facilitation of realistic acceptance of and adjustment to disability

8. improvement of functional communication skills and social interaction
9. facilitation of reentry to meaningful roles in family and community
10. facilitation of a balance between work, rest, and play.[46,56,59]

OCCUPATIONAL THERAPY EVALUATION

The occupational therapist begins the program with a thorough evaluation of the patient's deficits and assets to establish a baseline for progress. The evaluation process is continuous, beginning with simultaneous gross evaluation of motor, sensory, perceptual, and cognitive functions and their effects on simple self-care. It progresses to more formal and in-depth assessments of complex performance areas. A patient's performance of a simple self-care task can provide valuable screening information regarding ROM, sensorimotor functioning, perception, and cognition and identify problems for immediate attention.[48] Oral motor and swallowing functions should be assessed to determine the patient's ability to eat and take medication safely.

Motor Functions

The degree of hypertonicity in a patient with CVA should be evaluated (Chapter 10). The Brunnstrom test (Chapter 22) can be used to determine the stage of motor recovery, the presence of synergistic movement, and associated reactions. Abnormal movement patterns, the presence of primitive reflexes, abnormal motor patterns, abnormal coordination, righting reactions, equilibrium and protective reactions, and in general, the postural mechanism should be evaluated according to methods outlined by Bobath.[9,58]

Joint ROM may be measured or estimated, but the therapist should be aware that ROM often is limited by transient and variable degrees of hypertonicity at any given time. In recording joint ROM, the therapist must differentiate between apparent limitations caused by hypertonicity and actual limitations caused by structural changes.[19]

When the patient has achieved some voluntary control of movement, the therapist should evaluate the ability to perform selective movement. Spontaneous use of the affected extremities should be observed during testing and functional activities, because this ability is a good sign of improving sensorimotor status.

Muscle strength should be tested only if the patient has full selective movement and does not have abnormal tone. When there is hypertonicity, it is not possible to assess accurately the strength of muscles affected or muscles acting against those muscles that are hypertonic.[19]

Sensation

Senses of touch, superficial pain, temperature, and pressure, as well as stereognosis and proprioception should be tested.[59] Olfactory and gustatory sensation may be tested, because these senses are disturbed in some patients and often overlooked. Methods for evaluating sensation can be found in Chapter 13.

Perception

Body scheme and motor planning should be routinely evaluated. Tests for visual perception problems, such as hemianopsia and visual-spatial relationships, figure-ground perception, visual attention, and unilateral neglect, should be included in the battery of evaluation procedures. Methods for evaluating perception are described in Chapters 12 and 14.

Cognition

Cognitive skills such as memory, attention, initiation, planning and organization, mental flexibility and abstraction, insight and impulsivity, problem-solving skills, and ability to do calculations should be evaluated.[46] Methods for evaluating cognition are described in Chapter 15.

Psychosocial Factors

Through observation and interview of the patient, family members, friends, and other rehabilitation team members, the occupational therapist should ascertain the patient's vocational and recreational histories, role in the family and community, amount of family support, adjustment to disability, and frustration tolerance and coping skills.

Regressive behavior and functioning should be assessed because CVA can cause regression to less mature behaviors and coping strategies. The patient may deny the necessity to engage in apparently simplistic activities to regain motor, sensory, perceptual, cognitive, performance, and communication skills. Coping with the multitude of personal and social changes brought about by this catastrophic disability may affect the patient's ability to participate in his or her rehabilitation process. An evaluation by a neuropsychologist is often indicated to identify and direct treatment for depression. The rehabilitation team can develop strategies for dealing with motivation or adjustment difficulties.[56]

Communication and Oral Motor Function

An oral motor evaluation, carried out according to methods described in Chapter 11, may be necessary for many patients with CVA. Such an evaluation helps to determine the need for facilitation and inhibition of oral motor skills necessary for safe swallowing. A swallowing program is developed to address problem areas.

The occupational therapist should make an assessment of functional communication skills in the course of the evaluation process and treatment. The therapist can observe the patient's ability to interpret spoken and written language, ability to speak and write, difficulty with motor control of oral structures because of paralysis or mouth apraxia, difficulty with auditory perception and determining direction of auditory stimuli, and loss of hearing.[56]

If speech is affected, information about specific speech impairments should be gleaned from the evaluation by the speech pathologist. This specialist can recommend appropriate methods of adapting and modifying instruction to best suit the patient's deficits. The patient's attempts at nonverbal communication may be hampered by altered muscle tone and sensation, lack of movement, and facial paralysis.[56,58]

Performance Areas

Performance areas should be evaluated by actual performance of test items. Activities of daily living including self-care skills, home management skills, community living skills, mobility and transfer techniques, physical endurance, and work-related activities, when appropriate, should be included in the performance evaluation. It may take several weeks to complete the performance evaluation, which is an ongoing part of the treatment program. Methods of evaluating performance areas are described in Chapter 26.

TREATMENT
Motor Dysfunction
Motor retraining

The occupational therapy program may include one or a combination of the sensorimotor approaches to treatment such as the Brunnstrom (Chapter 22), Bobath (Chapter 24), and proprioceptive neuromuscular facilitation (PNF) (Chapter 23) approaches. The purposes of the motor retraining program are to facilitate normal movement and use of the affected side, develop more normal postural mechanisms, and inhibit abnormal reflexes and movement patterns.

Range of motion

The maintenance of joint ROM and prevention of deformity is an important early goal in the treatment program and should be continued indefinitely if a substantial amount of spontaneous voluntary movement is not regained. Improvement is achieved through positioning techniques such as those recommended by Bobath and passive, assistive, and self-administered ROM procedures.[9]

ROM exercises usually are carried out using principles of the selected treatment approach. In the Brunnstrom approach, positioning, passive movement through the synergy patterns, trunk and bilateral shoulder movements as described in Chapter 22, and the facilitating patterns of movement used in treatment all serve to maintain ROM.[13]

The Bobath approach uses bilateral upper extremity movement with clasped hands to release spasticity and maintain full passive or assisted shoulder flexion and scapula movement and to facilitate tone normalization. The patient grasps the affected hand with the sound hand. If tone is not excessive, the fingers can be interlaced with the hemiplegic thumb on top in some abduction. The patient is taught to begin the self ROM exercise by reaching forward and protracting the scapula before lifting the arms. This action serves to release the flexor spasticity and allows for scapula mobility before shoulder motion.[19] With elbows extended, the arms are then raised to the level of comfort. These exercises must be practiced many times during the day to maintain full pain-free shoulder ROM and scapular mobility.

The advantages of the Bobath exercise include an increased awareness of the affected arm as it is brought to midline and into the field of vision. Prevention of scapula and trunk retraction is facilitated.[19] Proper positioning and the patterns of movement used during treatment prevent loss of ROM. All the patterns of normal movement are incorporated into the motor retraining program. Upper extremity ROM is an integral part of the total treatment program.[20]

In the PNF approach, performance of antagonistic pairs of diagonal upper extremity patterns activates all muscle groups in the upper extremities. Ten repetitions of antagonistic diagonals maintain ROM of all joints of the arm. To perform ROM of the wrist and hand, the therapist grasps the side of the patient's thumb with the thumb and one finger of one hand. The patient's thumb is pulled into palmar abduction. The therapist places his or her fingers across the palmar surface of the patient's fingers in a diagonal direction. The patient's hand is then moved in partial diagonal patterns so that the forearm is supinated with wrist and finger flexion and pronated with wrist and finger extension.[39]

Shoulder pain and subluxation

"The shoulder is essentially a composite of seven joints, all moving synchronously and incumbent upon each other to ensure complete pain-free movement."[16] Any interference of this coordinated interaction of joints and muscles can result in pain and restriction of motion.[19,20]

Shoulder pain can be present during movement and/or when the patient is at rest. The patient with shoulder pain may have difficulty participating in the rehabilitation program and may be unable to concentrate on learning new skills. Fear or anticipation of pain may interfere with the therapist's attempts at ROM, muscle reeducation, and positioning of the extremity. Shoulder pain can be prevented with proper early management and treatment. Patients seen immediately after the CVA can receive instruction in positioning and ROM to prevent the development of shoulder pain. Nurses and family can be taught correct handling techniques to avoid injuring the weakened shoulder musculature.[19]

Intact scapular mobility is essential to maintain pain-free shoulder motion. Spasticity in the muscles that depress and retract the scapula is common following a CVA. This problem, in turn, prevents normal abduction and upward rotation of the scapula. When the glenohumeral joint is flexed or abducted and normal scapular motion does not take place, joint trauma results. Bicipital tendinitis, coracoiditis, brachial plexus traction, or supraspinatus tendinitis caused by compression of the ten-don between the humeral tuberosities and the acromion can occur from joint trauma.[16,19,20,46,58]

The Bobath,[9] Brunnstrom,[14] and PNF[39] approaches caution against the traditional passive ROM exercises to the shoulder. Tone of scapular muscles and scapula mobility must be assessed before moving the upper extremity. If the patient's scapula does not move sufficiently when the arm is passively lifted, trauma will occur and the patient will experience pain. Adequate scapula rotation must be achieved to ensure pain-free shoulder ROM.[20]

Reciprocal pulley exercises are contraindicated, because they are forced passive exercise and can cause joint pain and damage if there is inadequate scapula motion.[12,19,53] Shoulder pulleys should not be used for passive elevation of the affected arm. They force the internally rotated humerus upward, and there is not enough scapula rotation and shoulder external rotation for movement without joint trauma.[19]

Inappropriate exercise and incorrect handling of the upper extremity by professional staff during transfers, ambulation, bathing, and bed mobility activities are some of the causes of trauma to the shoulder joint.[19,46] Improper positioning of the arm can also contribute to the development of shoulder pain. In addition, patients with severe sensory loss or unilateral neglect may develop shoulder pain from inadvertently traumatizing the hemiplegic arm. For example, the affected arm could be left dangling at the side of the wheelchair or bumped into a door frame when entering or exiting a room.

In the past occupational therapists prescribed and applied arm slings to the patient for wear when the arm is in a dependent position for the purpose of preventing or reducing subluxation. Smith and Okamoto[54] reported that there are more than 22 hemiplegic sling designs. The benefits of such a sling are doubtful.[2,46] Bobath maintained that subluxation cannot be prevented if the muscles are weak and that slings contribute to poor positioning (i.e., sustained elbow flexion, humeral adduction), pain, swelling, and sensory deprivation.[9] Todd and Davies[58] stated that a sling should never be worn because it reinforces flexor spasticity and immobilizes the upper limb, both of which are factors contributing to shoulder pain.

Although the sling is not effective for reducing pain or preventing subluxation, there may be circumstances in which the use of a sling is beneficial to the patient. For example, a sling may provide reassurance for the patient who has severe pain and fears further pain on activity. Other patients with flaccid paralysis may find a sling helpful in supporting the upper extremity during community ambulation. Careful, ongoing monitoring and reevaluation are necessary when a sling is used.

Hand edema

Hand edema, resulting from fluid accumulation in the hand of the patient with hemiplegia, should be prevented. Lymphatic pumps located proximally and distally in the upper extremity are dependent on muscle tone and contraction for their function. The hypotonicity and inactivity of the hemiplegic upper extremity can result in faulty pumping action of the lymphatic system and subsequent hand edema.

Edema is most often evident on the dorsum of the hand. The skin loses its creases, especially over the PIP and DIP joints. The edema is soft and puffy initially and the tendons on the dorsum of the hand are not visible. Extended edema results in trophic skin changes (skin becomes shiny), the hand becomes hard, and there is joint stiffness and loss of ROM.

Edema can be prevented by elevation of the hand above the heart level to facilitate venous return. The hand can be propped on pillows at night and supported on a wheelchair arm or a distally elevated lapboard during the day when the patient is not involved in activity or treatment. Passive and active assisted ROM exercises help to prevent or reduce edema. Because immobilization contributes to the development of edema, splints and positioning devices should be closely monitored.

More aggressive techniques for edema reduction, which may be used by both physical and occupational therapists, are air splints, the Jobst pump, retrograde massage, elastic gloves,[46] centripetal wrapping of the fingers and hand with string, and immersion in a bucket of ice and water. Davies recommended the use of a small cock-up splint for the flaccid wrist and hand to prevent dependent positioning of the wrist in flexion.[19] The splint is held in place with an elastic bandage. Persistent wrist flexion contributes to edema because it prevents vascular pumping action.

Flexor spasticity of the UE and hand

Flexor spasticity in the hand musculature can result in strong, uncontrolled wrist flexion and a fisted position of the fingers (Fig. 41-2). This flexion can progress to contracture and deformity if not treated. Orthotic devices (splints) may be used to protect joints and prevent deformity, particularly if there is no active motion. The volar

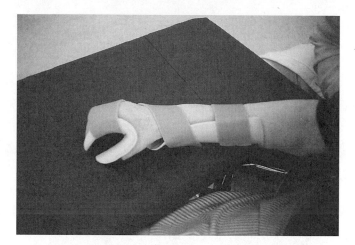

FIG. 41-3   Resting splint is used to position wrist and hand properly.

resting splint and the dorsal resting splint are frequently used to position the spastic hand (Fig. 41-3). It is essential that the splint be designed to support the wrist and fingers in the functional position. Todd and Davies[58] stated that splints can reduce sensory stimulation and decrease the need for activity. Splints must be closely monitored and frequently removed for ROM and muscle reeducation.

There are various splints that have been designed to inhibit flexor spasticity. However, the success of these splints in actually decreasing spasticity is controversial. No definitive study compares the long-term effects of various positioning devices on spastic hands of patients with hemiplegia.[37,38,41,55]

It is critical to reduce the abnormal hypertonicity in the upper extremity. Techniques to facilitate relaxation of spastic wrist and finger musculature followed by gentle, passive ROM may be adequate to prevent the flexion deformity of the hand if done regularly and followed by proper positioning of the hemiplegic upper extremity.[19] A wheelchair lapboard made of clear plastic or an arm trough may be used on the wheelchair to assist with proper UE positioning (Fig. 41-4).

Very early in the treatment program, the patient is taught to reduce the tone in the arm and around the scapula. The hands are clasped or held together and the patient is instructed to reach the clasped hand forward into scapular protraction before lifting the arms.[19] The patient is taught to do this movement many times throughout the day to inhibit abnormal tone and ensure pain-free shoulder ROM.

Proper positioning of the hemiplegic UE while the patient is in bed is important to aid in reducing spasticity. The affected arm should be positioned with the scapula in full protraction, shoulder in flexion up to 90°, elbow in extension, and fingers relaxed. It is preferable that the patient lie on the hemiplegic side because spasticity is reduced by elongation of the weak side.[19]

Attention must be paid to the effect of activity on the tone of the arm and hand, and frequent adjustments and

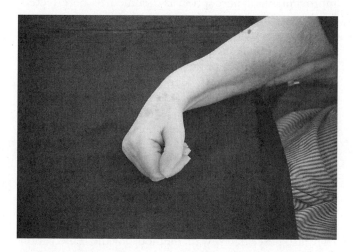

FIG. 41-2   Spastic hemiplegic wrist and hand with typical flexion posture.

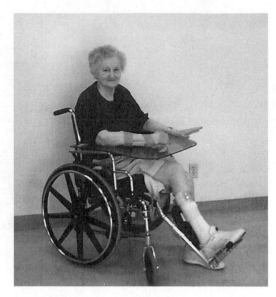

FIG. 41-4 Patient using lapboard to support hemiplegic arm while sitting in wheelchair.

repositioning may be necessary. Excessive effort, which contributes to increased spasticity, must be avoided. Patients can be taught to reduce their own spasticity, and family members can be instructed in how to assist.

Therapeutic activities

Early use of therapeutic activities enhances development of alertness, interest, and motivation and provides opportunities for socialization and communication. The use of therapeutic activities to enhance motor retraining is advocated in the Bobath,[9] Brunnstrom,[14] and PNF[39] approaches to treatment. Bobath advocated the close cooperation of the physical and occupational therapists in coordination of an integrated treatment program.[9] She recommended that occupational therapy could use bilateral activities with hands clasped such as pushing a roll or a ball to inhibit flexor spasticity while using the unaffected extremity in a functional task.

Activities that involve trunk rotation with weight-bearing on the affected arm, such as moving objects from one side of a bench to the other, are also useful to decrease tone and prevent associated reactions. Positioning of the sound arm well forward and in the field of vision is recommended during one-handed activities such as eating or sponge bathing at the wash basin.[9]

Eggers[24] described many very creative activities appropriate for the hemiplegic at each stage in the recovery process. Positioning, transfers, bilateral activities, unilateral activities, and activities for hand retraining are included in Eggers' work. All of the activities are directed to the inhibition of abnormal tone and reflexes and the facilitation of normal movement patterns.

Brunnstrom advocated the use of the limb synergies and other available movement patterns in ADL.[13] Activities such as sanding, sawing, using a carpet sweeper, and dusting furniture make use of movement patterns similar to the limb synergies. Symmetric bilateral activities facilitate the hemiplegic upper extremity and can elicit and reinforce extension. For the patient in the earlier stages of recovery, the hand can stabilize or hold objects while the unaffected hand does the skilled work. Activities for patients in more advanced stages of recovery should be designed to include combined movements of increasing complexity.[13]

In the PNF approach, activities are analyzed for the diagonal patterns. Activities of daily living and therapeutic activities that elicit desired diagonal patterns of movement can be used to reinforce motor learning.[39] When planning therapeutic activities, the therapist needs to take into account the patient's motor, sensory, perceptual, and cognitive dysfunctions. It is important for the patient to be successful at accomplishing the tasks. This goal can be achieved if the tasks are within his or her capabilities.

Sensory Reeducation

The occupational therapy program for the hemiplegic patient may include sensory reeducation and compensation techniques to remediate sensory dysfunction. Methods for sensory reeducation and compensation techniques are described in Chapter 13.

Perceptual Retraining

Occupational therapists have used perceptual retraining since the 1950s. They have focused on retraining specific perceptual skills and incorporating perceptual retraining into functional tasks such as ADL skills. Occupational therapists use perceptual training because performance of functional activities is assumed to be dependent upon perceptual skills and, conversely, perceptual deficits affect functional performance. Adaptation is dependent on intact perceptual processing, and a patient who has a perceptual disturbance will have difficulty adapting adequately to daily life.

Remediation of or compensation for perceptual deficits is assumed to improve functional performance, and improvement of perception is assumed to be effected through occupational therapy.[19] The relationship between perceptual deficits and functional performance has been demonstrated in several studies. The effectiveness of the various approaches to the remediation of perceptual deficits has not been well documented, however, and requires scientific investigation.[40]

Treatment of perceptual problems can be difficult and complex. The best results are obtained when the treatment is done on a daily basis. Zoltan, Siev, and Freishtat described four approaches that are used for perceptual training of the patient with hemiplegia.[64] These are the sensory integrative approach, the neurodevelopmental (Bobath) approach, the transfer of training approach, and the functional approach, described in Chapter 14. They also described several methods for the remediation of perceptual deficits.[64]

Cognitive Rehabilitation

Cognitive rehabilitation is an emerging field in which the neuropsychologist, speech pathologist, and occupational therapist have parts to play. Much of the effort in cognitive rehabilitation has been concerned with head injury patients. Cognitive rehabilitation is a complex, multidimensional process, which involves the patient and his or her human and nonhuman environment.[42,51] Methods of evaluation and treatment of selected cognitive dysfunctions are described in Chapter 15. For a detailed discussion of cognitive rehabilitation, see the references.[8,63,64]

Performance Areas

Training in ADL is a primary function of the occupational therapy service. Specific procedures are described in Chapters 24 and 26. Early in the rehabilitation process this training may include wheelchair mobility and transfer skills (Chapter 27) and simple self-care activities such as feeding, grooming, and oral hygiene. Training in more complex bathing and dressing skills might be added later.

As the patient progresses in independent performance in the area of self-maintenance, evaluation and training in appropriate home management activities, high level independent living skills, community reintegration skills, and vocational and leisure skills should be included in the ADL program. Driving and transportation are also addressed in a comprehensive occupational therapy program.

Affected limbs and the affected side of the body should be employed in ADL training as much as possible. Motor, sensory, perceptual, and cognitive deficits may influence the success of use of the affected limbs, however. The therapist should guide the affected limb through the motion of the task whenever possible to provide accurate sensorimotor information. The effect of the activity on frustration and muscle tone should be assessed.

Coordination and skill training in one-handed performance may be necessary when the dominant upper extremity is affected and a change of dominance is necessary or when motor recovery is so limited as to preclude any functional use of the affected arm. Such patients may have to rely on one-handed performance indefinitely.[9]

The patient must learn methods of stabilizing objects and equipment for one-handed performance. He or she must learn to use assistive devices and equipment adapted to ease functioning with one hand and improve safety. It is the role of the occupational therapist to acquire the necessary assistive devices and train the patient and the family or care giver in their use.

Home evaluation

As the patient nears discharge to home and community, the occupational therapist should be involved in a home evaluation (Chapter 26), and vocational or leisure skills potential should be explored. A living situation is recommended that accommodates the patient's needs. The occupational therapist, having evaluated self-care and home management skills performance, is the most qualified to estimate the patient's potential for independent living. Patients who have had a CVA range from those who can resume living independently to those who require continuous supervision and assistance. The outcome depends on the severity of the CVA, success in rehabilitation, mental status, and social factors.

Psychosocial Adjustment

An important role of the occupational therapist is to aid in the patient's adjustment to hospitalization and, more important, to disability. A patient and supportive approach by the therapist is essential. The therapist must be empathetic to the fact that the patient has experienced a devastating and life-threatening illness. Sudden and dramatic changes in life roles and performance have resulted. The therapist must be cognizant of the normal adjustment process and gear approach and performance expectations to the patient's level of adjustment. Frequently the patient is not ready to engage in rehabilitation measures with wholehearted effort until several months after onset of the disability.

Family education is extremely important throughout the treatment program. The family can be better equipped to assist their loved one with adjustment to disability if they have knowledge and understanding of the disability and its implications.

Many patients dwell on the possibility of full recovery of function and need to be made aware gradually that some residual dysfunction is very likely. The therapist may approach this probability by discussing what is known about prognosis for functional recovery from CVA in objective terms. This information may have to be reviewed many times with the patient before the patient begins to apply it to his or her own recovery and should be done in a way that is honest, yet does not destroy all hope.

The occupational therapy program should focus on the skills and abilities of the patient. The patient's attention should be focused, through the performance of activity, on his or her remaining and newly learned skills. Therapeutic group activities for socialization and sharing common problems and their solutions can be included.

The discovery that there are residual abilities and perhaps new abilities and success at performing many daily living skills and activities that were initially thought to be impossible can have a beneficial effect on the patient's mental health and outlook.

Treatment Gradation

Treatment of the motor dysfunction is directed toward the reintegration of the postural mechanism and the recovery of controlled, coordinated movement. The manner and speed with which treatment is graded depends on the patient, the rate of recovery, and the treatment approach. In general, inhibition and facilitation techniques should be decreased as voluntary control of motion is improved. The amount of assistance in exercise and activity should be decreased as control and coordination are gained. The difficulty of performance skills demanded can be increased as synergistic movement subsides, and isolated voluntary motion is possible.[47]

Treatment time and time spent in standing and ambulation activities can be gradually increased to improve endurance. The complexity and number of ADL can be increased as physical, perceptual, and cognitive functioning improves. The amount of assistance given during transfers and for all activities should be decreased as independence is increased.

SUMMARY

CVA is a complex disability that challenges the skills of professional health care workers. Although the number and effectiveness of approaches for the remediation of affected motor, sensory, perceptual, cognitive, and performance dysfunctions has increased considerably, many limitations in treatment remain. The occupational therapist must bear in mind that the degree to which the patient achieves treatment goals depends on the CNS damage and recovery, psychoneurologic residuals, psychosocial adjustment, and the skilled application of appropriate treatment by all concerned health professionals.

Some patients remain severely disabled in spite of the noblest efforts of rehabilitation workers, and others recover quite spontaneously with minimal help in a short period of time. Most benefit from the professional skills of occupational therapists and other rehabilitation specialists to achieve improvement of performance skills and resumption of meaningful occupational roles.

SAMPLE TREATMENT PLAN

This treatment plan is not a comprehensive one for the hypothetical patient. It deals with six of the identified problems. The reader is encouraged to add objectives and methods to make a more comprehensive plan.

CASE STUDY

Mr. S is a 59-year-old man who worked as a trucker until he suffered a CVA 6 weeks ago. He lives with his wife and teenage daughter in a modest, three-bedroom suburban home. He is their sole support.

Before the onset of CVA, Mr. S was a very hard worker and enjoyed working around the house doing repairs and gardening. Cooking and furniture refinishing were his hobbies.

His wife and teenage daughter are very loving but are exhibiting signs of oversolicitousness and denial of Mr. S's limitations and the potential residual disability. Mr. S is depressed and is expressing feelings of worthlessness because of the loss of his role as worker and breadwinner. He is beginning to sense his family's unrealistic attitude and feels he has to "play along" with them, which he resents; he would prefer to be open and get on with the business of dealing with life adjustments.

The CVA resulted in right hemiplegia and mild expressive aphasia. Mr. S is now able to ambulate with a quadruped cane under supervision. He walks slowly and occasionally loses his balance. He tolerates standing and walking activities up to 10 minutes. His right upper extremity exhibits beginning spasticity and some evidence of the flexor and extensor synergies, which can be elicited reflexly.

Mr. S has been in the occupational therapy program since the first week of hospitalization for maintenance of ROM, development of sitting balance, and training in simple self-care skills. He is now referred for improvement of the function of the right upper extremity, improvement of standing balance and tolerance, increased performance of self-care skills, and aid with adjustment to the disability.

TREATMENT PLAN

Personal data
Name: Mr. S
Age: 59
Diagnosis: CVA, 6 weeks after onset
Disability: Right hemiplegia, expressive aphasia

Treatment aims as stated in referral:
  Improve function of right limbs and body
  Improve standing balance and tolerance
  Improve performance of ADL

SAMPLE TREATMENT PLAN – cont'd

Other services

Physician: Supervision of rehabilitation team and provision of care

Nursing: Provision of nursing and supportive care; follow-through in self-care skills

Social service: Assistance in family and social adjustment

Speech therapy: Treatment of expressive aphasia

Physical therapy: Gait training and improvement in LE function

Frame of reference

Occupational performance

Treatment approaches

Bobath neurodevelopmental and rehabilitative

OT EVALUATION

Performance components

Sensorimotor
  Stage of motor recovery: Test
  Muscle tone: Test and observe
  Attempts at spontaneous use of involved upper extremity: Observe
  Reflexes/reactions: Test
  Standing tolerance: Observe
  Standing balance: Observe
  Walking tolerance: Observe
  Touch: Test
  Pain: Test
  Temperature: Test
  Stereognosis: Test
  Proprioception: Test

  Body scheme: Test
  Visual fields: Test
  Visual-spatial relationships: Test
Cognitive/Cognitive Integrative
  Judgment and reasoning: Observe
  Memory: Test and observe
  Motivation: Observe
  Problem solving: Test and observe
  Expression: Observe
Psychosocial/Psychological
  Adjustment to disability: Observe

Performance areas

Self-care: Test
Homemaking: Test

EVALUATION SUMMARY

Physical evaluation revealed ROM of upper extremity within normal limits except for shoulder flexion and abduction, which are limited by spasticity to 90°. Mr. S is unable to stand or walk without his cane and fatigues after 10 minutes of walking. He can sit in an armless chair without losing his balance. The right upper extremity shows beginning spasticity in flexor and extensor synergy patterns with greater tone in the flexor synergy. In the lower extremity, moderate spasticity in the extensor synergy pattern is present. Muscle tone is influenced by the asymmetric tonic neck and tonic labyrinthine reflexes.

Primary sensory modalities are intact but mild impairment of stereognosis and proprioception is present. Body scheme and motor planning are intact. All visual perceptual skills are within functional limits except that there is a right homonymous hemianopsia at 60°, which Mr. S compensates for without cuing.

Visual memory for demonstrated instructions is intact. There is some difficulty with memory for auditory instructions. Mr. S needs to have these instructions repeated and accompanied by demonstrated instructions. Judgment, reasoning, and problem-solving skills are adequate for daily living skills. Reading skills for everyday needs are accurate but slow. Mr. S has difficulty writing because he cannot use

the right dominant upper extremity. Mr. S's speech is limited but comprehensible for communication of basic needs. He has difficulty with word finding. With cues, questioning, and some use of pictures, it is possible to elicit Mr. S's ideas.

Mr. S is discouraged and shows some lack of motivation. He responds well to praise and encouragement. He has expressed feelings of worthlessness related to the loss of his role as worker. His family denies the extent of his limitations and is overanxious to help. Before his stroke, Mr. S was a kindly man who enjoyed working around the house, cooking, and refinishing antique furniture. Because of his age and disability, Mr. S has realized that he probably will not return to work and is considering retirement. He has expressed some interest in expanding his home and leisure activities to use his retirement purposefully.

In self-care, Mr. S is partially independent. He needs help with some dressing activities and transfers. In the OT clinic, Mr. S demonstrated ability to prepare a sandwich and pour juice while sitting, if all of the materials were brought to the table for him. Use of the stove has not been evaluated because of limited standing and walking tolerance. He shows ability to use assistive devices to enhance one-handed performance.

Mr. S attempts to use the right upper extremity when

confronted with bilateral tasks about 50% of the time. Limited voluntary movement makes success impossible at this time, however.

Assets

Intact sensation
Intact perception
Good cognitive functions
Positive attitude
Supportive family
Ability to learn new methods
Realistic outlook about limitations
Leisure interests

Problem list

1. Limited standing and walking tolerance
2. ADL dependence
3. Lack of selective movement in the right upper extremity
4. Limited scapula mobility and shoulder ROM
5. Right-sided spasticity and decreased postural reflex mechanism
6. Right visual field defect
7. Lack of coordination in nondominant (unaffected) upper extremity
8. Loss of worker role
9. Low sense of self-worth

PROBLEM 4: LIMITED SCAPULA MOBILITY AND SHOULDER ROM

Objective

Decrease spasticity and increase scapula mobility so that 120° shoulder flexion and abduction is possible

Methods

Bobath positioning techniques during sitting; clasps hands together with affected thumb on top and unaffected arm guides affected right arm into a position of full elbow extension with shoulder flexion and scapula protraction, arms on wheelchair lapboard or on table in this position when patient not engaged in activity

Following scapula mobilization by the therapist, patient's arm gradually brought into the reflex inhibiting pattern of scapula protraction, shoulder abduction, flexion, and external rotation, elbow extension, forearm supination, wrist and finger extension, and thumb abduction

Self-administered ROM; with hands positioned as described previously, patient to bring both arms down between knees; then move arms from side to side, rotating trunk, and gradually elevating arms to 90° shoulder flexion with elbows extended

Participation in activity group; using pegboard checkers and oversized checkerboard, play with another patient using the bilateral arm positioning pattern described previously; move the checkers by grasping them between the palms of his hands; also facilitates trunk rotation and looking over the entire visual field

Gradation

Decrease facilitation and assistance as spasticity declines and active motion improves

---

PROBLEM 7: LACK OF LEFT-HANDED COORDINATION

Objective

Improve left hand coordination so that Mr. S can write his name and address legibly and with ease

Method

Left-hand writing practice beginning with large round forms such as circles, ovals, and figure 8s performed in horizontal, vertical, and diagonal directions; may begin on chalkboard or large paper on table top

Gradation

Introduce straight lines and rectangular shapes. Progress to smaller paper with lines and to letters and then words; begin writing practice with right hand if recovery of function permits

---

PROBLEM 6: RIGHT VISUAL FIELD DEFECT

Objective

Patient to compensate spontaneously for visual field defect 80% of the treatment time

Methods

Patient to cover small (2 ft × 2 ft, or about 6 mm × 6 mm) table top with mosaic tiles (1 inch, or 2.5 cm); tiles placed

SAMPLE TREATMENT PLAN – cont'd

directly to right side of the body; table placed in front and slightly to left of the body; glue placed on left side of body; patient to reach across body to obtain tiles for placement on tabletop; affected arm positioned forward, used for weight-bearing on edge of wide chair; as right arm function improves, patient to reach for tiles with right hand; facilitates trunk rotation and visual attention to affected side

Room arranged so patient must look to affected side to get belongings, look to doorway for staff and visitors

Therapist to stand on affected side when talking to patient or giving instructions

PROBLEM 2: ADL DEPENDENCE

Objective
The patient to dress himself independently within 30 minutes

Method
Teach dressing techniques for pants, T-shirt, shirt, shoes, socks, and shorts, using Bobath methods for dressing.

Gradation
Begin with one garment, T-shirt; progress to shirt, then shorts, socks, pants, and shoes; progress to normal bilateral techniques as function improves

PROBLEM 1: LIMITED STANDING AND WALKING TOLERANCE

Objective
With a quadruped cane for support, the patient's balance to improve and standing tolerance to increase to 30 minutes

Methods
Light homemaking activities that require walking for short distances: meal preparation, table setting, and dusting, with supervision; grooming activities in a standing position under supervision

Gradation
Decrease supervision as balance and stability are gained

PROBLEM 9: LOW SENSE OF SELF-WORTH

Objective
The patient to achieve an increased sense of self-worth, expressing two positive things about self during group activities

Method
A group of 5 to 8 patients to meet biweekly for 1½ hours; the therapist to act as group facilitator; the group initially to be task-oriented; activities such as exercises to music, simple crafts, and cooperative meal preparation to be used

Gradation
Increase responsibility for planning the activities

Method
The group to move from the activity into discussion of the problems encountered during the activity, feelings about these, and solutions; the therapist to facilitate expansion of the discussion to include problems encountered beyond the activity and the treatment facility

Gradation
As group support and cohesiveness grow, discussion can include deeper feelings, and group members can act as facilitators

REVIEW QUESTIONS

1. Define CVA.
2. List three other dysfunctions that could accompany the motor dysfunction in hemiplegia.
3. List the disturbances that are likely to result from occlusion to the anterior cerebral artery, middle cerebral artery, posterior cerebral artery, and cerebellar arteries.
4. Which artery is most frequently affected in CVA?
5. Define *transient ischemic attack*.
6. Describe the dependence of motion on sensation in the normal sensorimotor process.

7. Besides the upper motor neuron paralysis of limbs and trunk after CVA, what other important motor disturbances can result?
8. List three poor prognostic signs for functional recovery.
9. List three good prognostic signs for functional recovery.
10. What differences in performance can be expected between persons with right and left hemiplegia? What accounts for these differences?
11. How does body scheme disorder interfere with rehabilitation?
12. How is training approached if there is a memory loss?
13. Describe apraxia. Give examples of apraxic behavior. How does it interfere with rehabilitation.
14. What is the difference between unilateral neglect and visual inattention?
15. Describe what is meant by lability. How can it be dealt with during a treatment session?
16. How does aphasia differ from dysarthria?
17. Describe four ways to aid effective communication with an aphasic patient.
18. What is the importance of comprehensive occupational therapy evaluation of patients with hemiplegia?
19. Describe two methods that are used to maintain ROM.
20. List four major elements of the occupational therapy program for hemiplegia. Describe the purposes of each.
21. How can occupational therapy assist with the psychosocial adjustment of the hemiplegic patient?

REFERENCES

1. Almli CR: Normal sequential behavioral and physiological changes throughout the developmental arc. In Umphred DA, editor: *Neurological rehabilitation,* St Louis, 1985, CV Mosby.
2. Andersen LT: Shoulder pain in hemiplegia, *Am J Occup Ther* 39:11, 1985.
3. Ayres AJ: Perceptual motor training for children. In *Approaches to the treatment of patients with neuromuscular dysfunction,* Proceedings of study course IV, Third International Congress, World Federation of Occupational Therapists, Dubuque, Iowa, 1962, Wm C Brown.
4. Banus BS, editor: *The developmental therapist,* Thorofare, NJ, 1971, Charles B Slack.
5. Bardach JL: Psychological factors in hemiplegia, *J Am Phys Ther Assoc* 43:792, 1963.
6. Baum B and associates: *Perceptual motor evaluation for head injured and neurologically impaired adults,* San José, 1983, Santa Clara County, Santa Clara Valley Medical Center.
7. Birch HG and associates: Perception in hemiplegia. I. Judgment of the vertical and horizontal by hemiplegic patients, *Arch Phys Med Rehabil* 41:19, 1960.
8. Bleiberg J: Psychological and neuropsychological factors in stroke management. In Kaplan PE, Cerullo LJ: *Stroke rehabilitation,* Boston, 1986, Butterworth.
9. Bobath B: *Adult hemiplegia: evaluation and treatment,* ed 2, London, 1978, William Heinemann Medical Books.
10. Bonner C: *The team approach to hemiplegia,* Springfield, Ill, 1969, Charles C Thomas.
11. Bounds JV, Wiebers DO, Whisnant JP: Mechanisms and timing of deaths from cerebral infarction, *Stroke,* 12:414-477, 1981.
12. Branch EF: The neuropathology of stroke. In Duncan PW, Badke MB: *Stroke rehabilitation: the recovery of motor control,* Chicago, 1987, Year Book Medical.
13. Brunnstrom S: Motor behavior in adult hemiplegic patients, *Am J Occup Ther* 15:6, 1961.
14. Brunnstrom S: *Movement therapy in hemiplegia,* New York, 1970, Harper & Row.
15. Buchwald J: General features of nervous system organization, *Am J Phys Med* 46:89, 1967.
16. Cailliet R: *The shoulder in hemiplegia,* Philadelphia, 1982, FA Davis.
17. Charness A: *Stroke/head injury: Rehabilitation Institute of Chicago procedure manual,* Rockville, Md, 1986, Aspen.
18. Chusid J: *Correlative neuroanatomy and functional neurology,* ed 19, Los Altos, Calif, 1985, Lange Medical Publications.
19. Davies PM: *Steps to follow: a guide to the treatment of adult hemiplegia,* New York, 1985, Springer-Verlag.
20. Davis J: Neurodevelopmental treatment. In Pedretti LW, Zoltan B, editors: *Occupational therapy practice skills for physical dysfunction,* ed 3, St. Louis, 1990, CV Mosby.
21. Delacato CH: Hemiplegia and concomitant psychological phenomena. I. *Am J Occup Ther* 10:157, 1956.
22. Delacato C, Doman G: Hemiplegia and concomitant psychological phenomena, *Am J Occup Ther* 11:186, 1957.
23. Duncan PW, Badke MB: Therapeutic strategies for rehabilitation of motor deficits. In Duncan PW, Badke MB: *Stroke rehabilitation: the recovery of motor control,* Chicago, 1987, Year Book Medical.
24. Eggers O: *Occupational therapy in the treatment of adult hemiplegia,* Rockville, Md, 1984, Aspen Systems.
25. Gilfoyle E, Grady A: Cognitive-perceptual-motor behavior. In Willard H, Spackman C, editors: *Occupational therapy,* ed 4, Philadelphia, 1971, JB Lippincott.
26. Granger C, Clark GS: Functional status outcomes of stoke rehabilitation, *Topics in Geriatric rehabilitation,* 9(3):72-80, Fort Lauderdale, Fl, 1994, Aspen.
27. Haberman S, Capildeo R, Rose FC: Risk factors for cerebrovascular disease. In Rose FC, editor: *Advances in stroke therapy,* New York, 1982, Raven Press.
28. Hague HR: An investigation of abstract behavior in patients with cerebral vascular accident. II. *Am J Occup Ther* 13:83, 1959.
29. Halper AS, Mogil SI: Communication disorders: diagnosis and treatment. In Kaplan PE, Cerullo LJ, editors: *Stroke rehabilitation,* Boston, 1986, Butterworth.

30. Hopkins HL: Occupational therapy management of cerebral vascular accident and hemiplegia. In Willard HS, Spackman CS, editors: *Occupational therapy,* ed 4, Philadelphia, 1971, JB Lippincott.

31. Horwitz B: An open letter to the family of an adult patient with aphasia, *Rehabil Lit,* 23:141, 1962.

32. Larson CB, Gould M: *Orthopedic nursing,* ed 9, St Louis, 1978, CV Mosby.

33. Levine RL: Diagnostic, medical and surgical aspects of stroke management. In Duncan PW, Badke MB, editors: *Stroke rehabilitation: the recovery of motor control,* Chicago, 1987, Year Book Medical.

34. Lieberman JS: Hemiplegia: rehabilitation of the upper extremity. In Kaplan PE, Cerullo LG, editors: *Stroke rehabilitation,* Boston, 1986, Butterworth.

35. Lorenze E, Cancro R: Dysfunction in visual perception with hemiplegia: relation to activities of daily living, *Arch Phys Med Rehab* 43:514, 1962.

36. MacDonald JC: An investigation of body scheme in adults with cerebral vascular accidents, *Am J Occup Ther* 15:75, 1960.

37. Mathiowetz V, Bolding DJ, Trombly C: Immediate effects of positioning devices on the normal and spastic hand measured by elecromyography, *Am J Occup Ther* 37:247, 1983.

38. McPherson JJ: Objective evaluation of a splint designed to reduce hypertonicity, *Am J Occup Ther* 35:189, 1981.

39. Myers B: *Proprioceptive neuromuscular facilitation, Unit III: Patterns and their application to occupational therapy,* Chicago, 1982, Rehabilitation Institute of Chicago (videotape).

40. Neistadt ME: Occupational therapy for adults with perceptual deficits, *Am J Occup Ther* 42:434, 1988.

41. Neuhaus BE and associates: A survey of rationales for and against hand splinting in hemiplegia, *Am J Occup Ther* 35:83, 1981.

42. Novack TA and associates: Cognitive stimulation in the home environment. In Williams JM, Long CJ, editors: *The rehabilitation of cognitive disabilities,* New York, 1987, Plenum Press.

43. Ogden LD: *Procedure guidelines for monitored self-care evaluation and monitored task evaluation,* Downey, Calif, 1981, Cardiac Rehabilitation Resources.

44. O'Leary SS: *Monitored showers during inpatient rehabilitation following cardiac events,* master's thesis, San José, Calif, 1986, San José State University.

45. Olson DA: Management of non-language behavior in the stroke patient. In Kaplan PE, Cerullo LJ, editors: *Stroke rehabilitation,* Boston, 1986, Butterworth.

46. Pelland MJ: Occupational therapy and stroke rehabilitation. In Kaplan PE, Cerullo LJ, editors: *Stroke rehabilitation,* Boston, 1986, Butterworth.

47. Perry C: Principles and techniques of the Brunnstrom approach to the treatment of hemiplegia, *Am J Phys Med* 46:789, 1967.

48. Rancho Los Amigos Hospital, Occupational Therapy Department: *OT evaluation guide for adult hemiplegia,* Downey, Calif, 1991, Los Amigos Research and Education, Inc. (LAREI).

49. Roth EJ: Medical complications encountered in stroke rehabilitation, *Physical Medicine and Rehabilitation Clinics of North America,* 2(3): 563-577, August, 1991.

50. Rubenstein E, Federman D, editors: Neurocerebrovascular diseases, New York, 1994, Scientific American, Inc.

51. Sbordone RJ: A conceptual model of neuropsychologically-based cognitive rehabilitation. In Williams JM, Long CJ, editors: *The rehabilitation of cognitive disabilities,* New York, 1987, Plenum Press.

52. Schlesinger B: *Higher cerebral functions and their clinical disorders,* New York, 1962, Grune & Stratton.

53. Sharpless JW: *Mossman's problem-oriented approach to stroke rehabilitation,* ed 2, Springfield, Ill, 1982, Charles C Thomas.

54. Smith RO, Okamoto GA: Checklist for the prescription of slings for the hemiplegic patient, *Am J Occup Ther* 35:91, 1981.

55. Snook JH: Spasticity reduction splint, *Am J Occup Ther* 33:648, 1979.

56. Spencer EA: Functional restoration. In Hopkins HL, Smith HD, editors: *Willard and Spackman's occupational therapy,* ed 8, Philadelphia, 1993, JB Lippincott.

57. Sutin JA: Clinical presentation of stroke syndromes. In Kaplan PE, Cerullo LJ, editors: *Stroke rehabilitation,* Boston, 1986, Butterworth.

58. Todd JM, Davies PM: Hemiplegia: assessment and approach. In Downie PA, editor: *Cash's textbook of neurology for physiotherapists,* Philadelphia, 1986, JB Lippincott.

59. Turner A: *The practice of occupational therapy,* ed 2, New York, 1987, Churchill Livingstone.

60. Van Deusen J: Unilateral neglect: suggestions for research by occupational therapists, *Am J Occup Ther* 42:441, 1988.

61. Wade JPH: Clinical aspects of stroke. In Downie PA, editor: *Cash's textbook of neurology for physiotherapists,* ed 4, Philadelphia, 1986, JB Lippincott.

62. Warren M: Relationship of constructional apraxia and body scheme disorders to dressing performance in adult CVA, *Am J Occup Ther* 35:431, 671, 1981.

63. Williams JM, Long CJ, editors: *The rehabilitation of cognitive disabilities,* New York, 1987, Plenum Press.

64. Zoltan B, Siev E, Freishtat B: Perceptual and cognitive dysfunction in the adult stroke patient, rev ed, Thorofare, NJ, 1986, Charles B Slack.

Traumatic Brain Injury

Katie Schlageter, Barbara Zoltan

Traumatic brain injury (TBI), sometimes referred to as the silent epidemic, has been little recognized by the general public despite ever-growing numbers of people suffering from this problem. There is less morbidity and mortality, and the number of those surviving severe brain injuries has increased because of continued improvement in the acute care of patients with traumatic brain injury. Therefore the management of patients with TBI has become an important issue not only to medical clinicians but also to society as a whole. TBI is estimated to cost billions of dollars per year for medical care and loss of productivity in the United States. Brain injury rehabilitation has been developed to meet the growing needs of this patient population.

The term traumatic brain injury refers to closed or open brain injuries. Other types of brain injuries include vascular damage such as aneurysms, metabolic disturbances such as anoxia or ischemia, and infections such as herpes simplex encephalitis.[19] The focus of this chapter is on traumatic brain injury in adults; however, the management of patients with other types of brain injuries is very similar.

The traumatic brain injured adult generally shows symptoms of highly diffuse damage resulting in a variety of clinical manifestations. No two patients have exactly the same symptoms. The traumatic brain injured patient may be emerging from coma and respond inconsistently and nonpurposefully to stimuli such as pain or a parent's voice. Another traumatic brain injured patient may be in a very agitated state. This type of patient may hit, grab, or strike out when overstimulated. This patient may be confused and have difficulty attending and following simple directions. On the other hand, a traumatic brain injured patient may be fully ambulatory with only minimal coordination deficits. This patient may be socially inappropriate, however, and exhibit higher level cognitive deficits such as impairments in abstract reasoning.

This diversity in clinical presentation differs substantially from other patient populations such as those who suffer a cerebral vascular accident (CVA) or a spinal cord injury (SCI) in which the damage tends to be localized to specific areas of the brain or levels of the spinal cord. In these patient populations the clinical presentations are more consistent and stereotyped from patient to patient. Treatment of the CVA and SCI patient is also usually more defined and predictable.

To give an overview of TBI rehabilitation, this chapter briefly outlines the incidence, pathophysiology, medical/surgical management, and evaluation of the severity of the injury. Additionally, this chapter describes the patient's clinical picture, including the physical, cognitive, behavioral, visual, perceptual, functional, and psychosocial aspects. Patients functioning at a beginning level are differentiated from those functioning at an intermediate or advanced level. Finally, the occupational therapy evaluation is reviewed and treatment ideas are provided. Specific emphasis is placed on describing contracture management related to spasticity, behavioral issues, visual deficits, and the vocational rehabilitation process because these areas are frequent problems in the TBI population and are seen less frequently in other patient populations.

INCIDENCE

The incidence of traumatic brain injury in the United States has continued to increase in the last few decades. More recently, however, there has been a noticeable decline in traumatic brain injuries. The current incidence for TBI in the United States is 130/100,000 per year, or for a populaton of 250 million people in the United States, an incidence of 325,000 cases of TBI per year.[61] The reduction in the number of traumatic brain injuries is attributed to a reduction in drunk driving, increased use of seat belts, airbags, motorcycle helmets, and increased public education on prevention of TBI.[56]

The leading causes of severe TBI are motor vehicle accidents and falls. TBI occurs more frequently in men

The editorial assistance of Carol McGough is greatly appreciated and the contributions of J. Dougal MacKinnon, Michelle Tipton-Burton, Jeff Englander, and Laurie Anderson are gratefully acknowledged.

than in women by a ratio of 3 to 1. The risk is greater among children 4 to 5 years old, males 15 to 24 years old, the elderly, and people who have had previous brain injuries. The mortality is higher in adults than in children. Most individuals who experience a TBI are from a lower socioeconomic status and are single. A high percentage of persons with TBI have a history of drug and alcohol abuse and/or a psychiatric history.[33]

PATHOPHYSIOLOGY

Traumatic brain injury can be caused by a penetrating injury (open) or a nonpenetrating injury (closed). Open brain injury typically is caused by a gunshot wound or fragments from exploding objects. Focal neurological symptoms and posttraumatic seizures are more common in penetrating injuries. Closed brain injury occurs when there are rotational acceleration and deceleration forces applied to the head. The momentum to the head causes diffuse shearing of white matter fiber. Closed brain injuries are often seen in patients who are involved in motor vehicle accidents. Both primary and secondary damage may result from a closed brain injury.

PRIMARY DAMAGE

During a closed brain injury, primary damage occurs at the time of injury. The damage is caused by localized contusions and diffuse axonal injury (DAI). Contusions, or bruises, are usually bilateral but asymmetric in their severity. Contusions occur in the frontal and temporal regions when the brain slides and strikes the rough skull. Localized contusions may also be found under areas of depressed skill fracture.[10] The closed brain injury may be associated with depressed skull fracture, intracerebral, subdural, or epidural hemorrhage or tentorial herniation.

DAI results from shearing forces that occur between the different components of the brain as a result of the rotational acceleration. This problem is seen most frequently in motor vehicle accidents (MVAs) when the vehicle stops. The corpus callosum and the brain stem are the most commonly affected areas.[1,3,10] DAI causes the widespread brain damage seen with these patients. When axonal damage is severe, coma is induced. On the other end of the spectrum, when the axonal fibers are stretched but not torn and most fibers escape permanent structural damage, a concussion, or brief loss of consciousness, can occur.[7]

SECONDARY DAMAGE

In addition to the primary damage sustained during a traumatic brain injury, secondary damage may evolve over time. Secondary effects include intracranial hematomas, cerebral edema, raised intracerebral pressure, hydrocephalus, intracranial infection, and posttraumatic epilepsy. Widespread hypoxic or ischemic brain damage can result from the secondary damage.[29] Diagnosis and treatment of these secondary changes during the acute phase of the injury are essential to minimize neurologic dysfunction and prevent further brain damage.

Refer to the references for a more detailed analysis and description of the mechanism and pathology of traumatic brain injury.

MEDICAL AND SURGICAL MANAGEMENT

Most important in the management of the TBI adult is to minimize the primary impact damage and prevent or treat secondary insults to provide the best possible recovery.[42] The medical and surgical management of a person who sustains a traumatic brain injury begins when the victim is rescued and brought into the emergency room. The patient with a severe brain injury may experience many complications. Major complications may include increased intracranial pressure, wound infection or osteomyelitis, pulmonary infections, hyperthermia, shock, and associated injuries or fractures.[12] Other potential medical complications include posttraumatic seizures, hydrocephalus, diabetes insipidus, inappropriate antidiuretic hormone secretion, heterotopic bone formation, and thrombophlebitis.[39]

On admission to the emergency room, the first concern is to establish an unobstructed airway, which may require suctioning, intubation, or tracheostomy. The patient may be in shock and may require intravenous fluids, plasma, blood transfusions, or vasopressor agents. The patient is evaluated for spinal and soft tissue injuries. Neuroradiological evaluation with magnetic resonance imaging (MRI) or computerized axial tomography (CT or CAT) scan is performed to help evaluate the extent of the damage and detect focal abnormalities. It may be difficult to evaluate the extent of the damage early after a brain injury, however. CT scans may not identify a diffuse type of injury to the brain. The neurosurgeon may have to perform an emergency craniotomy to reduce increased intracranial pressure or excise any demonstrated hematoma.[42]

Nutritional needs are usually initially treated with intravenous maintenance, which is adequate for the first few days after the injury. Parenteral nutrition (nasogastric tube, total parenteral nutrition) or enteral nutrition (gastrostomy tube) may be required to ensure that the patient receives adequate nutrition because of the patient's decreased level of awareness and impaired oral-bulbar status. If this approach is necessary, a nasogastric tube is inserted through the nose or a gastrostomy tube is surgically placed in the stomach.

Bowel and bladder function may be a management problem depending on the severity of the brain injury. The patient often is incontinent and may require catheterization. Later in the rehabilitation phase, as these functions start to return, a bowel and bladder program is initiated.

Posttraumatic epilepsy is also a common complication

of traumatic brain injury. Seizures may occur immediately at the time of injury to several years later. Prophylactic treatment with anticonvulsants in comatose patients should be started in the emergency room because data suggests that the risk of early epilepsy may be reduced by the administration of these medications.[6,29]

About 5% of all hospitalized brain injured patients develop late-onset seizures, which occur within the first year of injury in over 50% of the cases. The risk of late seizures (7 or more days after injury) is increased when the coma or posttraumatic amnesia lasts greater than 24 hours, the dura is penetrated, focal neurological signs are present, or seizures occur within the first week of injury. It is not clear, however, as to the extent that prophylactic anticonvulsants prevent late epilepsy. Additionally, there is no definite data that suggests how soon, if ever, the medication should be tapered and discontinued.[6] Side effects from the medications include cognitive impairments, which can further affect improvement in the patient's function.

After the initial evaluation and treatment (management in the emergency room and/or operating room), the patient is usually transferred to the intensive care unit (ICU). In the ICU, the patient is monitored for secondary complications such as those mentioned earlier. The clinical neurological status continues to be reassessed closely via the Glasgow Coma Scale, blood pressure, heart rate, body temperature, and intracranial pressure (ICP).[50] The patient is transferred to the acute care service or to a rehabilitation unit when the cardiovascular status, respiratory status, and neurological status have stabilized and there are no acute signs and symptoms of serious infection. The initial rehabilitation problem areas include nutrition, bowel and bladder dysfunction, joint range of motion, skin care, cardiorespiratory status, and cognitive status.

OCCUPATIONAL THERAPY (OT) IN THE ICU

After the patient has been medically stabilized and cleared by the physician, the occupational therapist begins the evaluation and treatment program. Treatment should start while the patient is in the ICU but should be closely coordinated with the physician, nursing staff, and the physical therapist. It is important for the therapist to be aware of the medical and surgical management problems and precautions before beginning the evaluation.

Usually a patient with an open brain injury or craniectomy defect greater than 5 cm by 5 cm requires a helmet before getting up for the first time to protect the open skull from further brain injury.[16] Blood pressure, pulse rate, and oxygen saturation rate should be closely monitored, and treatment should be withheld if they are not within the parameters established by the attending physician. This precaution is especially important when a patient is positioned in a wheelchair for the first time.

Those patients with an increase in ICP must be watched closely. The occupational therapy evaluation or treatment must stop if the ICP rises above the criteria established by the attending physician. Postural precautions for the patient with an increased ICP include slow changes in postural positioning, waiting about 5 minutes between changes to allow for ICP adaptations, and checking orthostatics. It is important to observe the patient after treatment to identify any delayed ICP responses.

The therapist should also be aware of any history of seizures. If seizures occur, the facility protocol is followed. The objective is to protect the patient from self-inflicted harm. The patient should be placed on his or her side if possible, and any objects near the patient removed. The nurse or physician should be contacted immediately, and the patient closely observed. The type of seizure, any associated abnormal head or body movements, the length of time, and what was occurring before the seizure should be reported.

Clinical observations such as changes in neurological status (including pupillary changes), diaphoresis (excessive sweating), vomiting, behavioral changes, changes in posture, and changes in respiratory pattern should continually be made as the occupational therapy evaluation and treatment are progressing. Any important changes warrant contacting the primary nurse and should be documented. Occupational therapy goals in the ICU include increasing functional endurance, establishing a bed and wheelchair positioning program, preventing contractures, and establishing a baseline cognitive status.

SEVERITY OF INJURY

It is essential to understand how severity of injury is assessed because management of TBI varies greatly depending on the degree of severity. There remains no absolute measure of severity of brain injury, but duration and depth of coma and length of posttraumatic amnesia (PTA) are the most accepted criteria.[21,29] The most dramatic recovery usually occurs during the first 6 months, but it is common opinion that neurological recovery can continue for years.

GLASGOW COMA SCALE

The method most used by critical care personnel to categorize the levels of consciousness following a traumatic injury to the brain is the Glasgow Coma Scale developed by Jennett and Teasdale.[29] This test is an attempt to quantify the severity of the brain injury, establish a baseline, and predict the outcome of the patient. The examiner using this scale assesses consciousness by three major areas: (1) motor responses, (2) verbal responses, and (3) eye opening. The patient is then rated and assigned the corresponding number of points for the best response elicited. The sum of these cumulative responses may be as low as 3 and as high as 15 (Table 42-1). A Glasgow Coma Scale rating less than 8 is usually predictive of poorer outcome. The Glasgow Coma Scale is usually performed 2 to 7 days after injury.

TABLE 42-1	Glasgow Coma Scale		ASSIGNED
EXAMINER'S TEST		**PATIENT'S RESPONSE**	**SCORE**
Eye Opening	Spontaneous	Opens eyes on own	4
	Speech	Opens eyes when asked to in a loud voice	3
	Pain	Opens eyes when pinched	2
	Pain	Does not open eyes	1
Best Motor Response	Commands	Follows simple commands	6
	Pain	Pulls examiner's hand away when pinched	5
	Pain	Pulls a part of body away when examiner pinches patient	4
	Pain	Flexes body inappropriately to pain (decorticate posturing)	3
	Pain	Body becomes rigid in an extended position when examiner pinches victim (decerebrate posturing)	2
	Pain	Has no motor response to pinch	1
Verbal Response (Talking)	Speech	Carries on a conversation correctly and tells examiner where he is, who he is, and the month and year	5
	Speech	Seems confused or disoriented	4
	Speech	Talks so examiner can understand victim but makes no sense	3
	Speech	Makes sounds that examiner can't understand	2
	Speech	Makes no noise	1

Reprinted with permission from Rosenthal M and associates: *Rehabilitation of the head-injured adult,* Philadelphia, 1984, FA Davis.

POSTTRAUMATIC AMNESIA

After the patient has emerged from coma, the best guide to the severity of the diffuse damage is the duration of posttraumatic amnesia. PTA is the length of time from the moment of injury until continuous memory returns.[42] There is considerable evidence that the duration of PTA correlates well with outcome. Russell and Smith,[30] who introduced the concept of PTA, demonstrated that longer PTAs were associated with worse cognitive and motor ability.[30] Usually a PTA of greater than 14 days is associated with a greater likelihood of moderate and severe disability (Table 42-2).

The most commonly accepted test to assess PTA is the Galveston Orientation and Amnesia Test (GOAT). The GOAT is a series of 10 questions that are given to a patient, usually on a weekly basis. The patient is then scored on a scale of 0 to 100. The patient is described as being out of PTA after the patient reaches a score of greater than 75.

TABLE 42-2	Duration of Posttraumatic Amnesia (PTA) and Severity of Injury	
	PTA DURATION	**SEVERITY**
	Less than 5 min	Very mild
	5 to 60 min	Mild
	1 to 24 hr	Moderate
	1 to 7 days	Severe
	1 to 4 weeks	Very severe
	More than 4 weeks	Extremely severe

Reprinted with permission from Rosenthal M and associates: *Rehabilitation of the head-injured adult,* Philadelphia, 1984, FA Davis.

FUNCTIONAL ASSESSMENT

Use of an assessment scale produces data used in clinical research, clinical evaluation, program evaluation, and prediction of outcome.[25] The needs of the individual facility or program determine which assessments are used at that particular facility. The following section reviews the most common assessment measures currently used in brain injury rehabilitation.

Glasgow Outcome Scale

The Glasgow Outcome Scale[26] consists of five global categories (death, persistent vegetative state, severe disability, moderate disability, and good recovery). The Glasgow Outcome Scale measures overall outcome but has been shown to have poor sensitivity to functionally significant changes.[26]

Disability Rating Scale

The Disability Rating Scale[25,49] is well established, brief, and easy to complete. This scale is effective in tracking general changes over recovery. The Disability Rating Scale was designed to be used with moderate to severe TBI in a rehabilitation setting.[49]

Functional Independence Measure

The Functional Independence Measure[23] is an 18-item, multidisciplinary assessment that is generally completed on admission and discharge from an inpatient program. The categories include self care, mobility, psychosocial function, and cognitive function. This assessment tool is used in many facilities throughout the United States.

BOX 42-1

LEVELS OF COGNITIVE FUNCTIONING

I **No Response** Patient appears to be in a deep sleep and is completely unresponsive to any stimuli presented to him.

II **Generalized Response** Patient reacts inconsistently and nonpurposefully to stimuli in a nonspecific manner. Responses are limited in nature and are often the same regardless of stimulus presented. Responses may be physiologic changes, gross body movements, and/or vocalization. Often the earliest response is to deep pain. Responses are likely to be delayed.

III **Localized Response** Patient reacts specifically but inconsistently to stimuli. Responses are directly related to the type of stimulus presented as in turning head toward a sound, focusing on an object presented. The patient may withdraw an extremity and/or vocalize when presented with a painful stimulus. He may follow simple commands in an inconsistent, delayed manner, such as closing his eyes, squeezing or extending an extremity. After external stimulus is removed, he may lie quietly. He may also show a vague awareness of self and body by responding to discomfort by pulling at nasogastric tube or catheter or resisting restraints. He may show bias by responding to some persons (especially family, friends) but not to others.

IV **Confused-Agitated** Patient is in a heightened state of activity with severely decreased ability to process information. He is detached from the present and responds primarily to his own internal confusion. Behavior is frequently bizarre and nonpurposeful relative to his immediate environment. He may cry out or scream out of proportion to stimuli even after removal, may show aggressive behavior, attempt to remove restraints or tubes or crawl out of bed in a purposeful manner. He does not, however, discriminate among persons or objects and is unable to cooperate directly with treatment effort. Verbalization is frequently incoherent and/or inappropriate to the environment. Confabulation may be present; he may be euphoric or hostile. Thus gross attention is very short and selective attention is often nonexistent. Being unaware of present events, patient lacks short-term recall and may be reacting to past events. He is unable to perform self-care (feeding, dressing) without maximum assistance. If not disabled physically, he may perform motor activities as in sitting, reaching, and ambulating, but as part of his agitated state and not as a purposeful act or on request necessarily.

V **Confused, Inappropriate, Nonagitated** Patient appears alert and is able to respond to simple commands fairly consistently. However, with increased complexity of commands or lack of any external structure, responses are nonpurposeful, random, or at best fragmented toward any desired goal. He may show agitated behavior, not on an internal basis (as in Level IV), but rather as a result of external stimuli, and usually out of proportion to the stimulus. He has gross attention to the environment, but is highly distractible and lacks ability to focus attention to a specific task without frequent redirection back to it. With structure, he may be able to converse on a social, automatic level for short periods of time. Verbalization is often inappropriate; confabulation may be triggered by present events. His memory is severely impaired, with confusion of past and present in his reaction to ongoing activity. Patient lacks initiation of functional tasks and often shows inappropriate use of objects without external direction. He may be able to perform previously learned tasks when structured for him, but is unable to learn new information. He responds best to self, body, comfort—and often family members. The patient can usually perform self-care activities with assistance and may accomplish feeding with maximum supervision. Management on the ward is often a problem if the patient is physically mobile, as he may wander off either randomly or with vague intention of "going home."

VI **Confused-Appropriate** Patient shows goal-directed behavior, but is dependent on external input for direction. Response to discomfort is appropriate and he is able to tolerate unpleasant stimuli (as NG tube) when need is explained. He follows simple directions consistently and shows carry-over for tasks he has relearned (as self-care). He is at least supervised with old learning; unable to maximally assist for new learning with little or no carry-over. Responses may be incorrect due to memory problems, but they are appropriate to the situation. They may be delayed and patient shows decreased ability to process information with little or no anticipation or prediction of events. Past memories show more depth and detail than recent memory. The patient may show beginning awareness of his situation by realizing he doesn't know an answer. He no longer wanders and is inconsistently oriented to time and place. Selective attention to tasks may be impaired especially with difficult tasks and in unstructured settings, but is now functional for common daily activities (30 min with structure). He shows at least vague recognition of some staff, has increased awareness of self, family, and basic needs (as food), again in an appropriate manner as in contrast to Level V.

VII **Automatic-Appropriate** Patient appears appropriate and oriented within hospital and home settings, goes through daily routine automatically, but frequently robotlike; with minimal to absent confusion, but has shallow recall of what he has been doing. He shows increased awareness of self, body, family, foods, people, and interaction in the environment. He has superficial awareness of, but lacks insight into his condition, demonstrates decreased judgment and problem-solving, and lacks realistic planning for his future. He shows carry-over for new learning, but at a decreased rate. He requires at least minimal supervision for learning and for safety purposes. He is independent in self-care activities

BOX 42-1—cont'd

and supervised in home and community skills for safety. With structure he is able to initiate tasks in social and recreational activities in which he now has interest. His judgment remains impaired, such that he is unable to drive a car. Prevocational or avocational evaluation and counseling may be indicated.

VIII **Purposeful and Appropriate** Patient is alert and oriented, is able to recall and integrate past and recent events and is aware of and responsive to his culture. He shows carry-over for new learning if acceptable to him and his life role and needs no supervision after activities are learned. Within his physical capabilities, he is independent in home and community skills, including driving. Vocational rehabilitation, to determine ability to return as a contributor to society (perhaps in a new capacity), is indicated. He may continue to show a decreased ability, relative to premorbid abilities, reasoning, tolerance for stress, judgment in emergencies, or unusual circumstances. His social, emotional, and intellectual capacities may continue to be at a decreased level for him, but are functional for society.

Original Scale, Levels of Cognitive Functioning, 1980. Acknowledgement of Rancho Los Amigos Medical Center, Downey, California, USA, Adult Brain Injury Service.

Community Integration Questionnaire

The Community Integration Questionnaire[62] has been recently developed for use with TBI individuals. The assessment addresses three areas: home, school/work, and psychosocial adjustment.

Rancho Los Amigos Scale of Cognitive Functioning

The Rancho Los Amigos Scale of Cognitive Functioning[48] is a behavioral rating system that assesses cognitive recovery (Box 42-1). This scale is frequently used by occupational therapists working with the TBI population and can assist therapists in communicating with each other regarding the patients' cognitive status. The scale does not assess physical recovery. Keep in mind that physical recovery does not correlate with the cognitive recovery of the TBI patient.

The Rancho Los Amigos scale uses the following eight levels: (1) no response, (2) generalized response, (3) localized response, (4) confused-agitated, (5) confused, inappropriate, nonagitated, (6) confused-appropriate, (7) automatic-inappropriate, and (8) purposeful-appropriate. This scale can be used at any time postinjury and in any treatment setting.

CLINICAL PICTURE OF PERSONS WITH TRAUMATIC BRAIN INJURY

The patient with a traumatic brain injury may show many different symptoms depending on the type of brain injury, severity, and location of the injury. The patient may have severe limitations in most of the areas listed below or the patient may have very subtle deficits, evident only in high level, complex activities.

PHYSICAL STATUS

The physical deficits encountered in patients with traumatic brain injury can vary from severe motor involvement (in one to four extremities) to full isolated control with minimally impaired coordination and muscle strength. Most patients seen by an occupational therapist exhibit deficits in one or more of the following areas: primitive reflexes, muscle tone, motor control, strength, posture, range of motion, sensation, endurance, and total body function. The occupational therapist must have a good theoretical knowledge of these physical deficits to design an effective treatment program.

Abnormal reflexes

Based on motor learning theory, ideas are changing regarding the evaluation and treatment of abnormal reflexes in the neurologically impaired adult. Typical reflexes seen in the low level TBI adult include the asymmetrical tonic neck reflex and the symmetrical tonic neck reflex. Treatment is focused not only on inhibiting these brain stem reflexes but also on replacing them with new motor programs to facilitate improvement in function.[9]

Abnormal muscle tone

Descriptions and definitions of muscle tone continue to be controversial. In the traumatic brain injured adult, muscle tone varies from hypotonus (flaccidity) to hypertonus (spasticity). When muscles are flaccid the resistance to passive movement is diminished and the stretch reflexes are dampened. When an entire upper extremity is hypotonic, such as in the early days postinjury, the arm appears floppy.

Spasticity

Spasticity is one of the most common and damaging physical problems encountered in the traumatic brain injured population. Spasticity may range from minimal to severe in any particular muscle or muscle group. The patient in coma may develop decorticate posturing (sustained contraction and posturing of both upper extremities (BUE) in flexion and the trunk and both lower extremities (BLE) in extension) or decerebrate posturing (sustained contraction and posturing of the trunk and extremities in extension) in the first days or weeks after injury. These postures generally diminish over time as the patient makes a neurological recovery. The patient emerging from coma usually exhibits severe spasticity throughout the body. Patients who are functioning at a higher cognitive level generally exhibit a combination of both hypotonicity (flaccidity) and hypertonicity (spasticity) throughout their bodies.

Spasticity fluctuates as a result of changes in the patient's position, volitional movement, medication, any infections or illness, an increase in pain or discomfort, or a change in emotions. Long-term consequences of spasticity include compromised function in activities of daily living (ADL), difficulty with transfers, difficulty in positioning the patient in bed or in the wheelchair, gait deviations, poor speech and breath control, painful spasms, and contracture formation.[40] See Chapter 10 for more information on spasticity evaluation.

Muscle weakness

Muscle weakness is a decrease in muscle strength without the presence of spasticity. When a TBI patient exhibits impaired strength in the upper extremities without spasticity, a manual muscle test is indicated. When muscle weakness is present in BUE, impaired coordination (both gross and fine motor control) will be evident and should also be included in the occupational therapy assessment.

Ataxia

Ataxia is an abnormality of movement and disordered muscle tone seen in patients with damage to the cerebellum or the sensory pathways. There is a close correlation between ataxia, hypotonia, and impaired sensation.[14] A patient may have ataxia of the total body, trunk, or upper and/or lower extremities. The normal flow of a smooth voluntary movement is destroyed by errors in the direction and speed of movement. The patient with ataxia has lost the ability to make small, minute adjustments that allow for smooth coordination of movement. Ataxia ranges from mild to severe and can be a substantial impediment to achieving a functional goal.

Clinically, the patient with truncal ataxia has a lack of postural stability in sitting and standing. The patient has difficulty maintaining the trunk in a stable position to free the upper extremities for activities. The patient generally attempts to compensate for this deficit by holding onto a fixed surface such a mat with one or both extremities and/or tensing or fixing the proximal muscles. If ataxia is present in the elbows and/or shoulders, movement impairments occur when the patient attempts to lift the upper extremities away from the body and off a stable surface such as a table. For example, when trying to bring food to the mouth, the upper extremity oscillates back and forth causing the food to spill.

Impaired motor control

Patients with traumatic brain injuries frequently experience impairments in motor control in both upper extremities as well as both lower extremities as a result of an imbalance in muscle tone and muscle weakness described previously. Usually one side of the body is more involved than the other. For instance, the patient may have minimal to moderate spasticity in the right upper extremity and require moderate assistance to incorporate the extremity in functional activities. The left upper extremity may exhibit muscle strength of grades 4 or 5 and minimally impaired gross and fine coordination.

Postural deficits

Postural deficits develop as a result of an imbalance in muscle tone throughout the body, impaired motor control, delayed or absent righting reactions and impaired vision, cognition, and perception. Postural impairments in the TBI population are similar to, but tend to be more complex than, the CVA population. Thorough knowledge of the patient's postural deficits allows the occupational therapist to position the patient in a wheelchair with the appropriate equipment to obtain an upright posture, maintain good postural alignment, and prevent postural deformities. An evaluation of the patient's posture is essential for initiating treatment of the trunk and upper extremities. Abnormal postures frequently exhibited in adults with moderate to severe traumatic brain injuries include the following:

Head/neck. Forward flexion or hyperextension. The head may be laterally flexed to one side. Lateral flexion of the neck often accompanies lateral flexion of the trunk.

Scapula. Scapula depression is common with elements of protraction, retraction, and/or downward rotation. There is frequently an imbalance of the scapular muscles, meaning some muscles are hypertonic and some are hypotonic.

Upper extremities. Bilateral involvement with asymmetry between sides or unilateral involvement may be seen, depending on the areas and severity of brain damage.

Trunk. Kyphosis, scoliosis, and loss of lordosis may all be present secondary to weak or spastic muscles (e.g., abdominals, spinals, paraspinals).

Pelvis. A posterior pelvic tilt usually exists, causing too much sacral sitting and facilitating the kyphosis just mentioned. Other common postural deviations include retraction of one side of the pelvis and a pelvic obliquity, in which one side of the pelvis sits lower than the other side.

Lower extremities. Severe extension patterns may be seen in both lower extremities in many patients who are in a persistent vegetative state. Other common postural deficits are hip adduction, knee flexion, plantar flexion, and inversion of the feet.

Limitations of joint motion

Loss of range of motion (ROM) is a common problem with the traumatic brain injured adult. In a TBI adult it is often difficult to distinguish between several possible causes of decreased range of motion: increased muscle tone, myostatic contracture, heterotopic ossification (HO), an undetected fracture or dislocation, pain, or lack of patient cooperation.[31] Treatment for loss of ROM may vary depending on the cause. Therefore, it is essential that the therapist determine the cause of the loss of ROM before beginning treatment.

Loss of sensation

Traumatic brain injured adults may have loss of light touch, sharp/dull differentiation, proprioception, kinesthesia, and/or stereognosis in the extremities. Additionally, loss of light touch and sharp/dull sensation may be evident in the face, and impaired senses of taste and smell may be observed as a result of cranial nerve involvement.

Decreased functional endurance

Decreased endurance and vital capacity are common sequelae of traumatic brain injury. Medical complications such as pneumonia or infections, as well as prolonged bed rest, also affect the patient's ability to participate in therapy programs. Increasing the patient's functional endurance is frequently a primary goal in the ICU or initial stages of rehabilitation.

Loss of total body function

Total body function skills are head and trunk control, sitting and standing balance, reaching, bending, stooping, and functional ambulation. A patient with severe physical involvement usually has poor sitting and standing balance. This patient may not even retain the ability to maintain the head in the upright position. The patient at a more advanced level exhibits more subtle deficits in areas such as bending to reach an item in a cupboard or stooping to pick up something on the floor. Total body function skills are necessary for performing both basic and advanced level ADL.

DYSPHAGIA

Traumatic brain injured patients may demonstrate dysphagia in any of the four stages of swallowing: oral pre-

paratory, oral, pharyngeal, and esophageal. There is a higher incidence of oral preparatory, oral, and pharyngeal stage dysphagia than esophageal stage dysphagia.[14] Typically, more than one abnormality in swallowing is observed (see Chapter 11).[35]

Additionally, the cognitive, behavioral, and linguistic problems evident in the TBI patient further complicate the ability to manage the intake of food and liquids.[37] The patient may not be able to attend long enough to obtain the required amount of nutrition. If impulsivity is a behavioral manifestation of the TBI, the patient will have difficulty monitoring the amount and rate of bringing the hand to the mouth, resulting in coughing and increasing the risk of aspiration.

COGNITIVE STATUS

Cognitive deficits, to varying degrees, are always evident in the TBI population. Frequently seen cognitive deficits are decreased levels of attention, impaired memory, impaired initiation, safety awareness, decreased ability to process information accurately, and difficulty with executive functions and abstract thinking.

Reduced attention and concentration

Reduced levels of attention and the inability to concentrate may seriously affect functional independence. Attentional deficits in varying degrees of severity are a common sequelae following brain injury. The patient with a brain injury often loses not only the ability to concentrate for any length of time, but also the ability to filter out distraction. Evidence of important deficits in attention and concentration are often noted for months or even years postinjury.

Impaired memory

Impaired memory is probably one of the most devastating problems the patient with a traumatic brain injury must face. There are several types of memory impairments, ranging from the inability to recall a few words just heard (immediate memory) to forgetting what happened in the last treatment session (short-term memory) to remembering events that occurred 24 hours ago or years before the injury (long-term memory). Although the severity differs with each patient, most patients have some level of memory impairment. This deficit is manifested in the inability to learn and carry over new tasks and contributes to confusion and inability to interact effectively with the environment.

Impaired initiation

Many persons who suffer a traumatic brain injury are able to complete a task or at least part of a task but may have difficulty in initiating the activity. This inability or difficulty in beginning the first actions, steps, or stages of a task can substantially affect the patient's ability to live independently. Frequently, the patient who has deficits in initiating does better in an inpatient rehabilitation setting than at home. Once home, in a less structured environment, the patient regresses (i.e., he or she is unable to get up in the morning without the established hospital routine).

Decreased safety awareness

The patient with a brain injury often displays unsafe behavior. This problem may be a result of impulsiveness, decreased insight into the disability, impaired judgment, or a combination of all of these. Decreased insight, disorientation, and impaired memory can contribute to the patient's inability to recognize limitations for specific situations or analyze the consequences of his or her actions. It is therefore imperative that all members of the treatment team assist the patient in structuring the environment and understanding the limitations to maximize relearning of appropriate, safe behavior.

Delayed processing of information

Most patients with a traumatic brain injury have some type of difficulty with processing visual and auditory information within a normal time frame. The delay may be only a few seconds or can persist for a few minutes. This problem needs to be kept in mind during all interactions with the patient. For instance, during a sensory evaluation, the patient may not respond quickly enough. The therapist may interpret that the patient has absent sensation when, in fact, the therapist did not allow the patient sufficient time to respond.

Impaired executive functions and abstract thinking

Executive function skills are composed of the ability to set goals, plan, and complete tasks effectively. This skill requires the patient to perform high level problem solving, reasoning, and judgment. Patients with brain injuries tend to analyze problems in concrete terms, interpreting all information at the most literal level. The ability to think abstractly and generalize knowledge and experience is usually considerably impaired. The patient may be able to recognize errors but unable to resolve the errors without external cuing. Furthermore, the patient may not be able to determine more than one solution to a problem. Functional independence, including appropriate social skills and successful return to work, demands the mastering and manipulation of these executive functions.[36]

BEHAVIORAL STATUS

Behavioral impairments are a natural part of the recovery from a traumatic brain injury although behavioral problems are disturbing both for the treatment team and the families. Behavioral management is an essential program in traumatic brain injury rehabilitation. A comprehensive behavioral management program should be established for any patient exhibiting behaviors that affect the treatment program. The goals of a comprehensive behavioral management program should include the following:

maintaining a safe environment through a multifaceted safety program; development and implementation of behavior management techniques; minimizing the use of all restrictive modalities; and providing an environment that enables patients to participate in a comprehensive treatment program and integrates caregivers into the rehabilitation process.[52]

Procedures that may need to be added to the behavior management program include one-to-one nursing care for the patient, psychotropic medication intervention, a safety policy, and a drug and alcohol abuse policy. One-to-one nursing care is especially important if the patient is at risk for harming self or others. Medications are required for the same reason although they are avoided whenever possible. A safety policy may include the use of a cubicle bed, alarm system, walkie-talkie, helmet, and a safety and positioning checklist for the wheelchair. The drug and alcohol policy is frequently necessary because it is well documented that many patients with traumatic brain injuries have preexisting alcohol/drug problems.[33]

It is a challenge for any professional to learn to work with someone with behavioral problems. It can be frustrating and at times frightening to deal with these deficits. Untrained staff frequently reinforce the patient's behavior through their own behavior. A first step in becoming more comfortable with working with an individual with behavioral problems is to understand why behavioral problems occur and how they manifest themselves.

Common behaviors observed in the traumatic brain injured population include agitation, combativeness, disinhibition, and refusal to cooperate. The patient who is unable to filter distractions becomes agitated in a noisy environment. A patient who is agitated may become combative and kick, bite, grab, or spit if not treated in the correct environment and not approached in an appropriate manner. This type of behavior may occur in isolation; however, some patients go through a period of combativeness in which they act this way for weeks or months during any interactions with staff. In this case, a strict behavior management program must be immediately established and enforced by all team members.

A disinhibited patient may lack awareness of the external environment and remove clothes in the treatment gym or flirt with the doctor. Other examples of socially inappropriate and disinhibited behavior are shouting obscenities or making indiscriminate sexual advances to a stranger in the community. Patients occasionally refuse to cooperate with the treatment team. Generally, the patient's lack of participation in therapy is organically based and is due to cognitive deficits such as lack of initiation and/or lack of insight into the disability. It is also important to differentiate between causes due to a cognitive impairment versus lack of interest in therapy. In the later case, the therapist needs to reanalyze the activities and find activities more appropriate and interesting to the patient.

The cognitive and behavioral aspects of a traumatic brain injury are complex and interrelated. It must be recognized that the behavior exhibited by the patient with a traumatic brain injury correlates significantly with the level of cognitive function. This chapter constitutes an overview of behavioral issues that pertain to the traumatic brain injured adult. Refer to Chapter 15 for more information on cognitive functions.

VISUAL STATUS

A disturbance in visual skills can profoundly affect daily life. Visual skills are closely related to attention, concentration, and judgment. People rely on vision indirectly in social and interpersonal interactions. The sense of sight assists in pragmatic activities such as turn-taking, identifying a speaker, and maintaining eye contact.

Visual deficits often become more obvious when they affect the successful completion of routine functional skills. Limited vision can affect daily activities in the areas of hygiene and grooming, kitchen skills, wheelchair mobility, and community activities. Likewise, the academic skills of reading and writing may be affected by visual problems. Oculomotor disturbances may result in disorders of tracking and scanning. Letters or words may jump around the page and the patient may constantly lose the place in the line of type. Motor skills can also be affected by vision. Both ambulation and eye-hand coordination activities use vision as a monitoring and feedback system. Finally, driving is a high level activity that integrates multiple visual skills. A driver is required simultaneously to process different types of visual information and coordinate the appropriate motor response at high speeds. A slight visual deficit can quickly compromise safety in most of the activities just discussed. Because vision affects function in so many areas, and because the ultimate goal in rehabilitation is to improve a patient's functional status, it is important to consider the role that the remediation of visual problems can play in a rehabilitation setting (see Chapter 12).

A traumatic brain injury may substantially affect a previously intact and functional visual system. Damage to the visual system following a traumatic brain injury is most likely the result of cranial nerve damage or direct trauma to the orbital content.[13,43] Visual problems frequently noted after a traumatic brain injury include the following: strabismus with diplopia, convergence insufficiency, accommodative dysfunction (blur up close), nystagmus, oculomotor dysfunction (poor tracking), field defects, reduced blink rate, and lagopthalmos (incomplete lid closure).[15]

PERCEPTUAL MOTOR SKILLS

The ability accurately to perceive and respond to people and objects within the environment is necessary for successful, independent function.[5] Disruption of various pathways within the central nervous system (CNS) can cause the brain injured patient to have difficulty with a multitude of perceptual-motor skills that previously were taken for granted. Depending on the nature and extent of damage, the impairment may involve visual, perceptual, and/or perceptual-motor skills. TBI patients may experience impairments in the following areas: praxis, body scheme, figure-ground, position in space, size and/or shape discrimination, unilateral spatial inattention, part-whole integration, or visual organization. The therapist usually is presented with a patient who has a constellation of problems. The therapist's job is to observe the patient's behavior carefully and interpret the reasons for impairments underlying abnormal responses.

It is also important to formulate an awareness of the cognitive functions and their relationship to perceptual-motor abilities. It is impossible to separate cognition from language, perception, or behavior, because all these areas are instrumental in the learning process. For example, the therapist who is evaluating praxis with a block design test can at the same time assess the cognitive strategy the patient uses to duplicate the design. Aside from analyzing only the perceptual skills, the cognitive functions of sequencing and problem solving also should be assessed. The person will fail to function optimally in any environment without the integration of visual, perceptual, and cognitive skills (see Chapters 12, 14 and 15).

PSYCHOSOCIAL FACTORS

The psychosocial aspects of brain injury are frequently overlooked but can be key components to the success of the patient's recovery process. It is important to know the family and social histories along with personality characteristics before the brain injury.

Family support is an important factor in dealing with the brain injured patient. It can determine the patient's level of motivation to achieve functional independence. Family and friends are an integral part of the rehabilitation process, especially in the beginning stages, because they may be able to elicit a response from the patient when no one else can.

Family role alterations and the patient's coping mechanisms for dealing with these role changes must be considered. The patient may go from being an extremely independent person to being totally dependent, which is frustrating and degrading. It is often difficult for family members to understand the uncontrolled behavior that they observe in their loved one. It is difficult for the patient and the family members or significant others to cope. No matter how cognizant the family and the patient are of the disability, it disrupts the family structure.

Previous educational status and values play an important part in the patient's progress toward independence. These factors must be incorporated into the long-term treatment plan. Eventual discharge plans must be set up to meet the needs of the patient. For example, a patient who had a learning disability before the brain injury and always had difficulty in school may not benefit from a traditional college program but rather from a disabled

BOX 42-2

POSSIBLE AREAS OF PERFORMANCE DEFICIT IN TBI

Self-care		**Transportation**	
Feeding	Dressing	Public modes	Driving
Hygiene	Grooming	**Community function**	
Bathing	Toileting	Shopping	Street safety
Mobility		Community facilities	
Bed	Wheelchair	**Work skills**	
Transfer skills	Functional ambulation	Prevocational activities	Work activities
Home management		**Leisure activities**	
Kitchen tasks	Housekeeping	Social activities	Sports, games, hobbies
Child care			
Communication			
Speech	Symbolic language		

students' program, directed toward the specific problem areas, at a community college.

FUNCTIONAL STATUS

A patient with a brain injury may have problems in all performance areas. Possible areas of deficit are listed in Box 42-2.

Functional disabilities cannot be separated from visual, cognitive, perceptual, sensory, motor, and behavioral problems. A problem in one of these areas can cause or contribute to the functional deficit. For instance, a kitchen activity requires a combination of skills, such as UE function, wheelchair mobility, figure-ground and form perception, visual scanning, sequencing, direction following, memory, safety awareness, and judgment. The person with a brain injury may struggle to put even the most basic components of the process together in some meaningful and orderly fashion.

It becomes extremely important, then, for the therapist to identify the underlying components that relate to the functional deficit so that the best treatment approach can be established. The therapist must have good observational skills and the ability to administer formal tests to help determine how to grade and structure the functional task to gain optimal results in performance.

OCCUPATIONAL THERAPY EVALUATION

Most of the evaluations used with the traumatic brain injured adult are the same as those used with other neurological diagnoses. Refer to Chapters 8 through 15 for more specific information on assessment of joint range of motion, muscle strength, motor control, dysphagia, sensation, vision, perception, and cognition. All of these assessments are applicable to the patient with a traumatic brain injury.

The therapist's approach to the evaluation is key to obtaining optimum results. For instance, when a patient exhibits severe attentional deficits, the evaluation can be given only in short segments, interspersed with rest periods or diversional activities. The therapist may not want to spend much time attempting to complete a formal evaluation. Instead, the therapist may complete parts of the evaluation via observation during ADL (e.g., muscle strength and sensation). Behavioral problems such as agitation or aggression also affect the evaluation process. Attempting to complete parts of the evaluation without an awareness of how to approach the patient may escalate the behavioral problem.

The environment in which the patient is assessed also substantially affects the results of the evaluation. Different environments elicit different responses in each patient. In general, a quiet environment allows for optimum concentration and attention to the task. This type of environment also positively affects other cognitive processes such as organization and processing speed. Conversely, the therapist may want to place the patient in a high stimulation environment to determine the patient's ability to attend selectively to the evaluation and tune out irrelevant information in the external environment.

Finally, the patient's level of comprehension and communication abilities complicate the interpretation of the patient's responses, especially when evaluating vision, perception, and cognition. It is important to be aware of possible deficits in those areas and to consult with the speech-language pathologist before initiating the evaluation whenever possible.

GUIDELINES FOR EVALUATION OF THE BEGINNING LEVEL PATIENT

When evaluating the beginning level patient (Rancho levels 1 to 3),[48] always evaluate the patient in a quiet, isolated environment. If the patient cannot be taken out of the room, close the curtain, turn off the TV and/or radio, close the door, and ask the family members to

BOX 42-3

EVALUATION AREAS FOR TBI (BEGINNING LEVEL)

PHYSICAL STATUS

ROM	Muscle tone
Motor control	Sensation
Oral/Motor control	

COGNITION/VISION/PERCEPTION

Level of alertness	Visual attention	Form and color perception	Response to sound
Visual saccades/pursuits	Visual neglect	Ability to follow directions	Ability to vocalize

watch quietly (unless a family member is asked to participate in the evaluation). It is important to maintain a quiet environment while performing the evaluation because the therapist will be looking closely for any changes in the patient's status.

Many evaluations have been developed for the beginning level patient. Many facilities have their own forms. A list of the areas to evaluate is given in Box 42-3.

A few of these areas can be evaluated according to protocols (passive range of motion and muscle tone). Evaluation of the beginning level patient (low consciousness patient) is generally completed by observing the patient's response to stimuli provided in an organized and meaningful fashion, however.[51] For example, when a family member walks into the room and says hello to the patient, does the patient open his or her eyes (response to auditory information, level of alertness)? Does the patient attempt to locate the family member and maintain fixation as the person walks into the room (visual saccades and pursuits)? Does the patient visually attend to the family member's face (visual attention)? The length of time the patient responds (able to maintain eyes open 2 minutes when family members are present), the quality of the response (poor visual pursuits), and the level of assistance (maximum assist to incorporate BUE into light hygiene tasks), give measurable information regarding the patient's status.

GUIDELINES FOR EVALUATION OF THE INTERMEDIATE AND ADVANCED LEVEL PATIENT

The intermediate to advanced level patients (Rancho Levels 4 to 8)[48] are able to complete many, if not all, parts of the occupational therapy evaluation. Cognitive impairments such as impaired attention span or behavioral issues such as decreased initiation may limit participation in standardized tests or established protocols.

Physical Status

Joint ROM, muscle strength, motor control, and total body function should be evaluated according to the facil-

ity or program protocol. As these areas are being assessed, the therapist should be aware of complications that are specific to traumatic brain injured adults, including heterotopic ossification, which is the abnormal growth of bone for no apparent reason. It occurs most commonly around the elbow and hip and can cause substantial loss of ROM at the joint. Warmth and/or swelling around a specific joint may be indicative of the beginning of the heterotopic ossification and should be reported to the attending physician immediately.

Fractures as well as soft tissue and peripheral nerve injuries may be present as a result of multiple trauma. Fractures should have been identified and treated before the occupational therapist initiates the evaluation. Consult the physician's orders in the medical chart to determine any precautions such as limitations in weight-bearing status or limitations in passive ROM in the joint or extremity. Peripheral nerve injuries are common in the traumatic brain injury population. If a peripheral nerve injury is suspected, a thorough evaluation should be completed.

Dysphagia

Assessment of the patient with TBI should include both a clinical (bedside) dysphagia assessment and a videofluoroscopy. The bedside exam will provide the therapist with information regarding the patient's cognitive ability, behavioral characteristics, and language functioning as they relate to the ability to manage food. The videofluoroscopy will provide information on the anatomy and physiology of the oral, pharyngeal, and esophageal stages of swallowing.[37]

Oral and pharyngeal functions of the adult with traumatic brain injury may be involved, affecting the patient's ability to eat a regular diet and drink thin and thick liquids. Cognitive-perceptual disorders, behavioral disorders, changes in posture, and self-feeding have all been implicated as contributing to swallowing disorders.[4] Most TBI patients exhibit problems in all of these areas. The evaluation and treatment of dysphagia are described in Chapter 11.

Cognition

It is often challenging to assess and treat patients at the intermediate and advanced levels of cognition. The deficits can be subtle and difficult to identify. Flexibility and creativity are required to accommodate for the patient's behavioral problems such as a denial of deficits.

When giving a cognitive assessment, it is important to consider factors that may affect the patient's performance on test items but may not be indicative of cognitive deficits. These factors include language problems such as aphasia, visual/perceptual deficits, medications, education, vocational and cultural background, and previous level of expertise with the task.[51]

Most therapists complete functional assessments to determine the patient's cognitive status. In a functional assessment the patient is observed during ADL, advanced ADL, or other activities such as an assembly task. For example, during a meal preparation activity of making soup, the therapist may observe any number of cognitive components including attention, memory, sequencing, ability to follow written and/or verbal instructions, safety, and judgment.

When evaluating the patient's cognitive status during ADL, measurement techniques that may be employed to grade the various skills include time (in minutes or seconds), number of errors or correct responses, the amount of assistance or cuing needed (supervised, minimal, moderate, or maximal), percentage of the task completed correctly, complexity of the task (simple versus complex or number of steps), and the environment (isolated, multistimulus).

Various cognitive assessments are used by occupational therapists. Two of these are the Rancho Los Amigos Scale of Cognitive Functioning[48] and the Allen Cognitive Level Test (ACL)[2], both of which assess the patient during functional activities. Occupational therapists also use standardized tests and measurements such as the Rivermead Behavioral Memory Test[63] and the Mini Mental State Exam[17] to determine the patient's level of cognitive functioning. These types of tests may also be given by a neuropsychologist or speech-language pathologist. In general, the neuropsychologist and the speech-language pathologist give most of the standardized tests to the brain injured patient. Each program varies across the country, however, and individual programs establish assessment responsibilities with regard to the various disciplines (see Chapter 15).

Behavior

All members of the team must work as a cohesive unit for behavioral intervention to be effective. Any team member may identify a behavior problem and alert the rest of the treatment team. The first steps in initiating a behavior management program are to evaluate a behavior problem and to implement behavior management meetings. A behavior symptom checklist or tracking form may need to be completed by each team member before the first meeting if the team is having difficulty identifying problematic behaviors, monitoring the frequency of the behavior, and determining the degree it interferes with each treatment session (Fig. 42-1).

SANTA CLARA VALLEY MEDICAL CENTER
Rehabilitation Center

BEHAVIOR CHECKLIST

Patient's Name__________ Room #__________
Date Begun__________

INSTRUCTIONS: The purpose of this checklist is to monitor both the FREQUENCY and INTERFERENCE (to what degree the behavior interfered with your session) of specific behaviors only. Please place your name, date, time, discipline, and length of session below. For FREQUENCY please estimate what percentage of time during your session the patient engaged in the specified behavior. For INTERFERENCE please estimate to what extent the behavior interfered with the session/shift.

STAFF NAME: __________ DISCIPLINE: __________
DATE: __________ TIME: __________ LENGTH OF SESSION/SHIFT: __________

BEHAVIOR TO BE MODIFIED: __________

FREQUENCY: (circle percentage of time behavior occurred)

0 10 20 30 40 50 60 70 80 90 100

INTERFERENCE: (circle extent behavior interfered with session/shift)

0 10 20 30 40 50 60 70 80 90 100
NONE MODERATELY GREATLY

BEHAVIOR TO BE MODIFIED: __________

FREQUENCY: (circle percentage of time behavior occurred)

0 10 20 30 40 50 60 70 80 90 100

INTERFERENCE: (circle extent behavior interfered with session/shift)

0 10 20 30 40 50 60 70 80 90 100
NONE MODERATELY GREATLY

COMMENTS: (describe situation)

FIG. 42-1 Behavior Checklist. (Reprinted with permission, Santa Clara Valley Medical Center, San José, Calif.)

During behavior management meetings, the patient's behavior is analyzed. The discussion should focus on the problematic behavior, which action, people, or words trigger the behavior, what happens to the patient after the behavior occurs (i.e., does the patient get what he or she wants?), what has been attempted to reduce the behavior, and the effect it has on the patient. The team decides on a behavior plan to assist the patient in reaching the behavioral goal. During the meeting, techniques (e.g., escapes, blocks, verbal responses) to be used for that particular patient may be demonstrated and practiced. Ongoing weekly behavioral management meetings should continue until the behavior is manageable or eliminated.

Vision

All adults with a TBI should undergo a vision screening, considering the high incidence of visual dysfunction.[8,15,47,55] When possible, visual skills should be evaluated early in the assessment process because early identification of visual deficits allows for more reliable information to be obtained in the overall team evaluation. Diplopia (double vision) or accommodative dysfunction, for example, could influence the results of neuropsychology or speech-language pathology assessments. Most important, a comprehensive vision treatment program can be designed by an optometrist and implemented by the occupational therapist.

A vision screening is a tool designed to identify potential visual deficits. Therapists are not allowed to diagnose conditions but can determine if the patient passes or fails a screening test based on certain criteria. This screening is a means to determine which patients require a referral to an optometrist or ophthalmologist for a complete evaluation. The optometrist or ophthalmologist can then recommend the appropriate treatment intervention.

The procedure for identifying patients with visual dysfunction includes clinical observations during other parts of the occupational therapy evaluation (e.g., head tilt, obvious eye turn, closing or covering one eye, bumping into walls) and completing a visual history questionnaire. The visual history questionnaire should contain an ophthalmologic history as well as specific questions regarding the use of glasses/contact lenses and current complaints (blurriness, dizziness, headaches, eyestrain, double vision, visual field loss).

Finally, a vision screening is completed. Common areas evaluated in a vision screening include visual attention, near/distance acuities, ocular movements such as range of motion, pursuits, saccades, and near point of convergence, ocular alignment, stereopsis (depth perception), and visual fields.[15] Criteria and procedures for referral to an optometrist or ophthalmologist should be developed by each facility and the referring doctor.

Perceptual Motor Function

The perceptual motor evaluation should be administered when the therapist has a clear understanding of the patient's cognitive, sensory, motor, and language status. A vision screening should precede the perceptual-motor evaluation. The evaluation should follow an established progression with motor planning evaluated before body scheme, which is evaluated before higher level discrimination skills (see Chapter 14).

Activities of Daily Living

The evaluation of ADL is thoroughly discussed in Chapter 26. Some occupational therapy assessments evaluate cognition through structured ADL or activity analysis. Cognition and ADL cannot be evaluated separately in the TBI population. In addition to formal assessments, many therapists have developed kitchen/homemaking evaluations and community evaluations that allow the therapist to assess systematically the visual, perceptual, cognitive, behavior, and motor components of the activity.

Driving

A comprehensive driving evaluation is an important part of the rehabilitation of the traumatic brain injured adult. At the end of the driving evaluation, the patient receives the results of the evaluation, feedback on the potential to become a safe driver, and suggestions for any follow-up training sessions required. The patient also receives recommendations regarding any vehicle modifications that are necessary to allow him or her to resume driving safely again.

Two types of assessments are required for the traumatic brain injured individual: a clinical assessment (evaluation of the patient's visual, cognitive, perceptual, and physical status as it relates to driving) and an on-road assessment. Both sections are essential for the TBI adult. Occasionally the patient fails the first section, but in the actual situation is able to compensate for deficits. Conversely, the patient may do well on the clinical assessment section but fail the on-road assessment.

Evaluating the patient on the road allows the driving instructor to determine if the patient has the potential to relearn to drive and to estimate the number of driver training lessons needed. The results from the on-road assessment may encourage the physician to report the patient to the department of motor vehicles. Many states require the physician to report to the department of motor vehicles any person who has had a lapse of consciousness or episodes of marked confusion resulting from neurological disorders; physicians are sometimes hesitant, however, to comply unless they have concrete evidence that the patient cannot drive safely.

The TBI patient frequently exhibits deficits that substantially affect the ability to drive safely. A few examples include impaired visual processing, deficits in figure-ground, and impulsivity. When visual processing is slowed, the patient hesitates during maneuvers and stops unsafely (e.g., in the middle of the road or at a corner) to allow adequate time to process visual information. A patient with figure-ground impairments may be unable to find traffic signs at intersections and may not be able to find the gearshift near the dashboard. An impulsive patient may respond aggressively rather than defensively. In addition, he or she may use poor judgment when driving and be unable to inhibit inappropriate responses[53] (see Chapter 26, section 2).

Vocational Rehabilitation

Employment outcomes for the TBI population have become major concerns for professionals working with this population. It has been well documented that the transition to return to work after a moderate to severe brain injury has not been very successful.[24,28,41] The high unemployment rates have been attributed to the adverse emotional, behavioral, and neuropsychological changes arising from injury. More recently, substance abuse has been identified as a major contributor to difficulty in initiating and maintaining employment.[34]

Various models have been developed to assist TBI adults to (re)enter the job market successfully. The supported employment model developed by Wehman and associates[59] is one of the current and most popular of these models. In the supported employment model, emphasis is placed on on-the-job training with support of a job coach as well as ongoing case management services.

Vocational rehabilitation of the TBI adult is a comprehensive process involving many disciplines including vocational counselors, vocational evaluators, case managers, job coaches, neuropsychologists, and therapists.

Vocational evaluations for the TBI adult are different from traditional vocational assessments in that traditional assessments do not provide the information necessary to ascertain whether or not an individual with a TBI has the potential to return to a job or enter the work force for the first time.

Specifically, the vocational assessment for the individual with a TBI must include assessment in actual work settings because psychometric tests and job simulations do not accurately determine work potential. The individual with a TBI is often able to compensate for deficits when working. Other adaptations that must be made when performing a vocational evaluation include an emphasis on identifying the patient's learning style, allowing for longer assessment periods because of cognitive deficits and slow motor responses, and varied assessment periods because of fatigue and inconsistent performance.[18]

Occupational therapists can play a variety of roles in the vocational rehabilitation of the TBI individual. The role is partially determined by the treatment model used at the facility and the occupational therapist's level of experience. In some settings the occupational therapist may be asked for a recommendation regarding the patient's ability to return to work. The occupational therapist may base the recommendation on observations of the patient's performance in ADL and estimate how that would translate into a work setting.

In other settings, the occupational therapist may complete a formal vocational evaluation. The evaluation should include an interview, formal testing, a physical capacity evaluation, observations on work behaviors, work samples, and an on-site assessment in the work environment. The written report should state results of these components and should summarize the patient's interests, strengths, and areas of deficits and concerns. The report should conclude with recommendations that state the patient's job goals and include a plan.

GENERAL PRINCIPLES OF OCCUPATIONAL THERAPY INTERVENTION

The principles and guidelines for occupational therapy intervention can be generalized for most patients with a traumatic brain injury, although the specific deficits may vary considerably. All patients require structured, normalized sensory input from their environment. This approach prevents behavioral outbursts or withdrawal, maximizes cognition, and facilitates learning.

The occupational therapist treating the traumatic brain injured patient must constantly observe, reevaluate, interpret behavior and response, and alter treatment accordingly. This patient population demands a great deal of flexibility and astute observation skills from the treating therapist.

When establishing a treatment plan, the therapist is faced with a long list of problems regarding the patient's physical, visual, cognitive, perceptual, behavioral, psychosocial, and ADL functioning. The therapist must place these problems in order of priority and set realistic goals for the patient. The therapist must analyze the treatment tasks and activities and structure the treatment sessions to facilitate maximal function.

Treatment strategies for each problem can vary, and a strategy must be chosen that is best for the patient. Common impairments already discussed can be treated during functional activities, table top activities, and with sensorimotor approaches. Most therapists who treat this population feel that a combination of therapeutic approaches with emphasis on functional activities are the most beneficial, however.

To facilitate carry-over of learned tasks and minimize patient confusion and agitation, constant communication must occur among team members. This aspect is more crucial in this patient population than any other. If the nursing staff approaches a behavioral issue one way and the therapists attempt to extinguish the behavior in another way, the patient will not make progress and may actually regress. A consistent, repetitive, and appropriately structured approach to the patient by all members of the treatment team yields optimal results.

GENERAL AIMS AND METHODS OF TREATMENT FOR THE BEGINNING LEVEL PATIENT

The aims of treatment for the beginning level patient are to increase the patient's level of response and overall awareness. Input must be well structured, broken down into simple steps, and enough time must be allowed for a response, which often is delayed during this phase of treatment.

Treatment at this stage can be grouped into six areas: sensory regulation, wheelchair positioning, bed positioning, casting and/or splinting, dysphagia management, and family and caregiver training. The treatments occur simultaneously to optimize the patient's progress. Each of the treatments affects and enhances the other treatments.

Sensory Regulation Program

After the patient has been evaluated, a baseline for treatment is established. Treatment of the beginning level patient should start as soon as the patient is medically stable. Treatment generally begins in the ICU. Often the patient has no response to pain, touch, sound, or sight or exhibits only a generalized response to pain. The goal of treatment is to increase the patient's level of awareness by trying to arouse the patient with controlled sensory input. Sensory regulation increases input into the reticular activating system, which increases arousal to the threshold necessary for responsiveness.[60]

Originally, a sensory stimulation program for traumatically brain injured patients consisted of providing the patient with individualized visual, auditory, tactile, olfactory, and gustatory stimulation. The therapist conducted the treatment sessions by presenting a stimulus such as a flashlight (visual stimulus) and attempting to elicit visual tracking. When working on auditory stimulation, the therapist would ring a bell, clap his or her hands, or give simple commands to the patient and observe the patient for a response. During olfactory stimulation, the therapist would place different odors under the patient's nose such as vanilla and banana. Again, the therapist would wait for the patient to respond in some way, such as opening the eyes. Gustatory stimulation is the controlled presentation of tastes. The therapist would present salty (sodium chloride solution), sweet (sucrose solution), bitter (quinine), and sour (vinegar or lemon juice) solutions onto the patient's tongue with a cotton swab. As with olfactory treatment, the therapist would note positive, negative, or no response and observe specific behaviors.

Sensory regulation has developed into a more functional approach over the years, although some therapists continue to provide sensory stimulation treatment as previously described. The rationale for changing the treatment to be more task specific is that it is believed that providing sensory stimulation in isolation is confusing for the patient. Also, with the changing health care environment, this type of approach allows the therapists to document changes in functional terms.

Sensory regulation treatment now incorporates presenting visual, auditory, tactile, and other senses into specific tasks such as rolling in bed. The patient is actively engaged in the activity as opposed to having the stimulus presented to the passive patient. In addition to the program being multisensory and meaningful, the treatments are usually brief (initially about 10 minutes) and incorporate both sides of the body. The modalities used are common, everyday tasks such as hygiene, bed mobility, turning on the radio, and playing checkers. The therapist continually observes the patient during the activity and documents any changes in behavior such as the patient turning the head in response to sounds, visual attention and visual tracking of the objects in the activity, physical responses (changes in breathing patterns, increases or decreases in muscle tone, voluntary use of the upper extremities, changes in posture), vocalizations (groans, sighs, one word), and following commands.

The Affolter concept, described in Chapter 25, is now commonly used as a treatment approach for eliciting the changes just described. This concept of providing tactile-kinesthetic input by guiding the patient through activities is a very functional way of helping the patient improve both physically and cognitively. The basic premise behind the Affolter concept is that learning must occur through interaction with the environment in a meaningful way. When using the Affolter approach, the therapist stands behind the patient, places his or her arms over the patient's arms and slowly, by giving different amounts of pressure, guides the upper extremities one at a time through an activity. Meaningful, everyday activities provide the opportunity for problems to develop. It is the

process of solving the new problems that facilitates cognitive and perceptual learning.[52]

Wheelchair Positioning Program

Seating and positioning is often a challenging task for therapists. Proper positioning assists in the prevention of skin breakdown and joint contractures, facilitates normal tone, optimizes cognition, improves behavior, and promotes safety. Effective seating and positioning requires a stable base of support at the pelvis, maintaining the trunk in midline and placing the head in an upright posture for functional upper extremity use (Fig. 42-2). A comprehensive wheelchair positioning program begins with a thorough evaluation that identifies the problems specific to that particular patient. Goals are determined and equipment is identified to alleviate the postural deficits and place the patient in good postural alignment. Positioning should occur in conjunction with neurodevelopmental and other treatment modalities.

Pelvis. Wheelchair positioning should begin at the pelvis because poor hip placement alters head and trunk alignment and influences tone in the extremities. A solid seat insert (½-inch plywood, 1-inch foam covered by vinyl) can be placed underneath the patient to facilitate a neutral to slight anterior tilt of the pelvis. A lumbar sup-

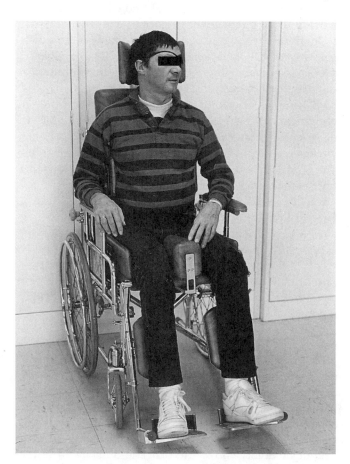

FIG. 42-2 Improved posture and trunk alignment is achieved with positioning devices.

port can also be used, in conjunction with the solid seat insert, to place the pelvis in the desired position and maintain a natural curve in the lumbar spine. A seat insert that is slightly wedged (the downward slope pointing toward the back of the wheelchair) can be used to flex the hips, to help inhibit extensor tone in the hip and lower extremities. A seat belt, angled across the pelvis, helps to maintain the desired position.

Trunk. Positioning the trunk occurs after the pelvis is properly positioned. A solid back insert (½-inch plywood, 1-inch foam covered by vinyl) or solid contoured back is placed behind the patient's back to facilitate a more erect posture of the spine. Lateral trunk supports can be employed to eliminate scoliosis while a chest strap or crossed chest straps (fabricated from stockinet and an open-cell, high-density foam padding material) decreases kyphosis, retracts the shoulders, and expands the upper chest. The pelvic position should be reevaluated if the therapist has difficulty maintaining the trunk in midline.

Lower extremities. Thigh pads placed along the lateral aspect of the thigh may be used to decrease lower extremity abduction, or an abductor wedge may be placed between the lower extremities just proximal to the knees to eliminate lower extremity adduction. Some patients with traumatic brain injuries exhibit hip flexion caused by spasticity, soft tissue contractures, or heterotopic ossification. In the case of spasticity, it may be possible to fabricate a positioning device out of open-cell, high-density foam padding material, which is placed over the knees and is strapped onto the footrests to lower the extremities to the cushion. A foot wedge is placed on top of the footplate if plantar flexion contractures are present in one or both feet. The foot is strapped into place to accommodate the contracture, equally distribute weight, and take the pressure off the ball of the foot.

Upper extremities. A full lap tray is generally used to support the upper extremities. The tray maintains the UEs on the same height surface and does not disturb trunk alignment. The upper extremities should be positioned with the shoulders in slight flexion and external rotation, the elbows in slight flexion, and the wrists and fingers in a functional position. This position is frequently difficult to achieve because of the severe spasticity and soft tissue contractures seen in this patient population. A hand splint or bivalved cast (shown later) may be used in conjunction with the lap tray to obtain the desired position.

Head. Attaining a neutral, midline head position is one of the most difficult tasks for the occupational therapist. The beginning level TBI patient usually has little to no active head control. Most head control devices are static positioning devices, for example, the U-shaped device,

fabricated out of a high-temperature thermoplastic and foam, that extends posteriorly and laterally. The head is kept from falling forward by a forehead strap. In head positioning, caution must always be taken to avoid overstressing the cervical area or causing excessive resistance to spastic neck musculature, which is often difficult to avoid with static devices. Reclining the patient back eliminates this problem. Although reclining the patient prevents good weight-bearing through the trunk and pelvis, it does not allow the patient to interact visually with the environment.

An alternative to static head positioning is using a dynamic head positioning device, which places the head in good alignment on the trunk and equally distributes pressure (unlike the head positioning devices previously mentioned). In addition, this type of device allows the patient to begin actively initiating head movements such as lateral rotation on command or in response to tracking an object or person in the environment visually (Fig. 42-3).

Wheelchair positioning is a process of constantly reevaluating and adapting the equipment to meet the changing needs of the patient. The devices should be removed gradually as the patient starts actively to control the body and to manipulate more aspects of the environment. The devices are slowly phased out or made less complicated, offering less support.

Patients may change rapidly and this constant change in status requires close monitoring, even after discharge from the hospital or after the patient has been discharged from occupational therapy. In long-term care, the patient should be reevaluated on a quarterly basis to determine the need for a change in the wheelchair positioning pro-

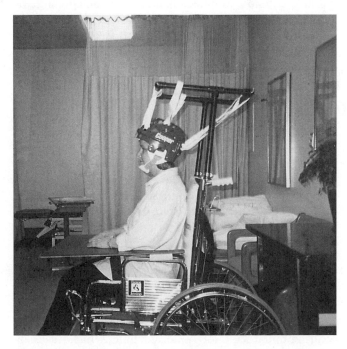

FIG. 42-3 Dynamic head control device.

gram. A patient may not require the devices while engaged in therapy, such as during wheelchair mobility or when facilitating head control.

It is critical to make a schedule for the amount of time the patient should be up in the wheelchair. Placing the patient up in the wheelchair longer than it can be tolerated may increase behavioral problems and decrease the patient's cognitive level.

Bed Positioning

Bed positioning is a crucial component of the total positioning program. The traumatic brain injured patient generally has bilateral involvement requiring a program for side-lying on both sides. The traditional bed positioning techniques used with CVA patients may need to be modified based on the bilateral involvement of the traumatic brain injured patient and any other complications such as a UE or LE cast, heterotopic ossification, fractures with open reduction, internal fixation devices, etc. A schedule for prone-lying may also be indicated during the day to maintain range of motion in hip and knee extension.

Another concern should be neuropathy. Compressive neuropathy occurs commonly following moderate or severe TBI. Neuropathy may occur as direct trauma to the nerve, but more commonly occurs as a consequence of orthopedic injury, spasticity, or improper positioning.[6]

Splinting and Casting

Splinting and/or casting may be indicated when (1) increased tone interferes with functional movement and ADL independence, (2) passive range of motion (PROM) limitations are evident, and (3) there is potential for soft tissue contractures. Splinting and casting are not required if PROM and wheelchair and bed positioning are sufficient to maintain ROM in the upper extremities. Serial casting is a more aggressive method of intervention than splinting but is frequently required in this patient group because of the severity of spasticity.

The goals of splinting and casting are to reduce abnormal tone or soft tissue tightness, increase or maintain PROM, increase the functional potential of the upper extremity, prevent skin breakdown (e.g., in the palmar surface of the hand) and simplify management of care for the beginning level patient (e.g., bathing, dressing, and performing bowel and bladder care).

The most commonly used splint for the beginning level patient is the stretch splint. This splint places the wrist and fingers in extension and abducts the thumb (Fig. 42-4). The stretch splint is a resting splint, which is worn when the patient is not involved in functional activities. Once the splint is fabricated a splint schedule must be established for the nursing staff or caregivers to follow. A typical splint schedule begins with 2 hours on and 2 hours off. The goal is generally to increase the wearing time to about 8 hours at a time, which varies, of course, from patient to patient.

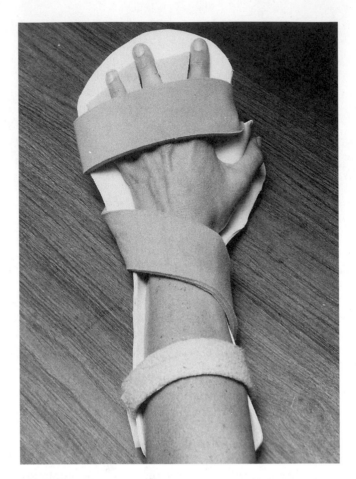

FIG. 42-4 Stretch splint.

Other splints that may be indicated for the brain injured patient include a wrist cock-up, which can be used to stabilize the wrist while working on improving finger prehension. A thumb opposition splint may be worn to facilitate palmar pinch or 3-point pinch. The splints are changed, modified, and eventually discontinued as the patient's motor control improves.

A casting program is implemented when other methods for managing spasticity are no longer effective or when the therapist is spending the majority of his or her time attempting to inhibit tone and maintain ROM. Factors that affect the success of a casting program include the onset date, the age of the patient, where the patient is living (hospital, skilled nursing facility, or home), and the patient's medical status (unstable intracranial pressure, febrile, IV lines, skin integrity). These factors help determine whether or not to cast, which type of cast to use, how many casts to fabricate, the length of time the cast is left on, and the length of time between the casts.

The most common UE casts are the (1) elbow cast which is used for loss of PROM in the elbow flexors; and (2) the wrist, thumb, and hand cast which is used for loss of PROM in the wrist, thumb, and/or finger flexors. Other variations of these casts include elbow and wrist casts, wrist and thumb casts, and individual finger casts. The type of cast fabricated depends on the patient's deficits and also on the philosophy of a particular therapist or facility.

Casts can be fabricated out of fiberglass or plaster. Fiberglass is more expensive but is more durable, lighter weight, is clean and easy to work with, and sets quickly. Fiberglass may be used with a patient who already has a painful shoulder to avoid causing further problems. Fiberglass is also ideal when casting an agitated patient who bends the elbow while the cast is being fabricated. Fiberglass sets so quickly that the cast does not usually have a chance to buckle if the patient begins to move. Plaster, on the other hand, is considerably less expensive and may be a more appropriate material for a skilled nursing facility. Plaster is effective for any patient who is not at risk for shoulder pain and is not agitated.

Casting is frequently performed in conjunction with motor point blocks. Blocks are the injection of a chemical substance (e.g., Lidocaine, Marcaine, or phenol) into the nerve or motor point, which temporarily blocks the innervation of the muscles. The purposes of motor point blocks are to diagnose underlying contractures, to improve the effectiveness of the serial casting, and to obtain quicker results. A block is given by the physician before initiating casting.

Indications for completion of the casting program include obtaining full PROM, reaching the initial goal (i.e., 0 to 45° wrist extension), or when the patient has reached a plateau (i.e., no significant improvement in PROM after two consecutive casts). When improvement has been made and the goal has been reached, the last cast is cut in half, the edges are finished, and it is used as a bivalved cast (Fig. 42-5). A wearing schedule is then established.[54]

The patient should never be placed in too many splints, casts, and positioning devices all at one time, because they are static tools to help the patient become more mobile. Splinting and casting are completed in progression, from initially breaking up the abnormal tone and reducing soft tissue contractures to aiding the patient to improve UE function.

Dysphagia

The patient emerging from coma is fed by a nasogastric tube or a gastrointestinal tube. There are no absolute criteria that determine when a patient is ready to begin eating by mouth. Many factors are taken into consideration. Refer to Chapter 11 for specific treatment procedures.

Family/Caregiver Training

Education of the family/caregivers starts the first time the professional meets them; however, the amount of information provided should be according to each person's ability to handle and process the information. Frequently, the familiar faces of the patient's relatives are among the first that the patient responds to when coming out of coma. Family/caregivers play an essential part

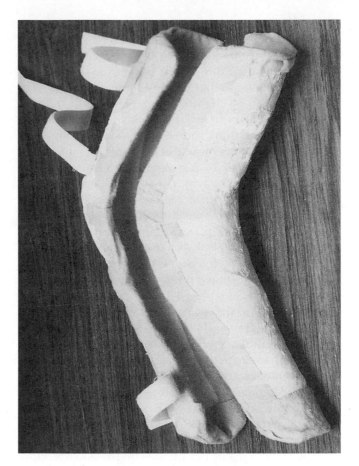

FIG. 42-5   Bivalved cast.

in eliciting the patient's responses and often play a large role in the sensory regulation program, bed positioning, and the ROM program. They are not always involved in wheelchair positioning initially, given the difficulty in transferring these patients and the precision that is required in correctly positioning them in the wheelchair.

TREATMENT OF THE INTERMEDIATE TO ADVANCED LEVEL PATIENT
Neuromuscular Impairments

The types of motor impairment present in the TBI patient are numerous. Weakness, spasticity, rigidity, soft tissue contractures, primitive reflexes, loss of postural reactions, and impaired sensation affect the patient's ability to perform activities independently and with normal motor control. The prerequisites for normal movement include normal postural tone, normal integration of flexor and extensor control (reciprocal innervation), normal proximal stability, and selective movement patterns.[27]

Although the program for each patient with TBI is individualized, the common principles of treatment are to progress proximal to distal, to establish symmetrical posture, to integrate both sides into activities, to encourage bilateral weight-bearing, and to introduce a normal sensory experience. A variety of treatment approaches, including neurodevelopmental treatment (NDT), proprioceptive neuromuscular facilitation (PNF), myofascial release, Rood techniques, and physical agent modalities can be effective for this patient population. In fact, successful treatment should employ more than one technique.

The trunk plays a major role in limb movements. Treatment of the trunk should focus on achieving alignment and stimulating muscle activity in the trunk. Alignment facilitates stability. A symmetrical posture also neutralizes the effects of gravity. Graded muscle activation of the dorsal and ventral trunk allows the patient to maintain a midline posture, weight shift out of that posture into all directions (e.g., scooting forward), move the lower trunk on a stable upper trunk, or move the upper trunk on a stable lower trunk. Once trunk control improves, treatment should progress to the upper extremities.

Treatment for the trunk and/or upper extremities should begin after problems have been identified. If a patient has soft tissue contractures and/or spasticity in a particular muscle or muscle group, appropriate treatment techniques may include NDT mobilizations and inhibitory techniques, myofascial release, and joint mobilizations. An example of an NDT mobilization is anterior pelvic tilt mobilization. The therapist sits in front of the patient. The patient begins in posterior pelvic tilt. The therapist places his or her thumbs on the anterior superior iliac spine and the fingers posteriorly on the iliac crests. During the mobilization, pressure is made upward and anteriorly with the thumbs and downward and posterior with the fingers. The direction to the patient is to "sit up tall."

Entirely different types of procedures would be used for the patient with low tone or weak muscles. In those patients, NDT, PNF, the Rood approach, or various physical agent modalities are often incorporated into treatment sessions. A PNF pattern that assists the patient to roll from supine to side-lying is UE D1 flexion (see Chapter 23). Facilitative techniques described by Rood such as tapping over the muscle belly or quick stretch can immediately stimulate the muscles (see Chapter 21). Carryover is usually noted when the techniques are used over a period of time. Neuromuscular electrical stimulation (NMES), a modality more frequently used with hand injuries, can also be used to stimulate many UE muscles or muscle groups including triceps, pronators, supinators, and wrist and finger extensors to enhance muscle strength, increase sensory awareness, and assist in motor learning and coordination.[11]

Many patients with TBI have fairly intact motor control. These patients ambulate independently and incorporate both upper extremities into functional activities. Closer observation, however, reveals subtle trunk and upper extremity deficits related to coordination and speed of movement. The treatment program for trunk control for these patients focuses on developing full isolated movements of the trunk and upper extremities, good dynamic standing balance for all activities including high reaching and bending to low surfaces, and the ability to shift weight naturally from one lower extremity to the other during activities. Upper extremity treatment programs are designed to increase scapular stability and improve fine motor control. A key component in treatment is improving the patient's speed while maintaining good coordination.

Ataxia is a common and frustrating problem that often develops early, persists into the late rehabilitation phase, and may remain permanently. Although various treatment methods have been tried, it is difficult to assess their long-term value. Weighting of body parts and the use of resistive activities appear to improve control during performance of tasks but show inconsistent carryover of control when the weights are removed. When applying weights to the patient, the therapist must carefully evaluate at which joint or joints the tremor originates. Applying weights to a patient's wrists when the tremor originates in the trunk or shoulders is ineffective.

Weighted eating utensils and cups are also used to compensate for ataxia in the upper extremities. These assistive devices are also limited in their effectiveness. Another alternative used more successfully in the lower extremities than the upper extremities is to wrap Theraband* in a figure eight pattern around the extremity during treatment. The Theraband gives increased proprioceptive feedback to the extremity.

Regardless of the types of motor control deficits, the therapist must continually evaluate the patient's response and alter techniques depending on the patient's response. Specific modalities and techniques used to obtain normal trunk and UE movement are limited only by the therapist's creativity. All treatment should be activity-based. Any prefunctional treatment techniques such as NDT mobilizations must be followed by an activity that is meaningful and which requires the same movement.

The evaluation of motor control and coordination is presented in Chapter 10. Chapters 21 through 24 address aspects of motor evaluation for the specific sensorimotor approaches to treatment. Davies[14] is an excellent resource for specific information on treatment techniques for individuals with traumatic brain injuries.

Cognitive retraining is generally accomplished through functional activities. In other words, the therapist treats the cognitive impairment in ADL, advanced ADL, and when using crafts or leisure activities. A functional approach is taken with these patients because of their confusion and difficulty with abstract concepts. The confused patient may become agitated when given sequence cards to put in order. The same sequencing

---

* Available from Sammons, Inc., P.O. Box 386, Western Springs, IL 60558-0386.

deficit may be addressed by having the patient assemble a footstool. The TBI patient may automatically understand the task and may participate for a longer period of time because it is familiar and makes sense to him or her.

Many of the activities found in the occupational therapy clinic storage cabinets will not challenge the TBI patients with high level cognitive deficits. These patients may become angry or bored if asked to work on a puzzle or craft project meant for a five-year-old or to make cookies for the second time. Planning, organization, and money management strategies can be reinforced by an activity such as planning a vacation. Another patient can work on attention span, frustration tolerance, and delays in processing information by playing with her child for an hour. Sequencing, organization, and problem solving can be addressed within the task of changing a washer in a dripping faucet. No matter which approach is used, the activity chosen for each patient should be age-appropriate, challenging, and of interest to that particular patient.

The use of computers in cognitive-perceptual training programs has become popular. The computer primarily uses visual and auditory stimulation and feedback. It does not provide adequate tactile and proprioceptive stimulation, which are vital sensory stimuli for training. Many therapists feel that computers have an integral place in cognitive-perceptual training but should be used in conjunction with other approaches.

Behavior

The types of intervention strategies employed to decrease and eliminate problem behaviors can be broken down into two categories: environmental and interactive. Occupational therapists play an important role in both areas.

Environmental interventions can be composed of anything that is altered in the environment to facilitate appropriate behaviors, inhibit unwanted behaviors, and maintain the safety of the patient. The first step in altering the environment is often to place the patient in a quiet, isolated room without a roommate. The shades are drawn, the television and radio are turned off, and the door is closed. All extraneous information on the walls is removed and extra furniture is taken out of the room.

Further steps may need to be taken such as one-to-one nursing care and a cubicle bed. One-to-one nursing care means that one nurse is assigned to only one patient for the entire shift. She sits in the bedroom with the patient, may also be with the patient during therapy, and is an integral part of implementing the behavioral management program. Typically, a nurse's aide performs this role. The insurance policy for a particular patient may not cover this expensive program.

A cubicle bed may be used in place of a standard hospital bed when patients are extremely agitated and at risk for falling out or crawling out of bed. A cubicle bed comprises a mattress, which sits on the floor, and four padded walls. Contraindications for the use of this bed include the patient who has an indwelling catheter or is on continuous nasogastric feedings. The patient must be able to be transferred from the floor to and from a wheelchair with assistance.

Alarm systems and walkie-talkies are other types of equipment systems that assist in maintaining patient safety. Alarm bracelets are attached to the patient or the wheelchair of a patient who is at risk for wandering off the floor or out of the building. The alarm sounds when the patient walks or propels the wheelchair past the alarm system. Walkie-talkies can be used with patients who are at risk for suddenly running away. One walkie-talkie is left at the nursing station. The other walkie-talkie is held by the staff member currently working with the patient. If the patient begins to walk or run away, the staff member can call for assistance.

Interactive interventions are the approaches that the staff and caregivers use to interact with the patient. Intervention strategies that can be implemented by the entire team include speaking in a calm, soothing, and concise manner to an agitated patient. Detailed explanations only increase the patient's confusion. Effective techniques for combative patients include keeping the bedroom door open when working with the patient and being aware of the patient in relation to oneself. When the patient exhibits lack of initiation, the therapist should physically assist the patient through the beginning of the activity or verbally cue the patient to begin the activity.[52]

Vision

Treatment alternatives for the traumatic brain injured adult with visual dysfunction include refraction, occlusion (patching and binasal occluders), prism lenses, vision exercises, environmental adaptations, and/or corrective surgery.

An optometrist or ophthalmologist can evaluate and prescribe glasses (refraction) for those patients who experience an accommodative dysfunction secondary to the brain injury. Although obtaining the correct glasses during the initial stages of rehabilitation is important, physiatrists may hesitate in having the patient purchase glasses soon after the injury because frequently the patient's eyes may improve, necessitating new glasses. Some insurance companies, especially Medicaid, will not pay for a second pair of glasses within a short time.

A common technique to eliminate double images is patching or occlusion. The patient wears a patch over one eye, which blocks the image or part of the image seen by the eye, therefore eliminating the diplopia. Patching is usually only a temporary intervention. Many patients and their families find the eye patch cosmetically unappealing, and it also inhibits the stimulus for making a binocular response.

Prism glasses or binasal occluders[20,58] may be prescribed by the optometrist for patients with intermittent or consistent diplopia caused by oculomotor nerve lesions. The prisms assist the eyes in fusing the images.

Prism glasses are not effective for all patients with diplopia, especially those with a substantial exotropia (outward eye turn). Binasal occluders encourage the malaligned eye to fixate centrally. The goal with the patient who has prisms or binasal occluders is eventually, in combination with vision training exercises, to decrease the diplopia and eliminate the need for the prism glasses.

Vision exercises consist of a series of activities designed to increase patients' awareness of their visual deficits, increase function while maximizing residual vision, and develop compensatory skills. Treatment usually progresses from monocular to binocular and follows a developmental progression: supine to sitting to standing. Exercises initially address basic skills such as visual attention, pursuits, and saccades, and may progress to more difficult skills such as fusion and stereopsis.[15]

Environmental adaptations can be used for a variety of visual deficits. Some are very simple to implement and can elicit immediate results. Compensatory strategies for visual field deficits include outlining work before beginning a task and using a colored border along one side of a page to facilitate efficient reading. Using large objects during treatment, appropriate task lighting, and contrast colors (e.g., marking the stove dials with red nail polish) are all adaptations that can be done for a loss of accommodation. If the patient has lost the ability to constrict the pupils, sunglasses should be worn whenever the patient is in bright light. If the patient has a vertical gaze paralysis and is unable to look up or down, objects should be placed within the patient's visual field.

Corrective surgery by an ophthalmologist may be indicated to align the eyes and eliminate double vision. Generally, the patient must be at least one year postinjury to allow for maximum improvement. The surgery is not always successful in eliminating the diplopia but can be warranted for cosmetic reasons.

Perceptual Training

Although occupational therapists use a variety of approaches in treating perceptual dysfunction, there are two classifications of perceptual training: adaptive and remedial. The adaptive approach is based on the theory that recovery results from the use of intact brain areas to perform functional activities in modified ways.[44] In an adaptive approach, the training of perceptual deficits occurs within activities of daily living. This approach is called functional training. For example, the patient is taught to compensate for or learn to alleviate the perceptual deficit by practicing dressing on a daily basis. In this approach there is repetitive practice of specific functional skills, such as transferring from a wheelchair, cooking a meal, or making change.

The functional approach includes compensatory training that involves making the patient aware of the problem and teaching the patient to work with the deficit. The patient learns to formulate a new scheme or strategy for performing the task. It can also involve adaptation of the environment to compensate for the patient's symptoms (setting the toothbrush and toothpaste out on the counter instead of in a crowded drawer) or adaptation of the patient's behavior.

Remedial approaches, on the other hand, are based on the theory that recovery is assumed to be the result of the reestablishment of disrupted synaptic connections or the growth of new ones. The remedial approach assumes that the adult brain is sufficiently elastic to repair and reorganize itself after injury.[45] Sensory integration,[5] neurodevelopmental treatment,[14] and transfer of training techniques are all examples of this approach. These approaches are described in Chapters 14 and 15.

Current research in motor learning and the neurobiology of learning suggests that both remedial and adaptive approaches are beneficial to the adult with brain injury, however, occupational therapists must first analyze how each patient learns and identify his or her level of learning.

Therapists should pursue functional training (adaptive approach) with patients who respond to their environment and situations at a very concrete level and are unable to transfer cognitive-perceptual learning to different situations.[45] These patients have a definite need for occupational therapy each time they are transferred to a new environment (i.e., rehabilitation to long-term care, long-term care to home) because they cannot transfer what they have learned to a new situation (new bedroom for example, or new clothes). On the other end of the spectrum, therapists should use a more remedial approach with those patients who function at a more abstract level. These patients are able to carry over a new technique learned (e.g., one-handed dressing) to a new situation.

Recent research supports the idea that those patients with diffuse injuries are extremely limited in their ability to transfer learning from table top activities such as puzzles and block designs to ADL. If the transfer of training approach is used, it will be more effective with patients who have localized brain lesions and relatively good cognitive skills.[45] Also, therapists seem to be moving toward a more functional and adaptive approach because health care trends have considerably shortened the lengths of stays in all settings. Occupational therapists no longer have the time to work on table top tasks. Instead, treatment is intensive and focused on increasing ADL independence.

The Affolter approach, described in Chapter 25, is a combination of both the remedial and adaptive approaches. Perhaps that is what makes it so successful in treating the TBI population. The Affolter technique allows the patient to interact with the environment, be presented with problems, and learn to solve the problems. The patient is always guided through meaningful, goal-oriented activities.

Self-care

ADL retraining improves the patient's functional independence. It is also a means to work on the patient's deficits within meaningful routine and familiar tasks. Hygiene or dressing activities must often be broken down into smaller segments to facilitate functional improvements because of the patient's cognitive, behavioral, and perceptual status. Backward chaining (having the patient complete the end of the task) and sequence cards are examples of ways to grade the activity to a particular patient's abilities.

A self-care program is usually fairly structured, with the patient following the same daily routine in the same environment. As the patient reaches a supervised level, more emphasis is placed on the patient's ability to complete the tasks if the routine is disrupted or altered in some way. For example, a different shower may need to be used one day and the patient's ability to adapt to a new location may be analyzed. Or, the clothes may not be in the patient's closet. He or she may need to figure out where to look for them.

The therapist must be aware of techniques that increase functional independence but cause the reinforcement of abnormal motor patterns. The therapist must constantly assess the techniques at each stage in recovery with other team members and decide whether the goal is to facilitate normal movement during ADL or to allow for independence in ADL with poor technique. In general, NDT principles such as normalizing tone and using both sides of the body are incorporated into self-care activities. The emphasis in treatment is to improve the quality of the patient's movements as well as to complete the task as independently as possible.

Compromising normal movements to obtain independence in a task is not usually advisable unless absolutely necessary, for example, if a patient was returning to live independently at the end of treatment and had to be able to complete all aspects of self-care by himself or herself. In this case the therapist would allow the patient to dress in whatever way necessary for safety and independence, but only after many attempts to facilitate normal movement.

Swallowing/Feeding

Treatment strategies for dysphagia generally follow the same guidelines as for other neurological impairments; however, strategies may be more complex or different in the TBI population based on bilateral involvement, the cognitive and behavioral issues, and the severe muscle tone that may affect the patient's posture.

Patients with TBI also exhibit frequent problems in feeding themselves. A feeding or dining program often begins in isolated areas such as the patient's bedroom or a quiet kitchen. Eating is graded to more social situations such as in the dining room with other patients or in the kitchen at home with the family.

Common pieces of adapted equipment such as a rocker knife, plate guard, or commuter mug may be introduced if a patient has difficulty with strength, coordination, or perceptual deficits. Introducing one item at a time may help with decreased attention and unilateral

neglect. If a patient is impulsive, the therapist may teach the strategy of placing the fork down after each bite to ensure that the patient chews and swallows completely before initiating the next bite.

Functional Mobility

Mobility training can be subdivided into bed mobility, transfer training, wheelchair mobility, and functional ambulation. Again, the NDT principles of bilateral involvement, equal weight-bearing, and tone normalization are used with these activities. Allowing the patient to compensate for a loss of function by grabbing a bedrail with one hand and rolling or standing on one leg to transfer allows the patient to function more independently earlier, but eventually affects the patient's ability to use the upper extremities and lower extremities normally six months or one year later. This problem occurs because the effort required to complete these activities with one arm or leg requires substantial effort and causes an increase in muscle tone. Over time, the increased effort can lead to typical hemiplegic postures, contractures, and gait deviations.

Bed mobility, wheelchair management, and functional ambulation

The bed mobility skills that the patient with brain injury may need to work on are scooting up and down in bed, rolling, bridging, moving from supine to and from a sitting position, and moving from a sitting position to and from a standing position. Wheelchair management includes the ability to manage wheelchair parts (e.g., removing a footplate) and to propel the wheelchair both indoors and outdoors on different surfaces. Only occasionally, with this patient population, does it include the ability to lift the wheelchair in and out of a car. The techniques used for bed mobility and wheelchair management are similar to those used with the CVA population but are adapted for those patients with bilateral involvement.

Functional ambulation refers to the patient's ability to walk during functional activities. Although physical therapists teach ambulation skills, the occupational therapist facilitates the carry-over of the techniques into daily living tasks such as getting dressed, preparing a meal, and mopping a floor. During the activities, the patient may do more than just walk (i.e., carry a plate, hold a purse, sweep with a broom, or carry a baby).

Transfers

Transfer training was described in Chapter 27. Cognitive, perceptual, and physical status affects the type of transfer used in training. Memory and limited carry-over of information require the technique and sequence to be consistent among all staff members treating the patient. It is preferable that transfers be practiced moving in either direction, if possible. Often a patient becomes proficient in a transfer with an approach to one side and is dismayed in a public rest room to discover that the particular approach is not possible. An additional reason for practicing transfers to both sides is that by doing so, more normal sensory input is provided by encouraging the patient to bear weight on both lower extremities and use the trunk muscles on both sides.

All family members/caregivers should be trained and cleared by an occupational therapist before transferring a patient alone. When the family/caregiver should be trained depends on the patient's functional level and the family's/caregiver's abilities. Training may take more than one session. Teaching transfers is only one of the many areas in which the therapist and the family/caregiver are involved. This ongoing relationship alleviates many of the family's/caregiver's and patient's fears and decreases the chance of failure during the first week at home.

Group Treatment

Most TBI programs use group treatment as a supplement to individual treatment. Group treatment provides learning experiences not available in individual occupational therapy (OT), physical therapy (PT), speech therapy (ST), or recreation therapy (RT). Group treatment provides structured social interactions in which patients can develop more appropriate psychosocial dynamics. Psychosocial deficits are one of the major barriers in the successful reintegration of the TBI individual back into the family and the community.

Groups allow individuals with brain injuries to receive feedback from their peers. Often patients become more aware of and make changes in their behavior in response to peer feedback.[32,38,46] Groups tend to be functionally based. Goals may include improvement in the following areas: self-monitoring conversations and behavior, executive functioning, functional money management skills, frequency of age-appropriate behavior, posture and gait patterns, functional memory, and socialization.[22]

Groups may be facilitated by one discipline but are frequently multidisciplinary. Examples of typical groups used in a TBI program are cognition group (OT/ST), functional mobility (OT/PT), community/reintegration (OT/RT), and dining group (OT/ST).

Home Management

As the patient gains increased skills and independence in dressing, feeding, and functional mobility, treatment is expanded to include kitchen and homemaking tasks. Homemaking tasks are dusting, sweeping, mopping, vacuuming, making the bed, doing laundry, and cleaning the kitchen and bathroom. Other home management activities include money management activities (balancing the check book, paying bills, and budgeting), home repairs, yard work, simple car repairs and maintenance such as washing the car and changing the oil. Examples of high level activities include planning a vacation, organizing a file cabinet, ordering from a catalog, and filing income tax.

It is important to determine the patient's interests and prior level of function in these areas before initiating treatment. Some patients make only simple meals using, at most, a microwave oven while others are gourmet cooks. Many adolescent TBI patients have little interest in cooking. For these patients, the goal is to determine whether or not they could safely and independently prepare simple hot and/or cold meals at home.

Some patients do not perform any other household activities except to make their own bed and possibly do their laundry. Attempting to work on activities they did not perform before their injury may only increase their agitation and affect their participation in occupational therapy.

As in other areas of treatment, training is graded to suit the patient's functional level. Beginning tasks might include simple sandwich or hot soup preparation. Depending on the patient's cognitive status, the therapist may place all food items on the table and have the patient verbally review the task before doing it for the first time. At the end of the session, the following day's activities can be discussed. A session such as this requires simple sequencing, organizing, and memory for the task. As the patient improves, more demands are made until the patient reaches the established long-term goals.

Total body function and endurance also are important aspects of home management activities. Standing endurance may be measured as well as the ability to bend to low shelves, reach high shelves, or kneel to clean a bathtub. Safety and judgment become key issues in the home setting. Analyzing the patient's ability to handle sharp utensils and use the stove can help the treatment team determine the patient's ability to be left unsupervised at home.

Child care is an area of treatment that is often overlooked. Family involvement is vital if a woman or man is to return effectively to his or her role as parent. Sensory overload is a common problem that must be handled when patients are involved with their children. Most people agree that sensory overload is a problem even for the parent who has not sustained a traumatic brain injury.

Gradually reintroducing the parent to the role in caring for the children should occur in occupational therapy sessions. The occupational therapist can also assist the parent in locating strollers, cribs, and child care equipment that can be handled more easily by the disabled adult.[57] Safely bathing a baby, preparing a meal while simultaneously caring for children, one-handed diapering techniques, and carrying a child are examples of the areas that might be covered by occupational therapy services.

Community Reintegration

In the rehabilitation process, the patient with a traumatic brain injury often reaches a maximal level of independence in the protected and structured atmosphere of the hospital or home and, when integrating back into the community, is faced with people, situations, and problems that have not yet been encountered. It is therefore vital that the occupational therapist incorporate community reintegration into the occupational therapy program before discharge.

Many facilities have developed community skills checklists to assist the therapist in providing a thorough community reintegration program. The training can begin with the basic skills involved in a simple purchase, that is, handling money or communicating needs. As the patient's cognitive, perceptual, and physical status changes, the therapist can help the patient progress to a more demanding activity or setting.

The transition of treatment from an initial setting, such as a hospital gift shop, to a community store not only demands skills in the areas listed but also presents new psychosocial issues with which the patient must deal. It is often of benefit for an appropriate family member/caregiver to accompany the therapist and the patient on a community trip. The family member can gain increased insight into the patient's level of functioning and into the way in which the outside world views the disability.

The therapist must be aware of the patient's and family's attitudes toward a community reintegration program. The therapist may become frustrated when a cooperative patient suddenly refuses to participate in the program. The patient may not feel ready for the outside world to view the disability. It is the therapist's responsibility to give the patient the support and guidance needed for the easiest transition possible.

Some occupational therapists work in transitional living centers for brain injured persons. As one of the final phases in the health care continuum, these programs are designed to develop daily life skills within the community. The patient lives initially within a supervised group home setting and progresses, if possible, to independence in an apartment. Although transitional living centers are thought to be effective by many professionals, they are costly. Based on the current climate in health care, more and more patients are discharged to home with therapy taking place in the home and community, in outpatient rehabilitation or day treatment programs.

Driver's Training

A specific number of hours of driver's training may be recommended as a result of the driving evaluation. If the patient must be referred to a community program, the person providing the training should be a driver instructor who also has experience in working with persons with traumatic brain injury (see Chapter 26, Section 2).

Vocational Training and Placement

Vocational training and placement of the patient with a brain injury are extended processes that require the involvement of an occupational therapist, vocational eval-uator, and other allied health professionals usually under the coordination of a vocational counselor. Each professional brings to the case a different expertise that is essential to successful job placement.

Discharge Planning

Planning for the patient's discharge from occupational therapy begins at the initial evaluation and continues until the last day of treatment. Components of discharge planning include a home/safety evaluation, equipment evaluation and ordering, family/caregiver training, and a home program. The treatment setting determines when and how the occupational therapist addresses these issues.

Home/safety evaluation

Areas of particular concern are the family/caregiver's ability to understand unsafe activities and to understand the longest reasonable time the patient should be left alone. In addition, the family/caregiver should be able to follow the appropriate steps during a seizure, understand how to evacuate the patient in case of emergency, and safely transfer the patient.[3] The patient's safety awareness and judgment are major concerns, especially if he or she will be left at home for any length of time. The patient's ability to handle sharp knives, use the stove, and remember to turn off the water, stove, and other appliances should be analyzed. Refer to Chapter 26, Section 1, for a detailed description of home evaluations.

Equipment evaluation and ordering

The time frame of an equipment evaluation varies depending on the treatment environment and the length of time since the injury occurred. In a rehabilitation unit or transitional living center, the equipment evaluation may not occur until close to discharge when the patient has made progress and the therapist can determine the appropriate equipment for that patient. If the patient is seen in an outpatient program, day treatment setting, or in the home, equipment should be evaluated immediately. For the patient who already owns equipment, a reassessment of the equipment should occur because some equipment may no longer be needed. For instance, the patient may have originally showered using a tub bench. If dynamic standing balance and safety awareness have improved sufficiently, the patient may be ready to stand to shower using a grab bar.

Family/caregiver training and home program

The participation of the family members/caregivers in the recuperation of the patient with a brain injury is extremely important. The family/caregiver should always be considered part of the treatment team. Constant communication between the therapist and the patient's family/caregiver aids in appropriate follow-through of the patient's newly acquired skills. Constant communication also provides feedback to the therapist and enables the family/caregiver to show the unique ways they solve a given problem. The family/caregiver often discovers methods that the therapist has never considered.

The extent of family/caregiver training depends on the level of the patient's disability, the family dynamics, and the discharge site. Training usually encompasses all areas of occupational therapy treatment (ADL, transfers, bed positioning and mobility, wheelchair positioning, splint/cast schedules, equipment, passive/self UE ROM) but may focus on specific areas of concern. A written home program and/or a videotape should be given to the patient upon discharge. The home program may include any or all of the areas just listed as well as specific activities for improving cognition, vision, perception, and UE motor control.

Home Health

There are some important differences in providing occupational therapy within the patient's home compared to other levels of care. The relationship between the therapist, the patient, and the family changes. The occupational therapist is a consultant as well as an invited guest. The occupational therapist has less control in the home, which means that the family unit is the key to successful treatment. If the family does not support or agree with the treatment goals, the goals will not be accomplished.

It is important to establish patient-focused goals with the patient and family. It is also essential to integrate the patient back into his community (i.e., school, church, work, friends). The therapist treats the patient for a short time so that assisting the patient's integration into the community helps ensure that the patient's improvement will be sustained long after discharge from therapy.

SUMMARY

Treatment of the brain injured adult is challenging and requires flexibility, stamina, and a great deal of creativity. Behavioral deficits frequently have a substantial impact on the treatment program. Most patients have a multitude of deficits. Goals should be interdisciplinary and established specifically to meet the needs of each patient. The treatment of the TBI population should be functionally based. Treatment provided within the context of activities has meaning for these patients, allows documentation of functional changes, and provides concrete evidence of improvement to third party payors.

 SAMPLE TREATMENT PLAN

This treatment plan is not a comprehensive one for the hypothetical patient. The reader is encouraged to add objectives and methods to make a more comprehensive plan.

CASE STUDY

KB is a 24-year-old male who sustained a gunshot wound to the head during an altercation 4 months ago. The bullet entered the left occipital area and traversed to the right temporal-parietal area. An emergency craniotomy and decompression were performed 1 week later. Craniotomy and debridement with removal of devitalized brain tissue, foreign bodies, and bone chips were performed 3 weeks after the injury.

KB was living in a city about 30 miles from the rehabilitation facility and had been married for 4 years. Presently he is divorced. He has a high school education and has worked as a bricklayer for 6 years. When initially interviewed by the occupational therapist, he stated that he would be returning to work "in a couple of weeks."

KB was referred to occupational therapy for evaluation and appropriate treatment to facilitate maximal function and independence.

TREATMENT PLAN

Personal data

Name: KB
Age: 24
Diagnosis: Traumatic brain injury
Disability: Motor, sensory, cognitive, visual, and perceptual dysfunction
Treatment aims as stated in the referral: Occupational therapy evaluation and treatment

Other services

Physiatrist: Supervision of the rehabilitation team and provision of care
Nursing: Nursing care and follow through in self-care skills
Physical therapy: Gait training, strengthening and coordination, mat mobility
Speech therapy: Cognitive and linguistic skills, academic skills retraining

SAMPLE TREATMENT PLAN – cont'd

Recreation therapy: Leisure time management
Psychology: Intelligence, memory testing, counseling
Social services: Community placement, financial arrangements

Frame of reference

Occupational performance

Treatment approaches

Rehabilitative, biomechanical, sensorimotor

OT EVALUATION

Performance components

Sensorimotor functioning
  ROM: Measure
  Muscle tone: Test and observe
  Motor control: Test and observe
  Hand function: Test and observe
  Total body function (head and trunk control, sitting and standing balance): Test and observe
  Sensation (touch, pain, temperature, stereognosis, proprioception): Test and observe
  Vision (visual attention, acuities, pursuits, saccades, near point of convergence, stereopsis, visual fields): Test and observe
  Perception (praxis, body scheme, form, size, figure-ground, position in space): Test and observe
Cognitive functioning
  Attention, memory, initiation, processing of information,

problem solving, planning and organization, mental flexibility: Test and observe
  Judgment: Observe
  Safety awareness: Observe
  Motivation: Observe
Psychosocial/Psychological functioning
  Coping skills: Observe
  Adjustment to disability: Observe
  Interpersonal relationships: Observe

Performance areas

Self-care: Test and observe
Mobility: Test and observe
Home management: Test and observe
Community skills: Test and Observe
Driving evaluation: Test and observe
Vocational evaluation: Test and observe

Evaluation Summary

KB has full isolated motion and normal strength in the right UE. He displays a moderate flexor pattern in the left UE with mild to moderate spasticity at the shoulder and elbow joints and wrist and finger flexors. With the left UE he is able to perform the following selective movements with fair quality: shoulder flexion to 90°, hand behind back, and hand to opposite shoulder. Incomplete motion is evident when performing hand behind head and wrist flexion and extension with the elbow relaxed. KB's passive ROM for BUE is within normal limits. His right hand functions normally. With the left hand, KB can perform gross grasp and lateral prehension, but these are weak. He is unable to put the prehension patterns to functional use. He is also unable to perform fine manipulative skills with the left hand.

All sensory modalities are intact in the right UE. In the left UE, impairment of superficial pain (pinprick) sensation is present. Proprioception and stereognosis are absent in the left UE. Visual saccades are slow and jerky and reduced to the left. KB has moderate difficulty with motor planning, as well as with figure-ground perception and perception of position in space. Body scheme deficits of poor right-left discrimination and unilateral left neglect also are present.

KB is oriented to person, place, and time. He is generally cooperative but exhibits a moderately impaired attention span in isolated environments. Impaired safety awareness,

judgment, and limited insight into his disability are apparent. He becomes extremely frustrated when unable to perform simple tasks.

KB requires moderate physical assistance for all dressing, hygiene, and grooming activities. He has a moderate dressing apraxia and moderately impaired position in space; that is, he puts on his shirt upside down or backwards or puts his shoes on the wrong foot, unless given cues by the therapist. He requires assistance with all fastenings. For feeding he requires moderate cues for attending to the task and to locate food on the left. He requires assistance for opening containers and cutting meat. Bed, chair, tub, and toilet transfers, as well as bed mobility, require moderate physical assistance and verbal cues to compensate for apraxia, difficulty with sequencing, and decreased perception of position in space and figure-ground perception.

KB requires maximal assistance for kitchen and community tasks. Driving and vocational evaluations are not indicated at this time secondary to the described deficits.

Assets

Good function of right upper extremity
Good motivation
Intact memory
Supportive family

SAMPLE TREATMENT PLAN – cont'd

Supportive employer and possibility for reemployment
Intact functional communication skills
Age

Problem list

1. Dependence in self-care
2. Dependent for functional mobility (i.e., transfers, bed mobility, and wheelchair management)
3. Sensory impairments
4. Lack of selective control of the left UE; moderate assistance to incorporate into ADL
5. Decreased left hand function
6. Visual dysfunction
7. Perceptual dysfunction
8. Cognitive deficits
9. Dependence in kitchen and community skills
10. Inability to drive
11. Unable to work

PROBLEM 1: DEPENDENCE IN SELF-CARE

Objective

Patient will perform UE dressing with supervision and assistance

Method

Daily ADL training in the patient's room with the door or curtain closed to reduce distraction; use of solid color shirts only (for figure-ground deficit) with clearly marked labels or adaptations as necessary. Guide patient through activity

Gradation

Decrease physical assistance until only verbal assistance is required. Begin with backward chaining techniques and gradually increase the patient's participation so that he begins the task himself by retrieving the clothes from his drawer. Expand to the use of print shirts and decrease the need for adaptations as the patient improves

---

PROBLEM 4: DECREASED LEFT UPPER EXTREMITY FUNCTION

Objective

Increase left upper extremity function sufficiently so it is a good functional assist to dominant right upper extremity

Method

NDT trunk mobilization, then trunk facilitation techniques to elicit normal trunk control. Weight-bearing and joint compression activities as needed to reduce spasticity in left UE and hand before active movement activities. Scapular stabilization exercises to facilitate control at the shoulder.

Bilateral work on the ball to elicit isolated elbow control. Activities with therapy putty for isolated wrist and hand movements as spasticity declines. Incorporate the left UE into functional activities such as washing the table, carrying a plate, folding towels

Gradation

Reduced need for adjunctive activities such as mobilization and facilitation before functional activities

---

PROBLEM 7: VISUAL DYSFUNCTION (POOR VISUAL SACCADES)

Objective

Increase visual scanning so that reading, driving, and community activities are possible

Method

Visual saccades exercises consisting of the Hart chart, finger saccades, yardstick reading pattern fixations, and games such as bingo and double solitaire. Reading using anchoring (cuing the patient where to begin the visual search) or red tape or marker. Incorporating visual saccades into functional activities such as locating an item on a shelf at the grocery store

Gradation

Vision exercises begin monocular (one eye at a time) and progress to binocular (two eyes at a time). Reduce the amount of anchoring and overall cuing required for effective scanning. Progress from visual saccades in an uncluttered environment to scanning a complex, high stimulus environment.

REVIEW QUESTIONS

1. What does TBI stand for?
2. What are the two major causes of severe traumatic brain injuries?
3. List four assessment scales used with the TBI population.
4. Name five major physical impairments that may be present in the patient with a traumatic brain injury.
5. Define ataxia.
6. List two components of a behavior management program.
7. List four psychosocial variables that influence the patient's behavior.
8. What are four activities of daily living that may be affected by a TBI?
9. List two measurement techniques that may be employed to grade the skills observed when performing a functional cognitive assessment.
10. List four areas that are commonly evaluated in a vision screening.
11. Why is it important for the TBI patient to complete an on-road driving assessment?
12. What is the goal of a sensory regulation program?
13. What is the purpose of proper wheelchair positioning?
14. What are the indications for splinting or casting in the TBI population?
15. Which cognitive deficits may be observed when a patient is given the task of changing a washer in a dripping faucet?
16. Should the occupational therapist pursue an adaptive or remedial approach to perceptual-motor treatment when a TBI patient functions at a concrete level?
17. Describe three areas that should be addressed during discharge planning.

REFERENCES

1. Adams JH and associates: Brain damage in fatal non-missile head injury, *J Clin Pathol* 33:1132-1145, 1980.
2. Allen CK: *Occupational therapy for psychiatric diseases: measurement and management of cognitive disabilities,* Boston, 1985, Little, Brown.
3. Anderson L: *NeuroCare patient safety assessment,* Concord, Calif, 1989, NeuroCare Rehabilitation without Walls.
4. Avery-Smith W, Dellarosa DM: Approaches to treating dysphagia in patients with brain injury, *Am J Occup Ther* 48(3):235-239, 1994.
5. Ayres AJ: *Sensory integration and learning disorders,* Los Angeles, 1972, Western Psychological Services.
6. Bachman DL: The diagnosis and management of common neurologic sequelae of closed head injury, *J Head Trauma Rehabil* 7(2):50-59, 1992.
7. Bakay L, Glasauer FE: *Head injury,* Boston, 1980, Little Brown.
8. Baker RS, Epstein AD: Ocular motor abnormalities from head trauma, *Surv Ophthalmol* 35(4):245-267, 1991.
9. Bly L: *NDT and motor learning theory,* paper presented at the Seventh Annual Interdisciplinary Bobath Symposium, San Francisco, Calif, April 22, 1994.
10. Bontke CF: Medical advances in the treatment of brain injury. In Kreutzer JS, Wehman P: *Community integration following traumatic brain injury,* Baltimore, 1990, Brookes.
11. Carmick J: Clinical use of neuromuscular electric stimulation for children with cerebral palsy. II. Upper extremity, *Phys Ther* 73(8):514-522, 1993.
12. Chusid JG: Correlative neuroanatomy and functional neurology, ed 19, Los Altos, Calif, 1985, Lange Medical.
13. Cohen M and associates: Convergence insufficiency in brain-injured patients, *Brain Inj* 3(2):187-191, 1989.
14. Davies PM: *Starting again,* Berlin, 1994, Springer-Verlag.
15. Efferson L: *Early intervention in identification and remediation of visual problems in traumatic brain injury,* paper presented at the Sixteenth Annual Santa Clara Valley Medical Center Head Trauma Conference, San José, Calif, April 10, 1993.
16. Englander J: Personal communication, October 4, 1993.
17. Folstein MF, Folstein SE, McHugh PR: Mini mental state: a practical method for grading the cognitive state of patients for the clinician, *J of Psych Res,* 12:189-198, 1975.
18. Fraser RT: Vocational evaluation, *J Head Trauma Rehabil* 6(3):46-58, 1991.
19. Fussey I, Giles GM, editors: *Rehabilitation of the severely brain-injured adult: a practical approach,* London, 1988, Croom Helm.
20. Gelstine N, Wetzel G: Binasal occluders: a viable alternative? *OT Week* 5(39):12-13, 1991, American Occupational Therapy Association.
21. Giles GM, Fussey I: Models of brain injury rehabilitation: from theory to practice. In Fussey I, Giles GM: *Rehabilitation of the severely brain-injured adult,* London, 1988, Croom Helm.
22. Goble L, Hier-Wellner S, Lee D: The role of community reintegration activities in a day treatment service, *Physical Disabilities Special Interest Section Newsletter* 12(3):7-8, 1989, American Occupational Therapy Association.
23. *Guide to the uniform data set for medical rehabilitation,* (Adult FIM), Version 4.0, Buffalo, NY 14214, 1993, Research Foundation, State University of New York at Buffalo.
24. Haffey WJ, Abrams DL: Employment outcomes for participants in a brain injury work reentry program: preliminary findings, *J Head Trauma Rehabil* 6(3):24-34, 1991.
25. Hall KM: Overview of functional assessment scales in brain injury rehabilitation, *NeuroRehabil* 2(4):98-113, 1992.
26. Hall KM, Cope DN, Rappaport M: Glasgow outcome scale and disability rating scale: comparative usefulness in following recovery in traumatic head injury, *Arch Phys Med Rehabil* 66:35-37, 1985.
27. Hulme JB: *Advanced problem solving: the interrelationship of trunk and limb function in abnormal movement patterns,*

paper presented at the Seventh Annual Interdisciplinary Bobath Symposium, San Francisco, Calif, April 23, 1994.

28. Jacobs HE: The Los Angeles head injury survey: procedures and preliminary findings, *Arch Phys Med Rehabil* 69:425-431, 1988.

29. Jennett B, Teasdale G: *Management of head injuries,* Philadelphia, 1981, FA Davis.

30. Katz DI: Neuropathology and neurobehavioral recovery from closed head injury, *J Head Trauma Rehabil* 7(2):1-15, 1992.

31. Keenan MA: The orthopedic management of spasticity, *J Head Trauma Rehabil* 2(2):62-71, 1987.

32. Klupt R, Baker E, Patsy D: The importance of functional activities on an inpatient brain injury unit, *Physical Disabilities Special Interest Section Newsletter* 12(3):6-7, 1989, American Occupational Therapy Association.

33. Kraus JF and associates: The incidence of acute brain injury and serious impairment in a defined population, *Am J Epidemiol* 119:186-201, 1983.

34. Kreutzer JS, Marwitz JH, Wehman PH: Substance abuse assessment and treatment in vocational rehabilitation for persons with brain injury, *J Head Trauma Rehabil* 6(3):12-23, 1991.

35. Lazarus CL: Swallowing disorders after traumatic brain injury, *J Head Trauma Rehabil* 4(4):34-41, 1989.

36. Lezak M: The problem of assessing executive functions, *Int J Psychol* 17:281-297, 1982.

37. Logemann JA: Evaluation and treatment planning for the head-injured patient with oral intake disorders, *J Head Trauma Rehabil* 4(4):24-33, 1989.

38. Lundgren CC, Persechino EL: Cognitive group: a treatment program for head injured adults, *Am J Occup Ther* 40(6):397-401, 1986.

39. MacKinnon JD: Personal communication, June 6, 1994.

40. Mann N: *Spasticity in traumatic brain injury,* paper presented at the Fifteenth Annual Santa Clara Valley Medical Center Head Trauma Conference, San José, Calif, April 18, 1992.

41. McMordie W, Barker S, Paolo T: Return to work after head injury, *Brain Inj* 4:57-69, 1990.

42. Miller JD: Early intervention and management. In Rosenthal M and associates: *Rehabilitation of the head-injured adult,* Philadelphia, 1984, FA Davis.

43. Neger RE: The evaluation of diplopia in head trauma, *J Head Trauma Rehabil* 4(2):27-34, 1989.

44. Neistadt ME: A critical analysis of occupational therapy approaches for perceptual deficits in adults with brain injury, *Am J Occup Ther* 44(4):299-304, 1990.

45. Neistadt ME: Perceptual retraining for adults with diffuse brain injury, *Am J Occup Ther* 48(3):225-233, 1994.

46. Oblender JM: Cognition groups in the rehabilitation of head injured adults, *Physical Disabilities Special Interest Section Newsletter* 12(3):5-6, 1989, American Occupational Therapy Association.

47. Padula WV: *Post-trauma vision syndrome caused by head injury: a behavioral vision approach for persons with physical disabilities,* Santa Ana, Calif, 1988, Optometric Extension Program.

48. Rancho Los Amigos Medical Center: *Levels of Cognitive Functioning,* Downey, Calif, 1980, Rancho Los Amigos Medical Center, Adult Brain Injury Service.

49. Rappaport M, Hall K, Hopkins H and associates: Disability rating scale for severe head trauma: coma to community, *Arch Phys Med Rehabil,* 63:118-123, 1982.

50. Rimel RW, Jane JA: Characteristics of the head-injured patient. In Rosenthal M and associates: *Rehabilitation of the head-injured adult,* Philadelphia, 1984, FA Davis.

51. Santa Clara Valley Medical Center: *Occupational therapy cognition competency,* San José, Calif, 1987, unpublished, Santa Clara Valley Medical Center.

52. Santa Clara Valley Medical Center: *Behavior management program policy and procedure manual,* San José, Calif, 1993, unpublished, Santa Clara Valley Medical Center.

53. Santa Clara Valley Medical Center Occupational Therapy Driving Program: *Driving related problems in neurological and progressive disorders,* San José, Calif, 1989, unpublished, Santa Clara Valley Medical Center.

54. Schlageter K, Tipton-Burton M: *Serial casting for the neurologically impaired adult,* paper presented at the Occupational Therapy Association of California Conference, San José, Calif, November 7, 1993.

55. Schlageter K and associates: Incidence and treatment of visual dysfunction in traumatic brain injury, *Brain Inj* 7(5):439-448, 1993.

56. Shilling M: A formula to estimate incidence, *Community Integration* 2(3):8-9, 1992.

57. Stewart C: Raising children from a wheelchair, *Physical Disabilities Special Interest Section Newsletter* 12(2):5-7, 1989, American Occupational Therapy Association.

58. Tassinari JD: Binasal occlusion, *J Behav Optom* 1(1):16-21, 1990.

59. Wehman P, Kreutzer JS, West M and associates: Return to work for persons with traumatic brain injury: a supportive employment approach, *Arch Phys Med Rehabil,* 71:1047-1052, 1990.

60. Westerman T: How I do it—head and neck: an objective approach to subjective testing for sensation of taste and smell, *Laryngoscope* 91:301, 1981.

61. Willer B, Abosh S, Dahmer E: Epidemiology of disability from traumatic brain injury. In Wood R: *Neurobehavioral sequelae of traumatic brain injury,* London, 1990, Taylor & Francis.

62. Willer B and associates: Assessment of community integration following rehabilitation for traumatic brain injury, *J Head Trauma Rehabil* 8(2):75-87, 1993.

63. Wilson B, Cockburn J, Baddeley A: *The Rivermead behavioural memory test,* Suffolk, England, 1985, Thames Valley Test Co.

Degenerative Diseases of the Central Nervous System

*Jean Hietpas, Merry Lee Hooks, Pat Atchison,
Lorraine Williams Pedretti, Guy L. McCormack*

Degenerative diseases are characterized by chemical changes and deterioration of neurons and supporting tissues.[15] This chapter discusses four degenerative diseases often seen in occupational therapy practice: multiple sclerosis, amyotrophic lateral sclerosis, Parkinson's disease, and Alzheimer's disease. Although these diseases are unrelenting and incapacitating, the occupational therapist can offer much in the form of supportive care, maintenance of physical abilities, compensatory measures, preventive measures against further complications, and retention of the quality of life.

Section 1   Multiple sclerosis

Jean Hietpas, Lorraine Williams Pedretti, Guy L. McCormack

Multiple sclerosis (MS) is a diffuse, chronic, slowly progressive disease of the central nervous system (CNS) characterized by the development of disseminated, demyelinated glial patches in the supporting tissue of the brain and spinal cord resulting in disruption of neurotransmission of the cerebrospinal nerves. The development of plaques or scar tissue on the myelin sheath or insulation of the nerve fibers leads to diversified symptoms. For this reason, MS is classified as a demyelinating disease.[1,4,23]

INCIDENCE

Multiple sclerosis is one of the most common neurologic diseases of young adults.[2] The figures vary, but in the United States about 350,000 persons are affected with multiple sclerosis and about 2 million world-wide. In areas of high incidence, 50 to 60 cases of MS are estimated per 100,000 of the population.[11,17] Reliable, definite statistics are difficult to obtain, because diagnosing multiple sclerosis is a process requiring time to collect and analyze with subjective, clinical, and objective laboratory data.[14]

Multiple sclerosis usually affects persons between the ages of 15 and 50. Females are affected more often than males at a ratio of nearly 3 : 2. It is interesting to note that geographic distribution of MS appears to be related to latitude. MS is most prevalent in North America, Europe, and Southern Canada between latitudes 65° and 40°.[13,17] The geographic distribution is dependent on where the individual spent the first 15 years of life, even if geographic relocation occurs after age 15. Caucasians are at higher risk for MS, and the incidence among Afro-Americans and Asians is lower.[13,25] Some evidence suggests that incidence of MS is related to socioeconomic conditions. Individuals are often well educated and establishing productive careers when symptoms first appear.[34]

ETIOLOGY AND PATHOPHYSIOLOGY

There is no known cause of multiple sclerosis, but three working hypotheses are under investigation. It is widely believed that MS may be an autoimmune disorder with stimulation of the immune system resulting in damage to the myelin sheath of the CNS. The body's immune system is unable to determine self from not self, and the body's own myelin cells are destroyed. Well-documented studies have led to the conclusion that a combination of a genetic susceptibility, perhaps coupled with environmental factors or triggers, results in the eventual acquisition of MS. The northern European gene pool and descendants seem to have a greater probability of acquiring descendants seem to have a greater probability of acquiring MS. Also, there is some evidence that certain viruses can cause demyelinative disorders. To date, however, no MS virus has been isolated.[2,3,7,13,21]

In acute cases of MS, demyelination occurs in a scattered fashion throughout the white matter located near the blood-brain barrier resulting in periventricular lesions. Immune cells called T lymphocytes or T cells mistake the myelin as something foreign and destroy it. The myelin sheath is broken down and chemically degraded, thus causing inflammation. Macrophages carry away the myelin debris, leaving scars or sclerotic plaque at certain sites.

In chronic cases, the increased demyelination can cause shrinkage of the cerebral hemispheres with widening of sulci and dilatation of the ventricles. The plaques of the demyelinated areas disrupt nerve transmission. In addition, unmyelinated axons conduct impulses more slowly and less efficiently because the electrical current is insufficient for depolarization. Eventually, formation of sclerotic plaques and enzymatic activity may disrupt neurotransmission in extensive locations.[20,23]

SIGNS AND SYMPTOMS

The signs and symptoms of MS depend on well-demarcated anatomic sites of the lesions in the brain and spinal cord. Onset of an exacerbation may be sudden, and symptoms may develop over a period of weeks. Clinical MS syndromes occur in various forms; the most common are related to the functions of the cerebrum, brain stem – cerebellum, and spinal cord. The manifestations include pyramidal, cerebellar, brain stem, sensory, bowel and bladder, visual, mental, and motor disturbances such as weakness, spasticity, intention tremors and ataxia, dysphagia, and dysarthria. Sensory symptoms vary from numbness and tingling to dysesthesia of specific sensory modalities such as temperature perception, light touch, and position sense.

Visual symptoms result from optic neuritis. Patients may experience blurring of vision, double vision, delayed blink reflex, nystagmus, ocular pain, decreased visual acuity, or blindness. Speech problems resulting from bulbar involvement may precipitate dysarthria and scanning speech. Urinary bladder and bowel symptoms include urinary incontinence, urinary retention, bowel incontinence, urinary urgency, and recurrent urinary tract infections. Sexual symptoms constitute varying degrees of impotence and decreased sensation in the genital area. Emotional and mental symptoms vary considerably. Depression is the most common problem and is often not diagnosed. Other symptoms include euphoria, intellectual deterioration, and emotional lability.[2,13,23,34]

MEDICAL MANAGEMENT

Medical management of MS remains empiric or symptomatic. Because of the occurrence of remissions and exacerbations, the course of treatment must respond to the needs of the patient. During exacerbations, patients are treated with bed rest and limited activity until symptoms subside. Steroid and hormone therapy is recommended during acute exacerbations. There is no evidence that long-term steroid therapy reduces the risk of relapse, however, and a risk of respiratory infections exists during the use of corticosteroids.

Immunosuppressive and diet therapy have been employed with some limited success. Antiinflammatory drugs are administered to reduce inflammation of the myelin sheath. Muscle relaxants are used to reduce spasticity. Anticholinergic drugs, intermittent catheterization, and in severe cases, indwelling or suprapubic catheterization is used for bladder management. Bowel complications are managed by adequate fluid intake, diet, digital stimulation, suppositories, and occasional enemas.*

The occupational therapist must be aware of which medications are being taken, what the intended effect is, and what the possible side effects are. The observations of the OT can be valuable to the medical team in titrating the dosage of medicines intended to manage spasticity, ataxia, emotional lability, and bladder control.

OT INTERVENTION

The severity and progression of multiple sclerosis varies from one person to the next. The disease is characterized by exacerbations and remissions of numerous CNS symptoms, resulting in temporary, transient, or permanent loss of function. Because of the variability, the occu-

---

* References 1,3,6,24,27,28,32.

pational therapy program must be individualized and based on the assessment of each patient. The physiologic changes and symptoms and psychological effects of the uncertainty of the disease course affect all areas of the patient's life.[8,19]

Occupational therapy for MS patients is concerned primarily with functional abilities. The goal is to maximize the person's physical, emotional, social, and vocational independence, quality of life, and productivity.[35] Occupational therapy focuses on the following seven areas:

1. energy conservation and work simplification methods
2. coordination and strength
3. ADL and assistive equipment/technology
4. home and community management
5. wheelchair and seating assessment
6. architectural modifications
7. sensation or vision loss compensation training[16,35]

OT EVALUATION

The course and symptoms of MS vary from time to time. Therefore, frequent reevaluation of the patient's status and treatment interventions is essential. Factors such as fatigue, temperature, mood, stress level, and time of day must be considered when evaluating the patient.[13]

The occupational therapy assessment for the MS patient should include evaluation of strength, physical endurance, range of motion (ROM), muscle tone, hand function, coordination, reflexes, and balance. The presence of tremor, ataxia, sensory loss, paresthesia, perceptual problems, and visual dysfunctions should be assessed. In some instances, a dysphagia and oral motor evaluation is indicated. A thorough evaluation of the person's activities of daily living (ADL), work, and leisure skills is necessary to assess the occupational function level. Cognitive and intellectual functions, mental status, behavior, communication level, emotional stability, and adjustment to disability are to be included in the psychosocial portion of the evaluation.[9,13,16,31,35]

OT GOALS

The overall goal of occupational therapy for the MS patient is to maintain the maximal level of function throughout the disease process. Specific objectives are as follows:

1. to increase or maintain ROM
2. to increase or maintain strength
3. to diminish abnormal spastic movement patterns
4. to prevent contractures, deformity, and decubiti
5. to facilitate maximal coordination and function of extremities
6. to maintain a maximal level of ADL
7. to maintain the ability to work and participate in leisure pursuits
8. to assist in psychosocial adjustment
9. to provide patient and family education and support[8,9,16,18,31]

TREATMENT METHODS

The selection of treatment methods for the MS patient depends on the symptoms, level of function, and patient's goals. The variability of the disease necessitates continual reestablishment of treatment goals and methods in response to therapy and changes in the patient's condition, home environment, and family situation.[13] The patient's identified problems are solved conjointly as a patient-therapist team. Life changes often necessitated by the disease must be made gradually with family support.[36]

Sensorimotor Dysfunction

Passive and active stretching and active ROM exercises should be performed several times a day to decrease spasticity, maintain joint mobility, and prevent contractures of the patient with MS. Engagement in daily living and leisure activities should be encouraged to help maintain joint mobility. Prolonged icing and inhibition techniques, and use of positioning to influence tone, can be used to reduce spasticity. The Bobath neurodevelopmental handling techniques using key points of control are used to reduce spasticity and enhance postural control.[9,13,16]

Strengthening exercises and activities are used to increase or maintain strength and flexibility. Exercises and activities done on the proprioceptive neuromuscular facilitation (PNF) diagonal patterns are helpful. Strengthening exercises are useful to increase strength of nonaffected muscle groups, to overcome spastic antagonists, and to prevent weakness secondary to disuse. Energy conservation techniques are taught to prolong strength, avoid fatigue, and enhance activity tolerance.[13]

Endurance for activities must be developed slowly and if heat sensitivity exists, the occupational therapist must be aware of increased body temperature and humidity. An aquatic exercise program with water temperature less than 82°F helps increase strength and endurance as long as spasticity does not increase with the cool temperature. Also, Yoga asanas or postures and tai chi exercises can promote flexibility, coordination, and stamina.

The occupational therapist should encourage the patient with MS to engage in activities that involve all extremities. Poor sensation, tremor, and incoordination can be discouraging and cause frustration in the performance of hand activities.[31] Coordination and stability may be improved by strengthening fixation musculature, adapting techniques for proximal stabilization, and facilitating proximal cocontraction.[13] Distal mobility can be superimposed on proximal stability as improvement occurs. The application of wrist weights often is used to increase proprioceptive feedback and decrease forearm tremor during upper extremity (UE) activity.[4,35] General coordination activities graded from gross to fine may be helpful.[13]

As in any treatment program, the effectiveness of treatment must be monitored and evaluated by its effect on the patient. Increased fatigue, spasticity, and frustration are undesirable and are indicators for analysis of their causes and possible changes in treatment media and methods.

Orthotic devices may be helpful for some patients with MS. A resting splint may be used in the presence of finger extensor weakness to allow the flexor tendons to remain at a functional length and prevent overstretching of the extensors. The wrist cock-up splint may be used for weak wrist extensors to place the hand in a functional position for activities and prevent overstretching of weak extensors. An antispasticity C-bar splint may be assistive to promote prehension and maintenance of the web space between the thumb and index finger. A mobile arm support may be useful to compensate for substantial weakness of the UEs.

A lightweight manual wheelchair, power wheelchair, or 3-wheeled power scooter may be indicated if ambulation becomes unsafe or if fatigue limits functional mobility. A wheelchair seating system provides postural support and assists in the prevention of pressure sores.[10]

Sensory problems are treated with a compensatory approach. Safety measures must be taught using visual feedback and increasing the patient's awareness of areas of sensory impairment. The patient and family need to be educated about the sensory deficits and how to employ safety techniques during routine ADL such as bathing, preparing meals, and nail care. Skin breakdown must be prevented by regular pressure relief, use of appropriate seating cushions, air or water mattresses, and daily skin inspection.[13,24]

Self-Care

Specific training in dressing, bathing, toileting, personal hygiene, and feeding can improve or maintain independence in ADL for the patient with MS.[13] The patient should be trained in suitable methods and advised about the need for special equipment and assistive devices. Such devices should be aesthetically pleasing and introduced only when absolutely necessary. Weighted or easy-to-grip silverware, a large-handled commuter mug with a lid, a plate guard or plate designed with a rim, and a nonskid mat may be helpful for feeding. Buttonhooks, reachers, sock aids, large-button shirts, elastic shoelaces, long-handled shoehorns, and Velcro closures may be useful for increasing dressing independence.[13,35]

The selection and use of assistive devices require a cooperative, problem-solving approach by both patient and therapist. Problems must be identified and alternative solutions explored. This process may require a trial-and-error approach, resulting in the adoption and discarding of various assistive devices.[35]

Home Evaluation

A home evaluation is necessary to assess the patient's ability to function maximally in the home environment. Occupational and physical therapists can make recommendations for equipment that improves safety and independence. Furniture may have to be rearranged or eliminated to allow easy mobility and access within the home. Grab rails and banisters may have to be installed to ensure the patient's safety on stairs and during toilet and tub transfers. When patients are renovating or building a home, occupational therapists can assist with architectural planning for wheelchair accessibility and ease of function in the home.[10,33]

Mobility

The ambulation ability of the patient with MS is likely to decrease as the disease progresses. Ambulation aids may progress from the use of a cane to forearm crutches and then a walker. Ultimately, acquisition of a wheelchair may be a necessary part of the rehabilitation program for some patients. The patient's current status and potential progression of the disease, as well as lifestyle and living environment, are important considerations in wheelchair selection. Generally a lightweight manual wheelchair allows for greater ease of use if UE function is sufficient to propel the wheelchair. Patients with UE impairment, truncal ataxia, fatigue, or poor endurance may find that a power wheelchair enhances their independence in functional mobility. Obtaining a wheelchair necessitates training in wheelchair mobility and transfers, which can be coordinated by occupational and physical therapists.[10,13]

Modifications of an automobile may be necessary if use of the right lower extremity (LE) makes it unsafe to operate a motor vehicle. Hand controls for driving can be recommended if UE function is good. Additional vehicle modifications that allow for increased mobility include either a van ramp or an electronic lift for wheelchairs.[10,36]

Communication

As tremor and incoordination increase, adaptations for communication become necessary for the patient with MS. Built-up pens, a universal cuff, a clipboard, a nonslip mat, magnifying devices, large-display calculators, tape recorders, an electric typewriter or a personal computer with a keyboard guard, a membrane keyboard, a voice-activated computer, or a screen enlargement program are devices that may be helpful for written communication. If severe dysarthria is present along with motor dysfunction, communication boards with scanners, page turners, speaker phones, and other telephone adaptations may be necessary.[13,26,33]

Leisure Skills

The use of previous leisure interests or the development of new ones can be helpful for satisfying intrinsic gratification needs, mental stimulation, and socialization for the patient. It is important to select leisure activities within the capabilities of the patient. Activities with the family or in a group can afford opportunities for socialization and support. The patient's activity configuration and interest history are important tools for discovering appropriate leisure activities.

Work Skills

A vocational evaluation may be necessary for patients whose capacities do not preclude employment. Whether the same employment can be continued or whether a change is necessary, the need for modifications of the workplace or work schedule can be determined by vocational evaluation. Psychological adjustment and perceptual and cognitive problems influence the feasibility for continued employment or reemployment.

A third of those with MS are only mildly affected and should have little or no problem continuing employment. Another third are moderately affected and may need job modifications such as distance of parking area to worksite, architectural barriers, and schedule modification. The ability to work not only contributes to the family economy, but also enhances self-esteem, maintains contact with work peers, and provides daily social interaction. The possibility of alternative jobs with the same employer can be explored as work tolerance and motor abilities decrease.[9,13,33]

Psychosocial Adjustment

To be informed of the diagnosis of MS is a critical and perhaps shocking event. It is well known that MS may lead to progressive disability, and it is generally regarded with dread and apprehension.[19,22,29] Some patients regard the news of the diagnosis with relief following a long period of diagnostic evaluation and unexpressed fears of mental dysfunction, brain tumor, and accusations of fabricating the symptoms.[22,33]

Initially, the patient with MS may feel that the future is hopeless and intolerable and may become depressed and despondent. Many patients rally and resolve to combat the disease, which now has a name and some known approaches to its management. The occupational therapist can be a valuable resource for helping the patient make the most of remaining capabilities and for giving appropriate advice, support, and treatment.[22,33] The occupational therapist must assist the patient in adjusting to the progression of the disability.[33] Stress management techniques can be taught by the occupational therapist. These techniques have both physical and psychological benefits.[12,35]

The therapist, patient, and family must bear in mind that a diagnosis of MS does not mean that there is going to be steady, rapid decline. Often there are long periods of remission, and the patient may remain stable for many years. The disease has a benign course in some patients, making it possible to retain complete or partial working capacity for many years after the initial diagnosis is made.[5,22,30]

Euphoria is a mental change associated with MS. The patient who is euphoric may overestimate abilities and underestimate the seriousness of problems and potential hazards, making safety awareness poor.[31] Denial is also part of the process of acceptance of the disease and may also contribute to poor safety awareness and unrealistic expectations for patients as well as the family members. Patients can benefit from the opportunity to talk about their concerns and fears with someone who is knowledgeable about MS. The National Multiple Sclerosis Society can supply the patient and family with current educational literature, research, and information about local support meetings. Group counseling techniques are suitable for some MS patients. Support of rehabilitation team members and neuropsychological or psychiatric intervention can be helpful.*

Treatment Precautions

Patients with MS should avoid fatigue, stress, heat, humidity, and chill.[28,30,31,36] Heavy resistance exercise and activity are contraindicated. Exercises should be planned in conjunction with physical therapy to avoid fatigue from the cumulative efforts of the patient.[35] Rest periods should be provided during evaluation and treatment. A daily schedule of rest and activity designed within the endurance level and capabilities helps to keep the patient at an optimal level of function. The therapist should be aware that euphoria, or a denial of the severity of the symptoms, and decline in function may result in a lack of acceptance of assistive devices, safety measures, and mobility aids.[31]

SUMMARY

Multiple sclerosis is a progressive, demyelinating CNS disease with onset usually between the ages of 15 to 50; women are affected more frequently than men. There is no known cause or cure. It is characterized by remissions and exacerbations and the CNS symptoms are diverse, depending on the areas of demyelination in the brain and spinal cord. Medical management is primarily symptomatic although corticosteroids, antiinflammatory drugs, and hormone therapy may be used during exacerbations.

The role of occpational therapy is to maintain and enhance functional abilities appropriate to the stage of the disease and the level of physical dysfunction. Treatment focuses on energy conservation and work simplification, coordination training and strengthening, ADL and assistive devices, home modification, appropriate work activities, wheelchair and seating assessment, and psychological adjustment.

Therapeutic exercise and activities, ADL, relaxation and aquatic exercises, coordination training, splinting, mobility training, communication, leisure skills, and work skills all may be used in the treatment program. Heavy resistive exercise is contraindicated, and fatigue, stress, heat, humidity, and chill are to be avoided.

---

* References 9, 16, 18, 19, 22, 29.

The patient with MS may live for years with a disease process that can progress slowly or rapidly. Many persons with MS enjoy long periods of remission during which they are relatively free of symptoms or disability.

The role of the occupational therapist is to enable the patient to live a life that is as meaningful and productive as possible given the stage of the disease and available physical capabilities.

Section 2   Amyotrophic lateral sclerosis

Lorraine Williams Pedretti, Guy L. McCormack

Amyotrophic lateral sclerosis (ALS), is a motor neuron disorder. It is also known as Lou Gehrig's disease and is the best known of the motor neuron disorders.[4,15] *Amyotrophic* refers to the neurogenic atrophy of muscles and *lateral sclerosis* refers to the hardness of the spinal cord felt at autopsy. Proliferation of astrocytes and scarring of the lateral columns of the spinal cord results in this hardness. Disease of the corticospinal tracts, which carry the axons of the premotor cells from the brain stem to the spinal cord, causes the scarring.[15] Although there is progressive degeneration of both upper and lower motor neurons in ALS, those that supply the ocular muscles and muscles concerned with voluntary control of bladder sphincters are spared. Sensory neurons and the autonomic nervous system are not affected.[8,15]

Clinical variants of ALS are (1) spinal muscular atrophy and (2) progressive bulbar palsy. In progresssive bulbar palsy, symptoms are confined to muscles innervated by the cranial nerves, resulting in dysphagia and dysarthria. Spinal muscular atrophy is characterized by lower motor neuron involvement only and is characazterized by weakness, atrophy, loss of reflexes, and fasciculation.[15]

INCIDENCE

In the United States amyotrophic lateral sclerosis is one of the most common neuromuscular disorders affecting adults.[10] The geographic distribution of the disease is about equal throughout the world.[12]

Epidemiologic data reveal that ALS occurs slightly more frequently in males than in females.[12] Most victims are between the ages of 40 and 70, with the average age of onset at 56.[11,12,14] Although ALS is distributed throughout the world, it occurs much more frequently among the people of Guam, the Mariana Islands, and other locales in the Western Pacific region.[3,9] Three forms of ALS are recognized: (1) the classic or sporadic, which accounts for about 90% of the cases in the United States;

(2) the Western Pacific form, which occurs in specific geographic locations and is relatively rare; and (3) a familial form, which accounts for about 10% of cases and is presumed to be hereditary.[9]

ETIOLOGY AND PATHOPHYSIOLOGY

The cause of ALS is unknown and there is no effective treatment. It is always fatal, with death usually occurring, on average, within 2 to 5 years of onset.[11,15] Some theories of its cause that have been proposed were a slow-acting virus infection, a toxic degeneration, an autoimmune reaction, hormonal abnormalities, circulating lead toxicity, and deficiency of a repair enzyme in the blood.[5,8] Studies of the Western Pacific type of ALS point to the possibility of some exogenous toxin peculiar to the region, or the absence of essential minerals, as possible causes.[9]

ALS is a bilateral, degenerative disease restricted to motor neurons primarily in the corticobulbar and corticospinal tracts and anterior horn cells of the spinal cord. The motor nuclei of the cranial nerves also are involved. Marked atrophy of distal muscles is characteristic. There is loss of muscle fibers and fascicles in the distribution of motor units with fasciculation and fibrillation of muscle.[10,15,18]

CLINICAL PICTURE

The initial symptoms are weakness in the upper and lower extremities, manifested at first by difficulty with activities requiring fine, coordinated movements such as typing or handling money. There is atrophy of the musculature of the hands and feet and fasciculations of distal muscle groups. Because ALS affects both the upper and lower motor neurons, signs of lower motor neuron dysfunction are associated with hyperreflexia and spasticity, characteristic of upper motor neuron disease.[15] Eventually, the accessory muscles of respiration are affected and the patient may experience dyspnea. Difficulties with swallowing and talking occur when there is bulbar involvement. Progressive muscle atrophy results in functional quadriplegia. There is no effect on mental capacities so the patient remains alert and aware of the disease process and its inevitable outcome.[11]

Other clinical manifestations depend on the variants of the disease. In *spinal muscular atrophy* only the lower motor neuron is involved and patients exhibit progressive weakening and wasting of distal musculature, loss of reflexes, and fasciculations. Atrophy can begin in either upper or lower extremities.[15] Patients with *progressive bulbar palsy* exhibit only symptoms of cranial nerve dysfunction such as difficulty in swallowing, coughing, speaking, and breathing. There is marked wasting of the musculature innervated by the cranial nerves, particularly the tongue.[5,15] In some patients with ALS, progressive involvement of the laryngeal and pharyngeal muscles produces dysphagia, aspiration problems, and respiratory insufficiency. This variation of ALS runs a rapid course, and the patient rarely survives more than 18 months from the onset of the symptoms.[6]

MEDICAL MANAGEMENT

There is no specific medical treatment for amyotrophic lateral sclerosis.[6,11,15] Treatment is symptomatic, with medications to decrease the discomfort of muscle spasms. Gastrostomy or esophagostomy for feeding and tracheostomy for breathing assistance may be used for patients with swallowing and/or breathing difficulties. Adequate nutrition and prevention of aspiration must be assured.[11] Tranquilizers and antidepressant drugs are used to alleviate anxiety and depression.[13]

OT INTERVENTION

The role of occupational therapy for patients with ALS is to maintain an optimal level of function during the relentless progression of motor impairment. The occupational therapy program addresses symptomatic care and includes graded exercise and activity, energy conservation and work simplification techniques, selection and management of appropriate ambulation aids and orthotics, and provision of assistive devices necessary for communication and self-care independence. In addition, psychological support for the patient and the family and family education are important elements of the occupational therapy program. The occupational therapist should work within a multidisciplinary team for a comprehensive approach to disease management.[6]

The complexity and progressive nature of ALS make each patient unique in terms of degree of weakness, rate of progression, and order and severity of clinical manifestations. Therefore each patient needs an individualized treatment program.

The progression of ALS may be classified into four clinical stages according to symptoms and level of func-

tion.[6] In the first stage, the patient is ambulatory and able to perform normal life activities, although mild discomfort or limitations of performance and endurance may be apparent. In the second stage, the patient is ambulatory with mild to moderate limitation of function. There is muscle imbalance, increased muscle fatigue caused by excessive energy expenditure, and decreased mobility and function. By the third stage the patient is using a wheelchair and is dependent in ADL. This stage is characterized by progressive weakness of axial muscles and deterioration of mobility and endurance. The patient is totally ADL-dependent and bedridden in stage four. Gastrostomy, tracheostomy, and some form of respiratory assistance may be needed.[6]

OT EVALUATION

The occupational therapy evaluation should include the assessment of muscle strength, muscle tone, active and passive ROM, ADL performance, and a home evaluation.[6] Activity tolerance and possible cranial nerve involvement also should be evaluated. The latter includes a dysphagia evaluation. Motor assessment for the use of nonvocal communication devices should be carried out when communication skills weaken.[17] Information from the evaluation of pulmonary function and gait should be obtained from physical and respiratory therapists. The evaluation results are used as a baseline for functional endurance and performance. From this baseline, progression of limitations can be measured and the treatment program modified.[6]

OT GOALS

The goals of the occupational therapy program are to (1) maintain strength, (2) prevent contractures, (3) reduce spasticity, (4) maintain independence in ADL, (5) facilitate psychosocial adjustment, and (6) provide family education and support.[16]

TREATMENT METHODS

Janiszewski and associates[6] outlined a multidisciplinary treatment program for each stage of ALS previously outlined.

In the first stage of the disease the patient should be taught work simplification and energy conservation methods. Mild aerobic exercise for uninvolved muscles may be helpful to maintain ROM and compensate for weakness in other muscles. Swimming and bicycling are recommended for general conditioning.[6] Progressive resistive exercises are not recommended because these usually cause cramping and fatigue. Fatigue should be avoided in any exercise or activity program because it seems to increase the rate of motor unit degeneration.[6,19] Simple assistive devices and orthotics may be provided.[6]

In the second stage of ALS, progressive atrophy of particular muscles is noted. Pain and discomfort from spasticity or pressure neuropathies may be present. Adaptive equipment and bracing are needed to support weak muscles and conserve energy. Such devices also can help to improve the patient's performance at home and at work. A cane, tripod, or quad cane, a rolling walker, and ankle-foot orthosis are necesary for ambulation.[6]

The treatment program for patients with ALS may include active ROM exercise to prevent contractures, active exercise and moderate activity to maintain strength, and teaching of positioning for comfort and function.[16,17] Exercise is monitored and patients are advised to have several brief exercise periods each day rather than a single strenuous exercise session. Swimming and limited bicycling are continued.[6]

In the third stage the patient is confined to a wheelchair for all or part of the time. A wheelchair with a reclining back, headrest, elevating padded legrests, padded armrests, safety belt, and lapboard may be necessary to accommodate the patient's increasing functional limitations and need for rest and special positioning. Active and passive ROM exercises and breathing exercises are included in the treatment program. Considerable psychological support is necessary for both patient and family.[6]

In the fourth stage of ALS, breathing and swallowing difficulties are common. Assistive techniques for breathing, coughing, and swallowing are employed. Breathing assistance by respirator or tracheostomy is used for some patients. Special feeding techniques and devices, as well as special diet, are introduced. Communication devices become necessary.[6]

Orthotics and Assistive Devices

Splints commonly used to prevent deformity and support weak musculature are the wrist cock-up splint, opponens splint, soft cervical collar, and ankle-foot orthosis.[6,19]

Some assistive devices that may be helpful are the long-handled comb, brush, and bath sponge; bath and shower chairs; grab bars in tub and around toilet; flexible shower hose; and raised toilet seat. Takai[17] recommended the padded drop-arm commode for use over the toilet while the patient is still ambulatory but has difficulty rising from a standard toilet seat.[17] For dressing, the long-handled shoe horn, sock aid, zipper pull, and buttonhook can be helpful. Clothing should be chosen for comfort as well as ease of putting on and removing.[2] Devices to ease home management tasks may be appropriate in the early stages of the illness.

Feeding can be managed with the assistance of a nonskid mat, plate guard, universal cuff, and cups with one or two handles. Food consistency must be modified to accomodate progressive difficulty with swallowing. In the intermediate stages of ALS, puréed foods are easier to manage than liquids. The patient must be allowed adequate time for eating because rushing increases the chances of choking. If eating is tiring, six small meals may be taken.[1]

When evaluating the patient for the use of assistive devices, the occupational therapist must consider the fatigue and frustration the patient experiences in using the device, its cost, appearance, acceptability to patient and family, and convenience of use. The stage of the disease, rate of progression, current motor status, endurance, and positioning are other important considerations in the selection and use of assistive devices. Whether the device is going to be helpful should be determined before it is ordered or fabricated, if possible.[17]

Communication

All patients with ALS ultimately become limited in communication. Problems with writing, using the telephone, speaking, or signaling for attention eventually arise. The occupational therapist should examine the problems and their causes and advise the patient about available alternatives. The patient needs reassurance that no matter how severe the communication difficulty, it is possible to convey needs and ideas to others. Different types of telephones are available such as the speaker phone, the automatic dialer, and the receiver holder. Communication boards, eye-gaze charts, electronic scanners, and personal computers are aids that can be used to augment communication.[17] As the patient loses more and more mobility, environmental control systems and attendant care may be necessary.[16]

Psychosocial Adjustment

Progressive muscular weakness creates feelings of hopelessness, discouragement, and despair.[19] Adjustment to the disease is especially difficult because of its progressive nature. Because no disability is static, adjustments must be made over and over again.[1] Reactive depression is common, but suicide is rare among patients with ALS.[6]

To facilitate psychosocial adjustment, the therapist must promote continued appropriate activity and exercise and provide support and encouragement.[19] Keeping the patient as active as possible and reducing dependency lessens depression and hopelessness and enhances self-image.[6] The provision of a concrete assistive device, for example, which makes an immediate change in performance has a positive psychological effect on the patient.[17] The maintenance or recovery of function has a good effect on self-esteem and improves the sense of independence. The occupational therapist can support the development of coping mechanisms and help both patient and family to confront a terminal illness.[16]

The pursuit of recreational and leisure skills should be encouraged for diversion, fitness, and a sense of personal gratification. Johnson[7] described an aquatic therapy program for a patient with ALS. The aquatics program was used to improve strength, ROM, and endurance. Functional ambulation and balance activities were facilitated by the buoyancy of the water. The program also allowed opportunity for recreation and socialization. The warm water was soothing and promoted muscle relaxation. The patient's feelings of self-esteem and well-being were improved by the program. Swimming is a very good multisystem conditioning activity.[7]

SUMMARY

ALS is a progressively disabling disease for which there is no known cause or cure. Rehabilitation efforts for these patients are directed toward maintaining performance at a level submaximal to the patient's endurance to save energy and avoid fatigue. Toward these ends, the patient is taught energy conservation and work simplification methods, is provided with orthotics and assistive devices, and is involved in an individualized graded exercise and activity program.[6]

Involvement of patient and family in the rehabilitation process is an essential part of the treatment program. Emotional support and encouragement of rehabilitation team members are necessary to help both patient and family deal with the progressive severity of the disability and terminal illness.

Section 3   Parkinson's disease

Merry Lee Hooks

The Decade of the Brain, 1990-2000, is a national commitment to do research about diagnosis, prevention, and treatment of diseases and disorders that originate in the brain.[20] Through computer technology this information is becoming immediately available to health care professionals and individuals who have Parkinson's disease. Polypharmacy, fetal tissue transplants, pallidotomy, thalamotomy, and the possibility of a genetic marker for people at risk of developing the disease offer a wide range of approaches to ameliorating human suffering. Research may result in elimination of the disease altogether. Although there is no good time to have Parkinson's disease, these next few years will offer more hope than any others in history.

Parkinson's disease is a disease of the basal ganglia. It results in a reduction in dopamine, serotonin, and norepinephrine. The symptoms are resting tremor, cogwheel rigidity, akinesia, bradykinesia, and impairment of the postural mechanism.[3] It is a neurodegenerative disease of aging with insidious onset and slow progression over many years.[30]

It is estimated that one million people, one of every 100 American men and women over the age of 50, share the condition known as Parkinson's disease. Each year 50,000 Americans join the ranks of people with Parkinson's disease. The average age of diagnosis is 57; it is rarely seen under age 30 and is more common after age 55.[31]

tal toxins.[3,8] Other possibilities that have been considered are arteriosclerosis, encephalitis, anoxia, and trauma or drugs. Genetic, immunologic, and infectious causes are also considerations.[8] Parkinson's disease may be a disease of multiple causes. The study of the interrelationships of host, agent, and environment may be significant in finding the cause(s) of Parkinson's disease.

Other related disorders, referred to as *Parkinsonism,* may be caused by factors such as viral infections, brain trauma, exposure to heavy metals, medications such as neuroleptics, antipsychotics, and methyldopa, and carbon monoxide or carbon disulfide gases. The most common cause of Parkinson'sism is drug treatment from neuroleptic therapy, a condition that is reversible.[30]

Parkinson's disease is a movement disorder caused by the unexplained loss of pigmented nerve cells of the substantia nigra. The death of these dopamine-producing cells causes progressively diminished neurotransmission projecting to the basal ganglia. The primary symptoms of Parkinson's disease reflect the gross disruption of normal striopallidal activity and are believed to be due in part to subsequent abnormalities in the motor circuit from the basal ganglia to the thalamus. This circuit is thought to be a reentrant pathway through which influences are returned to certain precentral and postcentral sensorimotor areas of the cortex after processing within the basal ganglia and thalamus.[33]

ETIOLOGY AND PATHOPHYSIOLOGY

The cause of Parkinson's disease is not known. One theory is that the disease may be caused by environmen-

MEDICAL MANAGEMENT

Parkinson's disease was the first degenerative disease of the CNS to be treated effectively by neurotransmitter replacement therapy.[18] The medications are designed to replace dopamine, act as dopamine agonists, act as anticholinergics, or enhance receptor sites of the dopaminergic system. Antioxidants may slow the progress of the disease.

The symptoms of a newly diagnosed person who is medically well-managed may not be readily apparent, and the individual may be able to continue to be active, to work, and to fulfill family, social, and community roles. This period of disease control may be from 4 to 8 years. As the disease progresses, however, increasing amounts of the dopamine precursor levodopa may lead to side effects. The person may experience waning of drug effect before the next dose or may describe the ON-OFF effect of the drug. Other potential problems are drug-related dystonia with sustained muscle contractions, twisting or repetitive movements or abnormal postures, and sudden, nonpurposeful movements known as peak-dose dyskinesia and end-of-dose dyskinesia.

The aging person may be more vulnerable to hallucinations and drug toxicity. Accurate and timely communication with the physician is crucial. Nurse practitioners are often helpful in reviewing medications with the client, family, or care partner. Medication diaries are available and recommended to track medications and their effects.

CLINICAL SIGNS: MOTOR DYSFUNCTION

Akinesia/Bradykinesia

These related terms generally refer to slowness and poverty of movement, difficulty with initiation and execution of willed and associated movements, and difficulty changing one motor pattern to another. Bradykinesia is the main motor symptom in Parkinson's disease and appears as a disorder in voluntary movement. It is considered partly responsible for dysfunction in posture and locomotion.[16,34]

Rigidity

Rigidity is manifested by increased resistance to passive movement of the limbs in any direction. It is characterized by an inability to relax and eliminate voluntary activation of muscles, increased limb stiffness, abnormal coactivation of agonist-antagonist muscle groups, and increased stretch reflexes.[16]

Tremor

A resting tremor is a reciprocal pattern of activation of agonist-antagonist muscle groups. The tremor is rhythmic, involuntary, and oscillatory.[3] The amount and intensity of tremor can be highly variable in the course of one day depending on factors such as alertness and emotional state.

Impairment of the Postural Mechanism

The postural mechanism controls the maintenance of the upright posture and protects the individual from falling secondary to postural perturbation. Vestibular, proprioceptive, and cerebellar mechanisms control posture and movement. Patients with an impaired postural mechanism take extra steps when pivoting during ambulation.[32] Marsden[17] made the following statements about the motor function of the basal ganglia:

1. Intact vision and kinesthesia allow slow movements to be executed by patients with Parkinson's disease, who operate by continuously checking progress.
2. Proprioceptive feedback, however, is not normal in Parkinson disease.
3. Although the dynamic component of the spinal monosynaptic stretch reflex machinery is unremarkable, static stretch reflexes and long-latency, perhaps transcortical stretch reflexes are exaggerated. Both abnormalities may contribute to rigidity.
4. Proprioceptive feedback also is used to generate anticipatory postural reflexes, which are lost or distorted in Parkinson disease.
5. Other postural reflexes, such as righting reactions and protective responses, also are lost in Parkinson's disease.[17]

CLINICAL PICTURE

The person with Parkinson's disease learns to function within the limitations of a "moving therapeutic window" provided by the medications. Early in the disease process, treatment may involve managing the tremor and preventing musculoskeletal changes, loss of mobility and independent living skills, pulmonary complications, or abnormal posture.

When OFF or in late-stage disease, functional problems may include a stooped posture and slow, shortened steps with a direct linear progression, as though on a narrow track. The shortened steps in a forward direction are known as *festination* and in a reverse direction as *retropulsion*. Turns, starts, stops, changes in direction, and backing up are challenges. Balance is impaired and falls are predictable in late-stage disease although people with Parkinson's disease are able to sustain a remarkable tolerance physically and psychologically for these falls. A study by Koller and associates[14] demonstrated that 38% of parkinsonian patients fell, and of those, 13% fell more than once a week. Broken bones, hospitalization, confinement to wheelchair, and fear of walking resulted from falls. The frequency of falling was correlated to the severity of the postural instability.[14]

The rhythm of movement is slowed or replaced by diminished amplitude. All aspects of motor expression mimic this loss of rhythm. Facial expression may not accurately reflect the state of feeling, and thought and speech may be slow, of diminished volume, and lacking inflection. Swallowing may be affected, and the person may have episodes of choking and drooling.

Use of the hands in functional activities reflects impairment of finger mechanoreceptor information. Reciprocal grip and lift in fine motor acts becomes ineffective and unbearably slow. Handwriting is micrographic. Activities such as cutting meat and buttoning reflect defective proprioception and movement. Reading may be difficult because the muscles of the eyes do not move in a coordinated fashion. The person with Parkinson's disease often complains of fatigue.[7] Forty percent of people with Parkinson's disease exhibit symptoms of depression and thirty percent show signs of dementia.[4] Social isolation and sedentary habits distinguish this population.

The activities of self-care are slow, deliberate processes for the person with Parkinson's disease. Indeed, living with a movement disorder is hard work because there are formidable obstacles to self-sufficiency. Yet people with Parkinson's disease are able to remain in the workforce; continue to enjoy family, friends, and community; and to live a normal lifespan.

For the newly diagnosed the process may be one of recognizing and communicating about the effect of the medications. For those who have had Parkinson's disease for a longer time, symptoms and mobility may vary throughout a 24-hour period. This fluctuating mobility slows and disrupts the day's routine and causes dramatic swings in the occupational function/dysfunction continuum.[21] Dynamic strength may be reduced by 10% to 30%.[22] Tightness and slowness may be present very early in the day but after medication, the symptom picture may change dramatically. With waning of medication effect, the patient may again become immobile. Postural instability is the major element in disability at home and at work, leading to premature retirement in many young patients.[5]

OT INTERVENTION

Occupational therapy intervention consists of (1) teaching the patient to accommodate to the symptoms, (2) providing guidelines to prevent musculoskeletal impairments, (3) grading activity to facilitate function despite fluctuating symptoms, and (4) adapting the environment to maximize sensory input and provide greatest effectiveness. Recent studies suggest the possibility that the unconscious component of proprioception is subject to faulty processing and integration within the basal ganglia and this underlying defect in the use of static proprioceptive information leads to errors in movement or judgment about the position of body parts in space.[28] For the hands to work, the shoulder must reach, the head must face the work, and postural support must be dynamic. The occupational therapist helps the patient with Parkinson's disease to remain mobile throughout the course of the disease. The patient must actively participate in therapy, and intervention should include purposeful activities in a structured environment.[11]

OT EVALUATION

A review of the neurologist's report and the results of the magnetic resonance imaging (MRI) are the crucial first steps in the evaluation process. After the chart review, the therapist is prepared to select the evaluation tools that will be most helpful in treatment planning.

A videotape recording is a useful evaluation tool. A recorded image of functional mobility including speed of movement, posture, balance, and functional use of the hands is useful as a baseline evaluation. A baseline videotape provides quantifiable information. The initial position of the patient for videotaping may be seated for hand movements such as writing a sentence, reaching to tie a shoe, and retrieving an offered object. Functional mobility should include rising from a chair, walking twenty feet, returning to the chair, turning around, backing up to the chair, and sitting down. The ADL Oriented Assessment-of-Mobility Scale is suitable for use with elderly people with dementia.[23]

Evaluation of physical dysfunction may include active and passive range of motion (ROM), strength, posture, and functional mobility. Degree and distribution of rigidity are subjective and best determined from the neurologist's report but most quickly noted in elbow and wrist movement (see Chapter 10). The evaluation should also include assessment of fatigue, depression, activity configuration, swallowing (see Chapter 11), cognitive status (see Chapter 15), knowledge about the disease, medications, and participation in support groups.

Assessment guidelines commonly used in evaluation of the client with Parkinson's disease are the Schwab and England ADL Scale,[29] the United Parkinson's Disease Rating Scale,[6] the Hoehn and Yahr Scale (Box 43-1),[9] the Fatigue Severity Scale,[7] the Neurobehavioral Cognitive Status Examination,[13] and Assessment of the Occupational Function/Dysfunction Continuum.[21] The Schenkman and Butler model for multisystem evaluation includes a videotaping protocol and specific treatment measures and guidelines[25] (Fig. 43-1).

OT GOALS

The goals of occupational therapy are as follows:
1. to develop a routine for performing the acts of self-care within the limitations of functional mobility
2. to educate and direct the performance of independent living skills through movement facilitation, therapeutic techniques, and sensory stimulation
3. to establish a repertoire of adaptive techniques and behaviors to stimulate movement
4. to establish an adaptive environment that accommodates immobility and maximizes sensory stimuli
5. to educate the individual, care partner, and family about Parkinson's disease and the process of habilitation
6. to develop a relationship with a support group

BOX 43-1

THE HOEHN AND YAHR SCALE

I   Unilateral involvement only, usually with minimal or no functional impairment.

II   Bilateral or midline involvement without impairment of balance.

III   First signs of impaired righting reflexes. Functionally restricted in his or her activities but can lead independent life. Disability mild to moderate.

IV   Severely disabled. Able to walk and stand unaided, but is markedly handicapped.

V   Confinement to bed or wheelchair unless aided.

From Hoehn MM, Yahr MD: Parkinsonism: onset, progression and mortality, *Neurology* 17:427-442, 1967. Reproduced with permission.

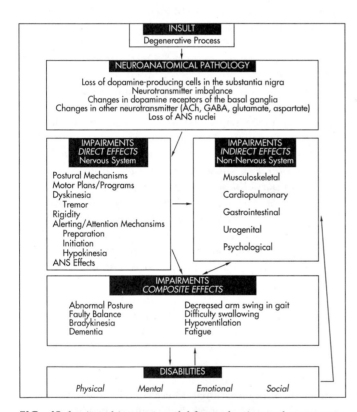

FIG. 43-1 A multisystem model for evaluation and treatment of patients with Parkinson's disease. (From Schenkman M, Butler RB: A model for multisystem evaluation treatment of individuals with Parkinson disease, *Phys Ther* 69(11):939, 1989. Reprinted from *Physical Therapy* with the permission of the American Physical Therapy Association.)

7.   to provide guidelines for habits that facilitate movement and good posture, such as stretching, relaxation, and cognitive and physical activity

TREATMENT METHODS

General principles of treatment include the following:

1.   The patient needs to understand the purpose of occupational therapy and believe this experience will improve his or her ability to function more independently.

2.   The patient needs to be comfortable with the therapeutic milieu and the sense of touch.[19]

3.   The patient needs to feel he or she will not fall.

When treating a patient with postural instability, the therapist should assist the patient in planning a motor response through prior information about the demands of the task. The therapist should then support the motor response through graded stimulation of functionally opposed muscles surrounding an individual joint or of muscles participating at opposite ends of the body (e.g., neck extensors with ankle flexors). The therapist enhances the feedback loop by intensifying a specific sensory input, or supplies cognitive input by discussing the patient's expected and actual response. Interference of conflicting stimuli is limited by having the patient practice a simple postural task within a structured environment.[12]

Routine for ADL

The patient's routine should begin with consistent medication times. People are usually in the OFF state very early in the day and need to take medication shortly after rising. Toileting facilities should be accessible and adapted to allow for compromised balance. Simple clothing and slippers need to be nearby, and the task of dressing should wait until the medication affects intricate and coordinated hand use. Throughout the day, the routine should reflect the state of mobility of the patient. During ON times, the patient performs the most demanding work. During OFF times the patient relies on a "user friendly" environment to accommodate symptoms. Stretching key muscles several times a day prevents muscle spasm, increases proprioceptive feedback, and retains active range of motion to help meet functional challenges such as those required in bed mobility and dressing.

The American Parkinson's Disease Association provides booklets on ADL, written by occupational therapists, free to patients. This information is extremely helpful in providing a home program of practical information about self-care, adaptive equipment, and clothing.[1]

Movement Facilitation

Carefully selected sensory stimuli help people focus on a movement task. Persons with Parkinson's disease call these *tricks*. A trick that frequently stops festination is to change the motor program in process. The therapist should ask the patient to stop and help to restore balance by placing his or her forearm in the patient's hand. The proprioceptive cues received from the patient's arm and hand supply the brain with sufficient information to facilitate upright and balanced posture.

To improve posture, pressure is provided at the foreshoulder and low back. This feedback elicits thoracic extension. The therapist can facilitate lateral weight shift by applying gentle pressure on the opposite hip with one hand while using his or her hip to touch the patient's adjacent hip. The patient is asked to straighten and take a deep breath and then told to step forward as long as the feet are taking long steps. The firmly spoken command "lift" or "toe up" often breaks the freezing, and saying "long stride" may help the individual to stride forward.

Motor Learning

Motor learning is concerned with "the acquisition of new skills with practice"[27] (see Chapter 7). Learned automatic movement patterns, such as reciprocal arm swings and lifting the eyes and head while walking, are affected by Parkinson's disease. Although it is not possible to relearn the automatic movements, the patient may be able to practice these movement patterns in a variety of settings.

To improve head position and facilitate thoracic extension, the patient should be taught to take deep breaths and feel the spinal column straighten. This movement pattern can be used at the computer, in the car, and in a seated or standing position. The therapist may encourage dynamic activities that demand visual tracking and upper body control.[2] Regulation horseshoes, kite flying, volleyball, and kneading bread dough are examples of activities that may involve the patient and that may be done standing or sitting.

Adaptive Techniques

The following can be used to enhance and facilitate movement: correct body mechanics, rhythm, and proprioceptive neuromuscular facilitation.

For example, to use correct body mechanics to stand up from a seated position, have the patient adjust forward in the chair, position the feet and hands, and chant "rock-two-three" with arm movements for each chant. A high stool is preferable to an overstuffed sofa or chair. A bar stool can be used at the work bench, computer, or

kitchen counter to help the patient continuously change position and prevent maladaptive posture while working with the hands and eyes.

Rhythm is effective to help continue movement toward end range. For example, the rhythm of walking is paced between a waltz and a march. Listening to music while walking helps to lengthen and heighten the stride of a person with Parkinson's disease. Handwriting can be practiced to music in a series of movement patterns. Writing a letter incorporates these varied patterns. A 10-week therapeutic handwriting program called *Callirobics** is used by the Washington University Program in Occupational Therapy and has met with success in improving the ability of clients with Parkinson's disease to write letters.[15]

Use of proprioceptive neuromuscular facilitation (PNF) movement patterns (see Chapter 23) are helpful for stretching and to keep kinesthetic memory intact for independent living. Drying off after bathing can be done using reciprocal extension/flexion patterns of the upper and lower body. The caregiver can participate in the activity by guiding the hands to the limits of movement, saying "push" for extension and "hold" for six seconds, and then directing the next pattern. Over time the verbal and tactile cues are withdrawn and timing and sequencing replaced by music of a waltz rhythm or a verbal chant the patient designs. For example: "Push to the corner, relax toward the floor; stretch for the shoulder, and a little bit more." The Schenkman model suggests a progression of treatment within sessions and over time as follows: (1) relaxation, (2) breathing exercises, (3) passive muscle stretching and positioning, (4) active ROM and postural alignment, (5) weight shifting, (6) balance responses, (7) gait activities, and (8) home exercises.[26]

Therapeutic Exercise

Rigidity of muscles that affect rotation profoundly restricts function. People with Parkinson's disease have difficulty turning in bed. Mat activities help with practice in lying down and getting up from the floor as well as rolling from side to side. Activities that require reaching across, looking over the shoulder, and turning the head stimulate vestibular and proprioceptive information and facilitate motor performance. Working in supine on a firm surface provides leverage, which may be lacking in a soft bed.

Rigidity also affects balance and the person with Parkinson's disease needs to practice slow stretching movements frequently. Tai chi, horseshoes, and volleyball combined with a short stretching program afterward may prevent muscle spasm. Balance practice may include imagery of cardinal directions of the compass with visual cues from imitating the therapist to lean north, south, east, and west and degrees between. It is helpful

---

* Callirobics, Box 6634, Charlottesville, VA 22906.

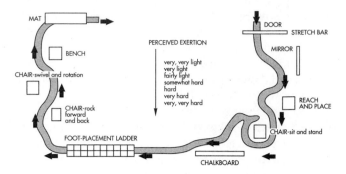

FIG. 43-2 Par course. Client performs functional movement patterns and is assisted to use techniques and practices learned in therapy. Therapist also encourages client to rate perceived exertion while using par course activities. (From Hooks ML, Oliver A: Nonpharmaceutical management of Parkinson's disease. Paper presented at the Parkinson's Institute, Dec. 8, 1993, Sunnyvale, Calif.)

to practice on a "balance beam" made with lines in the dirt or string on a lawn.

A functional par course for use by clients during routine visits to The Parkinson's Institute of Sunnyvale, California, was designed with stations correlated to functional tasks, which included facial expression, handwriting, functional mobility, and speech. Scoring of the stations was scaled similarly to the United Parkinson's Disease Rating Scale, numbers 0 to 4[6,10] (Fig. 43-2). On visits to the doctor, clients were able to spend fifteen minutes moving through the par course with the therapist's supervision and were able to participate actively in the process of measuring change.

Deep Breathing and Relaxation Techniques

Deep breathing and relaxation techniques raise the threshold at which the muscle is stimulated to contract. This approach may be used by the individual to prepare for stretching muscles that have become fatigued. Progressive muscle relaxation and imagery are helpful in preventing muscle tightness during the day. Often, people with Parkinson's disease have muscle spasms during the night. Stretching the large muscles of the shoulders, back, and hips frequently during the day and just before going to bed may alleviate this problem. A stretching program may be done with a towel several times a day to prevent build-up of metabolic by-products.

LONG-TERM CARE

Parkinson's disease is described as a disease of aging. It is not surprising, therefore, to find people with the disease in long-term care settings. Parkinson's disease is also a disease that isolates people if communication and movement are affected. Posture is frequently affected, leading to immobility and problems with self-image. The critical therapeutic goal is to prevent isolation while keeping the resident moving and talking.

The treatment plan may also need to address swallowing problems, and a videofluoroscopy exam may be ordered to rule out silent aspiration (see Chapter 11). Occupational therapy and speech therapy are effective as a team in addressing swallowing, feeding, and communication difficulties. Cotreatment with physical and speech therapy is ideal to encourage the resident to participate socially; walk to and from therapies, meals, and activities; and to be as active physically, intellectually, and socially as possible.

CARE PARTNERS

People with Parkinson's disease need to see themselves as others see them. The impaired motor/sensory system requires an objective observer to help translate the ever-changing picture of symptoms. The care-partner is a useful informant about drug effects and the real impact of the disease process on the partner. Through education, shared problem solving, and accurate communication with the doctor and other health care providers, the impact of the disease may be accommodated.

The partner may need to assist physically at one time or just provide a reminder at another. Psychological support may be sufficient one day and yet on another help may take the form of joining a support group together. The partner may find that the kind of help needed is motivation. Interest, imagination, and wonder stimulate activity. The care-partner may be called upon to be an active role model, surrounded with things to do, and to help make hobbies and interests available to the affected partner. If both partners make a goal of self-expression through activity, the motivation will follow.

The sense of time is affected for people with Parkinson's disease. There is slowness of thought as well as action. Being sensitive to this slowness is important. The partner may be able to give feedback to keep tasks flowing or to help plan a routine to accommodate the slowness. The basics are a balance of rest, exercise and activity, adequate diet, and emotional health.

Any good partnership has a quality of cooperation. In the book *Awakenings,* Oliver Sacks stated, "Love is the alpha and omega of being" and that the work of healing, or rendering whole, is first and last the business of love.[24]

SUPPORT GROUPS

The *Decade of the Brain*[20] continues to produce an outpouring of studies and scientific writing on the subject of Parkinson's disease. Much of this information may be gleaned from support groups and newsletters. A local library, physician's office, or community college may assist in making the Parkinson's Disease Information Exchange [computer] Network available for the support groups. Regular problem discussion and brainstorming sessions increase the knowledge base of the group, and social events help prevent isolation and inactivity. A forum for speakers may attract experts on a variety of subjects. An annual products and services fair is useful in making adaptive equipment and services available.

There are many video and audio exercise programs designed specifically for people with Parkinson's disease. A listing of these is available from the large support groups. The Young Parkinson's Support Network (YPSN)[1] is nationwide and is connected through a computer network.

SUMMARY: A PERSONAL NOTE

For ten years I taught a class called Parkinson's Disease Exercise and Activity through the Therapeutic Recreation Department of the City of San José, California, and West Valley Community College, Saratoga, California. Class members wrote an instructional booklet entitled *Comparing Notes — A Collection of Practical Tips and Solutions for People with Parkinson's Disease.* In addition to the monthly problem-solving process, which stimulated the development of the booklet, other group experiences were included such as the harvest and hobby showcases, holiday luncheons, skits, readings, limericks and lectures, the indoor parcourse, walking program, the telephone tree and buddy system, care-partners group, and the all-important seated volleyball game or horseshoes.

The group had its own library of resource books, videotapes, newsletters, and research information complete with index system and files. A consistent routine of therapeutic exercise was maintained, as well as activities for fun, function, and problem solving. The Peninsula Parkinson's Support Group, located at The Parkinson's Institute, Sunnyvale, California, and the Young Parkinson's Support Network of California helped us form relationships with other support groups in the area. Because of the longevity of the group, we were able to learn about one another as people. We also learned that people with Parkinson's disease are able to manage the disease process and their own lives through association with one another and intelligent behavior.

Section 4   Alzheimer's disease

Pat Atchison, Lorraine Williams Pedretti, Guy L. McCormack

In 1906 a German neurologist named Alois Alzheimer described a condition resulting in progressive intellectual deterioration in a 51-year-old woman.[31,37] Today Alzheimer's (AD) disease is refered to as senile dementia – Alzheimer type (SDAT) and is one of the most common forms of dementias.[14,19,42] Alzheimer's disease is a progressive, degenerative disease that is characterized by an insidious, irreversible loss of memory, cognitive impairment, speech and gait disturbances, disorientation, and changes in personality and behavior.[4,18,35]

Alzheimer's disease affects one person in every five over the age of 65.[38] It is estimated that four million Americans are afflicted with Alzheimer's disease and that this number will increase as the percentage of elderly over the age of 65 increases.[22] Females are diagnosed more frequently with this disease; however, gender difference may be due to womens longer lifespan and the frequency in which they seek medical attention.[42,51] It occurs with equal frequency in all racial, ethnic, and socioeconomic groups.[17,23]

ETIOLOGY

The cause of Alzheimer's disease is unknown, but there are several theories about causal factors. One theory suggests a deficiency of the neurotransmitter acetylcholine in the brain with large reductions in the frontal and temporal lobes.[15] Autopsies have shown that an enzyme catalyst needed for the production of acetylcholine is 70% to 90% below normal levels in the AD brain.[35] Another theory suggests that a slow-acting virus may be the cause.[31,36,38,46,47] A third theory suggests exogenous toxins such as aluminum, which have been found in concentration in dying neurons of AD patients, may have some causation or be an effect of the disease.[29,42,46] Head trauma may be another predisposing factor to Alzheimer disease in later life.[29,33]

Yet other studies hypothosize the presence of a protein, amyloid that causes destruction of blood vessels and neurons in the brain. Studies have shown a greater amount of destruction by this protein in the hippocampus and neocortex of the AD patient than in the normal aging brain.[31,36,40] It is the amyloid protein's presence and the correlation between Down's syndrome and AD that suggest a genetic link. Patients with Down's syndrome develop plaques and tangles identical to those found in AD.[30] Reisburg[44] stated that "One hundred percent of persons with Down's syndrome who survive into middle life develop a clinical and pathological condition identical to Alzheimer's disease!"[44]

It has also been hypothesized that the increased production of the beta amyloid protein in the brain of persons with AD has a direct link to chromosome 21.[5,27,46] Finally, studies have shown a familial correlation in early onset AD patients. It is believed that there is a single autosomal dominant pattern on chromosome 21 in families with multiple early onset AD victims.[5,13]

PATHOPHYSIOLOGY

Pathophysiology studies show that the brain of persons with AD undergoes atrophy, especially in the frontal and temporal lobes. Widening of sulci and narrowing of gyri result in a brain that is underweight. The cerebral ventricles are dilated, which causes pressure on the hippocampal formation. Histologic studies show loss of neurons in the cortex, nucleus basalis, and locus ceruleus. Other microscopic signs are senile plaques, which are ringlike structures resulting from gliosis; neurofibrillary tangles, which are coiled filaments twisted in helical configurations; and intraneuronal granulovacuolar degeneration, which signifies the formation of cavities within the cytoplasms of neurons.[12,14,15,32,50]

The clinical features of Alzheimer's disease may vary, and the course of the disorder may range from 5 to 25 years. The course of the disease is usually categorized in three stages.[1,23,25] In the initial stage the patient may be oriented, but begins to have difficulty with short-term memory. During this stage he or she may lose things, lack concentration, and experience mood changes. These changes are often subtle, may go unnoticed, or may merely be disregarded as fatigue.[11,16] The individual may deny difficulty with familiar tasks and try to cover up by confabulating. Recognition of limitations may cause depresion, anxiety, and frustration.[17,48]

In middle stage of AD, the individual begins to have difficulty with orientation and shows marked loss of memory. There is difficulty recognizing distant family members, remembering appointments, and retaining recently acquired information. The person may be unable to recall actions from yesterday, but can reminisce about events from long ago. Problems may surface with hygiene, dressing, eating, and speech. The individual with AD begins to become lost in familiar surroundings and the anxiety, frustration, and depression become more apparent.

Episodic bouts of irritability, aphasia, apraxia, neurologic movement disorders, inability to communicate effectively, sleep disturbances, and night wandering are manifested.[11,17,48] Symptoms may be magnified as the evening nears with increased pacing and wandering. This behavior is known as sundowning.[16] Such individuals need assistance in most of their activities of daily living, but can assist the caregiver.

As the disease progresses, patients have marked short- and long-term memory loss with constant disorientation to person, place, and time. They are unable to recognize close family members and more severe language deficits emmerge.[16,48] They become apathetic, unresponsive to stimuli, incontinent, prone to seizures, agitated, and may experience hallucinations. Increased frustration may lead to overreacting to minor events, which is termed castastrophic reaction.[16] Eventually they need assistance in all levels of care and require 24-hour supervision.[11,17]

In the final or terminal stage of Alzheimer's disease, patients are completely dependent in all aspects of daily living. They become apathetic and unresponsive to external stimuli except for facial grimacing.[48] They need to be fed and may be unable to swallow. Meaningful language and memory is absent with severe disorientation and marked agitation present.[17,48] There is little interaction with the physical environment, and motor function is decreased. They are generally bed- or chair-bound with incontinence of bowel and bladder.[16,48] Eventually, the patient may succumb to an infectious disease.[11]

MEDICAL MANAGEMENT

Presently the medical management tends to be experimental and symptomatic.[37] The use of acetylcholine precursors, cholinergic agonists, and cholinesterase inhibitors have been found to have some affects in early stage Alzheimer's disease; however, further research of their effectiveness is warranted. Phenothiazines (tranquilizers) are used to lessen the anxiety and restlessness associated with AD. These tranquilizers include Xanax, Ativan, Haldol, and Trilafon.[46,49] Antidepressants such as Norpramin and Elavil are other drugs commonly used. Medical management is also geared to help the patient function at an optimal level throughout the course of the disease, thus addressing maintenance of the patient's general health, independence, basic orientation, personal safety, and dignity.[1,11]

OT INTERVENTION

Alzheimer's disease profoundly affects the primary caregiver and all family members as well as the person with AD. If treatment is to be effective, the healthcare professional must consider the needs of all those involved.[28] The role of occupational therapy with persons with dementia focuses on self-care, independent living skills, and assessment of potential for continued employment if the patient is still in the early stages of the disease.[3] In addition, family education, behavior management, and support are also essential components of the occupational therapy program.

Occupational therapy provides a graded program of environmental modification and task simplification, which keeps pace with the patient's declining capacities. Such an approach allows the patient to maintain as much control over life as possible at each stage of the disease and to retain a sense of personal dignity. This structured environment also helps to manage stable behavior.[39] An important component of the occupational therapy program is to teach care givers how to manage the progressive incapacities of the patient to prevent institutionalization.[3]

OT EVALUATION

The purposes of the occupational therapy evaluation of a patient with AD are to assess the level of cognitive and motor functioning and to assess performance skills of self-care, home management, and leisure activities.[3] The occupational therapist administers tests of perceptual and cognitive abilities and observes for deficits of these functions during activity performance. Common cognitive evaluation tests used include the Mini-Mental State Examination (MMSE), Allen Cognitive Level Test (ACL), and the Cognitive Performance Test (CPT).[2,7,26] Evaluation of range of motion (ROM), coordination, equilibrium, muscle tone, gait, posture, and movement speed and rhythm are used to assess motor functioning.[52]

As the disease process continues and the patient loses the ability to communicate, evaluation tools that rely predominately on performance are warranted. A comprehensive evaluation of performance skills includes self-care assessments: feeding, swallowing, dressing, toileting, hair and nail care, bathing, shaving or make-up application, and mobility. Home management evaluation may include telephoning, meal preparation, doing laundry, housecleaning, gardening, and money management.[3,52] Two performance evaluations commonly used by occupational therapists include the Assessment of Motor and Process Skills test (AMPS) and the KTA (Kitchen Task Assessment).[10,41]

Performance of leisure skills is assessed through expressed interests, interest history, and observation of performance. If intervention is early, when cognitive impairment is minimal, evaluation of work skills is indicated. The therapist's skills may be needed to help assess the patient ability to continue driving and working. An assessment of environmental factors such as space, equipment, and objects should be a part of the occupational therapy evaluation to determine how the environment helps or hinders the patient's performance.[3,52] Recommendations for changes in space, equipment, and furniture arrangement to enhance the function and modify behavior of the patient may be made by the occupational therapist.

Data for the occupational therapy evaluation are obtained by interviewing the patient, family members, or caregivers. It is important that the therapist have a clear understanding of the patient's history before initiating the evaluation process. The therapist must always take into account that a diagnosis of AD can be established only during an autopsy and that other age-related processes may affect the patient's performance.

Performance skills are evaluated by observing the patient doing tasks. The performance observation yields information about those tasks that the patient performs easily, with moderate difficulty, or those that are not possible to perform. The occupational therapist determines factors that underlie dysfunctional performance. Careful consideration is given to the balance of activity in the patient's day. Too much activity may precipitate confusion or a catastrophic reaction, and too little activity may induce lethargy.[3]

The occupational therapy evaluation serves as a guide for selecting objectives and intervention strategies that are within the realm of the patient's and caregiver's capabilities. In addition, the evaluation may be used to determine the level of supervision or care the patient needs. The occupational therapy evaluation also can contribute valuable information for decision making about the feasibility of independent living and the need for attendant care or guardianship. Work evaluation can determine the feasibility of continued employment or the need for work adaptations. The effect of medical treatment on behavior can be assessed by controlled observation of patient performance in the occupational therapy clinic.[3]

OT GOALS

The goals of occupational therapy for the patient with Alzheimer's disease are (1) to improve or maintain functional capacities for as long as possible, (2) to maintain level of attention and memory, (3) to promote participation in activities that enhance physical and mental health, (4) to aid in socialization, (5) to increase patient comfort, and (6) to increase ease of activities for caregivers.[3,25] For the caregiver, the occupational therapist offers (1) support, (2) stress reduction, (3) training and education, (4) environmental adaptation, and (5) assistance with problem solving.[21,22]

TREATMENT METHODS
Activity Programs

Activities selected should be voluntary, relevant, and within the patient's physical and mental capacity, and should offer reasonable chance for success. The activity should never be childish or demeaning. Its purpose should be obvious to the patient. One way of grading activities for this population is by the degree of task involvement of the patient. Involvement can range from merely attending to a task that is presented, to initiating, planning, and executing an entire task independently. Activities most suitable for grading in this way are those involving several steps. To determine their suitability, activities must be analyzed for their physical, sensory, perceptual, and cognitive demands.[52]

Patients with Alzheimer's disease should be encouraged but not coerced to participate in an activity program. The therapist should use a structured approach with clear, concise instructions. The patient's habitual skills can be used advantageously. Although some habitual skills may be lost, the loss tends to be patchy while important abilities may be intact.[52] Active exercise, supervised activities of daily living (ADL), simple leisure activities related to past hobbies and interests, and structured social activities are useful for maintenance of physical and mental capacities.[3,25,52] Performance is sometimes better when rhythmic activities such as dancing and threading beads are used. Rhythmic walking may be done with more ease and instructions followed more accurately if given simply and in a rhythmic tone.[52]

As deterioration progresses, tasks must be analyzed to their component parts. Breaking down activities into more manageable steps allows for more success in functional activities. The more the activities are structured, the better the opportunity to maintain stable behavior.[39] It is then determined whether the patient with Alzheimer disease is capable of any part of the given task. In an activity group, each member may be assigned one part of a process so that the entire group completes a given activity.

Caregivers must avoid the tendency to take over all of the patient's activities, because this approach leads to inactivity and depression and hastens deterioration. The AD patient still feels the need to be productive and wants to have a sense of worth.[39,52] Continued engagement in activity has an influence on the patient's reality orientation.

Exercise, games, crafts, sensory stimulation, and rhythm activities may be used to maintain joint mobility, strength, mental alertness, and self-esteem. The debilitating effects of contractures, decubiti, fatigue, and depression can be forestalled by engaging the patient in activities at an appropriate level.[3] Zgola[52] offers several specific guidelines for activities, the activity program, and suitable environment and routine.

Environmental Modification

The occupational therapist can structure the environment to maximize the patient's performance. The environment should be kept predictable and familiar, consistent, and free of ambiguities.[4,25,52] The environment must be free from clutter to prevent agitation and to allow for optimal cue finding.[22] Furniture should have clear limits. Traffic areas should be free of obstacles.[3,25,52] Contrasting colors and textures can be used effectively to help the patients distinguish figures from background, as well as to decrease wandering by disguising doors and other environmental factors that may cause agitation.[4,20,25,52] Signs, photos, or drawings may be used to help identify rooms or objects. Areas that allow for interaction with the environment can be used for sensory integration and to decrease wandering by providing an area in which the patient with AD may safely explore the environment.[20]

Activities of Daily Living

As Alzheimer's disease progresses, the patient will require assistance with ADL. Simple assistive devices may make independent performance of some activities possible. Devices such as a tub seat or toilet rails may assist the caregiver in managing the patient with AD. Structuring the environment and cuing the patient during routine daily tasks such as washing and dressing allow the patient to participate in his or her own care. This task breakdown takes time to develop; however, once a routine is established the caregiver can get some relief and the patient will not be dependent in all aspects of ADL.[9,39]

Frequent orientation to time and place and frequent changes of activity may be helpful.[3,8,25] Arkin[6] suggests memory training in early Alzheimer's disease by means such as memory notebooks, sytematic teaching, and teaching prospective memory skills can improve function in ADL.

Patterning of social interactions and structuring is important for maintaining daily living skills. Activities should be broken down into very short steps. Instructions must be clear, concise, and brief. Verbal, visual, or physical prompting may help the patient to initiate and perform activities. Caregivers can be taught these methods for helping the patient initiate and sustain activity.[3,25]

Behavioral Control

It is important to eliminate sources of agitation and thus to avoid or reduce catastrophic reactions characteristic of this disease. These reactions may include a refusal to cooperate, outbursts of crying, stubbornness, and combative behavior.[24,25] Catastrophic reactions are caused by sensory or cognitive overload, misinterpretation of information, fatigue, or frustration over the inability to perform. They are generally excessive responses to minor situations. These reactions occur more frequently when the person becomes overwhelmed by personal limitations.[16,24] The patient is unable to modulate behavior; thus the therapist must try to reduce the reaction, which is done by getting the patient's attention, providing reassurance, and verbalizing what is happening.

Information must be given step-by-step, slowly and clearly. The patient must be able to see the therapist clearly. Activity and noise are reduced. Choice making is limited and reassuring touch without reastraints is used. Arguing should be avoided, and the therapist or caregiver should respond sympathetically to the patient's stress. Remove the patient to a calmer environment and use distraction to divert attention.[16,25]

The occupational therapist, the occupational therapy assistant, and the caregivers should take note of the kinds of stimuli or activity that provoke such reactions. The therapist may promote change in the caregivers approach and assist with improving communication through education. Human contact, social interaction, and frequent changes of activity may be helpful. Those responsible for treatment and care should use a calm, slow, and soft voice and allow adequate response time.[16,25,34] In a study by Baum[9] it was found that patients with Alzheimer's disease who were engaged in activities had fewer behavioral problems and could perform simple ADL tasks with less difficulty, but the caregiver had to structure the task.[9]

Family Education

The family should be made aware of the causes and handling of catastrophic reactions. It should be reinforced that their loved one is not in control of this behavior and it should not be personalized.[24] The occupational therapist can educate and train the family best in the home setting. Corcoran[21] describes an intervention process that involves five home visits in a three-month period by a registered occupational therapist. The first visit focuses on building rapport and establishment of goals, and the second visit focuses on the identification of environmental influences and behaviors. During this visit the occupational therapist educates the family members about dementia, models specific care activities, and uses the surroundings as a therapeutic tool. The caregiver and the therapist then develop a plan. On the third visit the plan is reviewed and implemented with discussion regarding its effectiveness.

On the fourth visit the occupational therapist starts to phase out of the position of control and allows the caregiver to develop his or her own skills. During the final visit the problem-solving process is reviewed and any final modifications are made.[21] In the final stages of the disease, the occupational therapist can contribute to patient safety and comfort by assisting caregivers with life maintenance functions. The therapist can instruct the caregiver in bed positioning, ROM exercises, dysphagia management, lifting and moving skills, and assistance with ADL. The use of touch, gentle speech, and tender loving care gives comfort to the patient.[3,25]

The rehabilitation team members must offer as much support as possible to the patient and the family. Recommendations for home modifications, safety factors, and handling catastrophic reactions need to be made at the appropriate time and with respect by members of the rehabilitation team. Determination of the caregiver's willingness and ability to care for the patient, the need for respite care, and potential plans for institutional placement must be handled by members of the rehabilitation team.[3,32]

Recommendations for the Therapist

Glickstein[28] offers several tips to healthcare professionals working with patients who have Alzheimer's disease. She recommends that therapists should be realistic and develop plans of action based on the patient's current level of function. Expectations that treatment can alter the course or outcome of the disease leads to frustration. It is important for the healthcare professional to work with others and to have ongoing reinforcement. The therapist should identify the patient's needs and all the barriers to fulfilling those needs.

Communication can be enhanced if the therapist addresses the patient directly by name and identifies self by name as well. Eye contact should be established with the patient before communication is attempted. The patient needs time to respond. Repetition is helpful and directions should be short and simple. The patient should not be offered choices unless he or she is capable of making a choice. Consistency of approach and of activities is very helpful in handling the patient with dementia.[28]

Day Care

The erratic behavior, irritability, poor judgment, and physical decline of patients with AD places a severe strain on family caregivers. Therefore, caregivers need options for assistance and respite. This relief comes in the form of an adult day-care center.[8] Day-care programs for patients with Alzheimer's disease and related disorders are increasing in number. Occupational therapists and occupational therapy assistants may be part of the staff of such programs. The purposes of day-care programs are to increase socialization, maintain physical and mental well-being, and promote reality orientation and task participation for the clients. In addition, the programs offer respite care to the primary caregiver and family members.[45]

Rudolph[45] describes a program that is open 3 days a week. This program accepts clients at all functional levels except those who are hazardous to themselves or others or are in need of constant attention and maximal physical assistance. The program includes a morning coffee time, which incorporates reality orientation activities such as reading and discussing the newspaper. Following this period, the clients are engaged in gross motor activity such as walking or simple chair exercises. The rest of the day includes relaxation and quiet time, music, entertainment, table games, and crafts. Clients also assist in preparing lunch and snacks. Participation in various activities is encouraged. Parallel programming allows clients at different functional levels to participate. The center provides nurturing and improved quality of life for the clients and their families.

Respite care has resulted in decreased depression in clients and families. The center serves as an interim step between home care and institutional placement.[45] Rabinowitz[43] described a day-care program on Saturdays only in New York City. This program uses activities such as reality orientation, reminiscence, exercises that use concrete objects such as an elastic jump rope for stretching, activities such as balloon toss, meal preparation, crafts, and structured games. Outdoor activities are sometimes used, and a special event such as pet therapy or a live concert is planned once a month.[43] Day-care programs also provide needed support systems for the care givers. Social workers, psychologists, and nursing staff may be available along with the occupational therapist to train and assist the family during stressful situations.

SUMMARY

In the treatment of patients with Alzheimer's disease and related disorders, the role of occupational therapy is to support, maintain, and improve the quality of life for the individual and the caregiver. The therapist must accept the progressive deterioration of the patient while providing intervention that stimulates maximal function in all phases of the disease process. The therapist must be one who cares about the patient and strives to make life as comfortable and fulfilling as possible in spite of the fact that the disease is incurable and decline is inevitable.

 SAMPLE TREATMENT PLAN

The following treatment plan is not a comprehensive one but a good initial sample for the hypothetical patient. It deals with five problems on the Problem List. The reader is encouraged to add objectives and methods to deal with the additional problems to make a more comprehensive plan.

CASE STUDY

Mr. D is a 30-year-old man who has multiple sclerosis, with onset 3 years ago. Since that time, there have been some short periods of remission, but generally a steady decline in function. Present symptoms are blurred vision, ataxia, upper extremity tremors, low physical endurance, limited standing tolerance, and occasional urinary incontinence.

Present functional limitations include difficulty with ambulation and transfers, meal preparation, writing, and feeding. He moves about his home with an ataxic gait while holding onto furniture, appliances, and doorframes.

Before onset of the disease, Mr. D worked as an inspector in a high-technology electronics factory. The job required long periods of standing, excellent visual acuity, and fine hand coordination. Mr. D has left the job and is being compensated by disability insurance.

Mr. D is single and has never been married. He lives in the home of his parents. His leisure activities were dating, dancing, sports, rock music, and computer activities. After the onset of the disease, he has tried to continue with the computer operation, but is having difficulty operating the keyboard and mouse control. He enjoys collecting rock music CDs and listening to sporting events on the radio and television.

Following the diagnosis of MS, Mr. D was in a reactive depression for several weeks. This depression lifted following prescription of an antidepressant medication in conjunction with early rehabilitation therapy. At this time, Mr. D demonstrates cheerfulness and a good sense of humor.

He was referred to occupational therapy for evaluation and training in ADL, equipment assessment and training, upper extremity management, vision loss compensation training, and exploration of leisure activities. Treatment precautions include avoidance of fatigue, stress, heat, and cold temperatures.

TREATMENT PLAN

Personal Data
Name: Mr. D
Age: 30
Diagnosis: Multiple sclerosis
Disability: Ataxia, tremors, poor vision

Treatment aims as stated in referral: Evaluation and training in ADL, equipment assessment and training, upper extremity management, vision loss compensation training, and exploration of leisure activities

OTHER SERVICES

Physician: Prescription of medication, oversee rehabilitation program, maintenance of general health
Physical therapy: Exercise for lower extremities, gait training with aids, safety in transfers
Social service: Family and patient counseling; assistance with financial arrangements for treatment. Contacts with community support groups.

Community social group: MS Society support group and education program

Frame of reference
Occupational performance

Treatment approach
Rehabilitative

SAMPLE TREATMENT PLAN – cont'd

OT EVALUATION

Performance components

Sensorimotor functioning
  Functional strength: Observe and test
  ROM: Test
  Physical endurance: Observe and interview
  Muscle tone: Test and observe
  Hand function: Test
  Coordination: Test and observe
  Involuntary movement: Observe
  Sensation: Test, observe, and interview
  Visual perception: Test and observe
  Functional visual acuity: Test and observe
Cognitive functioning
  Judgment: Observe

Safety awareness: Interview and observe
Motivation: Interview and observe
Intellectual functions: Observe
Psychosocial functioning
  Adjustment to disability: Observe
  Emotional stability, affect: Observe
  Coping skills: Observe
Interpersonal relationships: Observe and interview

Performance areas

Self-care: Observe and interview
Mobility: Test and observe
Home management: Test, observe, and interview
Leisure skills: Test, observe, and interview

EVALUATION SUMMARY

Evaluation of sensorimotor function revealed ataxia of the lower extremities with mild spasticity in hip flexor and adductor groups. Gait is unsteady because of ataxia. Upper extremity strength is good, but movement is affected by mild tremors especially when patient attempts to perform fine movements. Scores on the Jebsen Test of Hand Coordination were 3 standard deviations below the norm, showing a mild coordination disturbance. Passive ROM is within normal limits for all upper extremity joint motions. Physical endurance is limited to one half hour of moderate activity (e.g., standing or light bicycling) before he experiences fatigue and needs a rest.

Tests of sensation revealed that touch, pain, pressure, and thermal and proprioceptive senses are intact. Stereognosis is intact bilaterally. Accurate testing of visual perception was not possible because of blurred vision. Functional visual acuity is adequate for moving about in the environment, recognizing faces and large objects, and performing gross motor activities. Reading, identifying paper money, and working with small objects are not possible because of visual limitation.

According to the report of both Mr. D and his parents,

intellectual functioning is the same as before onset of illness. Mr. D is not always aware of potential hazards at home. He gets about by holding onto furniture, walls, and doorframes, which he believes is safe. He tends to overestimate his capabilities and resists the use of aids or assistance. He is well motivated for rehabilitation and seems to enjoy the socialization it offers him.

Mr. D is independent in dressing activities. He has some difficulty raising a full glass to his mouth and managing some types of food from hand to mouth. His responsibilities for meal preparation are minimal. His mother leaves a sandwich for him and he prepares coffee at lunchtime. He has some difficulty managing the placement of the coffee into the basket and pouring the water into the coffee maker while maintaining his balance.

He spends his time listening to music, attempting to operate his computer games, and listening to the television. He has difficulty with the computer because of his poor vision and incoordination for keyboard and mouse operation. Because of easy fatigability, he takes two or three short naps each day.

ASSETS

Good intelligence
Family support
Good family relationships
Comfortable living situation

Good sensation
Motivation
Good range of motion
Positive affect

PROBLEM LIST

  1. Ataxia
  2. Tremors

  3. Incoordination
  4. Lower extremity spasticity

5. Low physical endurance and standing tolerance
6. Difficulty with mobility and transfers
7. Poor safety awareness
8. Partial dependence in ADL
9. Not realistic about potential hazards and own abilities

10. Loss of social activities
11. Loss of work role
12. Loss of leisure skills

PROBLEMS 1, 6: ATAXIA, DIFFICULTY WITH MOBILITY AND TRANSFERS

Objective
Patient will use a front-wheel walker safely with minimal to moderate supervision

Method
Following gait training with the walker by a physical therapist, patient does clinic activities using the walker in performance of ADL. These activities include using the walker while making coffee and to ambulate to the kitchen table, bed, standing table, and stationary bike. Cues for safety and correct use of the walker are given by the therapist as required.

Educate parents about correct use of the walker and necessary supervision. Walker is to be taken home for moving about in the house during ADL following a home visit to assess patient's use of the walker in the home.

Gradation
Decrease verbal cues and supervision as safety awareness and correct procedure improve; introduce a wheelchair for mobility as function declines.

PROBLEM 5: LOW PHYSICAL ENDURANCE

Objective
Physical endurance for moderate activity will be maintained or increased from 30 to 40 minutes

Method
Stationary bicycle with no resistance for two 10-minute periods followed by 10 minutes of rest during the treatment

hour. Patient listens to music on personal radio while cycling. Patient stands at high table for two 10-minute periods during kitchen or grooming activities.

Gradation
Maintain same time schedule or increase time spent in activities if endurance allows.

PROBLEM 8: PARTIAL DEPENDENCE IN ADL

Objective
Increase safety and independence in lunch preparation, cleanup, and feeding

Method
To prepare lunch, patient uses walker with attached tray to gather prepared sandwich, dishes, and silverware and brings them to table. Soiled dishes and silverware are returned to the sink after he has eaten. Dishes are left in the

sink. He prepares the coffee by stabilizing his arm against the counter to fill the coffee basket and pour the water. He uses a broad-based, weighted cup with a lid and a long plastic straw.

Gradation
When function declines, Mrs. D will leave a thermos of coffee with a long straw. Use of a nonskid mat, plate guard, and weighted utensils may assist in feeding.

PROBLEM 12: LOSS OF LEISURE SKILLS

Objective
Patient will engage in meaningful leisure activities and initiate participation without cuing

Method
Explore possibility of computer use with enlarged screen and keyboard guards or an enlarged membrane keyboard or joystick operation. Use weighted wrist cuff to decrease tremors.

Organize music collection by artist or type of music. Cases can be color-coded with large stickers in geometric shapes.

Explore possibility of talking book services at local library.

Gradation
Increase passive activities such as listening to music, sports programs, and talking books.

REVIEW QUESTIONS

SECTION 1: MULTIPLE SCLEROSIS (MS)

1. Briefly describe the pathology of MS.
2. List three theories of the possible causes of MS.
3. Which psychological problem is sometimes associated with MS?
4. What is the overall goal of occupational therapy?
5. List the elements of the occupational therapy assessment.
6. Describe appropriate treatment procedures for maintenance or improvement of motor functioning.
7. List the treatment precautions.

REVIEW QUESTIONS

SECTION 2: AMYOTROPHIC LATERAL SCLEROSIS (ALS)

8. What is the pathology of ALS?
9. Describe the outstanding clinical manifestations.
10. How are speech and respiration affected in ALS?
11. Describe the stages of progression of ALS.
12. Describe the OT evaluation of a patient with ALS.
13. List six goals of OT for ALS.
14. How is treatment graded for ALS?
15. What are some alternatives for loss of verbal communication?

REVIEW QUESTIONS

SECTION 3: PARKINSON'S DISEASE

16. Which brain structures are affected in Parkinson's disease?
17. List six symptoms of Parkinson's disease.
18. Define the following terms: Bradykinesia, rigidity, tremor.
19. Is Parkinson's disease amenable to medications? What is their effect?
20. What is meant by moving therapeutic window?
21. How is function modulated within the therapeutic window?
22. What are the components of the occupational therapy evaluation?
23. List at least four goals of occupational therapy for patients with Parkinson's disease.
24. What are some rules for the routine for ADL?
25. Discuss some treatment methods and modalities that may be suitable for patients with Parkinson's disease.
26. What are some activities or exercises that can help reduce rigidity?
27. What is the role of a care partner?
28. How can support groups be helpful to the individual with Parkinson's disease?

REVIEW QUESTIONS

SECTION 4: ALZHEIMER'S DISEASE

29. What is the pathophysiology of Alzheimer's disease?
30. List the clinical features of the disease.
31. What is the characteristic progression?
32. What are the purposes of occupational therapy?
33. Describe what is meant by environmental modification.
34. List the elements of the occupational therapy evaluation.
35. What are the goals of occupational therapy?
36. Describe the principles of an activity program for Alzheimer's disease.
37. Define catastrophic reaction.
38. How can such reactions be managed?

REFERENCES

SECTION 1: MULTIPLE SCLEROSIS

1. Abissi C, Scheinberg L: Multiple Sclerosis: diagnosis and treatment, *Med Times* 7:109, 1981.
2. Allen I: The pathology of multiple sclerosis: fact, fiction and hypothesis, *Neurol Appl Neurobiol* 7:169, 1982.
3. Alter M, Yamoor M, Harshe M: Multiple sclerosis and nutrition, *Arch Neurol* 31:267, 1974.
4. Bahlin-Webb SR: A weighted wrist cuff, *Am J of Occup Ther* 40(5):363-4, 1986.
5. Beisel K: Multiple sclerosis—factors that affect activity performance: a patient survey. *Physical Disabilities Special Interest Section Newsletter* 6:1, 1983, American Occupational Therapy Association.
6. Blaivas JG: Management of bladder dysfunction in multiple sclerosis, *Neurol* 30:12, 1980.
7. Cole M, Ross RJ: Plaque of multiple sclerosis seen in computerized transaxial tomography, *Neurol* 27:360, 1977.
8. Ekberg PS: *Neurologist's perceptions of and referrals to occupational therapy for persons with multiple sclerosis,* San José State University, San José, Calif, 1985 (master's thesis).
9. Erickson RP, Lie MR, Wineinger MA: Rehabilitation in multiple sclerosis, *Mayo Clin Proc* 64:818-28, 1989.
10. Fellow SN: Wheelchair access: a privilege you deserve. In Wolf JK, editor: *Mastering multiple sclerosis: a guide to management,* Rutland, Vt, 1987, Academy Books.
11. Fischman HR: Multiple sclerosis: a new perspective on epidemiologic patterns, *Neurology* 32:864, 1982.
12. Foley FW and associates: Stress, multiple sclerosis and everyday functioning, *Neuro Rehabil* 3(4):57-66, 1993.
13. Frankel D: Multiple sclerosis. In Umphred DA, editor: *Neurological rehabilitation,* St Louis, 1990, CV Mosby.
14. Gilman S: The diagnosis of multiple sclerosis, *JAMA* 246(10):1122, 1981.
15. Gilroy I, Meyer JS: *Medical neurology,* ed 3, New York, 1979, Macmillan.
16. Harmon JE: *Multiple sclerosis: laying a foundation for occupational therapy,* Occupational Therapy Forum, October 4, 1991:4-9.

17. Kurland LT: The frequency and geographic distribution of multiple sclerosis as indicated by mortality surveys in the US and Canada, *Am J Hygiene* 55:457, 1952.

18. LaRocca NG, Kalb RC: Efficacy of rehabilitation in multiple sclerosis, *J Neuro Rehabil* 6:147-155, 1992.

19. LaRocca NG, Kalb RC, Foley FW, Caruso LS: Assessment of psychosocial outcomes, *J Neuro Rehabil* 7:109-116, 1993.

20. Leibowitz U, Kahana E, Altes M: Changing frequency of multiple sclerosis in Israel, *Arch Neurol* 29:197, 1973.

21. Lisak RP: Multiple sclerosis: evidence for immunopathogenesis, *Neurol* 30(2):99, 1980.

22. Matthews WB, Archeson ED, Batchelor JR, Weller RO: *McAlpine's multiple sclerosis,* New York, 1985, Churchill Livingstone.

23. Patzold V, Pocklington PR: Course of multiple sclerosis, *Acta Neurol Scand* 65(4):248, 1982.

24. Phair LS, Holland NJ: Nursing outcomes in multiple sclerosis, *J Neuro Rehabil* 7:131-7, 1993.

25. Poser CM: Epidemiology and genetics of multiple sclerosis. In Scheinberg LC, Holland NJ, editors: *Multiple sclerosis: a guide for patients and their families,* New York, 1987, Raven Press.

26. Post KM: Technology for people with multiple sclerosis, *Physical Disabilities Special Interest Section Newsletter* 12(4):3-6, 1989, American Occupational Therapy Association.

27. Rudick RA, Goodkin DE, Ransohoff RM: Pharmocotherapy of multiple sclerosis: current status, *Cleveland Clinic Journal of Medicine* 59:267-77, 1992.

28. Schapiro RT: *Symptom management in multiple sclerosis,* New York, 1994, Demos Publications.

29. Scheinberg LC, Smith CR: Rehabilitation of patients with multiple sclerosis, *Neuro Clin* 5:585-600, 1987.

30. Scheinberg LC, Smith CR: Signs and symptoms of multiple sclerosis: In Scheinberg LC, Holland NJ, editors: *Multiple sclerosis: a guide for patients and their families,* New York, 1987, Raven Press.

31. Spencer EA: Functional restoration: specific diagnosis. In Hopkins HL, Smith HD: *Willard and Spackman's occupational therapy,* ed 7, Philadelphia, 1988, JB Lippincott.

32. Tourtenotte WW: *Therapeutics of multiple sclerosis,* South Deerfield, Mass, 1981, Channing L Bete.

33. Turner A, editor: *The practice of occupational therapy,* ed 2, New York, 1987, Churchill Livingstone.

34. Weeks C: Multiple sclerosis: the malignant uncertainty, *Am J Nurs* 80(2):298, 1980.

35. Wolf B: Occupational therapy for patients with multiple sclerosis. In Maloney FP, Burks JS, Ringel SP, editors: *Interdisciplinary rehabilitation of multiple sclerosis and neuromuscular disorders,* Philadelphia, 1985, JB Lippincott.

36. Wolf JK: *Mastering multiple sclerosis: a guide to management,* Rutland, Vt, 1987, Academy Books.

REFERENCES

SECTION 2: AMYOTROPHIC LATERAL SCLEROSIS

1. Blount MN, Bratton C, Luttrell N: Management of the patient with amyotrophic lateral sclerosis, *Nurs Clin North Am* 14:157, 1979.

2. Brammell CA: Assistive devices for patients with neuromuscular diseases: the role of occupational therapy. In Maloney FP, Burks JS, Ringel SP, editors: *Interdisciplinary rehabilitation of multiple sclerosis and neuromuscular diseases,* Philadelphia, 1985, JB Lippincott.

3. Gilroy I, Meyer JS: *Medical neurology,* ed 3, New York, 1979, Macmillan.

4. Hopkins H: ALS: "Lou Gehrig's disease" still needs a cure, *FDA Consumer* 17(12):23, 1984.

5. Hudson AJ: Amyotrophic lateral sclerosis and its association with dementia, parkinsonism and other neurological disorders: a review, *Brain* 194:36, 1981.

6. Janiszewski DW, Carosico JT, Wisham LH: Amyotrophic lateral sclerosis: a comprehensive rehabilitation approach, *Arch Phys Med Rehabil* 64:304, 1983.

7. Johnson CR: Case report: aquatic therapy for an ALS patient, *Am J Occup Ther* 42:115, 1988.

8. Kraft G: Diseases of the motor unit. In Rosse C, Clawson DK: *The musculoskeletal system in health and disease,* New York, 1980, Harper & Row.

9. Kurland LT, Radhakrishnan K: An update of the epidemiology of Western Pacific amyotrophic lateral sclerosis. In Molgaard C, editor: *Neuroepidemiology, theory and method,* San Diego, 1993, Academic Press.

10. Lenox AC: When motor nerves die, *Am J Nurs* 4:540, 1983.

11. Miller BF, Keane CB: *Encyclopedia and dictionary of medicine, nursing and allied health,* Philadelphia, 1989, WB Saunders.

12. Molgaard CA: An introduction to neuroepidemiology. In Molgaard CA, editor: *Neuroepidemiology, theory and method,* San Diego, 1993, Academic Press.

13. Mulder DW: Treatment of anterior horn cell disease, *Modern Treatment* 3:243, 1966.

14. Mulder DW: Clinical limits of amyotrophic lateral sclerosis, *Adv Neurol* 36:151, 1982.

15. Rowland LP: Diseases of the motor unit. In Kandel ER, Schwartz JH, Jessell TM, editors: *Principles of neural science,* New York, 1991, Elsevier Science.

16. Spencer EA: Functional restoration: specific diagnosis. In Hopkins HL, Smith HD, editors: *Willard and Spackman's occupational therapy,* ed 8, Philadelphia, 1993, JB Lippincott.

17. Takai V: ADL and adaptive equipment for the ALS patient. *Physical disabilities special interest section newsletter* 6:2, 1983, American Occupational Therapy Association.

18. Wikstrom N and associates: Classic amyotrophic lateral sclerosis with dementia, *Arch Neurol* 39:681, 1982.

19. Zawodniak J: Recommended exercises and ambulation aids for people with ALS, *Physical disabilities special interest section newsletter* 6:2, 1983, American Occupational Therapy Association.

REFERENCES

SECTION 3: PARKINSON'S DISEASE

1. American Parkinson's Disease Association, Inc., 60 Bay Street, Suite 401, Staten Island, NY 10301, (800) 223-2732.

2. Boehme R: *Improving upper body control,* Tucson, Ariz, 1988, Therapy Skill Builders.

3. Cote L, Crutcher MD: The basal ganglia. In Kandel ER, Schwartz JH, Jessell TM: *Principles of neural science,* ed 3, New York, 1991, Elsevier.

4. Cummings JL: Depression and Parkinson's disease: a review. *Am J Psychiatry* 149(4):443, 448, 1992.

5. Fahn S: Concept and classification of dystonia. In Fahn S and associates, editors: Advances in neurology, *Dystonia* 50(2):1-8, 1988.

6. Fahn S and associates: The United Parkinson's Disease Rating Scale. In Fahn S, Marsden CD, Goldstein M, Calne CD, editors: *Recent developments in Parkinson's disease* ed 2, New York, 1987, Macmillan.

7. Friedman J, Friedman H: Fatigue in Parkinson's disease. *Neurology* 43:2016, 1993.

8. Gersten JW: Degenerative diseases of the central nervous system. In Kottke FJ, Lehmann JF: *Krusen's handbook of physical medicine and rehabilitation,* ed 4, Philadelphia, 1990, WB Saunders.

9. Hoehn MM, Yahr MD: Parkinsonism: onset, progression and mortality. *Neurology* 17:427-442, 1967.

10. Hooks ML, Oliver A: *Non-pharmaceutical management of Parkinson's disease.* Paper presented at The Parkinson's Institute, Dec. 8, 1993, Sunnyvale, Calif.

11. Jarus T: Motor learning and occupational therapy: the organization of practice, *Am J Occ Ther* 48:443, 1994.

12. Keshner EA, Cohen H: Current concepts of the vestibular system reviewed. I. The role of the vestibulospinal system in postural control, *Am J Occ Ther* 43:320-330, 1989.

13. Kiernan RJ, Mueller J, Langston JW, Van Dyke C: The neurobehavioral cognitive status exam: a brief but differentiated approach to cognitive assessment, *Ann Int Med* 107:4, 481–485, 1987.

14. Koller WC and associates: Falls and Parkinson's disease, *Clin Neuropharm* 12(2):98,1989.

15. Laufer L: *Handwriting exercises to music: callirobics,* Box 6634, Charlottesville, VA 22906, 1993.

16. Lee RG: Pathophysiology of rigidity and akinesia in Parkinson's disease, *Eur Neurol* 29(suppl 1):13,17, 1989.

17. Marsden CD: The mysterious motor function of the basal ganglia: the Robert Wartenberg lecture, *Neurology,* 32:515, 1982.

18. Marsden CD: Parkinson's disease, *Postgrad Med J* 68:538, 1992.

19. McCormack G: *Therapeutic use of touch: a treatment guide for the health care professional,* Tuscon, Ariz, 1991, Therapy Skill Builders.

20. National Advisory Neurological and Communicativbe Disorders and Stroke Council: *Decade of the brain: answers through scientific research, a report to Congress,* NIH Pub No 88-2957, Jan 1989.

21. Padilla R: *The generalist as specialist: applying the model of human occupation.* Paper presented to the Occupational Therapy Association of Calif, Santa Clara County Chapter, April, 1992.

22. Pedersen SW, Oberg B: Dynamic strength in Parkinson's disease, *Eur Neurol,* 33:97-102, 1993.

23. Pomeroy V: Development of an ADL oriented assessment-of-mobility scale suited for use with elderly people with dementia, *Physiotherapy,* 76(8):446-448, 1990.

24. Sacks O: *Awakenings,* New York, 1990, Harper-Perennial.

25. Schenkman M, Butler RB: A model for multisystem evaluation treatment of individuals with Parkinson's disease, *Phys Ther* 69(11):932-943, 1989.

26. Schenkman M and associates: Management of individuals with Parkinson's disease, *Phys Ther* 69:947,1989

27. Schmidt RA: Motor learning principles for physical therapy. In *Contemporary management of motor control problems, proceedings of the II step conference,* Alexandria, Va, 1991, Foundation for Physical Therapy.

28. Schneider JS, Diamond SG, Markham CH: Parkinson's disease: sensory and motor problems in arms and hands, *Neurol* 37:954, 1987.

29. Schwab RS, England AC: Projection technique for evaluating surgery in Parkinson's disease. In Gillingham FJ, Donaldson MC: *Third symposium on Parkinson's disease,* Edinburgh, 1969, E & S Livingstone.

30. Tanner CM: Occupational and environmental causes of Parkinsonism, *Occup Med* 7(3):511, 1992.

31. Washington H: Parkinson's disease, *Harvard Health Letter,* p 1, July 1993.

32. Weiner WJ: *Movement disorders: a comprehensive survey. Parkinson's disease,* Mt Kisco, NY, 1989, Futura.

33. Wichmann T, DeLong MR: Pathophysiology of parkinsonian motor abnormalities, *Advances in Neurology* 60:53-61.

34. Yanagisawa N, Fujimoto S, Tamaru F: Bradykinesia in Parkinson's disease: disorders of onset and execution of fast movement, *Eur Neurol* 29(suppl 1):19.

REFERENCES

SECTION 4: ALZHEIMER'S DISEASE

1. Aaron MM: Alzheimer's disease: care of the patient and her family, *The Female Patient* 8(11):36, 1983.
2. Allen C, Earhart C, Blue T: *Occupational therapy treatment goals for the physically and cognitively disabled,* Rockville, Md, 1992, American Occupational Therapy Association.
3. American Occupational Therapy Association: Occupational therapy services for Alzheimer's disease and related disorders, *Am J Occup Ther* 40:822, 1986.
4. American Psychiatric Association: Diagnostic and statistical manual of mental disorders, ed 3 rev, Washington, DC, 1987, The Association.
5. Anderton B: Genetics of Alzheimer's Disease: current status and future development of research. In Sinet P, Lamour Y, Christen Y, editors: *Genetics and Alzheimer's disease,* New York, 1988, Springer-Verlag.
6. Arkin S: Memory training in early Alzheimer's disease: An optimistic look at the field, *Am J Alz Care & Related Dis and Research,* July/Aug 1991.
7. Asher I: *An Annotated index of occupational therapy evaluation tools,* Rockville, Md, 1989, American Occupational Therapy Association.
8. Atchison P: Helping people with Alzheimer's and their families preserve independence, *OT Week* 8:16-17, 1994.
9. Baum C: The effect of occupation on behaviors of persons with senile dementia of Alzheimer's type and their carers, dissertation, St Louis, 1993, Washington University.
10. Baum C, Edwards D: Cognitive performance in senile dementia of the Alzheimer's type: the kitchen task assessment, *Am J Occup Ther* 47:431, 1993.
11. Beam IM: Helping families survive, *Am J Nurs* 84:229, 1984.
12. Berkow R, Fletcher A: *The Merck manual of diagnosis and therapy,* ed 15, Rahway, NJ, 1987, Merck Sharp and Dohme Research Laboratories, a Division of Merck and Co, Inc.
13. Boller F and associates: Biological markers of Alzheimer's disease, New York, 1989, Springer-Verlag.
14. Bowen DM: Accelerated aging or selective neuronal loss as an important cause of dementia, *Lancet* 8106(1):11, 1979.
15. Bowen DM: The biochemistry of cortical and subcortical neurons in Alzheimer's disease. In Glenner GG, editor: *Advancing frontiers in Alzheimer's disease research,* Austin, 1987, University of Texas Press.
16. Bowlby C: *Therapeutic activities with persons disabled by Alzheimer's disease and related disorders,* Gaithersburg, Md, 1993, Aspen.
17. Clayman C: *The American Medical Association encyclopedia of medicine,* New York, 1989, Random House.
18. Clayton T: *Taber's cyclopedic medical dictionary,* ed 15, Philadelphia, 1985, FA Davis.
19. Clive B: Dementia, depression, or grief? the differential diagnosis, *Geriatrics,* 45:37, 1990.
20. Cohen U, Weisman G: *Holding on to home: designing environments for people with dementia,* therapeutic environments workshop, Institute on Aging and Environment, Winston-Salem, NC, Feb 18, 1994.
21. Corcoran M: Management decisions made by caregiver spouses of persons with Alzheimer's disease, *Am J Occup Ther* 48:38, 1994.
22. Corcoran M, Gitlin L: Dementia management: an occupational therapy home-based intervention for caregivers, *Am J Occup Ther* 46:801, 1992.
23. Cybyk ME: Alzheimer's disease, *Nurs Times* 76:280, 1980.
24. Davis CM: The role of the physical and occupational therapist in caring for the victim of Alzheimer's disease. In Taira ED, editor: Therapeutic interventions for the person with dementia, *Phys Occup Ther Geriatr* 4:3,15, 1986.
25. Dorey MM: Alzheimer's disease the "new" old approach, *Phys Ther Forum* 4:32, 1985.
26. Duchek J: Assessing cognition. In Christiansen C, Baum C, editors: *Occupational therapy overcoming human performance deficits,* Thorofare, NJ, 1991, Slack.
27. Epstein C: Trisomic and transgenic mice in the study of the pathogenesis of Alzheimer's disease and Down's syndrome. In Sinet PM, Lamour Y, Christen Y: *Genetics and Alzheimer's disease,* New York, 1988, Springer-Verlag.
28. Glickstein JK: *Therapeutic intervention in Alzheimer's disease,* Rockville, Md, 1988, Aspen.
29. Grinspoon L: Alzheimer's disease. I and II. *The Harvard Mental Health Letter* 9:1, 1992.
30. Haynes A and associates: Alzheimer's disease and chromosome 21. In Boller F and associates, editors: Biological markers of Alzheimer's disease. New York, 1989, Springer-Verlag.
31. Hovaguimian T, editor: *Classification and diagnosis of Alzheimer's disease: an international perspective,* Toronto, Ont, 1989, Hogrefe & Huber.
32. Jackson-Klykken O: Brain function, aging and dementia. In Umphred DA, editor: *Neurological rehabilitation,* St Louis, 1985, CV Mosby.
33. Katzman R, Jackson JE: Alzheimer's disease: basic and clinical advances, *JAGS,* 39:516-525, 1991.
34. Kemp B: Eight methods family members can use to manage behavioral problems in dementia, *Top Geriatr Rehabil* 4:50-59, 1988.
35. Kent S: What causes Alzheimer's? *Geriatrics* 38:33, 1983.
36. Khachaturian Z: Cognitive changes in the aged: the need for further research. In Hovaguimian T, editor: *Classification and diagnosis of Alzheimer's disease: an international perspective,* Toronto, Ont, 1989, Hogrefe & Huber.

37. Mallison MB: Alzheimer's disease: theories and therapies, *Am J Nurs* 84:223, 1984.

38. Meyer E, Simpkins J, Yamamoto J, editors: *Novel approaches to the treatment of Alzheimer's disease,* New York, 1989, Plenum Press.

39. Morris A, Hunt G: *A part of daily life: Alzheimer's caregivers simplify activities and the home,* Bethesda, Md, 1994, American Occupational Therapy Association.

40. Nalbantoglu J: B-Amyloid protein in Alzheimer's disease, *Can J Neurol Sci,* 18:424, 1991.

41. Nygard L and associates: Comparing motor and process ability of persons with suspected dementia in home and clinic settings, *Am J Occup Ther* 48:689, 1994.

42. Powell L, Courtice K: *Alzheimer's disease: a guide for families,* rev ed, Reading, Mass, 1993, Addison-Wesley.

43. Rabinowitz E: Day care and Alzheimer's disease: a weekend program in New York City. In Taira ED, editor: Therapeutic interventions for the person with dementia, *Phys Occup Ther Geriatr* 4(3):95, 1986.

44. Reisberg B: *A guide to Alzheimer's disease for families, spouses, and friends,* New York, 1981, The Free Press.

45. Rudolph M: Alzheimer center replaces depression with dignity for clients and their families, *OT Week* 2(23):16, 1988.

46. Shapira J: Research trends in Alzheimer's disease, *J Geront Nurs* 20:4-9, 1994.

47. Singh V: Immunologic approach to therapy in Alzheimer's disease. In Meyer EM, Simpkins JW, and Yamamoto, J: *Novel approaches to the treatment of Alzheimer's disease,* New York, 1989, Plenum Press.

48. Steinke G: *Stages of Alzheimer's disease,* Palo Alto, Calif, 1984, Alzheimer's Disease and Related Disorders Association, Greater San Francisco Bay Area Chapter.

49. Steinke G: *The use of medications in Alzheimer's disease,* Palo Alto, Calif, 1988, Alzheimer's Disease and Related Disorders Association, Greater San Francisco Bay Area Chapter.

50. Sulkova R and associates: Clinical and neuropathological features in Alzheimer's disease, *Acta Neurol Scand* 65(suppl 90):294, 1982.

51. Volicer L and associates: Clinical management of Alzheimer's disease, Rockville, Md, 1988, Aspen.

52. Zgola J: *Doing things, a guide to programing activities for persons with Alzheimer's disease and related disorders.* Baltimore, Md, 1991, The Johns Hopkins University Press.

Index

Page numbers in *italics* indicate illustrations; page numbers followed by *t* indicate tables.